SOCIAL PSYCHOLOGY

SOCIAL PSYCHOLOGY

Handbook of Basic Principles

THIRD EDITION

Edited by
PAUL A. M. VAN LANGE
E. TORY HIGGINS
ARIE W. KRUGLANSKI

THE GUILFORD PRESS
New York   London

Library of Congress Cataloging-in-Publication Data

Names: Lange, Paul A. M. van, editor. | Higgins, E. Tory (Edward Tory),
   1946– editor. | Kruglanski, Arie W., editor.
Title: Social psychology : handbook of basic principles / edited by Paul A.
   M. Van Lange, E. Tory Higgins, Arie W. Kruglanski.
Description: Third edition. | New York : The Guilford Press, [2021] |
   Includes bibliographical references and index.
Identifiers: LCCN 2020006173 | ISBN 9781462543984 (cloth)
Subjects: LCSH: Social psychology.
Classification: LCC HM1033 .S637 2021 | DDC 302—dc23
LC record available at https://lccn.loc.gov/2020006173

About the Editors

Paul A. M. Van Lange, PhD, is Professor and Chair of Social Psychology at Vrije Universiteit Amsterdam, The Netherlands, and Distinguished Research Fellow at the University of Oxford, United Kingdom. His research focuses on human cooperation and trust. Dr. Van Lange has published over 200 articles in psychological and interdisciplinary journals. He is founding editor of *Current Opinion in Psychology* and *Current Research in Ecological and Social Psychology*, and is a past president of the Society of Experimental Social Psychology. Dr. Van Lange's work been recognized by the Kurt Lewin Medal from the European Association of Social Psychology, among other grants and awards. His website is *www.paulvanlange.com*.

E. Tory Higgins, PhD, is the Stanley Schachter Professor of Psychology at Columbia University, where he is also Professor and Director of the Motivation Science Center at the Columbia Business School. He is a Fellow of the American Academy of Arts and Sciences. Dr. Higgins has received the Distinguished Scientist Award from the Society of Experimental Social Psychology, the Anneliese Maier Research Award from the Alexander von Humboldt Foundation in Germany, the William James Fellow Award from the Association for Psychological Science, and the Award for Distinguished Scientific Contributions from the American Psychological Association, among other awards for his research, teaching, and mentoring.

Arie W. Kruglanski, PhD, is Distinguished University Professor of Psychology at the University of Maryland, College Park. He has published over 400 articles, chapters, and books on motivated social cognition. A Fellow of the American Psychological Association and the Association for Psychological Science, Dr. Kruglanski is cofounder of the National Consortium for the Study of Terrorism and Responses to Terrorism. He is a recipient of awards including the Research Scientist Award from the National Institute of Mental Health, the Donald T. Campbell Award from the Society for Personality and Social Psychology, and the Distinguished Scientific Contribution Award from the Society of Experimental Social Psychology.

Contributors

Lara B. Aknin, PhD, Department of Psychology, Simon Fraser University, Burnaby, British Columbia, Canada

Sara B. Algoe, PhD, Department of Psychology and Neuroscience, University of North Carolina at Chapel Hill, Chapel Hill, North Carolina

Xuechunzi Bai, BA, Department of Psychology, Princeton University, Princeton, New Jersey

Daniel Balliet, PhD, Department of Experimental and Applied Psychology, Vrije Universiteit Amsterdam, Amsterdam, The Netherlands

Joel Brockner, PhD, Columbia Business School, Columbia University, New York, New York

David S. Chester, PhD, Department of Psychology, Virginia Commonwealth University, Richmond, Virginia

Dov Cohen, PhD, Department of Psychology, University of Illinois at Urbana–Champaign, Champaign, Illinois

Dick de Gilder, PhD, Department of Organisation Sciences, Vrije Universiteit Amsterdam, Amsterdam, The Netherlands

Edward L. Deci, PhD, Department of Psychology, University of Rochester, Rochester, New York

C. Nathan DeWall, PhD, Department of Psychology, University of Kentucky, Lexington, Kentucky

Yarrow Dunham, PhD, Department of Psychology, Yale University, New Haven, Connecticut

Gerald Echterhoff, PhD, Department of Psychology, University of Münster, Münster, Germany

Naomi Ellemers, PhD, Faculty of Social and Behavioural Sciences, Utrecht University, Utrecht, The Netherlands

Jami Eller, BS, Department of Psychology, University of Minnesota, Minneapolis, Minnesota

Nicholas Epley, PhD, Booth School of Business, University of Chicago, Chicago, Illinois

Klaus Fiedler, PhD, Department of Psychology, Heidelberg University, Heidelberg, Germany

Eli J. Finkel, PhD, Department of Psychology and the Kellogg School of Management, Northwestern University, Evanston, Illinois

Susan T. Fiske, PhD, Department of Psychology, Princeton University, Princeton, New Jersey

Gráinne M. Fitzsimons, PhD, Department of Psychology and Neuroscience, Duke University, Durham, North Carolina

Ilona Fridman, PhD, Margolis Center for Health Policy, Duke University, Durham, North Carolina

Michele Gelfand, PhD, Department of Psychology, University of Maryland, College Park, Maryland

Francesca Gino, PhD, Harvard Business School, Boston, Massachusetts

Andrew H. Hales, PhD, Frank Batten School of Leadership and Public Policy, University of Virginia, Charlottesville, Virginia

Shihui Han, PhD, School of Psychological and Cognitive Sciences, Peking University, Beijing, China

Eddie Harmon-Jones, PhD, School of Psychology, The University of New South Wales, Sydney, Australia

Cindy Harmon-Jones, PhD, School of Psychology, The University of New South Wales, Sydney, Australia

Grit Hein, PhD, Department of Psychiatry, Psychosomatic and Psychotherapy, University of Würzburg, Würzburg, Germany

Miles Hewstone, DPhil, Department of Experimental Psychology, University of Oxford, Oxford, United Kingdom

E. Tory Higgins, PhD, Department of Psychology, Columbia University, New York, New York

Alexa D. Hubbard, PhD, Department of Psychology, New York University, New York, New York

Kurt Hugenberg, PhD, Department of Psychological and Brain Sciences, Indiana University, Bloomington, Indiana

Katarzyna Jasko, PhD, Institute of Psychology, Jagiellonian University, Krakow, Poland

Martha Jeong, PhD, Department of Management, The Hong Kong University of Science and Technology, Hong Kong

Tatum A. Jolink, BA, Department of Psychology and Neuroscience, University of North Carolina at Chapel Hill, Chapel Hill, North Carolina

David A. Kalkstein, PhD, Department of Psychology, Stanford University, Stanford, California

Michael Kardas, PhD, Booth School of Business, University of Chicago, Chicago, Illinois

Yoshihisa Kashima, PhD, Department of Psychology, University of Melbourne, Melbourne, Australia

Kerry Kawakami, PhD, Department of Psychology, York University, Toronto, Ontario, Canada

Arie W. Kruglanski, PhD, Department of Psychology, University of Maryland, College Park, Maryland

Nira Liberman, PhD, Department of Psychology, Tel Aviv University, Tel Aviv, Israel

Xi Liu, MA, Department of Psychology, University of Illinois at Urbana–Champaign, Champaign, Illinois

Angelika Love, DPhil, Department of Experimental Psychology, University of Oxford, Oxford, United Kingdom

Linda McCaughey, MSc, Department of Psychology, Heidelberg University, Heidelberg, Germany

Julia Minson, PhD, Center for Public Leadership, Harvard Kennedy School, Cambridge, Massachusetts

Emily Nakkawita, BS, Department of Psychology, Columbia University, New York, New York

Gandalf Nicolas, PhD, Department of Psychology, Rutgers, The State University of New Jersey, Piscataway, New Jersey

Michael I. Norton, PhD, Harvard Business School, Boston, Massachusetts

Ramona L. Paetzold, PhD, Department of Management, Mays Business School, Texas A&M University, College Station, Texas

David Pietraszewski, PhD, Max Planck Institute for Human Development, Berlin, Germany

Yanyan Qi, PhD, Chinese Academy of Sciences Institute of Psychology, Beijing, China

Harry T. Reis, PhD, Department of Psychology, University of Rochester, Rochester, New York

W. Steven Rholes, PhD, Department of Psychology, Texas A&M University, College Station, Texas

Richard M. Ryan, PhD, Institute for Positive Psychology and Education, Australian Catholic University, North Sydney, Australia; Department of Psychology, University of Rochester, Rochester, New York

Faith Shin, PhD, Department of Psychology, University of Illinois at Urbana–Champaign, Champaign, Illinois

Jeffry A. Simpson, PhD, Department of Psychology, University of Minnesota, Minneapolis, Minnesota

Deborah A. Small, PhD, The Wharton School, University of Pennsylvania, Philadelphia, Pennsylvania

Thomas Suddendorf, PhD, School of Psychology, University of Queensland, St. Lucia, Australia

Yaacov Trope, PhD, Department of Psychology, New York University, New York, New York

Kees van den Bos, PhD, Faculty of Social and Behavioral Sciences and School of Law, Utrecht University, Utrecht, The Netherlands

Gerben A. van Kleef, PhD, Department of Psychology, University of Amsterdam, Amsterdam, The Netherlands

Paul A. M. Van Lange, PhD, Department of Social Psychology, Vrije Universiteit Amsterdam, Amsterdam, The Netherlands

Nico W. Van Yperen, PhD, Department of Psychology, University of Groningen, Groningen, The Netherlands

Frank A. von Hippel, PhD, Department of Biological Sciences, Northern Arizona University, Flagstaff, Arizona

William von Hippel, PhD, School of Psychology, University of Queensland, St. Lucia, Australia

David Webber, PhD, Wilder School of Government and Public Affairs, Virginia Commonwealth University, Richmond, Virginia

Batia M. Wiesenfeld, PhD, Stern School of Business, New York University, New York, New York

Kipling D. Williams, PhD, Department of Psychological Sciences, Purdue University, West Lafayette, Indiana

Junhui Wu, PhD, Faculty of Psychology, Beijing Normal University, Beijing, China

Preface

The carriers of scientific development are ideas and theories. Ideas are what make us tick, what make us excited—and sometimes even make us smile. Ideas often capture something new, that presumably most people have not thought about before. Scientific ideas are also often constructive, in that they may bind and connect (often shared) observations into common *principles* that have the potential to contribute to scientific knowledge. As a classic illustration, if the idea is that people have a willful, conscious part and an unconscious part, and that the former often seeks to regulate the latter, then scientists not familiar with Freudian (or other) theorizing at the time should feel elated and energized; that is, at the time when psychology had just begun as new discipline, this must have been a crisp, inspiring idea that should have influenced the ways in which numerous scientists perceived, interpreted, and understood various forms of human behavior—from slips of the tongue in conversation to aggressive behavior.

Ideas are often primary building blocks for theories. Not every idea leads to a theory, but a theory cannot exist without ideas. Ideas are necessary but not sufficient to theoretical development and progress. More than ideas, theories get at the why and how of numerous phenomena and trace their implications for many situations. Theories thus organize a wide range of events and phenomena into coherent systems guided by common *principles*. Both statements were made in the preface of the *Handbook of Theories of Social Psychology* that we edited some years ago (Van Lange, Kruglanski, & Higgins, 2012). For example, the classic idea by Festinger (1954) that in the absence of objective criteria, people evaluate their opinions and abilities by comparing them to others' opinions and abilities is one that led to the development of a more comprehensive theory of social comparison. In later accounts, social comparison theory included not only self-evaluation (to use social information to define and evaluate oneself), a motive assumed by Festinger, but also other motives, such as self-enhancement (to use social information to provide self-serving evaluations) and self-improvement (to use social information to learn and improve) (see Suls & Wheeler, 2012; Wood, 1989).

Ideas should flourish in a world in which people do not sanction each other for lack of evidence, impossibility of testing, lack of novelty, or lack of application in the "real world." Sometimes "wild ideas" have a charm and are inspirational, for whatever reason, but are unlikely to make it to a theory. This is in part because theories are evaluated according to much more stringent criteria. Theories may be evaluated in terms of truth (and testability), abstraction, progress, and applicability, as these serve as the primary standards (TAPAS) for judging the merits (and limitations) of theories (Van Lange, 2013; see also Kruglanski, 2006).

We focus so much on ideas and theories because *Social Psychology* emphasizes *basic principles*. And basic principles are often the product of scientific ideas that may lead to theories if they do well in terms of the stringent criteria explicated in TAPAS. Basic principles are the glue between ideas and theories. They help a scientist to make ideas explicit to formalize them wherever possible, and often it is a set of basic principles that forms the beginnings of a new theory. Social psychology adopts an inclusive definition of a theory, and most theories tend to be "middle range" (Merton, 1949, p. 5) and hence "intermediate to minor working hypotheses" rather than grand theoretical edifices. Whether small or large in scope and reach, theories are grounded in basic principles.

Our handbook is grounded in the conviction that social psychology has a lot to offer in terms of basic principles. Yet basic principles have not always been made explicit in scientific writings. Therefore, as in previous editions of this handbook (Higgins & Kruglanski, 1996; Kruglanski & Higgins, 2007), we encouraged authors to explicate the basic principles that underlie their domains of research and theorizing. As the reader will see, the authors amply rose to the challenge. Along with the basic principles, the chapters often provide a state-of-the-art review of particular programs of research, and sometimes a review of well-established theories that have inspired multiple generations of researchers in social psychology and beyond.

This handbook comprises 30 chapters. Part I, *Principles in Theory*, includes 24 chapters that are categorized in terms of four levels of analysis: intrapersonal processes, interpersonal processes, intragroup processes, and intergroup processes. As the reader will see, although most chapters are relevant to multiple levels, it also true that the principles discussed in these chapters often focus on one of these levels. These chapters also capture multiple elements of biological, affective, cognitive, and motivational processes. This may in part reflect a growth in research and theorizing in social psychology, in that they more often than in the past combine motives; address cognition, motivation, and emotion; or seek bridges with broad perspectives such as evolutionary theory or neuroscience.

Furthermore, to highlight the idea that basic principles operate in distinct societal contexts, and that contexts illuminate the workings of these principles, Part II of this handbook is titled *Principles in Context*. Its six chapters address contexts of helping, law, negotiation, organization, political extremism, and sports. As the chapters illustrate, these are contexts in which basic principles of social psychology—whether they are linked to intrapersonal, interpersonal, intragroup, or intergroup processes—are very relevant. Clearly, this would also be true for many other contexts, such as a consumer context, an educational context, or an environmental context, but we felt that including these six contexts provides a broad spectrum of contexts in which people live their social lives, in which the actual, imaginary, or implied presence of others help us understand how and why basic principles of social psychology come alive.

The first and second editions of *Social Psychology: Handbook of Basic Principles* were edited by two of us (E. T. H. and A. W. K.), who invited the first editor (P. A. M. V. L.) to join in, and he enthusiastically agreed. The three of us had worked together on the two-volume *Handbook of Theories of Social Psychology*, and that had been a most inspiring and enjoyable venture. This handbook was similarly inspiring and enjoyable, not only because the editors work so well together, but also because the authors did a truly terrific job. It is, of course, impossible for the editors to produce and share a completely objective evaluation of the chapters. We are happy to leave that up to the readers, and hope that this handbook, like the previous ones, may be a source of scientific inspiration and enjoyment—just as it has been for us.

REFERENCES

Festinger, L. (1954). A theory of social comparison processes. *Human Relations, 7,* 117–140.
Higgins, E. T., & Kruglanski, A. W. (Eds.). (1996). *Social psychology: Handbook of basic principles* (1st ed.). New York: Guilford Press.

Kruglanski, A. W. (2006). Theories as bridges. In P. A. M. Van Lange (Ed.), *Bridging social psychology: Benefits of transdisciplinary approaches* (pp. 21–34). Mahwah, NJ: Erlbaum.

Kruglanski, A. W., & Higgins, E. T. (Eds.). (2007). *Social psychology: Handbook of basic principles* (2nd ed.). New York: Guilford Press.

Merton, R. K. (1949). *Social theory and social structure.* Glencoe, IL: Free Press.

Suls, J., & Wheeler, L. (2012). Social comparison theory. In P. A. M. Van Lange, A. W. Kruglanski, & E. T. Higgins (Eds.), *Handbook of theories of social psychology* (Vol. 2, pp. 460–482). Thousand Oaks, CA: Sage.

Van Lange, P. A. M. (2013). What we should expect from theories in social psychology: Truth, abstraction, progress, and applicability as standards (TAPAS). *Personality and Social Psychology Review, 17,* 40–55.

Van Lange, P. A. M., Kruglanski, A. W., & Higgins, E. T. (Eds.). (2012). *Handbook of theories of social psychology* (Vols. 1 and 2). Thousand Oaks, CA: Sage.

Wood, J. V. (1989). Theory and research concerning social comparison of personal attributes. *Psychological Bulletin, 106,* 231–248.

Contents

PART II. PRINCIPLES IN CONTEXT

PART I

Principles in Theory

INTRAPERSONAL LEVEL

Evolutionary Foundations of Social Psychology

William von Hippel
Frank A. von Hippel
Thomas Suddendorf

For over 200 million years, seed-producing plants called gymnosperms (which include pines, redwoods, and cypresses) were the most prevalent terrestrial flora on Earth (Beck, 1988). This dominance came to an end with the evolution of flowering plants (angiosperms), which had supplanted nearly all of the gymnosperms by the time the dinosaurs went extinct 65 million years ago (Soltis et al., 2018). The evolutionary pathway that made flowering plants so effective has parallels to our own ancestors' route to success; thus, we reflect on it briefly before discussing human evolution.

Because plants are rooted in place, reproduction requires that they overcome two challenges. First, they must find a way for sperm to meet egg. Gymnosperms evolved the capacity to release sperm-containing pollen into the air and thereby rely on the wind for fertilization (Beck, 1988). Airborne pollen was an important advance over the waterborne spores of older plants, but still a terribly inefficient mode of transport that requires massive overproduction of sperm to ensure that some will alight on the fertile eggs of the same species. Flowering plants evolved a novel approach to this problem by using nectar to attract insects and other animals to their flowers, that then serve as a far more efficient vector for bringing sperm to egg (Soltis et al., 2018).

The second reproductive challenge posed by a rooted lifestyle is that the soil directly under the parent is typically a poor place for a new seed because the parent is already established there, taking the lion's share of the available light, water, and nutrients. After fertilization, gymnosperms simply drop their seeds, with no capacity to spread them farther than they might blow in the wind. Flowering plants solved this problem by encasing their seeds in berries or fruit, thereby enticing animals to consume them, pass them through their digestive tracts, and eventually deposit the seeds elsewhere in a pile of fertilizing manure.

As can be seen in this brief description, flowering plants outcompeted gymnosperms via new forms of cooperation that allowed them to overcome their rooted nature via the mobility of animals. Their *mutualistic symbiosis* with pollinating insects resulted in much greater efficiency in fertilization, and their interdependence with fruit-eating animals led to much greater geographic distribution and success of their seedlings. This mutual dependence comes at a cost, as insects and other animals must be fed to entice them to play their role. Nonetheless, these costs are outweighed by the benefits, as flowering plants now dominate a landscape that for millions of years belonged to gymnosperms (Soltis et al., 2018).

The human success story is also one of interdependence (Balliet, Tybur, & Van Lange, 2016). In comparison with our chimpanzee cousins, we evolved to be much more cooperative with each other (see section on early hominin evolution). Our hypercooperativeness comes at a cost, but it provides enormous benefits that enabled our survival and eventual rise to the top of the food chain. Over the last few million years our interdependence has shaped nearly all aspects of our psychology. Indeed, the defining feature of our species—if we take our label *Homo sapiens* ("wise man") seriously—is an offshoot of our evolved sociality (Dunbar & Shultz, 2007). The pressures and opportunities that emerged with our increased cooperativeness appear to have been major forces that led to our impressive intelligence.

Given the important role sociality played in our evolution over the last few million years, there is a strong probability that our various motivational and cognitive processes were shaped by their effects on our ancestors' social success. As a consequence, when we consider these processes, an important question we should ask concerns how they interface with our sociality. One implication of this perspective is that any theory whose explanatory mechanisms concern only internal states—for example, people do X because it makes them happy, raises their self-esteem, or gives them a sense of confidence—may capture only part of the story (von Hippel & Buss, 2017). Such theories fail to address what is often a critical question: *Why* does X increase happiness, self-esteem, or confidence? If the feelings we evolved were shaped by the interpersonal consequences of our actions, happiness, self-esteem, confidence, and so forth, are not the ultimate cause of our behavior. Rather, those individuals who experience these feelings in appropriate circumstances have greater biological fitness. Hence, these feelings guide us toward outcomes that facilitate our survival and reproductive success (Buss, 2000; Cosmides & Tooby, 2000; von Hippel & Gonsalkorale, 2018).

The interpersonal nature of many internal states adds further complexity to research in social psychology, as evolutionary logic also dictates that processes that appear to be primarily or even entirely intrapersonal are likely to implicate others. To return to the examples of happiness, self-esteem, and confidence, all of these constructs are of great *inter*personal importance, even when they arise from events that do not appear to involve others (von Hippel & Trivers, 2011b). Consider, for instance, artists or scientists who work tirelessly to achieve mastery over their domain. From their perspective, their solitary efforts and sacrifices are driven by an intrinsic love of art or science (Deci & Ryan, 1975). From an evolutionary perspective, however, their proclivity to be intrinsically motivated in domains in which they have good prospects evolved because it enhanced their ancestors' success. Those with such a proclivity had greater chances of survival and reproduction than those without because they would have become more skilled and hence more valued as members of the small groups in which our ancestors resided. This evolutionary perspective clarifies that there are few purely intrapersonal processes, as *the ultimate outcome shaping many of our preferences, thoughts, and capabilities is their effect on others.*

Furthermore, and importantly, internal states are both outcomes and intermediaries. To return to happiness, self-esteem, and confidence, these are outcomes in that we evolved to feel positively when we meet our basic needs and when we achieve outcomes that others value, which motivates further efforts in these directions (Cosmides & Tooby, 2000; von Hippel & Gonsalkorale, 2018). As a consequence, such feelings also have communicative value, as their reliable association with success ensures that they signal our value to others. We are drawn to happy and confident people with high self-esteem because we interpret these traits as honest signals of competence and achievement (von Hippel & Trivers, 2011a).

The human success story is primarily one of sociality (Tomasello, 2014; von Hippel, 2018), and that is the focus of this chapter. Nonetheless, two more issues require consideration before we delve into our evolutionary past. First, although our cognitive system evolved largely to enhance our capacity to achieve our goals, evolution shaped many of our goals in advance of rather than through our cognitive processes. By way of example, a common misconception is that humans evolved a goal to have children, which in turn facilitates reproductive success. Such a preference for children is highly unlikely to have evolved, as the informational demands linking copulation to pregnancy were too challenging for our distant ancestors (Confer et al., 2010; Tooby & Cosmides, 1990). For the bulk of our evolutionary history, our ancestors, like other sexually reproducing animals, had no idea how to reproduce. Rather, it is far more likely that our ancestors evolved the predilection to enjoy sex and the subsequent tendency to feel nurturant to any offspring that resulted. Such a process would facilitate reproduction through our motivational system, essentially bypassing the cognitive demands required to understand mammalian reproduction.

Second, although our motivational and cognitive systems represent solutions to the challenges faced by our ancestors, their solutions were constrained by the prior challenges faced by *their* ancestors and the solutions they adapted. Evolution tinkers with existing traits rather than creating solutions de novo (with the exception of rare beneficial mutations; Jacob, 1977). A famous example of such historical constraints can be found in the human eye, which has a poor design in the sense that the receptor cell bodies and vascular structures lie between the light source and the photoreceptors (thereby obfuscating the information that is to be perceived). In contrast, the eyeball of an octopus does not have this problem, with receptor cell bodies and vascular structures located behind the photoreceptors as an intelligent bioengineer would undoubtedly have designed it (Fernald, 2000; Lamb, Collin, & Pugh, 2007). The recurrent laryngeal nerve is another example of a historical constraint, as it loops from the top of the neck down under the aortic arch in the chest, then back up to the voice box, which requires it to be several times longer than is necessary. The longer the neck, the bigger the waste, and in giraffes, this nerve is approximately 5 meters long, as it runs the entire length up and down the giraffe's throat in order to follow this earlier evolved pathway. The necks of sauropod dinosaurs were up to 14 meters long, suggesting that the recurrent laryngeal nerve was 28 meters

longer than necessary in these animals (Wedel, 2011). Like the giraffe and sauropods, we are stuck with an evolved nerve pathway that was efficient for an animal with an aortic arch near its larynx but increasingly inefficient as the distance between them grows.

How do such ancestral constraints manifest themselves in our modern psychology? Perhaps the clearest example can be found in research on the Wason (1968) selection task, in which people are asked to test a rule of the form "If *P,* then *Q.*" People typically perform very poorly on this task, most notably through their failure to search for disconfirmation (they fail to examine cases of "not-*Q*"). As Cosmides (1989) and her colleagues (Cosmides, Barrett, & Tooby, 2010) point out, however, problems in formal logic are evolutionarily novel for us, and hence are not framed in a manner that readily taps our innate abilities. When Cosmides reframed the Wason task in terms of social exchange (e.g., if you want to drink cassava juice, you must have a tattoo), people were much more likely to search for disconfirmation. This advantage did not emerge simply by reframing the problems in more familiar terms (e.g., everyone who eats cereal also drinks orange juice). As is clear from such examples, the study of human social cognition can benefit from a better understanding of our past and the challenges faced by our ancestors (e.g., Mercier & Sperber, 2011).

With this background in mind, we first consider basic evolutionary principles before turning our attention to our particular evolutionary history and how it might have forged our minds to work as they do.

Natural Selection, Sexual Selection, Genetic Drift, and the Founder Effect

Natural selection is an evolutionary mechanism proposed by Charles Darwin and Alfred Russel Wallace based on their observations of the following facts. Most species produce more offspring than can survive to adulthood, resulting in a great deal of pre-reproductive mortality, which Darwin (1859) referred to as the "struggle for existence." If all individuals were exactly the same, they would have an equal chance of survival, but individuals vary tremendously in their traits, and some of that variation is heritable. Some variants are better suited to their environment than others, resulting in greater survival and reproduction. Those individuals who survive to reproduce pass along their heritable beneficial traits to their offspring, which leads to population change over time as the beneficial traits become more common. Given enough accumulated change over time, populations—especially if isolated—can diverge from each other to form new species (Darwin, 1859). Natural selection is always occurring because the environment is constantly changing and resources are limited. A time lag between an evolutionary pressure (e.g., a change in climate) and an evolutionary response (e.g., a change in thermoregulation) gives rise to the concept of the *ghost of selection past*: The traits we see today evolved in response to past environmental conditions and do not necessarily reflect a response to current conditions (Tooby & Cosmides, 1990; see also Hawks, Wang, Cochran, Harpending, & Moyzis, 2007).

For sexually reproducing species, Darwin (1874) also proposed the evolutionary mechanism known as *sexual selection*. Conceptually, sexual selection is divided into intrasexual and intersexual processes. In most species, intrasexual selection takes the form of male–male competition, as males compete with each other for access to females. This one-sided competition emerges because females typically invest more energy in their offspring than males do, so males compete for access to the females' investment (Trivers, 1972). Although humans are no exception to this rule, because humans are a pair-bonding species (most people have only one long-term partner at a time), females also compete with each other for access to the best mate.

Nevertheless, the variability in our mitochondrial (maternally inherited) and Y-linked (paternally inherited) DNA suggests that humans have more female than male ancestors (Wilder, Mobasher, & Hammer, 2004). That finding, in turn, implies that more males than females were unsuccessful in their efforts to attract a partner. Thus, despite our pair-bonding nature, male–male competition is more intense than female–female competition in humans, just as it is in

most other animals. Because males compete with each other for reproductive access, they evolve traits that are beneficial in male–male competition, even if those traits have associated costs (Murphy et al., 2015). For example, sexual dimorphism may be a result of male–male competition, as larger bodies are costlier to build but more effective in physical contests with other males (Darwin, 1874; Lande, 1980).

Intersexual selection tends to take the form of female choice. Females evolve to prefer males with traits that increase success in contests with other males because females with such preferences tend to produce male offspring that themselves have greater mating success. Traits that are useful in intrasexual competition often signal good genes as well (e.g., genes that impart disease resistance or facilitate successful acquisition of the resources necessary to build a large body), and are preferred by females for the benefits they bring to offspring of both sexes. Sexual selection can act in opposition to natural selection, as in the case of traits such as bright coloration or long tails in male birds, which make them more vulnerable to predators (e.g., Andersson, 1982).[1]

Many other evolutionary mechanisms played important roles in the diversification of life, but two of these bear mention in this discussion of human evolution, the first of which is *genetic drift* (Hartl, Clark, & Clark, 1997). In a large population, gene frequencies are unlikely to change appreciably from one generation to the next. However, in a small population, gene frequencies can shift dramatically by chance alone. Consider a simple case in which there are two varieties of a gene (two alleles), whose consequences are neutral for survival and reproduction and hence vary randomly, like the toss of a coin. In a large population, the random process would ensure that both alleles remain common, but in a small population, chance alone can cause one allele to disappear through this process of genetic drift. Loss of alleles by genetic drift leads to constraints on evolutionary change because diversity in genes enables the variation in traits upon which natural selection operates.

Related to the concept of genetic drift is the *founder effect* (Hartl et al., 1997). When a new habitat is colonized (as happened innumerable times when hominins[2] migrated out of Africa) and the founding population is large, the founding population's genetic diversity likely reflects the genetic diversity of the population of origin. However, if a founding population is small, as was commonly the case, the genetic diversity of that founding population may be a small subset of the diversity of the population of origin. For example, the founding group of colonists might carry rare diseases, or rare eye or hair colors, which would lead to an abnormally large percentage of the population in future generations having these traits. Small founding populations thereby result in altered gene frequencies and the loss of ancestral alleles from the larger population of origin, leading to constraint on evolutionary potential.

Early Hominin Evolution

Many animals live in groups, as the numerous benefits of group living gave such animals a survival and reproductive advantage. Because many of those benefits (e.g., access to fertile mates, more eyes to watch out for predators) can be achieved in the absence of ongoing relationships among group members, living in a group per se does not require the ability to track and remember others. For example, wildebeest and fish gather in large numbers for mutual protection but do not appear to maintain knowledge of each other's personality or whereabouts. In contrast, many other animals, such as elephants and killer whales, know their fellow group members and show an interest in their whereabouts (Bates et al., 2008; Bigg, Olesiuk, Ellis, Ford, & Balcomb, 1990).

Primates not only know the members of their group but also have some knowledge of third-party relations. For instance, when an infant makes an alarm call, vervet monkeys look to the infant's mother, in apparent recognition of their relationship (Cheney & Seyfarth, 1990). Primates also maintain ongoing relationships with their fellow group members, often based on mutual grooming and support in conflict (e.g., De Waal, 2000; Dunbar, 1991). This interdependent form of sociality puts substantial demands on their cognitive abilities.

The mental challenges associated with cooperation and social coordination in such groups appear to have played an important role in the evolution of primate brains (Dunbar & Shultz, 2007; Frith & Frith, 2010). According to the *social brain hypothesis,* the evolution of primate intelligence was driven in large part by the challenges of group living rather than by challenges associated with the physical world (e.g., Byrne & Whiten, 1988; Humphrey, 1976; Jolly, 1966). Social challenges differ from physical ones in a variety of ways, but most of those differences reflect the fact that social goals often require a greater diversity of approaches and flexibility in responding due to changing social dynamics. For example, animals often attempt to manipulate each other to achieve a preferred outcome (Wheeler, 2009; Whiten & Byrne, 1988), but the targets of such social goals can change their behavior in response to such manipulation. For this reason, social success depends on flexibility in problem solving, as today's solution may no longer work tomorrow. As a consequence, the social brain hypothesis emphasizes that behavioral flexibility should be an important outcome of increased intelligence. Consistent with this possibility, problem-solving flexibility is associated with increased brain size across various species of primates (Reader & Laland, 2002; Street, Navarrete, Reader, & Laland, 2017).

Primates have been around for nearly 60 million years, but great apes are a relatively new addition to the Order, splitting off from the ancestors of small apes (i.e., gibbons) some 15.5 million years ago (Perelman et al., 2011). From this common ancestor, apes divided into the lineages leading to modern orangutans, gorillas, chimpanzees, and humans. The split between the line leading to chimpanzees and our own ancestry occurred about 6.5 million years ago (Perelman et al., 2011).

One prominent account of the event that set our lineage on a different path from that of chimpanzees centers on the tectonic movements that created the East African Rift Valley (Coppens, 1994; Kortlandt, 1972). The ongoing separation of the tectonic plates at this juncture led to a series of uplifts on the east side of the rift (Wichura, Bousquet, Oberhänsli, Strecker, &Trauth, 2011), with the result that the rain forests slowly dried out and were replaced by savannah. Our common ancestor with chimpanzees was arboreal, and judging from the ecology of modern chimpanzees, was probably safe from predation in the canopy (Boesch, 1991). In contrast, such an animal would have been relatively easy prey on the ground, as its comparatively slow speed and small size would have made it an easy target for the lions, leopards, saber-toothed cats, and other predators that hunted on the savannah (Hart & Sussman, 2005).

The shift from rain forest to savannah would have put extraordinary pressure on our ancestors, as they would have needed to learn or evolve new ways to find food and new ways to avoid predators. Modern savannah chimpanzees provide some clues about how our ancestors might have adapted to this environment, as the extant chimpanzees that live in similar environments travel in larger groups (Pruetz & Bertolani, 2009), use caves as shelters (Pruetz, 2007), occasionally use sharpened sticks to spear prey in tree hollows (Pruetz & Bertolani, 2007), and share with each other more readily than forest-dwelling chimpanzees (Pruetz & Lindshield, 2012). Similar responses to life on the savannah are likely to have played a role in the lives of our hominin ancestors.

Perhaps most notably, although modern chimpanzees are only occasional cooperators (Boesch, 1994; Gilby, 2006; Hare & Tomasello, 2004), reliable cooperation would have been essential for our ancestors to protect themselves from predators once they were away from the safety of the trees. The most efficacious solution to the increased risk of predation would have been the capacity to throw stones (Calvin, 1982; Isaac, 1987). Although clear evidence for projectile use only appears much later in the archaeological record, support for the possible early use of such a strategy can be seen in changes to the hands of *Australopithecus afarensis,* which enable better throwing and clubbing than the hands of chimpanzees (Marzke, 1983; Napier, 1993; Young, 2003). *Australopithecus* was also bipedal (Crompton et al., 2012), which led to a longer and more flexible waist, a critical trait for the bodily rotation required for strong throwing (Roach, Venkadesan, Rainbow, & Lieberman, 2013). Finally, the chest musculature of arboreal apes facilitates tree climbing and hence is more vertically aligned than is ideal for throwing (Roach et al., 2013).

Stones might not seem like much of a weapon, but the most important combat invention is the capacity to kill at a distance. Killing at a distance allows a large number of weaker individuals to simultaneously attack a stronger target from a position of relative safety. Driving away large predators with stones would likely have required the combined efforts of a group of hominins, so once our ancestors evolved the physical capacity to defend themselves by throwing, there would have been even greater pressure on them to evolve the psychological proclivity to cooperate.

Stone throwing would have also given our ancestors a tool with which they could enforce cooperation from recalcitrant group members, as uncooperative hominins could be safely and readily brought into line by stoning or the threat of stoning (Bingham, 2000). Furthermore, once our ancestors moved to the savannah, expulsion from the group would have been akin to a death sentence, as lone hominins on the grasslands are at much greater risk than lone hominins in the rain forest. Thus, ostracism would have become another highly effective tool for enforcing cooperation. Those hominins who evolved a strong and negative emotional reaction to ostracism would have done their utmost to avoid it, which would have enhanced their survival. Such an evolutionary pathway might explain why people today are so sensitive to rejection and ostracism (Williams, 2007).

Although we do not know when our ancestors began to rely on each other in such a manner, the result of these processes was dramatically increased cooperative inclinations and abilities in our lineage that are evident in many aspects of our psychology (see below). Our cooperative nature is also evident in our anatomy, most notably the whites of our eyes, which are much better at advertising the direction of our gaze than the brown eyes of other apes. The fact that we evolved white sclera suggests that it was to our ancestors' advantage to broadcast their intentions to their fellow group members, who were apparently more likely to facilitate their success than to disrupt it (Tomasello, Hare, Lehmann, & Call, 2007).[3]

The cooperativeness that we evolved to adapt to life on the savannah put increasing pressure on our intelligence, as interdependent group living demands sophisticated cognitive abilities to navigate complex alliances and social opportunities. The advantages of greater intelligence led to numerous changes in our brain, some of which manifested in the timing and rate of human development (Vrba, 1996). A common evolutionary mechanism for changes in morphology is through changes in the timing or pace of development (a concept known as *heterochrony*). The initiation or completion of the development of a trait might occur earlier or later, and development may slow down or speed up. In the case of hominins, development slowed down, enabling a longer period of brain development, as well as an extended period of learning during childhood and adolescence (Bogin, 1997; Sapolsky, 2017). This extended process of development made our species more reliant on a longer period of parental care than was the case for our ancestors (Hrdy, 2011).

By the time of *Homo erectus*—a hominin that appeared 2 million years ago and looks much more like a modern human than like a chimpanzee (Herries et al., 2020)—the evidence suggests that these social pressures and processes had led to the evolution of two important mental capacities. First, *Homo erectus* appears to have been able to envision unfelt needs. The clearest evidence for this capacity lies in the fact that the tools made by *Homo erectus* can be found at great distances from the sites at which they were quarried, suggesting that *Homo erectus* knew that the tools they made would be useful in the future and hence worth bringing along when they traveled (Shipton, 2013). Prior to *Homo erectus,* there is no evidence that our ancestors' tools were ever carried any great distance from the location at which they were made. Once *Homo erectus* was capable of envisioning potential future needs, it gained the advantages of increased preparation and long-term planning (Suddendorf & Corballis, 1997).

Homo erectus also appears to have invented division of labor. There are numerous pieces of evidence for this capacity, but the most common is butchering sites where groups of *Homo erectus* dismembered large and fast animals such as horses. These sites often reveal cut marks made by tools on upper limb bones, areas that are entirely denuded of flesh at carnivore kills. The frequency of these cut marks suggests that

Homo erectus made the kill and was not simply scavenging other animals' kills (Domínguez-Rodrigo, 2002). With their limited toolkit, it would have required the coordinated activities of a group of *Homo erectus* to hunt these animals successfully. Indeed, such achievements are far beyond the capacity of modern chimpanzees, which hunt in groups but lack central coordination and complex planning. As a consequence, chimpanzees do not hunt animals that are larger and stronger than themselves, nor do they show increased effectiveness in group hunting beyond the advantages provided by the sheer number of hunters (Newton-Fisher, 2007).[4]

There is also evidence for division of labor among *Homo erectus* at some of their tool production sites. For example, at a 1.2-million-year-old site in India, the manufacture of stone tools was partitioned into clusters, with spatial separation of different aspects of production (Shipton, 2013). The first step in the production of these stone tools is to knock "flakes" loose from larger stones, which are subsequently shaped into different tools. Evidence at this site suggests that flakes were knocked loose in one location, then retouched into their finished forms in another location. If one hominin were making each tool from start to finish, there would be no reason to separate the production of different stages into different locations (Shipton & Nielsen, 2015). Division of labor requires the capacity to envision the future; thus, it makes sense that division of labor appears to have emerged at approximately the same time as the ability to imagine unfelt needs.

Once *Homo erectus* developed these two important capacities, it would have experienced dramatic increases in effectiveness, with group outcomes now far exceeding the sum of individual efforts. From that point forward, the greatest potential threat to our hominin ancestors was no longer large predators, but rather the destructive capacity of other groups of hominins. With division of labor and future planning, only hominins could plan well enough and work together effectively enough to kill other groups of hominins reliably. As a consequence, although our ancestors had already evolved a strong inclination to cooperate with other members of their group, this disposition was unlikely to have extended to members of other groups that could have posed a deadly threat. Our own species, *Homo sapiens,* is certainly infamous for deadly intergroup conflict (Keeley, 1997; Thorpe, 2003), although we do not know whether this disposition extends back to earlier hominins.[4]

There is a great deal of evidence for *selective,* within-group cooperation in modern humans, but perhaps the clearest distinction is the one between humans and common chimpanzees. When levels of physical conflict within groups of small-scale human populations (that have no recourse to formal laws, police, etc.) are compared to those within chimpanzee groups, chimpanzees range from 150 to 550 times more likely than humans to resort to violence. In contrast, when between-group levels of violence are compared, rates of physical aggression are similar between human foragers and common chimpanzees (Wilson & Wrangham, 2003; Wrangham & Glowacki, 2012; Wrangham & Peterson, 1996).

This evolutionary history may explain why humans have such a strong proclivity to categorize people into ingroups and outgroups. The tendency to divide people into *us* and *them* based on even trivial preferences (Tajfel; 1982; Tajfel & Turner, 1979) may well have roots in an ancestral system that evolved to favor ingroup members (Schaller & Neuberg, 2012). Because members of other groups were sometimes an opportunity and sometimes a threat for our ancestors, the automatic disposition to favor the ingroup without necessarily being biased against outgroups (Brewer, 1999) might have been the most adaptive approach to intergroup relations. This logic is also consistent with numerous lines of evidence, beginning with Sherif, Harvey, White, Hood, and Sherif (1961), suggesting that outgroup hostility emerges with just the slightest sign of threat or competition (Riek, Mania, & Gaertner, 2006). Indeed, the well-known outgroup homogeneity effect can be eliminated or even reversed if outgroup members are depicted with angry expressions (Ackerman et al., 2006).

The tendency to be biased against outgroups was well established in social psychology prior to the advent of this evolutionary theorizing, but evolutionary scholars have also predicted previously undocumented sources of intergroup

friction. Potential for conflict was one source of animosity between ancestral groups, but it was not the only factor that drove groups apart. Parasites and pathogens have always been a major threat, and they appear to have played an important role in intergroup relations as well (Schaller & Neuberg, 2012). When people live in low-pathogen environments (e.g., high latitudes), there is little risk that other groups are a major source of disease, as there is little risk that they carry novel pathogens. But when people live in high-pathogen environments (e.g., the tropics), other groups may well carry novel pathogens to which one's own group has not gained immunity. This threat of pathogens is thought to be another source of ethnocentrism, as people would have learned to avoid members of other groups who made them sick. The end result of such pathogen-driven, intergroup avoidance is an increase in languages and religions among people who live in high-pathogen environments (e.g., close to the equator) because long-term separation results in linguistic and cultural divergence (Fincher & Thornhill, 2008a, 2008b). Such divergence, in turn, further isolates groups and reduces this biological threat.

Disease threats also led to cultural differences and active avoidance between groups based on local topography, such as between low-elevation societies that harbored malaria and adjacent mountain societies that did not (Webb, 2009). Indeed, it was the evolution of hypersociality and division of labor that led to pandemics in the first place, as people settled in large groups around water sources, which enabled vector-borne diseases such as malaria to cause widespread mortality, driving further cultural evolution.

Pathogen-driven ethnocentrism may also lead to emotions such as anger and disgust at cultural practices that diverge from one's own. Particularly when such practices concern norms regarding food preparation and sexual activities, unfamiliar practices can lead to new sources of disease transmission. Thus, the symbolic forms of prejudice that often focus on cultural differences, and that play an important role in various types of hostile intergroup relations, might have roots in habits that facilitated pathogen avoidance among our ancestors (Schaller & Neuberg, 2012). The relative importance of biological versus cultural evolution in the development of such forms of prejudice is an open question.

Uniquely Human Cognitive and Motivational Systems

Our social solution to the challenges of life on the savannah appears to have set our ancestors on a distinct path, with numerous consequences that are evident in our motivational and cognitive systems. The psychological domains most frequently proposed to set humans apart from our great ape cousins are language, foresight, theory of mind, intelligence, culture, and morality. Despite our unique abilities in each of these domains, in all of them other animals show more sophisticated competences than is often assumed. For instance, chimpanzees can maintain social traditions, solve problems through insight, and console others in distress (Suddendorf, 2013). Nevertheless, Suddendorf found that two major psychological features— one cognitive and the other motivational—kept reemerging as critical and distinctly human, transforming the abilities that are shared with other animals into the massively enhanced versions that characterize human functioning. First, humans have the unique capacity for *nested scenario building,* or the open-ended ability to imagine and reflect on different situations and embed them into larger narratives. Second, humans have an *urge to connect,* a strong and unique desire to link our scenario-building minds together, to exchange our experiences, reflections, and ideas. Together these two distinct features have profoundly altered our minds. Nonhuman animals have memory and some future-directed abilities, but only humans can use these capacities to make long-term plans, test them through mental simulations, embed them into larger narratives, and share them with others to recruit them to their cause.

As a consequence, humans rely on a uniquely flexible way to self-regulate. Through nested scenario building, we contemplate mutually exclusive possibilities and make contingency plans, envision the world from the perspectives of others, and even entertain entirely fictional scenarios (Redshaw & Suddendorf, 2016, 2020). Nested scenario building enables us to travel mentally through time, as it were,

and consider how events unfolded and, importantly, what the future might hold (Suddendorf & Corballis, 2007). This capacity enables us to prepare in prudent ways. Our current situations can be embedded into larger narratives, and by comparing alternative routes to the future we can deliberately select one plan over another— giving us a sense of free will and an advantage over creatures with more restricted imagination (Suddendorf, 2013).

Though tremendously potent, this mode of making decisions also burdens us with the responsibility for getting it right. The key to using these mental simulations effectively is our second distinct characteristic: our fundamental urge to link our minds together, to look to one another for useful information (Suddendorf, 2013; Tomasello, Carpenter, Call, Behne, & Moll, 2005). We regularly ask questions and give advice. This social approach allows us to take advantage of others' memory, insights, and plans to guide our own behavior. This social approach also allows us to bond over shared experiences and beliefs in our mutual pursuit of a *shared reality* (Higgins, 2019). We are deeply social animals because of this fundamental urge and capacity to wire our scenario-building minds together. And we are so powerful in groups because shared realities ensure that our goals are mutual and our strategies are complementary. We benefit from our accumulated, collective wit. Recently humans have taken this capacity to new levels, as we create ever larger networks of knowledge and information accumulated across generations and billions of people.

Most benefits are accompanied by associated costs, and nested scenario building along with an urge to connect are no exception in this regard. Constructing appropriate mental scenarios is resource intensive, and despite our best efforts we often get it wrong (Suddendorf, 2013; Tetlock & Gardner, 2016). For instance, we tend to exaggerate the impact of future successes and failures on how we will feel, resulting in affective forecasting errors (Wilson & Gilbert, 2003), though these biases may drive more future-directed decision making (Miloyan & Suddendorf, 2015; Morewedge & Buechel, 2013). Furthermore, it is not always obvious which problems are beneficial to simulate and ponder.

Some future events can be improved via planning, but there are many that we can do little about, and others (e.g., our own ultimate mortality) that are impossible to circumvent (Greenberg, Solomon, & Pyszczynski, 1997; Varki, 2009). Thus, it can be advantageous to foresee and hence forestall threats, but this capacity can also bring despair and misery. Anxiety disorders, depression, and suicidal tendencies are some of the more negative consequences of our capacity to generate complex mental scenarios regarding past and future events (Miloyan, Bulley, & Suddendorf, 2018).

The Evolution of Cultural Capabilities

The evolution of flowering plants revealed the superiority of a cooperative solution to the lack of mobility, and it also led to an explosion of new species in the coevolution between flowering plants and their insect pollinators. Insects now comprise the vast majority of animal life and flowering plants comprise the vast majority of plant life (Adams, 2009). Although many species of insects are capable of pollinating a wide variety of plants, specialists tend to outcompete generalists due to their greater efficiency (Waser & Ollerton, 2006). As a result, the symbiotic interaction between flowering plants and insect pollinators led to a massive increase in insects that specialized in retrieving the nectar from particular plants, and plants that adapted their morphology and developmental timing in concert with insect morphology and behavior. These new plants and insects created the conditions for the evolution of new herbivores, predators, and parasites; hence, the majority of terrestrial life on Earth owes its origins to the cooperative relationship that evolved between flowering plants and insects (Futuyma & Agrawal, 2009).

Again, we see parallels with the human success story. Our hypersociality led to an increase in brain size as we evolved greater intelligence to exploit our newly emerging social proclivities and capabilities. This increase in brain size, in turn, led to the creation of another niche on this planet: the cognitive niche (Pinker, 2010; Tooby & DeVore, 1987). Like the evolution of plant–insect mutualism, the creation of the cognitive niche also resulted in an explosion in evolution, but in this case only one generalist genus emerged from this process rather than countless specialist species. Why is that?

The answer to this puzzle can be found in our most important social strategy: cumulative culture (Baumeister, 2005; Dean, Kendal, Schapiro, Thierry, & Laland, 2012; Tennie, Call, & Tomasello, 2009; Tomasello, Kruger, & Ratner, 1993). Culture is our second inheritance system, beyond genetic inheritance, and it gives us extraordinary powers derived from our collective experience. Humans rely on social learning more than any other species, and one consequence of our dependence on social learning is the evolution of our incredible communicative capacities in the form of language (e.g., Pinker, 2010). Nested scenario building and an urge to wire our minds together led to the evolution of an open-ended communication system that allows us to exchange novel ideas, relay past, future, and fictional scenarios, and accumulate knowledge (Suddendorf, 2013). Whenever someone has a new idea, that person has the capacity to communicate that idea to others, with the result that people can learn from the experiences and innovations of others even in the complete absence of direct experience. That ability enables each generation to scaffold its innovations on the experiences and ideas of others, living and dead, which enables knowledge to accumulate over time. No other species can do this. The result of this process is that we are the greatest generalists on Earth, but at the same time we have all of the advantages of specialization.

Cultural learning enabled us to become specialists as we moved into every new environment, without requiring much in the way of further morphological or physiological evolution.[5] Consider, by way of example, the frequent story of European explorers who perished in environments that provided plenty of food, water, and shelter for the local indigenous population. The explorers were usually outfitted with more effective and modern tools than the local population, but they lacked the culturally accumulated capacity for exploiting the local environment and thus at times perished in a land of plenty (Henrich, 2015).

The incredible potential of cultural knowledge ensured that humans evolved special capacities and proclivities that facilitated social learning, which in turn enhanced the value of culture. The capacity for language is a clear example, as it enables much greater social learning than could ever be achieved by observation alone, but other abilities also play a role. Nested scenario building allows us to imagine other individuals' mental states (theory of mind) and the urge to connect drives us to understand and be understood (Suddendorf, 2013). These are important abilities for a cultural animal, as they enhance social learning. Deliberate teaching, for instance, requires reasoning about what the pupil does and does not know, as well as plotting how future experiences might change the pupil's knowledge or skills. This awareness about the minds of others also facilitates competition and cooperation. Indeed, perspective taking enhances the effectiveness of people's interactions across a wide range of domains (Galinsky, Maddux, Gilin, & White, 2008; Keysar, Barr, Balin, & Brauner, 2000; Stiller & Dunbar, 2007).

Humans also have a distinct tendency to *overimitate* or copy actions that appear to be of no use in problem solving (Nielsen & Tomaselli, 2010). The classic overimitation study by Horner and Whiten (2005) presented children and chimpanzees with a box that had a treat inside. Horner and Whiten demonstrated how to open the box but included some irrelevant actions that played no role in opening it. For example, they first poked a stick into a hole in the top of the box even though the only latch was on the side. When the box was opaque, and observers were unable to ascertain the relevance of the hole on the top, both children and chimpanzees copied all the actions and successfully opened the box. When the box was transparent, however, and it was obvious which actions were relevant and which were not, the chimpanzees only modeled the necessary actions and ignored the irrelevant ones. Human children, in contrast, continued to model the actions that were now obviously unnecessary. This overimitation plays an important role in social learning, as it ensures high-fidelity copying even when the learner does not understand the processes he or she is imitating. Overimitation also enables the maintenance of effective cultural practices, even if their original purpose might have been

forgotten or never fully understood (e.g., if the trial-and-error process that generated them resides in the distant past).

These unique human capacities and proclivities suggest that once they began to exploit the cognitive niche, culture itself became an increasingly important evolutionary force on our ancestors. It is important to keep in mind that the transfer of information and its accumulation is only adaptive when someone has valuable information to share. Human cultural transmission is so powerful largely because we are so innovative. Our capacity for nested scenario building allows us to imagine the functionality and aesthetics of different versions of tools before we make them, enabling us to envision and test solutions in our minds. Just as important as being creative problem solvers, and possibly even more so, our capacity for foresight enables us to realize when a solution is worth retaining (Suddendorf, Bulley, & Miloyan, 2018). Many animals use tools, and some even make tools to solve problems (Sanz, Call, & Boesch, 2013). But their tools do not appear to improve over time, as they discard them once they are finished with the task at hand, rather than retaining and potentially refining them for future use.

Foresight allows humans to ponder future situations in which the tool might again be useful, which can motivate us to retain the tool or share it with other group members (von Hippel & Suddendorf, 2018). The same foresight also allows us to ponder situations in which the tool might have weaknesses, which can motivate us to refine it further. These processes enabled humans to survive and thrive under incredibly diverse circumstances, and to become powerful predators despite the absence of outstanding biological weapons such as the massive musculature, teeth, and claws of the large cats that once threatened us on the savannah. As a consequence of these diverse processes, people have evolved extraordinary capacity for innovation. And because innovation is so critical for cumulative culture, innovative people are particularly valuable group members.

It is one thing to invent a new tool, but it is quite another to learn to use it properly. As tools become more complex, they often require highly specific skills to make them effective. Thus, the ability to acquire new skills would likely have had great adaptive value for ancestral hominins. For instance, the capacity to kill at a distance relies on the ability to throw accurately and with force, and that capacity can be leveraged further with the creation of new projectile weapons. Enhanced weaponry like a spear thrower and, later still, the bow and arrow, are only a powerful advance if people can acquire the motor skills to use them effectively. This potential bottleneck might seem like a physical problem rather than a mental one, but it is not. A key mental capacity that allows humans to hone new skills and benefit from cumulative culture is *deliberate practice,* the repetition of actions with the goal of enhancing future skills (Suddendorf, Brinums, & Imuta, 2016).

Deliberate practice presupposes an ability to think about future situations, and it develops similarly to other foresight skills in young children (Brinums, Imuta, & Suddendorf, 2018; Davis, Cullen, & Suddendorf, 2016). With the capacity for deliberate practice, humans gained the ability to shape their own future abilities. By deciding what to practice, people can elect to acquire skills that they foresee as being useful at a future point in time. The same logic applies to knowledge acquisition. We can study information that has no immediate value but that we assume will have future utility. Deliberate practice and information acquisition enabled our ancestors to change their future expertise and rapidly adapt to new circumstances. With deliberate practice we can teach ourselves.

Importantly, our urge to connect ensures that we also teach each other. As noted earlier, deliberate teaching tends to be based on reasoning about the minds of others. Teaching others tends to involve guided practice, instructions regarding deliberate practice, monitoring of progress, and correction of errors. Teaching and deliberate practice are closely associated and can be regarded as opposite sides of the same coin (Premack, 2007). Both can be employed to shape future capacities in intentional ways. Together with imitation, teaching oneself and each other are essential to the accumulation of human culture, and hence to the survival and reproductive success of the cultural animals we have become.

The combination of nested scenario building and the urge to connect their minds with each other enabled teaching and deliberate practice in our ancestors, which in turn gave them the possibility to *flexibly specialize* (Suddendorf, Brinums, & Imuta, 2016). Somewhat ironically, their generalist capacities enabled them to rapidly specialize in light of changing circumstances, even before the circumstances changed. We can shape our capacities according to what we foresee to be the most useful skills and knowledge in the future. This capacity unlocked the potential of our cognitive niche. It makes us capable of shaping the world to our design (a concept known as *niche construction*; Laland, Odling-Smee, & Feldman, 2000; Odling-Smee, Laland, & Feldman, 2003), while also shaping ourselves to fit the world. Biological evolution can only "look backward" in the sense that we evolve to fit past environments. In contrast, the capacity for flexible specialization allows us to change ourselves to fit a world that does not yet exist and can only be envisioned.

As we noted earlier, trade-offs are ubiquitous, and skills acquisition is no exception. The process of gaining expertise is time consuming, and not all people are equally suited to all tasks (that all-important variation in traits noted by Darwin). Thus, as the amount of knowledge and the number of potential skills multiplied, it became increasingly difficult to master all of them. Fortunately, individuals do not need to master all trades, as our sociality and interdependence enable us to benefit from each other's skills and knowledge. Not every member of our ancestral groups needed to be equally skilled at lighting a fire, making a spear, hunting, or weaving a basket. As long as a critical number of people were skilled in these activities, group members could share the rewards brought by these capacities; therefore, the pressure for division of labor intensified.

Play is rarely studied by social psychologists, but it is not hard to see that human development is a process of acquiring the capacities and skills that make one a valued group member. When children play with each other they not only learn social skills, they also learn about their gifts and their potential for different tasks (Suddendorf, 2013). Traits that set people apart are more likely to become part of their self-concept than traits they share with everyone else (Cooley, 1902/2011; McGuire, McGuire,

& Winton, 1979; McGuire & Padawer-Singer, 1976), particularly if these traits have positive value (von Hippel, Hawkins, & Schooler, 2001). From this perspective, one of the goals of childhood is to discover the domains in which you have good prospects, then develop skills in those areas, thereby allowing you to contribute most effectively as an adult group member.

Cooperative social groups that created complementary skills (i.e., that employed division of labor) eventually outcompeted other groups. Our sociality was the key to our success, but largely because our sociality redirected us onto an evolutionary pathway that happened to result in an extraordinary set of skills and proclivities. The cognitive capacity for nested scenario building combined with the motivation to connect our minds together led to dramatic changes in the way we communicate, understand and evaluate each other, solve problems, and cooperate. These processes provided us the necessary foundation to develop the technology, civilizations, and diversity that characterize human cultures. Just as the flowers and fruit of angiosperms created a coevolutionary explosion that led to a vast new array of species, our cognitive and motivational processes coevolved with our cultural capacities to create a population and technological explosion that has fundamentally altered our planet.

ACKNOWLEDGMENTS

Preparation of this chapter was facilitated by Grant No. DP160100942 from the Australian Research Council.

NOTES

1. Females often prefer features that are fitness neutral or detract from a male's chance of survival. Such preferences can be complex, multiply determined, and responsive to biases in female sensory systems (for reviews, see Fuller, Houle, & Travis, 2005; Kuijper, Pen, & Weissing, 2012; Zahavi & Zahavi, 1999).

2. *Hominin* is a term for modern humans and our extinct ancestors back to our common ancestor with chimpanzees. *Hominid* is a term for all existing and extinct great apes, including modern gorillas, orangutans, chimpanzees, and humans.

3. If broadcasting intentions was advantageous to the group but detrimental to the individual, it would have been highly unlikely to have evolved.

4. It is important to keep in mind that chimpanzees also lack the capacity to kill at a distance.

5. Although universal cooperation might have been beneficial to *Homo sapiens* as a species, evolution does not operate at the level of the species, and in fact competition is most intense with other members of the same species. Traits and behaviors that enhanced individual success were likely to propagate, and numerous opportunities made conflict with other groups advantageous to our ancestors (e.g., theft of portable wealth, expulsion of competitors from good hunting grounds or watering holes, mating opportunities; see Chagnon, 1988; Mathew & Boyd, 2011).

6. Some local adaptation occurs when people move into a new ecological niche, as they evolve the capacity to fight local pathogens, thermoregulate in a different climate, and so forth. Thus, different ethnic groups often have different blood markers, skin pigments, patterns of fat deposits, etc., that evolved in response to sustained local demands.

REFERENCES

Ackerman, J. M., Shapiro, J. R., Neuberg, S. L., Kenrick, D. T., Becker, D. V., Griskevicius, V., et al. (2006). They all look the same to me (unless they're angry) from out-group homogeneity to out-group heterogeneity. *Psychological Science, 17,* 836–840.

Adams, J. (2009). *Species richness: Patterns in the diversity of life.* Berlin, Germany: Springer.

Andersson, M. (1982). Female choice selects for extreme tail length in a widowbird. *Nature, 299,* 818–820.

Balliet, D., Tybur, J. M., & Van Lange, P. A. (2017). Functional interdependence theory: An evolutionary account of social situations. *Personality and Social Psychology Review, 21,* 361–388.

Bates, L. A., Sayialel, K. N., Njiraini, N. W., Poole, J. H., Moss, C. J., & Byrne, R. W. (2008). African elephants have expectations about the locations of out-of-sight family members. *Biology Letters, 4,* 34–36.

Baumeister, R. F. (2005). *The cultural animal: Human nature, meaning, and social life.* New York: Oxford University Press.

Beck, C. B. (1988). *Origin and evolution of gymnosperms.* New York: Columbia University Press.

Bigg, M. A., Olesiuk, P. F., Ellis, G. M., Ford, J. K. B., & Balcomb, K. C. (1990). Organization and genealogy of resident killer whales (*Orcinus orca*) in the coastal waters of British Columbia and Washington state. *Report—International Whaling Commission, 12,* 383–405.

Bingham, P. M. (2000). Human evolution and human history: A complete theory. *Evolutionary Anthropology, 9,* 248–257.

Boesch, C. (1991). The effects of leopard predation on grouping patterns in forest chimpanzees. *Behaviour, 117,* 220–242.

Boesch, C. (1994). Cooperative hunting in wild chimpanzees. *Animal Behaviour, 48,* 653–667.

Bogin, B. A. (1997). Evolutionary hypotheses for human childhood. *Yearbook of Physical Anthropology, 40,* 63–89.

Brewer, M. B. (1999). The psychology of prejudice: Ingroup love and outgroup hate? *Journal of Social Issues, 55,* 429–444.

Brinums, M., Imuta, K., & Suddendorf, T. (2018). Practicing for the future: Deliberate practice in early childhood. *Child Development, 89*(6), 2051–2058.

Buss, D. M. (2000). The evolution of happiness. *American Psychologist, 55,* 15–23.

Byrne, R. W., & Whiten, A. (1988). *Machiavellian intelligence: Social expertise and the evolution of intellect in monkeys, apes and humans.* Oxford, UK: Oxford University Press.

Calvin, W. H. (1982). Did throwing stones shape hominid brain evolution? *Ethology and Sociobiology, 3,* 115–124.

Chagnon, N. A. (1988). Life histories, blood revenge, and warfare in a tribal population. *Science, 239,* 985–992.

Cheney, D. L., & Seyfarth, R. M. (1990). *How monkeys see the world.* Chicago: University of Chicago Press.

Confer, J. C., Easton, J. A., Fleischman, D. S., Goetz, C. D., Lewis, D. M., Perilloux, C., et al. (2010). Evolutionary psychology: Controversies, questions, prospects, and limitations. *American Psychologist, 65,* 110–126.

Cooley, C. H. (1902). The looking-glass self. In J. O'Brien (Ed.), *The production of reality: Essays and readings on social interaction* (5th ed., pp. 126–128). Thousand Oaks, CA: Pine Forge Press. (Original work published 1902)

Coppens, Y. (1994). East side story: The origin of humankind. *Scientific American, 270,* 88–95.

Cosmides, L. (1989). The logic of social exchange: Has natural selection shaped how humans reason?: Studies with the Wason selection task. *Cognition, 31*(3), 187–276.

Cosmides, L., Barrett, H. C., & Tooby, J. (2010). Adaptive specializations, social exchange, and the evolution of human intelligence. *Proceedings of the National Academy of Sciences of the USA, 107,* 9007–9014.

Cosmides, L., & Tooby, J. (2000). Evolutionary psychology and the emotions. In M. Lewis & J. M. Haviland-Jones (Eds.), *Handbook of emotions* (2nd ed., pp. 91–115). New York: Guilford Press.

Crompton, R. H., Pataky, T. C., Savage, R., D'Août, K., Bennett, M. R., Day, M. H., et al. (2012). Human-like external function of the foot, and fully upright gait, confirmed in the 3.66 million year old *Laetolihominin* footprints by topographic statistics, experimental footprint-formation and computer simulation. *Journal of the Royal Society Interface, 9,* 707–719.

Darwin, C. (1859). *On the origin of the species by natural selection.* London: John Murray.

Darwin, C. (1874). *The descent of man, and selection in relation to sex* (2nd ed.). London: John Murray.

Davis, J. T. M., Cullen, E., & Suddendorf, T. (2016). Understanding deliberate practice in preschool aged children. *Quarterly Journal of Experimental Psychology, 69,* 361–380.

De Waal, F. B. (2000). Primates—a natural heritage of conflict resolution. *Science, 289,* 586–590.

Dean, L. G., Kendal, R. L., Schapiro, S. J., Thierry, B., & Laland, K. N. (2012). Identification of the social and cognitive processes underlying human cumulative culture. *Science, 335,* 1114–1118.

Deci, E. L., & Ryan, R. M. (1975). *Intrinsic motivation.* New York: Wiley.

Domínguez-Rodrigo, M. (2002). Hunting and scavenging by early humans: The state of the debate. *Journal of World Prehistory, 16,* 1–54.

Dunbar, R. I. (1991). Functional significance of social grooming in primates. *Folia Primatologica, 57,* 121–131.

Dunbar, R. I., & Shultz, S. (2007). Evolution in the social brain. *Science, 317,* 1344–1347.

Fernald, R. D. (2000). Evolution of eyes. *Current Opinion in Neurobiology, 10,* 444–450.

Fincher, C. L., & Thornhill, R. (2008a). Assortative sociality, limited dispersal, infectious disease and the genesis of the global pattern of religion diversity. *Proceedings of the Royal Society of London B: Biological Sciences, 275,* 2587–2594.

Fincher, C. L., & Thornhill, R. (2008b). A parasite-driven wedge: Infectious diseases may explain language and other biodiversity. *Oikos, 117,* 1289–1297.

Frith, U., & Frith, C. (2010). The social brain: Allowing humans to boldly go where no other species has been. *Philosophical Transactions of the Royal Society B: Biological Sciences, 365,* 165–175.

Fuller, R. C., Houle, D., & Travis, J. (2005). Sensory bias as an explanation for the evolution of mate preferences. *American Naturalist, 166*(4), 437–446.

Futuyma, D. J., & Agrawal, A. A. (2009). Macroevolution and the biological diversity of plants and herbivores. *Proceedings of the National Academy of Sciences of the USA, 106,* 18054–18061.

Galinsky, A. D., Maddux, W. W., Gilin, D., & White, J. B. (2008). Why it pays to get inside the head of your opponent: The differential effects of perspective taking and empathy in negotiations. *Psychological Science, 19,* 378–384.

Gilby, I. C. (2006). Meat sharing among the Gombe chimpanzees: Harassment and reciprocal exchange. *Animal Behaviour, 71,* 953–963.

Greenberg, J., Solomon, S., & Pyszczynski, T. (1997). Terror management theory of self-esteem and cultural worldviews: Empirical assessments and conceptual refinements. In M. P. Zanna (Ed.), *Advances in experimental social psychology* (Vol. 29, pp. 61–139). San Diego, CA: Academic Press.

Hare, B., & Tomasello, M. (2004). Chimpanzees are more skilful in competitive than in cooperative cognitive tasks. *Animal Behaviour, 68,* 571–581.

Hart, D., & Sussman, R. W. (2005). *Man the hunted: Primates, predators, and human evolution.* Boulder, CO: Westview Press.

Hartl, D. L., Clark, A. G., & Clark, A. G. (1997). *Principles of population genetics* (Vol. 116). Sunderland, MA: Sinauer Associates.

Hawks, J., Wang, E. T., Cochran, G. M., Harpending, H. C., & Moyzis, R. K. (2007). Recent acceleration of human adaptive evolution. *Proceedings of the National Academy of Sciences of the USA, 104,* 20753–20758.

Henrich, J. (2015). *The secret of our success: How culture is driving human evolution, domesticating our species, and making us smarter.* Princeton, NJ: Princeton University Press.

Herries, A. I., Martin, J. M., Leece, A. B., Adams, J. W., Boschian, G., Joannes-Boyau, R., et al. (2020). Contemporaneity of *Australopithecus, Paranthropus,* and early *Homo erectus* in South Africa. *Science, 368.*

Higgins, E. T. (2019). *Shared reality: What makes us strong and tears us apart.* New York: Oxford University Press.

Horner, V., & Whiten, A. (2005). Causal knowledge and imitation/emulation switching in chimpanzees (*Pan troglodytes*) and children (*Homo sapiens*). *Animal Cognition, 8,* 164–181.

Hrdy, S. B. (2011). *Mothers and others.* Cambridge, MA: Harvard University Press.

Humphrey, N. (1976). The social function of intellect. In P. P. G. Bateson & R. A. Hinde (Eds.), *Growing points in ethology* (pp. 303–313). Cambridge, UK: Cambridge University Press.

Isaac, B. (1987). Throwing and human evolution. *African Archaeological Review, 5,* 3–17.

Jacob, F. (1977). Evolution and tinkering. *Science, 196*(4295), 1161–1166.

Jolly, A. (1966). Lemur social behavior and primate intelligence. *Science, 153,* 501–506.

Keeley, L. H. (1997). *War before civilization.* New York: Oxford University Press.

Keysar, B., Barr, D. J., Balin, J. A., & Brauner, J. S. (2000). Taking perspective in conversation: The role of mutual knowledge in comprehension. *Psychological Science, 11,* 32–38.

Kortlandt, A. (1972). *New perspectives on ape and human evolution.* Amsterdam, the Netherlands: Stichting voor Psychobiologie.

Kuijper, B., Pen, I., & Weissing, F. J. (2012). A guide to sexual selection theory. *Annual Review of Ecology, Evolution, and Systematics, 43,* 287–311.

Laland, K. N., Odling-Smee, J., & Feldman, M. W. (2000). Niche construction, biological evolution, and cultural change. *Behavioral and Brain Sciences, 23,* 131–146.

Lamb, T. D., Collin, S. P., & Pugh, E. N., Jr. (2007). Evolution of the vertebrate eye: Opsins, photoreceptors, retina and eye cup. *Nature Reviews Neuroscience, 8,* 960–976.

Lande, R. (1980). Sexual dimorphism, sexual selection, and adaptation in polygenic characters. *Evolution, 34,* 292–305.

Marzke, M. W. (1983). Joint functions and grips of the *Australopithecus afarensis* hand, with special reference to the region of the capitate. *Journal of Human Evolution, 12,* 197–211.

Mathew, S., & Boyd, R. (2011). Punishment sustains large-scale cooperation in prestate warfare. *Proceedings of the National Academy of Sciences of the USA, 108,* 11375–11380.

McGuire, W. J., McGuire, C. V., & Winton, W. (1979). Effects of household sex composition on the salience of one's gender in the spontaneous self-concept. *Journal of Experimental Social Psychology, 15,* 77–90.

McGuire, W. J., & Padawer-Singer, A. (1976). Trait salience in the spontaneous self-concept. *Journal of Personality and Social Psychology, 33,* 743–754.

Mercier, H., & Sperber, D. (2011). Why do humans reason?: Arguments for an argumentative theory. *Behavioral and Brain Sciences, 34,* 57–74.

Miloyan, B., Bulley, A., & Suddendorf, T. (2018). Anxiety: Here and beyond. *Emotion Review, 11*(1), 39–49.

Miloyan, B., & Suddendorf, T. (2015). Feelings of the future. *Trends in Cognitive Sciences, 19,* 196–200.

Morewedge, C. K., & Buechel, E. C. (2013). Motivated underpinnings of the impact bias in affective forecasts. *Emotion, 13,* 1023–1029.

Murphy, S. C., von Hippel, W., Dubbs, S. L., Angilletta, M. J., Jr., Wilson, R. S., Trivers, R., et al.

(2015). The role of overconfidence in romantic de-sirability and competition. *Personality and Social Psychology Bulletin, 41,* 1036–1052.

Napier, J. R. (1993). *Hands.* Princeton, NJ: Princeton University Press.

Newton-Fisher, N. E. (2007). Chimpanzee hunting behavior. In W. Henke & I. Tattersall (Eds.), *Handbook of paleoanthropology* (pp. 1295–1320). Berlin, Germany: Springer.

Nielsen, M., & Tomaselli, K. (2010). Overimitation in Kalahari Bushman children and the origins of human cultural cognition. *Psychological Science, 21,* 729–736.

Odling-Smee, F. J., Laland, K. N., & Feldman, M. W. (2003). *Niche construction: The neglected process in evolution.* Princeton, NJ: Princeton University Press.

Perelman, P., Johnson, W. E., Roos, C., Seuánez, H. N., Horvath, J. E., Moreira, M. A., et al. (2011). A molecular phylogeny of living primates. *PLOS Genetics, 7,* e1001342.

Pinker, S. (2010). The cognitive niche: Coevolution of intelligence, sociality, and language. *Proceedings of the National Academy of Sciences of the USA, 107,* 8993–8999.

Premack, D. (2007). Human and animal cognition: Continuity and discontinuity. *Proceedings of the National Academy of Sciences of the USA, 104,* 13861–13867.

Pruetz, J. D. (2007). Evidence of cave use by savanna chimpanzees (*Pan troglodytesverus*) at Fongoli, Senegal: Implications for thermoregulatory behavior. *Primates, 48,* 316–319.

Pruetz, J. D., & Bertolani, P. (2007). Savanna chimpanzees, *Pan troglodytesverus,* hunt with tools. *Current Biology, 17,* 412–417.

Pruetz, J. D., & Bertolani, P. (2009). Chimpanzee (*Pan troglodytesverus*) behavioral responses to stresses associated with living in a savanna-mosaic environment: Implications for hominin adaptations to open habitats. *PaleoAnthropology, 2009,* 252–262.

Pruetz, J. D., & Lindshield, S. (2012). Plant-food and tool transfer among savanna chimpanzees at Fongoli, Senegal. *Primates, 53,* 133–145.

Reader, S. M., & Laland, K. N. (2002). Social intelligence, innovation, and enhanced brain size in primates. *Proceedings of the National Academy of Sciences of the USA, 99,* 4436–4441.

Redshaw, J., & Suddendorf, T. (2016). Children's and apes' preparatory responses to two mutually exclusive possibilities. *Current Biology, 26*(13), 1758–1762.

Redshaw, J., & Suddendorf, T. (2020). Temporal junctures in the mind. *Trends in Cognitive Sciences, 24,* 52–64.

Riek, B. M., Mania, E. W., & Gaertner, S. L. (2006). Intergroup threat and outgroup attitudes: A meta-analytic review. *Personality and Social Psychology Review, 10,* 336–353.

Roach, N. T., Venkadesan, M., Rainbow, M. J., & Lieberman, D. E. (2013). Elastic energy storage in the shoulder and the evolution of high-speed throwing in *Homo. Nature, 498,* 483–487.

Sanz, C. M., Call, J., & Boesch, C. (Eds.). (2013). *Tool use in animals: Cognition and ecology.* Cambridge, UK: Cambridge University Press.

Sapolsky, R. M. (2017). *Behave: The biology of humans at our best and worst.* New York: Penguin.

Schaller, M., & Neuberg, S. L. (2012). Danger, disease, and the nature of prejudice(s). *Advances in Experimental Social Psychology, 46,* 1–54.

Sherif, M., Harvey, O. J., White, B. J., Hood, W. R., & Sherif, C. W. (1961). *Intergroup conflict and cooperation: The Robbers Cave experiment.* Norman: University of Oklahoma Press.

Shipton, C. (2013). *A million years of hominin sociality and cognition: Acheuleanbifaces in the Hunsgi-Baichbal Valley, India.* Oxford, UK: Archaeopress.

Shipton, C., & Nielsen, M. (2015). Before cumulative culture. *Human Nature, 26,* 331–345.

Soltis, D., Soltis, P., Endress, P., Chase, M. W., Manchester, S., Judd, W., et al. (2018). *Phylogeny and evolution of the angiosperms: Revised and updated edition.* Chicago: University of Chicago Press.

Stiller, J., & Dunbar, R. I. (2007). Perspective-taking and memory capacity predict social network size. *Social Networks, 29,* 93–104.

Street, S. E., Navarrete, A. F., Reader, S. M., & Laland, K. N. (2017). Coevolution of cultural intelligence, extended life history, sociality, and brain size in primates. *Proceedings of the National Academy of Sciences of the USA, 114,* 7908–7914.

Suddendorf, T. (2013). *The gap: The science of what separates us from other animals.* New York: Basic Books.

Suddendorf, T., Brinums, M., & Imuta, K. (2016). Shaping one's future self: The development of deliberate practice. In S. B. Klein, K. Michaelian, & K. K. Szpunar (Eds.), *Seeing the future: Theoretical perspectives on future-oriented mental time travel* (pp. 343–366). London: Oxford University Press.

Suddendorf, T., Bulley, A., & Miloyan, B. (2018). Prospection and natural selection. *Current Opinion in Behavioral Science, 24,* 26–31.

Suddendorf, T., & Corballis, M. C. (1997). Mental time travel and the evolution of the human mind. *Genetic, Social, and General Psychology Monographs, 123,* 133–167.

Suddendorf, T., & Corballis, M. C. (2007). The evolution of foresight: What is mental time travel, and is it unique to humans? *Behavioral and Brain Sciences, 30,* 299–313.

Suddendorf, T., & Dong, A. (2013). On the evolution of imagination and design. In M. Taylor (Ed.), *The Oxford handbook of the development of imagination* (pp. 453–467). Oxford, UK: Oxford University Press.

Tajfel, H. (1982). Social psychology of intergroup relations. *Annual Review of Psychology, 33,* 1–39.

Tajfel, H., & Turner, J. C. (1979). An integrative theory of intergroup conflict. In W. G. Austin & J. Worchel (Eds.), *The social psychology of intergroup relations* (pp. 33–47). Monterey, CA: Brooks/Cole.

Tennie, C., Call, J., & Tomasello, M. (2009). Ratcheting up the ratchet: On the evolution of cumulative culture. *Philosophical Transactions of the Royal Society B: Biological Sciences, 364,* 2405–2415.

Tetlock, P. E., & Gardner, D. (2016). *Superforecasting: The art and science of prediction.* New York: Random House.

Thorpe, I. J. N. (2003). Anthropology, archaeology, and the origin of warfare. *World Archaeology, 35,* 145–165.

Tomasello, M. (2014). *A natural history of human thinking.* Cambridge, MA: Harvard University Press.

Tomasello, M., Carpenter, M., Call, J., Behne, T., & Moll, H. (2005). Understanding and sharing intentions: The origins of cultural cognition. *Behavioral and Brain Sciences, 28,* 675–691.

Tomasello, M., Hare, B., Lehmann, H., & Call, J. (2007). Reliance on head versus eyes in the gaze following of great apes and human infants: The cooperative eye hypothesis. *Journal of Human Evolution, 52,* 314–320.

Tomasello, M., Kruger, A. C., & Ratner, H. H. (1993). Cultural learning. *Behavioral and Brain Sciences, 16*(3), 495–511.

Tooby, J., & Cosmides, L. (1990). The past explains the present: Emotional adaptations and the structure of ancestral environments. *Ethology and Sociobiology, 11,* 375–424.

Tooby, J., & DeVore, I. (1987). The reconstruction of hominid evolution through strategic modeling. In W. G. Kinzey (Ed.), *The evolution of human behavior: Primate models* (pp. 183–237). Albany: State University of New York Press.

Trivers, R. (1972). Parental investment and sexual selection. In B. Campbell (Ed.), *Sexual selection and the descent of man* (pp. 136–179). Chicago: Aldine.

Varki, A. (2009). Human uniqueness and the denial of death. *Nature, 460,* 684.

von Hippel, W. (2018). *The social leap.* New York: HarperCollins.

von Hippel, W., & Buss, D. M. (2017). Do ideologically driven scientific agendas impede the understanding and acceptance of evolutionary principles in social psychology? In J. T. Crawford & L. Jussim (Eds.), *The politics of social psychology* (pp. 7–25). New York: Routledge.

von Hippel, W., & Gonsalkorale, K. (2018). Evolutionary imperatives and the good life. In J. P. Forgas & R. F. Baumeister (Eds.), *The social psychology of living well* (pp. 34–47). New York: Routledge.

von Hippel, W., Hawkins, C., & Schooler, J. W. (2001). Stereotype distinctiveness: How counterstereotypic behavior shapes the self-concept. *Journal of Personality and Social Psychology, 81,* 193–205.

von Hippel, W., & Suddendorf, T. (2018). Did humans evolve to innovate with a social rather than a technical orientation? *New Ideas in Psychology, 51,* 34–39.

von Hippel, W., & Trivers, R. (2011a). The evolution and psychology of self-deception. *Behavioral and Brain Sciences, 34,* 1–16.

von Hippel, W., & Trivers, R. (2011b). Reflections on self-deception. *Behavioral and Brain Sciences, 34,* 41–56.

Vrba, E. S. (1996). Climate, heterochrony, and human evolution. *Journal of Anthropological Research, 52,* 1–28.

Waser, N. M., & Ollerton, J. (Eds.). (2006). *Plant–pollinator interaction: From specialization to generalization.* Chicago: University of Chicago Press.

Wason, P. C. (1968). Reasoning about a rule. *Quarterly Journal of Experimental Psychology, 20,* 273–281.

Webb, J. L. A., Jr. (2009). *Humanity's burden: A global history of malaria.* Cambridge, UK: Cambridge University Press.

Wedel, M. J. (2011). A monument of inefficiency: The presumed course of the recurrent laryngeal nerve in sauropod dinosaurs. *Acta Palaeontologica Polonica, 57,* 251–256.

Wheeler, B. C. (2009). Monkeys crying wolf?: Tufted capuchin monkeys use anti-predator calls to usurp resources from conspecifics. *Proceedings of the Royal Society of London B: Biological Sciences, 276,* 3013–3018.

Whiten, A., & Byrne, R. W. (1988). Tactical deception in primates. *Behavioral and Brain Sciences, 11,* 233–273.

Wichura, H., Bousquet, R., Oberhänsli, R., Strecker, M. R., & Trauth, M. H. (2011). The Mid-Miocene East African Plateau: A pre-rift topographic model inferred from the emplacement of the phonolitic Yatta lava flow, Kenya. *Geologi-*

cal Society, London, Special Publications, 357,* 285–300.

Wilder, J. A., Mobasher, Z., & Hammer, M. F. (2004). Genetic evidence for unequal effective population sizes of human females and males. *Molecular Biology and Evolution, 21,* 2047–2057.

Williams, K. D. (2007). Ostracism. *Annual Review of Psychology, 58,* 425–452.

Wilson, M. L., & Wrangham, R. W. (2003). Intergroup relations in chimpanzees. *Annual Review of Anthropology, 32,* 363–392.

Wilson, T. D., & Gilbert, D. T. (2003). Affective forecasting. *Advances in Experimental Social Psychology, 35,* 345–411.

Wrangham, R. W., & Glowacki, L. (2012). Intergroup aggression in chimpanzees and war in nomadic hunter–gatherers. *Human Nature, 23,* 5–29.

Wrangham, R. W., & Peterson, D. (1996). *Demonic males: Apes and the origins of human violence.* New York: Houghton Mifflin Harcourt.

Young, R. W. (2003). Evolution of the human hand: The role of throwing and clubbing. *Journal of Anatomy, 202,* 165–174.

Zahavi, A., & Zahavi, A. (1999). *The handicap principle: A missing piece of Darwin's puzzle.* Oxford, UK: Oxford University Press.

CHAPTER 2

Approach Motivation and Emotion from a Biological Perspective

Eddie Harmon-Jones
Cindy Harmon-Jones

Biological perspectives concerned with approach motivation often consider it in relationship to rewards and incentives. Indeed, Elliot, Eder, and Harmon-Jones (2013, p. 308) wrote, "Most [perspectives] connect approach motivation to concepts of appetition, reward, and incentive, and connect avoidance motivation to concepts of aversion, punishment, and threat."

Panksepp (2013, p. 237), who provided one of the most influential biological perspectives on emotion and motivation, refers to this "general-purpose appetitive motivational system" as SEEKING (he capitalized his theoretical concepts to keep them distinct from layperson concepts). He further posited that the SEEKING system allows several other emotive systems to work effectively (e.g., CARE, LUST, PLAY), and that it causes animals to "become intensely interested in exploring their world, allowing them to find and eagerly anticipate all kinds of resources they need for survival, from water, food, sex and warmth to addictive drugs and social relationships" (p. 238). He further posited that

when fully aroused, the SEEKING urge fills the mind with eagerness and interest, and motivates organisms to move their bodies seemingly effort-

lessly in search of resources they need, crave, and desire. It sustains both mundane curiosity and sublime intellectual pursuits. When underactive for various reasons—from social defeat promoting chronic helplessness/stress or neural deficits of old age, depression can ensue. When overactive, which can arise from drug abuse, behavior can become excessive, guided often by psychotic delusions and manic thoughts. (p. 238)

Approach motivation involves a number of neural structures that go from the midbrain up to the medial frontal cortex. Although many scientists refer to the approach motivational system as a reward, pleasure, or reinforcement system, Panksepp (2013) posited that approach motivation is more involved in coaxing animals to move "energetically from where they are presently situated to the places where they can find and consume resources needed for survival" (p. 238). The neurochemical dopamine is critically involved in SEEKING, and it evokes a state of eagerness and anticipation, while mobilizing the frontal regions to engage in planning and execution of goal-directed behavior.

Other theoretical perspectives agree and posit that approach motivation is often aimed at seeking and acquiring resources needed for survival. These stimuli are often conceptualized as positive external goal objects (Lang & Bradley, 2008). Moreover, animals are proposed to experience positive affect when the approach motivational system is active.

However, research has challenged each of these principles and has suggested instead that (1) approach motivation is not invariably associated with positive affect but may be associated with negative affect; (2) approach motivation is not invariably evoked by positive stimuli; and (3) approach motivation may arise from other sources besides external goal objects. We review in this chapter theory and research that is supportive of these alternative principles of approach motivation.

A growing body of evidence suggests that approach motivation is more accurately defined as simply the urge or impulse to go toward (E. Harmon-Jones, Harmon-Jones, & Price, 2013). This definition purposefully omits the valence of stimuli toward which the urge is directed, and it also omits the requirement of an evoking stimulus. Although many theoreticians treat approach motivation as a stimulus-driven phenomenon (Lang & Bradley, 2008), approach motivation may also derive from internal processes at the state or trait level; that is, approach motivation may be an internal drive state that leads the organism to seek out stimuli with which to engage. In Panksepp's model (1998), SEEKING is the approach-motivated state that drives the organism to explore its surroundings with the potential to discover novel rewards. Similarly, humans and other organisms differ in their chronic drive to seek out rewards and pursue them (Carver & White, 1994).

Approach motivational states may be experienced as affectively negative. The common conception proposes that approach motivation is both evoked by pleasant stimuli and experientially positive (Lang & Bradley, 2008). However, current evidence challenges both ideas, as we elaborate below.

Before reviewing these main issues, we believe it important to explain our approach. The concept of motivation is a broad one, and it is studied at many levels of analysis. Whereas some theories of motivation focus the study of human motivation around consciously held goals, we believe that a complete conception of motivation includes unconscious processes (see

also Freud, 1900/1955; Hassin, 2013; Moskowitz & Grant, 2009). In fact, motivation is present in nonhuman animals, suggesting that consciousness is not necessary. Approach and avoidance behaviors appear to be basic to all organisms capable of movement. Even organisms as simple as worms move toward rewarding stimuli, such as food, and away from noxious stimuli, such as light (Schneirla, 1959). We assume that these fundamental motivational systems are continuous through all species, although they have been elaborated in more complex organisms that have a wider behavioral repertoire. Models of approach motivation that rely on uniquely human attributes such as goals, verbal thought, and cognitive framing are not fully adequate theories of motivation if similar processes could not apply to nonhuman organisms.

In addition, consciously held goals may be cold, cognitive concepts that are related to motivation but are not motivational urges themselves. In fact, motivational urges are often at odds with an individual's conscious goals. In this chapter, we equate motivation with impulses or urges to engage in behavior. These urges may mobilize attention, evoke cognitions, and involve planning, but an urgency to act is at the root of motivation (see also Woodworth & Schlosberg, 1954). On the other hand, motivation is not synonymous with behavior, as behavior may occur in the absence of an urge, and an organism may feel an urge to behave but not act on it. Competing motivations and situational limitations can prevent or compel other behaviors even when motivation is present. For example, if an organism moves toward a stimulus in an effort to escape, for example, when cornered, this would not reflect approach motivation but rather avoidance motivation.[1] Thus, measuring behavior is an imperfect proxy for the measurement of motivation, as behavior is not perfectly correlated with motivation.

As explained earlier, we define approach motivation as *the impulse to move toward*. This impulse is in the service of an overarching aim or goal that may be unconscious; it may be best accomplished by specific behaviors that cause the animal to move away at first, then later move toward the goal. We support this comprehensive and concise definition by reviewing evidence (1) that approach motivation may be experienced as a negative affective state; (2) that approach motivation may be experienced in response to negative stimuli; and (3) that stimuli are not necessary to produce approach motivation.

Principle 1: Approach Motivation Is Associated with Distinct Negative (and Positive) Affective States and Traits

Several conceptual models propose that positive affect reflects the experience of approach motivation, whereas negative affect reflects the experience of avoidance motivation (Cacioppo, Gardner, & Berntson, 1999; Lang & Bradley, 2008; Watson, Wiese, Vaidya, & Tellegen, 1999). However, approach motivation does not always feel subjectively positive, even when it is directed toward appetitive stimuli. Contrary to these conceptual models, research has revealed a more complex relationship between approach motivation and affective valence, and it suggests that approach motivation is associated with distinct positive and negative affective states and traits.

Psychophysiological Responses Associated with Approach Motivation

Before reviewing this research, however, we briefly review research using psychophysiological measures that have been found to be associated with approach motivation. We refer to these measures as evidence of approach motivation in the later portions of the chapter. The majority of the early research with these measures was based on the idea that approach motivation is associated with positive affect and not negative affect. However, research also suggests that these biological measures of approach motivation are associated with some negative affective states and traits.

Startle Eyeblink Modulation

One of the first biological variables found to support the idea of a link between approach motivation and positive affect is the startle eyeblink reflex. The startle eyeblink is part of the whole-body startle reflex; it is a defensive re-

flex that protects organisms from harm. It occurs in response to the quick onset of aversive, unexpected, and intense auditory, visual, or tactile stimuli. The startle reflex is modulated by the emotive significance of stimuli that are being processed at the same time as the startling event (Bradley, Codispoti, Cuthbert, & Lang, 2001; Vrana, Spence, & Lang, 1988).

In humans, the startle reflex is typically evoked by presenting individuals with a short burst of white noise (at approximately 100 decibels) with an abrupt onset (i.e., instantaneous rise time). In response, the muscle surrounding the eye, the orbicularis oculi, contracts.

The original research paradigm for linking the startle eyeblink response to approach motivation and emotion came from research and theory that views emotion as being organized along two primary dimensions: valence (positive to negative) and arousal (low to high; Lang, Bradley, & Cuthbert, 1990). According to the conceptual view guiding this research, appetitive/approach motivation is reflected by positive affective responses, whereas aversive/defensive motivation is reflected by negative affective responses. In both cases, arousal indexes the intensity of motivation. (Lang et al., 1990).

Research presented photographs differing in valence and arousal one at a time. In the midst of the presentation of some of these photographs, auditory startle probes were presented and electromyographic (EMG) responses from the orbicularis oculi were measured. Startle eyeblink responses were larger while viewing highly arousing negative pictures (e.g., threatening animals, mutilated bodies) and smaller while viewing highly arousing positive pictures (e.g., erotica, sports), compared to neutral pictures (e.g., Vrana et al., 1988).

According to the response-matching hypothesis, the magnitude of the startle response is determined by the degree to which the affective picture matches or mismatches the aversive motivation evoked by the startle stimulus. On the one hand, because arousing, negatively valenced photographs evoke aversive motivation that matches the aversive motivation evoked by the startle probe, these two aversive inputs should summate and cause a larger startle response. On the other hand, because arousing, positively valenced photographs evoke appetitive motivation that mismatches the aversive motivation evoked by the startle probe, this appetitive input should subtract from the aversive input and cause a smaller startle response. Thus, visual stimuli that evoke appetitive motivation should evoke smaller startle responses.

In support, much research has revealed that smaller startle responses occur during the viewing of appetitive (arousing positive) photographs. Further supporting the importance of the degree of approach motivation in driving these smaller startle responses during positive images, research has revealed that arousing positive images such as erotica, which are associated with more approach motivation, are associated with smaller startle responses than less arousing positive images such as sailboats, which are associated with low approach motivation (Gard, Gard, Mehta, Kring, & Patrick, 2007). Moreover, smaller startle responses occur during viewing of appetitive photographs for individuals who score higher in trait approach motivation (Hawk & Kowmas, 2003). Thus, the emotive modulated startle reflex is sensitive to both motivational direction and motivational intensity.

Asymmetrical Frontal Cortical Activity

Another psychophysiological measure found to be associated with approach motivation and emotion is asymmetrical frontal cortical activity. Research dating back to the 1930s has suggested that the left and right prefrontal cortices are involved in motivational and emotional processes, with the left frontal region involved in the experience and expression of approach motivation and emotion and the right frontal region involved in the experience and expression of withdrawal motivation and emotion (Goldstein, 1939). Studies revealed that persons who had sustained damage to the left frontal cortex were likely to develop symptoms of depression, whereas persons who had sustained damage to the right frontal cortex were likely to develop symptoms of mania (Robinson & Price, 1982). Manipulated suppression of activity in the right hemisphere (via injection of a barbiturate derivative, sodium amytal, into one of the internal carotid arteries) led to euphoria, whereas suppression of activity in the left hemisphere led to sadness (Perria, Rosadini, & Rossi, 1961).

These and other results suggested that with regard to emotive responses, the left and right frontal cortical regions worked in a reciprocal relationship, such that suppression of activity in one hemisphere was associated with an increased activity in the other hemisphere; that is, activity in the left frontal cortical region was associated with positive affect (or approach motivation), and activity in the right frontal cortical region was associated with negative affect (or withdrawal motivation). Similarly, research indicates that the left and right hemispheres are related to appetitive and avoidant behaviors, respectively, in a wide range of species (e.g., Vallortigara & Rogers, 2005).

In humans, these patterns of asymmetrical hemispheric activation associated with emotive variables are often specific to the frontal cortex. In much of this research, electroencephalography (EEG) has been used to measure asymmetrical frontal cortical activity, and the difference between right and left frontal cortical activity is often used as the primary dependent variable. The use of difference scores is consistent with the reviewed research using lesion and sodium amytal research, which suggests that when considering emotive responses, one hemisphere is inhibiting the other one (for a more thorough review of the neural mechanisms underlying this contralateral inhibition, see Schutter & Harmon-Jones, 2013).

In the EEG research on asymmetrical frontal cortical activity, one of the primary measures extracted from the EEG signal is power in the alpha frequency band. Alpha band power has been found to be inversely related to regional brain activity using hemodynamic measures (Cook, O'Hara, Uijtdehaage, Mandelkern, & Leuchter, 1998); increased brain activity is reflected by decreased alpha power (or alpha power suppression). In addition, this asymmetrical alpha power recorded over the frontal cortex and related to motivation/emotion variables most likely results from activity in the dorsolateral prefrontal cortex, as revealed in functional magnetic resonance imaging (fMRI) studies (Berkman & Lieberman, 2010), source localization of EEG signals (Pizzagalli, Sherwood, Henriques, & Davidson, 2005), and studies using transcranial magnetic stimulation (Schutter, 2009).

Research indicates that positive affective (or

approach-oriented) state emotional responses are associated with greater relative left frontal cortical activity. For example, when 10-month-old infants were shown photographs of a woman displaying a happy or sad facial expression, left frontal activation was increased to the happy expression (Davidson & Fox, 1982). Similarly, photographs that evoke basic motivational responses, such as erotica, produce greater left frontal activity compared to neutral photographs (Schöne, Schomberg, Gruber, & Quinn, 2016). In contrast, stimuli that evoke the withdrawal-related emotions of fear or disgust evoke greater right frontal activity (Davidson, Ekman, Saron, Senulis, & Friesen, 1990).

The Reward Positivity

Another psychophysiological measure found to be associated with approach motivation and emotion is the reward positivity (RewP), which is an event-related potential derived from the EEG. It is a positive-going electrical response that is larger in response to signals of rewarding outcomes (e.g., monetary gains) compared to losses (Proudfit, 2015). The RewP is associated with activation in a neural "reward" circuit involving the ventral striatum, medial prefrontal cortex/anterior cingulate cortex, orbital frontal cortex, amygdala, and caudate (Carlson, Foti, Harmon-Jones, & Proudfit, 2015).

Larger RewPs are associated with higher scores on approach motivation traits (Bress & Hajcak, 2013). In contrast, smaller RewPs are associated with lower scores on approach motivation traits, such as depressive tendencies (Foti & Hajcak, 2009).

The RewP is also influenced by the intensity of approach motivation. For example, perceived control over outcomes increases the intensity of approach motivation, as individuals are more motivated to approach if they believe that their efforts will influence whether they will acquire a reward. An experiment revealed that when participants were informed that they could influence their likelihood of receiving a reward by learning a mouse-click rule, they had larger RewP responses to reward signals compared to participants who were told that the rewards were random and did not depend on task performance (Mühlberger, Angus, Jonas, Harmon-Jones, & Harmon-Jones, 2017). Along with the trait re-

search, these results suggest that the RewP measures the intensity of approach motivation.

In summary, approach motivation has been found to be associated with physiological responses of (1) smaller startle eyeblink responses during the viewing of highly arousing and positive (appetitive) stimuli, (2) greater relative left frontal cortical activity at state and trait levels of measurement, and (3) the RewP.

The early research on these measures essentially confounded positive affect and approach motivation, as it assumed that the two constructs were perfectly related. Below we review evidence suggesting that some negative affects are associated with these biological measures because these negative affects are associated with approach motivation.

Anger and Approach Motivation

Research using the three psychophysiological measures we reviewed earlier has tested whether the emotion of anger is related to approach motivation. Anger is a subjectively unpleasant emotion (E. Harmon-Jones, 2004) that is nevertheless associated with urges to approach and attack (Plutchik, 1980). Offensive aggression appears to be motivated by anger-like affective responses, unlike defensive aggression which is motivated by fear (Blanchard & Blanchard, 1984). Evidence using a variety of paradigms suggests that anger is approach-related (Veenstra, Bushman, & Koole, 2018). For instance, both state and trait anger are correlated with behavioral approach sensitivity (Carver, 2004; E. Harmon-Jones, 2003). In addition, anger (and happiness) have been found to cause shorter delay to gait initiation, more forceful steps, and faster walking speeds (Fawver, Hass, Park, & Janelle, 2014), suggesting that anger increases approach-motivated behavior, even in the absence of a specific target.

With regard to the startle eyeblink response, research indicates that individuals who score high in trait anger also have smaller startle responses during viewing of arousing positive photographs (Amodio & Harmon-Jones, 2011). This same research also indicated that individuals who scored high in trait approach-oriented emotions, such as enjoyment, have smaller startle responses during viewing of arousing positive photographs (Amodio & Harmon-Jones,

2011), suggesting that anger bears similarities to approach-related positive affect in the effects on the startle response.

Researchers have also found that anger relates to greater relative left frontal cortical activity. In one study, reported trait anger was associated with higher left frontal activity and lower right frontal activity during a resting baseline in a sample of adolescents (E. Harmon-Jones & Allen, 1998). Other studies had similar results (e.g., Hewig, Hagemann, Seifert, Naumann, & Bartussek, 2004), even among men imprisoned for violent crimes (Keune et al., 2012). Moreover, research indicates that the relationship between anger and left frontal activity is not due to anger being experienced as subjectively positive (E. Harmon-Jones, 2004).

State anger also has been found to be related to increased relative left frontal activity. For example, individuals who were insulted had greater left frontal activity compared to individuals who received neutral feedback (Harmon-Jones & Sigelman, 2001). Furthermore, both reported anger and aggression were correlated with left frontal activity in the insult condition but not in the neutral condition. In another study, social rejection increased reported anger and relative left frontal cortical activity compared to social inclusion (Peterson, Gravens, & Harmon-Jones, 2011). Furthermore, a manipulated increase in relative left frontal cortical activity, via transcranial direct current stimulation, led to greater anger-related aggression (Hortensius, Schutter, & Harmon-Jones, 2012).

With regard to the RewP, evidence suggests that its magnitude is related positively with anger. In one study, manipulated state anger increased the relationship between self-reported liking of rewards and the RewP (Angus, Kemkes, Schutter, & Harmon-Jones, 2015). Another study revealed that individuals who score high in trait anger have larger RewPs in response to reward cues (Tsypes, Angus, Martin, Kemkes, & Harmon-Jones, 2019).

Taken together, this body of research provides support for Principle 1 by demonstrating that anger, although a negative affect, is associated with approach motivation. This research included state and trait studies of anger, as well as three different biological measures of approach motivation.

Jealousy and Approach Motivation

Jealousy typically involves three individuals, and it occurs when one of them perceives that another one (even if only imaginary) is a threat to the important dyadic relationship. This threatened loss often evokes feelings of jealousy, as well as other emotions, such as anger. Jealousy may motivate approach to protect the dyadic relationship or regain the lost relationship partner. Evidence suggests that jealousy relates to greater relative left frontal cortical activity (E. Harmon-Jones, Peterson, & Harris, 2009) and that manipulated increases in relative left frontal cortical activity increase self-reported jealousy (Kelley, Eastwick, Harmon-Jones, & Schmeichel, 2015). Moreover, 9-month-old infants also evidence greater relative left frontal cortical activity when jealous (Mize, Pineda, Blau, Marsh, & Jones, 2014). These results suggest that jealousy, a negative affective experience, is associated with approach motivation, further supporting Principle 1.

Sadness and Approach Motivation

Sadness appears to be a complex emotion that may be associated either with high or low approach motivation, depending on several variables. In Panksepp's (1998) model, human sadness is most closely related to the PANIC/ GRIEF system. In nonhuman animals, this system is activated when an infant is separated from its mother. The infant responds with distress vocalizations (crying) that function to restore proximity to the mother. This emotive response appears to be mediated by a decrease in endorphin release, and indeed, administration of opiates effectively prevents distress vocalizations (Panksepp, Herman, Connor, Bishop, & Scott, 1978). In humans and other animals, infants who are separated from their mothers first exhibit "protest" behavior, which includes crying, searching, and clinging to any maternal substitute. However, if proximity is not restored, this is followed by behavioral "despair," that is, lethargy, depression, and loss of interest (Bowlby, 1973). These states may be two strategies for problems of survival that have no apparent solution. The first is an approach-motivated response to vigorously expend energy in an attempt to restore the lost object or person, and the second is a reduction in approach to conserve the remaining energy in the hope that a solution presents itself (Thierry, Steru, Chermat, & Simon, 1984). Both of these states may be identified by the semantic label of "sadness," which is typically applied to an emotional response to an important loss. However, whereas *protest* is high in approach motivation, *despair* is characterized by a deficit in approach. Panksepp proposed that prolonged overactivation of the PANIC/GRIEF system causes psychological pain that inhibits SEEKING (Panksepp & Watt, 2011). Furthermore, the time course of sadness may influence its motivational characteristics, with an initial increase in approach followed by a decrease in approach.

Other evidence also suggests that sadness is an approach-related rather than avoidance-related emotional state. Emotions are often considered to be positive or negative in valence. *Affective valence,* whether an emotion is positive or negative, is often implicitly defined as whether the emotion is an experience that is liked or disliked. We (E. Harmon-Jones, Harmon-Jones, Amodio, & Gable, 2011) have tested this implicit assumption by creating self-report measures of attitudes toward emotions (and others have created implicit measures of these attitudes; Markovitch, Netzer, & Tamir, 2017). As expected, emotions referred to as positive (e.g., joy) are liked more than emotions referred to as negative (e.g., sadness). In addition, although the vast majority of individuals regard typical negative emotions as dislikable, individuals differ in the degree to which they dislike each negative emotion. Moreover, for approach-related emotions such as anger and joy, having a more positive attitude toward the emotion relates to reporting a stronger experience of the emotion (E. Harmon-Jones, Harmon-Jones, et al., 2011). In contrast, for avoidance-related emotions such as fear and disgust, having a more positive attitude toward the emotion relates to reporting a weaker experience of the emotion. For sadness, having a more positive attitude relates to reporting a stronger experience, suggesting that the relationship between attitude and experience is similar to the other approach-related emotions (E. Harmon-Jones, Harmon-Jones, et al., 2011).

The emotion of sadness also illustrates that an emotional state may feel subjectively unpleasant, even if the stimulus toward which it is directed is appetitive and approach related. This may reflect a curvilinear relationship between motivation and valence. For example, when organisms are moderately approach-motivated toward social connection, they may experience feelings of pleasant anticipation and liking or love, but when they are in a state of high approach social motivation due to deprivation or social loss, they may experience negative feelings of PANIC/GRIEF and separation distress (Panksepp, 1998). This is illustrated by research on social exclusion, a situation that produces the subjective feelings of sadness and anger (C. Harmon-Jones, Bastian, & Harmon-Jones, 2016). When individuals are socially rejected, they work harder to reconnect with others and rate others as more appealing (Maner, DeWall, Baumeister, & Schaller, 2007), suggesting that social exclusion produces an approach-motivated state. However, the threat of social exclusion may also reduce prosocial behavior when individuals believe that reestablishing connection is hopeless. When participants were informed that their personality profile suggested that they were likely to end their lives alone and friendless, they donated less money to a charity, were less helpful after an accident, and cooperated less in an economic game (Twenge, Baumeister, DeWall, Ciarocco, & Bartels, 2007). Taken together, these results suggest that sadness is an approach-related emotion but may be associated with either high or low approach motivation depending on a variety of factors. Thus, research on sadness also supports Principle 1 by revealing a negative affect that is associated with approach motivation.

Guilt and Approach Motivation

Guilt, another negative affect, has been proposed to motivate prosocial behavior, suggesting that it is associated with approach motivation (Maitner, Mackie, & Smith, 2006). The motivation behind prosocial behavior could be related to approach motivation in a dynamic manner that depends on timing and other variables. Indeed, research has revealed that when individuals were induced to experience guilt (for having supposedly behaved in a racially prejudiced manner), their reported guilt was associated with decreased relative left frontal cortical activity (Amodio, Devine, & Harmon-Jones, 2007). These results suggest that the immediate response to guilt may be a decrease in approach motivation. However, when these individuals were given an opportunity to engage in behavior that would reduce prejudice, reported guilt was associated with increased relative left frontal cortical activity and more interest in engaging in prejudice reduction. These results suggest that guilt is associated with an increase in approach motivation when opportunities for reparation exist. Much subsequent research has linked guilt—and shame, to a slightly lesser extent—with approach motivation (Leach & Cidam, 2015). Taken together, these studies on guilt suggest that it too supports Principle 1.

Principle 2: Approach Motivation Is Evoked by Negative (and Positive) Stimuli

In the previous section we discussed discrete negative emotions and their relationship with approach motivation. In this section we address stimuli that evoke approach motivation. For several decades, prominent theories have posited that approach motivation is evoked by positive or rewarding stimuli (Lang & Bradley, 2008). These theories are still widely accepted and continue to receive much research attention. However, other theories and research suggest a more complex relationship between approach motivation and the valence of the evoking stimuli, as we review below.

Anger–Evoking Stimuli as Triggers of Approach Motivation

One of the primary violations of the common relationship between approach motivation and positive stimuli concerns anger and aggression; that is, anger- and aggression-evoking stimuli, which are negatively valenced, often elicit approach motivation. In other words, organisms regard events that evoke anger and aggression as unpleasant or negative, but these stimuli still cause approach motivation. This connection between anger–aggression and approach motivation has been observed in a variety of settings and with a variety of organisms.

The blocking of movement toward goals,

which is a negatively valenced event, evokes aggression. This was recognized in the original frustration–aggression hypothesis of Dollard, Miller, Doob, Mowrer, and Sears (1939). The blocking or frustration of goal-directed activity evokes approach motivation as the organism attempts to regain the goal. More recent theories and research suggest that anger and aggression may be caused by the omission or termination of positive reinforcers (Rolls, 1999). Although positive reinforcers or rewards may be one source of approach motivation in the global context, the negative event of the omission or termination of expected rewards is the more specific or proximate cause of anger and aggression in such situations.

Furthermore, it is important to distinguish between offensive aggression, which is approach motivated and related to anger, and defensive aggression, which is avoidance motivated and related to fear. Defensive aggression is characterized by attack only when escape is impossible, punctuated by attempts to escape. In contrast, offensive aggression is characterized by attacks with no attempts to escape. In the laboratory, offensive aggression in rodents is most often provoked in the "resident-intruder paradigm," in which a smaller "intruder" is introduced into the home cage of a "resident" (Koolhaas et al., 2013). Resident mice will cross an electrified grid to attack an intruder (Lagerspetz, 1969), suggesting that the behavior is approach motivated because the animal is willing to undergo pain to engage in it.

Interestingly, evidence suggests that the approach motivation provoked by an offensive aggressive response may relieve depression (Wei et al., 2014). Rats were assigned to either normal living conditions or a depression-inducing conditions, with the latter induced through food and water deprivation, soiled cages, odors, continuous light, and other stressors. Half of the stressed rats were then subjected to a daily resident-intruder paradigm, during which most rats attacked and defeated the intruder (those who did not were excluded). The rats were then tested on three measures of depressive-like behavior: a task that measured liking for sucrose (loss of sensitivity to reward), a task that measured the degree to which they explore an open field (loss of interest), and a task that measured how long they would swim before giving up (despair). Stressed rats performed more poorly at these tasks. However, the stressed rats that had undergone the resident-intruder paradigm performed significantly better than those that had not, and over time recovered to levels similar to the unstressed rats. This suggests that angry approach may mobilize resources to overcome depression.

In human infants, anger evoked by negative stimuli is associated with approach motivation. In these studies, infants (2- to 8-month-olds) first learned to move one of their arms to see a picture of another baby's smiling face and hear happy music (Lewis, Sullivan, Ramsay, & Alessandri, 1992). Then, after the infants learned this association, they went through an extinction phase in which their arm movements did not "cause" the happy events. The termination of this positive reinforcer ("frustrating" event) caused most infants to display anger-like facial expressions.

Subsequent research extended this initial research by testing infants in this paradigm at age 5 months, then testing them again in a different situation at age 2 years (Lewis, Sullivan, & Kim, 2015). In this latter situation, the children's persistence at play was measured in response to an interruption of their play. Results revealed that the 2-year-olds' persistence was positively correlated with their anger responses at 5 months. These results further suggest that anger is related to approach motivation.

Taken together, the reviewed research support Principle 2 by suggesting that negative stimuli that evoke anger often evoke approach motivation. This evidence extends past research by suggesting that negative (as well as positive) stimuli evoke approach motivation.

Loss of Control as a Trigger of Approach Motivation

Loss of perceived control over outcomes, a negative event, may also cause approach motivation. According to the theoretical model that integrated reactance theory and learned helplessness theory (Wortman & Brehm, 1975), negative outcomes influence motivational responses depending on the importance of the outcome and the degree to which individuals expect to be able to control obtaining the outcome. If an individual expects to be able to control obtaining an outcome and the outcome is important but fails to be acquired, the individual will likely experience psychological reactance. The psychological reactance then motivates the individual to engage in increased effort to acquire the desired outcome. Indeed, the previously mentioned studies describing situations in which infants experienced frustration could be interpreted as loss-of-control situations.

In support of these ideas, research has revealed that individuals respond to brief experiences of lack of control with increased performance and persistence on challenging puzzles, but after repeated experiences of lack of control, they show decreased performance and persistence (Roth & Kubal, 1975). As predicted by the integrative model of reactance and learned helplessness, these initial increases in motivation (reactance) are followed by decreases in motivation if the lack of control persists (learned helplessness).

Other research testing this integrative model revealed that individuals who reported feeling more angry in response to an unsolvable puzzle performed better on a subsequent cognitive task compared to participants who reported feeling less angry (Mikulincer, 1988). These effects likely occurred because the reactance motivation caused by the loss of control manifested as anger, and this state increased approach motivation.

More recent research has revealed that low perceived control increases approach motivation (Greenaway et al., 2015). In this work, participants heard unpleasant sounds and either had no control or control over the sounds; in this latter condition, they pressed the keyboard spacebar to cause the sounds to be produced, and both conditions received the same number of sounds. Consistent with the prediction that loss of control would increase approach motivation, participants in the low-control, compared to the high-control, condition reported feeling more energized, capable, and so forth, and they also reported more motivation to pursue goals. A subsequent study replicated the effect of low control on increased approach motivation feelings. It is interesting to note that in this set of studies, participants did not explicitly lose control; they simply had low control. But even this low-control experience increased approach motivation on measures unrelated to that control task, suggesting that the approach motivation was not an explicit attempt to regain control on the task.

Taken together, these results illustrate that control deprivation, a negative stimulus situation, can increase approach motivation. As such, they provide further support for Principle 2 that negative stimuli can evoke approach motivation.

Cognitive Conflict as a Trigger of Approach Motivation

Several lines of theory and research have also suggested that cognitive conflict, broadly defined, has the potential to evoke approach motivation. The evoking stimulus in these situations is the negative stimulus situation of cognitive conflict.

Cognitive Dissonance Theory and Research

One line of theory and research suggesting that cognitive conflict evokes approach motivation is based on cognitive dissonance theory. The theory of cognitive dissonance (Festinger, 1957) proposed that individuals experience a negative affective state when they hold two or more cognitions that are in conflict with one another, that is, when one cognition implies that the other ought not to be true. The psychological discomfort motivates the individual to do cognitive work to resolve the inconsistency by changing cognitions to be more consistent with one another. The action-based model of dissonance (E. Harmon-Jones & Harmon-Jones, 2002; E. Harmon-Jones, Harmon-Jones, & Levy, 2015) was proposed to explain *why* holding conflicting cognitions causes discomfort. The model begins with the assumption that cognitions guide action, and that inconsistent cognitions are likely to have competing action tendencies. Thus, inconsistent cognitions would be expected to interfere with effective and unconflicted action, whereas by bringing cognitions more into alignment, effective action would be facilitated.

It follows from the action-based model that dissonance reduction is an approach-motivated process that enables an individual to carry out decisions and enact commitments. One of the first sets of tests of this model had participants believe they had either high or low choice to write a counterattitudinal statement. Writing a statement that is counter to one's beliefs is a common method of inducing dissonance in the laboratory, and dissonance reduction is shown when participants change their attitude to be more similar to the statement they wrote. Participants change their attitude more in the high- than in the low-choice condition because having low choice provides a justification for having engaged in the counterattitudinal behavior. In these studies, participants in the high-choice condition changed their attitude more and showed more relative left frontal cortical activation, which suggests increased approach motivation (E. Harmon-Jones, Gerdjikov, & Harmon-Jones, 2008; E. Harmon-Jones, Harmon-Jones, Fearn, Sigelman, & Johnson, 2008; E. Harmon-Jones, Harmon-Jones, Serra, & Gable, 2011).

Other dissonance-related studies have found patterns of neural activation consistent with the idea that dissonance is associated with increased approach motivation. In these studies, the free choice or difficult decision paradigm was used (Brehm, 1956). In this paradigm, participants make a decision between two equally attractive alternatives. Once they make the decision, they are committed to that course of action (decision), and they are approach-motivated to follow through with it. Dissonance would potentially manifest if they considered the positive aspects of the rejected alternative or negative aspects of the chosen alternative. However, individuals typically reduce dissonance by spreading of alternatives; that is, they have more positive attitudes toward the chosen alternative and more negative attitudes toward the rejected alternative after the decision as compared to prior to the decision. We suspect that this spreading of alternatives is self-generated and not the result of being provided an external solution (see E. Harmon-Jones, Harmon-Jones, Serra, & Gable, 2011, for neural evidence that supports this interpretation). In one study, activity in the left lateral prefrontal cortex after a difficult decision was associated with greater spreading of alternatives (Qin et al., 2011). Other studies have found that greater activity in the ventral striatum, a region associated with approach motivation, correlates with greater spreading of alternatives in a difficult decision paradigm (Kitayama, Chua, Tompson, & Han, 2013).

The magnitude of dissonance reduction is influenced by manipulations of approach motivation. In other studies using the difficult decision paradigm, left frontal cortical activation was manipulated using transcranial direct current stimulation (Mengarelli, Spoglianti, Avenanti, & Di Pellegrino, 2013) or neurofeedback (E. Harmon-Jones, Harmon-Jones, Fearn, et al., 2008). In both studies, dissonance reduction was greater in conditions with greater left frontal cortical activation. Another study using a mindset manipulation to induce an approach-related state (action orientation) after a difficult decision caused both greater dissonance reduction and greater left frontal cortical activity (E. Harmon-Jones, Harmon-Jones, Fearn, et al., 2008). Moreover, individuals who score higher in trait approach motivation engage in more dissonance reduction (C. Harmon-Jones, Schmeichel, Inzlicht, & Harmon-Jones, 2011). Taken together, these results show that dissonance reduction is an approach-motivated state and increases in approach motivation increase dissonance reduction. Thus, these results also support Principle 2, showing that situations that cause dissonance, an undesired state, trigger approach motivation.

Ego Depletion

Another line of inquiry that suggests cognitive conflict may evoke approach motivation is work on ego depletion and self-control. Initially, scientists proposed that the self-control mechanism functioned as a limited resource that was temporarily weakened by use (Muraven & Baumeister, 2000). One typical study revealed that dieters who were instructed to suppress their emotional reaction during a sad film subsequently ate more ice cream compared to dieters who were instructed to freely express their emotions during the film (Vohs & Heatherton, 2000). Conceptually similar results have been shown with a variety of manipulations of self-control and self-control failure.

Later research showed that in addition to weakening the control mechanism, exerting self-control increases the strength of impulsive

approach motivation. In one study, participants who had exerted self-control by suppressing their emotions reported higher approach motivation on Carver and White's (1994) scales (Schmeichel, Harmon-Jones, & Harmon-Jones, 2010, Study 1). Similarly, participants who exerted self-control engaged in more low-stakes gambles (Study 2) and had more perceptual sensitivity to symbols of reward (Study 3). Low-stakes gambles and perception of reward symbols should both be behaviors that reflect approach motivation but not inhibition, as there is no compelling reason to inhibit these behaviors.

Since these seminal studies, other evidence indicates that exerting self-control increases approach motivation. For example, chronic dieters who exerted cognitive control by attempting not to attend to words shown during the viewing of a film had increased activity in the nucleus accumbens when viewing photos of desirable foods compared to those who did not attempt to attend away from the words (Wagner, Altman, Boswell, Kelley, & Heatherton, 2013). Tasks that require cognitive control also have been shown to increase activity in the amygdala and reduce connectivity between the frontal cortex and amygdala, suggesting that depletion increases emotional reactivity (Wagner & Heatherton, 2012). Other evidence suggests that the increase in approach motivation following self-control may be stronger for those who are high in approach motivation at the trait level (Schmeichel, Crowell, & Harmon-Jones, 2016). Although the ego-depletion studies may bear some similarities to loss-of-control studies, we suspect they are tapping different psychological mechanisms, as loss-of-control situations often involve failure at a task, whereas ego-depletion situations do not. Together, these studies suggest that the exertion of self-control increases approach motivation, further supporting Principle 2 by demonstrating that the negative stimulus situation of cognitive conflict increases approach motivation.

Reactive Approach Motivation

Research also suggests that uncertainty and other threats may lead to an increase in approach motivation. A wide variety of threats may produce this *reactive approach* response, including romantic uncertainty, dissonance, economic worries, dilemmas, and goal conflicts (for a review, see McGregor, Prentice, & Nash, 2012). According to this perspective, all of these threats have the potential to interfere with one's goals and evoke a response of increased determination and goal striving. As such, these threats might also be thought of as frustrating events or situations evoking a loss of control.

For example, one experiment gave university undergraduate students 2 minutes to read a simple or complex and confusing passage about statistics, to manipulate anxious uncertainty (McGregor, Nash, Mann, & Phills, 2010). They then completed an implicit association task that measured the strength of association between the self and approach-related and avoidance-related words. Results revealed that students made to feel more anxious uncertainty (via reading the complex passage) had stronger implicit approach associations. Other studies have conceptually replicated this effect and revealed that anxious uncertainty increases relative left frontal cortical activation, particularly among individuals with high self-esteem (McGregor, Nash, & Inzlicht, 2009). These studies (as well as others reviewed earlier) suggest that the approach motivation occurs even in the absence of a concrete behavioral stimulus that provides a solution to the problematic situation. Thus, the organism shows increased approach motivation internally and not simply in response to some externally provided solution. In summary, a wide variety of negative stimulus situations evoke approach motivation, in support of Principle 2 and in contrast to past theories positing that approach motivation was only evoked by positive stimulus situations.

Principle 3: Approach Motivation Results from Many Causes in Addition to Goal Objects/Stimuli

The widely accepted contemporary view emphasizes that approach motivation is evoked by goals and other types of external stimuli (Lang & Bradley, 2008). However, approach motivation has a much wider array of causes. Approach motivation may arise due to internal

psychophysiological processes (e.g., drive states such as hunger and thirst; Hull, 1943), as well as other neurochemical and bodily activities. In other words, approach motivation and emotion may be initiated by processes, often non-conscious, occurring within the organism, and these processes motivate approach. Relatedly, individuals differ in their levels of approach motivation and emotions, and these individual differences may be the cause of approach-related motivation and emotion responses. We believe this principle is important to emphasize because it has not been widely integrated into theories of motivation that focus on end states, reference points, or goals (Lang & Bradley, 2008).

Panksepp's (1998) theory concurs with our position. His SEEKING system is an intrinsic motivational system that drives the organism to explore and search its environment for opportunities for incentives. It does not need to be triggered by positive external stimuli. The SEEKING system can be activated by drugs such as amphetamines that stimulate the dopaminergic system, as well as by other non-goal stimulation, such as changes in patterns of diurnal light (Panksepp, 1998; see also Butler & Harlow, 1954).

Below we provide support for Principle 3 by reviewing research demonstrating that chronic dispositions and bodily manipulations influence approach motivation.

Approach Motivation and Resting–Baseline Asymmetrical Frontal Cortical Activity

One body of evidence that suggests approach motivation and emotion may originate from sources other than external goal objects comes from research on asymmetrical frontal cortical activity. Some studies on the relationship between asymmetrical frontal cortical activity and emotive variables simply measured EEG while individuals sat resting in a chair, then correlated the resting frontal cortical asymmetry with other measures of traits related to motivation and/or emotion. For instance, individuals who score higher in depression have lower relative left frontal cortical activity (Thibodeau, Jorgensen, & Kim, 2006). Also, individuals who score higher in trait activated positive affect, trait approach motivation, and trait anger have greater relative left frontal cortical activity at resting baseline (E. Harmon-Jones & Gable, 2018). These results suggest that approach motivation has a trait component that may inspire approach urges in the absence of specific goals.

Other researchers have suggested that time of year and time of day may influence approach motivation. For example, asymmetrical frontal cortical activity has been found to relate to time of day and time of year, such that relative left front cortical activity during a resting-baseline session is lower during autumn mornings compared to other times (Peterson & Harmon-Jones, 2009). Along with past research suggesting that basal cortisol and self-reported mood vary with time of year and time of day, these results suggest that approach motivation levels may be influenced by these "background," nongoal stimuli. These results support Principle 3 by demonstrating some sources of approach motivation other than external stimuli.

Approach Motivation Evoked by the Body

The idea that emotional–motivational states are connected with facial expressions and body postures has a long history (Darwin, 1872/1965; James, 1894). The observation that physical responses correspond to emotional states led to facial feedback theories proposing that manipulating facial expressions can influence emotional reactions to stimuli (Laird, 1974) and produce emotional responses in the absence of other stimuli (Duclos et al., 1989).

Facial Expressions

Research has shown that manipulations of emotional facial expressions influence approach motivation. For example, genuine smiles (those that activate both the zygomaticus muscle in the cheek and the orbicularis oculi surrounding the eye) compared to social smiles (those that activate only the zygomaticus), created by covertly instructing participants to move individual facial muscles to form these smiles, produce greater relative left frontal cortical activity (Ekman & Davidson, 1993). In other words, activation of the facial muscles associated with genuine smiles evoked approach motivation, as measured neurally.

Other research had participants form facial expressions of joy, anger, fear, and disgust (Coan, Allen, & Harmon-Jones, 2001). Left frontal cortical activity was greater while participants made emotional expressions associated with approach motivation (anger and joy) compared to those associated with avoidance motivation (fear and disgust).

Another experiment manipulated levels of approach motivation by having participants make facial expressions of low-approach positive affect (satisfaction), high-approach positive affect (determination), or neutral affect (Price, Hortensius, & Harmon-Jones, 2013). Determination is a high-approach positive emotion that is typically experienced while striving to meet a challenge, whereas satisfaction is a low-approach positive emotion that is typically experienced while savoring a reward (C. Harmon-Jones, Schmeichel, Mennitt, et al., 2011). Participants in the determination facial expression condition had greater left frontal cortical activity compared to a resting baseline, but satisfaction and neutral facial expression conditions did not change relative to baseline. The facial expressions influenced self-reported emotions in the expected directions (e.g., the determined expression made participants report feeling more interested, strong, and determined).

Whole-Body Postures and Approach Motivation

Like facial expressions, whole-body postures have been shown to influence motivational direction and intensity. One experiment manipulated a "depressed posture" by having participants sit either in a hunched and stooped position (low approach) or with the spine erect and chest expanded (high approach; Riskind & Gotay, 1982). Participants then completed a measure of task persistence. Participants who had been assigned to the depressed posture showed less task persistence, suggesting that the depressed posture reduced approach motivation. Other studies have shown that this stooped posture slows recovery from negative mood experiences (Veenstra, Schneider, & Koole, 2017).

Research has also suggested that a simple supine posture may reduce approach motivation. This was expected because individuals often recline or lie flat on their backs while in post-goal states (e.g., after eating a delicious meal or accomplishing a goal). In one experiment, participants wrote an essay that would ostensibly be evaluated by another participant (E. Harmon-Jones & Peterson, 2009). While waiting to receive feedback, participants were asked to place their chairs in the reclined position or to sit upright. Participants then received insulting or neutral feedback. Participants who were insulted while sitting upright had greater relative left frontal cortical activity. However, those in the insulting feedback/supine condition and neutral feedback condition had less relative left frontal cortical activity than those in the insulting feedback/upright condition. These results suggest that the supine body posture reduced anger-related approach motivation.

In subsequent research, a leaning-forward body posture, while reaching forward as if to grasp a desired object, was used to increase approach motivation. Participants' resting EEG was measured while they maintained one of three postures: reclining, upright, or leaning and reaching forward. Results showed a linear trend, such that the reclining position showed the least left frontal cortical activity, leaning and reaching showed the most, and sitting upright fell between the two (Price & Harmon-Jones, 2011). These results supported the idea that the full-body posture assumed during high- and low-approach motivational states may influence an individual's state approach motivation in the absence of other stimuli. The whole-body posture itself was the triggering stimulus; it may have also created goal-directed thoughts in participants' minds. Future research is needed to test this possibility.

To test whether whole-body manipulations influence reactions to appetitive stimuli, participants were assigned to either reclining or leaning-forward postures while viewing appetitive dessert photos and neutral photos of rocks. In the leaning-forward condition, participants evidenced greater left frontal cortical activity in response to desserts compared to rocks, but in the reclining condition there was no difference in left frontal activity in response to desserts and rocks (E. Harmon-Jones, Gable, & Price, 2011). In this study, appetitive stimuli existed, but responses to them were moderated by whole-body posture, suggesting that approach-related body

postures may increase approach motivational responses to weakly appetitive stimuli.

Body posture may also influence startle eyeblink responses to appetitive stimuli. Participants were assigned to either a leaning-forward or a reclining posture, and they viewed appetitive photos of male–female couples in erotic situations or neutral photos of male–female couples (Price, Dieckman, & Harmon-Jones, 2012). When the stimuli were erotic, startle eyeblink responses were smaller in the forward-leaning condition than in the reclining condition, whereas when the stimuli were neutral photos of couples, startle responses did not differ between those in leaning and reclining postures. These results suggested that whole-body postures influence startle eyeblink responses to appetitive stimuli.

Other research has revealed that a supine body posture, which reduces approach motivation, also reduces cognitive dissonance reduction (E. Harmon-Jones, Price, & Harmon-Jones, 2015). Taken together, this research suggests that whole-body postures associated with low versus high approach motivation influence a wide array of approach-motivated responses, further supporting Principle 3.

Unilateral Hand Contractions and Approach Motivation

A number of studies have used movements of the left versus right hand to alter approach motivation. Activation of the motor cortex in one hemisphere (e.g., left) controls movement of the body on the opposite side (e.g., right). Because of this contralateral connection between the body and motor cortex, contraction of the right (left) hand should increase activity in the left (right) motor cortex. Moreover, connections between the motor cortex and ipsilateral frontal cortex suggests that cortical activation originating in the motor cortex may spread to the frontal cortex (E. Harmon-Jones, 2006).

Based on this physiology, research has tested whether right-hand contractions increase approach motivation by increasing left frontal cortical activation. In one example experiment, participants were instructed to squeeze a rubber ball with either the right or left hand for two 45-second intervals (E. Harmon-Jones, 2006).

They then squeezed the ball with the same hand while listening to a mildly positive radio broadcast on living options. Results revealed that participants who had contracted the right hand had greater activity in the left motor cortex and left frontal cortex than those who contracted the left hand. These results suggested that cortical activation spreads from the motor cortex to the frontal cortex of the same hemisphere. In addition, participants who had contracted the right hand reported greater activated positive affect to the radio broadcast (E. Harmon-Jones, 2006). These results suggest that unilateral motor contractions of the hand influence approach motivation and emotion.

Other research suggests that unilateral hand contractions can influence the anger-related approach motivation. In one experiment, participants wrote an essay on a controversial topic (Peterson, Shackman, & Harmon-Jones, 2008). They then squeezed a ball with either the right or left hand while they waited to receive feedback, ostensibly from another participant. They then received insulting feedback from the other participant. All participants then played a reaction-time game, during which they could "punish" the other participant with noise blasts. Those who squeezed the right hand delivered louder and longer blasts as expected, as well as showing greater left frontal cortical activity. Furthermore, right-hand contractions were associated with greater coherence between the left motor cortex and frontal regions, whereas left-hand contractions were associated with greater coherence between the right motor cortex and posterior regions (Peterson et al., 2008). With regard to the behavioral measures, participants who had contracted the right hand delivered louder and longer noise blasts than those who had contracted the left hand. These results support the idea that right-hand contractions increase approach-motivated left frontal cortical activity, anger, and aggression.

In summary, the evidence reviewed in this section has supported Principle 3 by pointing to chronic dispositions, times of the day and year, and various body movements and postures that influence approach motivation. All of these causes of approach motivation are not considered in many past theories of approach motivation that focused on end states, reference points, or goals (Lang & Bradley, 2008). Thus, approach motivation can be caused by a host of variables that are outside the domain of goals.

Summary and Discussion

The evidence we have reviewed suggests that several widely accepted principles of approach motivation and emotion need to be revised. That is, the revised principles are Principle 1: approach motivation is associated with discrete affects that are positive, as well as negative, in valence; Principle 2: approach motivation is evoked by positive, as well as negative, stimuli; and Principle 3: approach motivation has many causes in addition to goal objects and other external stimuli. We hope that our consideration of these other, relatively new principles will increase our conceptual understanding of approach motivation and emotion, and that they may benefit applications of theory and research on approach motivation.

ACKNOWLEDGMENT

This work was funded in part by a grant from the Australian Research Council (No. DP180102504).

NOTE

1. One way to address this example is to posit different levels of motivation (Scholer, Cornwell, & Higgins, 2019). According to this theoretical analysis, at the system level, the animal is avoiding danger, but at the strategic level, it is moving toward a safe location. This kind of theorizing posits that there can be approach and avoidance motivation at different levels at the same time. For example, rats that are more prevention-oriented will vigilantly approach a noxious-smelling threat (a bleach-soaked cotton ball) to bury it, thereby removing or avoiding a danger (Franks, Higgins, & Champagne, 2012). As we have argued elsewhere (E. Harmon-Jones & Harmon-Jones, 2019), we believe that the different "levels" are better described by separate concepts altogether rather than positing that they are different levels of motivation. *Motivation* is often defined as an urge or impulse to act and the organism's exertion of effort is often used as evidence of motivation. In the case of rats burying noxious-smelling

threats (Franks et al., 2012), rats with more of a prevention orientation may have been more likely to bury the "threat" because they "believed" they could not escape the noxious smell (even if they moved to a different but interconnected cage); that is, the rats may have believed that the only way to escape the smell was to bury it. These rats had to move toward (approach) the threat to bury it, but their moving toward the threat was not approach motivated in the sense of a motivational urge. If another organism had buried the threat, the rats would have likely been satisfied and not motivated to try to bury it again. In contrast, consider a rat being exposed to desired food. The rat is motivated to eat the food and will exert effort to eat it. If another rat started to eat the same small piece of food, the rat would likely be unsatisfied and might act aggressively to regain the lost food object. In other words, a behavior in which an organism moves toward or approaches is not necessarily motivated by approach; it may be motivated by avoidance. We prefer to call the behavior simply *behavior*; the motivation is a different matter.

REFERENCES

Amodio, D. M., Devine, P. G., & Harmon-Jones, E. (2007). A dynamic model of guilt: Implications for motivation and self-regulation in the context of prejudice. *Psychological Science, 18*, 524–530.

Amodio, D. M., & Harmon-Jones, E. (2011). Trait emotions and affective modulation of the startle eyeblink: On the unique relationship of trait anger. *Emotion, 11*, 47–51.

Angus, D. J., Kemkes, K., Schutter, D. J., & Harmon-Jones, E. (2015). Anger is associated with reward-related electrocortical activity: Evidence from the reward positivity. *Psychophysiology, 52*, 1271–1280.

Berkman, E. T., & Lieberman, M. D. (2010). Approaching the bad and avoiding the good: Lateral prefrontal cortical asymmetry distinguishes between action and valence. *Journal of Cognitive Neuroscience, 22*(9), 1970–1979.

Blanchard, D. C., & Blanchard, R. J. (1984). Inadequacy of pain-aggression hypothesis revealed in naturalistic settings. *Aggressive Behavior, 10*, 33–46.

Bowlby, J. (1973). *Attachment and loss: Vol. 2. Separation, anxiety and anger.* London: Hogarth Press and the Institute of Psycho-Analysis.

Bradley, M. M., Codispoti, M., Cuthbert, B. N., & Lang, P. J. (2001). Emotion and motivation: I. Defensive and appetitive reactions in picture processing. *Emotion, 1*(3), 276–298.

Brehm, J. W. (1956). Postdecision changes in the desirability of alternatives. *Journal of Abnormal and Social Psychology, 52*(3), 384–389.

Bress, J. N., & Hajcak, G. (2013). Self-report and behavioral measures of reward sensitivity predict the feedback negativity. *Psychophysiology, 50*, 610–616.

Butler, R. A., & Harlow, H. F. (1954). Persistence of visual exploration in monkeys. *Journal of Comparative and Physiological Psychology, 47*(3), 258–263.

Cacioppo, J. T., Gardner, W. L., & Berntson, G. G. (1999). The affect system has parallel and integrative processing components: Form follows function. *Journal of Personality and Social Psychology, 76*(5), 839–855.

Carlson, J. M., Foti, D., Harmon-Jones, E., & Proudfit, G. H. (2015). Midbrain volume predicts fMRI and ERP measures of reward reactivity. *Brain Structure and Function, 200*, 1861–1866.

Carver, C. S. (2004). Negative affects deriving from the behavioral approach system. *Emotion, 4*, 3–22.

Carver, C. S., & White, T. L. (1994). Behavioral inhibition, behavioral activation, and affective responses to impending reward and punishment: The BIS/BAS scales. *Journal of Personality and Social Psychology, 67*, 319–333.

Coan, J. A., Allen, J. J. B., & Harmon-Jones, E. (2001). Voluntary facial expression and hemispheric asymmetry over the frontal cortex. *Psychophysiology, 38*, 912–925.

Cook, I. A., O'Hara, R., Uijtdehaage, S. H. J., Mandelkern, M., & Leuchter, A. F. (1998). Assessing the accuracy of topographic EEG mapping for determining local brain function. *Electroencephalography and Clinical Neurophysiology, 107*, 408–414.

Darwin, C. (1965). *The expressions of the emotions in man and animals.* New York: Oxford University Press. (Original work published 1872)

Davidson, R. J., Ekman, P., Saron, C. D., Senulis, J. A., & Friesen, W. V. (1990). Approach–withdrawal and cerebral asymmetry: Emotional expression and brain physiology: I. *Journal of Personality and Social Psychology, 58*, 330–341.

Davidson, R. J., & Fox, N. (1982). Asymmetric brain activity discriminates between positive and negative affective stimuli in 10 month old infants. *Science, 218*, 1235–1237.

Dollard, J., Miller, N. E., Doob, L. W., Mowrer, O. H., & Sears, R. R. (1939). *Frustration and aggression.* New Haven, CT: Yale University Press.

Duclos, S. E., Laird, J. D., Schneider, E., Sexter, M., Stern, L., & Van Lighten, O. (1989). Emotion-specific effects of facial expressions and postures on emotional experience. *Journal of Personality and Social Psychology, 57*, 100–108.

Ekman, P., & Davidson, R. J. (1993). Voluntary smiling changes regional brain activity. *Psychological Science, 4*, 342–345.

Elliot, A. J., Eder, A. B., & Harmon-Jones, E. (2013). Approach–avoidance motivation and emotion: Convergence and divergence. *Emotion Review, 5*(3), 308–311.

Fawver, B., Hass, C. J., Park, K. D., & Janelle, C. M. (2014). Autobiographically recalled emotional states impact forward gait initiation as a function of motivational direction. *Emotion, 14*, 1125–1136.

Festinger, L. (1957). *A theory of cognitive dissonance.* Evanston, IL: Row, Peterson.

Foti, D., & Hajcak, G. (2009). Depression and reduced sensitivity to non-rewards versus rewards: Evidence from event-related potentials. *Biological Psychology, 81*, 1–8.

Franks, B., Higgins, E. T., & Champagne, F. A. (2012). Evidence for individual differences in regulatory focus in rats, *Rattus norvegicus. Journal of Comparative Psychology, 126*(4), 347–354.

Freud, S. (1955). *The interpretation of dreams* (J. Strachey, Ed. & Trans.). New York: Basic Books. (Original work published 1900)

Gard, D. E., Gard, M. G., Mehta, N., Kring, A. M., & Patrick, C. J. (2007). Impact of motivational salience on affect modulated startle at early and late probe times. *International Journal of Psychophysiology, 66*(3), 266–270.

Goldstein, K. (1939). *The organism: An holistic approach to biology, derived from pathological data in man.* New York: American Book.

Greenaway, K. H., Storrs, K. R., Philipp, M. C., Louis, W. R., Hornsey, M. J., & Vohs, K. D. (2015). Loss of control stimulates approach motivation. *Journal of Experimental Social Psychology, 56*, 235–241.

Harmon-Jones, C., Bastian, B., & Harmon-Jones, E. (2016). Detecting transient emotional responses with improved self-report measures and instructions. *Emotion, 16*, 1086–1096.

Harmon-Jones, C., & Harmon-Jones, E. (2019). A broad consideration of motivation, with a focus on approach motivation. *Psychological Inquiry, 30*(3), 132–135.

Harmon-Jones, C., Schmeichel, B. J., Inzlicht, M., & Harmon-Jones, E. (2011). Trait approach motivation relates to dissonance reduction. *Social Psychological and Personality Science, 2*, 21–28.

Harmon-Jones, C., Schmeichel, B. J., Mennitt, E., & Harmon-Jones, E. (2011). The expression of determination: Similarities between anger and approach-related positive affect. *Journal of Personality and Social Psychology, 100*, 172–181.

Harmon-Jones, E. (2003). Anger and the behavioural approach system. *Personality and Individual Differences, 35*, 995–1005.

Harmon-Jones, E. (2004). On the relationship of anterior brain activity and anger: Examining the role of attitude toward anger. *Cognition and Emotion, 18*, 337–361.

Harmon-Jones, E. (2006). Unilateral right-hand contractions cause contralateral alpha power suppression and approach motivational affective experience. *Psychophysiology, 43*, 598–603.

Harmon-Jones, E., & Allen, J. J. B. (1998). Anger and prefrontal brain activity: EEG asymmetry consistent with approach motivation despite negative affective valence. *Journal of Personality and Social Psychology, 74*, 1310–1316.

Harmon-Jones, E., & Gable, P. A. (2018). On the role of asymmetrical frontal cortical activity in approach and withdrawal motivation: An updated review of the evidence. *Psychophysiology, 55*, e12879.

Harmon-Jones, E., Gable, P. A., & Price, T. F. (2011). Leaning embodies desire: Evidence that leaning forward increases relative left frontal cortical activation to appetitive stimuli. *Biological Psychology, 87*, 311–313.

Harmon-Jones, E., Gerdjikov, T., & Harmon-Jones, C. (2008).The effect of induced compliance on relative left frontal cortical activity: A test of the action-based model of dissonance. *European Journal of Social Psychology, 38*, 35–45.

Harmon-Jones, E., & Harmon-Jones, C. (2002). Testing the action-based model of cognitive dissonance: The effect of action-orientation on postdecisional attitudes. *Personality and Social Psychology Bulletin, 28*, 711–723.

Harmon-Jones, E., Harmon-Jones, C., Abramson, L. Y., & Peterson, C. K. (2009). PANAS positive activation is associated with anger. *Emotion, 9*, 183–196.

Harmon-Jones, E., Harmon-Jones, C., Amodio, D. M., & Gable, P. A. (2011). Attitudes toward emotions. *Journal of Personality and Social Psychology, 101*, 1332–1350.

Harmon-Jones, E., Harmon-Jones, C., Fearn, M., Sigelman, J. D., & Johnson, P. (2008). Left frontal cortical activation and spreading of alternative: Tests of the action-based model of dissonance. *Journal of Personality and Social Psychology, 94*, 1–15.

Harmon-Jones, E., Harmon-Jones, C., & Levy, N. (2015). An action-based model of cognitive dissonance processes. *Current Directions in Psychological Science, 24*, 184–189.

Harmon-Jones, E., Harmon-Jones, C., & Price, T. F. (2013). What is approach motivation? *Emotion Review, 5*, 291–295.

Harmon-Jones, E., Harmon-Jones, C., Serra, R., &

Gable, P. A. (2011). The effect of commitment on relative left frontal cortical activity: Tests of the action-based model of dissonance. *Personality and Social Psychology Bulletin, 37*, 395–408.

Harmon-Jones, E., & Peterson, C. K. (2009). Supine body position reduces neural response to anger evocation. *Psychological Science, 20*, 1209–1210.

Harmon-Jones, E., Peterson, C. K., & Harris, C. R. (2009). Jealousy: Novel methods and neural correlates. *Emotion, 9*, 113–117.

Harmon-Jones, E., Price, T. F., & Harmon-Jones, C. (2015). Supine body posture decreases rationalizations: Testing the action-based model of dissonance. *Journal of Experimental Social Psychology, 56*, 228–234.

Harmon-Jones, E., & Sigelman, J. D. (2001). State anger and prefrontal brain activity: Evidence that insult-related relative left-prefrontal activation is associated with experienced anger and aggression. *Journal of Personality and Social Psychology, 80*, 797–803.

Hassin, R. R. (2013). Yes it can: On the functional abilities of the human unconscious. *Perspectives on Psychological Science, 8*(2), 195–207.

Hawk, L. W., & Kowmas, A. D. (2003). Affective modulation and prepulse inhibition of startle among undergraduates high and low in behavioral inhibition and approach. *Psychophysiology, 40*(1), 131–138.

Hewig, J., Hagemann, D., Seifert, J., Naumann, E., & Bartussek, D. (2004). On the selective relation of frontal cortical activity and anger-out versus anger-control. *Journal of Personality and Social Psychology, 87*, 926–939.

Hortensius, R., Schutter, D. J., & Harmon-Jones, E. (2012). When anger leads to aggression: Induction of relative left frontal cortical activity with transcranial direct current stimulation increases the anger–aggression relationship. *Social Cognitive and Affective Neuroscience, 7*(3), 342–347.

Hull, C. L. (1943). *Principles of behavior.* New York: Appleton-Century.

James, W. (1894). Discussion: The physical basis of emotion. *Psychological Review, 1*, 516–529.

Kelley, N. J., Eastwick, P. W., Harmon-Jones, E., & Schmeichel, B. J. (2015). Jealousy increased by induced relative left frontal cortical activity. *Emotion, 15*, 550–555.

Keune, P. M., van der Heiden, L., Várkuti, B., Konicar, L., Veit, R., & Birbaumer, N. (2012). Prefrontal brain asymmetry and aggression in imprisoned violent offenders. *Neuroscience Letters, 515*, 191–195.

Kitayama, S., Chua, H. F., Tompson, S., & Han, S. (2013). Neural mechanisms of dissonance: An fMRI investigation of choice justification. *NeuroImage, 69*, 206–212.

Koolhaas, J. M., Coppens, C. M., de Boer, S. F., Buwalda, B., Meerlo, P., & Timmermans, P. J. (2013). The resident–intruder paradigm: A standardized test for aggression, violence and social stress. *Journal of Visualized Experiments, 77*, e4367.

Lagerspetz, K. M. J. (1969). Aggression and aggressiveness in laboratory mice. In S. Garattini, & E. B. Sigg (Eds.), *Aggressive behavior* (pp. 77–85). New York: Wiley.

Laird, J. D. (1974). Self-attribution of emotion: The effects of expressive behavior on the quality of emotional experience. *Journal of Personality and Social Psychology, 29*, 475–486.

Lang, P. J., & Bradley, M. M. (2008). Appetitive and defensive motivation is the substrate of emotion. In A. Elliott (Ed.), *Handbook of approach and avoidance motivation* (pp. 51–66). New York: Taylor & Francis Group.

Lang, P. J., Bradley, M. M., & Cuthbert, B. N. (1990). Emotion, attention, and the startle reflex. *Psychological Review, 97*, 377–398.

Leach, C. W., & Cidam, A. (2015). When is shame linked to constructive approach orientation?: A meta-analysis. *Journal of Personality and Social Psychology, 109*, 983–1002.

Lewis, M., Sullivan, M. W., & Kim, H. M.-S. (2015). Infant approach and withdrawal in response to a goal blockage: Its antecedent causes and its effect on toddler persistence. *Developmental Psychology, 51*(11), 1553–1563.

Lewis, M., Sullivan, M. W., Ramsey, D. S., & Alessandri, S. M. (1992). Individual differences in anger and sad expressions during extinction: Antecedents and consequences. *Infant Behavior and Development, 15*, 443–452.

Maitner, A. T., Mackie, D. M., & Smith, E. R. (2006). Evidence for the regulatory function of intergroup emotion: Emotional consequences of implemented or impeded intergroup action tendencies. *Journal of Experimental Social Psychology, 42*(6), 720–728.

Maner, J. K., DeWall, C. N., Baumeister, R. F., & Schaller, M. (2007). Does social exclusion motivate interpersonal reconnection?: Resolving the "porcupine problem." *Journal of Personality and Social Psychology, 92*(1), 42–55.

Markovitch, N., Netzer, L., & Tamir, M. (2017). What you like is what you try to get: Attitudes toward emotions and situation selection. *Emotion, 17*(4), 728–739.

McGregor, I., Nash, K. A., & Inzlicht, M. (2009). Threat, high self-esteem, and reactive approach-motivation: Electroencephalographic evidence. *Journal of Experimental Social Psychology, 45*(4), 1003–1007.

McGregor, I., Nash, K., Mann, N., & Phills, C. E. (2010). Anxious uncertainty and reactive approach motivation (RAM). *Journal of Personality and Social Psychology, 99,* 133–147.

McGregor, I., Prentice, M., & Nash, K. (2012). Approaching relief: Compensatory ideals relieve threat-induced anxiety by promoting approach-motivated states. *Social Cognition, 30*(6), 689–714.

Mengarelli, F., Spoglianti, S., Avenanti, A., & Di Pellegrino, G. (2013). Cathodal tDCS over the left prefrontal cortex diminishes choice-induced preference change. *Cerebral Cortex, 25*(5), 1219–1227.

Mikulincer, M. (1988). Reactance and helplessness following exposure to unsolvable problems: The effects of attributional style. *Journal of Personality and Social Psychology, 54,* 679–686.

Mize, K. D., Pineda, M., Blau, A. K., Marsh, K., & Jones, N. A. (2014). Infant physiological and behavioral responses to a jealousy provoking condition. *Infancy, 19*(3), 338–348.

Moskowitz, G. B., & Grant, H. (Eds.). (2009). *The psychology of goals.* New York: Guilford Press.

Mühlberger, C., Angus, D. J., Jonas, E., Harmon-Jones, C., & Harmon-Jones, E. (2017). Perceived control increases the reward positivity and stimulus preceding negativity. *Psychophysiology, 54*(2), 310–322.

Muraven, M., & Baumeister, R. F. (2000). Self-regulation and depletion of limited resources: Does self-control resemble a muscle? *Psychological Bulletin, 126,* 247–259.

Panksepp, J. (1998). *Affective neuroscience: The foundations of human and animal emotions.* New York: Oxford University Press.

Panksepp, J. (2013). Cross-species neuroaffective parsing of primal emotional desires and aversions in mammals. *Emotion Review, 5*(3), 235–240.

Panksepp, J., Herman, B., Conner, R., Bishop, P., & Scott, J. P. (1978). The biology of social attachments: Opiates alleviate separation distress. *Biological Psychiatry, 13,* 607–618.

Panksepp, J., & Watt, D. (2011). Why does depression hurt?: Ancestral primary-process separation-distress (PANIC/GRIEF) and diminished brain reward (SEEKING) processes in the genesis of depressive affect. *Psychiatry: Interpersonal and Biological Processes, 74*(1), 5–13.

Perria, P., Rosadini, G., & Rossi, G. F. (1961). Determination of side of cerebral dominance with Amobarbital. *Archives of Neurology, 4,* 175–181.

Peterson, C. K., Gravens, L., & Harmon-Jones, E. (2011). Asymmetric frontal cortical activity and negative affective responses to ostracism. *Social Cognitive and Affective Neuroscience, 6,* 277–285.

Peterson, C. K., & Harmon-Jones, E. (2009). Circadian and seasonal variability of resting frontal EEG asymmetry. *Biological Psychology, 80,* 315–320.

Peterson, C. K., Shackman, A. J., & Harmon-Jones, E. (2008). The role of asymmetric frontal cortical activity in aggression. *Psychophysiology, 45,* 86–92.

Pizzagalli, D. A., Sherwood, R. J., Henriques, J. B., & Davidson, R. J. (2005). Frontal brain asymmetry and reward responsiveness: A source-localization study. *Psychological Science, 16*(10), 805–813.

Plutchik, R. (1980). *Emotion: A psychoevolutionary synthesis.* New York: HarperCollins.

Price, T. F., Dieckman, L., & Harmon-Jones, E. (2012). Embodying approach motivation: Body posture influences startle eyeblink and event-related potential responses to appetitive stimuli. *Biological Psychology, 90,* 211–217.

Price, T. F., & Harmon-Jones, E. (2011). Approach motivational body postures lean toward left frontal brain activity. *Psychophysiology, 48,* 718–722.

Price, T. F., Hortensius, R., & Harmon-Jones, E. (2013). Neural and behavioral associations of manipulated determination facial expressions. *Biological Psychology, 94,* 221–227.

Proudfit, G. H. (2015). The reward positivity: From basic research on reward to a biomarker for depression. *Psychophysiology, 52,* 449–459.

Qin, J., Kimel, S., Kitayama, S., Wang, X., Yang, X., & Han, S. (2011). How choice modifies preference: Neural correlates of choice justification. *NeuroImage, 55*(1), 240–246.

Riskind, J. H., & Gotay, C. C. (1982). Physical posture: Could it have regulatory or feedback effects on motivation and emotion? *Motivation and Emotion, 6,* 273–298.

Robinson, R. G., & Price, T. R. (1982). Post-stroke depressive disorders: A follow-up study of 103 patients. *Stroke, 13,* 635–641.

Rolls, E. T. (1999). *The brain and emotion.* Oxford, UK: Oxford University Press.

Roth, S., & Kubal, L. (1975). Effects of noncontingent reinforcement on tasks of differing importance: Facilitation and learned helplessness. *Journal of Personality and Social Psychology, 32*(4), 680–691.

Schmeichel, B. J., Crowell, A., & Harmon-Jones, E. (2016). Exercising self-control increases relative left frontal cortical activation. *Social Cognitive and Affective Neuroscience, 11*(2), 282–288.

Schmeichel, B. J., Harmon-Jones, C., & Harmon-Jones, E. (2010). Exercising self-control increases approach motivation. *Journal of Personality and Social Psychology, 99,* 162–173.

Schneirla, T. C. (1959). An evolutionary and developmental theory of biphasic processes underlying approach and withdrawal. In M. R. Jones (Ed.), *Nebraska Symposium on Motivation* (pp. 1–42). Lincoln: University of Nebraska Press.

Scholer, A. A., Cornwell, J. F., & Higgins, E. T. (2019). Should we approach approach and avoid avoidance?: An inquiry from different levels. *Psychological Inquiry, 30*(3), 111–124.

Schöne, B., Schomberg, J., Gruber, T., & Quirin, M. (2016). Event-related frontal alpha asymmetries: Electrophysiological correlates of approach motivation. *Experimental Brain Research, 234*(2), 559–567.

Schutter, D. J. L. G. (2009). Transcranial magnetic stimulation. In E. Harmon-Jones & J. S. Beer (Eds.), *Methods in social neuroscience* (pp. 233–258). New York: Guilford Press.

Schutter, D. J. L. G., & Harmon-Jones, E. (2013). The corpus callosum: A commissural road to anger and aggression. *Neuroscience and Biobehavioral Reviews, 37*, 2481–2488.

Thibodeau, R., Jorgensen, R. S., & Kim, S. (2006). Depression, anxiety, and resting frontal EEG asymmetry: A meta-analytic review. *Journal of Abnormal Psychology, 115*(4), 715–729.

Thierry, B., Steru, L., Chermat, R., & Simon, P. (1984). Searching–waiting strategy: A candidate for an evolutionary model of depression? *Behavioral and Neural Biology, 41*(2), 180–189.

Tsypes, A., Angus, D. J., Martin, S., Kemkes, K., & Harmon-Jones, E. (2019). Trait anger and the reward positivity. *Personality and Individual Differences, 144*, 24–40.

Twenge, J. M., Baumeister, R. F., DeWall, C. N., Ciarocco, N. J., & Bartels, J. M. (2007). Social exclusion decreases prosocial behavior. *Journal of Personality and Social Psychology, 92*(1), 56–66.

Vallortigara, G., & Rogers, L. J. (2005). Survival with an asymmetrical brain: Advantages and disadvantages of cerebral lateralization. *Behavioral and Brain Sciences, 28*(4), 575–588.

Veenstra, L., Bushman, B. J., & Koole, S. L. (2018). The facts on the furious: A brief review of the psychology of trait anger. *Current Opinion in Psychology, 19*, 98–103.

Veenstra, L., Schneider, I. K., & Koole, S. L. (2017). Embodied mood regulation: The impact of body posture on mood recovery, negative thoughts, and mood-congruent recall. *Cognition and Emotion, 31*(7), 1361–1376.

Vohs, K. D., & Heatherton, T. F. (2000). Self-regulatory failure: A resource-depletion approach. *Psychological Science, 11*(3), 249–254.

Vrana, S. R., Spence, E. L., & Lang, P. J. (1988). The startle probe response: A new measure of emotion? *Journal of Abnormal Psychology, 97*(4), 487–491.

Wagner, D. D., Altman, M., Boswell, R. G., Kelley, W. M., & Heatherton, T. F. (2013). Self-regulatory depletion enhances neural responses to rewards and impairs top-down control. *Psychological Science, 24*(11), 2262–2271.

Wagner, D. D., & Heatherton, T. F. (2012). Self-regulatory depletion increases emotional reactivity in the amygdala. *Social Cognitive and Affective Neuroscience, 8*(4), 410–417.

Watson, D., Wiese, D., Vaidya, J., & Tellegen, A. (1999). The two general activation systems of affect: Structural findings, evolutionary considerations, and psychobiological evidence. *Journal of Personality and Social Psychology, 76*, 820–838.

Wei, S., Ji, X. W., Wu, C. L., Li, Z. F., Sun, P., Wang, J. Q., et al. (2014). Resident intruder paradigm-induced aggression relieves depressive-like behaviors in male rats subjected to chronic mild stress. *Medical Science Monitor, 20*, 945–952.

Woodworth, R. S., & Schlosberg, H. (1954). *Experimental psychology.* London: Methuen.

Wortman, C. B., & Brehm, J. W. (1975). Responses to uncontrollable outcomes: An integration of reactance theory and the learned helplessness model. In L. Berkowitz (Ed.), *Advances in experimental social psychology* (Vol. 8, pp. 277–336). New York: Academic Press.

CHAPTER 3

Judgment and Decision Making
Basic Principles of Adaptive Behavior

Klaus Fiedler
Linda McCaughey

Research on judgment and decision making (JDM) has become one of the most prominent and fruitful fields of psychological science in general, and of social psychology in particular. This research focuses on the psychological processes and the (adaptive) strategies that underlie the formation of preferences, choices, and manifest actions, the consequences of which can be more or less likely to lead to positive or negative outcomes. On the one hand, these research topics are intrinsically normative in nature, as the goal always is to increase benefits and to decrease costs. On the other hand, at the descriptive level, judgments and decisions in real life, exposed to the influence of a social context and other factors, hardly ever adhere to normative standards, which are often complex and contestable. Accordingly, most empirical research is in one way or another concerned with biases and anomalies in decision making that deviate in distinct ways from classic normative standards due to environmental influences and human constraints.

Scope of JDM Research

At the practical level, a demand for applied JDM research arises in many domains of social life: in political voting decisions, financial investment, health-related risk, moral and ecological dilemmas, and legal decisions, to name just a few. At the theoretical level, JDM has been a center and fertilizer of innovation, inspiring not only research in social and cognitive psychology but also neighboring disciplines such as behavioral economics, neuropsychology, biology, and experimental philosophy. In social psychology, in particular, some of the most prominent contemporary topics relate to JDM work on risk taking, moral dilemmas, consumer choice, and heuristic inference schemes. Flagship journals—such as *Psychological Review* and *Journal of Experimental Psychology: General*—are replete with JDM contributions. And two of the most outstanding psychologists, Herbert Simon and Daniel Kahneman, received Nobel prizes in economics for groundbreaking work on JDM.

Origins and Sources

While the origins of modern JDM research can be found in hard-to-digest forerunner books by John von Neumann and Oskar Morgenstern (1944), Egon Brunswik (1956), or even Jacob Bernoulli (1713), a more intelligible history course may start with the key publications by

Herbert Simon (1982), Ward Edwards (1954), and Paul Meehl (1957).

The current state of the art in JDM research is best represented in several edited volumes that include Gilovich, Griffin, and Kahneman's (2002) collection of heuristics and biases articles, Arkes and Hammond's (1986) interdisciplinary reader, and Gigerenzer and Todd's (1999) work on "simple heuristics that make us smart," all of which document the work of the most influential researchers. These edited volumes are supplemented by compelling review articles, such as Slovic and Lichtenstein's (1971) review of Bayesian and regression approaches, Einhorn and Hogarth's (1978) insightful work on the illusion of validity, Simon's (1987) treatise on rationality, and Weber and Johnson's (2009) review on "mindful JDM."

JDM as a Popular Science

The wide interest in JDM was greatly enhanced by a number of best-selling popular science books, such as Gladwell's *Blink: The Power of Thinking without Thinking* (2005), Surowiecki's *The Wisdom of Crowds* (2004), Gigerenzer's *Gut Feelings: The Intelligence of the Unconscious* (2007), or Hogarth's *Educating Intuition* (2001). The open-minded, publicity-oriented strategy of leading decision researchers may have had its part in the success of this outstanding endeavor. Back in the 1970s, the decision research centers at Eugene, Oregon (with Kahneman, Tversky,

Slovic, Lichtenstein, and Fischhoff) and at Chicago (with Einhorn, Hogarth, Hoch, Klayman, and Loewenstein) were forward-looking enough to send out mailing lists to colleagues all over the world who could order a collection of articles from these strongholds of science.

Preview of Chapter Contents

This chapter is not meant as an alternative or rival to all these excellent publications. It rather constitutes an attempt to lay out the many commonalities between decision making and social psychology, that is, to portray JDM research from a deliberately social psychological perspective. Two conditions facilitate this goal. First, the subject matter of both disciplines is deeply involved in, and somehow co-responsible, for many societal challenges and current issues of public interest, such as migration, social security, ecological dilemmas, fake news, and many other challenges of the 21st century. Second, the theoretical and empirical research developments during the last decades of JDM and social psychology are intimately related, reflecting similar influences in the history of science. Table 3.1 illustrates these striking commonalities and offers an advanced organizer for the remainder of this chapter. The findings and concepts listed in Table 3.1 suggest an integrative perspective on some of the most important *basic principles.*

TABLE 3.1. Striking Parallels in Theoretical Developments, Empirical Research Topics, and Applied Domains Shared by the Subdisciplines of Decision Research and Social Psychology

Aspect	Parallel developments and related paradigms
Societal topics of public interest	Deep interest in the scientific analysis of reasoned action; conflict resolution; adaptive behavior; social, ecological and health-related dilemmas; forensic procedures; financial decision making; and marketing tools
Heuristics and biases	Adaptivity of heuristics; juxtaposition of heuristic and systematic cognition and action, as related to dual-process approaches
Affect and motivation	Emphasis on motivation and hedonic factors: loss aversion, hot stove effect, endowment effect, wishful thinking, unrealistic optimism
Asymmetry of self and others	Leading research paradigms dealing with self-reference effects: self-enhancement, psychological distance
Information search	Sampling approaches in decision research corresponding to social hypothesis testing approaches in social psychology

Definitions and Terminological Conventions

To create common ground in a book on basic principles, let us be explicit about some basic terms. Rather than using *rational, adaptive,* and *normative* as quasi-synonyms, let the term *rational* denote inferences based on good reasons, independent of an unequivocal normative criterion and a material payoff. Let the term *bias* denote any systematic response tendency, regardless of whether it reflects a biased cognitive process, a motivational tendency, or an adaptive strategy that is responsive to existing biases in the environment. Biases can be functional and highly adaptive and can reflect rational strategies.

A study by Olivola and Todorov (2010) may illustrate this point. A highly functional and adaptive strategy to predict binary outcomes from faces, such as predicting gun possession (yes vs. no) or sexual orientation (gay vs. straight), is to predict the more prevalent level of each dichotomy (e.g., to exhibit a bias to predict no gun possession and straight sexual orientation). Maximizing such a base-rate-driven bias produces the highest accuracy rates and affords a prime example of a rational strategy, whether used deliberately or not. Likewise, a "strategy" need not be conscious or deliberate; the tendency to infer truth from fluency can reflect a fully unconscious strategy (Dechêne, Stahl, Hansen, & Wänke, 2010).

Basic Principles of Decision Research from a Social Psychological Perspective

Applied Decision Research in the Public Interest

Let us illustrate the synergy of JDM and social psychology, and their joint responsibility as consultants of politicians and the public, with reference to three areas of applied science in the public interest: legal decision making, health-related risk management, and marketing behavior.

Forensic Decision Making

Existential decisions with serious consequences for the defendant, the victim, and the public are reached in court trials. Whether a defendant is guilty or innocent, whether he or she may ultimately lose his or her job, family, and reputation, depends on not just an objective assessment of physical evidence. Often, "soft evidence" needs to be relied on: verbal sophistication of testimony, social motives and conflicts of interest, or human memory in eyewitness reports, the reliability of which judges have to be able to estimate. Judges who are responsible for such existential legal decisions cannot abstain from a decision or vote for "indifferent," regardless of the degree of uncertainty that remains after all available evidence is evaluated. The resulting decisions are intricate and far from always correct, owing to the fallibility of verbal witness reports, unwarranted inferences from polygraph test results, or misidentifications of alleged perpetrators in eyewitness identification tasks and more.

The innocence project reports that 70% of 362 DNA exoneration cases (i.e., cases whose innocence became apparent after the legalization of DNA proofs) were convicted after eyewitness misidentification based on a decision task that is well known as a multiple-choice recognition task (*www.innocenceproject.org/dna-exonerations-in-the-united-states*). Witnesses have to identify a perpetrator in a panel of persons, which includes the suspect along with several other persons (of the same gender, race, and general appearance). They are bound to feel social pressure from prosecutors and police, being expected to identify a criminal whose guilt they may believe can only be demonstrated through their identification decision. They often fail to take into account the possibility that the suspect in the lineup may be innocent and thus unknown to them. In such a context, witnesses exhibit a marked response tendency to identify the suspect rather than indicate they cannot identify anyone beyond reasonable doubt, regardless of whether he or she is actually the perpetrator. This well-documented bias is further reinforced by the fact that memory of the original perpetrator is greatly degraded after a long retention interval and many intervening questions and retrieval attempts. Hence, the recognition decision is mainly driven by the vividly present faces in the lineup. Typically, witnesses "identify" the one person in the lineup who bears the highest resemblance to the original residing in a degraded memory. As a consequence, even under optimal conditions, when eyewitnesses reach identification hit rates of roughly 80%, they typically produce false-alarm rates (i.e., misidentification rates of innocent suspects) in the range of 40%. Thus, a typical, systemic feature in eyewitness identification settings is an intolerably high false-alarm rate that causes a good deal of harm and therefore calls for a corrective intervention.

Indeed, applied scientists developed decision aids that afford a remedy to the predominant bias in eyewitness identification. Using signal-detection analysis (SDA; Swets, Dawes, & Monahan, 2000) as a methodological tool, they arrived at a better understanding of the task, which then led to helpful interventions that greatly served to ameliorate the problem. SDA constitutes a prime example of a basic principle in JDM, a statistical decision theory.

Figure 3.1 portrays the statistical decision model that underlies SDA, illustrating a hit rate of 80% and a false-alarm rate of 40%. The assumption is that the memory strength varies as indicated by the two distribution curves. The horizontal distance between the black curve on the right (i.e., distribution of memory strength in witnesses exposed to lineups that actually include the perpetrator) and the dashed curve (i.e., distribution of memory strength when the suspect in the lineup is not the perpetrator) clearly indicate that memory is statistically sensitive to the discrimination between actually experienced perpetrators and innocent control persons. However, the overlap between both curves shows that discrimination performance is imperfect; some memories covered by the dashed curve produce stronger responses (toward the right end of the scale) than the weaker memory responses elicited by real perpetrators (covered by the black curve).

So, on the one hand, it is crystal clear from the statistical model that eyewitness performance cannot be perfect. The very overlap between curves highlights the fact that discriminability will sometimes fail, due to all kinds of influences that delimit human memory. In signal detection, *discriminability* corresponds

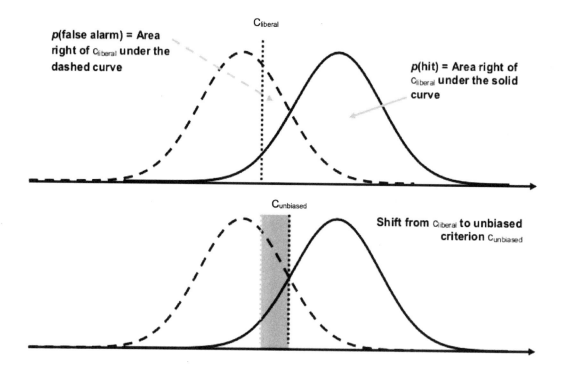

FIGURE 3.1. Signal-detection analysis of a strategy shift from a liberal response criterion $c_{liberal}$ to an unbiased criterion $c_{unbiased}$.

to the horizontal distance d' between the two distribution curves. This source of limited performance can hardly be eliminated by any decision aids. However, on the other hand, the model also reveals that independent of existing limits of discriminability, the resulting performance also depends to a notable extent on decision strategies that lend themselves to devising effective decision aids.

A strategy can be specified as a response *criterion c,* that is, as a critical threshold on the horizontal axis (dotted line) that a memory response must exceed to elicit an identification decision. Figure 3.1 includes two such response strategies. The liberal *criterion* $c_{liberal}$ in the upper chart is exceeded by roughly 80% of hits (area under the solid curve) and by roughly 40% of false alarms (area under the dashed curve), typical of the motivational and mnemonic conditions of the traditional eyewitness task. Assuming the same base rates of "guilty" and "innocent" lineups, it leads to a performance of (80% + 60%)/2 = 70% correct responses.

The other criterion $c_{unbiased}$ (lower chart) that corresponds to a more conservative strategy must inevitably produce lower percentages of both hits and false alarms because of the criterion shift to the right. Notably, however, the decrease in false alarms (from 40% to roughly 10%) is stronger than the decrease in hits (from 80 to 70%). This strategy shift not only reduced the intolerable rate of unjust convictions but also improved the overall accuracy, which is now (70 + 90%)/2 = 80%. Even when existing limitations of memory cannot be overcome in retrospect, merely changing the strategy can benefit the accuracy rate. Finding an effective decision aid then amounts to finding an intervention that induces more cautious, conservative responding (Wells et al., 1998)—a regulatory focus shift from a promotion to a more prevention focus (Higgins, 2012).

One such intervention that has already been implemented in legal practice is to present the lineup sequentially rather than simultaneously. A witness who has to make an independent recognition decision about each individually presented person in a lineup will be very cautious and refrain from making a premature identification, knowing that several alternative candidates will follow. Another remedy against too

liberal a criterion is to increase the number of persons in a lineup (Lindsay & Wells, 1985); not surprisingly, the uncertainty increases and induces a stricter criterion when a lineup includes 10 people rather than only five or six.

The improvement in accuracy is brought about by a procedural intervention that induces a mere criterion shift, replacing a liberal bias by a more conservative bias. Such an improvement is independent of rationality proper. Neither the eyewitnesses' memory strength nor their self-determined cognitive or metacognitive competence contribute to the accuracy gain. It is functional within a legal system that normally induces a liberal bias; the same intervention may be dysfunctional in case of a highly cautious witness with too conservative a response bias.

In any case, the statistical analysis of consequential forensic decisions reveals, as a basic principle, that accuracy can confound rationality and decision competence with response biases that may be functional or dysfunctional depending on the environment and should therefore always be evaluated in relation to it.

Health-Related Decisions and Risk Assessment

The same holds for health-related decisions. Swets and colleagues (2000) provide an impressive tutorial of how SDA can be used to maximize benefits and costs in health-related decisions. Let us assume that the HIV base rate in a population is $p(HIV) = .001$ (i.e., 0.1%). Assume further that the hit rate of the standard HIV test is perfect, $p(+|HIV) = 1.00$, such that all 100% of people who actually have the virus are tested positively and that the false-positive rate (people who tested positively but do not have the virus) is only $p(+|not\ HIV) = .01$ (i.e., 1%). Although this looks like a perfect test, the low HIV base rate implies that the posterior probability $p(HIV|+)$ that a positively tested person actually has the virus is less than 10%. This follows from the assumption of very low prior odds $\Omega_{prior} = p(HIV)/p(not\ HIV) = 0.001/0.999$, which render $p(not\ HIV)$ 999 times more likely than $p(HIV)$, whereas the likelihood ratio LR $= p(+|HIV)/p(+|not\ HIV) = 1.00/.01$ favors the HIV hypothesis only by the factor 100. Therefore, the posterior odds $\Omega_{post} = p(HIV|+)/p(not\ HIV|+)$ that the HIV hypothesis is true rather than false given a positive test are indeed only $\Omega_{post} = LR \cdot \Omega_{prior} = 100/999 \sim 1/10$. Such an odds ratio is fulfilled when $p(HIV|+)$ is slightly less than10%.

A similar impressive example of a false-positive risk in HIV screening is based on real data from a company's employees with a low HIV base rate of $p(HIV) = .003$ (Bloom & Glied, 1991). Even when a positive outcome on a typical screening test was followed up with a more conclusive (and expensive) confirmatory test to reduce the number of false positives, the expected rate of HIV after a positive result on both tests was as low as $p(HIV|++) = .13$. In other words, six out of seven people diagnosed as positive would be erroneously told they have HIV.

The elevated base rate of positive HIV tests is not a coincidence but presumably is motivated by liability law. The costs of false negatives can be immense (testers could be held responsible for missing a true case of HIV), but hardly any liability costs arise from false positives (no sanctions for unwarranted classification of HIV). Because of these unequal costs of false-negative and false-positive errors, tests are typically constructed to entail a rather liberal decision criterion. Holding the discriminability of a biochemical test constant, by merely changing the criterion (e.g., the color of a test serum for a positive test result), the likelihood that positively tested people do not have the virus can change radically, as a function of strategic response biases.

While the HIV example illustrates how decision strategies can be driven by cost-benefit considerations, it is instructive to understand the underlying logical principle, which can also be found in the Swet and colleagues (2000) article in *Psychological Science in the Public Interest*. Accordingly, the normatively optimal response criterion for diagnosing disease D is:

$$c_{optimal} = \frac{p(not\ D)}{p(D)} \times \frac{Benefit(correct\ rejection) + Cost(false\ positive)}{Benefit(hit) + Cost(false\ negative)}$$

Thus, the optimal criterion $c_{optimal}$ should be higher (i.e., more conservative) to the extent that the disease is more likely absent than pres-

ent, when the benefits of a correct rejection of the D hypothesis are higher than the benefits of a hit, and when false positives are more costly than false negatives. This optimal-criterion rule is extremely useful for decisions under risk, provided the base rates and the benefits and costs of the various outcomes can be reasonably estimated.

Marketing and Behavioral Finance

A third applied domain in which social psychology converges with decision research is marketing and financial investment. Making prudent financial decisions has become an important aspect of social intelligence. Even ordinary people with a modest income have to buy or rent an apartment, negotiate job offers, pay into retirement funds, or simply attempt to use their income optimally when making everyday consumer choices.

Again, subjective success and failure, satisfaction and dissatisfaction in the area of behavioral finance depend heavily on social psychological influences. For instance, consider the enigmatic endowment effect (Kahneman, Knetsch, & Thaler, 2005), that is, the discrepancy in the willingness to accept buying prices and selling prices. What people consider to be a fair buying price is lower than what they consider to be a fair selling price. This asymmetry (1) reduces the transaction rate and (2) leads to stabilized ownership because sellers see their goods as higher in value than do buyers, who do not yet possess the good. According to economists Morewedge and Giblin (2015, p. 339), "It creates market inefficiencies and irregularities in valuation such as differences between buyers and sellers," the economic impact of which is "consequential."

In a typical endowment experiment, like the one published by Van Boven, Dunning, and Loewenstein (2000) based on the original study by Kahneman, Knetsch, and Thaler (1990), participants are assigned one of two roles: sellers or buyers. Sellers are then endowed with a particular good, such as a coffee mug, and they are told it is their own possession, which can, however, later be sold (i.e., exchanged into money). Buyers are given the money and are shown the coffee mug that they will later have a chance to buy with their money. The canonical pattern of findings obtained is that the lowest acceptable selling prices were substantially and consistently higher ($5.40 and $6.37 in Experiments 1 and 2) than the highest acceptable buying prices ($1.56 and $1.85). Moreover, buyers' agents who did not negotiate for themselves but for the principal buyer were also reluctant to offer prices ($4.92 and $6.19 in Experiments 3 and 4) as high as those indicated by sellers ($6.83 and $7.38). Buyers' agents thus underestimate the value an object has for its owner. Still, the prices that agent buyers were willing to offer were higher than the prices indicated by principal buyers themselves, suggesting that ownership matters.

Consistent with these findings, Morewedge, Shu, Gilbert, and Wilson (2009) demonstrated that the endowment effect disappeared when buyers already owned an identical copy of the coffee mug they were offered to purchase and when brokers acted on behalf of buyers and sellers. These findings do not provide cogent support for the common explanation of the endowment effect in terms of loss aversion (van Dijk & van Knippenberg, 1998), that is, the notion that losses loom larger than gains.[1] Because selling entails losing and buying entails gaining an object, this principle alone might account for the endowment effect. However, the loss aversion account is incomplete because it misses the point that selling entails not only losing a piece of property but also gaining an amount of money, just as buying entails not only gaining a new piece of property but also losing the money

required for payment. In other words, loss aversion for possession has to be pitted against loss aversion for valence (money). Consistent with this distinction, Brenner, Rottenstreich, Sood, and Bilgin (2007) demonstrated an endowment effect for attractive goods (i.e., when possession loss aversion was stronger than valence loss aversion) but a reversed endowment effect for unattractive goods.

A growing body of evidence of this kind suggests that the endowment effect reflects a malleable process that can be moderated. For example, distinct emotions can moderate the endowment effect. In accordance with the chief appraisal function of depression (i.e., devaluing current states and desiring new states) and disgust (devaluing everything), the bias toward higher selling than buying prices producing the endowment effect was reversed under depression and disappeared in disgust (Lerner, Small, & Loewenstein, 2004).

Further support for this contention comes from Johnson, Häubl, and Keinan's (2007) query theory approach. Central to query theory (see Table 3.2) is the assumption that judgments and decisions are informed by retrieval of memorized information solicited in a kind of self-interrogation process. For instance, sellers and buyers in a trading situation would use queries such as "Why should I make the trade?" or "Why should I not make the trade?" While retrieved answers to the former query should refer to assets of the good and thereby support a higher price, the latter query should result in

TABLE 3.2. Query Theory Applied by Johnson et al. (2007) to Explaining Endowment Effects

Basic idea	Query principle	Queries trigger memory retrieval of evaluative information about decision options.
Premise 1	Decomposition	Decision makers decompose valuation into sequence of queries. First consider advantages of current status quo: Sellers first consider advantages of owning the object; buyers first consider disadvantages of transaction.
Premise 2	Prominence	Prefer the option that is superior on most important attributes.
Premise 3	Retrieval interference	Privileged retrieval of focal information comes along with retrieval inhibition for nonfocal information.
Premise 4	Impact of role or perspective	Therefore, sellers tend to retrieve information that boosts the value of the trading object, whereas buyers tend to retrieve information that serves to downplay the value.

downgrading arguments that serve to reduce the price.

For a sufficient account of the endowment effect, Johnson and colleagues (2007) introduced the (testable) assumption that sellers and buyers tend to ask the two queries in different order, and that early queries receive more weight than later queries. Sellers' higher price estimates reflect their tendency to first consider value-increasing aspects of the transaction, whereas buyers' lower estimates reflect their tendency to first consider value-decreasing reasons that speak against the transaction.

Summary

A synopsis of applied research in three areas—law, health, and financial decisions—illustrates the "symbiotic relation" between social psychology and decision research, whose joint role is to support rational decisions and actions in areas rife with social influences and to consult the public on "psychological science in the public interest." The sample of reviewed research highlights the importance of methodological tools (SDA and cost–benefit analysis based on it), as well as clearly spelled out theories (e.g., query theory).

Comparing Human Decision Making to Normative Standards

Early pioneers in JDM research emphasized existing analogies between human inferences and normative scientific methods (Kelley, 1967; Peterson & Beach, 1967; Sarbin, Taft, & Bailey, 1960). But the literature of the 1970s and subsequent decades was replete with demonstrations of judgments and decisions that deviated dramatically from normative prescriptions. Clinical expert judgments were shown to be inferior to actuarial models (Dawes, Faust, & Meehl, 1989; Goldberg, 1970); judges were insensitive to base-rate constraints and to regression (Tversky & Kahneman, 1971); laypeople's and experts' subjective confidence were ill calibrated; incontestable laws of probability and statistics were regularly violated. Experiments on heuristics and biases, and shortcomings and distortions of social judgment became leading research programs in JDM (Tversky & Kahne-

man, 1974) and in social cognition (Nisbett & Ross, 1978), respectively.

The upcoming pessimistic perspective on human rationality is best illustrated by Tversky and Kahneman's (1971) earliest paper, "Belief in the Law of Small Numbers." Both laypeople and scientists, despite their training, notoriously overestimate the reliability of small samples, expecting every random sample, however small, to resemble the population from which it is drawn. This naive neglect of Bernoulli's law of the large number contributes to a variety of unwarranted and superficial beliefs, such as the gambler's fallacy, which describes the (incorrect) judgment of an event as more likely the more other events have taken place since the last time that event occurred (e.g., judging it more likely for a coin to land as tails the more often it had previously landed as heads) (Tversky & Kahneman, 1971).

Heuristics and Biases

It is no exaggeration to say that psychology would not be the same without Tversky and Kahneman's (1974) groundbreaking work on heuristics and biases. Half a century later, heuristics and biases belong to the most basic principles of JDM. Heuristics are simple strategies for judging latent entities that do not lend themselves to direct perception or assessment, or are impossible to assess accurately, such as risk, truth, effective costs, diagnostic categorization, or predictions under uncertainty. Complete evidence about such latent entities is hardly ever available, and if it were, it would hardly be possible to process it all and to determine how much to weight each influence factor—a constraint that is recognized in the view of bounded rationality. In the face of these challenges, heuristics are good proxies to make informed guesses, relying on adaptive cues that are quite accurate under most conditions, though they can lead to distinct biases under some conditions. Table 3.3 gives an overview of most prominent heuristics, along with resulting biases and the standard references.

Consider, for example, the usefulness of the *availability* heuristic (Tversky & Kahneman, 1973) for judging frequency or probability. When estimating the probability of different causes of death, judges have no representative

TABLE 3.3. Synopsis of Prominent Heuristics and Biases

Heuristic	Description	Standard reference
Availability	Judgments of frequency or probability reflect the ease with which relative examples come to mind.	Tversky & Kahneman (1973)
Representativeness	Categorization depends on object's similarity with category (representativeness): conjunction fallacy, base-rate neglect, misconceived randomness.	Kahneman & Tversky (1972)
Anchoring	Quantitative judgments are biased toward initial anchors, subsequent adjustments are insufficient.	Tversky & Kahneman (1974)
Simulation	Mental simulations of situations are used as basis for likelihood estimates.	Kahneman & Tversky (1982)
Affect heuristic	Intuitive assessment of both risk and benefit biased in the same affect-congruent fashion.	Slovic & Peters (2006)
Recognition	If A is recognized but B is not, then A is inferred to be of higher value on the criterion in question.	Goldstein & Gigerenzer (2002)
Fluency	If A is retrieved more fluently than B, then A is inferred to be of higher value.	Hertwig, Herzog, Schooler, & Reimer (2008)

data arrays stored in memory. They can nevertheless make a reasonable estimate based on the ease with which memorized examples come to mind. Classes of events are judged to be frequent (infrequent) or likely (unlikely) if it is easy (difficult) to retrieve examples from memory or, should judges not engage in memory retrieval proper, if they believe it would be easy (difficult) to retrieve relevant examples. For example, as it is easier to retrieve cases of people dying from cancer or traffic accidents than people dying from a flash of lightning or from a poisonous spider, most people will correctly provide higher lethality estimates for cancer and traffic accidents than for lightning and spider bites. Thus, the *availability cue,* defined as subjective experience of memory accessibility, allows them to make reasonably accurate judgments even when they do not keep in memory an accessible epidemiological database.

The availability heuristic draws on the reversal of the well-known valid principle that the more frequently an item is encountered, the more easily it can be recalled later. Underlying the heuristic is the backward inference that the more easily an item can be recalled, the more frequently it must have been encountered. This may, however, produce systematic biases simply because frequency of exposure is not the only determinant of availability, and because

frequency of exposure itself might be distorted. Some causes of death may be easy to retrieve not because they are frequent but because they are frightening, or because one is exposed more often to them due to their being overrepresented in the media. For instance, dread risks (e.g., airplane crashes) are overrated for emotional reasons (Gigerenzer, 2004), or the rate of murder is overestimated relative to suicide (Combs & Slovic, 1979).

Another classic heuristic introduced by Tversky and Kahneman (1974) is the so-called *representativeness* heuristic, which describes the use of a target's representativeness of a category as a cue for categorization judgments. The similarity or typicality of the target and the category leads to judgments that neglects the base rate, and thus the general probability of any person belonging to that category. Similarly, representativeness makes very appealing the logically impossible judgment that the probability of two events or properties occurring together is higher than the probability of only one of those occurring. This is called the *conjunction fallacy* (Tversky & Kahneman, 1983), of which one memorable implication is that people are more confident in judging and in betting on more clearly specified subordinate categories compared to more abstract superordinate categories. Bar-Hillel and Neter (1993) provided their participants with sketches of a target person such as the following: "Writes letter home describing a country with snowy wild mountains, clean streets, and flower decked porches. Where was the letter written?" Based on this description, they more readily classified the target by, or bet on, the home country (Switzerland rather than Brazil) than the superordinate continent (Europe rather than Latin America). This constitutes a clear-cut conjunction fallacy; logically, one cannot be more certain about a specific country nested within a continent than about the embedding continent.

Another consequence with serious implications for moral and legal judgments is that causal explanations (e.g., of a crime) in terms of conjunctive causes (hostility ∧ alcohol ∧ provocation) often appear more plausible than explanations in terms of singular causes (e.g., provocation). In a study by Leddo, Abelson, and Gross (1984), such a conjunction effect in causal judgments generalized over many task conditions: simple and triple conjunctions, explanations of mundane and important actions, and across events of varying probability levels.

Perhaps the most intensively studied heuristic is *anchoring*. Quantitative judgments exhibit a pronounced bias toward the numerical value given as an unrelated cue before an estimation. For instance, checking the last two digits of one's social security number as a completely arbitrary anchor will influence how much money one is willing to bid for a bottle of wine and other consumer goods (Ariely, Loewenstein, & Prelec, 2003).These findings are very robust and have obvious relevance for actual negotiations or auctions, where buyers and bidders have been shown to be influenced by starting prices (Galinsky & Mussweiler, 2001; Orr & Guthrie, 2006). However, research has shown that this basic principle can be overridden by the dynamics of competitive negotiation in real auctions. Lower starting prices may serve to reduce the entry barriers and fuel competition between multiple bidders (Ku, Galinsky, & Murnighan, 2006). "Increased traffic" due to lower starting prices may thus eventually result in higher end prices. As a side effect of such an escalation process, the "traffic generated by lower starting prices can lead bidders to infer value in the item, thereby explaining previous findings that

traffic begets more traffic" (Ku et al., 2006, p. 975). Accordingly, the authors found that barriers that inhibit traffic (e.g., a misspelled item name) may eliminate the positive influence of low starting prices and reinstate the "normal" assimilation of end prices to starting prices.

Another applied area in which anchoring leads to astounding biases is that of legal judgments. The Englich and Mussweiler study (2001) showed that sentencing decisions were biased toward sentencing anchors shouted in the courtroom ("Two years in jail!").

Although it is common to point out the causal role of one specific heuristic in the genesis of particular biases, many naturally occurring biases can reflect the operation of two or more heuristics. Consider, for instance, the conjunction fallacy. The probability of a person being over 50 years of age *and* having a heart attack may appear higher than the probability of a person having a heart attack. Depending on the rhetoric used to interpret this bias, it may be attributed to the enhanced representativeness of A ∧ B, the availability of A ∧ B in memory, or to the *simulation heuristic,* that is, to the ease of mentally simulating A ∧ B.

Because mental simulation is greatly facilitated by knowledge of outcomes (e.g., of a football match), the famous hindsight bias (Fischhoff, 1975) can be covered under the simulation heuristic. From hindsight, the same known outcomes appear more likely than they were in a prediction task, before the outcomes were known.

From Heuristics and Biases to Dual-Process Theories

Analogous to the juxtaposition of biased heuristic judgments and normative models in JDM research, dual-process theories became a central topic in social cognition research. From earliest versions of the elaboration likelihood model (Petty & Cacioppo, 1986) or the heuristic–systematic model (Chaiken, Liberman, & Eagly, 1989) to recent versions such as the reflective–impulsive model (Strack & Deutsch, 2004), the common assumption of roughly 30 dual-process models is that humans can switch from a fast and error-prone heuristic processing mode to a slower, rule-based, and more effortful processing mode supposed to work in line with normative rules. Switching from impulsive to reflective processing, from thinking fast to thinking slow (Kahneman, 2011), from the peripheral to the central route (Petty & Cacioppo, 1986), or from System 1 to System 2 (Stanovich & West, 2000) is supposed to enable *Homo sapiens* to overcome the confines of heuristic reasoning.

There is a critical debate about the viability of dual-process theories, pointing out that counternormative biases persist in spite of deliberate reasoning attempts in System 2, that the border between System 1 and System 2 is hard to define (Keren & Schul, 2009), that most published findings to support dual-process assumptions can also be explained within a single system that is flexible enough to adapt its strategies to task conditions and processing goals (Kruglanski & Thompson, 1999), and that—if more than a single system must be assumed—it is hard to see why there should be exactly two.

However, while a huge literature revolves around qualitatively different cognitive processes and mechanisms on which judgments can be based, there is a conspicuous paucity of theorizing and experimental tests of specific mechanisms that underlie heuristics and biases (Fiedler & von Sydow, 2015). Almost 50 years after the Kahneman and Tversky's seminal papers, almost nothing is known about the similarity function used by the representativeness heuristic (Nilsson, Olsson, & Juslin, 2005) or about the assumed adjustment stage of the anchoring heuristic.

Some exceptional work on underlying mechanisms was conducted by social psychologists. Epley and Gilovich (2001) rediscovered the adjustment part of the anchoring hypothesis, demonstrating that insufficient adjustment is a plausible explanation of the anchoring bias in the case of self-generated anchors (e.g., estimating the freezing point of vodka evokes the generation of the freezing point of water as an anchor), but fails to explain the classic paradigm of external, random anchors, with which Mussweiler and Strack's (2001) selective accessibility account is consistent. It emphasizes the knowledge-priming function of anchors as underlying mechanism. For instance, a high-sentence anchor in a courtroom renders knowledge about severe crimes accessible, thus supporting

a severe sentencing decision. Other researchers (Wong & Kwong, 2000) point to numerical priming of high or low regions of a response scale as an underlying mechanism. Different mechanisms can coexist and are not mutually exclusive.

Regarding the availability heuristic, Schwarz and colleagues (1991) pitted the ease of retrieving relevant information against the number of items retrieved. When participants were to recall 12 self-assertive behaviors rather than only six, the number of recalled episodes of self-assertiveness increased, but ease of retrieval decreased. Consistent with Tversky and Kahneman's (1973) original account, they found that ease of retrieval dominated the number of items retrieved.[2] A recent meta-analysis by Weingarten and Hutchinson (2018) supports this often-replicated finding.

Summary

Heuristics are proxies, or rules of thumb, that allow people to assess frequencies and probabilities (availability or simulation heuristic), to draw categorization decisions (representativeness), or to estimate precise quantities (anchoring) in the absence of relevant data required to make evidence-based judgments in accordance with normative principles. Under many ordinary conditions, heuristics function pretty well. They are fast and frugal (Gigerenzer & Todd, 1999), offering adaptive judgments with minimal information and little effort expenditure. However, in specific situations that accentuate the deviation of heuristics from normative procedures, they lead to systematic distortions and illusions. Yet, as a basic principle, there is often no better alternative, or even any viable alternative to heuristic inferences, when information costs and lack of normative solutions are taken into account.

Affective and Motivational Approaches to Decision Making

A gamble that offers a 50% chance of winning $2,000 and a 50% chance of losing $500 should be considered very attractive with its expected value of $750. However, only 43% of Redelmeier and Tversky's (1992) participants were willing to play the gamble. Obviously, the reluctance to choose such an attractive lottery is due to the possibility of a loss. When participants could play the same gamble five times, making a loss in the total payoff very unlikely, the acceptance rate increased to 63%. That negative outcomes are judged more extremely than positive outcomes of the same absolute size has been noted for a long time, but different explanations have been offered (Higgins & Liberman, 2018; Scholer, Zou, Fujita, Stroessner, & Higgins, 2010; Zou, Scholer, & Higgins, 2014).

Asymmetry of Positive and Negative Experience

The asymmetry of positive and negative stimulation relates to a basic principle that Thorndike (1927) termed the *law of effect*. Organisms repeat sampling from pleasant categories but stop sampling stimuli from unpleasant categories, as illustrated in the hot stove effect (Denrell & March, 2001). We visit the same restaurants again when the food was tasty, but we avoid returning to a restaurant associated with sickness or bad service. As a consequence of such hedonic search, it is possible to correct for transient positive impressions, but the avoidance of negative sources precludes the correction of unwarranted negative impressions, leading to a persistent negativity bias (Denrell & Le Mens, 2012).

Experimental support for this hedonic principle comes from an ingenious experiment by Fazio, Eiser, and Shook (2004). In a computer game called BeanFest, participants engaged in feedback learning about the nutritional value of different beans (varying in shape and number of speckles). A clear-cut negativity effect consisted in avoiding beans that had been met with negative feedback (i.e., no nutritional value), and this avoidance generalized to other beans that resembled the hedonically negative beans in terms of shape and number of speckles. This idea inspired a highly influential computer-simulation approach by Denrell (2005) and Denrell and Le Mens (2012) that exerted a strong impact on recent decision research.

Prospect Theory

A different view of asymmetry between gains and losses is provided by the most prominent decision theory, prospect theory (Tversky & Kahneman, 1979), in which it is one of the most fundamental assumptions. A prospect describes the total utility $V = \Sigma \pi (p_i) \cdot v(x_i)$ of a decision option as a multiplicative function of the probabilities p_i and the values $v(x_i)$ of all its possible outcomes x_i. The subjective value function v is negatively accelerated (i.e., sublinear) both for gains and losses; that is, when an outcome x_i is doubled (e.g., a gain from +100 to +200, or a loss from –100 to –200) the subjective analogue $v(x_i)$ is less than doubled. Loss aversion means that the lower part (for losses) of the v function is steeper than the upper part (for gains). The decision weight function $\pi(p_i)$, which increases monotonically with increasing outcome probability p_i, is regressive, such that large probabilities are underweighted, whereas small probabilities are overweighted.

Overweighting of low-p probabilities has important practical implications. People buy expensive insurances because unlikely events are overrated (relative to their expected value), and they play lotteries as if they do not realize how extremely unlikely it is to win. The affective significance of dread risks is also consistent with prospect theory's assumption that low-p outcomes are overweighted. This well-established phenomenon was recently shown to be moderated by the so-called *description–experience gap* (Hertwig, Barron, Weber, & Erev, 2004), which has become a prominent research topic. Based on work by Weber, Shafir, and Blais (2004) on how animals experience probabilities (e.g., in partial reinforcement setups), they compared decisions under risk when prospects were described numerically (e.g., winning $100 or $0 at $p = 4\%$ and 96%, respectively) to decisions under uncertainty, when p was not described explicitly but had to be learned from experience (as in animal learning) from a series of random draws from an urn. The long delay with which a rare outcome was most likely experienced in the latter condition, if it was encountered at all, rendered low-p lotteries unattractive and thereby eliminated the overrating of low-p lotteries predicted by prospect theory.

Manipulating the broader experienced decision context can eliminate or even reverse the impact of loss aversion because the subjective value of an outcome was shown to depend on its relative position in a rank ordering (not sensitive to the absolute values) within the distribution of all possible outcomes (Walasek & Stewart, 2015). When we consider the debits and the credits of our bank account, we see that $100 is relatively high ranking among all debits (most of which are below $100) but relatively low ranking among all credits (because most credits are higher than $100). According to Walasek and Stewart (2004), loss aversion may simply reflect the higher relative rank of a debit than that of a credit of the same size. For an empirical test, they assessed the willingness to play a series of 64 lotteries, each of which offered a 50/50 chance of winning and losing a certain amount. The range of gains (up to +20 vs. +40) and losses (down to –20 vs. –40) was manipulated orthogonally, such that the relative rank of a gain of +30 (of a loss of –30) within a wide range was equivalent to a +15 gain (–15 loss) within a narrow range. As predicted on theoretical grounds, loss aversion was found when a wider range of gains than of losses gave a relatively higher rank to losses, but the opposite of loss aversion was obtained when the range was wider for losses than for gains.

Framing Effects

Both prospect theory's subjective functions, $v(x_i)$ and $\pi(p_i)$, produce characteristic framing effects that violate classic normative axioms stating that preferences should be independent of particular frames. This is illustrated nicely by the famous Asian disease problem (Tversky & Kahneman, 1981). Given two health programs to deal with a mysterious Asian disease, participants in a survival framing condition prefer a safe program that guarantees 200 surviving people for sure to a risky program (of the same expected value) that lets 600 people survive with a probability of one-third and nobody survive with a probability of two-thirds. Because the negatively accelerated $v(x_i)$ function implies that 600 survivors are worth less than three times 200 survivors, it would not be justified to accept a risky option that reduces the probability of an enhanced positive outcome to one-third. In contrast, when the same problem is framed in terms of losses, offering a choice between a certain option of 400 people dying for sure and a risky option of nobody dying with one-third and 600 people dying with a probability of two-thirds, the risky option appears more plausible. Now the negative accelerated $v(x_i)$ function implies that the additional loss is subjectively less severe than the objective increase from 400 to 600 people dying. Analogous findings were found in animal research by Lakshminarayanan, Chen, and Santos (2011) with capuchin monkeys, using apple pieces added or taken away to manipulate gains and losses. Technically, this subjective insensitivity to objectively increasing outcomes is generally called "risk-averse" in the gains domain and "risk-seeking" in the losses domain. This somewhat misleading terminology, however, should not prevent one from noting that when motivational states are manipulated, people with a promotion focus on positive goals (advancement, growth, accomplishment) tend to take more risk and to apply less conservative strategies than people with a prevention focus on negative goals (security, safety, and responsibility). This is evident from a vast body of research inspired by regulatory focus theory (Higgins, 2012).

Time Discounting

When two providers offer the same good for the same price but with a different delay, consumers will prefer the faster provider, who causes lesser delay. As a matter of principle, they are willing to pay more for faster delivery or, conversely, they expect a price discount for delayed delivery. Just like intolerance for delay of gratification in immature children, who forego a larger later reward to obtain a minor reward now (Metcalfe & Mischel, 1999), time discounting may reflect impatience and deficits of self-control, though it may be rationalized in terms of the utility of precious time resources.

Using query theory as a practical framework (see Table 3.3), Weber and colleagues (2007) pointed out an intriguing possibility to eliminate time discounting. They offered participants in a delay condition a choice between a $50 Amazon gift certificate right now and a gift in 3 months, the value of which varied between $50 and $100. In an acceleration condition, participants were offered a gift of $75 in 3 months that could be replaced by an immediate gift varying in value from $75 to $25. Query theory suggests that participants will ask two types of valuation questions—"Why should I consume now?" and "Why should I wait to get more?"—and, further, that queries concerning the status quo will be asked first. Thus, delay participants should start with queries about consuming now, whereas acceleration participants should first focus on queries about waiting. Due to a primacy advantage of the information prompted by the initial queries, impatient thoughts were more prominent, and time discounting was stronger in the delay condition than in the acceleration condition. When the query order was set experimentally, it was possible to eliminate the typical discounting effect by reversing the natural query order.

Asymmetries of Self-Referent and Other-Referent Judgments and Decisions

Unrealistic optimism (Regan, Snyder, & Kassin, 1995; Weinstein, 1980) refers to the tendency to overestimate one's own capabilities and to underestimate one's own weaknesses. If asked, people would concede that HIV has become a real danger, but they would also contend that their own probability of contracting HIV is negligible. They would claim to be less likely to be involved in a car accident and less affected by many risks than other persons. People are more prone to unrealistic optimism under promotion than under prevention focus (Grant & Higgins, 2003).

"I'm Better Than Average"

The belief "I am better than average" is so common that it is conceived to be neither a pathological self-deception nor a latent source of dissatisfaction. If anything, research on self-enhancement suggests that people who overestimate their capabilities (relative to objective measures) tend to be happy and satisfied with their life (Alicke & Sedikides, 2011; Taylor & Brown, 1988). This optimistic bias is also evident in change expectations (Dweck, 2012): People believe that their strengths, but not their weaknesses, determine their own future, while they expect other people's futures to depend on both their current strengths and their weaknesses (Steimer & Mata, 2016).

Many explanations have been offered for these self–other differences in risk assessment, drawing not only on self-serving motives (Leary, 2007) but also on rational ecological causes of apparently irrational optimism (Harris & Hahn, 2011). To give but one example, if the distribution of persons involved in a growing number of traffic accidents is left-skewed—most people have zero or only one accident, while the upper tail of the distribution shows very few people having more accidents—then the mean lies above the median, and the accident record of the majority of people is indeed better than average.

A refined theory that has greatly elucidated the debate about self–other asymmetries was presented by Moore and Healy (2008). Their first assumption is that all uncertain estimations are regressive; high percentages tend to be underestimated, whereas low percentages tend to be overestimated. However, because the strength of this regressive shrinkage is a direct function of unreliability, and unreliability increases with decreasing sample size, it follows that self-judgments are less regressive than other-judgments, simply because self-judgments rely on larger experience samples than judgments of others. Due to regression, people overestimate the low performance on difficult tasks but generally underestimate the high performance on easy tasks—the typical hard–easy effect (Juslin, Winman, & Olsson, 2000). Yet because regression effects increase with decreasing sample size, this pattern is more pronounced when judging others than when judging oneself. Thus, people underestimate others more than they do themselves on easy tasks, producing the impression that "I'm better than average." However, on difficult tasks, they come to believe that "I'm worse than average" (see also Galesic, Olsson, & Rieskamp, 2012).

Note in passing that self–other differences can be conceived as a specific case of the more general principle of social distance as influence on construal level. Analogous to temporal, spatial, and evidential distance (certain events vs. highly uncertain, far-fetched events), social distance is larger when judging others and outgroups than when judging the self or one's ingroup. Thus, regardless of the extent to which self–other differences reflect other causal influences, they may be inherently related to psychological distance in a broader sense.

Psychological Distance

Intensive social psychological research on construal-level theory has led to important insights about the influence of (temporal, spatial, social, and hypotheticality) distance on decision making. The basic principle seems to be well understood by now: From a distant perspective—for instance, when deciding for others or forming preferences for the far-away future—decision makers focus more on the desirability of the outcomes, and they give less weight to feasibility constraints compared to low-distance decisions (Liberman & Trope, 1998; Trope & Liberman, 2010), causing preferences to change when manipulations affect psychological distance. One straightforward implication of this basic principle says that the value of decision outcomes (i.e., their desirability) should be weighted more strongly from larger distance, whereas probabilities (i.e., feasibility constraints) should be given relatively more weight from shorter distance.

In a systematic test, Sagristano, Trope, and Liberman (2002) assessed how willing participants were to play, and how much money they would bid on across 20 different gambles (constructed from all combinations of five winning probabilities—.1, .3, .5, .7, .9—and four expected values—$4, $6, $8, $10), which they expected to play either immediately or in 2 months. The manipulation of temporal distance had the expected impact, with gambling preferences in 2 months depending more strongly on monetary payoffs (desirability) and to a lesser degree on winning probabilities (feasibility) than gambling preferences immediately after the session.

As a rule, decisions from a distal perspective are construed in more abstract and simplifying ways than from a proximal perspective. Thus, a decision about a holiday excursion next summer is based on an abstract account of the desirability of idealized clichés of different holiday locations. It is much less sensitive to feasibility issues such as time constraints, availability, and convenience of public transportation or weather conditions than the more concrete construal of decisions from a proximal perspective. Judgments based on high- versus low-level construal (of distal vs. proximal scenarios) differ systematically with regard to a variety of distinct phenomena. Compared to low-level construal, high-level construal reduces the dimensionality of mental representations, amplifies the correspondence bias in attribution, produces stronger halo effects, but enhances self-control and tolerance for delay of gratification (see Trope & Liberman, 2010).

Cognitive Ecological Approaches to Information Sampling

Implicit to traditional research on cognitive biases and shortcomings is the assumption that irrationality results from normatively inappropriate cognitive processes and bounded rationality conceived as a restriction of the human mind (Simon, 1982). Loss aversion and framing effects are conceived as deviations of subjective values and probabilities from their objective analogues; endowment effects appear to reflect irrational sentimental ownership relations; anchoring effects and frequency illusions are attributed to the priority of heuristic over systematic processes; and numerous biases (e.g., hot stove effect, unrealistic optimism) seem to reflect motivated cognition.

This focus on the human mind as origin of irrational judgments and decisions is so deeply entrenched in the social cognition literature that obvious alternative accounts were hardly ever noticed. Only recently, a novel perspective advocated in so-called *sampling theories* (Fiedler & Juslin, 2006; Fiedler & Kutzner, 2015; Le Mens & Denrell, 2011) suggests that alleged cognitive biases may already be inherent in the environmental samples that provide the input to cognitive and affective processes. To illustrate, consider again the case of the availability heuristic. A metacognitive inference from ease of retrieval to apparent frequency or probability is commonly assumed to underlie this judgment bias. However, from a sampling theory point of view, if individuals behave like "naive intuitive statisticians" (Juslin, Winman, & Hansson, 2007) who process given information uncritically but accurately, availability bias may originate in the environment. The rate of murder (vs. suicide) and of stereotypical (vs. counterstereotypical) behaviors may be overestimated because these available events are overrepresented in the media that provide the stimulus input for subjective judgments (Combs & Slovic, 1979). Seemingly biased estimates may perfectly represent the media input, which already exhibits the bias before any cognitive processes come into play; the retrieval process may be completely unbiased.

In a similar vein, judgments closely resemble the sample of available observations about the value of stocks (Unkelbach, Fiedler, & Freytag, 2007), the achievement of students (Fiedler, Freytag, & Unkelbach, 2007), or neutral stimulus attributes (Kareev, Arnon, & Horwitz-Zeliger, 2002). To use a term coined by Dawes and colleagues (1989), they behave like *actuarial decision makers,* sticking closely to the given sample statistics. They do it in a naive and uncritical way, though, taking sample contents for granted and hardly ever caring about the validity of the sampled information. Thus, even when samples stem from biased sources or selective information search, they follow the sample as if it were random and representative. This propensity to trust uncritically and follow the information given all the way to the utter inability to ignore it has been labeled *metacognitive myopia* (Fiedler, 2000, 2012; Salancik & Conway, 1975).

This calls into question the appropriateness of using standard normative measures to judge humanity's capacity for rational decision making. If humans' sensitivity to their environment drives some of the violations of normative standards, but this sensitivity or adaptivity to the environment also leads to our efficient functioning in a complex and uncertain world, a conception of rationality that does us more justice may be called for. One such conception is so-called *ecological rationality* (Todd, Gigerenzer, & ABC Research Group, 2011), which states that rationality should be judged by how well it is adapted to the environmental structure.

Unequal Sample Size

A sufficient condition for the occurrence of many prominent biases is the unequal size of samples about different persons or groups. We are fed with larger samples of observations that provide us with more opportunities to learn

about the self than about others, about ingroups than outgroups, about nearby familiar objects than about distant unfamiliar objects. As most observed behavior is positive due to normative influence, the environment provides us with more opportunities to learn about our own than about other people's positivity, and more opportunities to observe positive ingroup than outgroup behavior. No motivated bias is necessary to explain self-serving and ingroup-serving biases; the unequal size of environmental samples affords a sufficient account. The same minimal account is sufficient to explain the devaluation of minorities and illusory correlations (Kutzner & Fiedler, 2015). When 24 positive and 12 negative behaviors are observed in a majority compared to 12 positive and 6 negative behaviors in a minority, the larger sample allows for more complete learning of the high positivity rate in the majority than in the minority. Again, other influences may contribute to the relative devaluation of minorities, but sample size alone provides a sufficient condition.

Confirmation Bias

Confirmation biases in JDM (Nickerson, 1998), the tendency to verify rather than to falsify a social hypothesis, can simply be the result of unequal sample size. Positive testing alone (Klayman & Ha, 1987)—the strategy to gather more observations about the focal hypothesis than about alternative hypotheses—is sufficient to produce samples of unequal size. For instance, when interviewers are testing the hypothesis that the interviewee is an extravert rather than an introvert, more questions will refer to extraversion than to introversion, and vice versa. Because interviewees (like survey respondents) generally provide more confirming than disconfirming responses—reflecting a so-called "acquiescence bias" (Zuckerman, Knee, Hodgins, & Miyake, 1995)—a larger sample of mostly confirming evidence will support the focal rather than the alternative hypothesis. Thus, as already anticipated by Higgins and Bargh (1987), confirmation bias can be due to unequal sample size alone (Fiedler, Walther, & Nickel, 1999), regardless of whether other (motivational) influences may also be at work. Powell, Yu, DeWolf, and Holyoak (2017) showed that the attractiveness of four example products on Amazon depended not only on the mean rating but also the number of reviews on which those were based, with the number of reviews often weighted more heavily. Finally, it should be noted that positive testing is a rational strategy if hypotheses focus on rare events that are high in information value (Hendrickson, Navarro, & Perfors, 2016; Oaksford & Chater, 1994).

Output–Bound Sampling

Sample size is but one way in which selective or biased sampling can have a profound effect on judgments and decisions. A source of seriously flawed judgments and decisions is output-bound sampling in conditional reasoning tasks (Dawes, 2006; Fiedler, 2008). Diagnostic inferences or risk assessment tasks often call for the estimation of conditional probabilities, such as the probability of suicide given a patient who suffers from depression, p(suicide/depression), or the risk of a car accident given alcohol consumption p(accident/alcohol). Because conditional probabilities of effective outputs (accidents) given specific causal input conditions (alcohol) are often not available, judges often rely on the reverse output-bound conditionals, such as p(alcohol/accident), which may be available. This can lead to dramatic mistakes when base rates p(alcohol) and p(accident) are unequal. Because the base rate of accidents (suicide) is much lower than the base rate of alcohol consumption (depression), causal (input-bound) conditionals are much smaller than output-bound conditionals. According to Bayes' theorem, the ratio of the conditionals equals the ratio of base rates:

$$p(\text{accident}|\text{alcohol})/p(\text{alcohol}|\text{accident}) = p(\text{accident})/p(\text{alcohol})$$

In other words, when p(alcohol) is 10 times more likely than p(accident), then the output-bound conditional p(alcohol|accident) will overestimate the conditional p(accident|alcohol) to be inferred by the factor 10 (i.e., by 1,000%). For similar reasons, the hit rate p(positive test|HIV) that HIV-infected people are tested positively is about 15 times higher than the posterior probability p(HIV|positive test) that positively tested people have the virus (see Swets et al., 2000),

simply because the base rates differ dramatically: p(tested positively) > p(HIV).

Whereas the impact of sample size is only due to decreasing error in samples of increasing size, output-bound sampling creates systematic bias. In risk estimation, for instance, the criterion is typically a very rare event with a very low base-rate, say, p(HIV) < 1%. Imagine the task is to estimate the likelihood p(HIV/positive test) of HIV conditional on a positive test result. Output-bound sampling typically amounts to comparing the test result of a certain number of people who have HIV with roughly the same number of people without HIV. Such a sample dramatically overrepresents the low-probability criterion event. Despite the very low HIV base rate of < 1%, comparing roughly equal samples of HIV and non-HIV cases in an output-bound sample means to oversample the base rate of the criterion event by a factor of 50 or more!

Dawes (2006) provides a memorable example of the characteristic bias of output-bound sampling in legal context: Estimates of the likelihood of continued child abuse must be inflated when (output-bound) sampling concentrates on child abusers. Such a sample is, of course, more likely to include cases of continued abuse than a random sample from the entire population. In a similar vein, the #MeToo campaign might strongly overestimate the rate of sexual crime, as it deliberately solicits evidence for the criterion event to be estimated.[3] As a rule, an unbiased sample must conserve the base rate of the criterion event; an information search process that is contingent on the criterion (e.g., on HIV vs. non-HIV) can create a severe bias, unless the selected proportions exactly match the (typically unknown) base rates (see Fiedler, 2008, for a more elaborate discussion and simulation of this intricate problem).

Natural Sample Space and Environmental Structures

In actuality, though, information sampling does not adhere to these logical (Bayesian) rules but typically follows the intuition of what Gavanski and Hui (1992) called a "natural sample space." Accordingly, people spontaneously organize sample spaces (i.e., the set of all available stimuli) by naturally appearing and easy-to-encode categories. It is easy to judge specific attributes contingent on these categories. For instance, when people vary in two dimensions, gender and nose length, it is easier to organize stimuli and to conditionalize judgments by gender than by nose length. It is thus easier to estimate and compare nose length separately for different gender groups than it is to estimate the gender rates per nose length category. By the same token, physicians find it easier and they are better prepared to estimate p(positive test|HIV) than to estimate p(HIV|positive test), simply because grouping of patients by diagnosis (HIV vs. non-HIV) affords a more natural sampling space than grouping by test results. For illustration, in Figure 3.2, shape (circles vs. triangles) affords a more natural grouping than fill color (white vs. grey), making it easier to judge color as a function of shape than vice versa. As a basic principle, whether a task calls for judging $p(X|Y)$ or $p(Y|X)$, the mental representation will depend on whether X or Y affords a better Gestalt to organize the sample space.

In any case, the accuracy of judgments and the quality of decisions can dramatically depend on the validity, the selectivity, and the Gestalt-like organizational features of the environment:

1. Wicked environments may systematically conceal some information (e.g., negative product attributes in advertising; quality of rejected job applicants; Einhorn & Hogarth, 1978) but readily reveal other information (e.g., assets of consumer products; published studies).
2. Experience samples may be systematically biased toward pleasant sources and thereby ignore hedonically unpleasant sources (e.g., hot stoves or bad restaurants).
3. Normative constraints may further reinforce the bias toward more positive than negative information.
4. The conditional direction of sampled information depends on the alignment of decision goals (e.g., to assess a person's competence or to identify a competent person) and Gestalt-like properties of natural sample space (organized by person vs. by attribute).

And last but not least,

5. The size of information samples can greatly vary as a function of familiarity and social distance.

Overconfidence

Sampling biases can also be a problem in research and scientific reasoning. A telling example is overconfidence, one of the most prominent topics in the last half-century of decision research (Gigerenzer, Hoffrage, & Kleinbölting, 1991; Juslin, 1994). Calibration curves show that the percentage of correct responses on binary choice questions is typically lower than the judges' confidence, also expressed on a percentage scale. For instance, the actual correctness rate of items with a high confidence rate of 90% may be 70%, and given medium confidence of 80% responses, it may be 65%. Overconfidence is not confined to optimistic self-appraisals of laypeople; it also reduces the calibration of experts (McKenzie, Liersch,

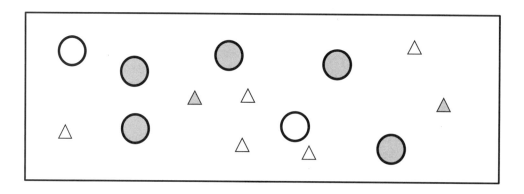

FIGURE 3.2. Illustration of natural sample space (see Gavanski & Hui, 1992).

& Yaniv, 2008), whose expertise may increase their confidence more than their accuracy.

Overconfidence is not only seen as a provocative challenge for applied decision research in medicine, economics, and politics, but is also considered strong evidence for motivational biases. Sampling approaches have shown that both assumptions may be unwarranted. On the one hand, meta-analyses have repeatedly shown that strong overconfidence effects are confined to studies in which researchers used intuitively sampled judgment tasks (Gigerenzer et al., 1991; Juslin, 1994). They disappeared or were greatly reduced in studies using representative samples of all tasks in a knowledge domain. Apparently, overconfidence is to some extent due to researchers' intuitive selection of tricky tasks, producing enhanced overconfidence effects.

On the other hand, the evidence for overconfidence also shrinks markedly when a regression artefact is controlled for (Erev, Wallsten, & Budescu, 1994). Because calibration curves almost always plot accuracy rates as function of confidence, high confidence ratings must regress to lower accuracy, just as very low confidence must regress to somewhat higher accuracy scores. By merely reversing the calibration curve and plotting confidence as a function of accuracy, evidence for underconfidence is apparent in the same data array as overconfidence (Erev et al., 1994): Items high on accuracy regress to lower confidence ratings, just as items low in accuracy regress to relatively higher confidence. Both ways to "cure" the overconfidence bias have nothing to do with wishful thinking or motivated reasoning; rather, they can be reduced to researcher biases in sampling knowledge tasks.

Conclusions

In a handbook of basic principles, the most appropriate format for presenting the conclusions consists of a clearly articulated list of basic principles, which we have presented in the preceding sections:

1. Clearly defined concepts (rationality, bias, positive testing, recognition heuristic) create common ground and foster scientific scrutiny in JDM research.

2. Methods tools (e.g., signal detection analysis) allow JDM researchers to make scientific inferences that go beyond common sense.

3. Strong JDM science is anchored in clearly spelled-out theories.

4. Applied and translational research on legal, health-related, and economic decisions testifies to the mutual inspiration and responsibility of JDM and social psychology.

5. Although judgment heuristics may deviate from normative rules and lead to systematic distortions and illusions under specific conditions, there is often no better alternative, or even any viable alternative to heuristic inferences, especially when information costs and weaknesses of normative solutions are taken into account.

6. Judgments and decisions are sensitive to distinct affective influences, positive–negative asymmetries (loss aversion), uncertainty aversion, time discounting, and distinct emotions.

7. Judgments and decisions depend in characteristic ways on psychological distance.

8. Sampling approaches highlight that biases can result from biased environmental samples, independent of any biased cognitive processes.

Outlook

After half a century of successful JDM research, with a huge impact on the growth of behavioral science in general, its future potential is no less promising. A glance at the most recent developments reveals that future approaches will certainly give more and more attention to the role of the environment in decision theory and practice (Thaler & Sunstein, 2008; Todd et al., 2011). Another stream of prominent future research that can be expected to unfold in the near future is "big data" and machine learning (Chen & Wojcik, 2016). These developments will not take place within the disciplinary confines of psychology but in the interdisciplinary interface of psychology, philosophy, computer science, mathematics, economics, and neuroscience (Frydman & Camerer, 2016). Last, but not least, it can be anticipated that the irresistible power of the digital revolution may lead to radical changes in the methods and theoretical perspectives used to study rational judgments, decisions, and actions.

ACKNOWLEDGMENT

The work underlying this chapter was supported by a grant provided by the Deutsche Forschungsgemeinschaft to Klaus Fiedler (No. FI 294/26-1).

NOTES

1. For a critical view on loss aversion, see Higgins and Liberman (2018) and Walasek and Stewart (2015).

2. Number of items became the dominant predictor, though, when attention was drawn to accessibility.

3. This overestimation (that would occur if one's only sources of occurrences and nonoccurrences were women's social media accounts) is very much intended by the campaign in order to counteract the preceding extreme underestimation due to crimes not being reported and the topic's being considered a taboo topic.

REFERENCES

Alicke, M. D., & Sedikides, C. (Eds.). (2011). *Handbook of self-enhancement and self-protection*. New York: Guilford Press.

Ariely, D., Loewenstein, G., & Prelec, D. (2003). "Coherent arbitrariness": Stable demand curves without stable preferences. *Quarterly Journal of Economics, 118*(1), 73–106.

Arkes, H. R., & Hammond, K. R. (1986). *Judgment and decision making: An interdisciplinary reader*. New York: Cambridge University Press.

Bar-Hillel, M., & Neter, E. (1993). How alike is it versus how likely is it: A disjunction fallacy in probability judgments. *Journal of Personality and Social Psychology, 65*(6), 1119–1131.

Bernoulli, J. (1713). *Ars conjectandi*. Impensis Thurnisiorum, fratrum.

Bloom, D. E., & Glied, S. (1991). Benefits and costs of HIV testing. *Science, 252,* 1798–1804.

Brenner, L., Rottenstreich, Y., Sood, S., & Bilgin, B. (2007). On the psychology of loss aversion: Possession, valence, and reversals of the endowment effect. *Journal of Consumer Research, 34*(3), 369–376.

Brunswik, E. (1956). *Perception and the representative design of psychological experiments* (2nd ed.). Berkeley: University of California Press.

Chaiken, S., Liberman, A., & Eagly, A. H. (1989). Heuristic and systematic information processing within and beyond the persuasion context. In J. S. Uleman & J. A. Bargh (Eds.), *Unintended thought* (pp. 212–252). New York: Guilford Press.

Chen, E. E., & Wojcik, S. P. (2016). A practical guide to big data research in psychology. *Psychological Methods, 21*(4), 458–474.

Combs, B., & Slovic, P. (1979). Newspaper coverage of causes of death. *Public Opinion Quarterly, 56,* 837–843.

Dawes, R. M. (2006). An analysis of structural availability biases, and a brief study. In K. Fiedler & P. Juslin (Eds.), *Information sampling and adaptive cognition* (pp. 147–152). New York: Cambridge University Press.

Dawes, R. M., Faust, D., & Meehl, P. E. (1989). Clinical versus actuarial judgment. *Science, 243,* 1668–1674.

Dechêne, A., Stahl, C., Hansen, J., & Wänke, M. (2010). The truth about the truth: A meta-analytic review of the truth effect. *Personality and Social Psychology Review, 14*(2), 238–257.

Denrell, J. (2005). Why most people disapprove of me: Experience sampling in impression formation. *Psychological Review, 112*(4), 951–978.

Denrell, J., & Le Mens, G. (2012). Social judgments from adaptive samples. In J. I. Krueger (Ed.), *Social judgment and decision making* (pp. 151–169). New York: Psychology Press.

Denrell, J., & March, J. (2001). Adaptation as information restriction: The hot stove effect. *Organization Science, 12*(5), 523–538.

Dweck, C. S. (2012). Implicit theories. In P. M. Van Lange, A. W. Kruglanski, & E. T. Higgins (Eds.), *Handbook of theories of social psychology* (pp. 43–61). Thousand Oaks, CA: SAGE.

Edwards, W. (1954). The theory of decision making. *Psychological Bulletin, 51*(4), 380–417.

Einhorn, H. J., & Hogarth, R. M. (1978). Confidence in judgment: Persistence of the illusion of validity. *Psychological Review, 85*(5), 395–416.

Englich, B., & Mussweiler, T. (2001). Sentencing under uncertainty: Anchoring effects in the courtroom. *Journal of Applied Social Psychology, 31*(7), 1535–1551.

Epley, N., & Gilovich, T. (2001). Putting adjustment back in the anchoring and adjustment heuristic: Differential processing of self-generated and experimenter-provided anchors. *Psycholological Science, 12,* 391–396.

Erev, I., Wallsten, T. S., & Budescu, D. V. (1994). Simultaneous over- and underconfidence: The role of error in judgment processes. *Psychological Review, 101*(3), 519–527.

Fazio, R. H., Eiser, J. R., & Shook, N. J. (2004). Attitude formation through exploration: Valence asymmetries. *Journal of Personality and Social Psychology, 87*(3), 293–311.

Fiedler, K. (2000). Beware of samples: A cognitive-ecological sampling approach to judgment bias. *Psychological Review, 107,* 659–676.

Fiedler, K. (2008). The ultimate sampling dilemma in experience-based decision making. *Journal of Experimental Psychology: Learning, Memory, and Cognition, 34,* 186–203.

Fiedler, K. (2010). The asymmetry of causal and diagnostic inferences: A challenge for the study of implicit attitudes. In J. P. Forgas, J. Cooper, & W. D. Crano (Eds.), *The psychology of attitudes and attitude change* (pp. 75–92). New York: Psychology Press.

Fiedler, K. (2012). Meta-cognitive myopia and the dilemmas of inductive-statistical inference. In B. H. Ross (Ed.), *The psychology of learning and motivation* (Vol. 57, pp. 1–55). San Diego, CA: Elsevier Academic Press.

Fiedler, K., Freytag, P., & Unkelbach, C. (2007). Pseudocontingencies in a simulated classroom. *Journal of Personality and Social Psychology, 92*(4), 665–677.

Fiedler, K., & Juslin, P. (2006). *Information sampling and adaptive cognition.* New York: Cambridge University Press.

Fiedler, K., & Kutzner, F. (2015). Information sampling and reasoning biases: Implications for research in judgment and decision making. In G. Keren & G. Wu (Eds.), *The Wiley–Blackwell handbook of judgment and decision making* (pp. 380–403). New York: Wiley.

Fiedler, K., & von Sydow, M. (2015). Heuristics and biases: Beyond Tversky and Kahneman's (1974) judgment under uncertainty. In M. Eysenck & D. W. Groome (Eds.), *Cognitive psychology: Revisiting the classical studies* (pp. 146–161). London: SAGE.

Fiedler, K., Walther, E., & Nickel, S. (1999). The autoverification of social hypothesis: Stereotyping and the power of sample size. *Journal of Personality and Social Psychology, 77,* 5–18.

Fischhoff, B. (1975). Hindsight is not equal to foresight: The effect of outcome knowledge on judgment under uncertainty. *Journal of Experimental Psychology: Human Perception and Performance, 1*(3), 288–299.

Frydman, C., & Camerer, C. F. (2016). The psychology and neuroscience of financial decision making. *Trends in Cognitive Sciences, 20*(9), 661–675.

Galesic, M., Olsson, H., & Rieskamp, J. (2012). Social sampling explains apparent biases in judgments of social environments. *Psychological Science, 23,* 1515–1523.

Galinsky, A. D., & Mussweiler, T. (2001). First offers as anchors: The role of perspective-taking and negotiator focus. *Journal of Personality and Social Psychology, 81*(4), 657–669.

Gavanski, I., & Hui, C. (1992). Natural sample spaces and uncertain belief. *Journal of Personality and Social Psychology, 63*(5), 766–780.

Gigerenzer, G. (2004). Dread risk, September 11, and fatal traffic accidents. *Psychological Science, 15*(4), 286–287.

Gigerenzer, G. (2007). *Gut feelings: The intelligence of the unconscious.* New York: Penguin.

Gigerenzer, G., Hoffrage, U., & Ebert, A. (1998). AIDS counselling for low-risk clients. *AIDS Care, 10*(2), 197–211.

Gigerenzer, G., Hoffrage, U., & Kleinbölting, H. (1991). Probabilistic mental models: A Brunswikian theory of confidence. *Psychological Review, 98*(4), 506–528.

Gigerenzer, G., & Todd, P. M. (1999). *Simple heuristics that make us smart.* New York: Oxford University Press.

Gilovich, T., Griffin, D., & Kahneman, D. (2002). *Heuristics and biases: The psychology of intuitive judgment.* New York: Cambridge University Press.

Gladwell, M. (2005). *Blink: The power of thinking without thinking.* New York: Little, Brown.

Goldberg, L. R. (1970). Man versus model of man: A rationale, plus some evidence, for a method of improving on clinical inferences. *Psychological Bulletin, 73*(6), 422–432.

Goldstein, D. G., & Gigerenzer, G. (2002). Models of ecological rationality: The recognition heuristic. *Psychological Review, 109*(1), 75–90.

Grant, H., & Higgins, E. T. (2003). Optimism, promotion pride, and prevention pride as predictors of quality of life. *Personality and Social Psychology Bulletin, 29,* 1521–1532.

Harris, A. J. L., & Hahn, U. (2011). Unrealistic optimism about future life events: A cautionary note. *Psychological Review, 118*(1), 135–154.

Hendrickson, A. T., Navarro, D. J., & Perfors, A. (2016). Sensitivity to hypothesis size during information search. *Decision, 3*(1), 62.

Hertwig, R., Barron, G., Weber, E. U., & Erev, I. (2004). Decisions from experience and the effect of rare events in risky choice. *Psychological Science, 15*(8), 534–539.

Hertwig, R., Herzog, S. M., Schooler, L. J., & Reimer, T. (2008). Fluency heuristic: A model of how the mind exploits a by-product of information retrieval. *Journal of Experimental Psychology: Learning, Memory, and Cognition, 34*(5), 1191–1206.

Higgins, E. T. (2012). Regulatory focus theory. In

P. M. Van Lange, A. W. Kruglanski, & E. T. Higgins (Eds.), *Handbook of theories of social psychology* (Vol. 1, pp. 483–504). Thousand Oaks, CA: SAGE.

Higgins, E. T., & Bargh, J. A. (1987). Social cognition and social perception. *Annual Review of Psychology, 38,* 369–425.

Higgins, E. T., & Liberman, N. (2018). The loss of loss aversion: Paying attention to reference points. *Journal of Consumer Psychology, 28,* 523–532.

Hogarth, R. M. (2001). *Educating intuition.* Chicago: University of Chicago Press.

Johnson, E. J., Häubl, G., & Keinan, A. (2007). Aspects of endowment: A query theory of value construction. *Journal of Experimental Psychology: Learning, Memory, and Cognition, 33,* 461–474.

Juslin, P. (1994). The overconfidence phenomenon as a consequence of informal experimenter-guided selection of almanac items. *Organizational Behavior and Human Decision Processes, 57*(2), 226–246.

Juslin, P., Winman, A., & Hansson, P. (2007). The naive intuitive statistician: A naive sampling model of intuitive confidence intervals. *Psychological Review, 114*(3), 678–703.

Juslin, P., Winman, A., & Olsson, H. (2000). Naive empiricism and dogmatism in confidence research: A critical examination of the hard–easy effect. *Psychological Review, 107*(2), 384–396.

Kahneman, D. (2011). *Thinking, fast and slow.* New York: Macmillan.

Kahneman, D., Knetsch, J. L., & Thaler, R. (1990). Experimental tests of the endowment effect and the Coase theorem. *Journal of Political Economy, 98,* 1325–1348.

Kahneman, D., Knetsch, J. L., & Thaler, R. H. (2005). Experimental tests of the endowment effect and the Coase theorem. In M. H. Bazerman (Ed.), *Negotiation, decision making and conflict management* (Vol. 1–3, pp. 92–115). Northampton, MA: Edward Elgar.

Kahneman, D., & Tversky, A. (1972). Subjective probability: A judgment of representativeness. *Cognitive Psychology, 3*(3), 430–454.

Kahneman, D., & Tversky, A. (1982). The simulation heuristic. In D. Kahneman, P. Slovic, & A. Tversky (Eds.), *Judgment under uncertainty: Heuristics and biases* (pp. 201–208). New York: Cambridge University Press.

Kareev, Y., Arnon, S., & Horwitz-Zeliger, R. (2002). On the misperception of variability. *Journal of Experimental Psychology: General, 131*(2), 287–297.

Kelley, H. H. (1967). Attribution theory in social psychology. In *Nebraska Symposium on Motivation* (Vol. 15, pp. 192–238). Lincoln: University of Nebraska Press.

Keren, G., & Schul, Y. (2009). Two is not always better than one: A critical evaluation of two-system theories. *Perspectives on Psychological Science, 4,* 533–550.

Klayman, J., & Ha, Y.-W. (1987). Confirmation, disconfirmation, and information in hypothesis testing. *Psychological Review, 94,* 211–228.

Kruglanski, A., & Thompson, E. (1999). Persuasion by a single route: A view from the unimodel. *Psychological Inquiry, 10,* 83–109.

Ku, G., Galinsky, A. D., & Murnighan, J. K. (2006). Starting low but ending high: A reversal of the anchoring effect in auctions. *Journal of Personality and Social Psychology, 90*(6), 975–986.

Kutzner, F. L., & Fiedler, K. (2015). No correlation, no evidence for attention shift in category learning: Different mechanisms behind illusory correlations and the inverse base-rate effect. *Journal of Experimental Psychology: General, 144*(1), 58–75.

Lakshminarayanan, V. R., Chen, M. K., & Santos, L. R. (2011). The evolution of decision-making under risk: Framing effects in monkey risk preferences. *Journal of Experimental Social Psychology, 47*(3), 689–693.

Le Mens, G., & Denrell, J. (2011). Rational learning and information sampling: On the "naivety" assumption in sampling explanations of judgment biases. *Psychological Review, 118*(2), 379–392.

Leary, M. R. (2007). Motivational and emotional aspects of the self. *Annual Review of Psychology, 58,* 317–344.

Leddo, J., Abelson, R. P., & Gross, P. H. (1984). Conjunctive explanations: When two reasons are better than one. *Journal of Personality and Social Psychology, 47*(5), 933–943.

Lerner, J. S., Small, D. A., & Loewenstein, G. (2004). Heart strings and purse strings: Carryover effects of specific emotions on economic transactions. *Psychological Science, 15*(5), 337–341.

Liberman, N., & Trope, Y. (1998). The role of feasibility and desirability considerations in near and distant future decisions: A test of temporal construal theory. *Journal of Personality and Social Psychology, 75,* 5–18.

Lindsay, R. C., & Wells, G. L. (1985). Improving eyewitness identifications from lineups: Simultaneous versus sequential lineup presentation. *Journal of Applied Psychology, 70*(3), 556–564.

McKenzie, C. R. M., Liersch, M. J., & Yaniv, I. (2008). Overconfidence in interval estimates: What does expertise buy you? *Organizational Behavior and Human Decision Processes, 107*(2), 179–191.

Meehl, P. E. (1957). When shall we use our heads instead of the formula? *Journal of Counseling Psychology, 4*(4), 268–273.

Metcalfe, J., & Mischel, W. (1999). A hot/cool-system analysis of delay of gratification: Dynamics of willpower. *Psychological Review, 106*(1), 3–19.

Moore, D. A., & Healy, P. J. (2008). The trouble with overconfidence. *Psychological Review, 115,* 502–517.

Morewedge, C. K., & Giblin, C. E. (2015). Explanations of the endowment effect: An integrative review. *Trends in Cognitive Sciences, 19*(6), 339–348.

Morewedge, C. K., Shu, L. L., Gilbert, D. T., & Wilson, T. D. (2009). Bad riddance or good rubbish?: Ownership and not loss aversion causes the endowment effect. *Journal of Experimental Social Psychology, 45*(4), 947–951.

Mussweiler, T., & Strack, F. (2001). The semantics of anchoring. *Organizational Behavior and Human Decision Processes, 86*(2), 234–255.

Nickerson, R. S. (1998). Confirmation bias: A ubiquitous phenomenon in many guises. *Review of General Psychology, 2*(2), 175–220.

Nilsson, H., Olsson, H., & Juslin, P. (2005). The cognitive substrate of subjective probability. *Journal of Experimental Psychology: Learning, Memory, and Cognition, 31*(4), 600–620.

Nisbett, R. E., & Ross, L. (1980). *Human inference: Strategies and shortcomings of social judgment.* Englewood Cliffs, NJ: Prentice-Hall.

Oaksford, M., & Chater, N. (1994). A rational analysis of the selection task as optimal data selection. *Psychological Review, 101*(4), 608–631.

Olivola, C. Y., & Todorov, A. (2010). Fooled by first impressions?: Reexamining the diagnostic value of appearance-based inferences. *Journal of Experimental Social Psychology, 46,* 315–324.

Orr, D. A. N., & Guthrie, C. (2006). Negotiation: New insights from meta-analysis (Vanderbilt Law and Economics Research Paper No. 06-12). *Ohio State Journal of Dispute Resolution, 21,* 597.

Peterson, C. R., & Beach, L. R. (1967). Man as an intuitive statistician. *Psychological Bulletin, 68*(1), 29–46.

Petty, R. E., & Cacioppo, J. T. (1986). *Communication and persuasion: Central and peripheral routes to attitude change.* New York: Springer-Verlag.

Powell, D., Yu, J., DeWolf, M., & Holyoak, K. J. (2017). The love of large numbers: A popularity bias in consumer choice. *Psychological Science, 28*(10), 1432–1442.

Redelmeier, D. A., & Tversky, A. (1992). On the framing of multiple prospects. *Psychological Science, 3*(3), 191–193.

Regan, P. C., Snyder, M., & Kassin, S. M. (1995). Unrealistic optimism: Self-enhancement or person positivity? *Personality and Social Psychology Bulletin, 21*(10), 1073–1082.

Sagristano, M. D., Trope, Y., & Liberman, N. (2002). Time-dependent gambling: Odds now, money later. *Journal of Experimental Psychology: General, 131*(3), 364–376.

Salancik, G. R., & Conway, M. (1975). Attitude inference from salient and relevant cognitive content about behavior. *Journal of Personality and Social Psychology, 32,* 829–840.

Sarbin, T. R., Taft, R., & Bailey, D. E. (1960). *Clinical inference and cognitive theory.* Oxford, UK: Holt, Rinehart & Winston.

Scholer, A. A., Zou, X., Fujita, K., Stroessner, S. J., Higgins, E. T. (2010). When risk-seeking becomes a motivational necessity. *Journal of Personality and Social Psychology, 99,* 215–231.

Schwarz, N., Bless, H., Strack, F., Klumpp, G., Rittenauer-Schatka, H., & Simons, A. (1991). Ease of retrieval as information: Another look at the availability heuristic. *Journal of Personality and Social Psychology, 61*(2), 195–202.

Simon, H. A. (1982). *Models of bounded rationality.* Cambridge, MA: MIT Press.

Simon, H. A. (1987). Rationality in psychology and economics. In R. M. Hogarth & M. W. Reder (Eds.), *Rational choice: The contrast between economics and psychology* (pp. 25–40). Chicago: University of Chicago Press.

Slovic, P., & Lichtenstein, S. (1971). Comparison of Bayesian and regression approaches to the study of information processing in judgment. *Organizational Behavior and Human Performance, 6*(6), 649–744.

Slovic, P., & Peters, E. (2006). Risk perception and affect. *Current Directions in Psychological Science, 15*(6), 322–325.

Stanovich, K. E., & West, R. F. (2000). Individual differences in reasoning: Implications for the rationality debate? *Behavioral and Brain Sciences, 23*(5), 645–665.

Steimer, A., & Mata, A. (2016). Motivated implicit theories of personality: My weaknesses will go away, but my strengths are here to stay. *Personality and Social Psychology Bulletin, 42,* 415–429.

Strack, F., & Deutsch, R. (2004). Reflective and impulsive determinants of social behavior. *Personality and Social Psychology Review, 8*(3), 220–247.

Surowiecki, J. (2004). *The wisdom of crowds: Why the many are smarter than the few and how collective wisdom shapes business, economies, societies, and nations.* New York: Doubleday.

Swets, J., Dawes, R. M., & Monahan, J. (2000). Psychological science can improve diagnostic decisions. *Psychological Science in the Public Interest, 1*(1), 1–26.

Taylor, S. E., & Brown, J. D. (1988). Illusion and well-being: A social psychological perspective on mental health. *Psychological Bulletin, 103*(2), 193–210.

Thaler, R. H., & Sunstein, C. R. (2008). *Nudge: Improving decisions about health, wealth, and happiness*. New Haven, CT: Yale University Press.

Thorndike, E. L. (1927). The law of effect. *American Journal of Psychology, 39*, 212–222.

Todd, P. M., Gigerenzer, G., & ABC Research Group. (2011). *Ecological rationality: Intelligence in the world*. New York: Oxford University Press.

Trope, Y., & Liberman, N. (2010). Construal-level theory of psychological distance. *Psychological Review, 117*(2), 440–463.

Tversky, A., & Kahneman, D. (1971). Belief in the law of small numbers. *Psychological Bulletin, 76*(2), 105–110.

Tversky, A., & Kahneman, D. (1973). Availability: A heuristic for judging frequency and probability. *Cognitive Psychology, 5*(2), 207–232.

Tversky, A., & Kahneman, D. (1974). Judgment under uncertainty: Heuristics and biases. *Science, 185*, 1124–1130.

Tversky, A., & Kahneman, D. (1979). Prospect theory: An analysis of decision under risk. *Econometrica, 47*(2), 263–291.

Tversky, A., & Kahneman, D. (1983). Extensional versus intuitive reasoning: The conjunction fallacy in probability judgment. *Psychological Review, 90*, 293–315.

Unkelbach, C., Fiedler, K., & Freytag, P. (2007). Information repetition in evaluative judgments: Easy to monitor, hard to control. *Organizational Behavior and Human Decision Processes, 103*(1), 37–52.

Van Boven, L., Dunning, D., & Loewenstein, G. (2000). Egocentric empathy gaps between owners and buyers: Misperceptions of the endowment effect. *Journal of Personality and Social Psychology, 79*(1), 66–76.

Van Dijk, E., & Van Knippenberg, D. (1998). Trading wine: On the endowment effect, loss aversion, and the comparability of consumer goods. *Journal of Economic Psychology, 19*(4), 485–495.

von Neumann, J., & Morgenstern, O. (1944). *Theory of games and economic behavior*. Princeton, NJ: Princeton University Press.

Walasek, L., & Stewart, N. (2015). How to make loss aversion disappear and reverse: Tests of the decision by sampling origin of loss aversion. *Journal of Experimental Psychology: General, 144*, 7–11.

Weber, E. U., & Johnson, E. J. (2009). Mindful judgment and decision making. *Annual Review of Psychology, 60*, 53–85.

Weber, E. U., Johnson, E. J., Milch, K. F., Chang, H., Brodscholl, J. C., & Goldstein, D. G. (2007). Asymmetric discounting in intertemporal choice—a query-theory account. *Psychological Science, 18*, 516–523.

Weber, E. U., Shafir, S., & Blais, A. R. (2004). Predicting risk sensitivity in humans and lower animals: Risk as variance or coefficient of variation. *Psychological Review, 111*(2), 430–445.

Weingarten, E., & Hutchinson, J. W. (2018). Does ease mediate the ease-of-retrieval effect?: A meta-analysis. *Psychological Bulletin, 144*(3), 227–283.

Weinstein, N. D. (1980). Unrealistic optimism about future life events. *Journal of Personality and Social Psychology, 39*(5), 806–820.

Wells, G. L., Small, M., Penrod, S., Malpass, R. S., Fulero, S. M., & Brimacombe, C. A. E. (1998). Eyewitness identification procedures: Recommendations for lineups and photospreads. *Law and Human Behavior, 22*(6), 603–647.

Wong, K. F. E., & Kwong, J. Y. Y. (2000). Is 7300 m equal to 7.3 km?: Same semantics but different anchoring effects. *Organizational Behavior and Human Decision Making, 82*, 314–333.

Zou, X., Scholer, A. A., & Higgins, E. T. (2014). In pursuit of progress: Promotion motivation and risk preference in the domain of gains. *Journal of Personality and Social Psychology, 106*, 183–201.

Zuckerman, M., Knee, C. R., Hodgins, H. S., & Miyake, K. (1995). Hypothesis confirmation: The joint effect of positive test strategy and acquiescence response set. *Journal of Personality and Social Psychology, 68*(1), 52–60.

CHAPTER 4

Construal Processes

Alexa D. Hubbard
David A. Kalkstein
Nira Liberman
Yaacov Trope

Humans have evolved a unique ability to mentally travel outside the here and now. We can contemplate the past, the future, counterfactual situations, other places, and other people's perspectives. However, these mental travels pose a central challenge: As the distance to the target of contemplation increases, the potential for variability within and surrounding that target also increases. For example, if I am preparing for the day, I can step outside to feel the weather—the temperature, the humidity, whether it is raining, and so forth—and use that information to decide what to wear that day. However, if I am thinking about preparing for a trip next month, I cannot simply step outside and know what the weather will be. It would be impossible to know all the details of the future weather in a distant place, and there are a variety of possibilities of what it could be, so it would be difficult to plan at the level of specific outfits. However, people are still easily able to imagine and plan for future vacations by considering certain features, such as the cost of the vacation, which are unaffected by details that are uncertain and liable to vary (e.g., the precise weather forecast). Or consider taking another person's perspective: If I see that someone has

stubbed their[1] toe, I can infer that they feel pain, and I can imagine that pain. But there will be uncertainty around the exact degree, localization, and nature of the pain that they feel compared to my own pain if I stub my toe. However, despite this uncertainty and the potential for their experience to vary from my own, humans are still easily able to consider, understand, and learn from the experiences of others.

How is it that humans are able to contemplate, learn from, and tailor their behavior toward distant events and objects even though that distance entails increasing the variability of possible details surrounding them? In this chapter, we advance the following theoretical framework: Humans overcome the psychological challenge of thinking about events that occur beyond the here and now by constructing abstract mental representations that remain stable as specific details of the event vary. This proposal builds on construal-level theory (CLT), which posits a basic relationship between abstraction and the ability to consider objects or events that are psychologically distant (i.e., removed from the here and now). Research in this tradition has shown that as psychological distance to a target increases, people rely on higher-level, more

67

abstract construals, whereas when psychological distance decreases, people rely on lower-level, more concrete construals (for reviews, see Liberman & Trope, 2008, 2014; Trope & Liberman, 2003, 2010).

In this chapter we elaborate and expand on several key principles that are foundational for CLT. The *first principle* is that increasing psychological distance to a mental target increases the variability in potential details surrounding that target. The *second principle* is that abstraction has evolved to deal with the variability. It does so by construing mental objects in terms of their commonalities while subordinating their variations. The *third principle* is that encountering or considering variability induces the mental process of abstraction as a way to manage all possibilities. Together, these three principles form the basis for CLT. In the first part of the chapter, we elaborate these key principles and review illustrative research. In the second part of the chapter we expand on how these principles are tied to additional research in memory, self-control, and social cognition.

Theoretical Principles

Principle 1: Psychological Distance Increases Potential Variability

Psychological distance refers to the extent that any target of thought is removed from the egocentric here and now on dimensions of time, space, social distance, or hypotheticality. Cognition involves constantly traveling along these dimensions, such as imagining your weekend plans, thinking about where you parked your car, taking your colleague's perspective, or thinking about a counterfactual outcome of an election.

The challenge of distances is that they are "epistemic barriers," in which increasing distance is necessarily accompanied by an increase in uncertainty (Gilead, Trope, & Liberman, 2019). As a target becomes removed from direct experience, we lose access to its concrete perceptual details. As a result, psychological distance carries with it some degree of uncertainty about these specifics. Moreover, as psychological distance increases, we lose access to even more details, which means that the variety of possibilities for these concrete details increases. As a result, psychological distance increases anticipation for variability of possible outcomes. For example, while I cannot know exactly what the interior design of the home down the block looks like, the range of possibilities is likely much narrower than the range of possibilities for what the interior design looks like for a home in a foreign and unfamiliar country.

In terms of goals and self-regulation this creates a challenge—pursuing distant outcomes entails regulating one's behavior in a way that is effective even when one faces a variety of possible future states of the world. For example, if I am commuting to work right now, I can be relatively certain about the traffic and how to deal with it. If I am considering my commute in the future, there is a wider range of options for what the traffic will be like and how I should deal with it. This example illustrates that when considering any outcome (in this case, getting to work), the psychological distance from it increases the potential for variability in the factors that could plausibly impact reaching it.

The same challenge of uncertainty and potential variability occurs in the social domain when considering another person's experience. I can be relatively certain about what I ate for breakfast this morning. But if I am trying to guess what a friend had for breakfast, there will be a wider variety of possibilities to consider—and thus more uncertainty. Therefore, in the social domain, distance operates as a cue to the degree of potential discrepancy between one's own circumstance and that of a target (Kalkstein, Hubbard, & Trope, 2018b).

A concluding point is that seemingly distinct distances—temporal, spatial, social, and hypotheticality—are interrelated and together form a common currency of psychological distance (Maglio, Trope, & Liberman, 2013). At a basic level, the experience of psychological distance operates in a similar way and has a similar impact on mental operation when it occurs along any of these four dimensions. The current framework emphasizes that the interrelation among distances is due to a shared relationship with variability; that is, it is a positive association in which an increase in any psychological distance means an increase in potential variability.

Principle 2: Abstraction Evolved to Manage Potential Variability

When encountering an object (a person, an event, situation, etc., real or imagined), *abstraction* is a cognitive process of making a distinction between aspects that are central for a given purpose and aspects that are incidental for it and therefore peripheral (Shapira, Liberman, Trope, & Rim, 2012). Objects that share the same central aspects but differ in their peripheral aspects are deemed equivalent to each other (with respect to the given purpose). Peripheral aspects are thus allowed to vary without changing how the object relates to the purpose. In contrast, variability in terms of the central aspects would change how the object relates to the purpose (Gilead et al., 2019).

For a given construal, the important aspects are the ones that define how a person responds to the mental object. For example, if you are trying to save money, you will likely choose a grocery store based on its prices. Variations in terms of price (e.g., price variations between a store at time point 1 vs. time point 2, or between store A and store B) will change how you respond. In contrast, peripheral aspects are the ones that have relatively less impact on how a person processes or responds to the mental object. For example, the exact location of the grocery store may be peripheral; you may walk slightly farther in light of the goal to save money.

The process of abstraction creates invariance through mental construal. High-level construals (i.e., abstract construals) place a single object in a class with other objects (e.g., construing specific grocery store A as "an affordable store"), or group several mental objects based on their commonalities (e.g., construing grocery stores A, B, and C as "affordable stores"). As can be seen in this example, abstraction identifies commonalities across variable mental objects; identification of these commonalities is based on their relevance to one's goal. In other words, stores A, B, and C may be quite variable (e.g., in terms of location, hours, and customer service). But abstraction omits the low-level details that vary in ways that are irrelevant for one's goal and unites them based on their goal-relevant similarities. This makes higher-level construals stable and invariant despite any degree of variability within lower-lev-el (less relevant) aspects. For example, changing the hours of the most affordable grocery store in my neighborhood will not affect my construal of it as my preferred store in light of my higher-level budgeting goals. In summary, abstraction distinguishes between which variability matters *for a given purpose* (i.e., changes to or variability among high-level aspects), and which variability does not matter for that purpose (i.e., changes to or variability among low-level aspects).

When abstraction occurs, the mind moves from a lower-level construal of a mental target (an object, event, action, situation, etc.) to a higher-level construal of that target. An example is taking the mental representation of the activity "exercise" as an input and construing it in terms of the more general concept of "improving health." Higher-level construals are more context independent. Improving health can manifest in various ways: choosing a salad in a restaurant, scheduling a checkup, or choosing to exercise. This means that high-level construals travel well across psychological distance, where contextual details are more likely to vary. As distance increases, and the uncertainty about how contextual details may vary increases, higher-level construals become increasingly important. For example, if I am considering my vacation in a year, and I don't have a location in mind yet, I won't know what specific exercises will be possible or what specific kinds of food will be available. But I can still maintain the high-level goal of being healthy during my vacation. In contrast, shifting downward from a more abstract construal to a more concrete construal would involve taking the input of "exercise" and construing it in terms of the more specific means of "running on a treadmill." Lower-level construals include more contextual features into their representation (e.g., the treadmill is at a gym). Returning to the example of the vacation, if I am making a plan to exercise during my vacation in a month but I don't know where I am going, I may not be able to make specific plans about the details of my exercise, so it makes sense to construe the goal in terms of "exercise" instead of something more specific. However, as the vacation approaches, and I know more about what options I have for exercise, moving to a lower-level construal will be functional for helping me plan for the specific activities (e.g., pack a bathing suit for swimming).

Note that abstraction is always a subjective and relative process, and it shifts according to one's goals. No external object is inherently high-level or low-level but is instead only high or low relative to other mental objects for a given purpose (Gilead et al., 2019). Say, for example, that you are more concerned with health goals than with budgeting: Then the store's inventory of certain health foods may take precedence over its prices. In other words, variation in terms of health food options might matter a great deal, while variations in price might matter relatively less. However, the opposite would be true for people who are more concerned about budgeting than with health. As this example illustrates, abstractness is not a feature of objects in the external world, but rather something that the mind imposes on external objects.

One of the key consequences of the process of abstraction is that it guides how a person responds to a situation in a range of ways. In other words, though it is a cognitive process, it guides not just how people think but also how they feel and act. The level at which a person is construing a target determines how the person responds to that target. For example, a higher-level construal that represents an object in terms of one's most important values, such as health, will lead one to choose a vegetable over a cookie. However, a construal that represents the object at a lower level in terms of its taste will choose a cookie over the vegetable. Note that in this example, the construal in terms of taste is low-level relative to the overall goal of improving health.

The current framework emphasizes that as construals become more abstract, they are capable of dealing with more variable contexts, and of identifying more variable means to the same end. In the following sections, we review three lines of research that demonstrate the importance of abstraction for identifying variability that is relevant for a given purpose, while subordinating irrelevant variability: (1) visual working memory, (2) time perception, and (3) categorization.

Visual Working Memory

Indirect evidence for the function of abstraction as a means to classify variability comes from work on how abstraction impacts visual working memory (VWM; Hadar, Luria, & Liberman, 2020). This study revealed that a lower level of construal impaired the ability to filter distractors in VWM. In the current framework, distractors correspond to low-level (i.e., task-irrelevant) features that may vary without impacting the important aspects of the task. When people had a less abstract mindset, they were less able to separate the irrelevant distractors from the targets.

Additional research has shown that inducing abstract processing via a power manipulation improved VWM (Hadar et al., 2020; for the relationship between power and abstraction, see Smith & Trope, 2006). The study used a typical task that involves testing the ability to detect changes to target items. The experiment displayed visual sources with less information—that entailed a higher signal-to-noise ratio (one changing target within a field of four total targets), compared to more information—that entailed a lower signal-to-noise ratio (one changing target within a field of eight total targets). The study revealed that inducing a sense of power increased ability to use VWM to detect change despite a lower signal-to-noise ratio. In other words, abstraction was putatively related to a greater ability to detect the meaningful variability—that is, whether a target had changed or remained the same, even in the face of a wider range of overall variability.

Time Perception

Research on time perception provides important indirect evidence for the relationship between variability and abstraction. Past work has shown that increasing the number of changes that happen in a situation increases the speed at which time is experienced (e.g., Block, 1989, 1990). Hansen and Trope (2013) examined the effect of construal level on time perception. Their research was built on the idea that adopting an abstract mindset reduces the number of variations that are perceived in a situation. Across three studies, they found that people in an abstract mindset perceived time as passing more slowly than did people in a concrete mindset. In two additional studies, they found that changes to low-level details speeded time perception for those in a low-level mindset, whereas changes to global features speeded time perception for those in the high-level mindset. This research provides important evidence for the idea that abstraction places greater weight on variation in high-level features, whereas concrete thinking places greater weight on variations in low-level features.

Categorization

Another field of research that explores the relationship between variability and abstraction is categorization. In a seminal paper on the psychology of categories, Rosch, Mervis, Gray, Johnson, and Boyes-Braem (1976, p. 382) assert, "The world consists of a virtually infinite number of discriminably different stimuli. One of the most basic functions of all organisms is the cutting up of the environment into classifications by which nonidentical stimuli can be treated as equivalent." These authors go on to argue that the abstraction of general categories that cover variable exemplars is a fundamental mental operation that allows people to organize the external world into cognitively and behaviorally useful units of representations. Through treating variable instances as exemplars of a general category, people are spared the mental work of generating unique predictions and action plans for each subtly different object or event they may encounter (see Murphy, 2010). The task of encountering each object or situation anew, without recognizing it as a case of a broader class, would make adaptive functioning nearly impossible given the seemingly infinite ways in which any two targets may differ from one another.

In general, the construction of categories is a cognitively efficient adaptation that humans have developed to simplify the massive complexity and variety of the external world. Categories serve as general knowledge on which people may draw on to understand both previously encountered and novel events or objects (Murphy & Medin, 1985). For example, suppose a young child has recently acquired the abstract category of "dog" and has learned that dogs are friendly creatures who slobber. The knowledge of this category and its typical characteristics would allow the child to infer much about a wide variety of new creatures as long as they are labeled as dogs. As a result, that child would

have a much stronger sense of how to interact with any new dog than if they had not acquired the abstract concept of "dog."

More generally, at their core, categories define and label variability. Lower-level categories include less variability among their members, whereas higher-level categories include more variability among their members. For example, there is less variability between various objects in the category "carrot" than in the category "vegetable." And there is more variability in the category "food" than there is in the category "vegetable." In this way, categories are general mental representations that partition the immense variability encountered in the external world into manageable and useful cognitive units.

Principle 3: Variability Prompts Abstraction

The third principle is that integrating across encountered or anticipated variability prompts abstraction. This principle follows from the first two principles, but it makes unique predictions. The first two principles dealt with the purpose of abstraction for processing variability in the world. In this final section, we review the idea that because abstraction is adaptive for managing variability, seeing or anticipating variability may begin the mental processes associated with abstraction. This principle further posits that when anticipating variability, the level of abstraction recruited will reflect the degree of predictability of the anticipated variability. More predictable forms of variability include a narrower range of possible outcomes, whereas less predictable forms of variability include a wider range of possible outcomes, and this wider range in turn requires a higher level of abstraction to manage it.

Structural Alignment

Support for the idea that integrating across variable inputs leads to abstraction comes from structural alignment theory (SAT; Gentner, 1983; Markman & Gentner, 1993). According to SAT, the process of comparing two or more distinct stimuli initiates a process of extracting an abstract and schematic representation of the underlaying structure of each. Structural alignment then works to identify commonalities across distinct stimuli that remain stable despite superficial or lower-level differences. For example, a structural alignment of a satellite and the moon might highlight the structural commonality that each orbits the earth. Through this process of structural alignment, the act of comparing distinct stimuli leads to the development of relational categories and, more generally, abstract schematic representations (e.g., Boroditsky, 2007; Christie & Gentner, 2010; Gentner & Namy, 1999, 2006; Gick & Holyoak, 1983; Kurtz, Boukrina, & Gentner, 2013; Markman & Gentner, 1993). Additional work indicates that increasing the variability between two objects in a comparison further promotes abstraction (Vendetti, Wu, & Holyoak, 2014).

Category Induction

Another example of variability prompting abstraction comes from research on distributed practice and category induction. A vast array of research has examined the role of massed versus distributed learning on long-term memory. While massed learning corresponds to learning something in one temporal context (e.g., studying for 3 hours in a row on a Monday), distributed (spaced) learning refers to learning the same thing, but spread out into variable temporal contexts (e.g., studying 1 hour per day on Monday, Wednesday, and Friday). In distributed learning, successful studying necessitates abstraction over these temporally variable contexts. This in turn helps to direct attention to the primary dimension, which is the content of study.

Recent research has tested whether distributed learning increases abstraction. Specifically, two studies tested the effect of distributed learning on inductive reasoning (i.e., generalization from observed cases to entire abstract categories; Vlach, Sandhofer, & Kornell, 2008). The researchers tested how well individuals could learn that a range of exemplars included members of different categories. Learning occurred with either massed (back-to-back) repetitions or spaced repetitions. They found, as predicted, that spaced repetitions facilitated learning of abstract categories compared to massed repetitions (see also Vlach, Ankowski, & Sandhofer, 2012).

Summary of Theoretical Principles: Variability Explains the Relationship between Abstraction and Psychological Distance

In this chapter, we build on CLT, which posits an essential relationship between psychological distance and abstraction. We do so by postulating three core principles that explain CLT in terms of a more basic relationship between abstraction and variability. The first principle states that distance is related to variability: As distance to a mental target increases, variability of possible specific details increases. The second principle states that abstraction is designed to manage this variability. The third principle states that considering variability prompts abstraction. Put together, these three principles lead to the conclusion of CLT, namely, that as psychological distance to a target increases, potential variability around details of that target increases, which in turn prompts the need to identify and extract sources of stability via abstraction. In other words, abstraction broadens the range of possibilities we can consider, which in turn broadens our scope to include more distant targets.

Empirical Evidence

In the first part of this chapter, we reviewed the three principles that form the theoretical basis of CLT. In the second part of the chapter we first provide further review of empirical evidence that relates these principles to existing research on CLT, then examine how these principles manifest in terms of how people store and apply information, how they make decisions, and how these processes are expressed in social contexts.

A diverse body of existing research provides evidence for the relationship between psychological distance and abstraction, which covers areas such as counterfactual thinking, memory, social cognition, communication, and morality (for a meta-analysis, see Soderberg, Callahan, Kochersberger, Amit, & Ledgerwood, 2015). For example, research has shown that people prefer to identify actions in terms of their ends rather than their means when they are more temporally distant (Liberman & Trope, 1998), spatially distant (Fujita, Henderson, Eng, Trope, &

Liberman, 2006), less likely (Wakslak, Trope, Liberman, & Alony, 2006), and socially distant (Liviatan, Trope, & Liberman, 2008). Construing an action in terms of its ends is functional for projecting it across greater distances wherein the means for completing that action become more uncertain. Consider the action of "locking the door." When I am currently engaging in the action, I can represent it in terms of how I will do it—for example, by "placing a metal key in a lock." However, when the action is psychologically distant, I may consider a wider range of ways that the action may be accomplished—for example, using a key card or a pin pad for a digital alarm system. Therefore, representing the action more abstractly, in terms of its end (i.e., "securing the house") provides a representation of the action that can remain stable, even as the contextual details around the action may vary.

As another example, temporal distance increases the relative weight people place on more abstract, aggregate information (e.g., average customer rating) compared to more concrete, individualized information (e.g., one specific customer review) when evaluating and making decisions about products (Ledgerwood, Wakslak, & Wang, 2010). In this example, when people imagine using a product in the more distant future, they tend to do so in a more decontextualized manner that allows for a variety of possibilities. This makes it useful to focus on more abstract information during evaluation (e.g., consensus rating), since it provides information that is more broadly applicable than does the specific experience of one reviewer.

An important question in learning and memory is the extent to which people generalize after they learn something. In this process, abstraction comes in as the ability to identify that event *A* is similar to event *B* even if their lower-level details diverge. Recent research examined how psychological distance impacts generalization (Ram, Struyf, Vervliet, Menahem, & Liberman, 2019). In these studies, participants underwent a learning phase that showed stimuli predicting outcomes. Whereas some participants saw stimuli that predicted a given outcome with low probability, others saw stimuli that predicted the outcome with high probability. Here, low probability corresponded to greater psychological distance to the outcome (i.e., it is more hypo-

thetical) than high probability to the outcome (i.e., it is less hypothetical). In terms of the present framework, the higher-probability condition corresponded to more certainty about the outcome and the lower-probability condition corresponded to more uncertainty. After the learning phase, generalization was tested by presenting identical stimuli, as well as a range of similar (but not identical) stimuli, and people rated their expectations for the outcome. During this test of generalization, people in the low-probability condition were more likely to expect the same outcome from similar, but not identical, stimuli.

This research provides evidence for the idea that initial exposure to psychological distance to an object (the outcome) led people to generalize more widely from that object. Ram and colleagues (2019) point out that there is variability inherent in distancing, and this calls for using broader generalization to maintain the applicability of one's prediction. This means knowing that stimulus *X* will lead to outcome *Y*, and generalizing to infer that stimulus *X'* may also lead to outcome *Y*. This is adaptive because as we extend beyond the here and now, we need to be able to understand that different things may predict the same outcomes, even if they are not identical to the things that predicted these outcomes in the past.

In addition to the effect that psychological distance has on abstraction, CLT posits a bidirectional relationship in which abstraction prompts the consideration of more distant objects (Trope & Liberman, 2010). We propose that variability is involved in this bidirectional relationship. Because abstract construals focus on stable features of mental objects and subordinate variability, they can apply to more distant situations, in which the details are variable, uncertain, or unknown. As an example, if I generate an abstract representation of my phone as a communication device, it fits a wide range of instantiations that extend across various psychological distances.

So far, we have sought to elaborate the three principles that form the basis of CLT and review research that illustrates this relationship. In the sections that follow we examine how the principles manifest in empirical work in terms of (1) memory, (2) decision making, and (3) social cognition.

Memory

A key area in which the relationship between abstraction and variability applies is in the domain of memory. Memory involves mental time travel, so it is no surprise that abstraction plays a role. Functionalist accounts of memory posit that memory exists to serve prospection (e.g., Schacter, Addis, & Buckner, 2007; Suddendorf, 2006). These theorists draw on evidence from neuroscience that memory systems highly overlap with systems responsible for simulation and propose that memories exist as the raw inputs for predictions about the future. These accounts emphasize that people construct simulations of anticipated future events by recombining concrete details of past experiences.

We posit that the memory-for-prospection process has a central problem in the form of uncertainty about details, to which we lose access when a target moves outside our direct experience. One source of uncertainty is in terms of how veridical our memories are, especially as they extend further into the past. A parallel source of uncertainty is in terms of what to expect in the future, especially as we try to simulate events that are further in the future. We therefore conclude that abstraction (i.e., moving to a higher level of construal that omits concrete details but maintains general meaning) is an essential part of the process of using our memories for prospection and prediction (see Liberman, Trope, & Rim, 2011). In this section, we cover evidence for this conclusion with research on (1) memory-based analogical comparison and (2) the effect of massed versus distributed practice on memory.

Memory-Based Comparison

Evidence for the role of abstraction in the process of using memories for prospection comes from research on memory-based comparison. One set of studies varied whether people made comparisons between two images presented simultaneously, or two images presented separately on two sequential trials (Kalkstein, Hubbard, & Trope, 2018a). While the simultaneous condition entailed comparing two sources in the same temporal context, the sequential condition entailed bridging representations across two separate (albeit proximal) temporal con-

texts. The experiments demonstrated that sequential comparison led people to construe the stimuli at a more abstract level than did simultaneous comparison. When two visual scenes were presented sequentially, people identified correspondences between objects in each scene based on their relational roles (e.g., they matched an umbrella in one scene with a newspaper in another because both occupied the role of protecting a girl from the rain). In contrast, when the scenes were presented simultaneously, people identified correspondences between objects in each based on their surface-level appearance (e.g., they matched an umbrella in one scene with a similar umbrella in another, even though they occupied different roles in the scene). In more general terms, when the source of comparison is removed from immediate experience, the comparison shifts to a higher level of abstraction.

From the current perspective, we argue that this shift toward more abstract processing when recalling the past is functional for prospection. Previous accounts of prospection suggest that people construct simulations of future scenarios by recombining specific details of past experience (Schacter et al., 2007). In contrast, this research suggests that abstraction facilitates simulation by constructing mental representations that omit concrete details rather than recombine them. Such decontextualized representations can then be used to prospect about future contexts whose details are unknown. In this way, abstraction may serve a critical role in linking memory to prospection.

The Distributed Learning Effect

The distributed learning effect demonstrates a link between contextual variability and long-term memory. Here, we elucidate this link by positing a role for abstraction in managing uncertainty and supporting long-term memory. The *distributed learning effect* refers to the phenomenon that memory retention for items studied across a set of spaced study phases is better than memory retention for items during one study phase, even if the total amount of study time is equivalent (Ebbinghaus, 1885; for a review, see Cepeda, Pashler, Vul, Wixted, & Rohrer, 2006). Distributed practice effects are important because they have been found in not only basic domains but also applied domains (e.g., foreign language learning: Bahrick & Phelps, 1987; surgical training: van Dongen, Mitra, Schijven, & Broeders, 2011; memorizing anatomical information: Dobson, Perez, & Linderholm, 2017).

Spaced repetitions correspond to variable temporal contexts, whereas massed study phases correspond to a single, stable context with limited variability. Studying across variable contexts leads to increases in the variability of low-level details around the targets that people are trying to learn. For example, if you are learning the meaning of new words in a foreign language, you are learning in a context that includes myriad peripheral details, such as the room you're in, the amount of daylight, your interoceptive state, and so forth. While increasing spaces between episodes of learning leads to decreasing similarity of those episodes (i.e., more variability in peripheral details), whatever remains that *is* similar across the episodes will be identified as stable and enduring. We posit that this is an instance of abstract processing, which is engaged to manage variability of low-level, context-bound details (see also Toppino & Gerbier, 2014). This abstract processing, in turn, may support better long-term memory for the targets at the test phase (i.e., by constructing representations of the targets that are robust to future contextual changes, including the contextual changes that occur in these studies between the learning phase and the test phase).

Decision Making

In addition to memory, abstraction can manage variability in the domains of decision making and self-control. The way people behave in response to a situation may be determined by how abstractly or concretely they construe the situation. When choosing how to act, an individual must manage a range of variable inputs and concerns. Abstraction facilitates making decisions that are in line with global concerns, which include more psychologically distal outcomes over more local concerns, which include only more proximal outcomes. In the following section, we review the relationship between abstraction and decision making in three domains:

(1) self-control, (2) decisions based on large versus small samples of information, and (3) exploration versus exploitation.

Self-Control

Self-control challenges are often defined by a conflict between an immediate temptation and a more global goal (e.g., Fujita, Trope, & Liberman, 2010; Kalkstein, Fujita, & Trope, 2018). One way to conceptualize self-control problems is the challenge of acting in line with global goals, despite the variability of interests and concerns that may influence any given decision about how to act. For example, a dieter may have the global goal of being healthy, but the specific smell when walking by the bakery may prompt an isolated desire to indulge in sweets, even though doing so would undermine their overall health goal. In this case, self-control entails adhering to one's health goals that are stable and enduring across various contexts. Failure means indulging in the momentary and contextual desire of consuming sweets.

Research within the CLT framework has shown that higher-level construals promote self-control by promoting structuring and prioritization of one's higher-level goals. Fujita and colleagues have manipulated level of construal and have shown that inducing a more abstract mindset leads to greater self-control in a range of domains, including reducing temporal delay discounting and changing food attitudes to align with dieting goals (Fujita & Carnevale, 2012; Fujita & Han, 2009; Fujita, Trope, Liberman, & Levin-Sagi, 2006). Furthermore, when people encounter a self-control dilemma, they choose to adopt a high-level construal (Nguyen, Carnevale, Scholer, Miele, & Fujita, 2019). One explanation for the way abstraction can promote self-control is that it creates a unifying policy that integrates across the range of variable concerns. This integration, and the resulting abstract policy, coordinates interests, so that an individual can act in line with their global goal.

Sampling Large versus Small Amounts of Information

When gathering information for a decision, it is optimal to rely on larger random samples of information because they are more representative and thus give rise to estimates that are more likely to generalize to a larger population or a different sample. The breadth of sampling has been found to impact the quality of decisions in financial and personal domains. For example, frequently checking investment outcomes splits information samples into smaller, less representative chunks. Relying solely on the most recent small chunk, without integrating it into a broader pattern, leads to underinvestment in relatively risky but high-paying alternatives (e.g., stocks) and overpreference for safe alternatives (e.g., bonds) (Benartzi & Thaler, 2007; Thaler, 1999). As another example, when people are learning about reward choice sets from small samples of their own direct experience compared to summary descriptions, they underweight the likelihood of rare events (Hertwig, Barron, Weber, & Erev, 2004).

Halamish and Liberman (2017) demonstrated in five experiments that psychological distance leads people to prefer larger samples of information before making a decision. In these studies, the decision was between two options that had different probabilities of a financial payout. The authors explain the effect in terms of desirability and feasibility: Gathering a larger sample of information may be more desirable (to make an optimal choice) than it is feasible (at the cost of time and cognitive resources). According to CLT, psychological distance promotes desirability concerns ("What do I want?") over feasibility concerns ("How I can get it?").

In the current account, obtaining more (vs. less) information may correspond to an anticipation of more (vs. less) variability. With greater psychological distance, people may anticipate a higher degree of variability in the outcome of choice. As a result, people may be motivated to obtain more information to extract a more generalizable estimate to protect against such uncertainty. This research reveals a relationship between psychological distance and choosing to sample more information; it also sets the stage for additional research on how larger or more variable samples themselves may promote higher levels of abstraction.

Exploration versus Exploitation

Many reward-based decisions can be framed in terms of staying in a local context, where the payoffs are certain (e.g., going to a nearby, familiar restaurant) versus venturing outside of the local context, where the payoffs are uncertain but include potential for higher reward than the current context affords (e.g., searching throughout the current and surrounding neighborhoods for a new restaurant). Traditionally, this is known as a trade-off between exploitation and exploration.

To exploit one's original local context is to take advantage of a known entity with a known value; it is a safe and certain choice (e.g., a restaurant that one knows is good enough). While relatively effortless to choose, the exploitation choice does involve a potential opportunity cost. To explore novel contexts is to gamble—to gain potentially higher rewards (e.g., a higher-quality restaurant) or risk potential losses (e.g., finding only lower-quality restaurants). There are many situations in which the expected value of exploration is greater than the expected value of exploitation. Yet despite this higher expected value, exploration likely involves the cost of time and resources, so exploration is not the default choice over exploitation.

What factors contribute to exploration over exploitation? Exploitation is based on choosing to stay in your local area, which entails less exposure to variability. Exploitation occurs when an individual chooses to stay put or chooses to stop exploring after an encounter with a negative short-term outcome, even when the possibility of a positive long-term outcome exists. In contrast, exploration is based on choosing to move beyond one's local area, which entails more exposure to variability. In theory, individuals who explore should have an abstract representation of the potential overall value to be gained, and this abstract representation can remain stable, even as they encounter variable experiences along the way to their ultimate goal.

Yudkin, Pick, Hur, Liberman, and Trope (2019) examined this question in a set of studies that used the Two Hills Game. The task involves uncovering tiles on a matrix that each have varying values. The participants start in a place on the matrix that is near one "hill" of value that corresponds to a local maximum. There is also another hill, which is farther away from the starting point, and corresponds to a global maximum. In order to arrive at the global maximum, participants must "explore," which includes traversing a valley of tiles that are lower in value than the local maximum, before gradually ascending to the global maximum. Exploitation was indexed by the likelihood of staying near the local maximum, whereas exploration was indexed by measuring the likelihood of leaving the area around the local maximum, as well as the overall points earned in the game. Across several studies, they found that greater psychological distance promoted more exploration. In addition, they found a correlation between level of construal, measured as a mindset before the task, and the degree of exploration, in which higher levels of construal were positively associated with amount of exploration.

One way to explain this relationship is that distance increases people's level of construal, which in turn allows them to mentally subordinate the variability that is irrelevant to their goal, while identifying and centering on variability that is relevant to their goal. Hence, construing the task at an abstract level encourages people to endure short-term experiences of low-value tiles in the "valley" by keeping them focused on the ultimate goal of eventual ascent to the global maximum that is meaningfully more rewarding.

Social Cognition

The ability to extract abstract commonalities across variable events and circumstances gives rise to humans' expansive social capabilities (Kalkstein et al., 2018b). At the most basic level, each individual necessarily has their own unique experience with the world. Furthermore, it is impossible to ever truly and fully know another person's inner experience. Yet despite such variability and lack of access to others' personal experiences, humans have a remarkable ability to learn from, share ideas with, and coordinate with one another. Drawing on the current framework, we argue that such sociality is made possible by abstract thought that renders idiosyncratic differences secondary to more general between-person commonalities. In the following section, we explore the relationship between abstraction and social cognition in four

domains: (1) causal attribution, (2) social learning, (3) communication, and (4) social diversity and creativity.

Social Causal Attribution

When engaging in social interactions or anticipating future ones, people are often trying to explain their own behavior and others' behavior, and make predictions based on those explanations. Classic theory and research on social judgment points to the role of abstraction in managing the high degree of variability in others' behaviors and uncertainty about potential causes of those behaviors (Fiske, 1993; Heider, 1944; Jones, 1972; Kelley, 1973). This uncertainty about causes corresponds to a wider range of possible options that could explain the behavior. For example, let's say you observe a woman who trips, and you are trying to explain her behavior. One possible explanation is a specific explanation based on a contextual detail: "The floor was slippery"; another explanation is a general one based on the person's disposition: "She is clumsy." The goal of causal social inferences is to make predictions about behavior that generalize to multiple contexts. In order to make a prediction, the causal inference must not only be adequate to describe the current behavior but also general enough to apply in new contexts.

From a CLT perspective, trait-level inferences are functional for making predictions, as they identify abstract qualities that are represented as enduring across variable contexts (e.g., you can imagine that a clumsy person will continue to make missteps even without knowing contextual specifics such as exactly what the misstep will be or how it will occur). Moreover, CLT predicts that with psychological distance, people shift from more specific, contextualized explanations (e.g., "She tripped because the floor was slippery") to more general, dispositional explanations (e.g., "She tripped because she is clumsy"). According to CLT, the classic *fundamental attribution error*, which is the tendency to make dispositional rather than situational attributions (Jones & Davis, 1965; Ross, 1977), would increase with increasing distance due to increased variability and uncertainty of the contextual details that may have given rise to the behavior.

One set of studies examined whether increasing psychological distance to a target scenario—by considering it in the future rather than the present—would prompt abstract processing and thus increase the weight of global traits in predicting and explaining behavior across situations that vary in time, location, or social context (Nussbaum, Trope, & Liberman, 2003). This research showed that temporal distance increased the level of trait-based attributions rather than situation-based attributions. In another study, people sought more information about global traits for the distant future than for the near future, and they also rated explanations of their own behavior as more global (applying to more situations) when the explanations were provided for distant rather than near outcomes. All these studies point to an overall preference for more global, consistent, trait-based explanations when the situations are distal compared to proximal (see also Henderson, Fujita, Trope, & Liberman, 2006; Rim, Uleman, & Trope, 2009).

The Kelley Covariation Model

As we noted earlier, the current framework is not the first to propose of a link between variability and social attribution. The Kelley covariation model seeks to explain how people make causal attributions based on multiple observations over time. It states that "an effect is attributed to the one of its possible causes with which, over time, it covaries" (Kelley, 1973, p. 108). The current framework builds on the covariation model by positing a role of abstraction in the process of identifying covariations. When a cause covaries with an effect over time, there are also things that inevitably do not covary with those two variables. If I see Robin being polite at work, at home, and at a party, Robin is covarying with being polite, while the locations are changing. I must not only track the covarying of Robin and "polite" but also subordinate the variability that is not relevant to my trait inference, which is the changing locations. Relatedly, if I hear 10 people say that a comedian is funny, that comedian covaries with being funny even as the people who evaluate her vary. In this case, the process of abstraction subordinates the dimension of who is evaluating the comedian and extracts a stable representation that the comedian is linked to the trait of being funny.

Finally, this model may apply to a situation as well. If I see 10 job candidates be polite in their job interview, then "job interview" and "polite" are covarying despite variability in the candidates. In this framework, we emphasize, there is a hierarchy in which the covarying factors are superordinate and other random variables are subordinate. Abstraction is the cognitive process that creates this hierarchy.

Social Reinforcement Learning

Evidence that people rely on trait information in order to generalize across contexts comes from a study on reinforcement learning and social decision making (Hackel, Doll, & Amodio, 2015) that investigated how people respond to reward information versus information that implied a trait in an economic game setting. The study showed that while people encode information about the reward value of other players in the game (i.e., the magnitude of money shared by a player across trials), they also encode trait-level information (i.e., generosity: the proportion of allotted money shared by a player across trials). Moreover, this study revealed that the trait-level information generalized more to new contexts more than did reward-level information. Specifically, participants preferred to interact in subsequent contexts with more generous players. Thus, the abstract trait concept guided people's preferences for interaction partners across variable contexts.

Social Learning

Social learning, the ability to vicariously learn from the experiences of others, is arguably the single greatest contributor to the richness and expansiveness of people's mental horizons (see Bandura, 1977; Boyd, Richerson, & Henrich, 2011). Through social learning, people gain exposure to an exponentially wider variety of experiences, events, and information than they could ever encounter on their own. Moreover, increasing the diversity of one's interaction partners creates more varied opportunities for learning, as it exposes that individual to an even wider array of ideas and experiences.

However, social learning also poses a challenge, in that it requires people to transfer information from one context (i.e., someone else's experience) to another that is potentially very different (i.e., one's own experience). Furthermore, as one's interaction partners become more distant and dissimilar, the possibility for their experiences to have occurred in vastly different contexts increases. Thus, at its core, social learning entails solving the problem of extracting general lessons that are applicable across variable circumstances.

Abstract thought is therefore foundational to social learning and to broadening the range of others from whom one can learn. One series of studies demonstrated that thinking abstractly increases the scope of others that people are willing to consider as sources for social learning. For example, people consider a broader range of others when they contemplate emulating traits rather than behaviors (traits are more abstract, as they encapsulate a variety of behaviors) (Kalkstein, Kleiman, Wakslak, Liberman, & Trope, 2016). This expansion in social scope afforded by abstraction is especially relevant in today's world of global interconnectedness. More than ever before, people are interacting with others from different and diverse contexts than their own. The ability to learn abstract lessons that generalize across a variety of contexts enables people to take advantage of the wealth of learning opportunities available through interacting with distant and diverse others (Kalkstein et al., 2018b).

As in other domains, the link between variability and abstraction in social learning is bidirectional. The challenge of transferring lessons from other people to the self leads people to engage in abstract thought that forms decontextualized representations of the lesson that are stable across variable contexts. Supporting this assertion, research has shown that people represent learned information at a more abstract level when they acquire it through social learning than when they acquire it through their own direct experience (Kalkstein et al., 2016). In addition, this research has shown that the more distant a model for social learning is, the more abstractly people construe the information learned from them (see also Hansen, Alves, & Trope, 2016). This occurs because distance operates as a cue to potential variability in circumstance. Since more distant models may occupy more discrepant circumstances, learners tend to represent their action and acquired information at a higher level to ensure its successful transfer to their own circumstance.

Moreover, research has also shown that when people apply information learned from more distant others, they do so by acting on higher-level representations of the information. For example, one set of studies showed that people were more likely to emulate a model by pursuing the same goal (but adopting different means) when the model was distant, but they were more likely to emulate the model by imitating specific movements when the model was near (Genschow, Hansen, Wanke, & Trope, 2019). This research shows that abstraction during social learning also impacts the application of learned information by providing a schema for emulation that permits flexibility in execution, which may be necessary if one's immediate environment is different than that of the model.

Communication

On the other end of the interaction, teachers and communicators are tasked with the challenge of sending out information in a way that is applicable to the context of their recipients. This challenge is exacerbated when communicators are attempting to reach audiences that are distant or diverse. As with social learning, a distance implies the potential that the audience inhabits a context very different from one's own. In this case, the communicator must account for a variety of possible contexts to ensure that the message is applicable to a distant receiver. To do so, communicators use more abstract language when communicating with more distant others (Joshi, Wakslak, Raj, & Trope, 2016). Similarly, when communicating with large and diverse audiences, communicators face the challenge of sending out a message that is applicable to the variable contexts and perspectives of all the people in the audience. Research has shown that communicators use more abstract language, discuss more abstract qualities of themselves (e.g., traits instead of behaviors), and use more high-level persuasive appeals (e.g., emphasize desirability of a product over its feasibility) when communicating to larger and more diverse crowds (Joshi & Wakslak, 2014). Overall, using abstract language to communicate with distant and diverse crowds is functional, as it sends messages that are more broadly applicable across the variable experiences of audience members. Finally, from our perspective, referential communication to an audience is likely to result in higher-level construal of the referent. Whether this will produce a shift toward the audience's evaluation of the referent (Echterhoff, Higgins, & Levine, 2009; Higgins, 2016) will depend on whether there is greater evaluative similarity to the audience at a high level of construal of the referent or greater similarity at a low level of construal.

Broader Implications

In this section, we briefly explore some broader implications of these principles. First, social diversity may affect processes of group decision making and creativity. Furthermore, abstraction may prompt preferences for social diversity and facilitate equitable application of justice principles. Finally, we discuss the implications for how people deal with variability of the climate—from typical seasonal changes to the consequences of global warming

Social Diversity and Inclusiveness

A central argument we have made throughout this chapter is that integrating across variable events or objects promotes abstraction. In the social domain, this suggests that exposure to diverse perspectives and cultures should facilitate abstract thought. While there is much debate around the effectiveness of group decision making, our perspective suggests that diverse groups may lead to more abstract decision making. However, we would only suspect such an outcome in cases in which the group actively integrates across diverse perspectives (Maznevski, 1994).

Indirect support for this comes from the finding that living abroad is related to increased creativity in problem solving and associations (Maddux & Galinksy, 2009). Given the link between abstraction and creativity (e.g., Polman & Emich, 2011), this finding is consistent with the hypothesis that exposure to diverse cultures promotes abstraction. Under our account, such a result would be expected, since living abroad entails living in a context that varies from one's own context. To the extent that individu-

als compare the two, we would expect them to develop more abstract understandings of each. Furthermore, this finding has implications for immigration in general, including migration of refugees. Such patterns increase the diversity of perspectives, cultural knowledge, customs, and so forth; abstraction may be recruited to extract high-level commonalities among groups in order manage this diversity.

Finally, abstract thinking may promote acceptance and preference for social diversity and inclusiveness. For example, research has shown that among conservatives, thinking abstractly is related to an increase in tolerance for non-normative groups (e.g., people who diverge from the majority in terms of sexual orientation or religion; Luguri, Napiere, & Dovidio, 2012). Abstract thinking is also related to endorsement of affirmative action, a precursor to social diversity (Fleischmann & Burgmer, 2019). In addition, psychological distance is related to a preference to apply justice principles universally rather than applying them based on individuating features of a target (Mentovich, Yudkin, Tyler, & Trope, 2016). Abstraction may be associated with preferences for certain forms of social diversity because it is able to extract variability that is important for the situation at hand (e.g., has this person been treated unfairly?) and subordinate variability that is irrelevant for that situation (e.g., a person's demographic characteristics).

Climate Change

These principles may have implications for how abstraction helps people manage environmental variability, both locally and globally. Moving from a consistent environment (e.g., a stable, temperate climate) to an environment that varies according to a pattern (e.g., seasonality) may require an increase in abstraction to facilitate planning and coordination to manage that variability. For example, within a local climate that includes both summer and winter months, a preagricultural community would need to plan for the shift in available food sources in the winter (see Van Lange, Rinderu, & Bushman, 2017). This kind of planning may be facilitated by abstraction: A range of food sources may be unified under the category of whether it can be preserved for winter, while other features of the food (e.g., its taste) may be subordinated. This process of abstraction and prioritization would then guide people toward acquiring preservable foods before winter rather than foods that are tasty but may rot (see also Kalkstein et al., 2018b).

Beyond seasonality, abstraction may be critical for unpredictable climate variability, namely, for finding ways to respond to the myriad variable consequences of the climate change crisis. Responding to climate change requires thinking beyond one's immediate local context and considering a wide variety of scenarios. For example, there is a great deal of uncertainty in predicting the severity and location of hurricanes 20 years from now. While we cannot yet predict exactly how climate change will impact future weather events, consensus has emerged that we are experiencing more variable and extreme weather events currently than in the past and that we can expect even more variable and extreme weather in the future. In order to plan and prepare for such events, we must identify policies and solutions that will be applicable across a range of possible natural disasters. These might include abstract procedures planned and enacted by governmental agencies to deliver aid to affected areas. They might be preventative measures, such as better initiatives to reduce carbon emissions, thus targeting the causes of climate change and perhaps alleviating the need to respond to myriad future calamities. In general, abstract thinking will be imperative for generating adaptive responses to the uncertain future we face because of climate change.

Conclusion

CLT proposes that abstraction is designed to manage targets at increasing levels of psychological distance. In this chapter, we have sought to elucidate the role of variability in this process, including variability of possibilities and the uncertainty therein. As psychological distance increases, variability increases, which in turn prompts the need for abstraction to manage that variability. We are proposing variability as a unifying factor that relates various psychological distances and highlighting abstraction as a unique cognitive adaptation that manages variability. In addition to connecting research

results across various domains, including memory, self-control, and social cognition, this proposal seeks to provide a theoretical basis for novel hypotheses in future research.

NOTE

1. Whenever the gender of a person is unknown in this chapter, we chose to use the singular "they/them" as the corresponding pronoun.

REFERENCES

Bahrick, H. P., & Phelps, E. (1987). Retention of Spanish vocabulary over 8 years. *Journal of Experimental Psychology: Learning, Memory, and Cognition, 13*(2), 344–349.

Bandura, A. (1977). *Social learning theory.* Englewood Cliffs, NJ: Prentice Hall.

Benartzi, S., & Thaler, R. (2007). Heuristics and biases in retirement savings behavior. *Journal of Economic Perspectives, 21*(3), 81–104.

Block, R. A. (1989). Experiencing and remembering time: Affordances, context, and cognition. *Advances in Psychology, 59,* 333–363.

Block, R. A. (1990). Models of psychological time. In R. A. Block (Ed.), *Cognitive models of psychological time* (pp. 1–35). Hillsdale, NJ: Erlbaum.

Boroditsky, L. (2007). Comparison and the development of knowledge. *Cognition, 102,* 118–128.

Boyd, R., Richerson, P. J., & Henrich, J. (2011). The cultural niche: Why social learning is essential for human adaptation. *Proceedings of the National Academy of Science of the USA, 108,* 10918–10925.

Cepeda, N. J., Pashler, H., Vul, E., Wixted, J. T., & Rohrer, D. (2006). Distributed practice in verbal recall tasks: A review and quantitative synthesis. *Psychological Bulletin, 132*(3), 354–380.

Christie, S., & Gentner, D. (2010). Where hypotheses come from: Learning new relations by structural alignment. *Journal of Cognition and Development, 11*(3), 356–373.

Dobson, J. L., Perez, J., & Linderholm, T. (2017). Distributed retrieval practice promotes superior recall of anatomy information. *Anatomical Sciences Education, 10*(4), 339–347.

Ebbinghaus, H. (1885). *Über das gedächtnis: untersuchungen zur experimentellen psychologie* [Memory: A contribution to experimental psychology]. Berlin, Germany: Duncker & Humblot.

Echterhoff, G., Higgins, E. T., & Levine, J. M. (2009). Shared reality: Experiencing commonality with others' inner states about the world. *Perspectives on Psychological Science, 4*(5), 496–521.

Fiske, S. T. (1993). Social cognition and social perception. *Annual Review of Psychology, 44,* 155–194.

Fleischmann, A., & Burgmer, P. (2019). Abstract thinking increases support for affirmative action. *Sex Roles.* [Epub ahead of print]

Fujita, K., & Carnevale, J. J. (2012). Transcending temptation through abstraction: The role of construal level in self-control. *Current Directions in Psychological Science, 21*(4), 248–252.

Fujita, K., & Han, H. A. (2009). Moving beyond deliberative control of impulses: The effect of construal levels on evaluative associations in self-control conflicts. *Psychological Science, 20*(7), 799–804.

Fujita, K., Henderson, M. D., Eng, J., Trope, Y., & Liberman, N. (2006). Spatial distance and mental construal of social events. *Psychological Science, 17*(4), 278–282.

Fujita, K., Trope, Y., & Liberman, N. (2010). Seeing the big picture: A construal level analysis of self-control. In R. Hassin, K. Ochsner, & Y. Trope (Eds.), *Self-control in society, mind, and brain* (pp. 408–427). New York: Oxford University Press.

Fujita, K., Trope, Y., Liberman, N., & Levin-Sagi, M. (2006). Construal levels and self-control. *Journal of Personality and Social Psychology, 90*(3), 351–367.

Genschow, O., Hansen, J., Wanke, M., & Trope, Y. (2019). Psychological distance modulates goal-based versus movement-based imitation. *Journal of Experimental Psychology: Human Perception and Performance, 45,* 1031–1048.

Gentner, D. (1983). Structure-mapping: A theoretical framework for analogy. *Cognitive Science, 7*(2), 155–170.

Gentner, D., & Namy, L. L. (1999). Comparison in the development of categories. *Cognitive Development, 14,* 487–513.

Gentner, D., & Namy, L. L. (2006). Analogical processes in language learning. *Current Directions in Psychological Science, 15*(6), 297–301.

Gick, M. L., & Holyoak, K. J. (1983). Schema induction and analogical transfer. *Cognitive Psychology, 15*(1), 1–38.

Gilead, M., Trope, Y., & Liberman, N. (2019). Above and beyond the concrete: The diverse representational substrates of the predictive brain. *Behavioral and Brain Sciences.* [Epub ahead of print]

Hackel, L. M., Doll, B. B., & Amodio, D. M. (2015). Instrumental learning of traits versus rewards: Dissociable neural correlates and effects on choice. *Nature Neuroscience, 18*(9), 1233–1235.

Hadar, B., Luria, R., & Liberman, N. (2019). Concrete mindset impairs filtering in visual working memory. *Psychonomic Bulletin and Review, 26,* 1917–1924.

Hadar, B., Luria, R., & Liberman, N. (2020). Induced social power improves visual working memory. *Personality and Social Psychology Bulletin, 46,* 285–297.

Halamish, V., & Liberman, N. (2017). How much information to sample before making a decision?: It's a matter of psychological distance. *Journal of Experimental Social Psychology, 71,* 111–116.

Hansen, J., Alves, H., & Trope, Y. (2016). Psychological distance reduces literal imitation: Evidence from an imitation-learning paradigm. *Journal of Experimental Psychology: Human Perception and Performance, 42*(3), 320–330.

Hansen, J., & Trope, Y. (2013). When time flies: How abstract and concrete mental construal affect the perception of time. *Journal of Experimental Psychology: General, 142*(2), 336–347.

Heider, F. (1944). Social perception and phenomenal causality. *Psychological Review, 51*(6), 358–374.

Henderson, M. D., Fujita, K., Trope, Y., & Liberman, N. (2006). Transcending the "here": The effect of spatial distance on social judgment. *Journal of Personality and Social Psychology, 91*(5), 845–856.

Hertwig, R., Barron, G., Weber, E. U., & Erev, I. (2004). Decisions from experience and the effect of rare events in risky choice. *Psychological Science, 15*(8), 534–539.

Higgins, E. T. (2016). Shared-reality development in childhood. *Perspectives on Psychological Science, 11*(4), 466–495.

Jones, E. E. (1972). *Attribution: Perceiving the causes of behavior.* Morristown, NJ: General Learning Press.

Jones, E. E., & Davis, K. E. (1965). From acts to dispositions the attribution process in person perception. *Advances in Experimental Social Psychology, 2,* 219–266.

Joshi, P. D., & Wakslak, C. J. (2014). Communicating with the crowd: Speakers use abstract messages when addressing larger audiences. *Journal of Experimental Psychology: General, 143*(1), 351–362.

Joshi, P. D., Wakslak, C. J., Raj, M., & Trope, Y. (2016). Communicating with distant others: The functional use of abstraction. *Social Psychological and Personality Science, 7*(1), 37–44.

Kalkstein, D., Fujita, K., & Trope, Y. (2018). Broadening mental horizons to resist temptation: Construal level and self-control. In D. de Ridder, M. Adriaanse, & K. Fujita (Eds.), *Routledge international handbook of self-control in health and well-being* (pp. 180–192). New York: Routledge.

Kalkstein, D. A., Hubbard, A. D., & Trope, Y. (2018a). Beyond direct reference: Comparing the present to the past promotes abstract processing. *Journal of Experimental Psychology: General, 147*(6), 933–938.

Kalkstein, D., Hubbard, A., & Trope, Y. (2018b). Expansive and contractive learning experiences: Mental construal and living well. In J. P. Forgas & R. F. Baumeister (Eds.), *The social psychology of living well* (pp. 223–236). New York: Routledge.

Kalkstein, D. A., Kleiman, T., Wakslak, C. J., Liberman, N., & Trope, Y. (2016). Social learning across psychological distance. *Journal of Personality and Social Psychology, 110*(1), 1–19.

Kelley, H. H. (1973). The processes of causal attribution. *American Psychologist, 28*(2), 107–128.

Kurtz, K. J., Boukrina, O., & Gentner, D. (2013). Comparison promotes learning and transfer of relational categories. *Journal of Experimental Psychology: Learning, Memory, and Cognition, 39*(4), 1303–1310.

Ledgerwood, A., Wakslak, C. J., & Wang, M. A. (2010). Differential information use for near and distant decisions. *Journal of Experimental Social Psychology, 46*(4), 638–642.

Liberman, N., & Trope, Y. (1998). The role of feasibility and desirability considerations in near and distant future decisions: A test of temporal construal theory. *Journal of Personality and Social Psychology, 75*, 5–18.

Liberman, N., & Trope, Y. (2008). The psychology of transcending the here and now. *Science, 322*(5905), 1201–1205.

Liberman, N., & Trope, Y. (2014). Traversing psychological distance. *Trends in Cognitive Sciences, 18*(7), 364–369.

Liberman, N., Trope, Y., & Rim, S. Y. (2011). Prediction: A construal-level theory perspective. In M. Bar (Ed.), *Predictions in the brain: Using our past to generate a future* (pp. 144–158). New York: Oxford University Press.

Liviatan, I., Trope, Y., & Liberman, N. (2008). The effect of similarity on mental construal. *Journal of Experimental Social Psychology, 44*, 1256–1269.

Luguri, J. B., Napier, J. L., & Dovidio, J. F. (2012). Reconstruing intolerance: Abstract thinking reduces conservatives' prejudice against non-normative groups. *Psychological Science, 23*(7), 756–763.

Maddux, W. W., & Galinsky, A. D. (2009). Cultural borders and mental barriers: The relationship between living abroad and creativity. *Journal of Personality and Social Psychology, 96*(5), 1047–1061.

Maglio, S. J., Trope, Y., & Liberman, N. (2013). The common currency of psychological distance. *Current Directions in Psychological Science, 22*(4), 278–282.

Markman, A. B., & Gentner, D. (1993). Structural alignment during similarity comparisons. *Cognitive Psychology, 25*, 431–467.

Maznevski, M. L. (1994). Understanding our differences: Performance in decision-making groups with diverse members. *Human Relations, 47*, 531–552.

Mentovich, A., Yudkin, D., Tyler, T., & Trope, Y. (2016). Justice without borders: The influence of psychological distance and construal level on moral exclusion. *Personality and Social Psychology Bulletin, 42*(10), 1349–1363.

Murphy, G. L. (2010). What are categories and concepts? In D. Mareschal, P. C. Quinn, & S. Lea (Eds.), *The making of human concepts* (pp. 11–28). Oxford, UK: Oxford University Press.

Murphy, G. L., & Medin, D. L. (1985). The role of theories in conceptual coherence. *Psychological Review, 92*(3), 289–316.

Nguyen, T., Carnevale, J. J., Scholer, A. A., Miele, D. B., & Fujita, K. (2019). Metamotivational knowledge of the role of high-level and low-level construal in goal-relevant task performance. *Journal of Personality and Social Psychology, 117*(5), 876–899.

Nussbaum, S., Trope, Y., & Liberman, N. (2003). Creeping dispositionism: The temporal dynamics of behavior prediction. *Journal of Personality and Social Psychology, 84*(3), 485–497.

Polman, E., & Emich, K. J. (2011). Decisions for others are more creative than decisions for the self. *Personality and Social Psychology Bulletin, 37*(4), 492–501.

Ram, H., Struyf, D., Vervliet, B., Menahem, G., & Liberman, N. (2019). The effect of outcome probability on generalization in predictive learning. *Experimental Psychology, 66*, 23–39.

Rim, S., Uleman, J. S., & Trope, Y. (2009). Spontaneous trait inference and construal level theory: Psychological distance increases nonconscious trait thinking. *Journal of Experimental Social Psychology, 45*(5), 1088–1097.

Rosch, E., Mervis, C. B., Gray, W. D., Johnson, D. M., & Boyes-Braem, P. (1976). Basic objects in natural categories. *Cognitive Psychology, 8*, 382–439.

Ross, L. (1977). The intuitive psychologist and his shortcomings: Distortions in the attribution process. In L. Berkowitz (Ed.), *Advances in experimental social psychology* (Vol. 10, pp. 173–220). New York: Academic Press.

Schacter, D. L., Addis, D. R., & Buckner, R. L. (2007). Remembering the past to imagine the future: The prospective brain. *Nature Reviews Neuroscience, 8*(9), 657–661.

Shapira, O., Liberman, N., Trope, Y., & Rim, S.

(2012). Levels of mental construal. In S. T. Fiske & C. N. Macrae (Eds.), *Handbook of social cognition* (pp. 229–250). New York: SAGE.

Smith, P. K., & Trope, Y. (2006). You focus on the forest when you're in charge of the trees: Power priming and abstract information processing. *Journal of Personality and Social Psychology, 90*(4), 578–596.

Soderberg, C. K., Callahan, S. P., Kochersberger, A. O., Amit, E., & Ledgerwood, A. (2015). The effects of psychological distance on abstraction: Two meta-analyses. *Psychological Bulletin, 141*(3), 525–548.

Suddendorf, T. (2006). Foresight and evolution of the human mind. *Science, 312*(5776), 1006–1007.

Thaler, R. H. (1999). Mental accounting matters. *Journal of Behavioral Decision Making, 12*(3), 183–206.

Toppino, T. C., & Gerbier, E. (2014). About practice: Repetition, spacing, and abstraction. In B. H. Ross (Ed.), *Psychology of learning and motivation* (Vol. 60, pp. 113–189). New York: Academic Press.

Trope, Y., & Liberman, N. (2003). Temporal construal. *Psychological Review, 110*(3), 403–421.

Trope, Y., & Liberman, N. (2010). Construal-level theory of psychological distance. *Psychological Review, 117*(2), 440–463.

Van Dongen, K. W., Mitra, P. J., Schijven, M. P., & Broeders, I. A. (2011). Distributed versus massed training: Efficiency of training psychomotor skills. *Surgical Techniques Development, 1*(1). Retrieved from *www.pagepress.org/journals/index.php/std/article/view/std.2011.e17.*

Van Lange, P. A. M., Rinderu, M. I., & Bushman, B. J. (2017). Aggression and violence around the world: A model of CLimate, Aggression, and Self-control in Humans (CLASH). *Behavioral and Brain Sciences, 40,* e75.

Vendetti, M. S., Wu, A., & Holyoak, K. J. (2014). Far-out thinking: Generating solutions to distant analogies promotes relational thinking. *Psychological Science, 25*(4), 928–933.

Vlach, H. A., Ankowski, A. A., & Sandhofer, C. M. (2012). At the same time or apart in time?: The role of presentation timing and retrieval dynamics in generalization. *Journal of Experimental Psychology: Learning, Memory, and Cognition, 38*(1), 246–254.

Vlach, H. A., Sandhofer, C. M., & Kornell, N. (2008). The spacing effect in children's memory and category induction. *Cognition, 109*(1), 163–167.

Wakslak, C. J., Trope, Y., Liberman, N., & Alony, R. (2006). Seeing the forest when entry is unlikely: Probability and the mental representation of events. *Journal of Experimental Psychology: General, 135,* 641–653.

Yudkin, D. A., Pick, R., Hur, E. Y., Liberman, N., & Trope, Y. (2019). Psychological distance promotes exploration in search of a global maximum. *Personality and Social Psychology Bulletin, 45*(6), 893–906.

CHAPTER 5

Motives Working Together

Value, Truth, and Control
in Goal Selection and Pursuit

E. Tory Higgins
Emily Nakkawita

A review of best-selling media today reveals broad popular interest in motivation and goal pursuit. Skim through the products offered by prominent online retailers and you will uncover thousands of items purported to reveal the secrets of motivation, enhance goal setting, and even broadcast one's interest in the topic through gear emblazoned with phrases such as "Goal Digger" (Etsy, 2018; Walmart, 2018). This area is not just interesting to the general public; researchers have explored the psychology of goal setting and striving for decades (for reviews, see Bargh, Gollwitzer, & Oettingen, 2010; Higgins & Scholer, 2015). Over the years, these topics have been studied across a range of academic domains, including philosophy, economics, and psychology. In social–personality psychology in particular, there has been an explosion of research on motivation over the last 20 years, leading to the creation of the international Society for the Science of Motivation (SSM).

Our purpose in this chapter is to describe the primary forces that motivate people, as well as to review theories and research that explain how these motives influence goal-directed behavior. We highlight three motivational principles regarding the distinct ways in which people want

to be effective: value (having desired results), control (managing what happens), and truth (establishing what's real). The importance to motivation of how these three ways of being effective *work together* is a fourth motivational principle. We provide both theoretical and empirical support for their status as primary motivational principles. We would like to begin by highlighting two general motivational assumptions that underlie our perspective on motivation. First, we suggest that the influence of motivation on human experience is *pervasive,* with important consequences for cognition, affect, and action. Although some scholars have proposed that "cold" cognitive and "hot" motivational processes reflect distinct systems (e.g., Metcalfe & Mischel, 1999), we share the perspective of those who argue that these domains are indelibly intertwined and synergistic (see, e.g., Kruglanski, 1996, Sorrentino & Higgins, 1986). Second, we posit that the mechanisms underlying motivated cognition and behavior *align with* and *build on* general principles established within the broader field of psychology (e.g., knowledge accessibility and activation; Eitam & Higgins, 2010, 2014; Higgins, 1996).

To achieve these aims, we begin by reviewing a range of perspectives on motivation. Then, we turn our attention to how motivation relates to goal selection and pursuit. In brief, we argue that there are three primary motives that animate human experience—value, control, and truth—and that these core motives *work together* in an integrated fashion to direct both *which* goals people take on and *how* these goals are pursued (see also Higgins, 2012).

What Is Motivation?

To begin with, what do we mean by "motivation"? What does it mean to be motivated? Historically, motivation has been broadly viewed in two ways—as an energizing force and as approach–avoidance tendencies. After briefly summarizing these viewpoints, we will propose a third, complementary definition that we consider useful.

Motivation as an Energizing Force

When asked to define motivation, many people describe it as a high-energy state. This conceptualization of motivation as "all-purpose energy" underlies a range of influential theories. Despite some differences in the hypothesized driver of motivation (e.g., biological needs vs. goal intentions), psychodynamic, behavioral, and Gestalt theorists considered motivation itself to be universal energy that creates tension within the individual and demands pursuit of the motivating need or goal. This idea of an energetic impulse is captured within Freud's (1957) conceptualization of instinctual energy, Hull's (1943) description of the "evocation of action" produced by a drive, and Lewin's (1944/1997) proposal that force is a "tendency to locomotion."

While we agree with the notion that motivation often manifests as energy directed at a task, this conceptualization does not reflect the reality that different goal pursuit strategies complement *different* motivational orientations (Higgins, 2012). Additionally, this definition fails to account for the differences in goal selection and pursuit when the goal in question is a desired versus undesired end state. For these reasons, defining motivation as "general-purpose" energy is limited at best and misleading at worst.

Motivation as Approach–Avoidance Tendencies

Motivation has also long been conceptualized as a set of distinct, conflicting tendencies to move toward desired reference points and away from undesired reference points, often described in terms of *approach* versus *avoidance*. A number of well-regarded approach–avoidance models that have risen to prominence can be broadly grouped into three categories.

First, conditioning theorists came to appreciate the fact that inhibitory avoidance tendencies conflict with excitatory approach tendencies. For example, Neal Miller (1959) recognized that Hull's (1932) "goal-gradient" effect, which suggested that people exhibit increasing effort as they approach a goal, might reverse for avoidance goals. After demonstrating such approach–avoidance conflict behavior through empirical research with rats, he revised the postulates within his stimulus–response model accordingly (Miller, 1959).

Second, a new group of theories based on cybernetic and control-process models also accounted for approach and avoidance behaviors. As an example, consider Miller, Galanter, and Pribam's (1960) test–operate–test–exit (TOTE) model, which posited that motivated behavior is produced through a series of feedback loops. Within each loop, an individual engages in approach or avoidance behaviors in sequential attempts to minimize his or her degree of mismatch with a desired state (for a more recent example of this perspective, see Carver & Scheier, 1981, 1998).

Finally, dynamic models such as John Atkinson's (1964) theory of achievement motivation reflected the interplay between approach and avoidance tendencies within a narrower context. According to Atkinson, all individuals with achievement goals experience a conflict between their hope for success and anxiety about failure, and resulting behavioral tendencies reflect the outcome of this excitation–inhibition conflict.

The prevalence of approach–avoidance theories is not surprising given how well the idea of movement toward or away from a goal corresponds with the phenomenological experience of motivated behavior. Indeed, the etymological root of the term *motivation* is the Latin word *movere,* which means "to move." But this itself is problematic, specifically because it suggests that motivation constitutes approach or avoidance movement when nonmovement is also motivated (e.g., suppression or inhibition), and monitoring, which plays a critical role in self-regulatory control, does not itself involve movement. Thus, once again, this viewpoint on motivation is limited.

Motivation as Having Preferences That Direct Choices

As an alternative, complementary definition of *motivation,* Higgins (2012, p. 24, original emphasis) suggested that what it means to be motivated is the following: "*to have preferences directing choices.*" This definition differs from the prior two, as these preferences reflect not only desired and undesired end states but also the *processes* of goal pursuit, including choices of which strategies and tactics to use in the goal pursuit.

It is important to clarify a few aspects of this proposal. First, the preferences described in the definition are not necessarily known or intentionally applied. On the contrary, these preferences may be unconscious, and their implementation may be relatively effortless (see Eitam & Higgins, 2014; Higgins & Eitam, 2014). Additionally, the term *choices* is used in a broad, systemic sense within this definition, as these choices (just like the preferences that drive them) are not necessarily intentional or even consciously accessible (see Huang & Bargh, 2014). Furthermore, these choices are not expressed only through action or behavior. As Bargh and colleagues (2010) pointed out in their chapter on goal pursuit, motivation may manifest itself cognitively or affectively. In fact, recent behavioral and neural work in the domain of motivated cognition suggests that motivational preferences are reflected in perception, attention, and memory (Hughes & Zaki, 2015).

The idea that perception may be influenced by motivational factors was highlighted by "New Look" theorists (Bruner & Goodman, 1947) who, in turn, were inspired by psychodynamic ideas. Research reveals that the preference for desired outcomes leads to an item of value being viewed as physically larger by people with a greater desire or need for that item. For example, children perceive coins as larger than identically sized cardboard discs, and *poor* children view the same coins as larger than do *rich* children (Bruner & Goodman, 1947; see also Dunning & Balcetis, 2013).

Memory is also affected by motivational factors. Research on *shared reality* reveals that communicators' memories will be biased by others' beliefs to the extent that the communicators are motivated to create a shared reality with them by tuning their message to match those others' beliefs (see Echterhoff, Higgins, & Groll, 2005; Echterhoff, Higgins, Kopietz, & Groll, 2008). This desire for shared reality involves both social relational and epistemic (i.e., truth-seeking) motives. Indeed, the effect of message tuning on memory disappears when the "others" are outgroup members with whom the communicators are *not* motivated to share reality (Echterhoff, Kopietz, & Higgins, 2013). The role that epistemic motives play within shared reality highlights another important point. While early theorists hypothesized that motivated cognition resulted from preferences related to desired end states (i.e., *value*), more recent research reveals that they also relate to motives for *truth* (e.g., Hughes & Zaki, 2015). The motive for truth is not the same as the motive for value. And each of these motives is different than the motive for control. Each of these motives provides a different answer to the question "What do people want?" Let us now consider how these three motives are different kinds of wants.

What Do People Want?

Higgins (2012, p. 41, original emphasis) made the following proposal about what it is that people want: "*to be effective in life pursuits.*" Once again, this proposal is not just about the end state of goal attainment. It is also about the processes involved in goal pursuit and includes strategies and tactics of goal pursuit. There are three general ways to be effective in life pursuits: (1) to be effective in having desired results, which is *value* effectiveness; (2) to be effective in managing what happens, which is *control* effectiveness; and (3) to be effective in establishing what is real, which is *truth* effectiveness. We consider next the historical support for each of these general motivational principles.

Value

People are effective in the domain of value when they experience desired end states and do not experience unwanted end states. As a result, *value motivation* is closely connected with the approach–avoidance conceptualization of motivation.

Value's role as a primary motivating force has long been recognized by philosophers, economists, animal behaviorists, and social psychologists, who have attempted to explain the motives that animate human (and, in some cases, nonhuman) experience. Below we review a range of perspectives that conceptualize motivation in value terms.

Drive Theories: Motivation to Satisfy Survival-Based Needs

Drive theories are rooted in the idea that survival is an evolutionary imperative (Darwin, 1909). In order for an organism to survive, appetitive biological drives such as hunger, thirst, and the desire to procreate must be satisfied; as a result, the value of food, water, and sex relates to the degree to which these are instrumental in satisfying a biological need or deficit (Woodworth, 1918).

Early conditioning theorists were inspired by this notion and, as a result, treated the need to satisfy biological drives as the primary force behind motivated behavior. In an attempt to reduce value to its most basic terms, these theorists suggested that *primary motivation* be defined as action evoked by the animal or person's need to satisfy appetitive drives (Hull, 1943).

Interestingly, not all need-satisfaction theories have focused on *biological* needs. Social needs have also received representation within the psychological literature for some time. For example, Abraham Maslow (1943) posited that once physiological and safety needs are sated, people seek to satisfy needs for love and esteem—both of which are inherently social. In the years since, researchers have explored a range of constructs related to the motive to establish and maintain positive, stable relationships with others, including needs for affiliation (Byrne, 1961; Shipley & Veroff, 1952), attachment (Bowlby, 1969), and belongingness (Baumeister & Leary, 1995). Though not directly reflecting "appetites," these social needs are certainly related to survival given that humans are social beings; social ineffectiveness threatens one's security and well-being.

Psychological Hedonism: Motivation to Approach Pleasure and Avoid Pain

Approximately 2,400 years ago, Aristippus described the hedonic principle to Socrates: "I beg to be enrolled amongst those who wish to spend their days as easily and pleasantly as possible" (Xenophon, 371 B.C.E./2018, II.1.13). Millennia later, in his writings on utility, Jeremy Bentham (1823, p. 169) dedicated a full chapter to a similar definition, proposing that "the motive in prospect, we see, is always . . . some pleasure, which the act in question is expected to be a means of continuing or producing: some pain which it is expected to be a means of discontinuing or preventing."

This principle offers several benefits in comparison to early drive theories. First, it aligns closely with the phenomenological experience of motivation; everyday life provides evidence for the notion that people wish to experience pleasure and avoid experiencing pain. Likely for this reason, the hedonic principle has received significant attention within lay conceptions of motivation, as captured within the notion of reward and punishment incentives, or "carrots" and "sticks." The hedonic principle also addresses a problem with drive theories—specifically, the fact that organisms sometimes behave in ways that contradict biological needs. As an extreme example, consider the problem of addiction: Injection drug users report very high levels of hunger and food insecurity, which are predicted by expenditures on drugs (Anema et al., 2010). This example highlights that, in some cases, urgent short-term needs that promote biological survival, such as the need for food, may be treated as subordinate to the motivation to engage in activities that produce pleasure.

By the middle of the 20th century, many motivational theories incorporated the influence of pleasurable and painful incentives. Kurt Lewin (1935) accounted for the powerful role of rewards and punishments in his field theory; by interacting with one's intrinsic interest in a goal, the resultant vectors produced by such incentives reflected the power of value motives to shape preferences and produce behavioral change. Later versions of drive theories also reflected the motivating role of incentives that were unrelated to the reduction of tissue deficits. For example, Clark Hull (1950) adapted his motivational model to reflect incentives' distinct contribution to action; this "value" factor represented the magnitude of the pleasure or pain inherent in the incentive. Additionally, in the years that followed, learning theorists built an entire body of work rooted in beliefs about approaching reinforcement and avoiding punishment.

As work on this topic advanced, research also revealed that pleasure and pain do not necessarily receive equal weighting in their influence over behavior. In their work on prospect theory, Kahneman and Tversky (1979) proposed that the desire to avoid a potential loss is more motivating than the desire for a potential gain of the same size (but see Higgins & Liberman, 2018).

What is clear from this (very brief) review is that for a very long time, hedonic experience has been considered to be a powerful contributor to the experience of value. Despite this fact, it is important to note that pleasure and pain are not the *only* factors involved in value effectiveness. Let us now consider (again, very briefly) several other drivers of value.

Value from Shared Standards: Motivation to Meet Personal and Social Reference Points

In addition to the sources of value we discussed earlier, people also derive value from meeting and exceeding reference points or standards. These standards are different from the needs described earlier because they are socially rather than biologically motivated; they reflect socially constructed beliefs about what is desirable or undesirable. In particular, standards considered especially relevant to value are shared beliefs that individuals hold with significant others and those that are normative within their culture (see Higgins, 2019).

The standards that we share with significant others at an interpersonal level are typically treated as *personal* standards. Research testing self-discrepancy theory (Higgins, 1987) has shown that these standards are used as a basis against which to evaluate one's *actual* self (i.e., a person's representation of the attributes and characteristics that he or she actually possesses). The theory posits two distinct sets of personal standards, or self-guides, to which this actual self is compared: the ideal self and the ought self. The *ideal self* is the representation of the characteristics that one ideally wants to possess (i.e., the hopes and aspirations for the type of person one might become), whereas the *ought self* is the representation of the characteristics that one ought to possess (i.e., the duties and responsibilities one should uphold). If a comparison between the actual self and an ideal or ought self-guide reveals a match between the two, the actual self is evaluated as having positive value; conversely, if this comparison reveals a discrepancy, the actual self is evaluated as having negative value.

In contrast with such personal standards, the standards of excellence that we share broadly with others in our society are often described simply as *values*. This term describes collective beliefs about which objectives are (or are not) worthy of desire, as well as which means of achieving these objectives are acceptable (see Merton, 1957). Such values are often defined at the societal or cultural level and include objectives, such as freedom, and means, such as procedural justice. These values guide behavior by functioning as a socially accepted standard.

Value Intensification: Engagement Strength as a "Signal Booster"

Until this point, our review of value has primarily focused on the *direction* of a value experience—whether it is associated with a positive or a negative motivational force. However, these forces also differ in *how* positive or *how* negative they are—their *intensity* (see Lewin, 1951). Importantly, the intensity of a motivational force—attraction or repulsion—can be strengthened without any impact on its direction by strengthening engagement in what one is doing. To be engaged "is to be involved, occupied, and interested in something" (Higgins, 2006, p. 442). Significantly, regardless of whether this stronger engagement is produced by the pursuit of the valued goal itself or by some other present activity, it can intensify the value experience of the goal pursuit. And when this stronger engagement is combined with hedonic factors that contribute a sense of direction to this value experience, this *directed* intensity yields a willingness to invest more effort or energy in an activity if that is needed for goal attainment (Scholer & Higgins, 2009). Contributors to engagement strength include opposition to interfering forces, overcoming personal resistance, use of proper means, and regulatory fit (Higgins, 2006); we discuss the latter in more detail later.

Control

Although value has received the greatest emphasis historically in the psychological literature, the motive for control has also appeared in several important theories. *Control motivation* is the desire to manage what happens, to have an effect on something. It describes the need to exert influence over oneself and others in order to either produce an effect or actively impede its occurrence. A person who is effective in the domain of control tends to be planful, organized, competent, autonomous, and generally interested in taking action. With this said, when not balanced by other motivational concerns, excessively strong control motivation may function to the detriment of the individual, predicting impulsivity and insufficient consideration of the right path forward (Cornwell, Franks, & Higgins, 2019).

Control effectiveness is fundamentally different from value effectiveness. Whereas value is primarily focused on the outcomes of goal pursuit, control is concerned with managing the process of goal pursuit. This motive for control can also overrule or outweigh value motives, as demonstrated in cases where pleasant outcomes are forgone in order to make things happen. Take the example of contrafreeloading, for instance, in which an animal that has free access to abundant food pellets chooses to exert itself to receive the very same food by repeatedly pressing a lever on a mechanical device (Osborne, 1977). Such phenomena show how control is a primary motive in its own right. Next, we review next several theories that highlight the importance of control motivation.

Psychodynamic Theories: Controlling Inner States

Sometimes people associate psychodynamic theories with value (i.e., pleasure and pain), but this neglects the theories' unique contributions to understanding control motives—particularly with regard to managing one's own inner states. According to Freud, the *ego* is primarily responsible for this process, balancing and controlling the competing motivational forces of the *id* (which basically cares about pleasure and pain) and the *superego* (which cares about standards from significant others and social norms; Freud, 1962). Freud believed that there can be emotional problems if either the id or the superego dominates. What is needed is the ego's management—control—of these inner dynamic forces.

Effectance Motivation: Controlling the External Environment

Control motivation pertains not just to inner states; people are also motivated to manage what happens in the world around them. In the early 20th century, Robert Woodworth (1940) introduced a new perspective on motivation, suggesting that rather than being motivated to *have* (i.e., to satisfy value-focused needs), organisms are primarily motivated to *do*:

> There is no more reason for saying that the muscles exist for the purpose of obtaining food than for saying that food is needed to supply energy for the muscles. . . . What we find in the young animal is activity directed toward the environment, along with the organic needs, and with no sign that one is more primitive and unlearned than the other. (p. 374)

Later, Robert White (1959) introduced a new theory of motivation based on *competence*, defined as the capability for effective interaction with one's environment. He proposed that organisms also experience a persistent need to produce an effect within their environment—naming this motive *effectance motivation*. Importantly, he drew attention to a way that this control-focused motive was qualitatively different from value: Whereas value motives are outcome-focused, with satisfaction occurring through reduction of a drive or satisfaction of a need, effectance motivation is process-focused, such that "satisfaction has to be seen as lying in a considerable series of transactions, in a trend of behavior rather than a goal that is achieved" (p. 322). Finally, White (1963) described how this need for competence is rooted in an evolutionarily adaptive tendency toward autonomous action, highlighting the primal importance to an organism of controlling its own fate and that of others.

Socially Acquired Control Motivation: Perspective Taking and Internalization

Although White (1963) briefly touched on social competence in his later writing, he proposed a conception of social control that was hierarchical and often antagonistic, based on needs for dominance, aggression, deference, and abasement. More recent work highlights a less competitive form of competence that develops through social interaction. In order to competently select and pursue their goals, people need to know what others want them to do and who they want them to *become*. By taking the perspective of these trusted others, people are able to infer the goals and standards that these people hold for them, learning in the process what counts as success versus failure. As an important example, consider the ideal- and ought-self-guides we introduced when we discussed value motivation. Higgins (e.g., 1991, 2019) posits that these self-guides are adopted by children (internalized) through social interactions with their caretakers: Children look to their parents to understand the ideal (aspirations) and ought (obligations) self-guides that function as goals to pursue and standards to follow. This requires that children take the perspective of their parents and accept as their own goals and standards those that their parents want for them. In doing so, these socially acquired self-guides become the goals and standards that will direct their future goal-pursuit efforts, even when the parents are not present. These internalized self-guides now control their choices.

Self-Determination Theory: Control via Autonomy

The connections White (1959) introduced between competence and autonomy have been expanded upon within Edward Deci and Richard Ryan's (2000) self-determination theory, which proposes that three specific needs underlie all goal-directed behavior. Two of these needs—autonomy and competence—reflect control motives. With this said, Deci and Ryan's conceptualization of *autonomy* is quite unique within the realm of motivation theories, so we focus on it here.

Autonomy refers to the need to experience volition by controlling one's own behavior, so that it integrates with one's sense of self (Deci & Ryan, 2000). Self-determination theory suggests that the experience of autonomy depends on the degree to which a person's behavior is motivated by varying levels of external control versus intrinsic motivation (Deci & Ryan, 1980). Interestingly, Deci and Ryan (2000) proposed that whereas the need for competence underlies all motivation, full autonomy must be experienced for an activity to be truly intrinsically motivated. Autonomous motivation is associated with a range of positive outcomes, including improved academic performance (Wang, 2008), greater intentions to engage in healthy behaviors (Pavey & Sparks, 2009), and increased well-being (Sheldon, Ryan, Deci, & Kasser, 2004).

Self-Efficacy Theory: Judgments of Personal Capability to Control

Albert Bandura (1977, 1982) also recognized that an important aspect of the human experience is the desire to create and manage what is happening in one's life. He and others have conducted extensive programs of research on perceptions of self-efficacy, which describe people's judgments of their "operative capabilities" in a given situation—the degree to which individuals believe that they have the capacity to organize their cognitions and behaviors to produce a desired effect in a particular context. Research on this topic has revealed that self-efficacy beliefs affect the goals we take on, the effort we expend in their pursuit, the degree to which we persist in the face of difficulty, and our success in achieving desired outcomes (Bandura, 1997; Schunk & DiBenedetto, 2016).

Perceived Agency: Control over Outcomes

Control effectiveness is also related to the experience of agency, in which individuals feel that they are responsible for causing the events that occur around them (Metcalfe & Greene, 2007). Though similar in nature, judgments of agency differ in an important way from self-efficacy beliefs: Whereas self-efficacy beliefs reflect the degree to which individuals believe they possess the capability to produce a specific response, perceptions of agency also reflect whether individuals believe they control the outcome itself.

Recent advances in research on metacognitive judgments of agency support distinguishing value and control as motives. For example, in a recent study using a video game paradigm within which experimenters manipulated both the rewards participants earned and the degree to which participants could effectively control the cursor, participants' ratings of "flow" closely tracked the rewards they earned (i.e., value), whereas agency (i.e., control) judgments reflected actual hit rates (Vuorre & Metcalfe, 2016; for more on control feedback, see Nafcha, Higgins, & Eitam, 2016).

As another example, motivation researchers have recently developed a Sense of Agency Scale that directly measures one's long-term, cross-contextual experience of control over one's mind, body, and actions (Tapal, Oren, Dar, & Eitam, 2017). Specifically, this scale allows researchers to measure both the sense of positive agency (the feeling that one is control) and the sense of negative agency (the feeling that one is *not* in control). Interestingly, positive and negative agency only appear to be moderately correlated, opening up an interesting possibility for future research on the different factors underlying control effectiveness (Tapal et al., 2017).

Truth

Finally, we turn our attention to the motive for truth, which, compared to value and control, has received relatively less attention as a distinct motive in psychology and other disciplines— although it has certainly not been ignored. *Truth motivation* captures how people want to understand better the world around them and establish what is real. It manifests in wanting to be accurate, to be consistent, to know the right path forward (both morally and practically), and to share what's real with others (Higgins, 2012).

Truth effectiveness is distinct from value effectiveness, as people will pursue truth even when it could lead to painful consequences, which includes being willing to die for what one believes to be the truth. Next, we review a range of theories that capture this third primary motive.

Need for Cognition: The Motivation to Think

To begin, the truth motive encompasses the need to think and understand. Maslow (1943) argued for the importance of cognitive needs, which drive learning, curiosity, exploration, and the search for meaning. In doing so, he clarified that "the desire to know and to understand are themselves conative, i.e., have a striving character, and are as much personality needs as the 'basic needs' we have already discussed" (p. 385). A decade later, Cohen, Stotland, and Wolfe (1955) conducted experimental research formally defining the *need for cognition,* defining it as a drive to "structure relevant situations in meaningful, integrated ways" (p. 291) and establishing it as a measurable individual difference distinct from the need for achievement. Years later, Cacioppo and Petty (1982) developed a Need for Cognition Scale, and found that people with a high (vs. low) need for cognition prefer more challenging problem-solving tasks and, despite expending more mental effort, do not report greater frustration or mental discomfort from having done so. Most recently, work on trait curiosity indicates that the motive to think, learn, and understand is associated with various positive outcomes, including increased well-being (Gallagher & Lopez, 2007) and a greater belief that one's life and goals are meaningful (Kashdan & Steger, 2007).

Cognitive Consistency Theories: Motivation to Experience Coherent Reality

The motive for truth effectiveness not only manifests in the desire to understand and structure cognitions about outside situations but also prompts people to ensure that their own cognitions and behaviors are consistent. One of the most influential theories regarding this need for consistency is Leon Festinger's (1957) cognitive dissonance theory. Festinger posits that people want to maintain and maximize the consistency of their cognitions because dissonance—incoherence among one's cognitions and behavior—is uncomfortable. As a result of wanting things to make sense, people attempt to reconcile inconsistencies by changing their cognitions (e.g., attitudes) or their behavior. Fritz Heider's (1958) balance theory of consistency has also been highly influential. It posits that all situations comprise entities (people or ideas) that are connected through positive or negative relations—sentiments (like or dislike) and units (entities that do or do not belong together). Heider theorized that people are motivated to maintain balance to establish order.

It should be noted that the existence of a *universal* need for cognitive consistency has recently been questioned (Kruglanski et al., 2018). Kruglanski and colleagues (2018) argue that effects typically attributed to dissonance reduction, for example, are better explained by an interaction between expectancies about different cognitive outcomes and the desirability of those outcomes. They note, for example, that individuals who hold unpleasant beliefs, for example, that they have a health problem, may actually welcome receiving inconsistent evidence. The motivation to change cognitions or behavior when there is inconsistency may also depend on the extent to which the cognitions involved in an inconsistency are beliefs that are shared with significant others (Rossignac-Milon & Higgins, 2018).

Lay Epistemics: Need for Closure

Arie Kruglanski's (1989, 1990) theory of lay epistemics posits that classification of an individual's epistemic motivations can be based on the person's disposition toward different types of closure. He suggests that people act as lay scientists by generating and evaluating hypotheses, and that this motivated process is prompted by discrepancies between their actual state and a desired epistemic state. In line with this theory, evidence reveals that people with a strong need for *nonspecific* closure tend to engage readily in truth seeking through hypothesis generation and testing but stop as soon as any plausible hypothesis is supported, as they are motivated to come to a "final" answer as quickly as possible. On the other hand, those

with a strong need for *specific* closure often remain within the hypothesis-generation phase until they find the particular epistemic "reality" they seek, at which point they stop seeking and even avoid alternative hypotheses.

Truth from Accessibility: Motivation to Reduce Uncertainty

In addition to needs for cognition and consistency, people are motivated to establish the truth about stimuli in cases of uncertainty. Beyond simply lacking information, both ambiguous information and vague information create a sense of uncertainty. A sense of certainty can be restored by categorizing such information in a way that expresses clarity about what it is (despite it being unclear). For example, research on accessibility reveals that the categorizations a person makes about another person's behavior are affected by which applicable mental categories are most *accessible* at the time of judgment, despite the level of accessibility (from priming or chronic accessibility) being independent of the properties of that person's behavior (Higgins, 1996). In one study (Higgins & Brendl, 1995), for example, participants were or were not primed with the construct "conceited." In a supposedly "unrelated" subsequent study, they then read a short story about a student named Sue. The story was written and tested to be highly vague, with most readers having no impression at all of what kind of person Sue was. Nonetheless, those participants who were primed with "conceited" *and* personally had "conceited" as a chronically accessible construct formed a clear impression that Sue was conceited. A construct with high accessibility is experienced as motivationally relevant (Eitam & Higgins, 2010), which increases the readiness to identify input as matching the construct, yielding certainty from accessibility and categorization even for highly vague input.

Shared Reality: Motivation to Co-Create and Socially Validate Truth

Similar to value, the motive for truth is also inherently social. Higgins and colleagues posit that humans have a fundamental need to co-construct and share their understanding of reality with others (Echterhoff, Higgins, & Levine, 2009; Hardin & Higgins, 1996; Higgins, 2016, 2019). This need is driven by both relational and epistemic motives, but here we focus on epistemic motives given our current focus on truth effectiveness. These epistemic motives reflect the need to establish meaning and achieve understanding of the world (Echterhoff & Higgins, 2017; Echterhoff et al., 2009).

Much of the research on shared reality has taken place within a "saying-is-believing" paradigm in which participants are asked to describe a target person's behaviors to an audience, with assessment of the valence of their memories of those behaviors taking place at a later time (e.g., Echterhoff et al., 2005, 2008; Higgins & Rholes, 1978). Participants first read a description of a target person (e.g., Michael) featuring ambiguous behaviors that might be evaluated either positively or negatively. They are then told that they need to describe Michael to members of an audience who know him, so that audience members will be able to guess the target. Next, the experimenter casually mentions that the audience members like or dislike Michael. At this point, participants describe Michael to the audience; typically, they "tune" the valence of their descriptions to match the attitude of the audience members, such that descriptions of Michael are positive when participants believe the audience likes him and are negative when participants believe the audience dislikes him. More importantly, though, when assessed after the primary task, even weeks later, participants' memories of Michael evaluatively match the "tuned" message—demonstrating the creation of a shared reality. These studies reveal that shared realities are created in cases in which audience-tuned messages are treated as the truth despite actually being distortions from reality. It is the shared message that is treated as real.

Although shared realities manifest in various stages of development (including shared practices, shared beliefs, and shared coordinated roles; see Higgins, 2016), here we would like to emphasize *shared relevance,* which is at the core of every shared reality (Higgins, 2019). When individuals share relevance with others, they share what is important or worthy of attention—what is motivationally relevant. This concept of motivational relevance will play an important role as we discuss next how goals are selected.

Motivations Working Together

The three primary motives we just reviewed—value, control, and truth as three general motivational principles—do not operate in isolation. A fourth motivational principle is that these motives *work together* to influence goal selection (deciding *what* goal to pursue and *why*) and the goal pursuit process (deciding *how* to pursue the goal).

Value, Truth, and Control in Goal Selection

Goal choice is driven by the *motivational relevance* of potential goals at any moment in time that determines accessibility (Eitam & Higgins, 2010). Specifically, goals are assessed in terms of value, truth, and control relevance. But before continuing, we need to address the question "What are goals?"

What Are Goals?

Goals are mental representations that comprise desired end states and their means of pursuit (Kruglanski et al., 2002; Shah & Kruglanski, 2000). Like other mental representations, goals vary in accessibility and may be activated either consciously or nonconsciously (e.g., through features within one's environment; Bargh, 1990). However, unlike *semantic* mental representations for which priming effects typically decay over time (Higgins, 1996), the activation of *goal* representations (particularly if co-activated with positive affect; see Custers, 2009) generally increases in strength until the goal is fulfilled (Förster, Liberman, & Higgins, 2005) or the goal is co-activated with negative affect (Aarts, Custers, & Holland, 2007). When activated, these representations appear to direct information processing about goal-relevant people (Chartrand & Bargh, 1996) and objects (Ferguson & Bargh, 2004). Furthermore, activation has been shown to produce cascading effects on behavioral intentions (Ferguson & Bargh, 2004), behavior

(Bargh, Chen, & Burrows, 1996), and mood resulting from perceived success or failure (Chartrand & Bargh, 2002).

Goal Types

Scholars have proposed a wide range of frameworks for categorizing goal types. Here we summarize two classification schemes that have received considerable attention.

Promotion versus Prevention Focus. Regulatory focus theory posits the existence of two distinct, independent self-regulatory systems: promotion and prevention (Higgins, 1997). The difference between promotion and prevention is primarily a distinction within the domain of *value,* although these orientations are also related to particular goal-pursuit strategies involving truth and control, as we discuss further in the section on goal pursuit.

Individuals with a promotion focus are concerned with the presence or absence of positive outcomes (gains and non-gains), such as the goals associated with one's ideal self-guides. Promotion goals relate to aspirations, nurturance, growth, and progress. In contrast, individuals with a prevention focus are concerned with the absence or presence of negative outcomes (non-losses and losses), such as the goals associated with one's ought self-guides. Prevention goals relate to safety, security, and responsibility.

Importantly, these two orientations are relatively independent: A person can have a strong promotion focus and weak prevention focus (i.e., promotion predominance), a strong prevention focus and weak prevention focus (i.e., prevention predominance), or be strong in both or weak in both. Additionally, while people tend to sustain a chronic, long-term regulatory focus that reflects the historical motivational relevance of promotion and prevention value, regulatory focus is a *state* that can also vary across situations.

Recently, the difference between promotion and prevention has been highlighted as a "story of 0." If one's current state were represented as a status quo "0," promotion- and prevention-focused individuals would view it in fundamentally different ways (Higgins, 2018b; Higgins

& Cornwell, 2016). Promotion-focused people are sensitive to the difference between "0" and "+1," with "+1" being experienced as a positive success (gain), and "0" (or anything below it) being experienced as a negative failure (non-gain). In contrast, prevention-focused people are sensitive to the difference between "0" and "–1," with "0" (or anything above it) being experienced as a positive success (non-loss) and "–1" being experienced as a negative failure (loss). What this means is that *neither* promotion-focused individuals *nor* prevention-focused individuals experience the state of "0" as neutral, as traditional approach–avoidance theorists might assume. Rather, promotion-focused individuals experience the maintenance of the status quo as a negative failure (non-gain), whereas prevention-focused individuals experience it as a positive success (non-loss).

In addition, the notion of goal *pursuit* implies that the pursuer is *not* yet experiencing the positive success of achieving the desired end state. Instead, the pursuer is currently experiencing some kind of negative failure (i.e., a discrepancy from the desired end state; see Higgins, 1987), with the kind of unsatisfactory state from negative failure varying by regulatory focus. Given that negative failures are experienced as nongains in the promotion system, the current state of an individual pursuing a promotion goal is likely to be represented as "0." In contrast, given that negative failures are experienced as losses in the prevention system, the current state of an individual pursuing a prevention goal is likely to be represented as "–1." More research is needed to identify the experienced reference points for promotion versus prevention goal pursuit (Higgins & Liberman, 2018).

Regulatory focus also influences the degree to which people take on different types of goals. For example, consider risky decision making. People with a prevention focus are generally risk-averse, with the goal of maintaining their satisfactory status quo. However, in cases of current loss, when a risky option offers the only opportunity to recover from the loss (i.e., restore a non-loss status quo), individuals with a prevention focus are more likely to choose the risky option than those with a promotion focus (Scholer, Zou, Fujita, Stroessner, & Higgins,

2010). Conversely, promotion-focused individuals, who tend to be relatively risk seeking, with the goal of making progress, choose the less risky option after they have made a significant gain (Zou, Scholer, & Higgins, 2014). In addition to these different goals that impact risk preferences, people with a promotion focus have task goals that prioritize speed versus accuracy, creative versus analytical thinking, and feelings versus reasons, with prevention-focused individuals preferring the opposite (Higgins & Cornwell, 2016).

Performance versus Mastery Goals. Another well-studied distinction is between performance- and mastery-oriented achievement goals (e.g., Ames & Archer, 1988; Elliott & Dweck, 1988; Nicholls, 1984). Performance goals are concerned with demonstrating sufficient ability in a particular domain, whereas mastery goals are associated with increasing the extent and scope of one's abilities over time. These orientations are associated with distinct implications for task choice. Whereas people with performance-oriented goals sacrifice actual learning to ensure that they are able to demonstrate their abilities, and select a level of task difficulty that maximizes displays of competence, people with mastery-oriented goals prioritize learning and growth, even if it means that their immediate performance suffers.

Recent work suggests the performance versus mastery distinction is even more useful when goals are further distinguished as approach- versus avoidance-focused performance or mastery goals, as both performance *and* mastery *avoidance* goals predict undesirable outcomes (Moller & Elliott, 2006). Conversely, whereas mastery approach goals appear to be associated with interest, performance approach goals offer unique benefits, including persistence and achievement (Senko, Hulleman, & Harackiewicz, 2011). This model highlights the dynamic interplay among value, truth, and control motives. When a performance goal is set, control trumps truth, as individuals take care to manage their goal pursuit to approach achievement or avoid self-evaluative failure. On the other hand, when a mastery approach goal is set, individuals embrace the truth of their current level of proficiency and forgo some immediate control to deepen their expertise.

How Are Goals Selected?

Most models of goal selection treat the process as rational, such as being guided by a maximization, "value × likelihood" analysis. For example, within their Rubicon model of action phases, Heckhausen and Gollwitzer (1987) propose that goal selection and pursuit take place within a sequential process comprising distinct phases, which are divided at a high level by deciding to take action—a step described as crossing a "psychological Rubicon." On one side of the Rubicon is the *predecisional* phase; on the other side are postdecisional phases (*preactional, actional,* and *postactional*; Gollwitzer, 1990; Heckhausen & Gollwitzer, 1987).

Regarding goal setting, let's consider the predecisional phase. According to Gollwitzer (1990), the predecisional phase is characterized by wishing and deliberating. Wishes represent desired and undesired outcomes, and deliberations take into account both the desirability and feasibility of each goal option. One crosses the Rubicon upon committing to a goal and transforming it into a specific intention.

Despite differences in their specifics, many models of goal setting account for the value of a given outcome (e.g., "desirability") in combination with the likelihood of achieving the outcome (e.g., "feasibility"; see Bargh et al., 2010). Traditionally, this conceptualization of goal selection has taken the form of subjective expected utility (SEU) models. These models posit a multiplicative relation between the subjective value of each potential outcome and the subjective probability of each outcome (often described as its likelihood or expectancy), and they typically assume that the potential outcomes are mutually exclusive and exhaustive (Higgins, Franks, Pavarini, Sehnert, & Manley, 2013). It is important to note that despite seemingly accounting for truth and control via expectancies, traditional SEU actually emphasizes only *value* calculations, as expectancies are considered to only moderate the degree to which an option is valuable (for more details on this point, see Higgins, 2012; Higgins et al., 2013).

Atkinson's (1964) theory of achievement motivation was similar to SEU models based on its reliance on a value × likelihood calculation to predict goal selection. However, Atkinson included a new variable (a relatively stable personality characteristic called the *motive to achieve*) and, more importantly, a special assumption that the incentive value of an activity and its expectancy of success are decimal values that sum to one. Implicit in this assumption is the concept that challenging activities, which have a lower likelihood of success, generate greater pride upon their achievement because they have higher value. As a result, the model predicts that goals of middling levels of difficulty are most likely to be selected because value × expectancy is highest at .5 × .5. This special assumption is noteworthy because, unlike traditional SEU, in which likelihood simply acts as a moderator for value's motivational force, here Atkinson suggests that expectancies relate to worth in their own right. Similarly, Higgins (2012) argued that high likelihood or expectancy has high truth effectiveness because it makes a future outcome real rather than imaginary.

In the ensuing years, Wigfield and Eccles (2000) developed a more complex take on an expectancy–value model of achievement motivation. What makes their model distinct is that both expectancies and values are affected by beliefs about the specific goals at hand. These include beliefs about one's ability to achieve this specific goal, which broadly relate to control effectiveness, with some truth involved as well.

Although SEU models seem to capture the phenomenology of how people evaluate goal options, reality may not be as straightforward as these theories suggest. For example, research reveals that expectancy judgments (i.e., the truth- and control-focused aspects of these theories) are affected by the desirability (i.e., value) of a potential outcome—motivated cognition. Specifically, the perceived likelihood of achieving an outcome—even a truly random outcome such as the draw of a card from a deck—has been shown to increase with the outcome's desirability in both grade school children (Marks, 1951) and college-age adults (Irwin, 1953). As another example, people who are hungry report greater expectancies of winning a food incentive in a drawing (Biner, Angle, Park, Mellinger, & Barber, 1995).

Additionally, more recent research has revealed that the probabilities inherent in these models are not perceived as rationally as the standard models have claimed. Higgins and colleagues (2013) have found that the very same information about a particular event's probability of occurrence is treated as more or less *real* (i.e., as more or less likely) depending on how that probability is *expressed*. In these studies, for *both* positive future events and negative future events involving two possible outcomes (*A* or *B*), events *expressed* with high likelihood language (80% *B*) produced stronger engagement in, and more intense evaluative judgments of, objects in the *present* than the *same* probable future event expressed with low likelihood language (20% *A*)—making, at the same time, a liked yogurt even more liked and a disliked yogurt even more disliked. When a high-likelihood expression was used for a future event (whether it was a positive or negative event), the event was treated as more "real" (i.e., high in truth), which strengthened engagement in the present while preparing for this real future event. This strengthened present engagement intensified the evaluations of the liked and disliked yogurts that were being tasted in the present.

How Are Goals Activated?

Until this point, we have focused on theoretical distinctions related to goal setting rather than on the specifics of how goals become active within the mind. However, in order for a goal to be "selected" in the sense that it guides behavior, it must be accessible and activated (Eitam & Higgins, 2010; Higgins, 1996; Higgins & Eitam, 2014). In the next section, we highlight two approaches to understanding how this process works.

"Direct Expression" Account. Early research on automaticity suggested that priming a social category would prompt the mental activation of stereotypical traits associated with the primed group (Bargh, 1994). Inspired by James's (1890/2007) "ideomotor" notion, Bargh and colleagues (1996) proposed that this activation might, in turn, trigger an unconscious goal to embody the trait within one's actions. To test this "direct expression" model and explore the effects of environmental stimuli on goal pursuit, Bargh and colleagues presented participants with primes (e.g., "Florida," "Bingo") that activated the mental representation of the social category "elderly," then measured the participants' subsequent walking behavior after the study was supposedly over. Notably, for most participants the social category "elderly" includes the information that they walk slowly, but "walk slowly" was not itself primed in the study. Spreading activation from "elderly" to "walk slowly" was expected to occur, such that "walk slowly" would be activated. This research supported a direct expression account: Compared to control participants not primed with "elderly," participants primed with "elderly" walked slowly while leaving the study, without any conscious awareness that the priming had influenced their subsequent action.

Despite Bargh and colleagues' (1996) original findings, this specific effect is not always found; across a wider range of studies, people primed with the concept "elderly" have *not* consistently appeared to adopt the goal of walking more slowly (Doyen, Klein, Pichon, & Cleeremans, 2012). One explanation for the inconsistencies is that behavioral priming may be affected by subtle factors of which the original researchers were unaware, such as variable features of the experimental setting and individual differences among participant samples. Such additional factors could make the "walk slowly" phenomenon appear and disappear. The implications of this possibility are considered next.

"Motivated Preparation to Interact" Account. Research exploring the motivational underpinnings of unconscious goal pursuit suggests one reason why these goal priming effects have not been consistently found. Cesario, Plaks, and Higgins (2006) proposed that people mentally represent members of social categories in the service of self-regulation, including preparing to interact with members of the social category. But preparation to interact with social category members would also be influenced by how one feels about them. Do you like them or dislike them? If you like them, then you use your knowledge of them to facilitate the interaction, to make it happen. But if you dislike them, then you use your knowledge of them to avoid interacting with them. This means that participants who like elderly adults should walk slowly after being primed with "elderly," as Bargh and colleagues (1996) found, in order to facilitate interacting with them, but those who dislike elderly adults should walk

quickly after being primed with "elderly" in order to avoid them. Both the predicted replication *and* the reversal were found by Cesario and colleagues (for further evidence supporting the "preparation to interact" account, see Cesario, Plaks, Hagiwara, Navarrete, & Higgins, 2010).

Motivational Relevance: Value, Truth, and Control in Goal Activation

Given the importance of value, truth, and control motives in goal selection, it is not surprising that these motives also contribute to a goal's mental *activation*. Specifically, Eitam and Higgins (2010) offer a motivational account for goal activation in their "relevance of a representation" ("ROAR") framework, positing that activation is driven by the *motivational relevance* of a goal representation. And the motivational relevance of a goal representation is a function of that goal's current relevance to value, truth, and control effectiveness.

Value, Truth, and Control in the Process of Goal Pursuit

Similar to the process of goal selection, the same three primary motives work together to influence *how* people pursue the goals they take on. At a high level, we propose that truth and control motives primarily drive the process of goal pursuit, as both motives are inherent in an effective goal pursuit journey—what has been referred to as "going in the right direction" (Higgins, 2018a). Below, we review several theories outlining how these motives work together in a complementary fashion to facilitate effective goal pursuit.

Cybernetic Theories: Control Process Models of Goal Pursuit

Cybernetic theories (Wiener, 1961) suggest that effective goal-directed behavior requires the integration of control, truth, and value. They posit that activity is produced through sequential feedback loops within which one's current state is compared to a desired end state reference point. When one's current state does not match this reference point, behaviors are undertaken to move oneself closer to the desired end state (i.e., reduce any discrepancy). Within these models, value is captured by the desired end state reference point; truth is captured by the monitoring feedback information (how am I doing?); and control is captured by the action taken to reduce any discrepancy.

Beyond the TOTE model described earlier in this chapter, Carver and Scheier's (1981, 1998) reference point model has been influential in describing how motives interact within the process of goal pursuit. In particular, this model highlights how control and truth motives work together to facilitate gathering and acting upon self-evaluative feedback at two levels. Within the first level of feedback, which concerns one's journey toward goal achievement, the person engages in comparison, contrasting *input* information about his or her current state with a *reference value* reflecting his or her desired state in search of discrepancies; when discrepancies are identified via error signals, an *output* is produced that drives action to minimize the mismatch. In addition to this first level of feedback, Carver and Scheier posit that a second layer of feedback tracks the speed at which discrepancies are reduced and manifests as positive affect (fast enough) or negative affect (not fast enough). This affect in turn impacts the urgency behind the output action.

Interestingly, this affective layer of feedback can produce effects that are not always helpful. For example, the positive feelings that arise when discrepancies are reduced faster than expected have been shown to produce "coasting" behavior, whereby the individual reduces effort in the goal-directed activity, particularly when the person is close to attaining the goal (Fulford, Johnson, Llabre, & Carver, 2010; Louro, Pieters, & Zeelenberg, 2007).

Regulatory Mode: Going in the Right Direction

Regulatory mode theory proposes that there are two basic, independent self-regulatory functions that work together to produce goal-directed activity (Higgins, Kruglanski, & Pierro, 2003; Kruglanski, Pierro, Mannetti, & Higgins, 2013; Kruglanski et al., 2000). *Assessment* is fundamentally related to truth motives, and it constitutes the motivation to compare and critically evaluate options in order to identify the right option. *Locomotion* is fundamentally re-

lated to control motives, and it constitutes the motivation to move away from the current state in order to effect change (Higgins, 2012; Kruglanski et al., 2013) Just like strength of promotion and prevention, strength of locomotion and assessment can vary across individuals as a chronic predisposition, as well as vary situationally.

Furthermore, assessment and locomotion are typically most effective when they constrain each other, such that neither is overly active or dominant (Higgins, 2018a; Pierro, Chernikova, Lo Destro, Higgins, & Kruglanski, 2018). For example, individuals who are too strong in assessment often experience greater regret and rumination as a result of failure, which can be detrimental to subsequent goal pursuit (Pierro et al., 2008). Strong assessment also appears to be associated with distress from the possibility of making the "wrong" decision (Chen, Rossignac-Milon, & Higgins, 2018). On the other hand, when individuals are too strong in locomotion, they may make impulsive decisions that lead to ineffectiveness in the domain of control (Mannetti et al., 2009). Strong locomotors are also known to engage in unwarranted self-flattery (Komissarouk, Chernikova, Kruglanski, & Higgins, 2018). That said, when they are both strong and well balanced, assessment and locomotion generally work together to promote effective goal pursuit in a variety of domains, such as grade point average (GPA; Kruglanski et al., 2000), retirement savings (Kim, Franks, & Higgins, 2013), and teamwork (Mauro, Pierro, Mannetti, Higgins, & Kruglanski, 2009).

Regulatory Fit: Aligning Motivational Orientations and Goal Pursuit Strategies

Research has also established that goal striving benefits from a match between individual motivational orientations and the strategic manner of goal pursuit—*regulatory fit* (Higgins, 2000). For example, individuals are more interested in doing an activity again later when the manner in which they originally did the activity was a fit, rather than a non-fit, with their motivational orientation toward that activity, such as doing an activity in a serious manner (fit) rather than in an enjoyable manner (non-fit) when they consider that activity to be important (Higgins, Cesario, Hagiwara, Spiegel, & Pittman, 2010). Doing an activity in a non-fit manner undermined interest in engaging in that activity again. Thus, for the activity that participants considered to be important, having them do it in an enjoyable manner actually subverted their interest in doing it again later. Lesson: Adding fun to an activity is not always a good idea.

In another study on regulatory fit, Avnet and Higgins (2003) had participants choose among different book lights using different decision-making strategies. Those participants who made their decision using a strategy that fit their regulatory mode orientation offered much more of their own money to buy their choice (which was, intentionally, the same for everyone). Locomotion-induced participants experienced fit when they used a progressive elimination strategy of removing one option at a time as they progressively considered different features of the book lights. In contrast, assessment-induced participants experienced fit when they used a full comparison strategy of critically comparing all of the options to one another for all of the book-light features before making any decision (see also Mathmann, Chylinski, de Ruyter, & Higgins, 2017).

There is evidence that the benefits of regulatory fit are wide-ranging. In the domain of health, for example, a field experiment testing the effects of promotion- versus prevention-focused messaging within a physical activity guide found that regulatory fit (eager messaging for promotion; vigilant messaging for prevention) resulted in increased activity (Latimer et al., 2008). Other recent research found that a fit between an exerciser's induced regulatory focus and the exercise environment—specifically, whether one counts up (fit for promotion) versus down (fit for prevention)—improved actual performance across a range of calisthenic exercises (Kay & Grimm, 2017).

In the domain of sports performance, Plessner, Unkelbach, Memmert, Baltes, and Kolb (2009) studied the performance of football (soccer) players in the German Football Association. In particular, these researchers examined the effects of regulatory fit between participants' chronic regulatory focus (i.e., whether these players generally tend to be ei-

ther prevention-focused or promotion-focused) and the regulatory focus of a given task, as framed by coaches' messaging. They found that prevention-focused players had more success in scoring goals during a shootout practice of five tries when the coach used a vigilant message ("Your obligation is not to miss more than two times") than an eager message ("Your aspiration is to score at least three times"). The opposite was true for the promotion-focused players.

Motivational Harmony: Effective Integration of Value, Truth, and Control Motives

A broader experience of fit has also been identified among individuals who indicate relatively equal and strong motivations to be effective in value, truth, and control (Cornwell et al., 2019; Higgins, Cornwell, & Franks, 2014). Cornwell and colleagues (2019) suggest that when there is a "proper mix" of all three motives, working together in a balanced way, a sense of fit between individuals and the world around them is created that manifests in a global feeling that life is going "right," which ultimately contributes to one's experience of happiness and meaning in life. They found that motivational harmony is positively associated with life satisfaction, balanced character strengths and virtues, and moral behavior.

Conclusion

In this chapter, we have reviewed a range of historical perspectives on the question of what motivates people, and discussed how the motivational principles of value, truth, and control, and the motivational principle of their *working together,* influence both goal selection and goal pursuit. We have described how different motivational orientations and strategies—both on their own and in combination with one another—appear to offer a range of benefits, as well as potential drawbacks. By understanding better how motivation works, people can apply the motivational principles to be more effective in goal selection and goal pursuit, thereby "going in the right direction" and experiencing "the good life" on a more regular basis.

REFERENCES

Aarts, H., Custers, R., & Holland, R. W. (2007). The nonconscious cessation of goal pursuit: When goals and negative affect are coactivated. *Journal of Personality and Social Psychology, 92*(2), 165–178.

Ames, C., & Archer, J. (1988). Achievement goals in the classroom: Students' learning strategies and motivation processes. *Journal of Educational Psychology, 80*(3), 260–267.

Anema, A., Wood, E., Weiser, S. D., Qi, J., Montaner, J. S., & Kerr, T. (2010). Hunger and associated harms among injection drug users in an urban Canadian setting. *Substance Abuse Treatment, Prevention, and Policy, 5*(1), Article No. 20.

Atkinson, J. W. (1964). *An introduction to motivation.* Princeton, NJ: Van Nostrand.

Avnet, T., & Higgins, E. T. (2003). Locomotion, assessment, and regulatory fit: Value transfer from "how" to "what." *Journal of Experimental Social Psychology, 39*(5), 525–530.

Bandura, A. (1977). Self-efficacy: Toward a unifying theory of behavioral change. *Psychological Review, 84*(2), 191–215.

Bandura, A. (1982). Self-efficacy mechanism in human agency. *American Psychologist, 37*(2), 122–147.

Bandura, A. (1997). *Self-efficacy: The exercise of control.* New York: Freeman.

Bargh, J. A. (1990). Auto-motives: Preconscious determinants of social interaction. In E. T. Higgins & R. M. Sorrentino (Eds.), *Handbook of motivation and cognition: Foundations of social behavior* (Vol. 2, pp. 93–130). New York: Guilford Press.

Bargh, J. A. (1994). The four horsemen of automaticity: Awareness, intention, efficiency, and control in social cognition. In R. S. Wyer, Jr. & T. K. Srull (Eds.), *Handbook of social cognition: Basic processes* (2nd ed., Vol. 1, pp. 1–40). Hillsdale, NJ: Erlbaum.

Bargh, J. A., Chen, M., & Burrows, L. (1996). Automaticity of social behavior: Direct effects of trait construct and stereotype-activation on action. *Journal of Personality and Social Psychology, 71*(2), 230–244.

Bargh, J. A., Gollwitzer, P. M., & Oettingen, G. (2010). Motivation. In S. T. Fiske, D. T. Gilbert, & G. Lindzey (Eds.), *Handbook of social psychology* (5th ed., Vol. 1, pp. 268–316). Hoboken, NJ: Wiley.

Baumeister, R. F., & Leary, M. R. (1995). The need to belong: Desire for interpersonal attachments as a fundamental human motivation. *Psychological Bulletin, 117*(3), 497–529.

Bentham, J. (1823). *An introduction to the principles of morals and legislation* (2nd ed., 2 vols.). London: Pickering.

Biner, P. M., Angle, S. T., Park, J. H., Mellinger, A. E., & Barber, B. C. (1995). Need state and the illusion of control. *Personality and Social Psychology Bulletin, 21*(9), 899–907.

Bowlby, J. (1969). *Attachment and loss: Vol. 1. Attachment.* New York: Basic Books.

Bruner, J. S., & Goodman, C. C. (1947). Value and need as organizing factors in perception. *Journal of Abnormal and Social Psychology, 42*(1), 33–44.

Byrne, D. (1961). Anxiety and the experimental arousal of affiliation need. *Journal of Abnormal and Social Psychology, 63*(3), 660–662.

Cacioppo, J. T., & Petty, R. E. (1982). The need for cognition. *Journal of Personality and Social Psychology, 42*(1), 116–131.

Carver, C. S., & Scheier, M. F. (1981). *Attention and self-regulation: A control-theory approach to human behavior.* New York: Springer-Verlag.

Carver, C. S., & Scheier, M. F. (1998). *On the self-regulation of behavior.* New York: Cambridge University Press.

Cesario, J., Plaks, J. E., Hagiwara, N., Navarrete, C. D., & Higgins, E. T. (2010). The ecology of automaticity: How situational contingencies shape action semantics and social behavior. *Psychological Science, 21*(9), 1311–1317.

Cesario, J., Plaks, J. E., & Higgins, E. T. (2006). Automatic social behavior as motivated preparation to interact. *Journal of Personality and Social Psychology, 90*(6), 893–910.

Chartrand, T. L., & Bargh, J. A. (1996). Automatic activation of impression formation and memorization goals: Nonconscious goal priming reproduces effects of explicit task instructions. *Journal of Personality and Social Psychology, 71*(3), 464–478.

Chartrand, T. L., & Bargh, J. A. (2002). Nonconscious motivations: Their activation, operation, and consequences. In A. Tesser, D. A. Stapel, & J. V. Wood (Eds.), *Self and motivation: Emerging psychological perspectives* (pp. 13–41). Washington, DC: American Psychological Association.

Chen, C. Y., Rossignac-Milon, M., & Higgins, E. T. (2018). Feeling distressed from making decisions: Assessors' need to be right. *Journal of Personality and Social Psychology, 115*(4), 743–761.

Cohen, A. R., Stotland, E., & Wolfe, D. M. (1955). An experimental investigation of need for cognition. *Journal of Abnormal and Social Psychology, 51*(2), 291–294.

Cornwell, J. F. M., Franks, B., & Higgins, E. T. (2019). The proper mix: Balancing motivational orientations in goal pursuit. *Journal of the Association for Consumer Research, 4*(1), 13–20.

Custers, R. (2009). How does our unconscious know what we want?: The role of affect in goal representations. In G. B. Moskowitz & H. Grant (Eds.), *The psychology of goals* (pp. 179–202). New York: Guilford Press.

Darwin, C. (1909). *The origin of species.* New York: P. F. Collier & Son.

Deci, E. L., & Ryan, R. M. (1980). The empirical exploration of intrinsic motivational processes. *Advances in Experimental Social Psychology, 13,* 39–80.

Deci, E. L., & Ryan, R. M. (2000). The "what" and "why" of goal pursuits: Human needs and the self-determination of behavior. *Psychological Inquiry, 11*(4), 227–268.

Doyen, S., Klein, O., Pichon, C.-L., & Cleeremans, A. (2012). Behavioral priming: It's all in the mind, but whose mind? *PLOS ONE, 7*(1), e29081.

Dunning, D., & Balcetis, E. (2013). Wishful seeing: How preferences shape visual perception. *Current Directions in Psychological Science, 22*(1), 33–37.

Echterhoff, G., & Higgins, E. T. (2017). Creating shared reality in interpersonal and intergroup communication: The role of epistemic processes and their interplay. *European Review of Social Psychology, 28*(1), 175–226.

Echterhoff, G., Higgins, E. T., & Groll, S. (2005). Audience-tuning effects on memory: The role of shared reality. *Journal of Personality and Social Psychology, 89*(3), 257–276.

Echterhoff, G., Higgins, E. T., Kopietz, R., & Groll, S. (2008). How communication goals determine when audience tuning biases memory. *Journal of Experimental Psychology: General, 137*(1), 3–21.

Echterhoff, G., Higgins, E. T., & Levine, J. M. (2009). Shared reality: Experiencing commonality with others' inner states about the world. *Perspectives on Psychological Science, 4*(5), 496–521.

Echterhoff, G., Kopietz, R., & Higgins, E. T. (2013). Adjusting shared reality: Communicators' memory changes as their connection with their audience changes. *Social Cognition, 31*(2), 162–186.

Eitam, B., & Higgins, E. T. (2010). Motivation in mental accessibility: Relevance of a representation (ROAR) as a new framework. *Social and Personality Psychology Compass, 4*(10), 951–967.

Eitam, B., & Higgins, E. T. (2014). What's in a goal?: The role of motivational relevance in cognition and action. *Behavioral and Brain Sciences, 37*(2), 141–142.

Elliott, E. S., & Dweck, C. S. (1988). Goals: An approach to motivation and achievement. *Journal of Personality and Social Psychology, 54*(1), 5–12.

Etsy. (2018, September 30). *Goal digger.* Retrieved September 30, 2018, from *www.etsy.com/market/goal_digger.*

Ferguson, M. J., & Bargh, J. A. (2004). Liking is for doing: The effects of goal pursuit on automatic evaluation. *Journal of Personality and Social Psychology, 87*(5), 557–572.

Festinger, L. (1957). *A theory of cognitive dissonance.* Stanford, CA: Stanford University Press.

Förster, J., Liberman, N., & Higgins, E. T. (2005). Accessibility from active and fulfilled goals. *Journal of Experimental Social Psychology, 41*(3), 220–239.

Freud, S. (1957). Instincts and their vicissitudes. In J. Strachey (Ed. & Trans.), *The standard edition of the complete psychological works of Sigmund Freud* (Vol. 14, pp. 113–138). London: Hogarth Press.

Freud, S. (1962). *The ego and the id* (J. Strachey, Trans.). New York: Norton.

Fulford, D., Johnson, S. L., Llabre, M. M., & Carver, C. S. (2010). Pushing and coasting in dynamic goal pursuit: Coasting is attenuated in bipolar disorder. *Psychological Science, 21*(7), 1021–1027.

Gallagher, M. W., & Lopez, S. J. (2007). Curiosity and well-being. *Journal of Positive Psychology, 2*(4), 236–248.

Gollwitzer, P. M. (1990). Action phases and mind-sets. In E. T. Higgins & R. M. Sorrentino (Eds.), *Handbook of motivation and cognition: Foundations of social behavior* (Vol. 2, pp. 53–92). New York: Guilford Press.

Hardin, C. D., & Higgins, E. T. (1996). Shared reality: How social verification makes the subjective objective. In R. M. Sorrentino & E. T. Higgins (Eds.), *Handbook of motivation and cognition: The interpersonal context* (Vol. 3, pp. 28–84). New York: Guilford Press.

Heckhausen, H., & Gollwitzer, P. M. (1987). Thought contents and cognitive functioning in motivational vs. volitional states of mind. *Motivation and Emotion, 11*(2), 101–120.

Heider, F. (1958). *The psychology of interpersonal relations.* Hillsdale, NJ: Erlbaum.

Higgins, E. T. (1987). Self-discrepancy: A theory relating self and affect. *Psychological Review, 94*(3), 319–340.

Higgins, E. T. (1991). Development of self-regulatory and self-evaluative processes: Costs, benefits, and trade offs. In M. R. Gunnar & A. Sroufe (Eds.), *Minnesota Symposium on Child Psychology* (pp. 125–165). Hillsdale, NJ: Erlbaum.

Higgins, E. T. (1996). Knowledge activation: Accessibility, applicability, and salience. In E. T. Higgins & A. W. Kruglanski (Eds.), *Social psychology: Handbook of basic principles* (pp. 133–168). New York: Guilford Press.

Higgins, E. T. (1997). Beyond pleasure and pain. *American Psychologist, 52*(12), 1280–1300.

Higgins, E. T. (2000). Making a good decision: Value from fit. *American Psychologist, 55*(11), 1217–1230.

Higgins, E. T. (2006). Value from hedonic experience and engagement. *Psychological Review, 113*(3), 439–460.

Higgins, E. T. (2012). *Beyond pleasure and pain: How motivation works.* New York: Oxford University Press.

Higgins, E. T. (2016). Shared-reality development in childhood. *Perspectives on Psychological Science, 11*(4), 466–495.

Higgins, E. T. (2018a). Going in the right direction: Locomotion control and assessment truth, working together. In C. E. Kopetz & A. Fishbach (Eds.), *The motivation–cognition interface: From the lab to the real world: A Festschrift in honor of Arie W. Kruglanski.* New York: Routledge.

Higgins, E. T. (2018b). What distinguishes promotion and prevention?: Attaining "+1" from "0" as non-gain vs. maintaining "0" as non-loss. *Polish Psychological Bulletin, 49*(1), 40–49.

Higgins, E. T. (2019). *Shared reality: What makes us strong and tears us apart.* New York: Oxford University Press.

Higgins, E. T., & Brendl, C. M. (1995). Accessibility and applicability: Some "activation rules" influencing judgment. *Journal of Experimental Social Psychology, 31*(3), 218–243.

Higgins, E. T., Cesario, J., Hagiwara, N., Spiegel, S., & Pittman, T. (2010). Increasing or decreasing interest in activities: The role of regulatory fit. *Journal of Personality and Social Psychology, 98*(4), 559–572.

Higgins, E. T., & Cornwell, J. F. M. (2016). Securing foundations and advancing frontiers: Prevention and promotion effects on judgment and decision making. *Organizational Behavior and Human Decision Processes, 136,* 56–67.

Higgins, E. T., Cornwell, J. F. M., & Franks, B. (2014). "Happiness" and "the good life" as motives working together effectively. In A. J. Elliot (Ed.), *Advances in motivation science* (Vol. 1, pp. 135–179). Waltham, MA: Academic Press.

Higgins, E. T., & Eitam, B. (2014). Priming . . . shmiming: It's about knowing when and why stimulated memory representations become active. *Social Cognition, 32*(Suppl.), 225–242.

Higgins, E. T., Franks, B., Pavarini, D., Sehnert, S., & Manley, K. (2013). Expressed likelihood as motivator: Creating value through engaging what's real. *Journal of Economic Psychology, 38,* 4–15.

Higgins, E. T., Kruglanski, A. W., & Pierro, A. (2003). Regulatory mode: Locomotion and assessment as distinct orientations. In M. P. Zanna (Ed.), *Advances in experimental social psychology* (Vol. 35, pp. 293–344). New York: Academic Press.

Higgins, E. T., & Liberman, N. (2018). The loss of loss aversion: Paying attention to reference points. *Journal of Consumer Psychology, 28*(3), 523–532.

Higgins, E. T., & Rholes, W. S. (1978). "Saying is believing": Effects of message modification on memory and liking for the person described. *Journal of Experimental Social Psychology, 14,* 363–378.

Higgins, E. T., & Scholer, A. A. (2015). Goal pursuit functions: Working together. In M. Mikulincer, P. R. Shaver, E. Borgida, & J. A. Bargh (Eds.), *APA handbook of personality and social psychology: Vol. 1. Attitudes and social cognition* (pp. 843–889). Washington, DC: American Psychological Association.

Huang, J. Y., & Bargh, J. A. (2014). The selfish goal: Autonomously operating motivational structures as the proximate cause of human judgment and behavior. *Behavioral and Brain Sciences, 37*(2), 121–135.

Hughes, B. L., & Zaki, J. (2015). The neuroscience of motivated cognition. *Trends in Cognitive Sciences, 19*(2), 62–64.

Hull, C. L. (1932). The goal-gradient hypothesis and maze learning. *Psychological Review, 39*(1), 25–43.

Hull, C. L. (1943). *Principles of behavior: An introduction to behavior theory.* New York: Appleton-Century-Crofts.

Hull, C. L. (1950). Behavior postulates and corollaries. *Psychological Review, 57*(3), 173–180.

Irwin, F. W. (1953). Stated expectations as functions of probability and desirability of outcomes. *Journal of Personality, 21*(3), 329–335.

James, W. (2007). *The principles of psychology* (Vol. 2). New York: Cosimo. (Original work published 1890)

Kahneman, D., & Tversky, A. (1979). Prospect theory: An analysis of decision under risk. *Econometrica, 47*(2), 263–291.

Kashdan, T. B., & Steger, M. F. (2007). Curiosity and pathways to well-being and meaning in life: Traits, states, and everyday behaviors. *Motivation and Emotion, 31*(3), 159–173.

Kay, S. A., & Grimm, L. R. (2017). Regulatory fit improves fitness for people with low exercise experience. *Journal of Sport and Exercise Psychology, 39*(2), 109–119.

Kim, H., Franks, B., & Higgins, E. T. (2013). Evidence that self-regulatory mode affects retirement savings. *Journal of Aging and Social Policy, 25*(3), 248–263.

Komissarouk, S., Chernikova, M., Kruglanski, A. W., & Higgins, E. T. (2018). Who is most likely to wear rose-colored glasses?: How regulatory mode moderates self-flattery. *Personality and Social Psychology Bulletin.* [Epub ahead of print]

Kruglanski, A. W. (1989). *Lay epistemics and human knowledge: Cognitive and motivational bases.* New York: Plenum.

Kruglanski, A. W. (1990). Motivations for judging and knowing: Implications for causal attribution. In E. T. Higgins & R. M. Sorrentino (Eds.), *Handbook of motivation and cognition: Foundations of social behavior* (Vol. 2, pp. 333–368). New York: Guilford Press.

Kruglanski, A. W. (1996). Motivated social cognition: Principles of the interface. In E. T. Higgins & A. W. Kruglanski (Eds.), *Social psychology: Handbook of basic principles* (pp. 493–520). New York: Guilford Press.

Kruglanski, A. W., Jasko, K., Milyavsky, M., Chernikova, M., Webber, D., Pierro, A., et al. (2018). Cognitive consistency theory in social psychology: A paradigm reconsidered. *Psychological Inquiry, 29*(2), 45–59.

Kruglanski, A. W., Pierro, A., Mannetti, L., & Higgins, E. T. (2013). The distinct psychologies of "looking" and "leaping": Assessment and locomotion as the springs of action. *Social and Personality Psychology Compass, 7*(2), 79–92.

Kruglanski, A. W., Shah, J. Y., Fishbach, A., Friedman, R., Chun, W. Y., & Sleeth-Keppler, D. (2002). A theory of goal systems. In M. P. Zanna (Ed.), *Advances in experimental social psychology* (Vol. 34, pp. 331–378). New York: Academic Press.

Kruglanski, A. W., Thompson, E. P., Higgins, E. T., Atash, M. N., Pierro, A., Shah, J. Y., et al. (2000). To "do the right thing" or to "just do it": Locomotion and assessment as distinct self-regulatory imperatives. *Journal of Personality and Social Psychology, 79*(5), 793–815.

Latimer, A. E., Rivers, S. E., Rench, T. A., Katulak, N. A., Hicks, A., Hodorowski, J. K., et al. (2008). A field experiment testing the utility of regulatory fit messages for promoting physical activity. *Journal of Experimental Social Psychology, 44*(3), 826–832.

Lewin, K. (1935). *A dynamic theory of personality: Selected papers* (D. K. Adams & K. E. Zener, Trans.). New York: McGraw-Hill.

Lewin, K. (1951). *Field theory in social science.* New York: Harper.

Lewin, K. (1997). Constructs in field theory. In K. Lewin (Ed.), *Resolving social conflicts and field theory in social science* (pp. 191–199). Washington, DC: American Psychological Association. (Original work published 1944)

Louro, M. J., Pieters, R., & Zeelenberg, M. (2007).

Dynamics of multiple-goal pursuit. *Journal of Personality and Social Psychology, 93*(2), 174–193.

Mannetti, L., Leder, S., Insalata, L., Pierro, A., Higgins, E. T., & Kruglanski, A. W. (2009). Priming the ant or the grasshopper in people's mind: How regulatory mode affects inter-temporal choices. *European Journal of Social Psychology, 39*(6), 1120–1125.

Marks, R. W. (1951). The effect of probability, desirability, and "privilege" on the stated expectations of children. *Journal of Personality, 19*(3), 332–351.

Maslow, A. H. (1943). A theory of human motivation. *Psychological Review, 50*(4), 370–396.

Mathmann, F., Chylinski, M., de Ruyter, K., & Higgins, E. T. (2017). When plentiful platforms pay off: Assessment orientation moderates the effect of assortment size on choice engagement and product valuation. *Journal of Retailing, 93*(2), 212–227.

Mauro, R., Pierro, A., Mannetti, L., Higgins, E. T., & Kruglanski, A. W. (2009). The perfect mix: Regulatory complementarity and the speed–accuracy balance in group performance. *Psychological Science, 20*(6), 681–685.

Merton, R. K. (1957). *Social theory and social structure.* Glencoe, IL: Free Press.

Metcalfe, J., & Greene, M. J. (2007). Metacognition of agency. *Journal of Experimental Psychology: General, 136*(2), 184–199.

Metcalfe, J., & Mischel, W. (1999). A hot/cool-system analysis of delay of gratification: Dynamics of willpower. *Psychological Review, 106*(1), 3–19.

Miller, G. A., Galanter, E., & Pribram, K. H. (1960). *Plans and the structure of behavior.* New York, NY: Henry Holt and Co.

Miller, N. E. (1959). Liberalization of basic S-R concepts: Extensions to conflict behavior, motivation, and social learning: Part I. In S. Koch (Ed.), *Psychology: A study of a science* (Vol. 2, pp. 196–292). New York: McGraw-Hill.

Moller, A. C., & Elliot, A. J. (2006). The 2 × 2 achievement goal framework: An overview of empirical research. In A. V. Mittel (Ed.), *Focus on educational psychology* (pp. 307–326). Hauppauge, NY: Nova Science.

Nafcha, O., Higgins, E. T., & Eitam, B. (2016). Control feedback as the motivational force behind habitual behavior. In B. Studer & S. Knecht (Eds.), *Progress in brain research: Vol. 229. Motivation: Theory, neurobiology and applications* (pp. 49–68). Amsterdam, the Netherlands: Elsevier.

Nicholls, J. G. (1984). Achievement motivation: Conceptions of ability, subjective experience, task choice, and performance. *Psychological Review, 91*(3), 328–346.

Osborne, S. R. (1977). The free food (contrafreeload-ing) phenomenon: A review and analysis. *Animal Learning and Behavior, 5*(3), 221–235.

Pavey, L., & Sparks, P. (2009). Reactance, autonomy and paths to persuasion: Examining perceptions of threats to freedom and informational value. *Motivation and Emotion, 33*(3), 277–290.

Pierro, A., Chernikova, M., Lo Destro, C., Hig-gins, E. T., & Kruglanski, A. W. (2018). Assess-ment and locomotion conjunction: How looking complements leaping . . . but not always. In J. M. Olson (Ed.), *Advances in experimental social psy-chology* (Vol. 58, pp. 243–299). Cambridge, MA: Academic Press.

Pierro, A., Leder, S., Mannetti, L., Tory Higgins, E., Kruglanski, A. W., & Aiello, A. (2008). Regula-tory mode effects on counterfactual thinking and regret. *Journal of Experimental Social Psychol-ogy, 44*(2), 321–329.

Plessner, H., Unkelbach, C., Memmert, D., Baltes, A., & Kolb, A. (2009). Regulatory fit as a deter-minant of sport performance: How to succeed in a soccer penalty-shooting. *Psychology of Sport and Exercise, 10*(1), 108–115.

Rossignac-Milon, M., & Higgins, E. T. (2018). Be-yond intrapersonal cognitive consistency: Shared reality and the interpersonal motivation for truth. *Psychological Inquiry, 29*(2), 86–93.

Scholer, A. A., & Higgins, E. T. (2009). Exploring the complexities of value creation: The role of engagement strength. *Journal of Consumer Psy-chology, 19*(2), 137–143.

Scholer, A. A., Zou, X., Fujita, K., Stroessner, S. J., & Higgins, E. T. (2010). When risk seeking be-comes a motivational necessity. *Journal of Per-sonality and Social Psychology, 99*(2), 215–231.

Schunk, D. H., & DiBenedetto, M. K. (2016). Self-efficacy theory in education. In K. R. Wentzel & D. B. Miele (Eds.), *Handbook of motivation at school* (2nd ed., pp. 34–54). New York: Routledge.

Senko, C., Hulleman, C. S., & Harackiewicz, J. M. (2011). Achievement goal theory at the crossroads: Old controversies, current challenges, and new di-rections. *Educational Psychologist, 46*(1), 26–47.

Shah, J. Y., & Kruglanski, A. W. (2000). Aspects of goal networks: Implications for self-regulation. In M. Boekaerts, P. R. Pintrich, & M. Zeidner (Eds.), *Handbook of self-regulation* (pp. 85–110). San Diego, CA: Academic Press.

Sheldon, K. M., Ryan, R. M., Deci, E. L., & Kasser, T. (2004). The independent effects of goal con-tents and motives on well-being: It's both what you pursue and why you pursue it. *Personality and Social Psychology Bulletin, 30*(4), 475–486.

Shipley, T. E., Jr., & Veroff, J. (1952). A projective measure of need for affiliation. *Journal of Experi-mental Psychology, 43*(5), 349–356.

Sorrentino, R. M., & Higgins, E. T. (1986). Motiva-tion and cognition: Warming up to synergism. In R. M. Sorrentino & E. T. Higgins (Eds.), *Hand-book of motivation and cognition: Foundations of social behavior* (pp. 3–19). New York: Guilford Press.

Tapal, A., Oren, E., Dar, R., & Eitam, B. (2017). The Sense of Agency Scale: A measure of consciously perceived control over one's mind, body, and the immediate environment. *Frontiers in Psychology, 8*, 1552.

Vuorre, M., & Metcalfe, J. (2016). The relation be-tween the sense of agency and the experience of flow. *Consciousness and Cognition, 43*, 133–142.

Walmart. (2018, September 30). Motivation. Re-trieved September 30, 2018, from *www.walmart. com/search/?query=motivation*.

Wang, F. (2008). Motivation and English achieve-ment: An exploratory and confirmatory factor analysis of a new measure for Chinese students of English learning. *North American Journal of Psychology, 10*(3), 633–646.

White, R. W. (1959). Motivation reconsidered: The concept of competence. *Psychological Review, 66*(5), 297–333.

White, R. W. (1963). Sense of interpersonal compe-tence: Two case studies and some reflections on origins. In R. W. White & K. F. Bruner (Eds.), *The study of lives: Essays on personality in honor of Henry A. Murray* (pp. 72–93). New York: Ather-ton Press.

Wiener, N. (1961). *Cybernetics: Or control and com-munication in the animal and the machine* (2nd ed.). Cambridge, MA: MIT Press.

Wigfield, A., & Eccles, J. S. (2000). Expectancy–value theory of achievement motivation. *Contem-porary Educational Psychology, 25*(1), 68–81.

Woodworth, R. S. (1918). *Dynamic psychology*. New York: Columbia University Press.

Woodworth, R. S. (1940). *Psychology* (4th ed.). New York: Holt.

Xenophon. (2018). *The memorabilia: Recollec-tions of Socrates* (H. G. Dakyns, Trans.) (Vol. 1177). Salt Lake City, UT: Project Gutenberg Literary Archive. (Original work published ca. 371 B.C.E.) Retrieved from *www.gutenberg.org/ files/1177/1177-h/1177-h.htm*.

Zou, X., Scholer, A. A., & Higgins, E. T. (2014). In pursuit of progress: Promotion motivation and risk preference in the domain of gains. *Journal of Per-sonality and Social Psychology, 106*(2), 183–201.

CHAPTER 6

Human Autonomy in Social Psychology
A Self-Determination Theory Perspective

Richard M. Ryan
Edward L. Deci

Human autonomy and self-determination are topics at the center of social psychologists' concerns, even if often as attributes being questioned or attacked. There are theories of obedience, reactance, external control, ego depletion, nonconscious priming, conformity, and the defensive management of terror, all of which reveal potential vulnerabilities in human choice and volition. There are also familiar frontal attacks on "free will," claims that all behavior is involuntary, and descriptions of the self and self-regulation as merely illusions created by our brains. Social psychologists, that is, have amply and often compellingly highlighted human susceptibilities to being controlled or manipulated, and have discussed myriad ways in which people show weakness of will, self-deception, incongruence, or are pawns to determinants of which they are unaware.

Yet when all the dust settles around such phenomena, a robust fact remains: People engage in some actions that they reflectively endorse and willingly do, and they distinguish these from behaviors that feel externally elicited, controlled, or pressured. This distinction between autonomous and controlled motivations goes beyond just phenomenal differences; it has functional importance. When people are auton-

omously motivated, they are more fully engaged and display higher-quality action—better persistence, better performance, and greater adaptive flexibility—than when controlled motives underpin their behavior. This is why organizational leaders, educators, health psychologists, clinicians, coaches, and other practitioners are constantly trying to recruit the volition and autonomy of the people with whom they work. Indeed, whether or not it is deemed illusory by some scientists, when it comes to achieving real-world outcomes, people's autonomy, sense of choice, and willingness matter.

Among current theoretical streams in social psychology, one has particularly focused on the issue of human autonomy or authentic volition. *Self-determination theory* (SDT; Ryan & Deci, 2017) supplies a thoroughgoing account of autonomy and self-regulation in every respect—philosophically, mechanistically, developmentally, and in terms of social and behavioral dynamics and consequences across domains and cultures (Ryan, Soenens, & Vansteenkiste, 2019). It is also a theory that accounts for many of the vulnerabilities highlighted in social psychological theories such as those to which we alluded earlier; that is, SDT is a theory of human volition that addresses not only how self-regulation is "designed," developed, and functionally exercised but also how it can be compromised and undermined by both situational and cultural factors.

In its social psychological aspect, SDT is particularly concerned with describing and predicting how social contexts impact human motivation, performance, and wellness. To do so, SDT begins with distinct assumptions that help to organize and focus its research on those aspects of social environments that are most functionally relevant to autonomous motivation and to wellness. Specifically, within SDT's "organismic view" (Ryan & Deci, 2017), people are seen as active organisms that have a set of intrinsic motivational propensities, in which experiences of autonomy, competence, and relatedness play a critical role. Correspondingly, SDT focuses on specific aspects of the environment that either frustrate or satisfy those needs, and thus disrupt or sustain, respectively, those propensities. As such, the theory is able to reliably predict the effects that social contexts have on the relative autonomy of motivation, and on people's behavioral performance and wellness. In short, SDT provides a theory about what is most important in social environments (namely, supports for basic human needs) with respect to promoting (or harming) optimal functioning. Although SDT focuses on multiple psychological needs, in this chapter we focus particularly on the basic need for *autonomy*. We do so for several reasons.

First, the issue of autonomy has enormous functional implications for people's quality of motivation, persistence, and performance, as SDT shows in studies of both play (Ryan, Rigby, & Przybylski, 2006) and work (Deci, Olafsen, & Ryan, 2017). Autonomy characterizes the quality of people's engagement, leading to better performance and higher satisfaction. The relation of autonomous motivation to positive outcomes is evident at both the level of specific activities or tasks and broader targets of measurement such as domains or vocations.

A second reason to focus on autonomy is that it is often misunderstood as a construct and has been more controversial than SDT's focus on needs for competence or relatedness. The very notion that people can behave with more or less autonomy challenges metapsychological per-

spectives that embrace naive reductionism or passive organism models (Ryan & Deci, 2006). The issue has also sparked controversies within cross-cultural psychology (see Yu, Levesque-Bristol, & Maeda, 2018) because of SDT's claim of the universality of basic needs, and the conflation by some theorists of autonomy with issues of independence and individualism.

A third, and perhaps primary, reason for this focus, however, is the strong evidence that social environments that support versus oppress autonomy impact not only people's motivation but also their wellness and flourishing (Ryan, Huta, & Deci, 2008) This is evident in main effects of autonomy on important outcomes, as well as the strong moderation by autonomy (and autonomy-related processes) of many phenomena within mainstream social psychology, from perfectionism (Nguyen & Deci, 2016) to ego depletion (Moller, Deci, & Ryan, 2006).

Autonomy in Social Psychology and in SDT

Autonomy within SDT is defined in terms of people acting with a full sense of willingness and volition. When autonomous, individuals endorse the actions they take, such that if they were to reflect on them, they would assent both to their behavior and its motives (Frankfurt, 2004). Autonomy is also an essential aspect of authenticity; when being authentic, one both authors one's actions and is congruently behind them (Ryan & Ryan, 2019). Research shows that whether measured in natural environments or in experimental settings, autonomy is manifest in behavior as greater persistence, task focus, and higher-quality performance, as well as more subjective vitality and positive experience (Ryan & Deci, 2008).

In addition to such phenomenological and behavioral data, the study of autonomy today extends to the differentiated neural processes activated in autonomous (vs. controlled) motivational states (see, e.g., Di Domenico & Ryan, 2017; Reeve & Lee, 2019b). For example, Reeve and Lee (2019a) recently reviewed studies indicating that autonomy is associated with striatum and anterior insular (AI) cortex activation, along with strong functional interactions between the two. As Ryan and Di Domenico

(2016) discuss, connectivity analyses have identified the AI as a critical node in the "salience network" (SN), which is thought to help focus attention to subjectively important events and mobilize neural resources for intentional behaving. Other findings from Di Domenico, Fournier, Ayaz, and Ruocco (2013; Di Domenico et al., 2018) suggest that need support allows better access to areas of the medial prefrontal cortex (PFC) in which self-related knowledge is accessed and informs autonomous behavior. Such patterned findings are, of course, just the beginnings of an emerging neuroscience of autonomy and control.

Autonomy and Perceived Locus of Causality

Within social psychology, SDT's concept of autonomy can be traced to the work of Heider (1958) and de Charms (1968). Heider argued that predicting social behaviors requires understanding the principles of "naive psychology," an important dimension of which was *personal versus impersonal causation* or perceiving whether the actions of people are intentional. Signs of personal causation include effort, motive, and equifinality in actions toward an end, among other indicators. Heider highlighted how notions of responsibility, credit, and blame are among the crucial social concepts that are intimately tied to perceptions of personal causation.

de Charms (1968) elaborated on Heider's concept of personal causation, differentiating it into two types. He argued that some intentional acts have an *internal perceived locus of causality* (IPLOC); people feel like "origins" of their action, and in which they are willingly engaged. Behaviors can also have an *external perceived locus of causality* (EPLOC) when people feel externally led or compelled to engage in them or feel more like "pawns." Particularly important, but often overlooked, in de Charms's theorizing was his observation that an IPLOC—the sense of being self-determined—is not merely a postbehavioral attribution. Instead he argued that people *directly* know when they are origins of their own actions—precisely because it is they who organize the actions. In SDT as well, an internal sense of volition and willingness is

understood as a salient dimension of human experience, not merely a cognitive appraisal based on inferences from external events (as, e.g., in Bem's [1967] attribution model).

SDT has expanded on de Charms's *perceived locus of causality* (PLOC) concept in multiple ways. On the personality functioning side, SDT describes a continuum of motivational types that vary in PLOC, including impersonal, controlled, and autonomous forms of motivation, and has explored the phenomenology, experiential and behavioral consequences, and neuropsychological underpinnings of these different forms of motivation. On the social psychology side, SDT has focused on the environmental and social conditions that affect people's PLOC; that is, the theory describes the social factors that support or undermine autonomous functioning.

Differentiating Motivation within SDT

Many psychological and economic theories treat motivation as essentially a unitary concept that differs mainly in amount. People have more or less motivation. SDT argues, however, that as, or even more, important than amount or intensity of motivation is what type of motivation is invigorating the behavior, as different types of motivation differ not only in source but also quality. SDT's differentiation of types of motivation thus allows researchers and practitioners to better predict qualities of behavior, learning, affect, and performance. In what follows, we review these subtypes of motivation and how each is related to the more general distinction between *autonomous* and *controlled* motivations.

Autonomy and Intrinsic Motivation

Intrinsic motivation refers to doing an activity because it is interesting or enjoyable. People have an inherent growth tendency and are oriented to take interest in their internal and external environments as part of their inclination toward learning and mastery. When free to do so, they gravitate toward behaviors that are intrinsically interesting, as seen in the way people spend leisure time in activities such as travel, sport, reading, and games.

When intrinsically motivated, people experience an IPLOC (de Charms, 1968), as the behavior they are doing is what they want to be doing at that moment. Intrinsic motivation is thus a prototype of autonomous motivation. In a practical sense, intrinsic motivation is an important class of behaviors, being so critically involved in learning and development, as well as people's revitalization. Yet although intrinsically motivated behaviors represent a prototype of autonomy, SDT recognizes that through integration, extrinsic motivations can also become self-regulated and fully autonomous.

Extrinsic Motivations and Their Relative Autonomy

Extrinsic motivation concerns people engaging in activities in order to obtain separable consequences. The behaviors are not done because they are rewarding in and of themselves, but instead are instrumental; that is, they are intended to accomplish or attain some other outcome. Although de Charms originally linked an IPLOC with intrinsic motivation and an EPLOC with extrinsic motivation, SDT's taxonomy allows that extrinsic motivations can be varied in their perceived causality or relative autonomy, some being autonomous and others more controlled (Ryan & Connell, 1989). For example, a person may be extrinsically motived because he or she is responding to external rewards or punishments, in which case he or she would have an EPLOC. But the person might also be extrinsically motivated to act in support of a personal value, in which case an IPLOC is more likely. Thus, Ryan, Connell, and Deci (1985) used the concept of *internalization* to formulate a more complete taxonomy of extrinsic motivation, suggesting that people can internalize and integrate extrinsic motivations to greater or lesser degrees. They specified four major types of regulation for extrinsic motivation that were said to vary in their sources and dynamics, as well as in their relative autonomy.

The first type is *external regulation,* which means that the regulation for the behavior is controlled by some external contingency, such as attempting to attain externally controlled rewards or avoid punishments. Here, the PLOC is likely to be highly external, as people are being regulated by an external contingency, and autonomy is low. External regulation was the primary focus of operant behaviorism, and

in agreement with behavioral theory, SDT predicts poor maintenance of behavior when external regulators are not in force. This is because external regulation represents a relative absence of internalization. Within external regulations are both approach and avoidance behaviors, as people approach rewards and avoid punishments controlled by others.

A second type of extrinsic motivation is *introjected regulation,* when a person acts from internal pressures and self-esteem contingencies. Introjection of values and behavioral regulations aims to protect or gain feelings of inclusion, approval, and self-worth and, on the avoidance side, to stave off guilt and feelings of self- or other disapproval. For example, if a student's parents have shown conditional regard for his or her performance as an athlete, he or she may internalize this as self-depreciation and guilt when he or she does not compete well. Introjection, then, is a form of internalization in which, although the contingency is "within" the person, the PLOC is still relatively external, as the experience is that of pressure *on* the self to be, act, or perform certain ways.

Introjection has been studied in SDT within many domains, from ego involvement in sports (e.g., Lonsdale & Hodge, 2011; Standage, Duda, & Pensgaard, 2005) to introjection of religious beliefs (Ryan, Rigby, & King, 1993). In SDT, research has further suggested that the development of introjection is connected with parental conditional regard and psychological control (e.g., Kanat-Maymon, Roth, Assor, & Raizer, 2016). Linking these ideas is recent work on *perfectionism,* an individual characteristic in which people hold high standards, are concerned about not making mistakes, and internalize stringent demands (Frost, Marten, Lahart, & Rosenblate, 1990). Much research shows that perfectionism is associated with ill-being, although there is controversy about whether there may be components of perfectionism that are more positive (Bong, Hwang, Noh, & Kim, 2014; Chang, Lee, Byeon, & Lee, 2015; Harvey et al., 2015; Hewitt & Flett, 1991; Thorpe & Netteelbeck, 2014). Nguyen and Deci (2016) hypothesized that when the pursuit of high standards is energized by controlled motivation, poorer outcomes should result. Their research with undergraduates supported this view, showing that perfectionism that was driven by controlled motivation (most notably introjection) predicted more anxiety and less learning progress, despite the salient internal pressure to succeed.

A third major type of extrinsic motivation is *identified regulation,* which results from a fuller form of internalization in which people have accepted the value and importance of the behaviors. Accordingly, they willingly engage in them out of a belief in their worth (rather than because of internal pressure or external demand). With identified regulation, the motivation is still extrinsic because the behavior is not done for interest or enjoyment but because it is instrumental to personally valued consequences. As such, the behaviors are relatively autonomous and the PLOC is relatively internal.

Identified regulations, even though they are experienced as relatively autonomous, can be more or less compartmentalized, or even well defended in a psychological sense (Ryan & Deci, 2017). Yet when fully integrated, the person's identifications and actions are congruent with his or her other values and beliefs, and there is an openness to contradictions and to awareness. Accordingly, the individual can be more wholehearted and less conflicted in acting. *Integrated regulation* describes a fourth type of extrinsic regulation that entails this further degree of assimilation and thus represents a fully autonomous expression of extrinsic motivation, with a strong IPLOC. Together, intrinsic motivation, identified regulation, and integrated regulation are often combined in research as *autonomous motivation,* and introjected and external regulations are combined as *controlled motivation.* Yet it is also important to recognize that each subtype of motivation has its own unique dynamics and consequences, beyond those associated with its relative autonomy (Litalien et al., 2017).

The internalization of extrinsic motivation is a lifespan process, as maturing individuals must grow into multiple roles, responsibilities, duties, and obligations that may not originally be intrinsically motivated. It complements the concept of *socialization,* which represents the attempts of authorities and groups to transmit values, norms, and behavioral regulations to individuals and to encourage compliance. As we review later, however, socializers differ in their effectiveness at fostering true internalization, just as they differ in supporting intrinsic motivation. In fact, different social situations tend to potentiate different forms of regulation, with some culling out people's greed, fears, or introjects and others inspiring more autonomous motives and goals. The taxonomy of motivation described within SDT, depicted in Figure 6.1, is thus applicable for any activity task or commitment, or at more general domain levels.

Effects of Autonomous Motivation

An enormous amount of research demonstrates that autonomous motivation is not only associated with but is also essential to a variety of positive outcomes (Ryan & Deci, 2017). This literature includes both experimental research and studies in applied fields, including parenting, education, work, sports, health care, religion, and even video games.

We cite just a few recent examples. In education, León, Núñez, and Liew (2015) showed that when students were more autonomously motivated for mathematics they engage in deeper processing of information and show more effort and persistence. This greater effort, in turn, accounts for the higher achievement outcomes associated with autonomy. In the field of psychotherapy, clients facing depression who were more autonomously motivated for treatment evidenced greater improvement, a finding across varied treatment approaches (Zuroff, Koestner, Moskowitz, McBride, & Bagby, 2012). In a medically supervised weight-loss program for morbidly obese patients, those who became more autonomously motivated for treatment displayed more weight loss and, more importantly, more sustained weight-loss-promoting behaviors (Williams, Grow, Freedman, Ryan, & Deci, 1996). In sports, Ntoumanis and colleagues (2014) found that more autonomously motivated athletes were more persistent, had more positive affect, and more interest in future task engagement. In the work domain, in a study of insurance employees, Guntert (2015) found that their intrinsic and identified motivations were related positively to job satisfaction and organizational citizenship, and negatively to turnover intentions.

Furthermore, autonomy appears to be a universal psychological need. For example, a meta-

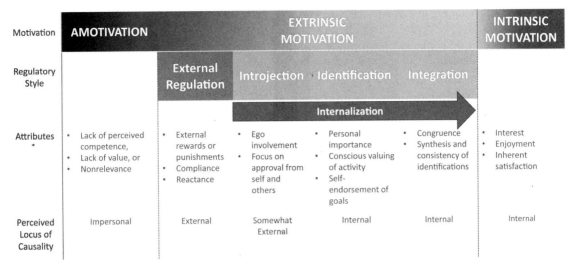

Motivation	AMOTIVATION	EXTRINSIC MOTIVATION				INTRINSIC MOTIVATION
Regulatory Style		External Regulation	Introjection	Identification	Integration	
			Internalization →			
Attributes •	• Lack of perceived competence, • Lack of value, or • Nonrelevance	• External rewards or punishments • Compliance • Reactance	• Ego involvement • Focus on approval from self and others	• Personal importance • Conscious valuing of activity • Self-endorsement of goals	• Congruence • Synthesis and consistency of identifications	• Interest • Enjoyment • Inherent satisfaction
Perceived Locus of Causality	Impersonal	External	Somewhat External	Internal	Internal	Internal

FIGURE 6.1. SDT's taxonomy of motivation. From the Center for Self-Determination Theory. Copyright © 2019. Reprinted by permission.

analysis by Yu and colleagues (2018) of studies done across the North America and East Asia showed that people's experience of autonomy need satisfaction was significantly related to well-being, and the magnitude of the relation did not differ between countries or cultures. Diener, Ng, Hartr, and Arora (2010) analyzed data from a global Gallup survey and found that across nations, autonomy was one of the strongest predictors of positive experience.

Autonomy, Subjective Vitality, and Ego Depletion

An excellent example of the importance of autonomy in motivational and wellness can be gleaned from the social psychological literature on ego depletion (Martela, DeHaan, & Ryan, 2016). The ego depletion phenomenon (e.g., Baumeister, Bratslavsky, Muraven, & Tice, 1998) emerged from the proposal that when people employ their self-control capacity, they are depleting a limited human resource. At about the same time as work on ego depletion began, within SDT we began working on a theory of factors that enhance or deplete vitality, or the energy available to the self (Ryan & Frederick, 1997). There are interesting points of convergence and divergence between these approaches to energy.

Ryan and Frederick (1997) argued that vitality is among the most salient and subjectively central aspects of human phenomenology. They defined *subjective vitality* as the perceived energetic resources available to the self, hypothesizing that this experience is systematically affected by both physical and psychological factors. In a series of studies, they showed how factors such as fatigue, pain, and illness result in lower subjective vitality. In addition, using varied methods, they showed that subjective vitality also covaries with basic psychological need satisfactions. Experiencing satisfaction of autonomy, competence, and relatedness predicted enhanced vitality, whereas need frustration diminished it (see also Martela et al., 2016).

Numerous experimental and field studies have further supported this framework. For example, Nix, Ryan, Manly, and Deci (1999) showed that people have more vitality when working on autonomously regulated tasks that when working under controlled conditions. In a field study within a nursing facility, Kasser and Ryan (1999) found that subjective vitality was predicted both by physical health and experiences of autonomy, and autonomy support from staff. Deci, LaGuardia, Moller, Scheiner, and Ryan (2006), showed how autonomy support in friendships predicts greater vitality, effects that also appear in domains such as work (e.g., Baard, Deci &, Ryan, 2004), sports (e.g., Bartholomew, Ntoumanis, Ryan, Bosch, & Thøgersen-Ntoumani, 2011), and education (e.g., Nie, Chua, Yeung, Ryan, & Chan, 2015), among many others.

Because SDT suggests that controlled (nonautonomous) motivation would diminish energy, it has a ready and semiconvergent explanation for many of the experimental studies done within the ego depletion framework (Martela et al., 2016). Usually in ego depletion paradigms, people are asked to exercise control over behavior without being given a rationale that would support their autonomous engagement. According to SDT, doing something for controlled motivations, which is the situation in ego deletion studies, is expected to be draining of energy relative to more autonomous motives that catalyze more energy and involve less conflict and need for inhibition.

Evidence has supported this hypothesized connection between ego depletion phenomena and SDT's model of vitality. For example, Muraven, Gagné, and Rosman (2008) had participants perform a brief, potentially depleting exercise (retyping a paragraph but omitting *e*'s and spaces). Participants in a controlling condition were pressured to do well on the task. Subsequently, all participants had to engage in another task requiring them to concentrate, performance at which was indicative of ego depletion. Results showed that those in the controlling condition performed worse, a relationship mediated by subjective vitality. Feeling controlled led to less subjective vitality, which in turn related to poorer performance at the later task. In another experiment, Muraven and colleagues similarly showed that subjective vitality mediated between more or less autonomy-supportive experimental condition and ego-depletion: People performing in autonomy-supportive environments experience more vitality, and thereby evidenced less ego-depletion. In still another relevant study, Muraven, Rosman, and Gagné (2007) reasoned that performance-contingent rewards for doing a task might undermine participants' autonomous motivation (see Deci, Koestner, & Ryan, 1999), resulting in greater ego depletion. Their experiemenical results supported this hypothesis. Finally, Mu-

raven (2008), rather than manipulating conditions of autonomy support, tried a different approach. Having placed a bowl of attractive cookies in front of participants, he asked them to complete a questionnaire that measured the relative autonomy of their motivation not to eat the cookies. Results showed that more autonomous reasons for abstaining predicted better performance on a subsequent task, again indicative of less depletion subsequent to "self-control."

In an illustrative study from a different laboratory, Kazén, Kuhl, and Leicht (2015) gave participants either autonomy-supportive or more "self-controlling" instructions to perform a difficult cognitive task, then measured both their quality of performance at a subsequent task and their blood glucose levels. Based on both *personality systems interaction* (PSI; Kuhl, 2000) as well as SDT, they predicted that self-controlling actions would deplete energy, and that autonomously motivated actions would not. Furthermore, based on a resource allocation model of self-control (Beedie & Lane, 2012), they suggested that blood glucose levels would follow the same patterns: Rather than being simply depleted by mental effort (Gailliot & Baumeister, 2007), the allocation of glucose to the brain would be governed by an appraisal of the import of the situation. Accordingly, in the autonomy supportive condition where value for the task was conveyed, blood glucose levels would be maintained or perhaps even increase. Results showed that, consistent with the ego depletion model, blood glucose levels of the self-controlling group decreased during the experiment. In contrast the more self-motivated group performed better on the subsequent task, and even more striking, showed an *increase* in blood glucose levels. Such findings provide evidence that performing tasks with autonomous regulation might not only maintain one's levels of energy but may also even increase them, at least short term.

A More Direct Test

Considering the act of making a choice as entailing regulatory effort, Baumeister and colleagues (1998) hypothesized that giving people a choice would be depleting, relative to not making a choice, a hypothesis seemingly opposed to what SDT would predict. To test their idea, Baumeister and colleagues (Study 2) created two groups of participants, a "high-choice group" and a "no-choice group." The high-choice group was, however, actually a pseudo-choice group: Its members were given a choice between two tasks, but then were told that it would "be very helpful to the experimenter" if they selected the first task, even though it was up to them. The no-choice group was simply told which task to do. We note, however, that this statement from the experimenter to the high-choice participants that "it would be helpful to the experimenter" if they would choose the first task had previously been shown to be a controlling condition that decreased intrinsic motivation (Pittman, Davey, Alafat, Wetherill, & Kramer, 1980). Thus (in our SDT view), the so-called "high-choice" condition in Baumeister and colleagues' study was really a subtlety controlling condition that was being compared to a no-choice condition. Findings showed that this "high-choice" condition (which we interpret as a controlling condition) resulted in greater depletion than no choice.

To clarify these findings, Moller and colleagues (2006) retested this issue and verified the SDT interpretation. Their experiment had three conditions: (1) a true-choice condition (with no pressure about what to choose); (2) a "controlling-choice" condition, which was the same one that Baumeister and colleagues had used and labeled the "high-choice" condition; and (3) a no-choice condition. As predicted, those in the "true choice" condition were more energized than those in the controlling-choice and no-choice conditions, confirming the effects of real choice as opposed to pseudo-choice.

In short, studies on subjective vitality and ego depletion are converging to suggest that type of motivation matters for depletion effects (Martela et al., 2016; Ryan & Deci, 2008). Ego depletion effects may often be mediated by changes in subjective vitality and moderated by motivational conditions that impact autonomy. Whereas external regulation and self-controlling motives can lead to depletion, more autonomous regulation of behaviors is less depleting, and in some cases, even energizing.

Summary

We have provided but a few examples of how SDT interfaces with social psychological themes, of which perfectionism and ego depletion are but two examples. Today hundreds of published studies attest to the robust positive effects of autonomous motivation on behavioral and wellness outcomes, many of which we recently comprehensively reviewed (Ryan & Deci, 2017). Rather than further review findings here, then, we move on to the critical questions raised within SDT concerning how social environments affect (i.e., support or diminish) autonomy.

Basic Psychological Needs in Growth, Integrity, and Wellness

Insofar as there are clear functional and well-being benefits to autonomous motivation, a fundamental question for social psychologists is what are the "causes" of autonomous functioning and how it can be "elicited." Starting from the classic behavioral view, one would seek to identify the environmental stimuli that control the occurrence of such behavior. SDT, being an organismic approach, addresses this question from a different vantage point, however. It assumes that human nature is *already* active or prone toward intrinsic motivation, internalization, and integration, and thus asks instead under what social conditions these prepotent aspects of our human nature express themselves, and under what conditions their expression is inhibited. SDT actually sees this as three questions: What are the psychological nutriments that are required for (1) *growth* (as represented in intrinsic motivation to learn and acquire masteries), (2) *integrity* (as represented in internalizing and integrating social regulations and values), and (3) *wellness* (as represented by individual and relational satisfaction and indicators of full functioning)? Considering these together the question is "What do people need to be vital and to thrive?"

Different mini-theories within SDT provide specific propositions and supporting evidence for the role of basic needs in these areas of growth, integrity, and wellness (Ryan & Deci, 2017), three of which are particularly relevant.

Cognitive evaluation theory (CET; Deci & Ryan, 1980a) specifies the psychological needs for autonomy and competence underlying intrinsic motivation as a prototype growth propensity; *organismic integration theory* (OIT; Ryan & Connell, 1989) specifies the role of autonomy, competence, and relatedness in internalization as a prototype of integrative processes; and *basic psychological needs theory* (BPNT; Ryan 1995) details how basic need satisfactions and frustrations predict psychological health and wellness—or, alternatively, illness. We thus briefly review these mini-theories that underpin the evidence base and claims that basic needs are essential to growth, integrity, and wellness.

Cognitive Evaluation Theory

CET (Deci & Ryan, 1980a, 1985), deals with how environments affect intrinsic motivation. It was initially formulated to explain the results of laboratory research on intrinsic motivation showing that rewards, especially monetary rewards, given for doing an interesting activity decreased people's intrinsic motivation for doing the activity (Deci, 1975). In CET, it was suggested that the rewards of certain types (Ryan, Mims, & Koestner, 1983) are readily perceived as controlling, leading to an EPLOC, thereby frustrating people's need for autonomy and diminishing their intrinsic motivation. A meta-analysis confirmed the undermining phenomenon and SDT's basic taxonomy of reward contingency effects on intrinsic motivation (Deci et al., 1999). Subsequent work using functional magnetic resonance imaging (fMRI) has not only replicated the undermining effect but also specified neural processes involved in the effect (see Reeve & Lee, 2019b). As one example of such research, Murayama, Matsumoto, Izuma, and Matsumoto (2010) showed that whereas nonrewarded participants showed maintained striatum and lateral PFC activations over two sessions of engagement with an interesting activity, those who were externally rewarded for engagement in the first session showed a significant decrease in activation in both areas in the second session, in which no rewards were administered. Striatal activation speaks to the experience of the task being rewarding, and the lateral PFC data are indicative of engagement. Thus, both the sense of enjoyment and task engagement are undermined by rewards.

CET addresses much more than the issue of reward effects. It argues further that *any* factors that detract from an IPLOC will diminish intrinsic motivation. Thus, threats of punishment, controlling deadlines and surveillance, evaluations, conditional regard, and other events that detract from autonomy can diminish intrinsic motivation, as would negative efficacy feedback or excessive difficulty. In contrast, social contexts that afford choice or reflection, as well as those that are optimally challenging, support autonomy and competence, and thereby enhance intrinsic motivation. As an example of a facilitating factor, experiments have shown that providing choice can enhance intrinsic motivation (e.g., Zuckerman, Porac, Lathin, Smith, & Deci, 1978), an effect that has been replicated across cultures (e.g., Bao & Lam, 2008), supported by meta-analyses (e.g., Patall, Cooper, & Robinson, 2008), and demonstrated within neuroscience research (Murayama et al., 2015). More generally, social contexts that respect autonomy help sustain intrinsic motivation. For example, in a longitudinal study of early- to mid-adolescent athletes, Joesaar, Hein, and Haggar (2012) found that when they perceived their coaches to be more autonomy supportive, they evidenced more intrinsic motivation 1 year later.

Furthermore, drawing on the work of White (1959), who spoke about a fundamental need for competence, Deci and Ryan (1980a) argued that both autonomy and competence are central to intrinsic motivation. Important here is that self-efficacy is not seen as sufficient for sustaining intrinsic motivation—autonomy is also required.

There is in fact a large literature detailing factors on both the facilitating and undermining sides of the ledger in CET, primarily focused on variations in autonomy and competence supports. Although relatedness satisfactions can enhance intrinsic motivation for many activities (e.g., Bao & Lam, 2008), this need has been less explored within CET. Yet it is clear that intrinsic motivation, a vital expression of our active human nature, is facilitated by supports for autonomy, competence, and (for many activities) relatedness (Ryan & Deci, 2000).

Organismic Integration Theory

OIT emerged after CET and is concerned with the differentiation of extrinsic motivation resulting from internalization and integration (Ryan & Connell, 1989). Earlier in this chapter we discussed the types of regulation—namely, external, introjected, identified, and integrated—that represent different degrees to which the perceived locus of causality has become internalized and thus the basis for autonomous extrinsic motivation. Beyond just describing these types of motivation, OIT argues that the process of internalization, moving people beyond external control toward self-regulation, is dependent on the support of all three basic psychological needs; that is, when socializers support autonomy, competence, and relatedness, they are more effective at promoting internalized motivation in others.

We cite just a couple examples. Chirkov and Ryan (2001) examined autonomy support of both teachers and parents, as well as the motivation and well-being of their high-school students in both Russia and the United States. Results indicated that the autonomy support of both teachers and parents contributed to students' identified motivation, and teachers' autonomy support contributed to students' intrinsic motivation. In a study of patients with diabetes, Williams and colleagues (2009) found that patients who perceived providers as more autonomy supportive were then more autonomously motivated to take the medications, resulting in greater adherence and higher quality of life.

As we noted, internalization is a key process in human development, as people have to take in the social practices, norms, and values around them. But in the SDT view, this is always a matter of degree. Most people behave in regulated ways, but not all behave with integrity—that is, with authenticity and congruence (Ryan & Ryan, 2019).

Basic Psychological Needs Theory

BPNT, yet another of SDT's current six mini-theories that is particularly relevant to this discussion, has a bearing on our third broad outcome of wellness. The core of BPNT is the proposal that there are fundamental psychological needs for autonomy, competence, and relatedness, the satisfaction of which promotes psychological wellness, and the frustration of which contributes to ill-being. Need thwarting, in extreme or chronic forms, both directly and indirectly contributes to various psychopathologies (Vansteenkiste & Ryan, 2013).

At this point, myriad cross-sectional and longitudinal studies have supported the important role of basic psychological need satisfaction for health and wellness across the world. For example, Chen and colleagues (2015) investigated need satisfaction and need frustration in samples from China, Peru, Belgium, and the United States. Each of the basic needs was uniquely related to greater subjective wellness across these samples, results that were not moderated by cultural membership. Church and colleagues (2013) surveyed participants from Venezuela, Philippines, China, Japan, and the United States using experience sampling and found across samples that SDT's basic need satisfaction predicted more openness, agreeableness, conscientiousness, and emotional stability, as well as less negative and more positive affect. Sheldon, Abad, and Omoile (2009) assessed Nigerian and Indian adolescents' perception of parent and teacher autonomy support and found in both samples that autonomy support predicted psychological need satisfaction in school, which in turn predicted greater life satisfaction.

These and many such studies support the universality premise of SDT. Yet it is important to delimit exactly what is universal in this formulation. Basic psychological needs in SDT are treated as *etic universals,* or as attributes or processes that can be empirically shown to have cross-cultural significance and validity. Specifically, the claim is that across development and cultures, satisfaction of these needs enhances wellness, and frustration of them hinders it. Yet SDT does not claim that these basic needs are *emic universals,* recognizing that even these basic needs vary in how they are valued, voiced, and expressed in different cultural contexts (Chirkov, Ryan, Kim, & Kaplan, 2003; Ryan & Deci, 2017). For example, although SDT posits that autonomy is a universal need, findings show that the way in which it is valued and supported varies across cultures (e.g., see Cheng, Shu, Zhou, & Lam, 2016; Marbell & Grolnick, 2013), and between genders within and across cultures (Weinstein, Legate, Al-Khouja, & Şengül, 2018). Studying the nuances of how internalization and autonomy are cultivated and hindered, and how these link with outcomes indicative of growth, integrity, and wellness within different cultures, is an active area of research within SDT.

Mindfulness as a Ground of Autonomy

From the outset of SDT, awareness has been postulated to be an important aspect of autonomous functioning (e.g., Deci & Ryan, 1980b). Awareness promotes integration and volitional behavior, and helps protect against defensiveness, which is a central component of controlled motivation. Furthermore, because autonomy, the wholehearted willingness to act, depends on congruence in motives, goals, and values, it is critically supported by such awareness, and specifically *mindfulness,* understood within SDT as nondefensive or open experience of what is occurring within and outside oneself (Deci, Ryan, Schultz, & Niemiec, 2015; Ryan & Rigby, 2015). Research shows that mindfulness is associated with autonomy both at trait and state levels of analysis (e.g., Brown & Ryan, 2003), suggesting that more mindful people act in more congruent ways.

Illustrating this is a study examining whether mindfulness could moderate people's reactions to a well-known social psychological phenomenon, namely, mortality salience effects. According to *terror management theory* (TMT; Greenberg, Pyszczynski, & Solomon, 1995) when people are reminded of mortality, especially if it is at the edge of their awareness, they tend to defend against those thoughts in ways that defensively protect their self-esteem and/or affirm the worldviews that keep them secure. This includes viewing ingroup members and others who share their values more positively and judging outgroup members more negatively.

SDT suggests that mindful awareness, which is conducive to more awareness and more access to self-endorsed choices and values, should buffer against such defensiveness. Across seven experiments, Niemiec and colleagues (2010) tested this idea. Assessing individual differences in mindfulness, they reported that more

mindful people were less likely to evidence worldview defense following mortality salience (MS) manipulations. This was mediated not by avoidance or suppression, but rather by fuller processing of the MS induction in the moment, resulting in less need for suppression after delay. In other words, greater awareness produced a more integrated response, whereas low mindfulness allowed the defensive processes postulated by TMT to operate out of awareness, and drive behaviors or attitudes the individual may not reflectively endorse.

Indeed, more autonomous integrated motivation has been shown in a number of ways to associated with not only greater awareness but also greater congruence between implicit and explicit processes. For example, Legault, Green-Demers, Grant, and Chung (2007) showed that persons with more autonomous motivations for acting without prejudice were more likely to show less racism on both implicit ad explicit assessments.

Autonomy in Close Relationships and Prosocial Behavior

Autonomy in Close Relationships

The most recent of SDT's six mini-theories is *relationships motivation theory* (RMT). *Relatedness,* one of the three fundamental psychological needs, is critical to explain people's motivation to be close to others and to disclose to and care for others. Yet one of the important propositions of RMT is that satisfaction of the autonomy need is as fully important to the satisfaction of the relatedness need as is warmth or involvement per se. In order to have a high-quality close relationship, people need to feel fully volitional about being in the relationship and to feel that the other is volitionally and autonomously involved as well; that is, high-quality dyadic relationships require mutuality of autonomy between the two parties in a relationship (Deci et al., 2006). Furthermore, data show that the act of giving support to others turns out to enhance one's own wellness, through greater satisfaction of inherent psychological needs.

Autonomy in Prosocial Behavior

The satisfactions of giving have been further explored within SDT. For example, Weinstein and Ryan (2010) reported four studies of helping behavior and its motivations using varied methods. An event sampling study examined the effects of helping others on psychological need satisfaction, subjective well-being, vitality, and self-esteem. Findings showed that helping per se had at most a weak positive effect on well-being outcomes, whereas, as expected within SDT, when the helping was autonomously motivated, these positive effects were substantially more robust. In another study, experimental participants played a dictator game in which they were given money that they could donate or not donate to another participant, without the other knowing about the donor's choices. Some donors were in a choice condition in which they decided how much to give, whereas others were in a "yoked" condition, and were told to donate specified amounts. Only those in the choice condition showed enhanced need satisfaction and wellness as a function of giving. Two additional experiments showed that autonomous helping enhanced the wellness of the helper (whereas controlled helping did not), and that the *recipients* of help showed greater positive affect, vitality, and self-esteem when the helper's motivation was autonomous.

These and other studies (Gagné, 2003; Martela & Ryan, 2016) highlight that helping others volitionally and practicing benevolence can be inherently satisfying, leading to increased wellness in the helper, an effect mediated by the satisfaction of basic needs. Assembling a review of related studies, Ryan and Deci (2017) summarized that people appear to find need satisfaction in prosocial behaviors, which in turn help sustain this deeply evolved propensity of human nature (see Ryan & Hawley, 2017).

But do they find satisfaction in harming others, aggression, or violence? Legate, DeHaan, Weinstein, and Ryan (2013) reported results of experiments meant to demonstrate the converse point to that found by Weinstein and Ryan (2010). They asked participants to inflict social pain on an experimental confederate by excluding that person. They found that although most people followed instructions to exclude, these participants also experienced their compliance as nonautonomous and need thwarting, resulting in distress. Przybylski, Ryan, and Rigby (2009) showed that violence in video games did

not motivate players, and further that postgame increases in violence from games was largely the effect of frustrating the need for competence (Przybylski, Deci, Rigby, & Ryan, 2014). These and other experiments in SDT suggest that people do not typically derive basic satisfaction from antisocial acts; rather, it is more likely that they become more aggressive, competitive, and antisocial under need thwarting conditions.

Wealth, Economics, and Basic Needs

A basic premise within SDT is that satisfaction rather than frustration of basic psychological needs is critical for wellness. Of course, many SDT studies show this in proximal social contexts such as parent–child relationships, workplaces, classrooms, clinical encounters, and friendships. But it is also true that large-scale societal factors affect issues related to autonomy, competence, and relatedness. For example, poverty may well have its negative effects because it diminishes autonomy and competence experiences. People with lower socioeconomic status (SES) often have fewer intrinsic job satisfactions, higher stress, more emotional exhaustion, and lower vitality, all reflective of low psychological need satisfaction on a day-to-day basis. Thus, basic needs could be among the most important mediators in the relations between wealth, wealth inequality, and the flourishing of citizens.

Consistent with this, González, Swanson, Lynch, and Williams (2016) examined basic need satisfaction in a sample of U.S. workers. They found that autonomy, competence, and relatedness need satisfactions mediated between SES and physical and mental health, even when they controlled for other variables known to affect health, such as age, physical activity, and smoking. Interesting, too, the higher people's SES, the less their gains in wealth were associated with basic need satisfaction. This converges with evidence that as wealth exceeds moderate levels, the strength of its positive effects on well-being substantially weaken (Kasser, 2002).

Di Domenico and Fournier (2014) went further to examine whether, beyond SES, *income inequality* might itself frustrate basic needs. They assumed it would frustrate needs by increasing insecurity and by making more salient social comparisons and completion. To test this, they assessed both income and perceived SES, and in addition gathered data on wealth inequality in the geographic area surrounding each participant's home, as predictors of their health and wellness. All three predictors were relevant: Greater income, higher perceived SES, and lower inequality predicted greater health and well-being. Again, it was shown that the basic need satisfactions of autonomy, competence, and relatedness substantially mediated these relations. Such results help to explain the observations of Wilkinson and Pickett (2011) and other scholars who have highlighted how income disparities can diminish the well-being of people at all levels of income within a society.

Capabilities, Basic Psychological Needs, and Wellness

A number of economic theorists and philosophers such as Sen (2000) and Nussbaum (2000) have forwarded what is called the *capabilities approach,* emphasizing how specific social conditions are necessary to support individuals' ability to experience a "good life." Societies with the most flourishing citizens are, in this perspective, those that provide for and facilitate people's abilities and opportunities to pursue "that which they have reason to value."

Nussbaum (2000) proposed 10 capabilities that she viewed as essential: (1) reasonable life expectancy; (2) bodily health; (3) bodily integrity, including freedom of movement and freedom from violence; (4) ability to use imagination, senses, and thought; (5) freedom to experience and express emotions; (6) practical reason; (7) affiliation, including the freedom to live with others, and respect for relational choices; (8) appreciation and accessibility of other species; (9) opportunities for play; and (10) sense of control over the environment, both political and material. Nussbaum argues that people with these capabilities have more likelihood of thriving, and that furthermore, the lack of these capabilities undermines flourishing. Anand and colleagues (2009) created a survey assessment of Nussbaum's capabilities. Linking this with BPNT, DeHaan, Hirai, and Ryan (2016) hypothesized not only that capabilities

would predict well-being but also that this relation would be substantially mediated by SDT's basic psychological needs. Surveying participants from the United States and India, DeHaan and colleagues showed that Nussbaum's capabilities were significantly related with vitality, happiness, meaning in life, and overall life satisfaction, and as predicted, satisfaction and frustration of SDT's basic needs largely mediated these associations.

Together, such studies point to an important new direction in self-determination theory research (see Ryan, Ryan, Di Domenico, & Deci, 2019), namely, the influence of *pervasive environments* on people's needs, wellness, and performance. Pervasive environments include cultural norms and mores, economic structures and constraints, and political and legal rights and privileges. SDT is moving beyond the study of proximal social environments to inquire into the mechanisms through which broad societal structures influence the basic psychological needs satisfactions and frustrations of individuals. Pathways of effects are expected to be both direct and mediated by the autonomy supportive versus controlling styles and value sets of authorities and influencers in proximal contexts who help transmit and maintain pervasive influences.

Conclusions

Autonomy is both a salient human experience and a mode of functioning that yields more effective performance and greater wellness. It is distinct both phenomenally and neurologically from regulation by external forces or by internal pressures such as ego involvement or introjection. We have reviewed considerable research showing the positive consequences of autonomy on growth, as represented by intrinsic motivational processes; on integrity, as shown in studies of internalization and authenticity; and on wellness, as shown in research on mental health and psychopathology. We have suggested that autonomy and its positive consequences are supported by developmental and interpersonal contexts that afford greater opportunities for people to satisfy basic psychological needs for autonomy, competence, and relatedness. We have also pointed to a voluminous body of research showing the importance of autonomous motivation across domains including health care, education, sport, psychotherapy, technology use, work, and parenting, among others (see Ryan & Deci, 2017, for comprehensive reviews). Beyond such proximal interpersonal contexts, we have further reviewed how more pervasive social contexts such as economic and political systems can afford more or less support for people's basic psychological needs, thereby impacting thriving at population levels.

From these theoretical formulations and findings several principles can be derived, including the following:

1. Intentional actions vary in the extent to which they are autonomous or controlled.
2. The greater the autonomy, the greater the engagement and commitment, leading behaviors to be better performed and sustained.
3. Social environments impact autonomy, with controlling elements undermining and autonomy supportive elements facilitating autonomy.
4. Because autonomy represents a basic psychological need, the positive effects of autonomy are apparent across developmental periods from infancy to old age, and across cultures, both individualistic and collectivistic.

Although in this chapter we have focused primarily on autonomy, these four principles are consistent with SDT's six mini-theories and the formal propositions in each concerning motivation, basic psychological needs satisfaction and frustration, and wellness, as detailed in Ryan and Deci (2017).

We described at the outset that, in our view, social psychologists have long been shadow boxing with the phenomena of autonomy, will, and choice. SDT brings these phenomena out of the shadows and into the light of careful theory and extensive empirical study, so they can be understood as human capacities that are widely expressed, and yet pervasively vulnerable. Autonomy is clearly a critical issue for everyday practitioners across applied domains and, in a more overarching way, a core concern in global wellness, as it is affected by political regimes, cultures, and economies.

REFERENCES

Anand, P., Hunter, G., Carter, I., Dowding, K., Guala, F., & Van Hees, M. (2009). The development of capability indicators. *Journal of Human Development and Capabilities, 10*(1), 125–152.

Baard, P. P., Deci, E. L., & Ryan, R. M. (2004). Intrinsic need satisfaction: A motivational basis of performance and well-being in two work settings. *Journal of Applied Social Psychology, 34,* 2045–2068.

Bao, X.-H., & Lam, S.-F. (2008). Who makes the choice?: Rethinking the role of autonomy and relatedness in Chinese children's motivation. *Child Development, 79*(2), 269–283.

Bartholomew, K. J., Ntoumanis, N., Ryan, R. M., Bosch, J., & Thøgersen-Ntoumani, C. (2011). Self-determination theory and diminished functioning: The role of interpersonal control and psychological need thwarting. *Personality and Social Psychology Bulletin, 37*(11), 1459–1473.

Baumeister, R. F., Bratslavsky, E., Muraven, M., & Tice, D. M. (1998). Ego depletion: Is the active self a limited resource? *Journal of Personality and Social Psychology, 74,* 1252–1265.

Beedie, C. J., & Lane, A. M. (2012). The role of glucose in self-control. *Personality and Social Psychology Review, 16,* 143–153.

Bem, D. J. (1967). Self-perception: An alternative interpretation of cognitive dissonance phenomena. *Psychological Review, 74*(3), 183–200.

Bong, M., Hwang, A., Noh, A., & Kim, S. I. (2014). Perfectionism and motivation of adolescents in academic contexts. *Journal of Educational Psychology, 106*(3), 711–729.

Brown, K. W., & Ryan, R. M., (2003). The benefits of being present: Mindfulness and its role in psychological well-being. *Journal of Personality and Social Psychology, 84*(4), 822–848.

Chang, E., Lee, A., Byeon, E., & Lee, S. M. (2015). Role of motivation in the relation between perfectionism and academic burnout in Korean students. *Personality and Individual Differences, 82,* 221–226.

Chen, B., Vansteenkiste, M., Beyers, W., Boone, L., Deci, E. L., Van der Kaap-Deeder, J., et al. (2015). Basic psychological need satisfaction, need frustration, and need strength across four cultures. *Motivation and Emotion, 39*(2), 216–236.

Cheng, R. W. Y., Shu, T. M., Zhou, N., & Lam, S. F. (2016). Motivation of Chinese learners: An integration of etic and emic approaches. In R. B.

King & A. B. I. Bernardo (Eds.), *The psychology of Asian learners* (pp. 355–368). Singapore: Springer.

Chirkov, V. I., & Ryan, R. M. (2001). Parent and teacher autonomy-support in Russian and U.S. adolescents: Common effects on well-being and academic motivation. *Journal of Cross-Cultural Psychology, 32*(5), 618–635.

Chirkov, V. I., Ryan, R. M., Kim, Y., & Kaplan, U. (2003). Differentiating autonomy from individualism and independence: A self-determination theory perspective on internalization of cultural orientations and well-being. *Journal of Personality and Social Psychology, 84*(1), 97–110.

Church, A. T., Katigbak, M. S., Ching, C. M., Zhang, H., Shen, J., Arias, R. M., et al. (2013). Within-individual variability in self-concepts and personality states: Applying density distribution and situation-behavior approaches across cultures. *Journal of Research in Personality, 47*, 922–935.

de Charms, R. (1968). *Personal causation: The internal affective determinants of behavior.* New York: Academic Press.

Deci, E. L. (1975). *Intrinsic motivation.* New York: Plenum Press.

Deci, E. L., Koestner, R., & Ryan, R. M. (1999). A meta-analytic review of experiments examining the effects of extrinsic rewards on intrinsic motivation. *Psychological Bulletin, 125*, 627–668.

Deci, E. L., La Guardia, J. G., Moller, A. C., Scheiner, M. J., & Ryan, R. M. (2006). On the benefits of giving as well as receiving autonomy support: Mutuality in close friendships. *Personality and Social Psychology Bulletin, 32*, 313–327.

Deci, E. L., Olafsen, A. H., & Ryan, R. M. (2017). Self-determination theory in work organizations: The state of a science. *Annual Review of Organizational Psychology and Organizational Behavior, 4*, 19–43.

Deci, E. L., & Ryan, R. M. (1980a). The empirical exploration of intrinsically motivated behavior. In L. Berkowitz (Ed.), *Advances in experimental social psychology* (Vol. 13, pp. 39–80). New York: Academic Press.

Deci, E. L., & Ryan, R. M. (1980b). Self-determination theory: When mind mediates behavior. *Journal of Mind and Behavior, 1*(1), 33–43.

Deci, E. L., & Ryan, R. M. (1985). *Intrinsic motivation and self-determination in human behavior.* New York: Plenum Press.

Deci, E. L., Ryan, R. M., Schultz, P. P., & Niemiec, C. P. (2015). Being aware and functioning fully: Mindfulness and interest taking within self-determination theory. In K. W. Brown, J. D. Creswell, & R. M. Ryan (Eds.), *Handbook of mindfulness* (pp. 112–129). New York: Guilford Press.

DeHaan, C., Hirai, T., & Ryan, R. (2016). Nussbaum's capabilities and self-determination theory's basic psychological needs: Relating some fundamentals of human wellness. *Journal of Happiness, 17*(5), 2037–2049.

Di Domenico, S. I., & Fournier, M. A. (2014). Socio-economic status, income inequality, and health complaints: A basic psychological needs perspective. *Social Indicators Research, 119*(3), 1679–1697.

Di Domenico, S. I., Fournier, M. A., Ayaz, H., & Ruocco, A. C. (2013). In search of integrative processes: Basic psychological need satisfaction predicts medial prefrontal activation during decisional conflict. *Journal of Experimental Psychology: General, 142*, 967–978.

Di Domenico, S. I., Fournier, M. A., Rodrigo, A. H., Dong, M., Ayaz, H., & Ruocco, A. C. (2018). Need fulfillment and the modulation of medial prefrontal activity when judging remembered past, perceived present, and imagined future identities. *Self and Identity, 17*(3), 259–275.

Di Domenico, S. I., & Ryan, R. M. (2017). The emerging neuroscience of intrinsic motivation: A new frontier in self-determination research. *Frontiers in Human Neuroscience, 11*, 145.

Diener, E., Ng, W., Hartr, J., & Arora, R. (2010). Wealth and happiness across the world: Material prosperity predicts life evaluation whereas psychological prosperity predicts positive feeling. *Journal of Personality and Social Psychology, 99*, 52–61.

Frankfurt, H. G. (2004). *The reasons of love.* Princeton, NJ: Princeton University Press.

Frost, R. O., Marten, P., Lahart, C., & Rosenblate, R. (1990). The dimensions of perfectionism. *Cognitive Therapy and Research, 14*(5), 449–468.

Gagné, M. (2003). The role of autonomy support and autonomy orientation in prosocial behavior engagement. *Motivation and Emotion, 27*(3), 199–223.

Gailliot, M. T., & Baumeister, R. F. (2007). The physiology of willpower: Linking blood glucose to self-control. *Personality and Social Psychology Review, 11*(4), 303–327.

González, M. G., Swanson, D. P., Lynch, M., & Williams, G. C. (2016). Testing satisfaction of basic psychological needs as a mediator of the relationship between socioeconomic status and physical and mental health. *Journal of Health Psychology, 21*(6), 972–982.

Greenberg, J. R., Pyszczynski, T., & Solomon, S. (1995). Toward a dual-motive depth psychology of self and social behavior. In M. H. Kernis (Ed.), *Efficacy, agency, and self-esteem* (pp. 73–99). New York: Springer.

Guntert, S. T. (2015). The impact of work design, autonomy support, and strategy on employee outcomes: A differentiated perspective on self-determination at work. *Motivation and Emotion, 39*(1), 74–87.

Harvey, B., Milyavskaya, M., Hope, N., Powers, T. A., Saffran, M., & Koestner, R. (2015). Affect variation across days of the week: Influences of perfectionism and academic motivation. *Motivation and Emotion, 39*(4), 521–530.

Heider, F. (1958). *The psychology of interpersonal relations*. New York: Wiley.

Hewitt, P. L., & Flett, G. L. (1991). Perfectionism in the self and social contexts: Conceptualization, assessment, and association with psychopathology. *Journal of Personality and Social Psychology, 60*, 456–470.

Joesaar, H., Hein, V., & Haggar, M. (2012). Youth athletes' perceptions of autonomy support from the coach, peer motivational climate, and intrinsic motivation in sport settings: One-year effects. *Psychology of Sport and Exercise, 13*, 257–262.

Kanat-Maymon, Y., Roth, G., Assor, A., & Raizer, A. (2016). Controlled by love: The harmful relational consequences of perceived conditional positive regard. *Journal of Personality, 84*, 446–460.

Kasser, T. (2002). *The high price of materialism*. Cambridge, MA: MIT Press.

Kasser, V. M., & Ryan, R. M. (1999). The relation of psychological needs for autonomy and relatedness to health, vitality, well-being and mortality in a nursing home. *Journal of Applied Social Psychology, 29*, 935–954.

Kazén, M., Kuhl, J., & Leicht, E. M. (2015). When the going gets tough . . . Self-motivation is associated with invigoration and fun. *Psychological Research, 79*(6), 1064–1076.

Kuhl, J. (2000). The volitional basis of personality systems interaction theory: Applications in learning and treatment contexts. *International Journal of Educational Research, 33*(7), 665–703.

Legate, N., DeHaan, C. R., Weinstein, N., & Ryan, R. M. (2013). Hurting you hurts me too: The psychological costs of complying with ostracism. *Psychological Science, 24*(4), 583–588.

Legault, L., Green-Demers, I., Grant, P., & Chung, J. (2007). On the self-regulation of implicit and explicit prejudice: A self-determination theory perspective. *Personality and Social Psychology Bulletin, 33*(5), 732–749.

León, J., Núñez, J. L., & Liew, J. (2015). Self-determination and STEM education: Effects of autonomy, motivation, and self-regulated learning on high school math achievement. *Learning and Individual Differences, 43*, 156–163.

Litalien, D., Morin, A. J. S., Gagné, M., Valle-

rand, R. J., Losier, G. F., & Ryan, R. M. (2017). Evidence of a continuum structure of academic self-determination: A two-study test using a bifactor-ESEM representation of academic motivation. *Contemporary Educational Psychology, 51*, 67–82.

Lonsdale, C., & Hodge, K. (2011). Temporal ordering of motivational quality and athlete burnout in elite sport. *Medicine and Science in Sports and Exercise, 43*(5), 913–921.

Marbell, K. N., & Grolnick, W. S. (2013). Correlates of parental control and autonomy support in an interdependent culture: A look at Ghana. *Motivation and Emotion, 37*(1), 79–92.

Martela, F., DeHaan, C. R., & Ryan, R. M. (2016). On enhancing and diminishing energy through psychological means: Research on vitality and depletion from self-determination theory. In E. R. Hirt, J. J. Clarkson, & L. Jia (Eds.), *Self-regulation and ego control* (pp. 67–85). New York: Elsevier.

Martela, F., & Ryan, R. M. (2016). The benefits of benevolence: Basic psychological needs, beneficence, and the enhancement of well-being. *Journal of Personality, 84*(6), 750–764.

Moller, A. C., Deci, E. L., & Ryan, R. M. (2006). Choice and ego-depletion: The moderating role of autonomy. *Personality and Social Psychology Bulletin, 32*(8), 1024–1036.

Muraven, M. (2008). Autonomous self-control is less depleting. *Journal of Research in Personality, 42*(3), 763–770.

Muraven, M., Gagné, M., & Rosman, H. (2008). Helpful self-control: Autonomy support, vitality, and depletion. *Journal of Experimental Social Psychology, 44*(3), 573–585.

Muraven, M., Rosman, H., & Gagné, M. (2007). Lack of autonomy and self-control: Performance-contingent rewards lead to greater depletion. *Motivation and Emotion, 31*(4), 322–330.

Murayama, K., Matsumoto, M., Izuma, K., & Matusumoto, K. (2010). Neural bases of the undermining effect of monetary rewards on intrinsic motivation. *Proceedings of the National Academy of Sciences of the USA, 107*(49), 20911–20916.

Murayama, K., Matsumoto, M., Izuma, K., Sugiura, A., Ryan, R. M., Deci, E. L., et al. (2015). How self-determined choice facilitates performance: A key role of the metromedial prefrontal cortex. *Cerberal Cortex, 25*(5), 1241–1251.

Nguyen, T.-V. T., & Deci, E. L. (2016). Can it be good to set the bar high?: The role of motivational regulation in moderating the link from high standards to academic well-being. *Learning and Individual Differences, 45*, 245–251.

Nie, Y., Chua, B. L., Yeung, A. S., Ryan, R. M., & Chan, W. Y. (2015). The importance of autonomy support and the mediating role of work motivation for well-being: Self-determination theory in a Chinese work organization. *International Journal of Psychology, 50*(4), 245–255.

Niemiec, C. P., Brown, K. W., Kashdan, T. B., Cozzolino, P. J., Breen, W. E., Levesque, C. S., et al. (2010). Being present in the face of existential threat: The role of trait mindfulness in reducing defensive responses to mortality salience. *Journal of Personality and Social Psychology, 99,* 344–365.

Nix, G., Ryan, R. M., Manly, J. B., & Deci, E. L. (1999). Revitalization through self-regulation: The effects of autonomous versus controlled motivation on happiness and vitality. *Journal of Experimental Social Psychology, 35,* 266–284.

Ntoumanis, N., Healy, L. C., Sedikides, C., Duda, J., Stewart, B., Smith, A., et al. (2014). When the going gets tough: The "why" of goal striving matters. *Journal of Personality, 82*(3), 225–236.

Nussbaum, M. C. (2000). *Women and human development: The capabilities approach.* Cambridge, UK: Cambridge University Press.

Patall, E. A., Cooper, H., & Robinson, J. C. (2008). The effects of choice on intrinsic motivation and related outcomes: A meta-analysis of research findings. *Psychological Bulletin, 134,* 270–300.

Pittman, T. S., Davey, M. E., Alafat, K. A., Wetherill, K. V., & Kramer, N. A. (1980). Informational versus controlling verbal rewards. *Personality and Social Psychology Bulletin, 6,* 228–233.

Przybylski, A. K., Deci, E. L., Rigby, C. S., & Ryan, R. M. (2014). Competence-impeding electronic games and players' aggressive feelings, thoughts, and behaviors. *Journal of Personality and Social Psychology, 106*(3), 441–457.

Przybylski, A. K., Ryan, R. M., & Rigby, C. S. (2009). The motivating role of violence in video games. *Personality and Social Psychology Bulletin, 35*(2), 243–259.

Reeve, J., & Lee, W. (2019a). Motivational neuroscience. In R. M. Ryan (Ed.), *The Oxford handbook of human motivation* (2nd ed., pp. 355–372). New York: Oxford University Press.

Reeve, J., & Lee, W. (2019b). A neuroscientific perspective on basic psychological needs. *Journal of Personality, 87*(1), 102–114.

Ryan, R. M. (1995). Psychological needs and the facilitation of integrative processes. *Journal of Personality, 63*(3), 397–427.

Ryan, R. M., & Connell, J. P. (1989). Perceived locus of causality and internalization: Examining reasons for acting in two domains. *Journal of Personality and Social Psychology, 57,* 749–761.

Ryan, R. M., Connell, J. P., & Deci, E. L. (1985). A motivational analysis of self-determination and self-regulation in education. In C. Ames & R. E. Ames (Eds.), *Research on motivation in education: The classroom milieu* (pp. 13–51). New York: Academic Press.

Ryan, R. M., & Deci, E. L. (2000). Intrinsic and extrinsic motivations: Classic definitions and new directions. *Contemporary Educational Psychology, 25,* 54–67.

Ryan, R. M., & Deci, E. L. (2006). Self-regulation and the problem of human autonomy: Does psychology need choice, self-determination, and will? *Journal of Personality,74*(6), 1557–1585.

Ryan, R. M., & Deci, E. L. (2008). From ego depletion to vitality: Theory and findings concerning the facilitation of energy available to the self. *Social and Personality Psychology Compass, 2*(2), 702–717.

Ryan, R. M., & Deci, E. L. (2017). *Self-determination theory: Basic psychological needs in motivation, development, and wellness.* New York: Guilford Press.

Ryan, R. M., & Di Domenico, S. I. (2016). Distinct motivations and their differentiated mechanisms: Reflections on the emerging neuroscience of human motivation. In S. Kim, J. Reeve, & M. Bong (Eds.), *Recent developments in neuroscience research on human motivation: Advances in motivation and achievement* (Vol. 19, pp. 349–369). Bingley, UK: Emerald Group.

Ryan, R. M., & Frederick, C. M. (1997). On energy, personality and health: Subjective vitality as a dynamic reflection of well-being. *Journal of Personality, 65*(3), 529–565.

Ryan, R. M., & Hawley, P. (2017). Naturally good?: Basic psychological needs and the proximal and evolutionary bases of human benevolence. In K. W. Brown & M. R. Leary (Eds.), *The Oxford handbook of hypo-egoic phenomena* (pp. 205–222). New York: Oxford University Press.

Ryan, R. M., Huta, V., & Deci, E. L. (2008). Living well: A self-determination theory perspective on eudaimonia. *Journal of Happiness Studies, 9*(1), 139–170.

Ryan, R. M., Mims, V., & Koestner, R. (1983). Relation of reward contingency and interpersonal context to intrinsic motivation: A review and test using cognitive evaluation theory. *Journal of Personality and Social Psychology, 45*(4), 736–750.

Ryan, R. M., & Rigby, C. S. (2015). Did the Buddha have a self?: No-self, self, and mindfulness in Buddhist thought and Western psychologies. In K. W. Brown, J. D. Creswell, & R. M. Ryan (Eds.), *Handbook of mindfulness: Theory, research, and practice* (pp. 245–265). New York: Guilford Press.

Ryan, R. M., Rigby, C. S., & King, K. (1993). Two types of religious internalization and their relations to religious orientations and mental health.

Journal of Personality and Social Psychology, 65(3), 586–596.

Ryan, R. M., Rigby, C. S., & Przybylski, A. (2006). The motivational pull of video games: A self-determination theory approach. *Motivation and Emotion, 30*(4), 347–364.

Ryan, R. M., Ryan, W. S., Di Domenico, S. I., & Deci, E. L. (2019). The nature and the conditions of human flourishing: Self-determination theory and basic psychological needs. In R. M. Ryan (Ed.), *The Oxford handbook of human motivation* (2nd ed., pp. 89–110). New York: Oxford University Press.

Ryan, R. M., Soenens, B., & Vansteenkiste, M. (2019). Reflections on self-determination theory as an organizing framework for personality psychology: Interfaces, integrations, issues and unfinished business. *Journal of Personality, 87*, 115–145.

Ryan, W. S., & Ryan, R. M. (2019). Toward a social psychology of authenticity: Exploring within person variations in self-disclosure, transparency and congruence using self-determination theory. *Review of General Psychology, 23*(1), 99–112.

Sen, A. (2000). *Development as freedom*. New York: Anchor Books.

Sheldon, K. M., Abad, N., & Omoile, J. (2009). Testing self-determination theory via Nigerian and Indian adolescents. *International Journal of Behavioral Development, 33*(5), 451–459.

Standage, M., Duda, J. L., & Pensgaard, A. M. (2005). The effect of competitive outcome and task-involving, ego-involving, and cooperative structures on the psychological well-being of individuals engaged in a co-ordination task: A self-determination approach. *Motivation and Emotion, 29*(1), 41–68.

Thorpe, E., & Netteelbeck, T. (2014). Testing if healthy perfectionism enhances academic achievement in Australian secondary school students. *Journal of Educational and Developmental Psychology, 4*(2), 1–9.

Vansteenkiste, M., & Ryan, R. M. (2013). On psychological growth and vulnerability: Basic psychological need satisfaction and need frustration as a unifying principle. *Journal of Psychotherapy Integration, 23*(3), 263–280.

Weinstein, N., Legate, N., Al-Khouja, M., & Şengül, S. (2018). Relations of civil liberties and women's health satisfaction around the globe: The explanatory power of autonomy. *Journal of Health Psychology.* [Epub ahead of print]

Weinstein, N., & Ryan, R. M. (2010). When helping helps: Autonomous motivation for prosocial behavior and its influence on well-being for the helper and recipient. *Journal of Personality and Social Psychology, 98*(2), 222–244.

White, R. W. (1959). Motivation reconsidered: The concept of competence. *Psychological Review, 66*, 297–333.

Wilkinson, R. G., & Pickett, K. E. (2011). *The spirit level: Why greater equality makes societies stronger*. New York: Bloomsbury Press.

Williams, G. C., Grow, V. M., Freedman, Z. R., Ryan, R. M., & Deci, E. L. (1996). Motivational predictors of weight loss and weight-loss maintenance. *Journal of Personality and Social Psychology, 70*(1), 115–126.

Williams, G. C., Patrick, H., Niemiec, C. P., Williams, L. K., Divine, G., Lafata, J. E., et al. (2009). Reducing the health risks of diabetes: How self-determination theory may help improve medication adherence and quality of life. *Diabetes Educator, 35*(3), 484–492.

Yu, S., Levesque-Bristol, C., & Maeda, Y. (2018). General need for autonomy and subjective well-being: A meta-analysis of studies in the US and East Asia. *Journal of Happiness Studies, 19*(6), 1863–1882.

Zuckerman, M., Porac, J., Lathin, D., Smith, R., & Deci, E. L. (1978). On the importance of self-determination for intrinsically motivated behavior. *Personality and Social Psychology Bulletin, 4*, 443–446.

Zuroff, D. C., Koestner, R., Moskowitz, D. S., McBride, C., & Bagby, R. M. (2012). Therapist's autonomy support and patient's self-criticism predict motivation during brief treatments for depression. *Journal of Social and Clinical Psychology, 31*(9), 903–932.

INTERPERSONAL LEVEL

CHAPTER 7

The Biological Foundations and Modulation of Empathy

Grit Hein
Yanyan Qi
Shihui Han

Empathy is one of the core processes that connect humans and allow us to feel with and to understand others' emotional states. Reflecting its importance, empathy has been investigated in many different fields and contexts. In the first part of our chapter, we summarize how empathy is conceptualized and defined in different fields of psychology and introduce a model of empathy that combines these approaches with novel findings from social neuroscience. In the second part of our chapter, we review and discuss evidence of the biological foundations of empathy on the neural level. Finally, we summarize evidence for modulations of empathic neural processes, mainly in the light of intergroup processes.

What Is Empathy?

The term *empathy* is used in many different fields, with a broad range of meanings (Hein, 2014). Often, even the definitions of empathy within one field are far from consistent. For example, social psychology has offered different definitions of empathy that depend on the focus of research. Some researchers provide rather broad definitions of empathy, as does Hoffman (1981, p. 44), who sees empathy as "an affective response appropriate to someone else's situation rather than one's own." According to Hoffman, perceived distress in the other can elicit "empathic distress" or "sympathetic distress." The latter is the basis for altruistic motivation that mainly aims to relieve one's own distress. Note that other models of prosocial behavior predict that distress mainly results in withdrawal but not helping (e.g., Batson, 2014; see below), contradicting Hoffman's assumption.

Other influential definitions have emphasized the conceptual difference between empathy and sympathy (Eisenberg & Miller, 1987). *Empathy* is defined as "an affective state that stems from the apprehension of another's emotional state or condition, and that is congruent with it" (Eisenberg & Miller, 1987, p. 91). *Sympathy* is defined as "an emotional response stemming from another's emotional state or condition that is not identical to the other's emotion, but consists of feelings of sorrow or concern for another's welfare" (Eisenberg & Miller, 1987, p. 92). According to these definitions, empathy in its pure form does not induce a prosocial motivation. With further cognitive processing, it can turn into sympathy, personal distress, or a combination of both (Eisenberg, 2000). Prosocial behavior is negatively correlated with personal distress, and positively associated with sympathy (Eisenberg & Miller, 1987). Sympathy can derive from not only empathy but also cognitive perspective taking.

While these models define empathy as an affective response (Eisenberg & Miller, 1987; Hoffman, 1981), other authors conceptualize empathy as a multidimensional construct that contains both cognitive and affective processes. A prominent example of the multidimensionality approach is the work by Davis (1980, 1983), which dissects empathy in four different dimensions: (cognitive) perspective taking, empathic concern, fantasy, and personal distress. Davis developed subscales to measure individual differences in these four dimensions and assumes that these individual differences account for differences in trait empathy.

Yet another conceptual approach is offered by Batson and associates, who hold that perceiving a person is in need can induce empathy or "empathic concern," or personal distress. *Empathic concern* is defined as an other-oriented response congruent with the perceived distress experienced by another person (Batson, Turk, Shaw, & Klein, 1995). It is elicited by adopting another's perspective and requires valuing the other's welfare (Batson, Eklund, Chermok, Hoyt, & Ortiz, 2007). An impressive series of experiments demonstrated that empathic concern motivates helping behavior toward the person in need, even if it is costly for the helper (Batson, 2014). By contrast, personal distress is a self-centered stress response that motivates withdrawal rather than helping. For example, a person experiencing mainly distress when seeing a handicapped person struggling to get on the bus will take the back door in order to avoid the other in need of help.

Definitions of empathy in clinical contexts stress the importance of "empathic accuracy" or the empathic reaction that resembles the other's emotions as closely as possible (Rogers, 2013). At the same time, the empathizer needs to be fully aware that the empathic reaction represents the other's emotional state but not the emotions of the empathizer. The focus of attention in clinical fields is the use of empathy as a therapeutic tool, and its concrete impact on the other in need, in this case, the client. Thus, in the definition by Rogers, and in its clinical application, the term *empathy* clearly refers to a prosocial motivation, in contrast to models that define empathy as a "neutral" apprehension of another's emotional state (e.g., Eisenberg & Miller, 1987; see below for similar definitions).

More recent work has also considered the cost for the empathizer (Maslach, 2003). One impressive example is the cost reflected in *burnout,* a complex of symptoms related to fatigue and depression that is often seen in caretakers. Witnessing another person in need can elicit different motivational states (Van Lange, 2008), including empathy and personal distress (e.g., Batson, 2014). It is unclear which of these motivational states leads to burnout (i.e., whether burnout stems from empathy or from personal distress; see Klimecki & Singer, 2012, for a similar point).

In last decades, empathy has been investigated extensively in social neuroscience. Social neuroscience studies aim to elucidate the biological foundations of empathy, both on neural and hormonal levels. Definitions of empathy used in neuroscience research are inspired by the empathy concepts from social, clinical, and developmental psychology we outlined earlier, but they also incorporate neuroscience findings. *Empathy* is defined as the affective sharing of the emotions of others (Figure 7.1). In line with Eisenberg and Miller (1987) and Batson (2014), it is assumed that empathy as such is not other-oriented in the sense of a prosocial motivation. Sharing the other's emotions can reveal the other person's "weak spot" (i.e., information that can also be used to harm the other person). Considering this potential "dark side" of empathy, empathy should be distinguished from sympathy (Eisenberg & Miller, 1987) or empathic concern (Batson, 2014; i.e., feeling of concern for the other that incites the motivation to improve the other's welfare). Empathy can transform into not only sympathy but also personal distress (i.e., a self-centered state that motivates withdrawal from the suffering person rather than prosociality; see Figure 7.1).

Moreover, as in definitions of empathy from clinical psychology (Rogers, 2013), it is assumed that empathy requires a differentiation between one's own emotions and emotions of others (Cuff, Brown, Taylor, & Howat, 2016). In the case of empathy, the person needs to be aware that the felt emotions are induced by ob-

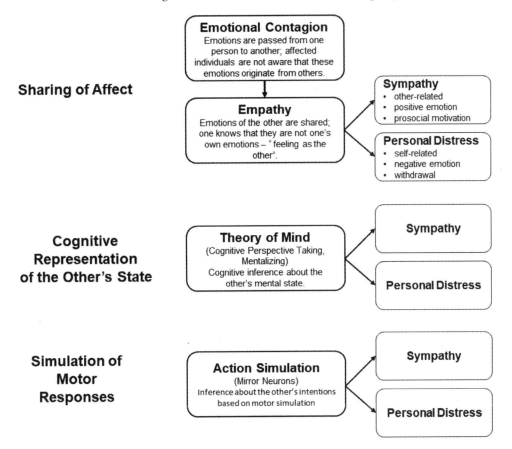

FIGURE 7.1. Routes of understanding others. Empathy is only one of the processes that allows us to understand others. This model assumes that emotional contagion is a precursor of empathy. Theoretically, empathy can be differentiated from theory of mind and action simulation, and there is neural evidence supporting this division. Practically, however, the different processes are tightly linked and commonly activated simultaneously.

serving the other's emotional state, and not by an event directly happening to the empathizer (e.g., "I am sad for a friend who is getting divorced, knowing that my sadness is related to her situation and independent of my own relationship"). This differentiates empathy from emotional contagion (i.e., a state in which emotions are passed from one individual to the other, but the person is not aware that the felt emotions originate from the state of the other; see Figure 7.1; see also Singer & Hein, 2012).

Besides the incorporation of existing concepts of empathy from social and clinical psychology, neuroscientific findings have added new aspects. One aspect is to differentiate

among empathy, cognitive perspective taking (also known as "theory of mind" or "mentalizing") and action simulation. Cognitive perspective taking connotes a person's ability to cognitively represent the mental states of others, including their affective states, without necessarily becoming emotionally involved (Figure 7.1, central portion). *Action simulation* refers to a process that mirrors the motor response of another individual that, again, does not necessarily include a simulation of emotions (Figure 7.1, bottom center portion). By contrast, an empathic response always means an affective response that is derived from sharing the feelings of the other, in line with definitions from social psychology that conceptualize empathy mainly as an affective state (Eisenberg & Miller, 1987; Hoffman, 1981). Based on social neuroscience evidence, it is plausible to differentiate between processes that involve the sharing of affect (empathy), cognitive perspective taking, and action simulation because there is evidence that these processes correlate with activations in distinct brain regions.

In more detail, it has been proposed that empathy is mainly correlated with activation in the anterior insula (AI), and cognitive perspective taking is mainly correlated with activation of the ventral temporoparietal junction (TPJ; Kanske, Böckler, Trautwein, Parianen Lesemann, & Singer, 2016; Kanske, Böckler, Trautwein, & Singer, 2015). Action simulation has been linked to the so-called "mirror neuron" system that mainly involves inferior parietal (IP) and ventral premotor cortices (Molenberghs, Cunnington, & Mattingley, 2009; Reynolds et al., 2015; Rizzolatti & Craighero, 2004).

Discovered in the monkey brain, mirror neurons describe a group of motor neurons that fired whenever the animal observed the moving arm of the experimenter (Rizzolatti & Craighero, 2004). Neuroscience studies in humans have shown that observing a movement elicits neural activation in brain regions that are also involved in the processing of active motor responses (see Hardwick, Caspers, Eickhoff, & Swinnen, 2018, for a recent meta-analysis). Motor information (e.g., facial expression, body language) are important for understanding others (Gallese, 2009; Iacoboni, 2009), and given that they are motor neurons, mirror neurons contribute to inferring the other's state based on such action-related cues.

However, there is evidence that the mirror neuron system is activated when people are processing others' facial muscle movements, while brain regions related to emotion processing (e.g., the insula cortex) are activated when people are instructed to infer emotions (Jabbi & Keysers, 2008). This indicates that mirror neurons are neither necessary nor sufficient for affective sharing of others' emotions (i.e., the process that is defined as empathy in Figure 7.1; see Singer & Hein, 2012, for a similar point). That said, there is meta-analytic evidence that shows activation of the TPJ for empathy-related

processes (Bzdok et al., 2012) and that parts of the mirror neuron system are activated by empathy paradigms (Bird et al., 2010; Lamm, Decety, & Singer, 2011).

Such evidence implies that empathy, cognitive perspective taking, and action simulation may recruit different neural regions but often operate in concert. The interactions between the different routes probably depend on situational contexts and on an individual's ability to empathize, mentalize, or simulate the other's actions. For example, empathy might be the dominant route for inferring others' emotional states in people with strong empathic abilities, while strong "mentalizers" first activate the brain regions related to theory of mind, and people who are particularly good in motor simulation might first recruit parts of the mirror neuron system. Given the close interactions among empathy, theory of mind, and action simulation, it is plausible to assume that sympathy or personal distress can originate from all three processes, and not just from empathy (Figure 7.1; see Eisenberg & Miller, 1987, for a similar point regarding empathy and theory of mind). In other words, sharing the affect of the other (empathy), generating a cognitive representation of the other's state (theory of mind), or simulating the other's actions can transform into sympathy and a resulting prosocial motivation, or into personal distress, inciting self-centered withdrawal (Figure 7.1).

The Biological Foundations of Empathy

The biological basis of empathy has been investigated on the neural level. Most studies that investigate the neural correlates of empathy have focused on empathy for the pain of another person (for reviews, see Hein & Singer, 2008; Lamm et al., 2011; Shamay-Tsoory & Lamm, 2018; Wondra & Ellsworth, 2015; Zaki, Wager, Singer, Keysers, & Gazzola, 2016). To study empathy for another's pain, participants were presented with pictures of faces expressing pain (e.g., Lamm, Batson, & Decety, 2007; Saarela et al., 2006; Sheng & Han, 2012) or body parts in painful positions (e.g., Cheng et al., 2007; Gu & Han, 2007; Lamm et al., 2007; Xu, Zuo, Wang, & Han, 2009). Other studies combined the observation of painful stimulation to others and the experience of self-pain (Eidelman-Rothman et al., 2016; Hein, Engelmann, Vollberg, & To-bler, 2016; Hein, Silani, Preuschoff, Batson, & Singer, 2010; Rütgen, Seidel, Riečanský, & Lamm, 2015; Rütgen, Seidel, Silani, et al., 2015; Singer et al., 2004, 2006). Here the participants inside the scanner experienced more or less painful shocks via an electrode attached to the back of their hands and observed a person sitting next to them in the scanning room in the same situation. Cues of different colors indicated to the participants both the painful and nonpainful nature and the intensity of the stimulation administered to the other person. This setup allowed the localization of brain regions involved in the processing of firsthand pain and brain regions associated with the processing of pain experienced by the other person. There is evidence that brain structures such as the AI, parts of the cingulate cortex, and often also the inferior frontal gyrus (IFG) are commonly activated when participants experience pain stimulation themselves and observe pain stimulation in others (de Waal & Preston, 2017; Gonzalez-Liencres, Shamay-Tsoory, & Brüne, 2013; Lamm et al., 2011; Singer & Lamm, 2009; Walter, 2012). Brain responses to others' pain in the AI and cingulate cortex were found to correlate with questionnaires that assess empathic states (Hein, Engelmann, et al., 2016; Hein et al., 2010; Yao et al., 2016), and to predict prosocial motivation, for example, a person's willingness to endure pain in order to help another person (Hein, Engelmann, & Tobler, 2018; Hein, Engelmann, et al., 2016; Hein, Morishima, Leiberg, Sul, & Fehr, 2016).

The results of studies using different paradigms such as faces with painful expressions and body parts in painful positions have partly confirmed these findings (Cheng et al., 2007; Saarela et al., 2006). However, meta-analyses (Lamm et al., 2011) also have shown differences in neural activations between empathy measured with "picture paradigms" (i.e., pictures of faces) and "cue paradigms" (i.e., cues indicating painful stimulation of self or other) (see Figure 7.2). In addition to activating the AI and anterior cingulate cortex (ACC), pictures of body parts in painful situations activated parts of the so-called "mirror neuron system,"

the neural structures related to sensory–motor functions and action understanding (IP/ventral premotor cortices). By contrast, cues indicating the other's pain activated areas associated with mentalizing or "theory of mind" (precuneus, ventral medial prefrontal cortex, superior temporal cortex, and TPJ). These findings bolster the claim that there are different neural routes allowing one to understand and predict others' actions, feelings, and beliefs (Figure 7.1). Empathy is only one of these routes that in many situations operate in concert with theory of mind and the mirror neuron system.

Some studies have extended the investigation of empathic brain responses to the domain of social pain, such as social exclusion (Masten, Morelli, & Eisenberger, 2011; Mischkowski, Crocker, & Way, 2016; Nordgren, Banas, & McDonald, 2011; Novembre, Zanon, & Silani, 2014) and vicarious embarrassment (Hawk, Fischer, & Van Kleef, 2011; Krach et al., 2011; Laneri et al., 2017). In Masten and colleagues' (2011) study, participants in the functional magnetic resonance imaging (fMRI) scanner observed one person who was excluded by two others. Later on, participants could write e-mails to offer help or comfort to the excluded person. When seeing someone being excluded, participants who scored high on a trait empathy questionnaire displayed activation in AI and cingulate cortex, in addition to activations typically related to mentalizing (e.g., medial prefrontal cortex [mPFC]). Krach and colleagues (2011) presented participants with cartoons and descriptions of scenes depicting a protagonist in a possibly embarrassing situation. The results showed that the observation of vicarious embarrassment activated the AI and cingulate cortex.

In addition to physical pain and social pain, neuroscience studies have investigated empathic responses related to others' experience of touch (Keysers et al., 2004; Lamm, Silani, & Singer, 2015; Schaefer, Heinze, & Rotte, 2012) and taste (Jabbi, Swart, & Keysers, 2007; Wicker et al., 2003). There is evidence that the observation of touch and the firsthand experience of touch activate similar regions in the somatosensory cortex (Keysers et al., 2004; Schaefer et al., 2012). For example, in a study by Jabbi and colleagues (2007), participants watched video clips showing people sampling pleasant and un-

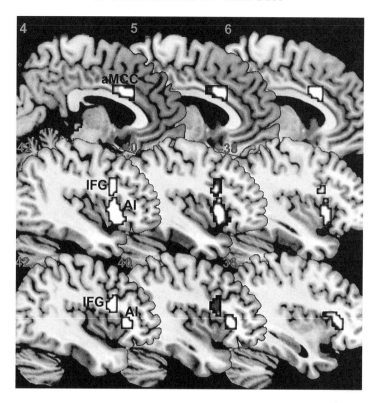

FIGURE 7.2. Common activation (conjunction) for the picture-based and cue-based empathy paradigms. aMCC, anterior medial cingulate cortex; AI, anterior insular cortex; IFG, inferior frontal gyrus. With kind permission from C. Lamm.

pleasant tastes, and then experienced the different tastes themselves. In line with the results of empathy for pain, Jabbi and colleagues found neural activation in AI cortex when people passively watched disgust in another person, and when they were disgusted themselves (see also Wicker et al., 2003).

The studies summarized here have examined the neural correlates of empathy mainly in the domains of negative emotions such as pain, social exclusion, and disgust. However, there are neuroscience studies that extend this focus to positive emotions (Morelli, Lieberman, & Zaki, 2015; Lockwood, Apps, Roiser, & Viding, 2015; Morelli, Sacchet, & Zaki, 2015), such as sharing others' happiness about winning money (Mobbs et al., 2009), other positive events (e.g., winning a scholarship; Lockwood et al., 2015; Perry, Hendler, & Shamay-Tsoory, 2011), or positive emotion (Jabbi et al., 2007).

Perry and associates (2011) used vignettes to introduce a person matching the participant's gender, then presented sentences describing everyday-life positive or negative events happening to that person. Sharing the other's distress was related to activations in the insula and regions related to "mentalizing," such as superior temporal cortex and mPFC. Sharing the other's joy revealed similar but weaker activations in these brain regions. In the Mobbs and colleagues (2009) study, participants in the fMRI scanner witnessed similar or dissimilar others winning or losing money in a TV show. Seeing a similar other winning money correlated with increased activation in the nucleus accumbens, a brain region that was also activated when the participants won money themselves.

These results have been taken as evidence that empathy with the state of the other person is based on a simulation of his or her neural response by the empathizer's brain (i.e., the activation of brain regions that are also active during the empathizer's firsthand experience of the positive or negative emotion) (Hein & Singer, 2008; Singer & Lamm, 2009). However, the interpretation of the neural overlap between empathic and self-experienced emotions is heavily debated, in particular regarding its meaning for underlying psychological processes (Zaki & Ochsner, 2012). Sharing of neural substrates does not necessarily indicate similarity of the psychological processes that underlie empathic and firsthand experience because the involved brain regions are also activated in many other contexts. For example, the AI and cingulate cortex, two regions that were found to show overlapping activations for empathic and nociceptive pain, are both known to track changes in aversive arousal. Thus, the neural overlap might reflect such unspecific common processes rather than psychological processes that are shared by empathic and nociceptive pain (Decety, 2010; Yamada & Decety, 2009; Zaki et al., 2016).

Elucidating the neural processing of empathic reactions in relation to self-experienced states requires the use of new methods and paradigms. Neural overlap should be assessed based on multivariate pattern classification methods that, for example, classify empathic reactions based on nociceptive pain responses in an independent sample (Zaki et al., 2016). New paradigms should systematically investigate the experimental conditions that elicit neural commonality between empathic responses and firsthand experiences. For example, as outlined below, the neural empathic response is known to be modulated by a number of social factors, including group membership (Han, 2018; Hein et al., 2010; Xu et al., 2009). However, it is unclear whether such social modulation is also found in the processing of nociceptive pain. A similar modulation of empathic and self-pain-related neural responses by the same social factors would indicate that a shared neural coding for empathic and firsthand experience reflects similarity in psychological processes. Differences in the impact of social modulation on empathic and firsthand processes would challenge simulation accounts. At least it would be unlikely that empathy involves the psychological simulation of firsthand experience. Given the importance

of social modulators for testing these questions, next we review evidence for social modulation of empathy in intergroup contexts.

Modulation of Empathy by Intergroup Processes

While empathy provides a psychological basis for social interactions, it is not rigid and has to be adjusted in response to social demands. Evidence for flexibility of empathy comes from early social neuroscience research that has shown evidence that how the brain responds to others' pain is influenced by the involvement of observers' cognitive endeavor such as attention (Gu & Han, 2007) and perceived fairness of others (Singer et al., 2006). To date, there has been increasing interest in modulations of empathy by intergroup relationships due to the desire to understand ingroup favoritism—a widely acknowledged feature of social behavior rooted in human evolution (Efferson, Lalive, & Fehr, 2008). To favor ingroup over outgroup members characterizes our prosocial behavior but conflicts with some of the contemporary cultural norms, such as individual equality and philanthropy, that discourage discrimination of others by social markers. As empathy plays a key role in prosocial behavior, to probe how empathy is modulated by intergroup processes opens a window for understanding biases in social behavior.

Intergroup processes include the processing of novel social cues that drive classification of other individuals into ingroup and outgroup, generate prejudice and attitude biases, modify emotional responses to others' need, and lead to discrimination of social behavior. In real-life situations, people quickly sort others into different social categories in terms of age, gender, and ethnicity/race, using facial cues, skin tone, and so forth, and racial categorization of others creates one of the most novel intergroup relationships between oneself and others that determine how we act upon others' demand (Kawakami, Amodio, & Hugenberg, 2017; Zhou et al., 2020). Besides the widely documented racial discrimination in clinical treatment (Drwecki, 2015) and school harassment (Bucchianeri, Eisenberg, & Neumark-Sztainer, 2013), racial biases in behavior have been reported in empirical studies and have been related to racial ingroup bias in empathy. For example, after reading a passage involving a Black or a White defendant in a criminal case, White students reported greater feelings of empathy for the target and assigned more lenient punishments to a White than to a Black defendant (Johnson et al., 2002). When asking nursing professionals (mainly Whites) to watch videos of Black and White patients' genuine facial expressions of pain and to provide pain treatment decisions, their pro-White empathy biases to patients' pain expressions can predict their pro-White pain treatment biases (Drwecki, Moore, Ward, & Prkachin, 2011). These behavioral findings implicate a favor of the neural underpinnings of empathy for same-race rather than other-race pain.

An early fMRI study examined racial ingroup bias in empathic neural responses scanned Asian and White college students who were presented with video clips showing faces of Asian and White models who received either painful (needle penetration) or nonpainful (touched with a cotton bud) stimulation applied to their left or right cheeks (Xu et al., 2009). Participants were asked to judge whether the model in each video clip was feeling pain during scanning and also to rate each model's pain intensity and their own unpleasantness induced by others' suffering after scanning. It was found that watching painful compared to nonpainful stimulations applied to the models activated the ACC and supplementary motor area (ACC/SMA) and the inferior frontal (IF)/AI cortex in all participants. Interestingly, while participants reported comparable feelings of perceived pain in others and their own unpleasantness induced by perceived pain of same-race and other-race models, the brain activity showed evidence for racial ingroup bias (i.e., the ACC/SMA activation was significantly decreased in response to painful stimulations applied to other-race rather than same-race models in both Chinese and White students. Thus, racial ingroup bias in empathic brain activity was evident even when self-report failed to show racial ingroup bias in empathy, possibly due to the influence of social desirability on self-report of one's own feelings.

Is racial ingroup bias in empathic neural responses a universal phenomenon? This has now been tested in a number of laboratories in several countries using different types of stimuli. For instance, an fMRI study scanning Whites in Australia reported greater activity in the ACC, AI, and somatosensory cortices in response to video clips showing painful (vs. nonpainful) stimulation to White rather than Asian faces (Contreras-Huerta, Baker, Reynolds, Batalha, & Cunnington, 2013). Viewing video clips of painful (vs. nonpainful) stimulation applied to Black and to White hands also activated the left AI more strongly in response to same-race rather than other-race models in Blacks and Whites in Italy (Azevedo et al., 2013). While these researchers reported evidence for modulations of sensory–motor and affective components of empathy by racial relationships between observers and targets, other researchers also found evidence for racial ingroup bias in cognitive component of empathy. For example, it was found that viewing video clips of dynamic physical or social suffering of Black and White models resulted in greater activity relative to same-race rather than other-race pain in the precuneus and TPJ in Blacks and Whites in South Africa (Fourie, Stein, Solms, Gobodo-Madikizela, & Decety, 2017). Photos showing naturalistic visual scenes depicting either Blacks or Whites in a painful or a neutral situation induced stronger mPFC activity in response to same-race rather than other-race pain in Blacks in the United States, and the mPFC activity predicted participants' greater altruistic motivation for their racial ingroup (Mathur, Harada, Lipke, & Chiao, 2010). The TPJ and mPFC are the key nodes of the theory-of-mind network (Schurz, Radua, Aichorn, Richlan, & Perner, 2014). Overall, these fMRI results indicate that racial ingroup bias in empathic neural responses is evident in multiple nodes of the empathy network underlying sensory–motor, affective, and cognitive processes involved in empathy for others' pain. In addition, the racial ingroup bias in empathic neural responses is not characteristic of a specific society. Instead, it reflects a universal neural strategy in multiple ethnic groups that facilitates understanding and sharing emotional states of same-race individuals and provides one of the psychological and neural bases of ingroup favoritism during human evolution (Efferson et al., 2008).

Besides the aforementioned fMRI findings, electroencephalography (EEG) research also revealed the time course of greater empathic neural responses to same-race than to other-race pain. By recording EEG from Chinese students when they made racial identity judgments on Asian and White faces, researchers found increased amplitude of a positive component at 128–188 milliseconds (P2) after stimulus onset over the frontal/central regions in response to painful (vs. neutral) expressions of Asian but not White faces (Sheng & Han, 2012). The P2 amplitude to pain (vs. neutral) expressions can predict both unpleasantness induced by perceived pain expressions and empathic concern and is thus believed to manifest early neural activity underlying empathy for pain. There was also evidence that the amplitude of a following negative N2 activity (200–300 milliseconds) was decreased (or also positively shifted) by pain versus neutral expressions of Asian (but not White) faces. Similar patterns of modulations of the P2 and N2 amplitudes to others' pain by racial relationships were replicated in Chinese and White participants (Han, Luo, & Han, 2016; Sessa, Meconi, & Han, 2014; Sheng, Han, & Han, 2015; Sheng, Lui, Zhou, Zhou, & Han, 2013). These results demonstrate that interracial relationships between targets and onlookers modulate empathic neural responses quite early in the processing stream. The early neural responses favoring understanding and sharing emotional states of same-race individuals possibly influence later process of decision making to generate ingroup favoritism in social behavior.

Another line of research has examined the impact of intergroup processes on empathy by manipulating ingroup–outgroup relationships based on participants' life experiences. In one study, soccer fans were scanned when viewing a fan of their favorite team (vs. a rival team) experience pain (Hein et al., 2010). It was found that the left AI showed increased activity when soccer fans witnessed ingroup compared to outgroup members' pain. Moreover, the ingroup bias in the insular activity predicted the extent of participants' ingroup favoritism in subsequent costly helping (i.e., the extent to which a participant was willing to receive a painful shock in order to save the other person from pain). Another fMRI study indicated a similar effect that witnessing failure of the favored team or success of the rival team activated the

ACC and insula (Cikara, Bruneau, & Saxe, 2011). Interestingly, these studies also indicated activation in the reward system, including the nucleus accumbens and ventral striatum, when participants viewed outgroup members' suffering or failure, indicating distinct patterns of modulations of empathy and reward systems by intergroup processes.

Given that empathic neural responses are sensitive to intergroup relationships based on both racial identity and mini-group (e.g., soccer team) identity, researchers have tested whether mini-group relationships can overcome racial relationships to reduce racial ingroup bias in empathy. To clarify this question is of practical importance because, if mini-group relationships built temporarily can override racial relationships in modulating empathic neural responses, mini-group manipulation implicates a potential intervention of racial bias in prosocial behavior. This idea was tested in an early event-related potential (ERP) study that employed the minimal group paradigm to examine empathic neural responses in a mixed-group relationship context (Sheng & Han, 2012). Chinese participants were assigned to a team that included both Asian and White faces to compete with another team that also included Asian and White faces. This design allowed researchers to evaluate whether racial ingroup bias in empathy can be reduced by including other-race individuals in one's team. Interestingly, the ERP results showed that while racial ingroup bias in the P2 amplitude to painful (vs. neutral) expressions was evident for opponent team faces, participants showed increased P2 amplitude in responses to painful (vs. neutral) expressions of both same-race and other-race faces from the fellow team. It seems that ingroup membership defined by mini-group relationship can override interracial relationship to enhance empathy for other-race pain. However, another fMRI study manipulating both interracial and mini-group relationships found significant racial ingroup bias in ACC and insular activity in response to others' pain but did not observe reliable minimal group effects on empathic neural responses (Contreras-Huerta et al., 2013). Future work is required to further examine how different intergroup relationships interact with each other to modulate empathy for other's pain and related prosocial behavior.

Taken together, there is now increasing evidence for influences of intergroup processes on empathic neural responses to others' pain. The impact of intergroup relationships on empathy can be observed when individuals perceive same-race and other-race pain or fellow-team and opponent-team suffering. The same pattern of modulations of empathy by racial and minigroup relationships implicate that similar downregulation mechanisms are possibly engaged, though this has to be clarified in future work. The modulation of empathic neural responses by ingroup–outgroup relationships reflects the sensitivity of empathy to social contexts and its flexible role in supporting prosocial behavior depending on the targets of social interactions. Empathy as a social function can be adjusted to adapt to appropriate social communication and behavior.

Conclusions

Empathy is a multifaceted function and a key concept in various fields. Reviewing empathy and its neurobiological foundations has provided insights that can be summarized in four statements. First, empathy can be distinguished from emotional contagion and is one route for understanding others. The other routes are theory of mind (cognitive perspective taking) and action simulation (mirror neurons). There is evidence that these different routes recruit distinct neural networks but often work in concert. Second, empathy is an other-oriented state. However, it only elicits a prosocial motivation if it is transferred into sympathy. Alternatively, empathy can result in personal distress that results in withdrawal rather than prosociality. Third, regarding the biological foundations of empathy, there is evidence for overlapping neural networks for empathic and firsthand experiences. Based on this evidence, it has been suggested that empathic reactions derive from a simulation of firsthand experiences. Fourth, we conclude that empathy is strongly modulated by social factors, in particular by group membership.

ACKNOWLEDGMENTS

This work was supported by the German Research Foundation (to Grit Hein; HE 4566/5-1 and HE 4566/3-1), the National Natural Science Foundation of China (to Shihui Han; Projects 31661143039, 31421003, and 31470986), and the Joint Training Program of the University of Chinese Academy of Sciences (to Yanyan Qi).

REFERENCES

Azevedo, R. T., Macaluso, E., Avenanti, A., Santangelo, V., Cazzato, V., & Aglioti, S. M. (2013). Their pain is not our pain: Brain and autonomic correlates of empathic resonance with the pain of same and different race individuals. *Human Brain Mapping, 34*(12), 3168–3181.

Batson, C. D. (2014). *The altruism question: Toward a social-psychological answer.* New York: Psychology Press.

Batson, C. D., Eklund, J. H., Chermok, V. L., Hoyt, J. L., & Ortiz, B. G. (2007). An additional antecedent of empathic concern: Valuing the welfare of the person in need. *Journal of Personality and Social Psychology, 93*(1), 65–74.

Batson, C. D., Turk, C. L., Shaw, L. L., & Klein, T. R. (1995). Information function of empathic emotion: Learning that we value the other's welfare. *Journal of Personality and Social Psychology, 68*(2), 300–313.

Bird, G., Silani, G., Brindley, R., White, S., Frith, U., & Singer, T. (2010). Empathic brain responses in insula are modulated by levels of alexithymia but not autism. *Brain, 133*(5), 1515–1525.

Bucchianeri, M. M., Eisenberg, M. E., & Neumark-Sztainer, D. (2013). Weightism, racism, classism, and sexism: Shared forms of harassment in adolescents. *Journal of Adolescent Health, 53*(1), 47–53.

Bzdok, D., Schilbach, L., Vogeley, K., Schneider, K., Laird, A. R., Langner, R., et al. (2012). Parsing the neural correlates of moral cognition: ALE meta-analysis on morality, theory of mind, and empathy. *Brain Structure and Function, 217*(4), 783–796.

Cheng, Y., Lin, C.-P., Liu, H.-L., Hsu, Y.-Y., Lim, K.-E., Hung, D., et al. (2007). Expertise modulates the perception of pain in others. *Current Biology, 17*(19), 1708–1713.

Cikara, M., Bruneau, E. G., & Saxe, R. R. (2011). Us and them: Intergroup failures of empathy. *Current Directions in Psychological Science, 20*(3), 149–153.

Contreras-Huerta, L. S., Baker, K. S., Reynolds, K. J., Batalha, L., & Cunnington, R. (2013). Racial bias in neural empathic responses to pain. *PLOS ONE, 8*(12), e84001.

Cuff, B. M., Brown, S. J., Taylor, L., & Howat, D. J.

(2016). Empathy: A review of the concept. *Emotion Review, 8*(2), 144–153.

Davis, M. H. (1980). Individual differences in empathy: A multidimensional approach. *Dissertation Abstracts International, 40*(7-B), 3480.

Davis, M. H. (1983). Measuring individual differences in empathy: Evidence for a multidimensional approach. *Journal of Personality and Social Psychology, 44*(1), 113–126.

de Waal, F. B., & Preston, S. D. (2017). Mammalian empathy: Behavioural manifestations and neural basis. *Nature Reviews Neuroscience, 18*(8), 498–509.

Decety, J. (2010). The neurodevelopment of empathy in humans. *Developmental Neuroscience, 32*(4), 257–267.

Drwecki, B. B. (2015). Education to identify and combat racial bias in pain treatment. *AMA Journal of Ethics, 17*(3), 221–228.

Drwecki, B. B., Moore, C. F., Ward, S. E., & Prkachin, K. M. (2011). Reducing racial disparities in pain treatment: The role of empathy and perspective-taking. *Pain, 152*(5), 1001–1006.

Efferson, C., Lalive, R., & Fehr, E. (2008). The co-evolution of cultural groups and ingroup favoritism. *Science, 321,* 1844–1849.

Eidelman-Rothman, M., Goldstein, A., Weisman, O., Schneiderman, I., Zagoory-Sharon, O., Decety, J., et al. (2016). Prior exposure to extreme pain alters neural response to pain in others. *Cognitive, Affective, and Behavioral Neuroscience, 16*(4), 662–671.

Eisenberg, N. (2000). Emotion, regulation, and moral development. *Annual Review of Psychology, 51*(1), 665–697.

Eisenberg, N., & Miller, P. A. (1987). The relation of empathy to prosocial and related behaviors. *Psychological Bulletin, 101*(1), 91–119.

Fourie, M. M., Stein, D. J., Solms, M., Gobodo-Madikizela, P., & Decety, J. (2017). Empathy and moral emotions in post-apartheid South Africa: An fMRI investigation. *Social Cognitive and Affective Neuroscience, 12*(6), 881–892.

Gallese, V. (2009). Motor abstraction: A neuroscientific account of how action goals and intentions are mapped and understood. *Psychological Research, 73*(4), 486–498.

Gonzalez-Liencres, C., Shamay-Tsoory, S. G., & Brüne, M. (2013). Towards a neuroscience of empathy: Ontogeny, phylogeny, brain mechanisms, context and psychopathology. *Neuroscience and Biobehavioral Reviews, 37*(8), 1537–1548.

Gu, X., & Han, S. (2007). Attention and reality constraints on the neural processes of empathy for pain. *NeuroImage, 36*(1), 256–267.

Han, S. (2018). Neurocognitive basis of racial ingroup bias in empathy. *Trends in Cognitive Sciences, 22*(5), 400–421.

Han, X., Luo, S., & Han, S. (2016). Embodied neural responses to others' suffering. *Cognitive Neuroscience, 7*(1–4), 114–127.

Hardwick, R. M., Caspers, S., Eickhoff, S. B., & Swinnen, S. P. (2018). Neural correlates of action: Comparing meta-analyses of imagery, observation, and execution. *Neuroscience and Biobehavioral Reviews, 94,* 31–44.

Hawk, S. T., Fischer, A. H., & Van Kleef, G. A. (2011). Taking your place or matching your face: Two paths to empathic embarrassment. *Emotion, 11*(3), 502–513.

Hein, G. (2014). Empathy and resilience in a connected world. In M. Kent, M. C. Davis, & J. W. Reich (Eds.), *The resilience handbook: Approaches to stress and trauma* (pp. 144–155). New York: Routledge.

Hein, G., Engelmann, J. B., & Tobler, P. N. (2018). Pain relief provided by an outgroup member enhances analgesia. *Proceedings of the Royal Society of London B: Biological Sciences, 285,* 20180501.

Hein, G., Engelmann, J. B., Vollberg, M. C., & Tobler, P. N. (2016). How learning shapes the empathic brain. *Proceedings of the National Academy of Sciences of the USA, 113*(1), 80–85.

Hein, G., Morishima, Y., Leiberg, S., Sul, S., & Fehr, E. (2016). The brain's functional network architecture reveals human motives. *Science, 351,* 1074–1078.

Hein, G., Silani, G., Preuschoff, K., Batson, C. D., & Singer, T. (2010). Neural responses to ingroup and outgroup members' suffering predict individual differences in costly helping. *Neuron, 68*(1), 149–160.

Hein, G., & Singer, T. (2008). I feel how you feel but not always: The empathic brain and its modulation. *Current Opinion in Neurobiology, 18*(2), 153–158.

Hoffman, M. L. (1981). The development of empathy. In J. P. Rushton & R. M. Sorrentino (Eds.), *Altruism and helping behavior: Social, personality, and developmental perspectives* (pp. 41–63). Hillsdale, NJ: Erlbaum.

Iacoboni, M. (2009). Imitation, empathy, and mirror neurons. *Annual Review of Psychology, 60,* 653–670.

Jabbi, M., & Keysers, C. (2008). Inferior frontal gyrus activity triggers anterior insula response to emotional facial expressions. *Emotion, 8*(6), 775–780.

Jabbi, M., Swart, M., & Keysers, C. (2007). Empathy for positive and negative emotions in the gustatory cortex. *NeuroImage, 34*(4), 1744–1753.

Johnson, J. D., Simmons, C. H., Jordav, A., Ma-
cLean, L., Taddei, J., Thomas, D., et al. (2002).
Rodney King and OJ revisited: The impact of
race and defendant empathy induction on judicial
decisions. *Journal of Applied Social Psychology,
32*(6), 1208–1223.

Kanske, P., Böckler, A., Trautwein, F.-M., Parianen
Lesemann, F. H., & Singer, T. (2016). Are strong
empathizers better mentalizers?: Evidence for independence and interaction between the routes of
social cognition. *Social Cognitive and Affective
Neuroscience, 11*(9), 1383–1392.

Kanske, P., Böckler, A., Trautwein, F.-M., & Singer,
T. (2015). Dissecting the social brain: Introducing
the EmpaToM to reveal distinct neural networks
and brain–behavior relations for empathy and
Theory of Mind. *NeuroImage, 122,* 6–19.

Kawakami, K., Amodio, D. M., & Hugenberg, K.
(2017). Intergroup perception and cognition: An
integrative framework for understanding the
causes and consequences of social categorization.
Advances in Experimental Social Psychology, 55,
1–80.

Keysers, C., Wicker, B., Gazzola, V., Anton, J.-L.,
Fogassi, L., & Gallese, V. (2004). A touching
sight: SII/PV activation during the observation
and experience of touch. *Neuron, 42*(2), 335–346.

Klimecki, O., & Singer, T. (2012). Empathic distress
fatigue rather than compassion fatigue?: Integrating findings from empathy research in psychology
and social neuroscience. In B. Oakley, A. Knafo,
G. Madhavan, & D. S. Wilson (Eds.), *Pathological altruism* (pp. 368–383). New York: Oxford
University Press.

Krach, S., Cohrs, J. C., de Echeverría Loebell, N. C.,
Kircher, T., Sommer, J., Jansen, A., et al. (2011).
Your flaws are my pain: Linking empathy to vi-
carious embarrassment. *PLOS ONE, 6*(4), e18675.

Lamm, C., Batson, C. D., & Decety, J. (2007). The
neural substrate of human empathy: Effects of
perspective-taking and cognitive appraisal. *Journal of Cognitive Neuroscience, 19*(1), 42–58.

Lamm, C., Decety, J., & Singer, T. (2011). Meta-
analytic evidence for common and distinct neural networks associated with directly experienced
pain and empathy for pain. *NeuroImage, 54*(3),
2492–2502.

Lamm, C., Silani, G., & Singer, T. (2015). Distinct
neural networks underlying empathy for pleasant
and unpleasant touch. *Cortex, 70,* 79–89.

Laneri, D., Krach, S., Paulus, F. M., Kanske, P.,
Schuster, V., Sommer, J., et al. (2017). Mindfulness meditation regulates anterior insula activity during empathy for social pain. *Human Brain
Mapping, 38*(8), 4034–4046.

Lockwood, P. L., Apps, M. A., Roiser, J. P., & Vid-

ing, E. (2015). Encoding of vicarious reward prediction in anterior cingulate cortex and relationship with trait empathy. *Journal of Neuroscience,
35*(40), 13720–13727.

Maslach, C. (2003). *Burnout: The cost of caring.* Los
Altos, CA: ISHK.

Masten, C. L., Morelli, S. A., & Eisenberger, N. I.
(2011). An fMRI investigation of empathy for
"social pain" and subsequent prosocial behavior.
NeuroImage, 55(1), 381–388.

Mathur, V. A., Harada, T., Lipke, T., & Chiao, J. Y.
(2010). Neural basis of extraordinary empathy
and altruistic motivation. *NeuroImage, 51*(4),
1468–1475.

Mischkowski, D., Crocker, J., & Way, B. M. (2016).
From painkiller to empathy killer: Acetamino-
phen (paracetamol) reduces empathy for pain. *Social Cognitive and Affective Neuroscience, 11*(9),
1345–1353.

Mobbs, D., Yu, R., Meyer, M., Passamonti, L., Seymour, B., Calder, A. J., et al. (2009). A key role for
similarity in vicarious reward. *Science, 324,* 900.

Molenberghs, P., Cunnington, R., & Mattingley, J.
B. (2009). Is the mirror neuron system involved
in imitation?: A short review and meta-analysis.
Neuroscience and Biobehavioral Reviews, 33(7),
975–980.

Morelli, S. A., Lieberman, M. D., & Zaki, J. (2015).
The emerging study of positive empathy. *Social
and Personality Psychology Compass, 9*(2), 57–
68.

Morelli, S. A., Sacchet, M. D., & Zaki, J. (2015).
Common and distinct neural correlates of personal and vicarious reward: A quantitative meta-
analysis. *NeuroImage, 112,* 244–253.

Nordgren, L. F., Banas, K., & MacDonald, G. (2011).
Empathy gaps for social pain: Why people underestimate the pain of social suffering. *Journal
of Personality and Social Psychology, 100*(1),
120–128.

Novembre, G., Zanon, M., & Silani, G. (2014). Empathy for social exclusion involves the sensory-
discriminative component of pain: A within-sub-
ject fMRI study. *Social Cognitive and Affective
Neuroscience, 10*(2), 153–164.

Perry, D., Hendler, T., & Shamay-Tsoory, S. G.
(2011). Can we share the joy of others?: Empathic
neural responses to distress vs joy. *Social Cognitive and Affective Neuroscience, 7*(8), 909–916.

Reynolds, J. E., Thornton, A. L., Elliott, C., Williams,
J., Lay, B. S., & Licari, M. K. (2015). A systematic
review of mirror neuron system function in developmental coordination disorder: Imitation, motor
imagery, and neuroimaging evidence. *Research in
Developmental Disabilities, 47,* 234–283.

Rizzolatti, G., & Craighero, L. (2004). The mirror-neuron system. *Annual Review of Neuroscience, 27,* 169–192.

Rogers, C. R. (2013). A theory of therapy and personality change: As developed in the client-centered framework. In R. J. Morris (Ed.), *Perspectives in abnormal behavior* (pp. 341–351). New York: Pergamon Press.

Rütgen, M., Seidel, E.-M., Riečanský, I., & Lamm, C. (2015). Reduction of empathy for pain by placebo analgesia suggests functional equivalence of empathy and first-hand emotion experience. *Journal of Neuroscience, 35*(23), 8938–8947.

Rütgen, M., Seidel, E.-M., Silani, G., Riečanský, I., Hummer, A., Windischberger, C., et al. (2015). Placebo analgesia and its opioidergic regulation suggest that empathy for pain is grounded in self pain. *Proceedings of the National Academy of Sciences of the USA, 112*(41), E5638–E5646.

Saarela, M. V., Hlushchuk, Y., Williams, A. C., Schürmann, M., Kalso, E., & Hari, R. (2006). The compassionate brain: Humans detect intensity of pain from another's face. *Cerebral Cortex, 17*(1), 230–237.

Schaefer, M., Heinze, H.-J., & Rotte, M. (2012). Embodied empathy for tactile events: Interindividual differences and vicarious somatosensory responses during touch observation. *NeuroImage, 60*(2), 952–957.

Schurz, M., Radua, J., Aichhorn, M., Richlan, F., & Perner, J. (2014). Fractionating theory of mind: A meta-analysis of functional brain imaging studies. *Neuroscience and Biobehavioral Reviews, 42,* 9–34.

Sessa, P., Meconi, F., & Han, S. (2015). Double dissociation of neural responses supporting perceptual and cognitive components of social cognition: Evidence from processing of others' pain. *Scientific Reports, 4,* Article No. 7424.

Shamay-Tsoory, S., & Lamm, C. (2018). The neuroscience of empathy—from past to present and future. *Neuropsychologia, 116*(Part A), 1–4.

Sheng, F., & Han, S. (2012). Manipulations of cognitive strategies and intergroup relationships reduce the racial bias in empathic neural responses. *NeuroImage, 61*(4), 786–797.

Sheng, F., Han, X., & Han, S. (2015). Dissociated neural representations of pain expressions of different races. *Cerebral Cortex, 26*(3), 1221–1233.

Sheng, F., Liu, Y., Zhou, B., Zhou, W., & Han, S. (2013). Oxytocin modulates the racial bias in neural responses to others' suffering. *Biological Psychology, 92*(2), 380–386.

Singer, T., & Hein, G. (2012). Human empathy through the lens of psychology and social neuroscience. In F. B. M. de Waal & P. F. Ferrari (Eds.),

The primate mind: Built to connect with other minds (pp. 158–174). Cambridge, MA: Harvard University Press.

Singer, T., & Lamm, C. (2009). The social neuroscience of empathy. *Annals of the New York Academy of Sciences, 1156*(1), 81–96.

Singer, T., Seymour, B., O'Doherty, J., Kaube, H., Dolan, R. J., & Frith, C. D. (2004). Empathy for pain involves the affective but not sensory components of pain. *Science, 303,* 1157–1162.

Singer, T., Seymour, B., O'Doherty, J. P., Stephan, K. E., Dolan, R. J., & Frith, C. D. (2006). Empathic neural responses are modulated by the perceived fairness of others. *Nature, 439,* 466–469.

Van Lange, P. A. (2008). Does empathy trigger only altruistic motivation?: How about selflessness or justice? *Emotion, 8*(6), 766–774.

Walter, H. (2012). Social cognitive neuroscience of empathy: Concepts, circuits, and genes. *Emotion Review, 4*(1), 9–17.

Wicker, B., Keysers, C., Plailly, J., Royet, J.-P., Gallese, V., & Rizzolatti, G. (2003). Both of us disgusted in my insula: The common neural basis of seeing and feeling disgust. *Neuron, 40*(3), 655–664.

Wondra, J. D., & Ellsworth, P. C. (2015). An appraisal theory of empathy and other vicarious emotional experiences. *Psychological Review, 122*(3), 411–428.

Xu, X., Zuo, X., Wang, X., & Han, S. (2009). Do you feel my pain?: Racial group membership modulates empathic neural responses. *Journal of Neuroscience, 29*(26), 8525–8529.

Yamada, M., & Decety, J. (2009). Unconscious affective processing and empathy: An investigation of subliminal priming on the detection of painful facial expressions. *Pain, 143*(1–2), 71–75.

Yao, S., Becker, B., Geng, Y., Zhao, Z., Xu, X., Zhao, W., et al. (2016). Voluntary control of anterior insula and its functional connections is feedback-independent and increases pain empathy. *NeuroImage, 130,* 230–240.

Zaki, J., & Ochsner, K. N. (2012). The neuroscience of empathy: Progress, pitfalls and promise. *Nature Neuroscience, 15*(5), 675–680.

Zaki, J., Wager, T. D., Singer, T., Keysers, C., & Gazzola, V. (2016). The anatomy of suffering: Understanding the relationship between nociceptive and empathic pain. *Trends in Cognitive Sciences, 20*(4), 249–259.

Zhou, Y., Gao, T., Zhang, T., Li, W., Wu, T., Han, X., et al. (2020). Neural dynamics of racial categorization predicts racial bias in face recognition and altruism. *Nature Human Behaviour, 4*(1), 69–87.

CHAPTER 8

Social Bonds

A New Look at an Old Topic

Sara B. Algoe
Tatum A. Jolink

Contact with other humans is a biological imperative. This is obviously true for survival at birth. It is less obviously true in adulthood. Yet being socially isolated, whether objectively or subjectively, predicts earlier death (Holt-Lunstad, Smith, Baker, Harris, & Stephenson, 2015; Rico-Uribe et al., 2018), as does having lower *quality* of social relationships, whether assessed via one meaningful relationship, such as a spouse (e.g., King & Reis, 2012), or considering one's entire social network (Holt-Lunstad, Smith, & Layton, 2010). These are not trivial effects: The risk for death from poor social relationships is the same as that from smoking 15 cigarettes per day and is greater than that of obesity (Holt-Lunstad & Smith, 2012; Holt-Lunstad et al., 2015), with the latter two factors widely recognized as important risk factors for health and longevity (e.g., Samet, 1990; Wang & Beydoun, 2007). It stands to reason, then, that forming and maintaining social bonds is a central task of human survival. As it turns out, social psychologists are uniquely well suited to illuminate the basic mechanisms that support this central task.

In this chapter, we define a *social bond* as a close, intimate relationship that holds two people together. To illustrate the phenomenon, the presence of a strong social bond may be observed in (1) a reaction of "distress when separated," (2) willingness to "spend energy to get together again," and (3) demonstrations of "positive contact behavior upon reunion" (de Waal, 1986, p. 463). Critical to this chapter, social bonds are the end products of a cumulative social bonding *process*; these end product relationship types are often between parents and children, romantic relationship partners, and good friends. However, as social psychologists, we recognize the power of situations. Specifically, we study—and here bring attention to—situations that represent *bonding opportunities*; these momentary opportunities can happen between anyone—including strangers—and should cumulatively influence the strength of the overall bond at any one time it is assessed. (Evidence from scores of studies that obtain daily self-reports lead to the conclusion that even romantic partners fluctuate in the degree to which they would say they are "bonded" with their partner from one day to the next.) Taking this situation-based approach, we aim to identify the behaviors and tasks of everyday life that may most rapidly promote connections with other people, especially those other people who are the very best for us.

In this chapter, our first goal is to provide some basic principles that can guide a program of research in this area, and in fact have guided mine (S. B. A.). Next, we use three areas of research to illuminate how these principles inform theory development. Finally, because we suggest that the study of factors that *promote* social bonds has received limited attention in recent years, we briefly call attention to bodies of literature that have developed in the past two decades—picking up steam over the past 10 years—that will usefully inform theory and evidence going forward.

Principle 1: The Presence and Promotion of Connection

In the 1950s and 1960s, Mary Ainsworth, John Bowlby, and Harry Harlow conducted groundbreaking research that highlighted the value of warm maternal connection in the healthy development of the infant (Ainsworth, 1964; 1969; Ainsworth & Boston, 1952; Ainsworth & Bowlby, 1954; Bowlby, 1958; Harlow, 1958; Harlow, Dodsworth, & Harlow, 1965; Harlow & Zimmerman, 1959). Whereas Ainsworth was dependent on naturalistic observation to document and understand the impact of parents on healthy child development (e.g., separation of the child and mother due to illness; Ainsworth & Boston, 1952), Harlow worked with monkeys, so was able to conduct experiments that manipulated the presence and type of a maternal figure. These experiments vividly illuminate the concept of a social bond, as well as its value.

At the time Harlow was conducting these experiments, the prevailing theory in psychology and sociology for why infants become attached to their mothers (parent figure) was behaviorism: A child has primary drives that include hunger, and affection toward a mother only developed secondarily because of a learned association between getting that need met and the mother providing the food. Harlow put this to the test by isolating infant macaque monkeys from their real mothers starting within 12 hours after their birth and building surrogate "mothers" with feeding capabilities. Critically, one of the surrogate mothers was made from chicken wire and the other was wrapped in a soft terrycloth cover; both were in the cage with each infant monkey, but only one had food: Half the infants received milk from a nipple on the mother made from wire, and the other half from the mother made from cloth. In stark contrast to the behaviorists' prediction, regardless of where the milk was coming from, the infants quickly developed a strong preference for the cloth mother. The infants ate the food from the wire mother, but they craved more than food: They spent substantially more time on the cloth mother, and it was just as much time as those infants who were receiving their food from the cloth mother. Harlow concluded from these studies that the presence of comfort is a primary rather than secondary need (Harlow, 1958; Harlow & Zimmerman, 1959).

Much further than this, however, subsequent experiments documented that when presented with a strange, anxiety-inducing situation, infants would retreat to the inanimate cloth rather than the wire mother for comfort, and when they could be in the safe, secure presence of the cloth mother—either physically touching her or even if she was merely visible (but inaccessible)—the young monkeys showed significantly reduced emotional distress compared to control conditions. Not only that, once they calmed down through contact comfort with their inanimate cloth mother, they would start to *explore*; in contrast, the infants with no contact comfort in that strange situation were immobilized with fear and distress (Harlow, 1958; Harlow & Zimmerman, 1959; human infants demonstrate similar behavior; see Arsenian, 1943). Finally, revealing some of the more dramatic consequences for not only healthy development but also survival, infant monkeys raised in total social isolation for the first 6 or 12 months of their lives were reintroduced to the social group. Not only did these previously isolated monkeys not play well with other monkeys, which stunts the opportunity to learn important life skills (see Harlow & Harlow, 1965), they were more aggressive toward and subsequently rejected by the other monkeys. Harlow concluded, "Placed in a free living situation, most of these animals [reared in isolation] would be driven off or eliminated before they could have an opportunity to learn to adapt to the group" (Harlow, Dodsworth, & Harlow, 1965, p. 96).

Of course, the elegance of these experiments is their ability to strip away all the other behavioral and emotional signals within repeated interaction with a live parental figure—the mere presence of physical comfort and warmth, always there when needed, was sufficient to initiate these divergent developmental consequences. Human research between parents and children has since added great richness and corroboration to these basic conclusions (Bowlby, 2008; Fraley, 2002; McLaughlin, Sheridan, & Nelson, 2017; Nelson, 2007; Ranson & Urichuk, 2008). Children with psychologically warm, behaviorally responsive, and safe parent figures tend to develop into psychologically healthy, successful, and physically healthy adults. Beyond getting one's physical needs met, like a roof over one's head or food, moments of bonding cumulatively influence one's ability to survive threats and learn about the environment; once bonded, partners themselves—like parents, lovers, and friends—keep one out of risk for danger (e.g., by proactively warning about a threat in the environment) and provide opportunities for growth (e.g., by teaching new skills).

It is with this backdrop that we fast-forward to the contemporary social psychological literature on relationships. This field predominantly studies relationships between adults. In contrast to parents and their offspring, adult social networks are made up of a wide array of voluntary relationships, all with varying degrees of bond (e.g., Clark & Mills, 2012). Recognizing the value of close connections, researchers have investigated a broad range of interpersonal behaviors that occur within them; many behaviors help prevent decline in relationships (e.g., fighting respectfully: Gottman, 1994), help a person not get kicked out of a social group (e.g., embarrassment: Keltner & Anderson, 2000; guilt: Baumeister, Stillwell, & Heatherton, 1994), or help maintain the status quo (e.g., equity: Utne, Hatfield, Traupmann, & Greenberger, 1984). However, we hope we have demonstrated from the brief review of the animal and child literature that it is especially worthwhile to identify and understand yet another type of interaction: those that create the connection in the first place. In everyday life, what are the situations that actively and directly *promote*—not merely maintain or prevent from declining—these social bonds? Understanding these kinds of moments may bring the next-generation return on investments for uncovering the myriad pathways through which high-quality relationships impact health. The focus of this chapter is thus the *presence* of bonding opportunities.

Principle 2: Situations Matter

Although of course bonded relationships develop over time, perhaps best illustrated by the profound distress exhibited upon losing a close other (e.g., Bowlby, 1982a, 1982b; Harlow & Zimmermann, 1959; Keyes et al., 2014), as social psychologists, we argue that situations—momentary opportunities for bonding—matter (Reis, 2008). They matter for developing the bonded relationship in the first place and for getting reconnected when it inevitably goes awry. As examples, typical bonding situations we discuss more extensively below are shared laughter, kindness, expressed gratitude, and affectionate touch.

In this chapter, we highlight the critical need for researchers to drill down into the features of a situation most likely to create the bond. For example, as we will demonstrate later, on their own, a given factor such as "laughter," "touch," or "oxytocin" does not promote bonds, but it is only in the right context that they do. Touch, after all, can be painful (Stith, Smith, Penn, Ward, & Tritt, 2004), and oxytocin can cause aggression (De Dreu & Kret, 2016). Instead, these are general tools that the body uses for a wide variety of purposes; as social psychologists, we can and should identify the specific contexts in which the body uses them for promoting bonds.

Principle 3: It Takes Two

By definition, a bond happens between two people. This means that the thoughts, feelings, behavior, and biology of each person can come into play in the situation. As such, there is much room for theoretical specification and substantial opportunity for the generation of hypotheses. To this end, our work is guided by a foundational model in the close relationships literature (Reis & Shaver, 1988). The model specifically considers the construct of intimacy but is instructive in a general sense via the detail with which it elaborates on what can be gained by considering social interactions between two people as a dynamic, transactional *interpersonal process*. Broadly, person *A* enacts a behavior, which is interpreted by person *B*, who then re-acts, responds, or simply, behaves; this, in turn, is interpreted by person *A*.

Although the interpersonal process model of intimacy (Reis & Shaver, 1988) acknowledged individual differences (e.g., cognitive working models of attachment might act as a filter through which the partner's behavior is interpreted), it did not emphasize biological factors as potential individual differences. In this chapter, given more recent integrative research showing the powerful ways in which the body influences the mind and behavior (Booth, Granger, Mazur, & Kivilghan, 2006; Bosch & Young, 2018), we feel it is important to explicitly bring biology into play as well, in part because evidence suggests that momentary bonding opportunities—the most powerful, especially—are deeply ingrained from our evolutionary history (e.g., Finkel & Eastwick, 2015; Fletcher, Simpson, Campbell, & Overall, 2015; Hrdy, 2001; Wilson, 2004). As such, the biopsychosocial systems to support bonding would have co-evolved, with the behavioral and subjective psychological responses recruiting from biological foundations when the right situation arises.

As one example of this, although oxytocin is notoriously difficult to link to *general* social–emotional behaviors across various types of relational situations (Graustella & MacLeod, 2012), early work emphasized its role in facilitating specific dyadic bonds (Williams, Carter, & Insel, 1992). So, building from the theory that expressions of gratitude represent an opportunity for a grateful person to promote a bond with a kind benefactor (Algoe, 2012), Algoe and Way (2014) found indirect but suggestive evidence that dispositional oxytocin is associated with greater frequency and quality of behavioral gratitude expressions toward a romantic partner, as well as more positive subjective psychological responses to expressing gratitude in real time that may (1) create momentary feelings of closeness, as well as (2) reinforce the bonding behavior. Other work suggests that circulating oxytocin influences perceptions of bonding-relevant behavior (Algoe, Kurtz, & Grewen, 2017). Specifically, greater oxytocin is associated with greater perceptions of a partner's responsiveness and greater experienced love toward that partner following the partner's expression of gratitude to the self. In short, fuller understanding of the mechanisms through which humans form and sustain social bonds will come from considering deeply rooted biological processes of each member of the dyad.

Principle 4: Seeking High-Quality Dyadic Partners

Harlow's (1958) infant monkeys were attracted to and sought time with the inanimate cloth mothers compared to the wire mothers. Having anyone matters (Holt-Lunstad et al., 2015), but having people who are good fits *for you* adds further value (Bell & Ainsworth, 1972; Kane, McCall, Collins, & Blascovich, 2012). This implies that we (humans) should instinctually look for and be sensitive to signals from those other people who might be good for us: Do they understand, validate, and care about us? Can we tell that they are motivated to look out for our best interests? Do they like us? Are we similar to them (to facilitate understanding)? Do we *want* to see them and spend time with them, or do we feel anxious about the prospect of losing them?

As many social psychologists are aware, Fiske and colleagues have robustly documented that people do evaluate social interaction partners on at least two general social dimensions—whether people are warm/sociable and whether people are competent/assertive (Fiske, 2018). Here, however, we draw attention to more precise indicators of dyad-specific potential, highlighting the dynamic between person *A* (i.e., judge) and person *B* (interaction partner). Indeed, abundant research shows that the judge's evaluations of an interaction partner's responsiveness to the self—that is, how understanding, validating, and caring the partner is toward the judge (Reis, Clark, & Holmes, 2004); how trustworthy the interaction partner is (Rempel, Holmes, & Zanna, 1985); whether there is reciprocal liking (Eastwick, Finkel, Mochon, & Ariely, 2007); whether one perceives similarity (Montoya, Horton, & Kirchner, 2008); whether the interaction partner is thought to be inclined to approach positive outcomes on the judge's behalf (Impett et al., 2010; Visserman, Righetti, Impett, Keltner, & Van Lange, 2018); and whether the partner is perceived to be committed to the judge (Agnew, Van Lange, Rusbult, & Langston, 1998) all forecast higher-quality bonds. These are all measured as evaluations of specific social interaction partners' relational orientation toward the self, not as general impressions of how those people would act toward anyone. In summary, plenty of research shows that we evaluate others on interpersonal dimensions that would (and do) forecast whether they could be a good relationship partner.

Principle 5: Bonding Opportunities Span Relationship Types

Like many other scholars, we assume these processes are learned throughout the developmental trajectory, not only in parent–child dyadic systems but also among siblings and friends in childhood and early adolescence, then built on into adulthood (Balliet, Tybur, & Van Lange, 2017; Hazan & Shaver, 1994; Raley, Crissey, & Muller, 2007). The literature on the attachment system for both children and adults is abundant, and romantic (i.e., sexual) bonds are the stereotypical version of a social bond in adults. So these specific processes might be the first that researchers consider (e.g., Muise, Giang, & Impett, 2014; Simpson, Collins, Farrell, & Raby, 2015), and they would not be wrong to do so. However, peer social groups regulate one's ability to learn new cognitive and social skills (e.g., through play; de Waal & Preston, 2017; Ginsburg, 2007; Tamis-LeMonda, Shannon, Cabrera, & Lamb, 2004) and access to resources (de Waal, 1989), so opportunities for bonding across relationship type would have been evolutionarily advantageous (e.g., stronger social skills may facilitate development of other skills, access to resources). Indeed, although we believe the type of relationship will dictate the frequency and impact of any given event, the situations we describe below are more general-purpose tools that momentarily increase connection regardless of relationship type.

Principle 6: Easier to Observe Naturalistically in Ongoing Relationships

Probabilistically, because people interact with people they know more frequently than with people they don't know, these situations happen most often with others with whom they have

regular interaction. Moreover, many scholars have laid the theoretical foundation for the case that because already-close relationships are more meaningful than those with most neighbors, coworkers, and certainly strangers, the situations themselves are more meaningful, intense, and, we emphasize, perhaps better prototypes of the phenomenon of interest than those between people who are not already invested in one another's welfare (Berscheid & Ammazzalorso, 2001; Clark & Mills, 1993; Reis, Collins, & Berscheid, 2000; Rusbult & Van Lange, 2008). As researchers who take the empirical approach of uncovering what happens naturalistically prior to imposing constraints of experimental design, then, we see (and have experienced) substantial advantages to studying the phenomenon of interest as it unfolds between people who know and are invested in one another, and who have regular interactions (also see Crocker, 2011). This might be roommates, good friends, or romantic partners.

Of course, there is different value in studying people at zero acquaintance, including the greater measurement variance because people have no expectation of how the person will act nor investment in them. Moreover, zero acquaintance is a great way to test hypotheses about the influence of bonding moments on the trajectory of a new relationship. Theoretically, however, in many cases, studying strangers may limit what can be known by producing smaller effect sizes, changing the meaning of a gesture, or—because they will not see one another again—limit ability to test for longer-term impact. In summary, relationship type is a not-to-be-overlooked tool for theory testing.

Principle 7: Time Matters

Following from the prior section, "regular interaction" implies "ongoing relationship." We have advocated for zooming in on the details of a given interaction, but, of course, one interaction—and the feeling one has when walking away from it—shapes the next. This includes possible influence on the likelihood, frequency, or quality of a subsequent interaction. For example, people we get along with better are simply more attractive to be around, which might influence how much time we spend with those people (e.g., Kirchler, 1988), and good inter-actions on earlier occasions set the stage for a smoother interaction on future occasions (e.g., Van Lange, Ouwerkerk, & Tazelaar, 2002).

The specific implication from the concept of *promoting bonds* is to grow closer together over time. As such, adding a temporal perspective opens opportunities for predictions about tra-jectories (e.g., Algoe, 2019), as well as temporal dynamics (e.g., Chow et al., 2005). For example, we have already discussed how bonds develop over time, and the implication is growth in the quality of the relationship (e.g., Algoe, Fred-rickson, & Gable, 2013). However, the reality of the time course of life and relationships is that situational factors may cause stress for one or both members of the relationship (e.g., a new job for one person, getting fired, a chronic ill-ness, a house fire, an emergency in the extended family), or they may simply drift apart. As such, the value of naturalistic bonding opportunities such as sharing a laugh, feeling grateful, or a playful touch is to break through that monotony or stress and momentarily reconnect the pair, thereby resetting the trajectory.

Principle 8: Nature Provides

We argue that the most common moments ob-served in nature (below we review laughter, kindness, and touch) are likely to be central to the regulation and promotion of bonds precisely because they are so common in social life (cf. Wilson, 2004). As we have discovered, it is often more complicated than it looks at first blush (see Principle 2). As social psychologists, figuring out the specific mechanisms that contribute to bonding (rather than producing backfiring ef-fects, for example; Algoe & Zhaoyang, 2015) is key to unlocking understanding of downstream consequences of close social bonds. One of us (S. B. A.) was once told by a friend who is an inventor that his best inventions come from carefully identifying what works well in nature, then adapting it. Likewise, everyday social be-haviors and situations that have stood the test of time—across species and cultures, the more common, the better—stand to provide the big-gest yield.

We note that for a time in social psychology, there was a push for counterintuitive findings

(e.g., Krueger & Funder, 2004). Instead, the approach we advocate is to ask, what are the situations that happen so frequently in daily life and seem so central to the fabric of high-functioning relationships that they are empiri-cally overlooked, perhaps because people think it might be boring or "we already know that"? Do we? For example, when Algoe proposed that gratitude facilitates high-quality relationships, she got feedback from people inside and outside academia that we must already know that (one friend gave a blank look and said, "Duh"); yet no evidence for that proposition existed, and the extant, well-cited theoretical account would not have predicted most of what is now known about the role of gratitude in social life, sup-ported by her early theorizing (Algoe, Haidt, & Gable, 2008). And when Kurtz proposed what it was about situations involving laughter that *best* promotes social connections (reviewed below), she and Algoe went on to review the literature assuming they would find plenty of evidence linking laughter in general and rela-tionship quality, but instead they found a couple of correlations from early studies and an exten-sive body of literature on the related but quite distinct topic of humor (Kurtz & Algoe, 2015). We believe there is much more to gain from tak-ing a close look at everyday behaviors as they play out in the context of ongoing relationships and that the next three sections illuminate this point.

How Theory Development Plays Out in Practice

Throughout the following three subsections we describe social behaviors deeply engrained in social life across species: exerting effort on behalf of non-kin (sometimes studied as "altru-ism" or "prosocial behavior" or simply "kind-ness"), touch, and laughter. For each, we show how use of the eight basic principles we de-scribed earlier can help get to the core of the situations under which these broad categories of behavior are most likely to promote a bond, and the value of studying both members of the dyad. The first behavior we discuss is first because we believe that most dyadic evidence regards the momentary bonding opportunities (so much, in fact, that there is good evidence for two steps of a temporal process: what types of "kind gestures" cause gratitude in a recipient, and how a recipient's expression of gratitude for kind gestures circles back to the original benefactor); the latter two behaviors—touch and laughter—have been well studied for other outcomes (e.g., emotion regulation or socially *relevant* acoustic properties, respectively), yet here we focus on bonding-specific evidence that is known and what more can be learned from application of the previously discussed principles. Across the set, when evidence is available, we show how isolating environmental, biological, behavioral, and psychological mechanisms of opportunities ripe for bonding helps distinguish them from their close cousins, and why it matters.

Frequent Social Behavior: Expending Personal Resources on Someone Else's Behalf; Translation to Bonding: Situations That Produce Gratitude

For more than a century, scientists, anthropologists, mathematicians, and philosophers have been intrigued by the puzzle of why one person would ever expend energy or resources in ways that would facilitate the survival (and therefore reproductive fitness) of non-kin; that is, given finite resources, logically, one should only help or be kind to people most likely to help one pass on one's own genes; that is, genetic relatives or sexual/parenting mates. Yet across the animal kingdom, examples of "helpful" behavior toward non-kin abound. An elegant explanation for such effects emerged in the theory of reciprocal altruism (Trivers, 1971), following documentation across the animal kingdom that, actually, patterns emerge wherein favors are exchanged for favors. On the one hand, exchange partners like these are not to be ignored—they are essential to moving through the economy of daily life. Having a person who can be trusted not to "cheat" by defaulting on an obligation to help certainly will (must) facilitate survival.

But contemporary social psychology shows that, at least in humans, beyond exchange there is another qualitatively different type of relationship that can emerge from repeated interactions with another person: one that is communal (Clark & Mills, 1979, 2012). Early experiments documented that people have (at least) two different expectations about interpersonal norms:

Sometimes people do things for others because they assume the other person will do something for them in return, which is considered an exchange-based relationship, whereas at other times, people do things for others because they care about the other's needs and welfare—that is, they give *noncontingently*—which is a communal-based relationship (Clark & Mills, 1993; Mills & Clark, 1982). When people perceive they are operating with communal relationship norms, for example, they did something "just because," it is actually offensive if their relationship partner repays them: Benefactors operating on communal norms *liked the recipient less* if the recipient repaid the benefactor (Clark & Mills, 1979, Study 1). This distinction between types of relational norms matters because it is the communal relationship partners who will likely watch out for their close others and are most likely to be there for them when the going gets tough. Consistent with Basic Principle 5, above, although some relationship types are characteristically more communal than others (e.g., on average people are more communal with friends than with strangers) experiments between strangers document that anyone can be momentarily communal, that is, within a situation (Clark & Mills, 1993; Clark, Mills, & Corcoran, 1989). And consistent with Basic Principle 4, above, we assume it would be evolutionarily advantageous to be sensitive to cues about whether another party is such a person.

The key way to know whether someone is going to be a high-quality, communal relationship partner is to perceive him or her as being *responsive* to the self (Laurenceau, Barrett, & Pietromonaco, 1998; Reis et al., 2004). Responsive people act in ways that show they understand, validate, and care about the needs and preferences of the other person (Reis et al., 2004), and communal relationship partners are responsive to needs, by definition (Clark & Mills, 1979). Indeed, Reis and colleagues have argued that *perceiving* responsiveness in a social interaction partner—whether that partner is a robot, a therapist, friend, or lover—is foundational to fostering these much-needed close and intimate relationships (Birnbaum et al., 2016; Kleiman, Kashdan, Monfort, Machell, & Goodman, 2015; Shelton, Trail, West, & Bergsieker, 2010).

Putting these interpersonal theories together

with functionalist theories of emotion (Fredrickson, 1998; Keltner & Haidt, 1999; Tooby & Cosmides 1990), Algoe and colleagues (2008; Algoe, 2012) proposed that the emotion of gratitude is an evolved detection and response system to readily identify good social partners, then to promote a connection with those people. Here, by "good potential relationship partners," we mean people who have just demonstrated a willingness and ability to provide a thing of value to the recipient, without wanting anything in return (i.e., because they care); that is, the benefactor is communally responsive rather than seeking an exchange. These types of situations trigger the emotion of gratitude (Algoe, Gable, & Maisel, 2010; Algoe et al., 2008; Tesser, Gatewood, & Driver, 1968; Visserman et al., 2018). Notably, gratitude can arise from a wide variety of responsive gestures from another person, including sacrificing one's own wishes to go along with what a romantic partner wants to do, helping someone out of a jam, providing emotional support during a difficult time, giving a gift, arranging a fun event, making the person a special meal, and more. Algoe and colleagues argue that the emotional response of gratitude is a signal that there is something notable about that situation and this person in particular. Even if one is already in a relationship, gratitude momentarily reminds one of what one loves about the partner (Algoe et al., 2010); with a stranger, gratitude opens one's eyes to the positive qualities of the benefactor (Algoe & Haidt, 2009; Algoe et al., 2008).

In turn, when that signal is given about the good potential partner, Algoe and colleagues (2008) contend that gratitude does a second thing: It binds the grateful person more closely to this potential partner. This is because gratitude is a positively valenced emotional response to the situation. Emotions have been long considered as evolved adaptive responses to commonly recurring situations across millennia (Darwin, 1872; Keltner & Haidt, 1999; Tooby & Cosmides, 1990). They remain in existence to the extent that they continue to prove useful for survival, and serve to mobilize the body—mind, behavior, and biological responses—in a coordinated effort to take advantage of the situation (in the case of positive emotions such as gratitude) or solve the problem (in the case of negative emotions such as fear or anger). The

situation identified by a gratitude response is that the environment has just presented a person who might make a great (i.e., survival-promoting) relationship partner; the coordinated response serves to draw the grateful person and benefactor into that relationship (i.e., binding). Indeed, several studies suggest changes in the way grateful people think about and act toward their benefactors that would support both momentary and downstream bonds (e.g., Algoe & Haidt, 2009; Algoe et al., 2008; Bartlett, Condon, Cruz, Baumann, & DeSteno, 2012; Bartlett & DeSteno, 2006; Gordon, Impett, Kogan, Oveis, & Keltner, 2012; Kubacka, Finkeneaur, Rusbult, & Keijsers, 2011; Tsang, 2006), and other work shows that experienced gratitude toward a benefactor forecasts future reports of having a good relationship with that benefactor (e.g., the next day [Algoe et al., 2010] or next month [Algoe et al., 2008]).

Taking into account that these are likely to be ongoing relationships, the previous theorizing begged the question of whether gratitude has implications for the other person, too: Does it really shore up the relationship by drawing in the other person? If so, the beneficial social consequences are not just for the person experiencing the gratitude; gratitude helps promote a high-quality bond with the person who originally signaled that he or she values and is invested in the outcomes of the grateful person. For example, measured gratitude in one person is associated with a romantic partner's improved relationship connection from the prior day (Algoe et al., 2010), and a new friend's report of time spent with the grateful person a month later (Algoe et al., 2008). Additionally, building on the idea that it is likely the behavior of the grateful person that most reliably draws a benefactor further in to the relationship, and evidence that the most immediate and frequently reported consequence from feeling grateful is expressing it (e.g., Algoe & Haidt, 2009), many researchers have been using expressions of gratitude to test downstream consequences for the benefactor. These studies show that expressing further draws in the person who chose to be nice in the first place, by making him or her more likely to do nice things for the grateful person in the future (e.g., Grant & Gino, 2010; Rind & Bordia, 1995).

Yet, does this promote the bond, in the sense of making the benefactor him- or herself feel more satisfied in the relationship over time? Recent work zooming in on the situations in which one person's gratitude is expressed to another has helped reveal mechanisms for this process, too. Specifically, theory suggests that grateful people convey mutual responsiveness back toward their benefactors—that they understand, *validate*, and care about their benefactors, too (Algoe, 2012). Notably, this prediction is for a qualitatively different response than if the (grateful) person were merely expressing *joy* over the positive outcome from the situation; evidence suggests that joyful people engage in celebratory broadcasting of their own personal positive feelings ("Look at this cool sweater!"; Algoe & Haidt, 2009; also see Gable, Reis, Impett, & Asher, 2004). In one recent set of studies of couples as they actually expressed gratitude to one another live in our lab, we predicted that responsiveness would be conveyed to a benefactor by a grateful person drawing attention to the behavior that likely caused the gratitude in the first place, that is, by calling out the praiseworthiness of the benefactor's actions. Indeed, even after taking into account how much positivity was expressed about the benefit itself (e.g., "It made me happy" or "I loved it," akin to expressing the closely related emotion of joy), the extent to which the grateful person called out the praiseworthiness of his or her partner's behavior (e.g., "I feel like you're really good at that" or "It shows how responsible you are") was robustly associated with the benefactor's perception of the grateful person's responsiveness, as well as the benefactor's positive and loving feelings after the interaction (Algoe, Kurtz, & Hilaire, 2016). From across the literature, it is now clear that the grateful person's benefactor-oriented motivations and behavior can trigger the benefactor's perceptions that the grateful person understands, validates, and cares about him or her, too; in turn, this is precisely the perception from walking away from the interaction that should (and does) forecast a better future relationship with the grateful person (Algoe et al., 2013; Algoe & Zhaoyang, 2015).

Although much of the mechanistic work for gratitude in an interpersonal process involves people in close relationships, these ecologically valid and meaningful data added richness to understanding *how* altruistic/prosocial/kind gestures could promote all kinds of relationships, as well as to the literature on gratitude in general. Prior to 2008, gratitude studies had relied on economic principles of exchange: Person *A* does something intentionally (contrasted with *incidentally*) for person *B*, the level of its value to person *B* combined with person *A*'s effort/investment determines person *B*'s level of gratitude, and person *B*'s gratitude would determine *whether* person *B* repays person *A*'s effort in addition to the *level* of repayment (e.g., Tesser et al., 1968). Studies were typically conducted between strangers (e.g., Bartlett & DeSteno, 2006) and in fact, because people already in close (e.g., romantic) relationships were already connected, some might have argued that research in such a context would be less informative (e.g., McCullough, Kilpatrick, Emmons, & Larson, 2001). Instead, the evidence that has accumulated pushes back on that assumption. For example, using experience sampling between people in ongoing relationships, we demonstrated that *despite* the strong current or potential bond, the situations matter (Algoe et al., 2008, 2010). In other work, it was precisely because participants in ongoing relationships had experiences to draw from and the impact would be meaningful that we were able to get more ecologically valid understanding of what happens during expressed gratitude and its potential downstream consequences for the relationship (e.g., Algoe et al., 2013; 2017). Since showing these relational consequences within ongoing relationships and the communal principles underlying our theoretical approach, researchers have expanded the types of dependent measures used in stranger-based interactions, beyond repayment, showing that grateful people behaviorally mimic benefactors (Jia, Lee, & Tong, 2015), conform to their benefactors' goals (Jia, Tong, & Lee, 2014), and choose to spend time with the benefactor (Bartlett et al., 2012). All are more consistent with bids for affiliation or connection than with exchanging resources.

It is important to note that in his theory of reciprocal altruism, Trivers (1971) gave roles to psychological mechanisms for reciprocity that included gratitude and liking. Nothing we have said really negates the things he said at the time—very little evidence was available. However, it adds both richness and predictive power to incorporate contemporary social psychological understanding of relationships as well as emotions to understand what transpires in the moments when one person does something kind for another: The gesture is evaluated for not only whether it benefits the self but also for the *type of relational intentions* of the benefactor—does it take into account the needs and preferences of the recipient and does the giver expect to get something from doing it? This distinction, in turn, should predict the positively valenced emotion of gratitude better than the negatively valenced emotion of indebtedness (Algoe & Stanton, 2012). Gratitude helps a person go beyond normatively expected exchange scripts to promote a qualitatively different type of relationship: a communal, more intimate, social bond, in which both members care about and watch out for the other person. In terms of survival, even beyond having someone to trade favors with, having someone who is motivated to watch your back and help you grow is a better value.

Frequent Social Behavior: Touch; Translation to Bonding: Affectionate Touch

The first interpersonal gesture humans encounter upon entering the world is touch. Then, across the lifespan, touch peppers our days, flavoring interactions between lovers, between friends, and from parents to children, doctors to patients, and salespeople to consumers. Touch, abundant throughout the entire animal kingdom, is often functional for survival, but some touch is *social* (Dunbar, 2010). For example, dolphins engage in a social behavior called "flipper-rubbing," affiliative touch that is posited to reestablish bonds following conflict (Tamaki, Morisaka, & Taki, 2006). Moreover, functional grooming is commonly observed in nonhuman primates, but a name exists for frequent intraspecies grooming that is social: *allogrooming*. In fact, primate species spend as much as 20% of their waking hours socially grooming—more time than is hygienically necessary (Dunbar, 1991; Lehmann, Korstjens, & Dunbar, 2007).

Within human childhood, researchers have concluded that touch is necessary for the child's survival and development for more obvious functional reasons (e.g., carrying: Feldman, Weller, Sirota, & Eidelman, 2003; feeding: Feldman, Keren, Gross-Rozval, & Tyano, 2004), as well as being integral to the "social, cognitive, and physical development" of a healthy child (Hertenstein, 2002, p. 70). As such, touch has been relatively well studied in this type of relationship, with researchers documenting a wide variety of functional touches (e.g., carrying: Anisfeld, Casper, Nozyce, & Cunningham, 1990; kissing, hugging, and patting: Landau, 1989) that coordinate biopsychosocial systems within the child. For example, touch regulates emotion in infants (Hertenstein & Campos, 2001), certain kinds of mother's touch elicit positive affect in infants (Stack & Muir, 1990), and touch from a caregiver can spur behavior changes in the infant, such as promoting or hindering exploratory behavior (Hertenstein & Campos, 2001; Moszkowski, Stack, & Chiarella, 2009). Finally, touch can regulate an infant's biological responses, such as down-regulating cortisol reactivity when infants are distressed (e.g., during a simulated maternal deprivation paradigm; Feldman, Singer, & Zagoory, 2010) or up-regulating vagal activity (e.g., through massage therapy of preterm infants; Field, 1998). Touch is relevant to the sociocognitive and physical development of a child and continues to functionally regulate broader social life (e.g., peers) during adolescence and beyond (Diamond, 2000; Field, 2010).

Throughout the child and adult literature, however, one kind of touch stands out as doing more: affectionate touch. *Affection* is a positive emotional state of fondness or liking directed toward someone (Floyd, 2006). Affectionate *touch* is its physical manifestation. It can be used in times of comfort or playfulness and may include pats on the back, hugging, kissing, stroking, and cuddling. In the adult literature, emerging evidence in relationship science has accrued on the *intrapersonal* benefits—psychological and physical—of affectionate touch (e.g., emotion regulation, risk for rhinovirus [common cold] infection; Cohen, Janicki-Deverts, Turner, & Doyle, 2015; Debrot, Schoebi, Perrez, & Horn, 2013, 2014; Holt-Lunstad, Birmingham,

& Light, 2008), but here we focus on how it can contribute to social bonding—the potential *interpersonal* benefits, using the basic principles to guide theorizing about how it presents a momentary opportunity for bonding in everyday life.

Indeed, evidence suggests that cumulatively over time, affectionate touch either marks or actually causes high-quality relationships (for a review, see Jakubiak & Feeney, 2017). For example, as in childhood, affectionate touch in adulthood signals secure attachment and felt security within a relationship (Jakubiak & Feeney, 2016). In a sample of dating college students, frequency of affectionate touch was positively correlated with both the individual's and his or her partner's satisfaction with the relationship (Gulledge, Gulledge, & Stahmann, 2003). For married couples, perceptions of how much a partner enacts affectionate touch corresponds with greater feelings of liking, love, and general relationship satisfaction (Dainton, Stafford, & Canary, 1994). A specific instantiation of touch—cuddling—is perceived as a nurturing (and nonsexual) aspect of romantic relationships (van Anders, Edelstein, Wade, & Samples-Steele, 2013). Finally, couples assigned to a "kissing" intervention for 6 weeks experienced better relationship satisfaction at the end of the study compared to couples who did not undergo the intervention (Floyd et al., 2009). The question of this section is, how do the momentary consequences of affectionate touch add up for long-term bonds? What happens in the moment?

Recall that our definition of affectionate touch stipulates that affection is directed from one person (person *A*) toward another (person *B*). In turn, we suggest that in the moment it occurs, affectionate touch feels *intimate*. While empirical evidence is just catching up, theory has long posited that affectionate touch is part of the intimacy process (Brennan, Wu, & Loev, 1998; Reis & Shaver, 1988), and Thayer (1986) even called affectionate touch the "gatekeeper of intimacy . . . the final bond between people" (p. 24). Physical proximity and touch are often assessed in subjective evaluations of intimacy (Burgoon, Buller, Hale, & DeTurck, 1984) or in psychometric measurements of intimacy and closeness (e.g., kissing; Berscheid, Snyder, &

Omoto, 1989; Waring, 1984), and receiving affectionate touch (or the relationship in which it is experienced) is often interpreted as intimate (Debrot et al., 2013; Hertenstein, Verkamp, Kerestes, & Holmes, 2006). Intimacy has long been hailed as foundational to relationship quality (Reis & Shaver, 1988; Reis et al., 2004). These moments of intimacy are the proposed mechanism through which affectionate touch contributes to the relational bond over time.

Affectionate touch implies someone will be there, both physically near and emotionally close (e.g., Coan, Schaefer, & Davidson, 2006; Jakubiak & Feeney, 2016), yet, importantly, research on its role in the bonding process is just beginning. Most studies on affectionate touch, while they are dyadic, focus only on the participant's report of his or her partner's affection toward him or her (e.g., how frequent, how affectionate). But this is just one side of the coin. What prompts person *A* to enact affectionate touch in the first place? For example, initial evidence reveals that affectionate touch is more likely in situations when people perceive their partner as being responsive to the self (Jolink, Chang, & Algoe, 2020). And what are the various manifestations of affectionate touch in everyday life? Does affectionate touch prompted by compassion, for instance, lead to the same interpersonal consequences—for partner *A*, partner *B*, or both—as affectionate touch triggered by a moment of playfulness? Is perceived intimacy the proximal mechanism through which all such moments solidify a bond between the two people? Additionally, the majority of studies on affectionate touch rely on recall of the frequency of touch provided the previous day or week, or daily diaries monitoring daily self-reported affectionate touch. Contrary to work on gratitude and laughter as described earlier and discussed next, very little work on touch has tested this behavior in action using real-time observations in the laboratory (though see Jakubiak & Feeney, 2019). We believe there is much to be learned. And given the pervasiveness of touch in everyday relationships, it is worth learning.

Intriguingly, uncovering these basic mechanisms may lead to deeper understanding of why good relationships are good for health. For example, in the "kissing" study we described earlier, couples in the intervention group also had reduced psychological stress and serum cholesterol compared to couples in the control condition (Floyd et al., 2009). Very early evidence is surfacing on the protective role affectionate touch may have on one's physical health—perhaps by way of improved relationship quality (Floyd & Riforgiate, 2008; Grewen, Anderson, Girdler, & Light, 2003; Holt-Lunstad et al., 2008). This preliminary evidence recalls Harlow's (1958) conclusions about the value of affectionate connection for survival, even beyond physical nourishment: "We were not surprised to discover that contact comfort was an important basic affectional or love variable, but we did not expect it to overshadow so completely the variable of nursing; indeed, the disparity is so great as to suggest that the primary function of nursing as an affectional variable is that of insuring frequent and intimate body contact of the infant with the mother. Certainly, man cannot live by milk alone" (p. 677).

Frequent Social Behavior: Laughter; Translation to Bonding: Shared Laughter

A final fascinating behavior that shows up across mammalian species, including rats (Panksepp & Burgdorf, 1999, 2003) and apes (Berntson, Boysen, Bauer, & Torello, 1989; Vettin & Todt, 2005), is laughter. In human children, laughter typically develops by around 4 months of age (Sroufe & Wunsch, 1972) and by adulthood becomes such a frequent behavior that some estimates suggest people laugh an average of 18 times per day (Martin & Kuiper, 1999; Provine & Fischer, 1989). People laugh in all kinds of situations and at a wide variety of stimuli. For example, people may laugh when amused, nervous, or embarrassed.

However, one factor stands out in the data and guides theorizing of many researchers: Laughter is social (Scott, Lavan, Chen, & McGettigan, 2014). People are more likely to laugh when another person is present than when alone (Nwokah, Hsu, Dobrowolska, & Fogel, 1994; Provine & Fischer, 1989). Early researchers examining when laughter occurs in speech and conversations theorized important social affiliative signaling cues that come from laughter (see review in Gervais & Wilson, 2005). In fact, drawing from situations in which laughter occurs in rat

pups and chimpanzees, one widely endorsed conclusion is that naturally occurring, spontaneous laughter signals a nonserious situation that is safe (e.g., Gervais & Wilson, 2005; Wood & Niedenthal, 2018), with common examples that include teasing or play fighting; in turn, this facilitates growth via play, thereby facilitating the healthy development of children (Ginsburg, 2007) as well as adults (Panksepp & Biven, 2012). Although this may be one important consequence of an individual's social laughter, and may even *indirectly* promote bonds, this is not a direct route to bonding from laughter.

Moreover, recent work has started to uncover the rich array of social signaling that comes from laughter; it is a remarkable tool for the regulation of social life. For example, some researchers have focused on laughter that involves different facial musculature (e.g., Keltner & Bonanno, 1997); others document the impact of vocalized (vs. nonvocalized) laughter on eliciting positive emotion in the perceiver (Bachorowski & Owren, 2001), while still others have focused on the acoustic properties of vocalized laughter. This latter category reveals the complexity of this social behavior; for example, whereas some research has focused on the signal value of spontaneous (rather than fake) laughter (Bryant & Aktipis, 2014), other research shows that social status can be conveyed by laughter (Oveis, Spectre, Smith, Liu, & Keltner, 2016); finally, a compelling social functions account of laughter suggests distinct acoustic properties of laughs that convey reward, affiliation, and dominance for regulation of key social situations (Wood, Martin, & Niedenthal, 2017; Wood & Niedenthal, 2018). However, this rich body of research does not employ methods that empirically address the situations involving laughter that help people *connect* with one another in the moment, and that may cumulatively influence the strength of the bond between the two people.

Therefore, interested in the question of how laughter facilitates relationships, we took a different tack; to do so, we drew from several literatures to focus on a specific situation: when two people are laughing together. This is because, in addition to laughter being social in general, an interesting feature is that it tends to be contagious (Chapman & Wright, 1976; Provine, 1992; Smoski & Bacorowski, 2003). Though researchers call this phenomenon by different names, the point is that one person's behavior involuntarily draws out the same behavior in the social partner. Of course, there will be situations in which this does not happen (e.g., when someone else is laughing at one's own expense), and researchers have documented that shared laughter is more likely to happen when one knows the other person better (Smoski & Bachorowski, 2003); we return to this later. Intriguingly for our research question, outside observers from all societies can judge the strength of a social bond between people laughing together (i.e., whether friends or strangers), merely based on hearing an audio clip (Bryant et al., 2016). For now, the question is, psychologically, what happens for the people in that moment as they laugh together? Is shared laughter an opportunity for bonding?

Three different literatures lead to the prediction that the people will see themselves as more similar to one another—even if momentarily—after sharing laughter, and a wide body of literature suggests that perceived similarity makes people feel more connected and closer (Montoya et al., 2008). First, spontaneous laughter in particular is believed to be rewarding to both the laugher and the person who hears (or elicits) the laugh (Wood & Niedenthal, 2018), and this has implications for connection: Reward is experienced as positively valenced affect, which implies that in the moments it is experienced, the worldviews of both individuals are broadened (e.g., scope of attention; Fredrickson & Branigan, 2005); in turn, this can make the other person seem more similar to the self (Johnson & Fredrickson, 2005; Waugh & Fredrickson, 2006). Second, laughter is often caused by humorous, unique situations that are defined as involving "benign violations" of expectations (McGraw & Warren, 2010), so laughing together at the same situation would naturally imply that two people see the world in the same way—that they are like-minded. The third conjecture comes from the neuroscientific literature that focuses on the contagion of laughter, with researchers positing a role for sensory–motor simulation (e.g., McGettigan et al., 2015) or mirror neurons (Rizzolatti & Craighero, 2004), with one researcher suggesting the process creates a "shared manifold of intersubjectivity" (Gallese, 2003) between the two people;

that is, the two are experiencing the world in the same way. Relative to unshared laughter, then, laughing together is expected to trigger the perception of similarity with the other person. And due to the violation of expectations that triggers a laugh (McGraw & Warren, 2010), the information in these shared moments should be particularly salient, so that people sharing laughter should also see themselves as more similar than people sharing different pleasant experiences.

Indeed, several studies now provide evidence that shared laughter uniquely promotes social bonds and that, moreover, a key mechanism for this effect is the influence of shared laughter on perceptions of similarity with the other person. In one study, romantic couples talked about how they first met, which generated a lot of laughter (Kurtz & Algoe, 2015). To take a snapshot of the role of laughter in the couple's social bond, each person's laughter throughout the conversation was coded, and moments when both were laughing simultaneously were quantified separately from moments when either member of the couple was laughing alone. Consistent with the prediction, the proportion of time the partners spent laughing together was significantly positively associated with the extent to which the participant reported greater self–other overlap (as a proxy for perceived similarity; see the Inclusion of Other in Self Scale; Aron, Aron, & Smollan, 1992). This was true even when taking into account the extent to which either or both members of the couple laughed independently during the conversation, thereby supporting the prediction about the unique situational features involving laughter most likely to facilitate bonding (Kurtz & Algoe, 2015).[1] Though that study was correlational, another study used a zero-acquaintance paradigm to address causality. During a purported Web-based video chat with someone they thought was another participant (but who was actually a prerecorded confederate), participants were randomly assigned to view stimuli that (1) elicited shared laughter with the confederate (i.e., the other "participant"), (2) elicited laughter to the same degree as the first condition but was not shared with the confederate (who was watching the same stimuli), or (3) elicited shared, mildly pleasant affect with the confederate. Immediately after the experience, participants in the shared laughter condition reported perceiving greater similarity between themselves and the partner compared to participants in the other two conditions. In turn, the increase in perceived similarity led to increased liking and interest in affiliating with the zero-acquaintance person (Kurtz & Algoe, 2017). This experiment provides the first evidence of which we are aware that shared laughter causally improves a key mechanism for promoting bonds.

Whereas other work has posited several indirect routes through which laughter could promote relationships, or might *facilitate* social life in important ways (Oveis et al., 2016; Wood et al., 2017), in this review we focus on situations that may directly promote bonds in the moments they are occurring. Relevant to Basic Principle 6, we first studied shared laughter in existing dyads, where we assumed we would see frequent and spontaneous (i.e., prototypical) laughter, then shifted to zero-acquaintance pairs to provide the first test of our causal hypotheses (Kurtz & Algoe, 2015, 2017). At the same time, given the small number of studies focusing on dyadic laughter, we believe much more work is needed on the role of shared laughter in creating momentary social connections and its implications for the long-term functioning of high-quality social relationships. For example, shared laughter might amplify positive emotions or, in some situations, decrease negative emotions, which would be two additional mechanisms through which shared laughter could bring people closer together (see Kurtz & Algoe, 2017).

One question is about the situations most likely to give rise to shared laughter in the first place. We predict that shared laughter is more likely to occur when people feel safe, perhaps because both people perceive the situation is safe and spontaneously break out laughing at precisely the same time or, more likely, we suspect, because one person's spontaneous laugh gives a signal that it is a safe and playful situation (e.g., Wood & Niedenthal, 2018) that then works as a behavioral bid or invitation for the other person to join in. When this happens, both people get a momentary boost from the connection. While the current evidence does not take into account what the two people are laughing at, we do assume the behavior of laughter

builds on biological architecture for bonding and provides a signal—even if brief—of similarity. This means that laughing at a sexist joke with a boss or colleague—even if involuntary and explicitly disavowed—likely makes the two people feel momentarily more similar than if no shared laughter occurred. This means laughter may be helpful in creating common ground in situations where people are negotiating social standing and group membership. Regardless of the relationship type, our analysis of the behavior of laughter suggests certain situations in which it likely directly facilitates bonds; in turn, these moments of shared laughter in ongoing relationships can set the stage for what comes next.

Are There Downsides?

As we stated at the outset, in this chapter we have focused on situations—both general behaviors (e.g., laughter) and the contextual features of those situations (e.g., shared laughter)—most likely to *promote* social bonds because we believe these situations have been relatively neglected in the empirical literature on relationships, yet provide great opportunity for understanding how people get into (and then sustain) close social bonds. Along the way, our focus on what promotes bonds helps illuminate features of situations that might make an ostensibly beneficial behavior, such as laughter, undermine the opportunity for bonding, such as laughing at another person's expense. Another example is when one person does something kind for another: When the beneficiary thinks the benefactor wants something in return for his or her actions, it may yield the negative emotion of indebtedness rather than the positive, bond-promoting experience of gratitude (Watkins, Scheer, Ovnicek, & Kolts, 2006); that is, one of our goals in this chapter is to show that through careful theorizing and rigorous empirical work, we can unseat assumptions to identify features of situations that optimize connections.

That said, there is much more to do. Certain individual differences or situations, such as low self-esteem, having an insecure attachment style, or feeling unsafe in the moment, may make these situations harder to come by or cause them to backfire. Moreover, much more work is needed with both members of the dyad. For example, we have a pretty good understanding of what happens when expressions of gratitude go well (e.g., Algoe et al., 2013, 2016, 2017; Williams & Bartlett, 2015), but what happens when one person thanks another and the person being thanked has a negative reaction? What if that person conveys that the other person is *wrong to be grateful* for some reason? Such moments of misplaced gratitude may arise if the benefactor did the kind thing for different reasons than the grateful person assumed, or because he or she has different norms about what is expected in this particular relationship (e.g., an exchange norm, expecting reciprocity, rather than a communal norm, in which the benefit was provided noncontingently). Similarly, affectionate touch can be met with distress or negative affect, especially if it is perceived as a sexual initiation cue by women who experience sexual pain (Curtis, Eddy, Ashdown, Feder, & Lower, 2012; Hinchliff, Gott, & Wylie, 2012). Empirically testing such boundaries would help to refine theoretical understanding of opportunities for creating bonds from these moments.

Finally, this focus on moments of connection is not to overlook the fact that (1) it is risky to try to create new relationships (e.g., one might get rejected) and (2) once bonded (i.e., once one is in a trusted, high-quality relationship with another), then negative personal and interpersonal consequences can loom larger. For example, negative emotions can be more intense regarding people we care about; these include jealousy, hurt from a betrayal of trust, and sadness at the loss of a loved one. Nonetheless, the preponderance of evidence suggests that, on balance, it is worth the risk because of the myriad long-term benefits that come from high-quality bonds.

Implications of Reconsidering the Concept of "Promoting Bonds" and Mechanisms for the Promotion of Bonds

Though social psychologists have long studied the basic features of situations that bring people together or drive people apart (e.g., Tajfel & Billig, 1974; Walster, Aronson, Abrahams, & Rottman, 1966), in this chapter we wanted to take a fresh look at the concept of a bond. To do so, we integrated literature from across species and considered both the interpersonal process as it unfolds for each member of the dyad in real time and the cumulative impact such moments may have over time in ongoing relationships. We think this is an especially useful time in the field to do this because of evidence we reviewed earlier that has been strongly influenced by two fundamental theoretical perspectives that have emerged in the relationships literature in the last 15–20 years and, we believe, should really enhance researchers' ability to develop rich theory and strong hypotheses regarding the *promotion of bonds*.

One of these theoretical perspectives is at least partially reflected in de Waal's (1989) observation that bonded individuals are willing to exert effort to spend time with their bondmates; that is, they *approach* the other. In the social psychological literature, Gable and her colleagues have drawn attention to the appetitive social goals system as an important motivational system underlying social interactions (e.g., Gable & Gosnell, 2013; Gable & Impett, 2012; Gable & Reis, 2001; Gable, Reis, & Elliot, 2003). Now, evidence from a range of studies shows that when people do things for social approach goals—that is, because they want a good social outcome—as opposed to avoiding a bad outcome, they have better personal and relational outcomes on a wide range of dimensions (see Gable & Impett, 2012). Like acknowledging that Harlow's infant monkeys would simply rather spend time in the positive presence of their cloth-monkey mothers, we believe that researchers interested in how humans form and maintain social bonds will make the fastest gains by explicitly acknowledging the role and value of these motivational—and likely biological—distinctions between motivations to avoid bad outcomes and to approach good outcomes from interacting with others.

A second, yet related, topic is the work of Fredrickson and colleagues on positively valenced emotional states (e.g., Fredrickson, 1998; 2013; Fredrickson, Cohn, Coffey, Pek, & Finkel, 2008; Kok et al., 2013), which highlights the core cognitive changes and functional value of positive relative to negative valence in situations. As we mentioned in the previous paragraph, seeking positive emotional states might drive some opportunities for bonding. Moreover, positive emotions that result from social interactions may both facilitate the momentary connection between the two people and lay the groundwork for the building of that social relationship over time (e.g., Waugh & Fredrickson, 2006). Explicitly acknowledging that other people are key sources of positive emotions and incorporating theorizing about positive emotions into predictions has led us to more rapid progress in considering what makes for high-quality, close relationships in our own work, and in the topics we have reviewed here (also see Algoe, 2019).

In closing, there is insurmountable evidence that social bonds are critical to survival. The basic principles we have offered are intended to serve as a guide to selecting research questions, developing theory, and testing hypotheses about the features of one-time social interactions that cumulatively help humans develop and maintain high-quality social bonds. We believe that further illumination of the specific situations and mechanisms through which humans directly *promote bonds,* in turn, will open doors to discovering additional pathways to health through relationships that go well beyond considering deficits that come from the lack of bonds (e.g., Luo, Hawkley, Waite, & Cacioppo, 2012) or from broken bonds (Sbarra & Coan, 2017); this might include the possibility that spending time alone *increases* cumulative metabolic load relative to spending time in the presence of a trusted partner (cf. Beckes & Coan, 2011), potential physiological benefits of affectionate touch (e.g., Holt-Lunstad et al., 2008), and more. In short, taking a closer look the concept of a bond, and what it means to promote it, stands to open new avenues of inquiry that will inform basic understanding of close relationships and may ultimately lead to fuller understanding of why these close relationships can lead to longer life.

NOTE

1. In fact, in some models, this "solo laughter" was significantly *negatively* associated with perceived self–other overlap with the partner after statistically taking into account the shared laughter in

the conversation (Kurtz & Algoe, 2015). This negative association suggests a potential "dark side" to certain situations involving laughter and reinforces our message that it is important to identify the specific features of the situations involving these ostensibly positive behaviors (e.g., laughter) that optimize opportunities for bonding.

REFERENCES

Agnew, C. R., Van Lange, P. A., Rusbult, C. E., & Langston, C. A. (1998). Cognitive interdependence: Commitment and the mental representation of close relationships. *Journal of Personality and Social Psychology, 74*(4), 939–954.

Ainsworth, M. D. (1964). Patterns of attachment behavior shown by the infant in interaction with his mother. *Merrill–Palmer Quarterly of Behavior and Development, 10*(1), 51–58.

Ainsworth, M. D. (1969). Object relations, dependency, and attachment: A theoretical review of the infant–mother relationship. *Child Development, 40,* 969–1025.

Ainsworth, M. D., & Boston, M. (1952). Psychodiagnostic assessments of a child after prolonged separation in early childhood. *British Journal of Medical Psychology, 25*(4), 169–201.

Ainsworth, M. D., & Bowlby, J. (1954). Research strategy in the study of mother–child separation. *Courrier, 4,* 105–131.

Algoe, S. B. (2012). Find, remind, and bind: The functions of gratitude in everyday relationships. *Social and Personality Psychology Compass, 6*(6), 455–469.

Algoe, S. B. (2019). Positive interpersonal processes. *Current Directions in Psychological Science, 28*(2), 183–188.

Algoe, S. B., Fredrickson, B. L., & Gable, S. L. (2013). The social functions of the emotion of gratitude via expression. *Emotion, 13*(4), 605–609.

Algoe, S. B., Gable, S. L., & Maisel, N. C. (2010). It's the little things: Everyday gratitude as a booster shot for romantic relationships. *Personal Relationships, 17*(2), 217–233.

Algoe, S. B., & Haidt, J. (2009). Witnessing excellence in action: The "other-praising" emotions of elevation, gratitude, and admiration. *Journal of Positive Psychology, 4*(2), 105–127.

Algoe, S. B., Haidt, J., & Gable, S. L. (2008). Beyond reciprocity: Gratitude and relationships in everyday life. *Emotion, 8*(3), 425–429.

Algoe, S. B., Kurtz, L. E., & Grewen, K. (2017). Oxytocin and social bonds: The role of oxytocin in perceptions of romantic partners' bonding behavior. *Psychological Science, 28*(12), 1763–1772.

Algoe, S. B., Kurtz, L. E., & Hilaire, N. M. (2016). Putting the "you" in "thank you": Examining other-praising behavior as the active relational ingredient in expressed gratitude. *Social Psychological and Personality Science, 7*(7), 658–666.

Algoe, S. B., & Stanton, A. L. (2012). Gratitude when it is needed most: Social functions of gratitude in women with metastatic breast cancer. *Emotion, 12*(1), 163–168.

Algoe, S. B., & Way, B. M. (2014). Evidence for a role of the oxytocin system, indexed by genetic variation in CD38, in the social bonding effects of expressed gratitude. *Social Cognitive and Affective Neuroscience, 9*(12), 1855–1861.

Algoe, S. B., & Zhaoyang, R. (2015). Positive psychology in context: Effects of expressing gratitude in ongoing relationships depend on perceptions of enactor responsiveness. *Journal of Positive Psychology, 11*(4), 399–415.

Anisfeld, E., Casper, V., Nozyce, M., & Cunningham, N. (1990). Does infant carrying promote attachment?: An experimental study of the effects of increased physical contact on the development of attachment. *Child Development, 61,* 1617–1627.

Aron, A., Aron, E. N., & Smollan, D. (1992). Inclusion of other in the self scale and the structure of interpersonal closeness. *Journal of Personality and Social Psychology, 63*(4), 596–612.

Arsenian, J. M. (1943). Young children in an insecure situation. *Journal of Abnormal and Social Psychology, 38*(2), 225–249.

Bachorowski, J. A., & Owren, M. J. (2001). Not all laughs are alike: Voiced but not unvoiced laughter readily elicits positive affect. *Psychological Science, 12*(3), 252–257.

Balliet, D., Tybur, J. M., & Van Lange, P. A. (2017). Functional interdependence theory: An evolutionary account of social situations. *Personality and Social Psychology Review, 21*(4), 361–388.

Bartlett, M. Y., Condon, P., Cruz, J., Baumann, J., & DeSteno, D. (2012). Gratitude: Prompting behaviours that build relationships. *Cognition and Emotion, 26*(1), 2–13.

Bartlett, M. Y., & DeSteno, D. (2006). Gratitude and prosocial behavior: Helping when it costs you. *Psychological Science, 17*(4), 319–325.

Baumeister, R. F., Stillwell, A. M., & Heatherton, T. F. (1994). Guilt: An interpersonal approach. *Psychological Bulletin, 115*(2), 243–267.

Beckes, L., & Coan, J. A. (2011). Social baseline theory: The role of social proximity in emotion and economy of action. *Social and Personality Psychology Compass, 5*(12), 976–988.

Bell, S. M., & Ainsworth, M. D. S. (1972). Infant crying and maternal responsiveness. *Child Development, 43*(4), 1171–1190.

Berntson, G. G., Boysen, S. T., Bauer, H. R., & Torello, M. S. (1989). Conspecific screams and laughter: Cardiac and behavioral reactions of infant chimpanzees. *Developmental Psychobiology, 22*(8), 771–787.

Berscheid, E., & Ammazzalorso, H. (2001). Emotional experience in close relationships. In G. J. O. Fletcher & M. S. Clark (Eds.), *Blackwell handbook of social psychology: Interpersonal processes* (pp. 308–330). Oxford, UK: Blackwell.

Berscheid, E., Snyder, M., & Omoto, A. M. (1989). The Relationship Closeness Inventory: Assessing the closeness of interpersonal relationships. *Journal of Personality and Social Psychology, 57*(5), 792–807.

Birnbaum, G. E., Mizrahi, M., Hoffman, G., Reis, H. T., Finkel, E. J., & Sass, O. (2016). What robots can teach us about intimacy: The reassuring effects of robot responsiveness to human disclosure. *Computers in Human Behavior, 63,* 416–423.

Booth, A., Granger, D. A., Mazur, A., & Kivlighan, K. T. (2006). Testosterone and social behavior. *Social Forces, 85*(1), 167–191.

Bosch, O. J., & Young, L. J. (2018). Oxytocin and social relationships: From attachment to bond disruption. *Current Topics in Behavioral Neurosciences, 35,* 97–117.

Bowlby, J. (1958). The nature of the child's tie to his mother. *International Journal of Psycho-Analysis, 39,* 350–373.

Bowlby, J. (1982). Attachment and loss: Retrospect and prospect. *American Journal of Orthopsychiatry, 52*(4), 664–678.

Bowlby, J. (1983). *Attachment and loss: Vol. 1. Attachment.* New York: Basic Books. (original work published 1969)

Bowlby, J. (2008). *A secure base: Parent–child attachment and healthy human development.* New York: Basic Books.

Brennan, K. A., Wu, S., & Loev, J. (1998). Adult romantic attachment and individual differences in attitudes toward physical contact in the context of adult romantic relationships. In J. A. Simpson & W. S. Rholes (Eds.), *Attachment theory and close relationships* (pp. 248–256). New York: Guilford Press.

Bryant, G. A., & Aktipis, C. A. (2014). The animal nature of spontaneous human laughter. *Evolution and Human Behavior, 35*(4), 327–335.

Bryant, G. A., Fessler, D. M., Fusaroli, R., Clint, E., Aarøe, L., Apicella, C. L., et al. (2016). Detecting affiliation in colaughter across 24 societies. *Proceedings of the National Academy of Sciences of the USA, 113*(17), 4682–4687.

Burgoon, J. K., Buller, D. B., Hale, J. L., & DeTurck, M. A. (1984). Relational messages associated with nonverbal behaviors. *Human Communication Research, 10*(3), 351–378.

Chapman, A. J., & Wright, D. S. (1976). Social enhancement of laughter: An experimental analysis of some companion variables. *Journal of Experimental Child Psychology, 21*(2), 201–218.

Chow, S. M., Ram, N., Boker, S. M., Fujita, F., Clore, G., & Nesselroade, J. (2005). Capturing weekly fluctuation in emotion using a latent differential structural approach. *Emotion, 5*(2), 208–225.

Clark, M. S., & Mills, J. R. (1979). Interpersonal attraction in exchange and communal relationships. *Journal of Personality and Social Psychology, 37*(1), 12–24.

Clark, M. S., & Mills, J. R. (1993). The difference between communal and exchange relationships: What it is and is not. *Personality and Social Psychology Bulletin, 19*, 684–691.

Clark, M. S., & Mills, J. R. (2012). A theory of communal (and exchange) relationships. In P. A. M. Van Lange, A. W. Kruglanski, & E. T. Higgins (Eds.), *The handbook of theories of social psychology* (Vol. 2, pp. 232–250). Thousand Oaks, CA: SAGE.

Clark, M. S., Mills, J. R., & Corcoran, D. M. (1989). Keeping track of needs and inputs of friends and strangers. *Personality and Social Psychology Bulletin, 15*(4), 533–542.

Coan, J. A., Schaefer, H. S., & Davidson, R. J. (2006). Lending a hand: Social regulation and the neural threat response to threat. *Psychological Science, 17*, 1032–1039.

Cohen, S., Janicki-Deverts, D., Turner, R. B., & Doyle, W. J. (2015). Does hugging provide stress-buffering social support?: A study of susceptibility to upper respiratory infection and illness. *Psychological Science, 26*(2), 135–147.

Crocker, J. (2011). Presidential address: Self-image and compassionate goals and construction of the social self: Implications for social and personality psychology. *Personality and Social Psychology Review, 15*(4), 394–407.

Curtis, Y., Eddy, L., Ashdown, B. K., Feder, H., & Lower, T. (2012). Prelude to a coitus: Sexual initiation cues among heterosexual married couples. *Sexual and Relationship Therapy, 27*(4), 322–334.

Dainton, M., Stafford, L., & Canary, D. J. (1994). Maintenance strategies and physical affection as predictors of love, liking, and satisfaction in marriage. *Communication Reports, 7*(2), 88–98.

Darwin, C. (1872). *The expression of emotions in animals and man.* London: Murray.

Debrot, A., Schoebi, D., Perrez, M., & Horn, A. B. (2013). Touch as an interpersonal emotion regulation process in couples' daily lives: The mediating

role of psychological intimacy. *Personality and Social Psychology Bulletin, 39*(10), 1373–1385.

Debrot, A., Schoebi, D., Perrez, M., & Horn, A. B. (2014). Stroking your beloved one's white bear: Responsive touch by the romantic partner buffers the negative effect of thought suppression on daily mood. *Journal of Social and Clinical Psychology, 33*(1), 75–97.

De Dreu, C. K., & Kret, M. E. (2016). Oxytocin conditions intergroup relations through upregulated in-group empathy, cooperation, conformity, and defense. *Biological Psychiatry, 79*(3), 165–173.

de Waal, F. B. (1986). The integration of dominance and social bonding in primates. *Quarterly Review of Biology, 61*(4), 459–479.

de Waal, F. B. (1989). Food sharing and reciprocal obligations among chimpanzees. *Journal of Human Evolution, 18*(5), 433–459.

de Waal, F. B., & Preston, S. D. (2017). Mammalian empathy: Behavioural manifestations and neural basis. *Nature Reviews Neuroscience, 18*(8), 498–509.

Diamond, L. M. (2000). Passionate friendships among adolescent sexual-minority women. *Journal of Research on Adolescence, 10*(2), 191–209.

Dunbar, R. I. (1991). Functional significance of social grooming in primates. *Folia Primatologica, 57*(3), 121–131.

Dunbar, R. I. (2010). The social role of touch in humans and primates: Behavioural function and neurobiological mechanisms. *Neuroscience and Biobehavioral Reviews, 34*(2), 260–268.

Eastwick, P. W., Finkel, E. J., Mochon, D., & Ariely, D. (2007). Selective versus unselective romantic desire: Not all reciprocity is created equal. *Psychological Science, 18*(4), 317–319.

Feldman, R., Keren, M., Gross-Rozval, O., & Tyano, S. (2004). Mother–child touch patterns in infant feeding disorders: Relation to maternal, child, and environmental factors. *Journal of the American Academy of Child and Adolescent Psychiatry, 43*(9), 1089–1097.

Feldman, R., Singer, M., & Zagoory, O. (2010). Touch attenuates infants' physiological reactivity to stress. *Developmental Science, 13*(2), 271–278.

Feldman, R., Weller, A., Sirota, L., & Eidelman, A. I. (2003). Testing a family intervention hypothesis: The contribution of mother–infant skin-to-skin contact (kangaroo care) to family interaction, proximity, and touch. *Journal of Family Psychology, 17*(1), 94–107.

Field, T. (1998). Massage therapy effects. *American Psychologist, 53*(12), 1270–1281.

Field, T. (2010). Touch for socioemotional and physical well-being: A review. *Developmental Review, 30*(4), 367–383.

Finkel, E. J., & Eastwick, P. W. (2015). Attachment and pairbonding. *Current Opinion in Behavioral Sciences, 3,* 7–11.

Fiske, S. T. (2018). Stereotype content: Warmth and competence endure. *Current Directions in Psychological Science, 27*(2), 67–73.

Fletcher, G. J., Simpson, J. A., Campbell, L., & Overall, N. C. (2015). Pair-bonding, romantic love, and evolution: The curious case of *Homo sapiens. Perspectives on Psychological Science, 10*(1), 20–36.

Floyd, K. (2006). *Communicating affection: Interpersonal behavior and social context.* New York: Cambridge University Press.

Floyd, K., Boren, J. P., Hannawa, A. F., Hesse, C., McEwan, B., & Veksler, A. E. (2009). Kissing in marital and cohabiting relationships: Effects on blood lipids, stress, and relationship satisfaction. *Western Journal of Communication, 73*(2), 113–133.

Floyd, K., & Riforgiate, S. (2008). Affectionate communication received from spouses predicts stress hormone levels in healthy adults. *Communication Monographs, 75*(4), 351–368.

Fraley, R. C. (2002). Attachment stability from infancy to adulthood: Meta-analysis and dynamic modeling of developmental mechanisms. *Personality and Social Psychology Review, 6*(2), 123–151.

Fredrickson, B. L. (1998). What good are positive emotions? *Review of General Psychology, 2*(3), 300–319.

Fredrickson, B. L. (2013). Positive emotions broaden and build. In P. Devine & A. Plant (Eds.), *Advances in experimental social psychology* (Vol. 47, pp. 1–53). San Diego, CA: Academic Press.

Fredrickson, B. L., & Branigan, C. (2005). Positive emotions broaden the scope of attention and thought-action repertoires. *Cognition and Emotion, 19*(3), 313–332.

Fredrickson, B. L., Cohn, M. A., Coffey, K. A., Pek, J., & Finkel, S. M. (2008). Open hearts build lives: Positive emotions, induced through loving-kindness meditation, build consequential personal resources. *Journal of Personality and Social Psychology, 95*(5), 1045–1062.

Gable, S. L., & Gosnell, C. L. (2013). Approach and avoidance behavior in interpersonal relationships. *Emotion Review, 5*(3), 269–274.

Gable, S. L., & Impett, E. A. (2012). Approach and avoidance motives and close relationships. *Social and Personality Psychology Compass, 6*(1), 95–108.

Gable, S. L., & Reis, H. T. (2001). Appetitive and aversive social interaction. In J. Harvey & A. Wenzel (Eds.), *Close romantic relationships: Maintenance and enhancement* (pp. 169–194). Mahwah, NJ: Erlbaum.

Gable, S. L., Reis, H. T., & Elliot, A. J. (2003). Evidence for bivariate systems: An empirical test of appetition and aversion across domains. *Journal of Research in Personality, 37,* 349–372.

Gable, S. L., Reis, H. T., Impett, E. A., & Asher, E. R. (2004). What do you do when things go right?: The intrapersonal and interpersonal benefits of sharing positive events. *Journal of Personality and Social Psychology, 87*(2), 228–245.

Gallese, V. (2003). The roots of empathy: The shared manifold hypothesis and the neural basis of intersubjectivity. *Psychopathology, 36*(4), 171–180.

Gervais, M., & Wilson, D. S. (2005). The evolution and functions of laughter and humor: A synthetic approach. *Quarterly Review of Biology, 80*(4), 395–430.

Ginsburg, K. R. (2007). The importance of play in promoting healthy child development and maintaining strong parent–child bonds. *Pediatrics, 119*(1), 182–191.

Gordon, A. M., Impett, E. A., Kogan, A., Oveis, C., & Keltner, D. (2012). To have and to hold: Gratitude promotes relationship maintenance in intimate bonds. *Journal of Personality and Social Psychology, 103*(2), 257–274.

Gottman, J. M. (1994). *What predicts divorce?: The relationship between marital processes and marital outcomes.* Hillsdale, NJ: Erlbaum.

Grant, A. M., & Gino, F. (2010). A little thanks goes a long way: Explaining why gratitude expressions motivate prosocial behavior. *Journal of Personality and Social Psychology, 98*(6), 946–955.

Graustella, A. J., & MacLeod, C. (2012). A critical review of the influence of oxytocin nasal spray on social cognition in humans: Evidence and future directions. *Hormones and Behavior, 61*(3), 410–418.

Grewen, K. M., Anderson, B. J., Girdler, S. S., & Light, K. C. (2003). Warm partner contact is related to lower cardiovascular reactivity. *Behavioral Medicine, 29,* 123–130.

Gulledge, A. K., Gulledge, M. H., & Stahmann, R. F. (2003). Romantic physical affection types and relationship satisfaction. *American Journal of Family Therapy, 31*(4), 233–242.

Harlow, H. F. (1958). The nature of love. *American Psychologist, 13*(12), 673–685.

Harlow, H. F., Dodsworth, R. O., & Harlow, M. K. (1965). Total social isolation in monkeys. *Proceedings of the National Academy of Sciences of the USA, 54*(1), 90–97.

Harlow, H. F., & Harlow, M. K. (1965). The affectional systems. *Behavior of Nonhuman Primates, 2,* 287–334.

Harlow, H. F., & Zimmermann, R. R. (1959). Affectional responses in the infant monkey. *Science, 130*(3373), 421–432.

Hazan, C., & Shaver, P. R. (1994). Attachment as an organizational framework for research on close relationships. *Psychological Inquiry, 5*(1), 1–22.

Hertenstein, M. J. (2002). Touch: Its communicative functions in infancy. *Human Development, 45*(2), 70–94.

Hertenstein, M. J., & Campos, J. J. (2001). Emotion regulation via maternal touch. *Infancy, 2*(4), 549–566.

Hertenstein, M. J., Verkamp, J. M., Kerestes, A. M., & Holmes, R. M. (2006). The communicative functions of touch in humans, nonhuman primates, and rats: A review and synthesis of the empirical research. *Genetic, Social, and General Psychology Monographs, 132*(1), 5–94.

Hinchliff, S., Gott, M., & Wylie, K. (2012). A qualitative study of heterosexual women's attempts to renegotiate sexual relationships in the context of severe sexual problems. *Archives of Sexual Behavior, 41*(5), 1253–1261.

Holt-Lunstad, J., Birmingham, W. A., & Light, K. C. (2008). Influence of a "warm touch" support enhancement intervention among married couples on ambulatory blood pressure, oxytocin, alpha amylase, and cortisol. *Psychosomatic Medicine, 70*(9), 976–985.

Holt-Lunstad, J., & Smith, T. B. (2012). Social relationships and mortality. *Social and Personality Psychology Compass, 6*(1), 41–53.

Holt-Lunstad, J., Smith, T. B., Baker, M., Harris, T., & Stephenson, D. (2015). Loneliness and social isolation as risk factors for mortality: A meta-analytic review. *Perspectives on Psychological Science, 10*(2), 227–237.

Holt-Lunstad, J., Smith, T. B., & Layton, J. B. (2010). Social relationships and mortality risk: A meta-analytic review. *PLOS Medicine, 7*(7), e1000316.

Hrdy, S. B. (2001). Mothers and others. *Natural History, 110*(4), 50–62.

Impett, E. A., Gordon, A. M., Kogan, A., Oveis, C., Gable, S. L., & Keltner, D. (2010). Moving toward more perfect unions: Daily and long-term consequences of approach and avoidance goals in romantic relationships. *Journal of Personality and Social Psychology, 99*(6), 948–963.

Jakubiak, B. K., & Feeney, B. C. (2016). A sense of security: Touch promotes state attachment security. *Social Psychological and Personality Science, 7*(7), 745–753.

Jakubiak, B. K., & Feeney, B. C. (2017). Affectionate touch to promote relational, psychological, and physical well-being in adulthood: A theoretical model and review of the research. *Personality and Social Psychology Review, 21*(3), 228–252.

Jakubiak, B. K., & Feeney, B. C. (2019). Hand-in-hand combat: Affectionate touch promotes relational well-being and buffers stress during conflict. *Personality and Social Psychology Bulletin, 45*(3), 431–446.

Jia, L., Lee, L. N., & Tong, E. M. W. (2015). Gratitude facilitates behavioral mimicry. *Emotion, 15*(2), 134–138.

Jia, L., Tong, E. W., & Lee, L. N. (2014). Psychological "gel" to bind individuals' goal pursuit: Gratitude facilitates goal contagion. *Emotion, 14*(4), 748–760.

Johnson, K. J., & Fredrickson, B. L. (2005). "We all look the same to me": Positive emotions eliminate the own-race bias in face recognition. *Psychological Science, 16*(11), 875–881.

Jolink, T. A., Chang, Y.-P., & Algoe, S. B. (2020). *Perceived partner responsiveness forecasts behavioral intimacy via affectionate touch.* Manuscript under review.

Kane, H. S., McCall, C., Collins, N. L., & Blascovich, J. (2012). Mere presence is not enough: Responsive support in a virtual world. *Journal of Experimental Social Psychology, 48*(1), 37–44.

Keltner, D., & Anderson, C. (2000). Saving face for Darwin: The functions and uses of embarrassment. *Current Directions in Psychological Science, 9*(6), 187–192.

Keltner, D., & Bonanno, G. A. (1997). A study of laughter and dissociation: Distinct correlates of laughter and smiling during bereavement. *Journal of Personality and Social Psychology, 73*(4), 687–702.

Keltner, D., & Haidt, J. (1999). Social functions of emotions at four levels of analysis. *Cognition and Emotion, 13*(5), 505–521.

Keyes, K. M., Pratt, C., Galea, S., McLaughlin, K. A., Koenen, K. C., & Shear, M. K. (2014). The burden of loss: Unexpected death of a loved one and psychiatric disorders across the life course in a national study. *American Journal of Psychiatry, 171*(8), 864–871.

King, K. B., & Reis, H. T. (2012). Marriage and long-term survival after coronary artery bypass grafting. *Health Psychology, 31*(1), 55–62.

Kirchler, E. (1988). Marital happiness and interaction in everyday surroundings: A time-sample diary approach for couples. *Journal of Social and Personal Relationships, 5*(3), 375–382.

Kleiman, E. M., Kashdan, T. B., Monfort, S. S., Machell, K. A., & Goodman, F. R. (2015). Perceived responsiveness during an initial social interaction with a stranger predicts a positive memory bias one week later. *Cognition and Emotion, 29*(2), 332–341.

Kok, B. E., Coffey, K. A., Cohn, M. A., Catalino, L. I., Vacharkulksemsuk, T., Algoe, S. B., et al.

(2013). How positive emotions build physical health: Perceived positive social connections account for the upward spiral between positive emotions and vagal tone. *Psychological Science, 24*(7), 1123–1132.

Krueger, J. I., & Funder, D. C. (2004). Towards a balanced social psychology: Causes, consequences, and cures for the problem-seeking approach to social behavior and cognition. *Behavioral and Brain Sciences, 27*(3), 313–327.

Kubacka, K. E., Finkenauer, C., Rusbult, C. E., & Keijsers, L. (2011). Maintaining close relationships: Gratitude as a motivator and a detector of maintenance behavior. *Personality and Social Psychology Bulletin, 37*(10), 1362–1375.

Kurtz, L. E., & Algoe, S. B. (2015). Putting laughter in context: Shared laughter as behavioral indicator of relationship well-being. *Personal Relationships, 22*(4), 573–590.

Kurtz, L. E., & Algoe, S. B. (2017). When sharing a laugh means sharing more: Testing the role of shared laughter on short-term interpersonal consequences. *Journal of Nonverbal Behavior, 41*(1), 45–65.

Landau, R. (1989). Affect and attachment: Kissing, hugging, and patting as attachment behaviors. *Infant Mental Health Journal, 10,* 59–69.

Laurenceau, J. P., Barrett, L. F., & Pietromonaco, P. R. (1998). Intimacy as an interpersonal process: The importance of self-disclosure, partner disclosure, and perceived partner responsiveness in interpersonal exchanges. *Journal of Personality and Social Psychology, 74*(5), 1238–1251.

Lehmann, J., Korstjens, A. H., & Dunbar, R. I. M. (2007). Group size, grooming and social cohesion in primates. *Animal Behaviour, 74*(6), 1617–1629.

Luo, Y., Hawkley, L. C., Waite, L. J., & Cacioppo, J. T. (2012). Loneliness, health, and mortality in old age: A national longitudinal study. *Social Science and Medicine, 74*(6), 907–914.

Martin, R. A., & Kuiper, N. A. (1999). Daily occurrence of laughter: Relationships with age, gender, and Type A personality. *Humor, 12,* 355–384.

McCullough, M. E., Kilpatrick, S. D., Emmons, R. A., & Larson, D. B. (2001). Is gratitude a moral affect? *Psychological Bulletin, 127*(2), 249–266.

McGettigan, C., Walsh, E., Jessop, R., Agnew, Z. K., Sauter, D. A., Warren, J. E., et al. (2015). Individual differences in laughter perception reveal roles for mentalizing and sensorimotor systems in the evaluation of emotional authenticity. *Cerebral Cortex, 25*(1), 246–257.

McGraw, A. P., & Warren, C. (2010). Benign violations: Making immoral behavior funny. *Psychological Science, 21*(8), 1141–1149.

McLaughlin, K. A., Sheridan, M. A., & Nelson, C. A. (2017). Neglect as a violation of species-expectant experience: Neurodevelopmental consequences. *Biological Psychiatry, 82*(7), 462–471.

Mills, J., & Clark, M. S. (1982). Exchange and communal relationships. *Review of Personality and Social Psychology, 3,* 121–144.

Montoya, R. M., Horton, R. S., & Kirchner, J. (2008). Is actual similarity necessary for attraction?: A meta-analysis of actual and perceived similarity. *Journal of Social and Personal Relationships, 25*(6), 889–922.

Moszkowski, R. J., Stack, D. M., & Chiarella, S. S. (2009). Infant touch with gaze and affective behaviors during mother–infant still-face interactions: Co-occurrence and functions of touch. *Infant Behavior and Development, 32*(4), 392–403.

Muise, A., Giang, E., & Impett, E. A. (2014). Post sex affectionate exchanges promote sexual and relationship satisfaction. *Archives of Sexual Behavior, 43*(7), 1391–1402.

Nelson, C. A. (2007). A neurobiological perspective on early human deprivation. *Child Development Perspectives, 1*(1), 13–18.

Nwokah, E. E., Hsu, H. C., Dobrowolska, O., & Fogel, A. (1994). The development of laughter in mother–infant communication: Timing parameters and temporal sequences. *Infant Behavior and Development, 17*(1), 23–35.

Oveis, C., Spectre, A., Smith, P. K., Liu, M. Y., & Keltner, D. (2016). Laughter conveys status. *Journal of Experimental Social Psychology, 65,* 109–115.

Panksepp, J., & Biven, L. (2012). *The archaeology of mind: Neuroevolutionary origins of human emotions.* New York: Norton.

Panksepp, J., & Burgdorf, J. (1999). Laughing rats?: Playful tickling arouses high frequency ultrasonic chirping in young rodents. In S. Hameroff, D. Chalmers, & A. Kazniak (Eds.), *Toward a science of consciousness III* (pp. 231–244). Cambridge, MA: MIT Press.

Panksepp, J., & Burgdorf, J. (2003). "Laughing" rats and the evolutionary antecedents of human joy? *Physiology and Behavior, 79*(3), 533–547.

Provine, R. R. (1992). Contagious laughter: Laughter is a sufficient stimulus for laughs and smiles. *Bulletin of the Psychonomic Society, 30*(1), 1–4.

Provine, R. R., & Fischer, K. R. (1989). Laughing, smiling, and talking: Relation to sleeping and social context in humans. *Ethology, 83*(4), 295–305.

Raley, R. K., Crissey, S., & Muller, C. (2007). Of sex and romance: Late adolescent relationships and young adult union formation. *Journal of Marriage and Family, 69*(5), 1210–1226.

Ranson, K. E., & Urichuk, L. J. (2008). The effect of parent–child attachment relationships on child biopsychosocial outcomes: A review. *Early Child Development and Care, 178*(2), 129–152.

Reis, H. T. (2008). Reinvigorating the concept of situation in social psychology. *Personality and Social Psychology Review, 12*(4), 311–329.

Reis, H. T., Clark, M. S., & Holmes, J. G. (2004). Perceived partner responsiveness as an organizing construct in the study of intimacy and closeness. In D. J. Mashek & A. Aron (Eds.), *Handbook of closeness and intimacy* (pp. 201–225). Mahwah, NJ: Erlbaum.

Reis, H. T., Collins, W. A., & Berscheid, E. (2000). The relationship context of human behavior and development. *Psychological Bulletin, 126*(6), 844–872.

Reis, H. T., & Shaver, P. (1988). Intimacy as an interpersonal process. In S. Duck, D. F. Hay, S. E. Hobfoll, W. Ickes, & B. M. Montgomery (Eds.), *Handbook of personal relationships: Theory, research and interventions* (pp. 367–389). Chichester, UK: Wiley.

Rempel, J. K., Holmes, J. G., & Zanna, M. P. (1985). Trust in close relationships. *Journal of Personality and Social Psychology, 49*(1), 95–112.

Rico-Uribe, L. A., Caballero, F. F., Martín-María, N., Cabello, M., Ayuso-Mateos, J. L., & Miret, M. (2018). Association of loneliness with all-cause mortality: A meta-analysis. *PLOS ONE, 13*(1), e0190033.

Rind, B., & Bordia, P. (1995). Effect of server's "thank you" and personalization on restaurant tipping. *Journal of Applied Social Psychology, 25*(9), 745–751.

Rizzolatti, G., & Craighero, L. (2004). The mirror-neuron system. *Annual Review of Neuroscience, 27,* 169–192.

Rusbult, C. E., & Van Lange, P. A. (2008). Why we need interdependence theory. *Social and Personality Psychology Compass, 2*(5), 2049–2070.

Samet, J. M. (1990). The 1990 Report of the Surgeon General: The health benefits of smoking cessation. *American Review of Respiratory Disease, 142*(5), 993–994.

Sbarra, D. A., & Coan, J. A. (2017). Divorce and health: Good data in need of better theory. *Current Opinion in Psychology, 13,* 91–95.

Scott, S. K., Lavan, N., Chen, S., & McGettigan, C. (2014). The social life of laughter. *Trends in Cognitive Sciences, 18*(12), 618–620.

Shelton, J. N., Trail, T. E., West, T. V., & Bergsieker, H. B. (2010). From strangers to friends: The interpersonal process model of intimacy in developing interracial friendships. *Journal of Social and Personal Relationships, 27*(1), 71–90.

Simpson, J. A., Collins, W. A., Farrell, A. K., & Raby, K. L. (2015). Attachment and relationships across time: An organizational-developmental perspective. In V. Hayas & C. Hazan (Eds.), *Bases of adult attachment* (pp. 61–78). New York: Springer.

Smoski, M., & Bachorowski, J. A. (2003). Antiphonal laughter between friends and strangers. *Cognition and Emotion, 17*(2), 327–340.

Sroufe, L. A., & Wunsch, J. P. (1972). The development of laughter in the first year of life. *Child Development, 43*(4), 1326–1344.

Stack, D. M., & Muir, D. W. (1990). Tactile stimulation as a component of social interchange: New interpretations for the still-face effect. *British Journal of Developmental Psychology, 8,* 131–145.

Stith, S. M., Smith, D. B., Penn, C. E., Ward, D. B., & Tritt, D. (2004). Intimate partner physical abuse perpetration and victimization risk factors: A meta-analytic review. *Aggression and Violent Behavior, 10*(1), 65–98.

Tajfel, H., & Billig, M. (1974). Familiarity and categorization in intergroup behavior. *Journal of Experimental Social Psychology, 10*(2), 159–170.

Tamaki, N., Morisaka, T., & Taki, M. (2006). Does body contact contribute towards repairing relationships?: The association between flipper-rubbing and aggressive behavior in captive bottlenose dolphins. *Behavioural Processes, 73*(2), 209–215.

Tamis-LeMonda, C. S., Shannon, J. D., Cabrera, N. J., & Lamb, M. E. (2004). Fathers and mothers at play with their 2- and 3-year-olds: Contributions to language and cognitive development. *Child Development, 75*(6), 1806–1820.

Tesser, A., Gatewood, R., & Driver, M. (1968). Some determinants of gratitude. *Journal of Personality and Social Psychology, 9*(3), 233–236.

Thayer, S. (1986). History and strategies of research on social touch. *Journal of Nonverbal Behavior, 10*(1), 13–27.

Tooby, J., & Cosmides, L. (1990). The past explains the present: Emotional adaptations and the structure of ancestral environments. *Ethology and Sociobiology, 11*(4–5), 375–424.

Trivers, R. L. (1971). The evolution of reciprocal altruism. *Quarterly Review of Biology, 46*(1), 35–57.

Tsang, J. A. (2006). Gratitude and prosocial behavior: An experimental test of gratitude. *Cognition and Emotion, 20,* 138–148.

Utne, M. K., Hatfield, E., Traupmann, J., & Greenberger, D. (1984). Equity, marital satisfaction, and stability. *Journal of Social and Personal Relationships, 1*(3), 323–332.

van Anders, S. M., Edelstein, R. S., Wade, R. M., & Samples-Steele, C. R. (2013). Descriptive experiences and sexual vs. nurturant aspects of cuddling between adult romantic partners. *Archives of Sexual Behavior, 42*(4), 553–560.

Van Lange, P. A., Ouwerkerk, J. W., & Tazelaar, M.

J. (2002). How to overcome the detrimental effects of noise in social interaction: The benefits of generosity. *Journal of Personality and Social Psychology, 82*(5), 768–780.

Vettin, J., & Todt, D. (2005). Human laughter, social play, and play vocalizations of non-human primates: An evolutionary approach. *Behaviour, 142*(2), 217–240.

Visserman, M. L., Righetti, F., Impett, E. A., Keltner, D., & Van Lange, P. A. M. (2018). It's the motive that counts: Perceived sacrifice motives and gratitude in romantic relationships. *Emotion, 18*(5), 625–637.

Walster, E., Aronson, V., Abrahams, D., & Rottman, L. (1966). Importance of physical attractiveness in dating behavior. *Journal of Personality and Social Psychology, 4*(5), 508–516.

Wang, Y., & Beydoun, M. A. (2007). The obesity epidemic in the United States—gender, age, socioeconomic, racial/ethnic, and geographic characteristics: A systematic review and meta-regression analysis. *Epidemiologic Reviews, 29*(1), 6–28.

Waring, E. M. (1984). The measurement of marital intimacy. *Journal of Marital and Family Therapy, 10*(2), 185–192.

Watkins, P., Scheer, J., Ovnicek, M., & Kolts, R.

(2006). The debt of gratitude: Dissociating gratitude and indebtedness. *Cognition and Emotion, 20*(2), 217–241.

Waugh, C. E., & Fredrickson, B. L. (2006). Nice to know you: Positive emotions, self–other overlap, and complex understanding in the formation of a new relationship. *Journal of Positive Psychology, 1*(2), 93–106.

Williams, J. R., Carter, C. S., & Insel, T. (1992). Partner preference development in female prairie voles is facilitated by mating or the central infusion of oxytocin A. *Annals of the New York Academy of Sciences, 652*(1), 487–489.

Williams, L. A., & Bartlett, M. Y. (2015). Warm thanks: Gratitude expression facilitates social affiliation in new relationships via perceived warmth. *Emotion, 15*(1), 1.

Wilson, E. O. (2004). *On human nature.* Cambridge, MA: Harvard University Press.

Wood, A., Martin, J., & Niedenthal, P. (2017). Towards a social functional account of laughter: Acoustic features convey reward, affiliation, and dominance. *PLOS ONE, 12*(8), e0183811.

Wood, A., & Niedenthal, P. (2018). Developing a social functional account of laughter. *Social and Personality Psychology Compass, 12*(4), e12383.

CHAPTER 9

Understanding the Minds of Others
Activation, Application, and Accuracy of Mind Perception

Nicholas Epley
Michael Kardas

In 2011, the Marist Institute for Public Opinion asked over 1,000 randomly selected Americans to indicate which of five superpowers they would want most: invisibility, teleportation, flight, time travel, or reading others' minds. Although most movie superheroes possess one of the first three, most Americans opted for one of the last two: time travel and mind reading tied for the top spot, each selected by 28% of respondents. This is somewhat ironic because thousands of psychology experiments have documented the many ways in which most people already possess an ability to read the minds of others, whereas not one experiment has identified even a single person with any of the other superpowers. Most people are readily able to make inferences about another person's thoughts, beliefs, attitudes, motivations, intentions, and other mental states, with at least some above-chance accuracy. Mind reading is a superpower that most already possess.

Indeed, the human brain stands out in the animal kingdom for its relatively large cerebral cortex (Herrmann, Call, Hernández-Lloreda, Hare, & Tomasello, 2007; Jerison, 1971), an adaptation that enables the sophisticated social cognition necessary to function effectively in large social groups (Dunbar, 1993). These neu-

rons are not involved in any sort of supernatural psychic activity but instead are involved in the routine kind of mind reading that people do many times a day when wondering what others think, believe, feel, or want. By 2 years of age, human toddlers are similar to our nearest primate relatives in their ability to reason about physical objects, but they stand out for their ability to reason about others' mental states (Herrmann et al., 2007). If a human toddler, for instance, watches another person reach for a glass of water but miss it, then he or she is likely to recognize that another person *wants* a drink or *feels* thirsty and so will pick up the glass and hand it to the person. You can do this all day long in front of a chimpanzee without ever being handed a glass of water.

This almost magical ability to go beyond a mere observation of behavior to infer an underlying mental state allows us to understand what another person is doing in the present, to predict another person's behavior in the future, and to arrive at a shared understanding of reality (Echterhoff, Higgins, & Levine, 2009; Hudson, Nicholson, Ellis, & Bach, 2016; Wegner, 2002). By age 4, human children have developed a fairly sophisticated set of beliefs that explains both their own and others' actions in terms of

163

underlying mental states (Frith & Frith, 2005). These beliefs about how minds work are often referred to by psychologists as a theory of mind (Leslie, 1987; Saxe & Kanwisher, 2003). Because mental states cannot be observed directly, most human beings merely presume that behaviors are guided by unobserved mental states, hence developing a "theory" of how others' minds work. By adulthood, most people define others' minds in terms of two fundamental abilities (Gray, Gray, & Wegner, 2007; Haslam & Loughnan, 2014): the ability to think (including reasoning, planning, and exercising) and to feel (including experiencing pain, pleasure, and complicated emotions such as regret and joy). Developing a theory of mind and then applying it to our understanding of both our own and others' actions makes mind perception possible. It is also one of the features that make human beings unique. We are mind readers.

Here we cover the basic psychological processes that comprise what may be the human brain's most impressive capacity. Engaging with the mind of another person requires this capacity to be activated. The factors that govern activation can explain both anthropomorphism and dehumanization. Once activated, at least three basic processes guide the inferences people make about others' mental states and capabilities: egocentrism, stereotyping, and behavioral inference. These processes can work both in isolation and in coordination with each other, based on the information people have available to them at the time of judgment. Each process provides some accuracy but also some systematic error. Understanding these processes can provide wisdom, enabling people to increase their insight into the minds of others and helping to avoid some inferential mistakes that can lead to misunderstanding and conflict.

Processes of Mind Perception: Activation and Application

Having a capacity and using it effectively are two very different things. Most psychological research on human capacities attempts to understand how psychological processes get used in everyday life. Two questions are primary. First, what activates a given capacity, such as the capacity to think about another's mind? A

person might walk down a busy city sidewalk without ever thinking about the thoughts or intentions of a single passerby. As William James (1890/1990) correctly noted over a century ago, "My thinking . . . is for doing" (p. 669); hence, our theory of mind should be activated only if it is motivationally relevant for some potential action. Second, once a person is thinking about the mind of another person, what guides the application of this capacity in daily life? What processes enable people to get outside of their own minds and make inferences about invisible mental states in the minds of others, ranging from family to friends to complete strangers?

Ultimately these questions matter because our inferences about other people can guide our behavior toward them. You act differently toward a person you trust than toward a person you don't trust. You blame a person you believe harmed another on purpose more intensely than a person who harmed another by accident (Malle & Bennett, 2002). And you'll engage a stranger in conversation if the person seems interested in talking but avoid it if the person seems uninterested. Because these mental state inferences guide behavior, the accuracy of mind perception is also critical for identifying potential mistakes people might make that have important consequences for social interaction. In this chapter we cover what psychologists currently know about the activation and application of mind perception, ending with implications for interpersonal understanding *and* misunderstanding.

Activating Mind Perception

The human brain contains a wide array of capacities that get activated only when they are useful. Vision is useful for perceiving the physical world, and sighted people activate their visual system by opening their eyes when navigating the physical world. Mind perception is useful for perceiving the social world, and is therefore activated by goals to explain, understand, or predict others' actions (Koster-Hale & Saxe, 2013). These goals typically arise when there is interdependence between one person and another. Situations that increase the interdependence between the self and others should therefore increase the tendency to consider another person's mental states, whereas situations that decrease interdependence should decrease the tendency.

Sometimes cues to interdependence can come from subtleties in behavior. You might not give any thought to a passerby on the sidewalk until he looks directly at you, at which point you might wonder why he is interested in you. People tend to look at the things they are thinking about and think of the things they are looking at, so attending to another person's eye gaze is a good cue for what that person might be thinking about. Direct eye gaze also signals interpersonal connection and engagement that can activate approach-oriented neural systems (Hietanen, Leppänen, Peltola, Linna-Aho, & Ruuhiala, 2008). Being looked at directly can therefore trigger mind perception processes. In one experiment, for instance, participants saw an experimenter drop a heavy TV onto his hand in a staged accident (Bavelas, Black, Lemery, & Mullett, 1986). In one condition, the experimenter looked directly at the participant while showing a pained expression. In another condition, the experimenter looked slightly away, showing the same pained expression. Videotaped recordings indicated that the participants showed more concern for the accident when they were looked at directly, suggesting more sensitivity to another's mind when engaged by a direct eye gaze. In another experiment (Khalid, Deska, & Hugenberg, 2016), participants evaluated another person's mental capacities based only on a photograph, presented with either a direct gaze or an averted gaze. These pictured targets were perceived to be less mindful—less capable of thinking and feeling—when presented with averted gaze than with direct gaze. It is often said that "eyes are the window to the soul," but these results suggest that eyes are also a trigger for our tendency to think about, and therefore recognize, another mind standing right before our eyes.

More blatant signals of interdependence also show similar tendencies to activate mind perception processes. If, for instance, you are about to meet a new roommate, then you probably want to know something about this person's beliefs, attitudes, and preferences. Consistent with this, people who expect to interact with another person in the future are more likely to seek information about another person's mental states—his or her preferences, interests, attitudes, or desires—than when they are not expecting to interact again (Douglas, 1984, 1990). Similarly, the need to understand and attend to another person's mental states is stronger when you are in a real interaction with another person compared to just imagining being in an interaction. Consistent with this, participants in one experiment believed they were more likely to reject unsuitable romantic partners in a hypothetical situation than they actually were when in the midst of a real interaction with the unsuitable partner (Joel, Teper, & MacDonald, 2014). This occurred at least partly because participants were more sensitive to the pain of hurting another person's feelings in a real interaction than in a hypothetical interaction. Others' feelings might be top of mind when you're interacting with them, but out of mind when you're only imagining an interaction.

Understanding another's mind gives a person the ability to cooperate, coordinate, connect, and share reality with that person. This means that being motivated to understand another's behavior, or to connect with another person, should also trigger people to think about the minds of others. Research indicates that those who are interested in connecting with others are more likely to attend to others' emotions (Pickett, Gardner, & Knowles, 2004), adopt another person's psychological perspective (Knowles, 2014), and attribute a mind to nonhuman animals or gadgets (Epley, Akalis, Waytz, & Cacioppo, 2008; Epley, Waytz, Akalis, & Cacioppo, 2008). Diminishing the motivation to connect with others, such as by being reminded of friends, can diminish the degree to which people attribute mental capacities of thinking and feeling to outgroup members (Waytz & Epley, 2012) and to nonhuman animals (Bartz, Tchalova, & Fenerci, 2016).

Needing to explain others' behavior can likewise trigger people to think about others' minds. When a person acts exactly as you expect, you shrug your shoulders and move on. However, when a person behaves unexpectedly, then additional thinking is prompted to try to understand the behavior. Often this additional thinking shifts attention to another's mind. What was he *thinking*? Why did she *want* to do that? Unpredictable and unexpected behavior triggers people to think about the minds of others, increasing attention to mental states and even increasing the tendency to attribute human-like mental capacities to animals or objects (Waytz et al., 2010). In one experiment on gift giving (Zhang & Epley, 2012), the amount of thought a gift giver was presumed to have put into a gift affected the recipient's evaluation only when it was a gift that really needed to be explained—specifically, when the recipient received a bad gift (vs. good gift) from a friend (vs. a stranger).

Once one is interacting with another person, the motivation to connect can also activate mind perception processes. One example involves power and social status. Having power allows a person to act independently, without constraints imposed by others. Lacking power, in contrast, requires a person to operate under constraints, and hence requires coordination with others in order to achieve one's goals. Several experiments demonstrate how this can affect the activation of mind perception. Those in positions of high power, for instance, tend to be less accurate when inferring others' interests and attitudes (Keltner & Robinson, 1997), less likely to adopt another's psychological perspective (Galinsky, Magee, Inesi, & Gruenfeld, 2006; Gordon & Chen, 2013; but see Schmid Mast, Jonas, & Hall, 2009), and less likely to experience empathy for another's misfortune (Van Kleef et al., 2008). High status similarly creates a sense of disconnection and independence from others, and the effects of status appear similar to the effects of power on mind perception. Feeling like you are of high status, for instance, can increase attention to your own goals, interests, and desires, while decreasing attention to those same mental states in others, creating what one group of researchers described as "solipsistic social cognitive tendencies" (Kraus, Piff, Mendoza-Denton, Rheinschmidt, & Keltner, 2012).

These tendencies may vary, however, depending on more precise details of a person's status that might heighten motivation to attend to very specific mental states. If a person's status or power is perceived as illegitimate, then others' anger may be especially relevant to a high-power person who is concerned about losing his or her position, whereas a leader's fear may be especially relevant to a low-power person in this same situation. Several experiments

support this possibility, demonstrating that those in illegitimate high-power positions detect anger more quickly (and more accurately) than those in legitimate high-power positions, whereas those in illegitimate low-power positions detect fear more accurately (Stamkou, Van Kleef, Fischer, & Kret, 2016). Social contexts that require coordination with others trigger attention to others' mental states, and sometimes to very specific mental states, whereas contexts that reduce the need for coordination can lead people to overlook the minds of others.

That mind perception processes are triggered by personal motivation makes it clear that thinking about others' mental states requires at least some deliberate attention and effort in order to be utilized. Over time, as with any effortful process, repeated practice can create a less effortful habit. As people age, the ability to consider another's thoughts in the midst of an interaction becomes easier and more automatic (Epley, Morewedge, & Keysar, 2004). People in cultures in which interdependence is especially prominent, such as those with a history of highly interdependent agrarian practices (Talhelm et al., 2014), may also consider others' perspectives more readily than do people from independent cultures (Leung & Cohen, 2007; Wu & Keysar, 2007). As Markus and Kitayama (1991, p. 229) note about interdependent cultures, "The requirement is to 'read' the other's mind and thus to know what the other is thinking or feeling." Even growing up in a family with siblings, which may generally increase the need for coordination and attention to others, seems to increase the likelihood of attending to other minds in social interactions compared to growing up in a family without siblings (Jenkins & Astington, 1996; Lewis, Freeman, Kyriakidou, Maridaki-Kassotaki, & Berridge, 1996; McAlister & Peterson, 2007; Perner, Ruffman, & Leekam, 1994).

Mind perception enables effective coordination with others, comprehension and understanding of others' behavior, and also prediction of how others are likely to behave. A person's mind perception processes are therefore activated by the interdependent demands of the context a person is in, the goals of a person within that context, and the person's behavioral history. Understanding how mind perception is activated enables an understanding of when people are likely to be sensitive to others' thoughts, beliefs, and attitudes, and when they likely to overlook others' minds almost completely.

Applying Mind Perception: Processes of Egocentrism, Stereotyping, and Behavioral Inference

The ability to go beyond observable characteristics to make inferences about another's invisible mental states is among the brain's greatest strengths. Once activated, what are the processes that people use in order to make inferences about others' minds? Like many great abilities, mind perception is not enabled by a single process but instead comprises several different processes that are used in varying degrees depending on the information we have about another person, and on our own processing capacity and motivation. Three distinct processes have received the most empirical attention by psychological scientists: egocentric simulation, stereotyping, and behavioral inference.

Egocentric Simulation

"The only true voyage of discovery," Proust (1923/1993, p. 343) wrote, "would be not to visit strange lands but to possess other eyes, to behold the universe through the eyes of another." No person will ever be able to actually take Proust's voyage into the mind of another person, but many have noted that you don't need to travel very far to find a good source of inspiration. You can simply use your own mental experience as a guide to another's. If a meal tastes disgusting to you, then it is reasonable to presume that others will find it to be disgusting, too (Dawes & Mulford, 1996). In one of the earliest papers introducing the concept of a theory of mind, Nicholas Humphrey (1986, pp. 71–72) described this as the bedrock process guiding mind perception: "We could . . . imagine what it's like to be [others] because we know what it's like to be ourselves [and] make sense of [others'] behavior by projecting what I know about my mind into them." Humphrey was not exactly describing a new idea. Decades before, Bertrand Russell (1948) hypothesized that people use themselves as analogy to explain others'

actions. Centuries before that, Immanuel Kant (1781/1953, p. 180) simply took this process for granted as common sense: "It's obvious that if anyone x wants to represent a thinking being y to himself he has to put himself in y's place, as it were substituting his own subject for y's."

Less obvious are the numerous ways in which using oneself as guide for others manifests itself in everyday judgment. For instance, people tend to overestimate the extent to which their own emotions are visible to others, mainly because people's own emotions are so clear to themselves (Gilovich, Savitsky, & Medvec, 1998). In conversation, listeners likewise tend to interpret another's message in a way that is consistent with their own egocentric perspective on the situation (Keysar, Barr, Balin, & Brauner, 2000; Kruger, Epley, Parker, & Ng, 2005). Speakers may do the same, assuming that their intentions are clearer to listeners than they actually are, an egocentric bias that can become problematic in social interaction if one's "obviously" sarcastic joke is interpreted as sincere (Keysar & Barr, 2002), or if one's intentionally harmless teasing is mistaken as a malicious insult (Kruger, Gordon, & Kuban, 2006). People also use their own behavior as a guide to others' likely behavior, such that people tend to assume that others will act in a way that is relatively similar to the way they personally would act (Ross, Greene, & House, 1977). Those who cheat on a test, for instance, assume that others are more likely to cheat than do those who do not cheat on the same test (Katz, Allport, & Jenness, 1931). People may also project their own experience onto others, assuming that others will feel something relatively similar to their own experience after hearing a joke, seeing a movie, or experiencing an event. In one experiment, for instance, participants predicted how willing they would be, and how much they would need to be paid, to dance in front of their large class to Rick James's iconic funk song "Superfreak" (Van Boven, Loewenstein, Welch, & Dunning, 2012). These participants facing a purely hypothetical choice overestimated how willing they would be to dance compared to a group that actually faced this choice in front of a real classroom full of students, and also underestimated how much they would need to be paid in order to dance. As a result, people also overestimated how willing other people would be to dance when facing an actual choice, and also underestimated how much people would need to be paid to do it (Van Boven, Loewenstein, & Dunning, 2005).

Of course, adult human beings are not entirely egocentric. As people age, they quickly and sometimes painfully learn that their own perspective might be unique and that others do not see the world exactly as they do. Whereas young children make relatively egregious perspective-taking errors, often failing to attribute false beliefs to others (Baillargeon, Scott, & He, 2010), adults make perspective-taking errors that seem relatively less severe. This is not because adults outgrow their tendency to start with an egocentric default in judgment, but because adults become more adept at correcting their egocentric default when they are aware that another person's perspective might differ from their own (Epley, Keysar, Van Boven, & Gilovich, 2004; Epley, Morewedge, & Keysar, 2004; Tamir & Mitchell, 2013). This egocentric correction process documented across age may also characterize the cross-cultural differences that emerge in mind perception, with those from interdependent cultures being more likely to correct an egocentric default rather than failing to rely on it at all (Wu & Keysar, 2007).

Cognitive processes such as egocentric projection can also be moderated by a person's motivational state. The motive to connect to another person, or to distance oneself, seems to explain why people project their own personality traits—and presumably mental states as well—onto other people (Machunsky, Toma, Yzerbyt, & Corneille, 2014). Some research also suggests that basic motives of self-protection and mate search may also lead to more sophisticated patterns of egocentric projection (Maner et al., 2005). Feeling threat may make people hypervigilant for signs of danger from threatening others, increasing the likelihood of seeing anger in outgroup faces. Likewise, men who are actively seeking women for a romantic relationship may be more vigilant to signs of reciprocal interest than men who are not, increasing the likelihood of perceiving sexual arousal in women's faces. A person's goals can guide the information to which he or she attends, at least in some cases affecting the processes used to understand the minds of others.

Stereotyping

Mental state inferences are complicated, composed of multiple processes that interact in order to render a judgment about another person's inner life. Other minds can sometimes be blank slates onto which we project our own, using the previously discussed process of egocentric simulation. But we often know considerably more than nothing about the people we are trying to understand. Others can be police officers or parolees, teachers or students, conservatives or liberals. These categories activate beliefs about groups that can then provide information about another individual's attitudes, beliefs, or other mental states. Learning that someone is a member of a conservative political party, for instance, gives you some information about his or her likely attitudes on social and economic issues. These *stereotypes*—defined simply as "a set of beliefs about the personal attributes of a group of people" (Ashmore & Del Boca, 1981, p. 16)—comprise a second process by which people infer others' mental states.

It is reasonable to use oneself as a guide to others who are relatively similar to us, but it is less reasonable when others clearly differ from us. The perceived similarity of another person to the self therefore moderates the use of an egocentric default in social judgment, which is corrected or even replaced by using stereotypes or other individuating information in its place. In one experiment, university students tended to use their own attitudes as a guide to the attitudes of students from their own university, but they relied on stereotypes as a guide to the attitudes of students from a dissimilar university (Ames, 2004a, 2004b). Specifically, students from Columbia University predicted what percentage of fellow Columbia students and University of California, Berkeley students would agree to a series of statements, along with indicating their own agreement with each statement. Berkeley students are perceived as being politically liberal, with a long history of social activism. The statements were either consistent with the liberal stereotype of Berkeley students ("Do you engage in political protests at least once a year?") or inconsistent with the stereotype ("Do you think capital punishment is ever an acceptable policy?").

Results indicated that participants' own views were highly correlated with the views they expected of their fellow Columbia University students. In contrast, participants' own views were not correlated with predictions of the dissimilar outgroup's views—that is, of Berkeley students. Instead, participants presumed that Berkeley students held views relatively consistent with the common stereotype of these students. By measuring participants' own beliefs, as well as group stereotypes, this researcher was able to confirm that participants relied on egocentrism when understanding the mind of a similar other but relied on a group-based stereotype when understanding the mind of a dissimilar other.

Perceived similarity on one dimension can even moderate the use of an egocentric default on what might be seen as a completely unrelated dimension. If you are feeling cold because you have been standing in cold weather for a long time, then it's easy to presume that concerns about the cold are top of mind for other people as well. One series of experiments, however, found, that this projection occurred when people were making inferences about someone from the same political party but not when reasoning about someone from an opposing political party (O'Brien & Ellsworth, 2012). Kant's (1781/1953) "obvious" mechanism for understanding the minds of others seems not to be employed in cases in which another person's mind seems obviously different from one's own. In these cases, the stereotypes that allow people to identify the differences between themselves and others also guide their inferences about the minds of dissimilar others.

Behavioral Inference

Both egocentrism and stereotyping are relatively indirect sources of information about the mind of another person. A person may gain somewhat more direct insight by watching another's behavior and then working backward to a corresponding inference about a person's underlying mental states and experience (Jones, 1979). When a manager yells at an employee, it is easy to infer that the manager felt angry and intended to change the employee's behavior. When a person votes for a candidate, it is easy to presume the voter likes the chosen candidate. When someone is crying, then his or her suffering is obvious.

A person's behavior can provide such a strong cue to mental experience that egocentrism and stereotyping are quickly supplanted by behavioral inference when someone else can be observed directly. In one experiment, for instance, participants who watched a White or Black person being interviewed for 15 seconds showed strong evidence of using ethnic stereotypes to think about the person's characteristics. After 12 minutes of an interview, however, no evidence of stereotypic thinking could be detected (Kunda, Davies, Adams, & Spencer, 2002).

Recognizing the value of another person's behavior as a guide to his or her mental experience may be somewhat obvious, but the attributional process that people go through to understand the meaning of behavior is a nuanced, multistep causal analysis that moves from perceptions of others' mental states to inferences about others' stable traits and dispositions (Gilbert & Malone, 1995; Heider, 1958; Van Overwalle, Van Duynslaeger, Coomans, & Timmermans, 2012). Most behavior, after all, is somewhat ambiguous. Was the question asked during an interview hostile or earnest? Is a coworker giving the boss honest praise or insincere flattery? In order to understand what a behavior might mean for underlying mental states, its nature first has to be interpreted and characterized by a perceiver so as to remove inherent ambiguity (Trope, 1986). This characterization can then lead to an automatic inference of a corresponding mental state consistent with one's characterization of the action. If a coworker's praise is perceived as unjustified, then the coworker is presumed to be insincere and engaging in attempted flattery. If a person votes for a political candidate, then the voter is generally presumed to like the chosen candidate (even if the perceiver personally dislikes the candidate; Miller & Nelson, 2002).

If mental states are inferred directly from behavioral cues, then the cues most closely related to actual mental experience should also be the most powerful in guiding mind perception. One such cue is a person's voice, through speech. The human voice evolved as a tool to communicate the content of one's own mind to others, and vice versa (Pinker & Bloom, 1990).

Beyond the obvious semantic content present in language, speech also contains paralinguistic cues including intonation, pace, and cadence that may all be used as cues to others' mental states. *Intonation* (variance in pitch) may reflect the process of thinking as it is occurring. A pause in speech may be interpreted as thinking or deliberation. And a rising tone may signal enthusiasm, whereas a falling tone signals sadness. The paralinguistic cues appear to be at least somewhat accurate, as several experiments demonstrate that people can predict another person's thoughts and emotions more accurately when they can hear another person speak compared to reading the same content in text or simply observing the person's nonverbal cues (Bond & DePaulo, 2006; Hall & Schmid Mast, 2007; Ickes, 2003; Kruger et al., 2005; Mehrabian & Wiener, 1967; Zaki, Bolger, & Ochsner, 2009).

Beyond conveying the content of his or her mind—what a person may be thinking or feeling—a person's voice may also convey the actual presence of a person's mind—that another person is *capable* of thinking or feeling. Just as you might infer the presence of biological life in another person by watching for variance in motion (i.e., movement), so too might you infer the presence of mental life by listening for variance in paralinguistic cues that would suggest a lively, active, and thoughtful mind. Changes in the tone or pace of one's speech (*intonation* and *cadence,* respectively) can reveal the presence of conscious experience as it is occurring. Consistent with this possibility, potential job candidates in one experiment were perceived to be more mindful—more thoughtful, intelligent, and rational—when potential employers heard the candidate's "elevator pitch" compared to when they read a written pitch or read a transcript of the spoken pitch (Schroeder & Epley, 2015). Even a person with an opposing political viewpoint is perceived to be more mindful when you hear the other person explain his or her beliefs compared to reading the same content, or reading a written explanation of the other person's viewpoint (Schroeder, Kardas, & Epley, 2017).

Although nonverbal cues are considerably less diagnostic than verbal cues, people nevertheless rely on them to infer underlying mental states. Some of these cues are quite obvious, such as facial or bodily expressions that communicate emotions or intentions. Other cues, however, are considerably subtler. Eye movements, for instance, are also used to infer emotions and intentions (Baron-Cohen, Jolliffe, Mortimore, & Robertson, 1997; Wesselmann, Cardoso, Slater, & Williams, 2012). Around the world, people report that "shifty eyes" are a clear sign that another person is lying (Global Deception Research Team, 2006), even though empirical evidence suggests that eye movements do not provide accurate signals to honesty. Other facial cues, such as a more feminine appearance, increase perceived trustworthiness even in children as young as 3 years of age (Jessen & Grossmann, 2016; see Todorov, 2017, for a review). These judgments from nonverbal cues tend to be triggered automatically, producing consistent impressions from another's face or body with as little as 39-millisecond exposure to another person's face (Bar, Neta, & Linz, 2006; Willis & Todorov, 2006). Some researchers suggest that rapid mental state inferences are a core component of human social intelligence, producing rapid inferences about others with above-chance accuracy that can be used to make critical split-second judgments (Ambady & Weisbuch, 2010). These inferences, however, can also produce systematic errors that lead to significant interpersonal misunderstanding and undermine the quality of social relationships (Epley, 2014).

Research on basic processes of egocentrism, stereotyping, and behavioral inference make it clear that mind perception is guided by multiple processes operating in different contexts, sometimes alone or in concert with each other, based on the cues available at the time of judgment. When the implications of another person's behavior are clear, corresponding inferences from observed behavior are likely to drive judgment. When lacking clear behavioral cues, people may resolve ambiguity by using either stereotypes or egocentric simulations, depending on what is known about the target, sometimes correcting an automatic egocentric inference based on additional information that might be known about a target. Given this complexity, the field currently lacks a comprehensive account of mind perception that accommodates all of the varying contexts and conditions in which mental state inferences are made.

Consequences of Mind Perception

People try to understand others' minds in order to interact more effectively with them in the present, or to more accurately predict others' behavior in the future. Mind-perception processes are therefore aimed at answering two basic questions about others' minds (Epley & Waytz, 2010). First, does "it" have a mind? Understanding how people attribute mental states to others helps explain the related processes of anthropomorphism and dehumanization. *Anthropomorphism* arises when people attribute human-like minds to nonhuman agents, whereas *dehumanization* arises when people fail to attribute a human-like mind to other human beings. Second, what state is another's mind in? The specific attributions people make about others' mental states inherently raise complicated questions about the degree to which mental state inferences are accurate versus inaccurate. Understanding the processes that enable mind perception allows precise predictions about when mental state inferences will be relatively accurate versus relatively inaccurate. Perhaps of most interest for everyday life, mind perception processes can also create systematic errors that undermine the quality of interpersonal relationships, while also pointing the way to more effective strategies for understanding others.

Anthropomorphism and Dehumanization

Scientists may vigorously debate which capacities make us uniquely human, but almost everyone else has a fairly clear intuition that personhood is defined not by the presence of particular physical features, such as opposable thumbs or bipedalism, but rather the presence of mental features. For instance, Article 1 from the United Nations Universal Declaration of Human Rights states, "All human beings are born free," indicating a capacity for autonomy, and "are endowed with reason and conscience," indicating a sophisticated capacity for thinking. One of the earliest philosophical definitions defined a person as "an individual substance of a rational nature" (Boethius, sixth century C.E.),

a view reinforced by John Locke, who likewise defined a person as "an intelligent being that has reason and reflection" (quoted in Farah & Heberlein, 2007, p. 37). And when psychologists ask people in surveys to identify uniquely human features, they consistently focus on the presence of a human-like mind capable of thinking and feeling (Demoulin et al., 2004; Gray et al., 2007; Haslam, 2006). Attributing human-like mental capacities to other agents is therefore the essence of anthropomorphism (Epley, Waytz, & Cacioppo, 2007). *Failing* to attribute human-like mental capacities to other people, thereby conceptualizing them as more similar to a nonhuman animal or object, is the essence of dehumanization (Haslam, 2006).

The processes of mind perception discussed earlier can therefore help to explain both anthropomorphism and dehumanization. For instance, egocentric projection of one's own mental states onto others is moderated by the perceived similarity of others to the self. Research indicates that people are more likely to anthropomorphize nonhuman agents when they are perceived to be similar to human beings either in physical appearance or in bodily movements (Aggarwal & McGill, 2007; Eddy, Gallup, & Povinelli, 1993; Johnson, Slaughter, & Carey, 1998). In one series of experiments, nonhuman animals, robots, and even plants were perceived to have a more human-like mind when they moved at a human-like pace (Morewedge, Preston, & Wegner, 2007). Hummingbirds, with their fast and erratic motion, seem relatively neurotic and thoughtless. Sloths, perpetually stuck in what seems to us like slow motion, were described by the first naturalist ever to study them as clearly mindless creatures: "Slowness, stupidity, neglect of own body, and even habitual sadness, result from this bizarre and neglected conformation" (quoted in Gould, 1998, pp. 380–381). Similar findings have emerged in perceptions of other humans. When normal human motion is shown in slow motion or sped up compared to normal speed, the person seems less thoughtful or rational, consistent with dehumanizing another person by attributing diminished mental capacities to them (see also Caruso, Burns, & Converse, 2016).

Anthropomorphism and dehumanization can also be moderated by the motivations that activate mind perception processes, such as the motivations to connect with another agent, or to explain and understand another agent's behavior. Feeling lonely or isolated can increase the likelihood of believing in anthropomorphized religious agents such as a god, or can increase the likelihood of attributing humanlike mental characteristics to pets (Aydin, Fischer, & Frey, 2010; Bartz et al., 2016; Epley, Akalis, et al., 2008; Epley, Waytz, et al., 2008). Inversely, thinking about anthropomorphized pets can also satisfy relational needs, increasing well-being and diminishing the psychological pain that can follow social rejection (McConnell, Brown, Shoda, Stayton, & Martin, 2011). When thinking about other human beings, feeling socially connected to members of one's ingroup, and hence feeling little motivation to connect to others, can increase the tendency to dehumanize outgroup members (Waytz & Epley, 2012). Similarly, being motivated to explain another agent's behavior—for example, because it behaves unpredictably—increases the tendency to anthropomorphize a nonhuman agent. In one experiment, an alarm clock outfitted with wheels that rolls around after pressing its snooze button twice was more likely to be perceived as having "a mind of its own" when its behavior was described as relatively unpredictable compared to when its behavior was described as relatively predictable (Waytz et al., 2010). Similar effects seem to emerge when evaluating other people as well. When people behave in a way that violates social norms, observers are more likely to explain this unusual behavior by appealing to a person's underlying mental states as explanation. When someone goes with the flow and behaves as the norms dictate, then people are less likely to attribute behavior to a person's mental states (Uttich & Lombrozo, 2010). More research is needed, however, to firmly establish a link between indifference to explaining another's actions and dehumanization.

Finally, cues that reveal the presence of mind, such as paralinguistic cues in voice, have also been linked to anthropomorphism and dehumanization. One experiment demonstrated that a simulated self-driving vehicle seemed more mindful—better able to sense its environment, and more intelligent—when it was able to speak to the driver in a human voice than when it contained no voice (Waytz, Heafner, & Epley, 2014). In another experiment, people were more likely to believe that computer-generated writing was actually created by a person when they heard the content read by a human voice than when they read the exact same content in text (Schroeder & Epley, 2016). When evaluating other people, the presence of voice seems to be humanizing, and its absence is dehumanizing. Job candidates giving an elevator pitch (a brief description of their qualifications for a job) were judged to be more mindful—more thoughtful, rational, and intelligent—when a hypothetical employer heard the candidate's pitch than when they read a text-only transcript of exactly the same content, or read the candidate's written elevator pitch (Schroeder & Epley, 2015). In another experiment conducted on the weekend before the 2016 U.S. Presidential election, voters who were explaining why they were voting for an *opposing* political candidate seemed less mindful—less thoughtful, rational, and intelligent—when evaluators read the voter's written explanation or read a transcript than when they heard the voter's explanation in his or her own voice (Schroeder et al., 2017). Cues that convey the presence of mind are humanizing, with their presence producing anthropomorphism when evaluating nonhuman agents and their absence producing dehumanization when evaluating other human beings. Perceptions of another's mind matter in these cases because they have the power to award or deny aspects of personhood, along with the rights, responsibilities, and status that come with it.

Accuracy, Bias, and Confidence

The main goal of trying to infer other people's thoughts, beliefs, attitudes, or other mental states is to understand them better, allowing you to interpret their current behavior appropriately and also to predict their future behavior before they actually do it. How accurately we can understand the minds of others is therefore of primary interest. Actually assessing accuracy, however, turns out to be extremely complicated, as many different paradigms are utilized, involving predictions of a wide variety of mental states. The standard experimental methods typically involve having one person self-report the mental state being predicted, then having a perceiver predict that mental state. One spouse, for instance, might be asked to report his or her attitudes on a range of issues, while the other spouse predicts these responses. Or in what is known as the "empathic accuracy paradigm" (Ickes, 2001), two people could have a conversation, after which one person goes back through the video and notes what he or she was thinking or feeling at specific points in time, while the other person predicts those thoughts or feelings at the same points in time. Accuracy may also be assessed across a range of different targets, with accuracy then indexed either by averaging the targets' ratings together and comparing them against a perceiver's predicted average (known as *generalized accuracy*), or by correlating a perceiver's predictions for each target with the actual evaluations made by each target (known as *dyadic accuracy*).

Despite this complexity, several broad conclusions emerge from existing research. First, accuracy tends to be better than chance but far from perfect. For instance, one meta-analysis reported results from experiments in which people were asked to predict how much others in a group liked them (Kenny & DePaulo, 1993). These groups ranged from close acquaintances who had worked together over time to participants who had just met in a short get-to-know-you session. The average correlation between predicted and actual liking was .18, significantly greater than zero but also dramatically lower than a perfect correlation of 1. In summarizing this literature, David Kenny (1994, p. 159) wrote, "People seem to have just a tiny glimmer of insight into how they are uniquely viewed by particular other people." In the empathic accuracy procedure described in the preceding paragraph, accuracy is calculated as the percentage of others' thoughts predicted correctly, which can range from 0 to 100%. Accuracy rates here are typically around 20%, again higher than chance but also far from perfection. Accuracy tends to be a little higher when predicting friends or romantic partners, but not markedly so, averaging around 30% (as reported by Ickes & Hodges, 2013). These results, along with many others (Epley, 2014), make it clear that people are not clueless when it comes to understanding the minds of others, but

they are also not psychic savants. Other people are complicated creatures to understand, with mental states that have to be inferred rather than directly observed. Understanding the minds of others is therefore an extremely challenging task. Accuracy rates reflect this challenge.

Second, accuracy rates vary systematically based on the mind perception process utilized by perceivers. The processes of egocentrism, stereotyping, and behavioral inference described earlier all provide some systematic understanding of others but also create predictable biases in judgment that can lead to systematic misunderstanding. Consider egocentrism. Assuming that others' minds match one's own can lead to systematic egocentric biases in judgment. People tend to assume, for instance, that others' attitudes, knowledge, beliefs, and emotional experience is at least somewhat similar to one's own (Krueger, 1998; Krueger & Clement, 1994; Ross et al., 1977). This can create systematic accuracy when others' mental states are indeed similar to one's own, such as when predicting the attitudes of a spouse (Hoch, 1987) but can lead to systematic error when another's perspective is quite different from one's own (Epley & Caruso, 2008). In general, people have difficulty recognizing when their own perspective is truly unique, which means that it is difficult for most people to correct an egocentric bias when it is appropriate to do so (e.g., Kruger et al., 2005).

Stereotyping likewise yields both a predictable mix of accuracy, bias, and error (see Jussim, 2012, for a comprehensive review). Knowledge about groups of others—that is, stereotypes—is often based on either direct or indirect observations of behavior and therefore contains at least some degree of accuracy about members of these groups. People have some sense of how attitudes might differ between old and young people, conservatives and liberals, or mothers and fathers because they have interacted with people from these groups, observed them indirectly, or heard from others about members of these groups. Accuracy is considerably lower when predicting the mental states of individual members of these groups, but higher when predicting the average ratings of members from these groups (Jussim, 2012). To the extent that stereotypic knowledge contains some genuine accuracy, relying on stereotypes even when judging individuals should increase accuracy compared to avoiding stereotype knowledge. Stereotypes lead perceivers astray, not surprisingly, when judging someone who has relatively counterstereotypical views (Lewis, Hodges, Laurent, Srivastava, & Biancarosa, 2012). However, because groups are defined by the attributes that make them differ from each other rather than those that make them similar to each other, the attributes that come most readily to mind when thinking about groups tend to exaggerate the actual differences between them simply due to regression to the mean. In one experiment, for instance, men and women predicted how accurate members of each group would be in a variety of mind-reading tasks that require interpersonal sensitivity, a highly accessible component of gender stereotypes (Eyal & Epley, 2017). Although women tended to perform slightly better than men on some of these tests, people predicted that these differences would be dramatically larger than they actually were.

Likewise, inferences from behavior can yield predictably accurate inferences to the extent that the available behavioral cues provide valid information about a target's mental states but can also yield predictable errors when the behavioral cues are misleading. As reviewed earlier, a person's voice gives meaningful cues to the presence of a person's mind, at least compared to text that is inherently more ambiguous. People tend to be better able to infer another's thoughts and feelings when they hear another person speaking compared to when they read the very same content in text alone (Zaki et al., 2009). Targets who are more "readable"— that is, who more transparently express their thoughts and feelings—also yield higher accuracy rates among perceivers (Ickes & Hodges, 2013). And as anyone who has ever acted in theater knows well, targets who are instructed to exaggerate their emotional expressions yield higher accuracy rates among perceivers than targets who simply show their genuine emotions, who in turn yield higher accuracy rates than targets asked to suppress their emotional experience (Zhou, Majka, & Epley, 2017). Relying on observed behavior to infer corresponding mental states, however, can lead to predictable

mistakes. People may infer that accidental outcomes were actually intended (Kelemen & Rosset, 2009; Rosset, 2008), or assume that a person's attitudes match his or her behavior even when the behavior was coerced by the context the person was in (Gilbert & Malone, 1995).

Accurate mind perception through egocentrism, stereotyping, or behavioral inferences stems from the correspondence between the cues derived from these processes and the actual attributes of the target being judged. Although this correspondence can often be known by the scientists conducting these experiments, it is not so clearly known to the people participating in these experiments, or to people judging others in their everyday lives. Accuracy may vary from one context to another based on the quality of cues available to a perceiver, but the perceiver's confidence in his or her judgment often seems insensitive to this variability, and also tends to outstrip his or her actual accuracy (Realo et al., 2003). For instance, participants in one experiment were asked to predict their romantic partner's level of self-worth, self-rated abilities, and activity preferences on three separate measures. People predicted their partner's responses perfectly accurately between 30 and 40% of the time, on average, but these same people *estimated* that they had predicted their partner's responses perfectly accurately roughly 80% of the time (Swann & Gill, 1997). This gap between confidence and accuracy actually *increased* the longer these romantic couples had been together. In another experiment, romantic partners (most of them married) predicted how their partner would answer a series of attitude statements (Eyal, Steffel, & Epley, 2018). Participants predicted their partners' answers a little better than chance guessing alone, answering an average of 4.9 statements out of 20 exactly correctly when chance was 2.7. However, these partners *believed* they had estimated 12.6 out of 20 exactly correctly. People do not seem to know how little they know about others.

These results collectively suggest that the key to enabling accurate understanding of another person is to utilize judgment strategies that provide more accurate cues to the other's mental states, but that people themselves may not recognize when they are using an effective strategy and when they are not. Perhaps the most effective way to understand the mind of another person is to get his or her perspective on a situation directly, either by being in exactly the same situation that another person is in and then relying on egocentric simulation as a guide, or by obtaining more accurate behavioral cues by directly asking another person to report what is on his or her mind—strategies we will refer to as "perspective getting" (Eyal et al., 2018). But if people's confidence in judgment is not sensitive to the actual accuracy of their judgment, then they may undervalue these effective strategies.

Emerging research is consistent with this. In one experiment, participants were asked to predict their own mental states in the future. Specifically, to predict how much they would like another person after meeting him or her. Participants thought they would be better able to predict their own minds if they learned demographic information about the person they would be meeting, rather than by talking to another person who had just spent time interacting with this same person (Gilbert, Killingsworth, Eyre, & Wilson, 2009). However, participants were actually more accurate when they learned the impression of the person who had just met with the target. In another experiment (Zhou et al., 2017), people were asked to predict another person's emotional experience while watching a series of 50 photographs. Participants could either choose to "read" the other person's behavior while watching a videotape of the person's facial expressions or get the person's perspective directly by seeing the photographs the other person was seeing. Results indicated the highest accuracy when participants actually got the other person's perspective by viewing the pictures the other person was seeing, yet participants tended to assume that watching the other person's facial expressions would systematically increase their accuracy. Finally, in the most straightforward method of increasing accuracy yet tested (that we know of), romantic couples in one condition of the experiment described in the previous paragraph (Eyal et al., 2018) were allowed to ask their partner to verbally answer the attitude statements they would later be asked to predict, essentially interviewing their partner about his or her attitudes before predicting those same attitudes. Results indicated that participants in this "perspective getting"

condition were dramatically more accurate in predicting their partners' responses than those in the control condition, but participants' beliefs about their accuracy were identical in these two conditions. Perhaps the most reliable way to understand the mind of another person is either to be in their shoes, experiencing the world as they are directly, or asking them to reveal their mind to you directly through language. Just don't expect that the people you might be advising to use these strategies will believe you.

Conclusion

Another person's mind is the most sophisticated system you are ever going to think about. Many aspects of social life would be much easier if others' minds were simpler to understand. Lacking a direct conduit into another person's mental experience, we have reviewed the indirect mechanisms that enable human beings to reason about each other's minds, and the motivational triggers that set these indirect mechanisms in motion. The basic processes that guide the activation and application of mind perception help to explain related phenomena of anthropomorphism and dehumanization, predict both systematic accuracy and error in judgments of others, and also identify both ineffective and effective strategies for understanding others better. Understanding these basic processes will not turn others' minds into open books, but we do hope it will help the one superpower you might already possess work just a little bit more effectively than it might otherwise.

REFERENCES

Aggarwal, P., & McGill, A. L. (2007). Is that car smiling at me?: Schema congruity as a basis for evaluating anthropomorphized products. *Journal of Consumer Research, 34,* 468–479.

Ambady, N., & Weisbuch, M. (2010). Nonverbal behavior. In S. T. Fiske, D. T. Gilbert, & G. Lindzey (Eds.), *Handbook of social psychology* (5th ed., pp. 464–497). Hoboken, NJ: Wiley.

Ames, D. R. (2004a). Inside the mind reader's tool kit: Projection and stereotyping in mental state inference. *Journal of Personality and Social Psychology, 87,* 340–353.

Ames, D. R. (2004b). Strategies for social inference:

A similarity contingency model of projection and stereotyping in attribute prevalence estimates. *Journal of Personality and Social Psychology, 87,* 573–585.

Ashmore, R. D., & Del Boca, F. K. (1981). Conceptual approaches to stereotypes and stereotyping. In D. L. Hamilton (Ed.), *Cognitive processes in stereotyping and intergroup behavior* (pp. 1–35). Hillsdale, NJ: Erlbaum.

Aydin, N., Fischer, P., & Frey, D. (2010). Turning to God in the face of ostracism: Effects of social exclusion on religiousness. *Personality and Social Psychology Bulletin, 36,* 742–753.

Baillargeon, R., Scott, R. M., & He, Z. (2010). False-belief understanding in infants. *Trends in Cognitive Sciences, 14,* 110–118.

Bar, M., Neta, M., & Linz, H. (2006). Very first impressions. *Emotion, 6,* 269–278.

Baron-Cohen, S., Jolliffe, T., Mortimore, C., & Robertson, M. (1997). Another advanced test of theory of mind: Evidence from very high functioning adults with autism or Asperger syndrome. *Journal of Child Psychology and Psychiatry, 38,* 813–822.

Bartz, J. A., Tchalova, K., & Fenerci, C. (2016). Reminders of social connection can attenuate anthropomorphism: A replication and extension of Epley, Akalis, Waytz, and Cacioppo (2008). *Psychological Science, 27,* 1644–1650.

Bavelas, J. B., Black, A., Lemery, C. R., & Mullett, J. (1986). "I show how you feel": Motor mimicry as a communicative act. *Journal of Personality and Social Psychology, 50,* 322–329.

Bond, C. F., Jr., & DePaulo, B. M. (2006). Accuracy of deception judgments. *Review of Personality and Social Psychology, 10,* 214–234.

Caruso, E. M., Burns, Z. C., & Converse, B. A. (2016). Slow motion increases perceived intent. *Proceedings of the National Academy of Sciences of the USA, 113,* 9250–9255.

Dawes, R. M., & Mulford, M. (1996). The false consensus effect and overconfidence: Flaws in judgment or flaws in how we study judgment? *Organizational Behavior and Human Decision Processes, 65,* 201–211.

Demoulin, S., Leyens, J.-P., Paladino, M.-P., Rodriguez-Torres, R., Rodriguez-Perez, A., & Dovidio, J. (2004). Dimensions of "uniquely" and "nonuniquely" human emotions. *Cognition and Emotion, 18,* 71–96.

Douglas, W. (1984). Initial interaction scripts: When knowing is behaving. *Human Communication Research, 11,* 203–219.

Douglas, W. (1990). Uncertainty, information-seeking, and liking during initial interaction. *Western Journal of Communication, 54,* 66–81.

Dunbar, R. I. (1993). Coevolution of neocortical size, group size and language in humans. *Behavioral and Brain Sciences, 16,* 681–694.

Echterhoff, G., Higgins, E. T., & Levine, J. M. (2009). Shared reality: Experiencing commonality with others' inner states about the world. *Perspectives on Psychological Science, 4,* 496–521.

Eddy, T. J., Gallup, G. G., Jr., & Povinelli, D. J. (1993). Attribution of cognitive states to animals: Anthropomorphism in comparative perspective. *Journal of Social Issues, 49,* 87–101.

Epley, N. (2014). *Mindwise: Why we misunderstand what others think, believe, feel, and want.* New York: Knopf.

Epley, N., Akalis, S., Waytz, A., & Cacioppo, J. T. (2008). Creating social connection through inferential reproduction: Loneliness and perceived agency in gadgets, gods, and greyhounds. *Psychological Science, 19,* 114–120.

Epley, N., & Caruso, E. M. (2008). Perspective taking: Misstepping into others' shoes. In K. D. Markman, W. M. P. Klein, & J. A. Suhr (Eds.), *The handbook of imagination and mental simulation* (pp. 295–309). New York: Psychology Press.

Epley, N., Keysar, B., Van Boven, L., & Gilovich, T. (2004). Perspective taking as egocentric anchoring and adjustment. *Journal of Personality and Social Psychology, 87,* 327–339.

Epley, N., Morewedge, C. K., & Keysar, B. (2004). Perspective taking in children and adults: Equivalent egocentrism but differential correction. *Journal of Experimental Social Psychology, 40,* 760–768.

Epley, N., & Waytz, A. (2010). Mind perception. In S. T. Fiske, D. T. Gilbert, & G. Lindzey (Eds.), *The handbook of social psychology* (5th ed., pp. 498–541). New York: Wiley.

Epley, N., Waytz, A., Akalis, S., & Cacioppo, J. T. (2008). When we need a human: Motivational determinants of anthropomorphism. *Social Cognition, 26,* 143–155.

Epley, N., Waytz, A., & Cacioppo, J. T. (2007). On seeing human: A three-factor theory of anthropomorphism. *Psychological Review, 114,* 864–886.

Eyal, T., & Epley, N. (2017). Exaggerating accessible differences: When gender stereotypes overestimate actual group differences. *Personality and Social Psychology Bulletin, 43,* 1323–1336.

Eyal, T., Steffel, M., & Epley, N. (2018). Perspective mistaking: Accurately understanding the mind of another requires getting perspective, not taking perspective. *Journal of Personality and Social Psychology, 114,* 547–571.

Farah, M. J., & Heberlein, A. S. (2007). Personhood and neuroscience: Naturalizing or nihilating? *American Journal of Bioethics, 7,* 37–48.

Frith, C., & Frith, U. (2005). Theory of mind. *Current Biology, 15,* R644–R645.

Galinsky, A. D., Magee, J. C., Inesi, M. E., & Gruenfeld, D. H. (2006). Power and perspectives not taken. *Psychological Science, 17,* 1068–1074.

Gilbert, D. T., Killingsworth, M. A., Eyre, R. N., & Wilson, T. D. (2009). The surprising power of neighborly advice. *Science, 323,* 1617–1619.

Gilbert, D. T., & Malone, P. S. (1995). The correspondence bias. *Psychological Bulletin, 117,* 21–38.

Gilovich, T., Savitsky, K., & Medvec, V. H. (1998). The illusion of transparency: Biased assessments of others' ability to read one's emotional states. *Journal of Personality and Social Psychology, 75,* 332–346.

Global Deception Research Team. (2006). A world of lies. *Journal of Cross-Cultural Psychology, 37,* 60–74.

Gordon, A. M., & Chen, S. (2013). Does power help or hurt?: The moderating role of self–other focus on power and perspective-taking in romantic relationships. *Personality and Social Psychology Bulletin, 39,* 1097–1110.

Gould, S. J. (1998). Can we truly know sloth and rapacity? In *Leonardo's mountain of clams and the diet of worms: Essays on natural history* (pp. 375–391). New York: Three Rivers Press.

Gray, H. M., Gray, K., & Wegner, D. M. (2007). Dimensions of mind perception. *Science, 315,* 619.

Hall, J. A., & Schmid Mast, M. (2007). Sources of accuracy in the empathic accuracy paradigm. *Emotion, 7,* 438–446.

Haslam, N. (2006). Dehumanization: An integrative review. *Personality and Social Psychology Review, 10,* 252–264.

Haslam, N., & Loughnan, S. (2014). Dehumanization and infrahumanization. *Annual Review of Psychology, 65,* 399–423.

Heider, F. (1958). *The psychology of interpersonal relations.* New York: Wiley.

Herrmann, E., Call, J., Hernández-Lloreda, M. V., Hare, B., & Tomasello, M. (2007). Humans have evolved specialized skills of social cognition: The cultural intelligence hypothesis. *Science, 317,* 1360–1366.

Hietanen, J. K., Leppänen, J. M., Peltola, M. J., Linna-aho, K., & Ruuhiala, H. J. (2008). Seeing direct and averted gaze activates the approach–avoidance motivational brain systems. *Neuropsychologia, 46,* 2423–2430.

Hoch, S. J. (1987). Perceived consensus and predictive accuracy: The pros and cons of projection. *Journal of Personality and Social Psychology, 53,* 221–234.

Hudson, M., Nicholson, T., Ellis, R., & Bach, P. (2016). I see what you say: Prior knowledge of other's goals automatically biases the perception of their actions. *Cognition, 146,* 245–250.

Humphrey, N. (1986). *The inner eye.* London: Faber and Faber.

Ickes, W. (2001). Measuring empathic accuracy. In J. A. Hall & F. J. Bernieri (Eds.), *Interpersonal sensitivity: Theory and measurement* (pp. 219–241). Mahwah, NJ: Erlbaum.

Ickes, W. (2003). *Everyday mind reading: Understanding what other people think and feel.* Amherst, MA: Prometheus Books.

Ickes, W., & Hodges, S. D. (2013). Empathic accuracy in close relationships. In J. A. Simpson & L. Campbell (Eds.), *Handbook of close relationships* (pp. 348–373). New York: Oxford University Press.

James, W. (1990). *The principles of psychology.* Chicago: Encyclopedia Britannica. (Original work published 1890)

Jenkins, J. M., & Astington, J. W. (1996). Cognitive factors and family structure associated with theory of mind development in young children. *Developmental Psychology, 32,* 70–78.

Jerison, H. J. (1971). More on why birds and mammals have big brains. *American Naturalist, 105,* 185–189.

Jessen, S., & Grossmann, T. (2016). Neural and behavioral evidence for infants' sensitivity to the trustworthiness of faces. *Journal of Cognitive Neuroscience, 28,* 1728–1736.

Joel, S., Teper, R., & MacDonald, G. (2014). People overestimate their willingness to reject potential romantic partners by overlooking their concern for other people. *Psychological Science, 25,* 2233–2240.

Johnson, S., Slaughter, V., & Carey, S. (1998). Whose gaze will infants follow?: The elicitation of gaze-following in 12-month-olds. *Developmental Science, 1,* 233–238.

Jones, E. E. (1979). The rocky road from acts to dispositions. *American Psychologist, 34,* 107–117.

Jussim, L. (2012). *Social perception and social reality: Why accuracy dominates bias and self-fulfilling prophecy.* New York: Oxford University Press.

Kant, I. (1953). *Critique of pure reason.* New York: Macmillan. (Original work published 1781)

Katz, D., Allport, F. H., & Jenness, M. B. (1931). *Students' attitudes: A report of the Syracuse University reaction study.* Syracuse, NY: Craftsman.

Kelemen, D., & Rosset, E. (2009). The human function compunction: Teleological explanation in adults. *Cognition, 111,* 138–143.

Keltner, D., & Robinson, R. J. (1997). Defending the status quo: Power and bias in social conflict. *Personality and Social Psychology Bulletin, 23,* 1066–1077.

Kenny, D. A. (1994). *Interpersonal perception: A social relations analysis.* New York: Guilford Press.

Kenny, D. A., & DePaulo, B. M. (1993). Do people know how others view them?: An empirical and theoretical account. *Psychological Bulletin, 114,* 145–161.

Keysar, B., & Barr, D. J. (2002). Self-anchoring in conversation: Why language users don't do what they "should." In T. Gilovich, D. Griffin, & D. Kahneman (Eds.), *Heuristics and biases: The psychology of intuitive judgment* (pp. 150–166). Cambridge, UK: Cambridge University Press.

Keysar, B., Barr, D. J., Balin, J. A., & Brauner, J. S. (2000). Taking perspective in conversation: The role of mutual knowledge in comprehension. *Psychological Science, 11,* 32–38.

Khalid, S., Deska, J. C., & Hugenberg, K. (2016). The eyes are the windows to the mind: Direct eye gaze triggers the ascription of others' minds. *Personality and Social Psychology Bulletin, 42,* 1666–1677.

Knowles, M. L. (2014). Social rejection increases perspective taking. *Journal of Experimental Social Psychology, 55,* 126–132.

Koster-Hale, J., & Saxe, R. (2013). Theory of mind: A neural prediction problem. *Neuron, 79,* 836–848.

Kraus, M. W., Piff, P. K., Mendoza-Denton, R., Rheinschmidt, M. L., & Keltner, D. (2012). Social class, solipsism, and contextualism: How the rich are different from the poor. *Psychological Review, 119,* 546–572.

Krueger, J. (1998). On the perception of social consensus. In M. P. Zanna (Ed.), *Advances in experimental social psychology* (Vol. 30, pp. 163–240). San Diego, CA: Academic Press.

Krueger, J., & Clement, R. W. (1994). The truly false consensus effect: An ineradicable and egocentric bias in social perception. *Journal of Personality and Social Psychology, 67,* 596–610.

Kruger, J., Epley, N., Parker, J., & Ng, Z. W. (2005). Egocentrism over e-mail: Can we communicate as well as we think? *Journal of Personality and Social Psychology, 89,* 925–936.

Kruger, J., Gordon, C. L., & Kuban, J. (2006). Intentions in teasing: When "just kidding" just isn't good enough. *Journal of Personality and Social Psychology, 90,* 412–425.

Kunda, Z., Davies, P. G., Adams, B. D., & Spencer, S. J. (2002). The dynamic time course of stereotype activation: Activation, dissipation, and resurrection. *Journal of Personality and Social Psychology, 82,* 283–299.

Leslie, A. M. (1987). Pretense and representation: The origins of "Theory of Mind." *Psychological Review, 94,* 412–426.

Leung, A. K., & Cohen, D. (2007). The soft embodiment of culture: Camera angles and motion through time and space. *Psychological Science, 18,* 824–830.

Lewis, C., Freeman, N. H., Kyriakidou, C., Maridaki-Kassotaki, K., & Berridge, D. M. (1996). Social influences on false belief access: Specific sibling influences or general apprenticeship? *Child Development, 67,* 2930–2947.

Lewis, K. L., Hodges, S. D., Laurent, S. M., Srivastava, S., & Biancarosa, G. (2012). Reading between the minds: The use of stereotypes in empathic accuracy. *Psychological Science, 23,* 1040–1046.

Machunsky, M., Toma, C., Yzerbyt, V., & Corneille, O. (2014). Social projection increases for positive targets: Ascertaining the effect and exploring its antecedents. *Personality and Social Psychology Bulletin, 40,* 1373–1388.

Malle, B. F., & Bennett, R. E. (2002). *People's praise and blame for intentions and actions: Implications of the folk concept of intentionality* (Technical Reports of the Institute of Cognitive and Decision Sciences, No. 02-2). Eugene, OR: Institute of Cognitive and Decision Sciences.

Maner, J. K., Kenrick, D. T., Becker, D. V., Robertson, T. E., Hofer, B., Neuberg, S. L., et al. (2005). Functional projection: How fundamental social motives can bias interpersonal perception. *Journal of Personality and Social Psychology, 88,* 63–78.

Markus, H. R., & Kitayama, S. (1991). Culture and the self: Implications for cognition, emotion, and motivation. *Psychological Review, 98,* 224–253.

McAlister, A., & Peterson, C. (2007). A longitudinal study of child siblings and theory of mind development. *Cognitive Development, 22,* 258–270.

McConnell, A. R., Brown, C. M., Shoda, T. M., Stayton, L. E., & Martin, C. E. (2011). Friends with benefits: On the positive consequences of pet ownership. *Journal of Personality and Social Psychology, 101,* 1239–1252.

Mehrabian, A., & Wiener, M. (1967). Decoding of inconsistent communications. *Journal of Personality and Social Psychology, 6,* 109–114.

Miller, D. T., & Nelson, L. D. (2002). Seeing approach motivation in the avoidance behavior of others: Implications for an understanding of pluralistic ignorance. *Journal of Personality and Social Psychology, 83,* 1066–1075.

Morewedge, C. K., Preston, J., & Wegner, D. M. (2007). Timescale bias in the attribution of mind. *Journal of Personality and Social Psychology, 93,* 1–11.

O'Brien, E., & Ellsworth, P. C. (2012). More than skin deep: Visceral states are not projected onto dissimilar others. *Psychological Science, 23,* 391–396.

Perner, J., Ruffman, T., & Leekam, S. R. (1994). Theory of mind is contagious: You catch it from your sibs. *Child Development, 65,* 1228–1238.

Pickett, C. L., Gardner, W. L., & Knowles, M. (2004). Getting a cue: The need to belong and enhanced sensitivity to social cues. *Personality and Social Psychology Bulletin, 30,* 1095–1107.

Pinker, S., & Bloom, P. (1990). Natural language and natural selection. *Behavioral and Brain Sciences, 13,* 707–727.

Proust, M. (1993). *In search of lost time: Vol. V. The captive and the fugitive* (D. J. Enright, Ed.). New York: Modern Library. (Original work published 1923)

Realo, A., Allik, J., Nolvak, A., Valk, R., Ruus, T., Schmidt, M., et al. (2003). Mind-reading ability: Beliefs and performance. *Journal of Research in Personality, 37,* 420–445.

Ross, L., Greene, D., & House, P. (1977). The "false consensus effect": An egocentric bias in social perception and attribution processes. *Journal of Experimental Social Psychology, 13,* 279–301.

Rosset, E. (2008). It's no accident: Our bias for intentional explanations. *Cognition, 108,* 771–780.

Russell, B. (2009). Analogy. In *Human knowledge: Its scope and limits* (pp. 482–486). New York: Routledge. (Original work published 1948)

Saxe, R., & Kanwisher, N. (2003). People thinking about thinking people: The role of the temporo-parietal junction in "theory of mind." *NeuroImage, 19,* 1835–1842.

Schmid Mast, M., Jonas, K., & Hall, J. A. (2009). Give a person power and he or she will show interpersonal sensitivity: The phenomenon and its why and when. *Journal of Personality and Social Psychology, 97,* 835–850.

Schroeder, J., & Epley, N. (2015). The sound of intellect: Speech reveals a thoughtful mind, increasing a job candidate's appeal. *Psychological Science, 26,* 877–891.

Schroeder, J., & Epley, N. (2016). Mistaking minds and machines: How speech affects dehumanization and anthropomorphism. *Journal of Experimental Psychology: General, 145,* 1427–1437.

Schroeder, J., Kardas, M., & Epley, N. (2017). The humanizing voice: Speech reveals, and text conceals, a more thoughtful mind in the midst of disagreement. *Psychological Science, 28,* 1745–1762.

Stamkou, E., Van Kleef, G. A., Fischer, A. H., & Kret, M. E. (2016). Are the powerful really blind to the feelings of others?: How hierarchical concerns shape attention to emotions. *Personality and Social Psychology Bulletin, 42,* 755–768.

Swann, W. B., Jr., & Gill, M. J. (1997). Confidence and accuracy in person perception: Do we know what we think we know about our relationship partners? *Journal of Personality and Social Psychology, 73,* 747–757.

Talhelm, T., Zhang, X., Oishi, S., Shimin, C., Duan, D., Lan, X., et al. (2014). Large-scale psychological differences within China explained by rice versus wheat agriculture. *Science, 344,* 603–608.

Tamir, D. I., & Mitchell, J. P. (2013). Anchoring and adjustment during social inferences. *Journal of Experimental Psychology: General, 142,* 151–162.

Todorov, A. (2017). *Face value: The irresistible influence of first impressions.* Princeton, NJ: Princeton University Press.

Trope, Y. (1986). Identification and inferential processes in dispositional attribution. *Psychological Review, 94,* 237–258.

Uttich, K., & Lombrozo, T. (2010). Norms inform mental state ascriptions: A rational explanation for the side-effect effect. *Cognition, 116,* 87–100.

Van Boven, L., Loewenstein, G., & Dunning, D. (2005). The illusion of courage in social predictions: Underestimating the impact of fear of embarrassment on other people. *Organizational Behavior and Human Decision Processes, 96,* 130–141.

Van Boven, L., Loewenstein, G., Welch, E., & Dunning, D. (2012). The illusion of courage in self-predictions: Mispredicting one's own behavior in embarrassing situations. *Journal of Behavioral Decision Making, 25,* 1–12.

Van Kleef, G. A., Oveis, C., Van Der Löwe, I., LuoKogan, A., Goetz, J., & Keltner, D. (2008). Power, distress, and compassion: Turning a blind eye to the suffering of others. *Psychological Science, 19,* 1315–1322.

Van Overwalle, F., Van Duynslaeger, M., Coomans, D., & Timmermans, B. (2012). Spontaneous goal inferences are often inferred faster than spontaneous trait inferences. *Journal of Experimental Social Psychology, 48,* 13–18.

Waytz, A., & Epley, N. (2012). Social connection enables dehumanization. *Journal of Experimental Social Psychology, 48,* 70–76.

Waytz, A., Heafner, J., & Epley, N. (2014). The mind in the machine: Anthropomorphism increases trust in an autonomous vehicle. *Journal of Experimental Social Psychology, 52,* 113–117.

Waytz, A., Morewedge, C. K., Epley, N., Monteleone, G., Gao, J. H., & Cacioppo, J. T. (2010). Making sense by making sentient: Effectance motivation increases anthropomorphism. *Journal of Personality and Social Psychology, 99,* 410–435.

Wegner, D. M. (2002). *The illusion of conscious will.* Cambridge, MA: MIT Press.

Wesselmann, E. D., Cardoso, F. D., Slater, S., & Williams, K. D. (2012). To be looked at as though air: Civil attention matters. *Psychological Science, 23,* 166–168.

Willis, J., & Todorov, A. (2006). First impressions: Making up your mind after a 100-ms exposure to a face. *Psychological Science, 17,* 592–598.

Wu, S., & Keysar, B. (2007). The effect of culture on perspective taking. *Psychological Science, 18,* 600–606.

Zaki, J., Bolger, N., & Ochsner, K. (2009). Unpacking the informational bases of empathic accuracy. *Emotion, 9,* 478–487.

Zhang, Y., & Epley, N. (2012). Exaggerated, mispredicted, and misplaced: When "it's the thought that counts" in gift exchanges. *Journal of Experimental Psychology: General, 141,* 667–681.

Zhou, H., Majka, L., & Epley, N. (2017). Inferring perspective versus getting perspective: Underestimating the value of being in another's shoes. *Psychological Science, 28,* 482–493.

CHAPTER 10

Shared Reality

Motivated Connection and Motivated Cognition

Gerald Echterhoff
E. Tory Higgins

Shared reality is ubiquitous. We are incessantly confronted with situations that evoke and demand judgments, beliefs, and emotional responses about a vast variety of objects, topics, or issues. Within the stream of events and information impinging on us on a daily basis, boosted by global networks and technology, we need to select and focus on what we feel is worthy of attention and find ways to regulate our thinking, feelings, and actions in the environment while coordinating with others. Achieving confident evaluations and judgments is thus a constant challenge, especially when the incoming information is novel, complex, or ambiguous. A key means for coping with this challenge is to create a shared reality with others, which can briefly be characterized as a motivated commonality of inner states about a target (Echterhoff & Higgins, 2017; Echterhoff, Higgins, & Levine, 2009; Higgins, 2019).

Humans are profoundly motivated to create shared realities with others (Higgins, 2011, 2019), and our world is virtually brimming with opportunities for doing so. For instance, when people meet a new employee at their workplace, they tend to form their impressions of the newcomer jointly with their colleagues, and they feel more confident in their impressions when others agree. People take into account the views of others, especially significant others (Andersen & Chen, 2002; Andersen & Przybylinski, 2018), to appraise experiences and events, and to coconstruct or verify views about various types of issues (Hardin & Higgins, 1996). Shared reality allows us to evaluate other people or groups; to form political, moral, or religious convictions (Heiphetz, 2018); and even to develop and maintain a sense of who we are and what we want (Higgins, 1996b; Sullivan, 1953). Furthermore, shared-reality creation comes with another immense benefit for members of an "ultrasocial" species (Campbell, 1983; Tomasello, 2014b): When we create a shared reality with others, we connect with them, we establish or strengthen our social relationships (Rossignac-Milon, Bolger, Zee, Boothby, & Higgins, in press) and thus fulfill our fundamental need for belonging (Baumeister & Leary, 1995).

The role of shared reality in the achievement of these needs becomes starkly apparent in instances in which people are deprived of the opportunity for social sharing. The detrimental effects of such deprivation on people's sense of confidence and feelings of connectedness can be found in short-term interactions, long-term social relations, and group processes. When current interaction partners withhold an expected shared reality, such as in the classical conformity studies by Asch (1951, 1956), people are left uncertain, uncomfortable, even physically agitated. Furthermore, when a close or intimate relationship dissolves, individuals lose an important source of shared reality that previously allowed them to validate their judgments, feelings, opinions, and even their self-concept (Slotter, Emery, & Luchies, 2014; see also Rossignac-Milon & Higgins, 2018b). Such consequences explain why the breakdown of a romantic relationship constitutes a highly distressing life event. And when people do not create a shared reality with others, for example, when they keep a secret from someone, they suffer because they cannot achieve epistemic and relational needs (see Liu & Slepian, 2018). Finally, exclusion from a group threatens the excluded member's needs for belongingness, meaning, and self-esteem (see Williams, 2009). Conversely, the defection of a group member to an outgroup is most disconcerting for remaining members with a high need for the group's shared reality (Mannetti, Levine, Pierro, & Kruglanski, 2010).

Beyond individual motivation, shared reality also has significant adaptive value for human sociality. Relations between humans are characterized by the need for cooperation (i.e., obligatory interdependence), which involves the exchange of information, support, or resources (Brewer, 1997; Tomasello, Melis, Tennie, Wyman, & Herrmann, 2012). Cooperation, which is essential to the evolutionary success and adaptiveness of humans (Henrich & Henrich, 2007; Tomasello, 2009), requires mutual trust (Axelrod, 1984; McAllister, 1995). As McAllister aptly put it, "Under conditions of uncertainty and complexity, requiring mutual adjustment, sustained effective coordinated action is only possible where there is mutual confidence or trust" (1995, p. 25). Interpersonal trust is both a key factor and consequence of experienced shared reality. Groups, which have been portrayed as "bounded communities of mutual trust" (Brewer, 1999), can achieve fundamental goals and outcomes to the extent that group members rely on a shared reality (Levine, 2018).

Accounts emphasizing the social nature of our representations of reality have been around for decades in psychology and the social sciences (e.g., Asch, 1951; Cooley, 1964; Festinger, 1950; Heider, 1958; Lewin, 1947; Mead, 1934; Moscovici, 1981; Newcomb, 1959; Schachter, 1959; Sherif, 1935; Turner & Oakes, 1997). Given the long history of these accounts, explicit theorizing about "shared reality" is relatively young. The conceptual framework was developed mainly in the 1990s (Hardin & Higgins, 1996; Higgins, 1992, 1999). Since then, the critical role of shared reality in many phenomena of psychology has been increasingly recognized. According to the Web of Science, the total number of publications with the term *shared reality* in the title or abstract has roughly doubled every 5 years since 1998.

The first stage of research was primarily devoted to the interpretation of existing findings on conversational meaning making, social interaction, attitude formation, social influence, and self-regulation through the lens of the initial theory of shared reality (Hardin & Higgins, 1996). Here, shared reality was broadly understood as consensual social verification, which confers a sense of objectivity, validity, and generality on individual experiences.

In the second stage, beginning around 2005, a more specific concept of shared reality was primarily employed to explain experimentally induced effects of communication on communicators' memory in the saying-is-believing paradigm (for a review, see Echterhoff, Higgins, & Levine, 2009). In this paradigm, participants are given evaluatively ambiguous behavioral information about a target person, such as a set of behaviors that could be characterized as either "stubborn" or "persistent" (Higgins & Rholes, 1978). The ambiguity of the stimulus information is critical because it triggers epistemic needs for uncertainty reduction that can be achieved by shared-reality creation (Pierucci, Echterhoff, Marchal, & Klein, 2014). Participants are asked to describe the target person to an audience who knew the target person and already had a positive or negative opinion of him. Those who communicated with an audience who liked (vs. disliked) the target described him in a more positive (vs. negative) way—evaluatively tuning the message toward the audience's attitude. Important-ly, participants' subsequent free recall of the target's behaviors is evaluatively distorted in the direction that matches the evaluative tone of their audience-tuned message. This *audience-tuning memory bias* has been conceptualized as the communicators' subjective creation of a shared reality with their audience (Echterhoff, Higgins, & Levine, 2009; Higgins, 1992).

The free-recall test in these studies probes participants' accessible knowledge about the communication topic. Accessible knowledge is the basis for many other cognitive processes, such as the formation of judgments, beliefs, and attitudes (Higgins, 1996a; Wyer & Srull, 1989). Hence, the audience-tuning memory bias reflects a profound influence on how communicators construct their social reality (see Echterhoff & Hirst, 2009). Below we discuss findings illuminating the principles and processes underlying this form of shared reality.

In recent years, research on shared reality has deepened and branched out, for instance, regarding a differentiated analysis of epistemic mechanisms and functions afforded by shared reality (Echterhoff & Higgins, 2017), and insights into building blocks of shared reality, including shared attention (Shteynberg, 2015, 2018), shared relevance and interest (Higgins, 2016, 2019; Tomasello, 2014a), and inferences of others' inner states (Heleven & Van Overwalle, 2018; Keysers & Gazzola, 2007; Semin, 2007). Simultaneously, the notion of shared reality has been explicitly applied to fields spanning close relationships, secrecy, health, conflict, politics, morality, religion, organizational change, and leadership, which are showcased in a Special Issue in *Current Opinion in Psychology* (Echterhoff & Higgins, 2018a). These extensions and diversifications mark the third stage of shared-reality research.

The next section is devoted to the terminology and conceptualization of shared reality. In the subsequent section, we identify basic principles involved in shared-reality processes; specifically, motivated connection and motivated cognition. We illustrate these principles in research on communication effects on memory, close relationships, and intergroup relations. In the final section we outline perspectives for future research.

Shared Reality: Conceptualization and Terminology

People are fundamentally motivated to create shared realities. *Shared reality* has been defined as the motivated and experienced commonality of inner states about target objects or issues (Echterhoff & Higgins, 2017, 2018b; Echterhoff, Higgins, & Levine, 2009). Inner states can represent interest in a target in a given context, as well as judgments, feelings, beliefs, or evaluations of a target (Higgins, 2016, 2019). The experience of commonality allows individuals to perceive such inner states as reflecting the "true" or "real" qualities of the target: how relevant it is, how we should feel about it or think about it (see Echterhoff, 2010). Shared reality thus captures an individual's experience of interpersonal commonality that produces sufficient confidence in his or her inner states (e.g., judgments, attitudes, feelings) about some target and makes him or her experience that truth as being shared with others (i.e., one is not alone in one's experience of the world). This shared reality experience, in turn, allows individuals to regulate their responses to that target (e.g., approach or avoidance) and work together in responding to that target.

A close examination of the term *shared* reveals different possible meanings (Thompson & Fine, 1999). A first possible meaning is "communicated or disclosed to others." This meaning focuses on the process whereby speakers make their internal personal reactions, for instance, about a new colleague at work, known to others. In this sense, the fact that something is shared implies that one person becomes aware of *what* another person believes or feels about an issue, but it does not require that the two hold the same beliefs or judgments about the issue. As such, this meaning does not capture a commonality of inner states, which is critical to shared reality.

According to a second meaning, *shared* means "divided up into portions," such as when we say that a task is shared among different people. This meaning refers to the division of cognitive labor or of responsibilities for different subdomains of a task. In this sense, the term implies that there is a joint task or project, and that each of the participating individuals is responsible for his or her specialized part in the task. What this meaning of *shared* emphasizes is the collaborative nature of information being "shared" between persons. Note, however, that this meaning highlights the *differences* between the individuals concerned with a common task. As in the first case, it is *not* required that the individuals have the same inner state about a target referent or have something in common (other than working on the same task or project).

In contrast, a correspondence or commonality between inner states about the world *is* implied in a third sense of the term, "partaking in a consensus," which applies to expressions such as "sharing an opinion." This possibility designates a state in which the views of at least two individuals are consensual or in common. Note that this meaning can merely refer to an objective condition that can be identified by an outside observer rather than to the feeling of sharedness experienced by the individuals holding the same view. Thus, in this third sense, people may hold similar or identical views without being aware of each other's view or subjectively experiencing a commonality of views.

There is also a fourth possible meaning of *shared*—"held and experienced in common." In this case, the individuals involved *do* perceive their inner states as being in agreement. When we say, for instance, that "*A* shares *B*'s interest in contemporary classical music," we imply that person *A* experiences a commonality between the inner state of *B* and her or his own inner state about a target referent. This fourth meaning of *shared* is essentially consistent with the conceptualization of shared reality outlined earlier.

Subjective experience is critical for understanding not only "sharedness" but also the term *reality*. From a psychological perspective, what matters is people's *experience* of what is real (Brickman, 1978). The motivation to achieve this experience is so strong that people can prefer objectively less rather than more accurate knowledge if the former produces a stronger subjective sense of knowing or *establishing what is real* (Higgins, 2012). This greater striving for the subjective experience rather than objectively verifiable knowledge of reality is epitomized by the power of political and religious ideologies (see also Jost, Ledgerwood, & Hardin, 2007).

The concern with reality construal raises a classical issue that has been contemplated by scholars in philosophy, psychology, and the neurosciences for a long time. How do people, given the constructive operation of the human mind, determine whether their perceptions and knowledge of something are real? Humans are equipped with cognitive and neural mechanisms, such as comparing predicted and actual sensory input, that tell them whether their mental models are sufficiently consistent with external stimulus conditions (Frith, 2007). They also use various cues to infer whether their memories stem from the perception of the world or from other sources such as imagination or information from others (Johnson & Raye, 1981). In contrast, shared-reality theory focuses on processes that are different from or subsequent to such low-level cognitive monitoring of their perceptions and inferences. For instance, when members of a work team meet a new colleague, they try to find out what kind of person the newcomer is, whether she is outgoing, trustworthy, committed, or open-minded, allowing them to evaluate the newcomer, predict her actions, and regulate interactions with her. Thus, the question is not whether the observed events (i.e., the newcomer's behaviors) are real, that is, whether the team members trust their perception and memory of the newcomer's behaviors as real (vs. made up or imagined). Rather, the task concerns the attributes and qualities of the target entity and the meaning of the observed events, that is, how the team members think about, categorize, judge, and evaluate the newcomer based on their perceptions and observations.

In summary, the conceptualization of shared reality provides a distinctive perspective on reality construction. The current theory has enhanced the precision, differentiation, integration, and testability of the concept of shared reality, and it affords distinctions between shared reality and related concepts such as common ground, informational social influence, alignment with norms, empathy, perspective taking, and socially distributed knowledge (see Echterhoff & Higgins, 2017; Echterhoff, Higgins, & Levine, 2009). For example, *common ground* involves shared background knowledge, which permits or at least facilitates conversation. However, common ground, as it is typically used in the literature, does not require that the communication partners experience shared judgments or evaluations of the topic of the conversation. For instance, when an employer and employees negotiate a new business plan, they would typically need to ground their understanding of what the business refers to (e.g., specific measures for reducing labor costs). Via grounding, they would establish a shared reference of the term *business plan*. However, this achievement of common ground on the meaning of *business plan* does not mean that employers and employees agree in their judgments or evaluations about the plan. For common ground, shared reference is sufficient. In contrast, for shared reality, shared reference is needed, but it is not sufficient. Rather, shared reality additionally requires common judgments, attitudes, or evaluations, which include sharing the opinion that the plan is worthy of their attention (shared relevance).

Furthermore, when two people experience having a shared reality, that shared reality is about, or in reference to, something in the world. This *aboutness* (i.e., being about a target entity; Higgins, 1998) distinguishes shared reality from other types of social commonalities (Echterhoff, Higgins, & Levine, 2009). For instance, empathy per se is not shared reality. For example, a woman could be sad about her dog passing away, and another person could see her sadness and empathically feel sad (see Hatfield, Cacioppo, & Rapson, 1994). Yes, the sad feeling is being shared, but not the reality of the dog passing away. Shared reality begins with shared relevance—sharing that something in the world is important, is worthy of attention. What is shared is that the dog passing away is a significant event, and the shared experience is *about* the event of the dog passing away. You do not need to have the same emotional reaction to the event; indeed, it is highly unlikely that you do. It is enough that you share the experience that this event is significant. The shared reality is about the dog passing away being a significant event in the world—not the sadness per se. Aboutness is a critical feature of shared-reality creation.

Shared-reality creation builds on processes that help individuals to infer the referent of the other's inner state, as well as the approximate content of the other's inner states (mentalizing, perspective taking). While shared reality as such is uniquely human (Higgins, 2019), some building-block processes such as shared reference or shared attention have been documented for nonhuman animals (for research on such processes in domesticated dogs, see Johnston, Byrne, & Santos, 2018). First, shared reality requires mechanisms that allow people to infer the target referent of their sharing partner's inner state, such as the referent of another person's feeling. One basic mechanism, also found among some nonhuman species (Shepherd, 2010), is to follow the direction of someone else's eye gaze (Csibra & Volein, 2008; Tomasello, 2008). Eye-gaze following, together with imputing intentionality to the other person, allows people to identify the referent of another person's interest or attention and to allocate shared interest in an object (Baron-Cohen, 1995; Butterworth & Jarrett, 1991). Other mechanisms include following someone else's pointing movements or manipulations of objects (Clark, 2003; Tomasello, 2008) and interpreting verbal utterances as referring to an object (Clark & Marshall, 1981).

Furthermore, shared-reality creation requires processes that allow people to become aware of or infer someone else's inner state. Research suggests several mechanisms by which this can be accomplished (e.g., Higgins & Pittman, 2008; Malle & Hodges, 2005). For instance, people draw on various nonverbal cues (e.g., facial expression, body movements, and gestures) to intuit their feelings, needs, and intentions. They infer others' mental states, such as others' beliefs and attitudes, based on mechanisms such as conscious reasoning, unconscious simulation, and theory of mind (e.g., Leslie, Friedman, & German, 2004); causal theories and schemas (e.g., Heider, 1958; Malle, 1999); or projection of their own inner states (Keysar & Barr, 2002; Nickerson, 2001). Neuroscientific research has made substantial strides at identifying brain mechanisms involved in the inference of and reasoning about other people's inner states, primarily, beliefs, judgments, and goals (Heleven & Van Overwalle, 2018; Molenberghs, Johnson, Henry, & Mattingley, 2016).

All of these processes facilitate the subjective creation of shared reality with another person but do not satisfy the definitional criteria of shared reality (see Echterhoff, Higgins, & Levine, 2009): They merely serve the *inference* of another person's judgments or beliefs but do not imply that two individuals hold or endorse the same judgment or belief. Being able to infer another person's inner state does not mean that I share the inner state with that person.

The Intrinsic Motivation to Create Shared Reality

Creating shared realities with others is critically important for humans to fulfill major needs. But it must be emphasized that creating shared realities with others is intrinsically motivating (Higgins, 2019). It is not simply an instrumental tool in the service of other needs. It is motivating for its own sake. It is something that humans want to do and, indeed, need to do. It can be considered an evolutionary characteristic of humans given that other human characteristics that are considered to be evolutionary (e.g., language, use of complex tools) require creating shared realities with others (e.g., Henrich, 2016). Notably, shared-reality creation is so strongly associated with achieving critical ends for humans that even if it began as an instrumental means, there would have been the kind of means–ends fusion that made shared-reality creation intrinsically motivating a very long time ago (see Kruglanski et al., 2018).

Shared reality is an experience with others about something in the world. Because it is about the world we live in with others, it directly relates to self-regulation and social regulation in the world. This is why shared reality is so important. The motivation to create shared realities is basic to humans for two major reasons. The first reason is that humans don't want to live alone in the world. They want to share the world with others (Baumeister & Leary, 1995). They want companionship. A sense of connection and companionship derives from sharing our experiences about the world with others. The second reason is that humans want to experience their beliefs, judgments, or feelings about the world as representing something real. When we create shared realities with others about something in the world, that thing is experienced as being real—the objective truth

(see Hardin & Higgins, 1996). In other words, shared reality allows us to feel confident that our judgments, evaluations, or beliefs about issues are truthful and valid.

These two reasons for wanting to create shared reality with others constitute two basic motives underlying the shared-reality creation motivation: *motivated connection* and *motivated cognition*. The first motive is essentially relational, while the second is essentially epistemic (see Echterhoff, Higgins, & Levine, 2009). Each of these motivations is special. First, the motivated connection via shared reality is special because the connection is sharing *the truth about the world*: connecting to others about what *really* matters in the world, what the world is *really* like, what is the *right* way to respond to it and deal with it (Higgins, 2019). Second, the motivated cognition of shared reality is special because the cognition about the world is *shared with others*: cognitions that are shared with significant others, with fellow community members, teammates, and companions (Higgins, 2019).

In addition to being special in these ways, motivated connection and motivated cognition constituting shared reality are special in being *synergistic*—each contributes to the other. Thus, we propose the following two principles of the interplay of motivated connection and motivated cognition in shared reality:

- *Principle 1:* Experiencing with others truth about the world (the perceived reality that satisfies motivated cognition) contributes to our experience of closeness with them, thereby satisfying motivated connection (Hardin & Conley, 2001; Rossignac-Milon & Higgins, 2018b).
- *Principle 2:* Having others verify or co-construct our experience of the world (sharing our experience that satisfies motivated connection) transforms that experience from being subjective to being objective, thereby becoming *the* truth and satisfying motivated cognition.

By this account, shared-reality creation encompasses a special kind of motivated connection and motivated cognition, and their relation to one another. When shared reality is created, people experience these special kinds of connection and truth, and their interrelation. Interestingly, the experience of trust also involves an interrelation between connection and truth—having faith that one can depend and rely on another person for the truth. Thus, experiencing shared reality with someone can induce trust in that person.

Furthermore, the experience of connection is intensified by metaperceptions of my own role in others' experience of shared reality: Because others experience a shared reality through my social verification of their feelings, beliefs, and concerns, and this shared reality makes their feelings, beliefs, and concerns feel more real to them, they are likely to feel connected to me and to perceive me as significant. All of this contributes to achieving my need for significance (see Kruglanski et al., 2013).

To sum up, motivated connection and motivated cognition are basic principles of shared-reality motivation. In this chapter, we discuss these two basic principles of shared-reality motivation and present evidence for how they function, and for how motivated connection and motivated cognition have both benefits and costs for self-regulation and social regulation, as reflected in our judgments and memory, feelings, opinions, social practices, close relationships, and intergroup relations—the shared reality trade-offs for humans. There is a good news story for humans from our motivation to create shared reality with others. But there is a bad news story as well (Higgins, 2019).

The Principle of Motivated Connection

According to the principle of motivated connection, a commonality of inner states about an issue or topic helps people to feel connected with others who share their inner state. Thus, shared-reality creation allows people to experience connectedness, belonging, and companionship. In the following, we illustrate this principle with examples and findings on shared reality in communication, social relationships, and intergroup relations.

Let us begin with a straightforward demonstration of the role of motivated connection in

audience-tuning effects on memory. In a study using the saying-is-believing paradigm (Higgins & Rholes, 1978), Pierucci, Klein, and Carnaghi (2013) manipulated the desire for communicating with the audience. This manipulation was based on a pretest in which participants were presented with pictures of potential interaction partners and indicated their desire to communicate with each of them. Participants were asked to describe an ambiguous target to an audience that either liked or disliked the target (audience attitude manipulation). Messages and recall were aligned with the audience's attitude when the audience was a person who qualified as a likable communication partner, that is, a partner with whom participants were highly motivated to communicate. In contrast, these effects did not emerge when the audience was a person who did not qualify as a likable communication partner, that is, a partner with whom participants had little desire to communicate.

Thus, when participants in Pierucci and colleagues (2013) were not motivated to connect with their audience, they did not bother to tune their message to the audience's attitude, and they did not create a shared reality with their audience, as indicated by the absence of the audience–attitude effect on memory. Interestingly, there was no evidence that participants' epistemic trust differed between the communication–desire conditions. Thus, the observed differences in audience tuning of the message and the memory bias were apparently driven by differences in motivated connection. Without motivated connection, there would be no grounds for motivated cognition to affect memory processes in an audience-congruent way (for a similar case regarding cognitive consistency effects, see Rossignac-Milon & Higgins, 2018a). This interpretation is consistent with the notion that motivated connection and motivated cognition operate synergistically in shared-reality creation.

A study by Echterhoff, Lang, Krämer, and Higgins (2009) suggests that the motivated connection inherent to shared reality also depends on status differences. These authors employed the saying-is-believing paradigm in the context of organizational personnel assessment. Student participants described an employee's behaviors to either an equal-status audience (a student temp) or a high-status audience (a company board member). The high-status audience was perceived as possessing higher domain-specific expertise, that is, professional competence in the assessment of employees. The message description was tuned to both audiences. However, and importantly, the audience-tuning memory bias was found only in the equal-status condition. The participants in Echterhoff, Lang, and colleagues reported lower affiliative-relational motivation toward the high-status audience than the equal-status audience. According to our analysis, the lack of motivated connection with the high-status audience curbed people's motivation to create a shared reality with them. Because they felt more distant to the company board member (vs. the student temp worker), they refrained from creating a shared reality. Furthermore, message tuning toward the higher-status audience was particularly strong among participants scoring high on Authoritarianism and Social Dominance Orientation. This finding suggests that these participants' message tuning was driven to a greater extent by strategic ingratiation or compliance goals rather than connecting to the audience via shared reality.

There are, of course, audience characteristics other than the distance within an organizational hierarchy that affect the motivation to connect with the audience via shared reality. A key characteristic suggested by the literature on intergroup processes is the audience's social category or group membership. Features of the audience related to social category, including group membership, have been manipulated in several audience-tuning studies (Echterhoff, Higgins, & Groll, 2005, Experiments 2 and 3; Echterhoff, Higgins, Kopietz, & Groll, 2008, Experiment 1; Echterhoff, Kopietz, & Higgins, 2017, Experiment 1; Echterhoff et al., 2017, Experiments 1a and 1b; Kopietz et al., 2009). For instance, communicators with a German background were paired with either a German or Turkish audience (Echterhoff et al., 2008, Experiment 1; Echterhoff et al., 2017, Experiment 1; Echterhoff et al., 2017, Experiments 1a, 2, and 3). Regarding educational background as another social category difference, Echterhoff and colleagues (2005, Experiments 2 and 3) had students communicate with either a fel-

low student or a hairdresser trainee. In all studies, as in previous audience-tuning studies, the audience's attitude was manipulated (positive vs. negative). According to the principle of motivated connection, communicators should be more motivated to make a shared-reality connection with an audience from their own group (i.e., from the same social category) than with an audience from an outgroup (i.e., from a different social category).

These intergroup communication studies found that the *messages* were tuned to the audience's attitude regardless of the audience's social category. Thus, at the overt, verbal level, communicators appeared to connect to their outgroup audience by tailoring their messages to the audience's attitude. However, no evidence for a shared-reality connection with the outgroup audience was found for the audience-tuning *memory* bias. When the audience's social category matched the participants' own social category (e.g., when German communicators talked to a German audience), the evaluative tone of participants' recall was aligned with the evaluative tone of their audience-tuned message, revealing the audience-tuning memory bias. In stark contrast, no such memory effect was found when the audience's social category did not match the participants' own social category (e.g., when German communicators talked to a Turkish audience).

Given these results, message tuning toward an outgroup audience was presumably motivated by goals other than connecting via shared reality, such as compliance with conversational rules, politeness, or egalitarian norms. This is not to say, however, that epistemic motives and motivated cognition were irrelevant in these studies. Rather, as outlined earlier, motivated connection and motivated cognition operate synergistically in shared-reality creation. We elaborate on the role of motivated cognition in intergroup audience-tuning studies in a subsequent section.

So far, we have distinguished communication settings or study conditions in which motivated connection was generally high or low. However, motivated connection may also vary with concurrent events and relevant updating information. For instance, after communicators have started to create a shared reality with an audience, they may lose their sense of connection with their audience. This loss of connection may also restrict or rescind their achievement of shared reality with their audience.

Imagine, for example, an employee who recently joined the branch of a large organization and is now being interviewed over the phone by a friendly representative at the organization's headquarters (HQ) about a new team in the branch. The employee has not yet formed a clear impression of that team, but she notices that the HQ representative apparently views it favorably. Because the representative is an ingroup member and acts in a friendly manner, she wants to connect with him via shared reality. She hence starts creating a shared reality, depicting the team's performance rather positively. But now imagine that after a few minutes, the employee realizes that the representative she actually had talked to was not the person she thought he was; that is, her audience-tuned messages were not received by the intended audience but, instead, by a different person. Realizing this failure should impede the sense of shared-reality creation, which in turn should eliminate the audience-tuning memory bias.

A similar scenario was examined by Echterhoff and colleagues (2013, Experiments 2 and 3). Would an emergent shared reality dissolve when communicators feel that they did not connect with the intended audience? The disconnection was achieved by telling communicators after a while that their audience-tuned message had been erroneously delivered to a different audience, not to the intended audience. According to a shared-reality account, the audience-tuning memory effect should be diminished or even eliminated when communicators realize that the presumed connection with the audience was not created.

In Experiments 2 and 3 by Echterhoff and colleagues (2013), participants first learned about the attitude of an audience, encoded the original target material, and tuned their messages to their audience. According to previous research, participants typically have created a shared evaluation or judgment with the audience at this point. Then, participants in the audience-change condition were informed that their message was erroneously delivered to a different audience (specifically, an outgroup member in

Experiment 2, an ingroup member in Experiment 3). Participants in a control condition (no audience change) were told that their message had been transmitted to the intended audience. The findings from both studies showed that the audience-tuning memory bias disappeared when participants learned that they did not connect with the intended audience. It did not matter whether the new, unintended audience was from the participants' ingroup or outgroup. According to an alternative explanation, learning about the erroneous message delivery might create a sense of frustration and negative mood, which could affect memory (Eich & Macauley, 2000). But no effects of audience change on participants' mood were found.

These findings suggest that communicators' creation of shared reality with their audience requires the experience of a sustained personal connection with the audience. For this experience, the group membership of the new, unintended audience is not critical. Rather, what matters is the sense of a continuing connection with the audience. When a personal connection turns out to be absent or falsely assumed, communicators abandon the shared reality they have started to achieve. In this case, a motivated connection through a shared reality is not feasible.

Further evidence on the role of motivated connection in shared reality comes from studies by Sinclair and colleagues on the social tuning of attitudes (Huntsinger, Sinclair, Kenrick, & Ray, 2016; Sinclair, Lowery, Hardin, & Colangelo, 2005; Skorinko et al., 2015; for reviews, see Sinclair & Lun, 2010; Skorinko & Sinclair, 2018). These researchers found that participants' own attitudes about a stigmatized outgroup (e.g., African Americans or homosexuals) can automatically align with the ostensible attitude of an interaction partner, specifically, an experimenter endorsing egalitarian beliefs. The endorsement of egalitarian beliefs was typically signaled by the egalitarian pun "eracism" (a composite of *erase* and *racism*) printed on the experimenter's T-shirt. The effect on attitudes was assessed with implicit, response-latency measures. By aligning their attitudes with the experimenter's attitude, the participants achieve a common inner state (i.e., attitude) with the interaction partner about an outgroup. In some studies, the strength of participants' affiliative motivation toward the experimenter was manipulated (Sinclair et al., 2005), while in other studies it was measured (Huntsinger et al., 2016, Experiments 1 and 2). Affiliative motivation was manipulated, for instance, by having the experimenter behave in a friendly, welcoming (vs. unfriendly, unwelcoming) manner toward participants. Consistent with the notion of motivated connection in shared reality, the alignment of participants' implicit attitudes with the experimenter's egalitarian attitude was stronger when participants' affiliative motivation was high (vs. low).

Subsequent social-tuning research suggests that motivated connection may be generally higher for people who are more (vs. less) oriented toward maintaining relationships with their ingroup members. Specifically, Skorinko and colleagues (2015) compared attitudinal alignment between participants from a collectivistic and individualistic culture (Experiment 1), or between participants from the same culture (either from the United States in Experiment 2, or from Hong Kong in Experiment 3) who were primed with either a collectivistic or with an individualistic mindset. The experimenter, with whom participants interacted, wore a T-Shirt reading "People don't discriminate, they learn it" (vs. a blank T-shirt), thus ostensibly endorsing an antidiscrimination view. The mindset was induced by presenting participants with a narrative about a warrior who, faced with a difficult decision, opts for a self-interested decision (individualistic prime) or for a family-interested decision (collectivistic prime). Across the three studies, the researchers found that participants with a collectivistic cultural background or a temporarily induced collectivistic mindset aligned their attitudes toward homosexuals and African Americans (Blacks) with the experimenter's antidiscrimination view. In contrast, this effect was not found, or even reversed, for participants with an individualistic cultural background or an individualistic mindset. This pattern was found on both implicit attitude measures and explicit self-report measures.

Overall, the findings on social tuning of attitudes suggest that the magnitude of such shared-reality creation depends on participants' willingness or their need to affiliate and connect with the partner. According to this analysis, motivated connection is satisfied by creating a shared view about the (social) world. This is precisely what is expressed by the principle of motivated connection.

This rationale implies that people should prefer to affiliate with individuals who offer or afford experiences of shared reality to a greater (vs. lower) extent, and this preference should be boosted by increased affiliative needs. Research on the sharing of idiosyncratic, subjective experiences, referred to as "I-sharing" is consistent with this reasoning (Huneke & Pinel, 2016; Pinel, Long, Landau, Alexander, & Pyszczynski, 2006; for a review, see Pinel, 2018). In contrast to I-sharing, Me-sharing is based on a similarity or commonality of objective features, such as hometown, cultural background, or personality traits.

In several studies, Pinel and colleagues found that participants responded to an I-sharer (vs. Me-Sharer) with stronger feelings of closeness and a greater desire for affiliation, as well as more prosocial behaviors and helping intentions (Huneke & Pinel, 2016). Further illuminating the role of motivated connection, Pinel and colleagues (2006, Experiment 5) manipulated the feeling of existential loneliness, which typically triggers the need to reaffiliate and experience social connectedness. Participants in the loneliness condition wrote about a time during which they felt existentially isolated, whereas participants in two control conditions wrote about boredom or their morning routine. In a subsequent chat room simulation, participants interacted with (1) a partner who shared spontaneous subjective choices to a great extent (but shared objective self-features to a low extent) and (2) a partner who shared spontaneous subjective choices to a low extent (but shared objective self-features to a high extent). Participants finally indicated their liking and sympathy for their interaction partners. Participants who needed (vs. did not need) social connectedness due to the loneliness priming expressed more closeness toward and desire to affiliate with the I-sharer (vs. the Me-sharer). Taken together, people want to affiliate and feel connected with others who share (vs. do not share) their subjective inner states about something, and this motivated connection via shared reality is enhanced when affiliative needs are high (vs. low). Again, these findings epitomize the principle of motivated connection.

The Principle of Motivated Cognition

According to the principle of motivated cognition, people can achieve common inner states about an issue or topic, learn what is real about the world, via shared reality. The more we believe that someone has valid and reliable information about something that we do not have, and the more we are willing to learn from this someone, the more motivated we are to create shared reality with that person. In other words, the sharing of experiences with others allows people to achieve sufficiently valid judgments, feelings, or beliefs about a given topic or issue. Lack of confidence regarding one's judgment or belief about a target opens the door for shared-reality creation (Echterhoff & Higgins, 2017). This notion is broadly consistent with the logic of informational influence (Deutsch & Gerard, 1955), as demonstrated in classical experimental studies by Sherif (1935) or Baron, Vandello, and Brunsman (1996), and research on others perceived as epistemic authorities (Kruglanski et al., 2005).

The extent to which individuals' feelings, beliefs, and judgments are influenced by others (i.e., informational influence) can vary in strength depending on an individual's self-ascribed epistemic authority, as illustrated by famous independent thinkers (e.g., Darwin, Einstein, Freud). In our epistemic-process model of shared reality in communication (Echterhoff & Higgins, 2017), such self-ascribed epistemic authority affects one of three epistemic inputs, that is, Judgment of the Communicator (JC). The likelihood of the communicator's shared-reality creation with an audience increases with increasing strength of other, socially rooted epistemic inputs, such as Judgment of Audience (JA) and Message of Communicator (MC). As we elaborated in that paper, the need for shared-reality creation is reduced with increasing strength of input JC. When self-ascribed epistemic authority is particularly strong, input JC can more easily override the potential influence from other inputs that contribute to shared reality. In this case, individuals may prefer disagreement over shared reality and feel they can tolerate unshared reality.

Analogous to the previous section, we illustrate the principle of motivated cognition with examples and findings on shared reality in interpersonal communication, social relationships, and intergroup relations. We begin with studies on the role of epistemic motivation in the spontaneous tuning of attitudes by Lun, Sinclair, Whitchurch, and Glenn (2007), which complement the findings on motivated connection in this phenomenon (see the previous section). In these studies, the strength of participants' epistemic confidence in their own attitudes was either measured (via the cognitive accessibility of attitudes; Lun et al., 2007, Experiment 1) or experimentally manipulated via a sentence completion task (Lun et al., 2007, Experiment 2). Findings revealed that alignment with the experimenter's egalitarian attitude was stronger when participants were in a state of low (vs. high) epistemic certainty.

The research on audience-tuning effects shows that communication can have consequences for communicators' own cognition, biasing their memory for the original information about the topic in a way that matches their audience's attitude (Higgins & Rholes, 1978; McCann & Higgins, 1992; see also Chiu, Krauss, & Lau, 1998). The motivational backdrop for such cognitive adjustments is the epistemic need that results from uncertainty about how to judge and evaluate a target object. Such uncertainty can be rooted in the perceiver's own subjective confidence in his or her judgments in a given domain (top-down confidence) and in the features of the stimulus (bottom-up confidence), specifically, its ambiguity, vagueness, and novelty. While top-down and bottom-up processes interact in the experience of uncertainty, it can be relatively more perceiver-based or stimulus-based.

The stimulus material about a target person's behavior in the classic "saying-is-believing" paradigm (Higgins & Rholes, 1978) was carefully designed to be evaluatively ambiguous. This was achieved by using input information about a target person's behaviors that could be characterized in evaluatively opposite ways, such as some behaviors that could be characterized as either "persistent" or "stubborn." By making the original target information (i.e., the features of the stimulus) ambiguous, communicators' confidence in their own judgments decreases, which in turn increases their motivation to reduce uncertainty via shared-reality creation.

In many studies on audience-tuning effects and on social tuning of attitudes, the shared-reality partner was another student or the experimenter, and participants had known neither of these partners before. According to our rationale, finding effects on memory and attitudes with these partners testifies to the potency of motivated cognition. When people are faced with ambiguous or novel information regarding an issue they care about, they tend to seize current opportunities for creating a shared reality with another person, even if they are unfamiliar with that person and know little about him or her.

The role of perceiver's confidence (top-down confidence) in the motivated adjustment of memory for the target person is revealed by a study by Kopietz, Hellmann, Higgins, and Echterhoff (2010, Experiment 2). Participants' epistemic needs were manipulated via their confidence in their own judgment. Before participants engaged in the communication task, they were asked to provide judgments and impressions about characters on the basis of depictions open to multiple interpretations, and then received feedback about their ability to form reliable social judgments. The material for manipulating perceiver confidence in Kopietz and colleagues (Experiment 2) consisted of several ambiguous pictures depicting social interactions from the Multi-Motive Grid (Sokolowski, Schmalt, Langens, & Puca, 2000). Participants selected one out of five brief statements that they thought best described the characters in the scene. Shortly afterward, participants received bogus performance feedback, which was designed to induce participants to have either high or low confidence in their social judgments. In brief, participants in the low-confidence/high-epistemic need condition were told that relative to other test takers, their ability to form reliable social judgments and impressions was *below* average, and that they should not feel too confident about their own social judgments. In contrast, participants in the high-confidence/

low-epistemic need condition were told that relative to other test takers, their ability to form reliable social judgments and impressions was *above* average, and that they could feel confident about their own social judgments.

Results showed that participants in the high-confidence/low-epistemic need condition felt significantly more confident about the accuracy of their judgments of other people than did participants in the low-confidence/high-epistemic need condition. According to the shared-reality account, participants in this latter condition should be more motivated to achieve a confident judgment via shared reality and to adjust their knowledge to the audience's position. The results supported this prediction. Whereas participants in the low-confidence/high-epistemic need condition tuned their messages to the audience's attitude, participants in the high-confidence/low-epistemic need condition did not. From a shared-reality perspective, participants in the latter condition were sufficiently confident in their own judgment that they did not tune their messages to their audience. Additional results suggested that participants with initially low confidence in their own judgment increased their confidence by tuning their message to the audience's evaluation of the target.

Motivated cognition in shared reality can also be driven by the ambiguity of the stimulus material (bottom-up uncertainty). Relevant to this issue, Pierucci and colleagues (2014) examined the role of evaluative ambiguity of the original stimulus information in the audience-tuning effect on memory. These researchers employed a workplace scenario to study whether shared-reality creation depends on the confidence of inner states afforded by the stimulus material. To this end, they varied the presence of definite outcome information about an event involving potential sexual harassment of a female employee by her supervisor. When definite outcome information is absent (vs. present), the perceived ambiguity of the stimulus material is high (vs. low).

A notorious feature of sexual harassment is the ambiguity of the surrounding behaviors (Pryor & Day, 1988), which elicits epistemic uncertainty and, hence, the likelihood of seeking epistemic certainty through shared reality.

Sexual harassment often develops gradually, from subtle acts (e.g., benevolent sexist utterances) to more blatant forms of harassment. The ambiguity of sex-related behaviors is greater at the beginning of a potential harassment episode but is resolved when the potential harasser performs blatant acts of harassment. To model these characteristics in their stimulus material, Pierucci and colleagues (2014) created a scenario describing interactions between a female employee, who was the potential harassment victim, and a male supervisor, who was the potential harasser and target person.

The experiment was ostensibly about impression formation based on others' testimonies. The stimulus material contained the same number of harassment-consistent and harassment-inconsistent behaviors. Participants wrote their message about the supervisor (the target person) to an audience who was a female colleague of the potential victim who had either a positive or negative attitude toward the supervisor. To manipulate stimulus-based ambiguity, the researchers created two versions of the scenario: One version contained brief outcome information revealing unambiguous harassment (known-outcome condition). Specifically, participants in this condition learned that the supervisor finally offered a promotion in exchange for sexual favors. In this condition, the stimulus-based ambiguity should be low. The other version of the scenario did not contain the outcome information (unknown-outcome condition). In the absence of outcome information, the ambiguity of the stimulus material should be high. A free-recall memory test was administered after a delay of one week.

Pierucci and colleagues (2014) argued that participants in the unknown-outcome (vs. known-outcome) condition should feel more uncertain regarding the evaluation of the supervisor's behaviors. Thus, the motivation to reduce uncertainty via shared reality should be lower, if not absent, in the known-outcome condition. In other words, motivated cognition via shared reality should be greater in the unknown-outcome (vs. known-outcome) condition. There was no alternative, non-shared-reality goal for audience tuning in the known-outcome condition; thus, participants should be unlikely to tune their messages to the audience.

The researchers also measured participants' trust in their audience.

Supporting predictions, participants in Pierucci and colleagues' (2014) study aligned their messages and memory with their audience's evaluation in the unknown-outcome (i.e., high-uncertainty) condition but not in the known-outcome (i.e., low-uncertainty) condition. Similar to the high-confidence/low-epistemic need participants in Kopietz and colleagues (2010, Experiment 2), participants in the known-outcome condition did not even tune their messages to the audience's attitude. Participants' epistemic uncertainty was higher in the unknown-outcome condition than in the known-outcome condition. This finding is consistent with the notion that participants who did not know the outcome experienced higher epistemic needs, which is conducive to motivated cognition via shared reality. Furthermore, in the unknown-outcome condition, there was a significant positive correlation between participants' trust in the audience and both the magnitude of the audience-tuned message bias and the magnitude of the audience-congruent memory bias. Hence, the extent to which participants under high-epistemic need aligned their messages and their memory with the audience's attitude was associated with how much they trusted their audience. In contrast, these correlations were nonsignificant, and significantly lower, in the known-outcome condition. All in all, the results suggest that stimulus-based uncertainty triggered motivated cognition for creating shared judgments about the potential harasser with the audience.

Motivated cognition can also depend on features of the audience, specifically, the audience's epistemic expertise or epistemic authority (Kruglanski et al., 2005). The role of this factor has been studied in situations in which, by default, communicators regard their audience as inappropriate for achieving shared reality. As we described earlier, communicators typically refrain from creating shared reality with an audience who is a member of a stigmatized outgroup (see Echterhoff et al., 2005, 2008). Echterhoff and colleagues (2017, Experiment 2) examined whether the audience-tuning memory bias, reflecting shared-reality creation, might emerge with an outgroup audience under conditions that support motivated shared-reality cognition. Echterhoff and colleagues wanted to create such conditions by having participants communicate about a topic that fell into the outgroup audience's specific areas of expertise.

In the study by Echterhoff and colleagues (2017, Experiment 2), participants with a German background communicated with a Turkish audience. In the audience's ingroup target condition, the target person was also Turkish. In the audience's outgroup target condition, the target person was German, as in the previous studies by Echterhoff and colleagues (2005, 2008). The fact that the Turkish audience's group membership matched the target's group membership should enhance the German communicators' perception of the Turkish audience's specific epistemic expertise about a Turkish target. This, in turn, should increase the German communicators' willingness to create a shared reality with the outgroup Turkish audience.

As in other studies (Echterhoff et al., 2008, Experiment 1; Echterhoff et al., 2017, Experiment 1a), there was no evidence for the audience-tuning memory bias with the Turkish audience when the target person was German. In other words, communicators did not create a shared reality with the outgroup audience when there was a mismatch between the target person's group membership (German) and the audience's group membership (Turkish). In contrast, when the target person was another Turk (audience's ingroup), the German communicators *did* create a shared reality with the Turkish audience, indicated by the audience-tuning memory effect.

Regarding the underlying motivated cognition process, additional data showed that Germans' epistemic trust in the Turkish audience's judgment of the specific target person was boosted when the target's group membership was shifted from German to Turkish. In terms of lay epistemic theory (Kruglanski, Orehek, Dechesne, & Pierro, 2010), the communicators apparently perceived the outgroup audience as an epistemic authority when the topic was a target from the audience's own group.

In a subsequent study, Echterhoff and colleagues (2017, Experiment 3) found that the epistemic motivation for shared reality was also enhanced by having (German) participants

communicate with a three-person audience of (Turkish) outgroup members, who had the same attitude toward the target person. Social influence from group consensus can be powerful (Asch, 1956; Erb & Bohner, 2010). From our perspective, this is because a consensus among group members signals an existing shared reality within the group (Conley, Rabinowitz, & Matsick, 2016). An existing shared reality is a readily available source of epistemic confidence and allows the disambiguation of ambiguous information about a target issue (see Higgins, Echterhoff, Crespillo, & Kopietz, 2007).

To test these predictions, Echterhoff and colleagues (2017, Experiment 3) informed German participants that the audience consisted of three outgroup members (Turks), who held the same attitude toward the target person. Ostensibly, the consensual view was reached *independently*, which should prevent perceptions of a biased shared reality within the audience group (Hausmann, Levine, & Higgins, 2008; Wilder, 1990). Thus, the three-person audience exhibited a high epistemic consensus in their judgment of the target person. As in Echterhoff and colleagues (2017, Experiment 2), the target person's group membership either matched or did not match the audience's group membership (Turkish). It was found that the memory bias was significantly greater when the Turkish outgroup *audience* had high (vs. low) epistemic expertise about the target person due to matching group membership. Importantly, with the multiperson audience, the memory bias was obtained even with a target for whom the Turkish audience group had *no* specific epistemic expertise (i.e., a German target). Thus, the epistemic input from the consensual judgment of a multiperson audience was sufficiently strong to compensate for the lack of the audience's target-specific epistemic expertise. Taken together, the findings by Echterhoff and colleagues (2017, Experiments 2 and 3) demonstrate how motivated shared-reality cognition can be induced in communication with an audience who is otherwise not perceived as a trusted shared reality partner.

Conclusion and Future Perspectives

Major psychological principles play out in ways that have both upsides and downsides. There are always trade-offs. Shared reality is no exception. Both the motivated connection principle and the motivated cognition principle of shared reality have trade-offs. There is a good news story and a bad news story. In each case, we begin with the good news story.

- *Motivated connection, the good news.* A father takes his infant daughter outside to the park. He sits down on a bench and holds her on his lap. They both look around. Suddenly the daughter grabs her father's shirt and points excitedly at something on a branch above them. She checks whether he now looks in the same direction. When he does and then smiles, she smiles broadly, and then his smile broadens as well. This kind of event between parents and their infants is common for humans. It is so common that it can be taken for granted. No big deal. But it *is* a big deal because it makes us human and not some other animal. The parent and child are sharing that this object on the tree is worth receiving attention—they share its relevance (Higgins, 2019; see also Liszkowski, 2018; Shteynberg, 2015). And, in this case, they also share how to feel about it. It is something to smile about; it connects them in a special way.

This is the initial phase of shared-reality development called *shared feelings.* Following this phase, toddlers acquire *shared practices,* such as how their family and community eat and dress; preschoolers acquire *shared self-guides,* such as accepting as their own goals for themselves, the goals that their significant others (e.g., mom, dad) have for them (i.e., internalization); and schoolers acquire *shared coordinated roles,* such as learning the different roles and rules for working with teammates to play a sport (see Higgins, 2016, 2019). In all of these phases, shared-reality creation is enriching children's connections to others about the world in which they live—connecting with caretakers and significant others, with their family and community, and with teammates. This enrichment of human connections from shared reality creation continues throughout our lives (e.g., Levine, 2018; Pinel, 2018; Rossignac-Milon & Higgins, 2018b).

- *Motivated connection, the bad news.* The motivational connectedness from shared reality creation has at least two major downsides. First, there is the downside of shared self-guides.

As just mentioned, preschoolers accept as their own goals and standards the goals and standards that their significant others have for them (internalization). They are motivated to attain these shared goals and follow these shared standards even when the significant others are not present (without surveillance). And this is true for adults as well. This has the upside to individuals of strengthening their motivation to attain their goals and follow their standards. However, when individuals fail to meet these goals and standards, they suffer emotionally (see Reznik & Andersen, 2007; Shah, 2003). And the stronger the shared self-guide, the more they suffer emotionally from failure to meet it (Higgins, 2019; Newman, Higgins, & Vookles, 1992). This is a downside because the internalized goals and standards can be unrealistic or overdemanding.

The second major downside from motivational connectedness relates to the fact that shared reality creates strong social identities and ingroups (see Higgins, 2019; Hogg & Rinella, 2018). This has the benefit of strengthening the interconnectedness among members of ingroups. However, it also produces conflict between ingroups and outgroups (e.g., Stern & Ondish, 2018). If your ingroup's shared reality is the objective truth—the whole truth and nothing but the truth—then members of another group who do not accept your shared reality must be stupid or crazy. Disconnection with outgroup members is the result. Their unshared reality makes them potentially dangerous people who need to be avoided or even harmed and obliterated. Indeed, atrocities against outgroups are notoriously committed in the name of truth (ideological, religious or social; Harris, 2005; Kruglanski & Fishman, 2009).

- *Motivated cognition, the good news.* We mentioned earlier that the "supposedly simple" act of an infant getting a caretaker to share the relevance of something happening is profoundly human in its motivation to create a shared reality. It relates to some other phenomenon that seems rather straightforward but really is profoundly human: communicating to others about something you know that they do not, and asking others to communicate to you something they know that you do not. It is the not-so-simple role of teacher and learner. An early form of this would be an infant knowing something is happening on the tree above that is worthy of attention and communicating this to the co-present caretaker. That interaction could be considered as an instruction situation, with the infant being the teacher and the caretaker being the learner. A clearer case is an infant looking over at someone to learn how to respond to an event from his or her reaction to what just happened (shared feelings; see Higgins, 2016). And an even clearer case is the "naming period," when children recognize that older people know the names of things in the world that they do not know, and communicate to them, usually by pointing to something, that they would like them to tell them the name—asking them as teacher to share reality with them as learner (see Harris, 2012; Higgins, 2019). This motivated cognition involving teacher–learner shared reality is what allowed humans to develop complex tools, language, and culture more generally (see Henrich, 2016). Although we experience it as just part of everyday life, it is a very big deal (Higgins, 2019).

Shared-reality motivated cognition has another major upside. What matters to humans is that the knowledge they have is a shared reality (Hardin & Higgins, 1996). The knowledge could be arbitrary, like the different names in different languages for the same four-legged, furry animal that barks and fetches sticks (*dog*; *chien*; *Hund*), or fictional, such as treating paper "money" as something of real value beyond its material value. Still, such shared realities have allowed humans to cooperate in ways that otherwise would not be possible, such as in linguistic communication and financial exchanges that facilitate trade and commerce (Harari, 2015). Our close relationships, especially, provide opportunities to create and maintain shared meaning systems about the world (Andersen & Przybylinski, 2018). Individuals who are in basically satisfying relationships maintain a sense of life's meaning even when dealing with unexpected events (Murray, Lamarche, & Seery, 2018). Thus, shared-reality motivated cognitions, even when they are arbitrary or fictional, contribute to humans experiencing their life as meaningful, as making sense.

• *Motivated cognition, the bad news.* It is ironic that the research that historically provided the best illustration of the strength of people's motivation to create shared reality with others

also provides convincing evidence of how motivated cognition can be problematic. In Sherif's (1935, 1936) classic research on norm formation using the "autokinetic effect," different groups of individuals change their judgment of the distance that a light moved so as to converge upon a shared norm about the distance of its movement. Different groups construct different shared realities, and then each group sticks with their norm. As we noted earlier, this can be good news because the shared reality can facilitate interpersonal cooperation. However, there is a potential downside if that shared belief is false. And it *is* false in Sherif's study because the light was actually stationary—it did not move at all.

This is also the case for Asch's (1956) classic study on matching different line options to a standard line, in which participants will agree with the unanimous judgment of other members of their group, even when that judgment is *false*. The good news is that some participants do so because they trust the other group members and are willing to concede the inaccuracy of their own judgment. The bad news is that participants ultimately end up expressing a judgment that is false.

In the "saying-is-believing" paradigm (Higgins & Rholes, 1978), communicators modify what they say about the behaviors of a target person (originally named *Donald*) to match evaluatively their audience's attitude toward Donald. Such audience tuning has the advantage of creating a shared reality with the audience about Donald, which can make the communicators feel closer to their audience (Rossignac-Milon & Higgins, 2018b). However, the audience tuning is distorting the original information about Donald. In the condition in which the audience supposedly dislikes Donald, this means that the message description of Donald is negatively distorted. When communicators create a shared reality with the audience, their personal attitude toward Donald also turns more negative. Poor Donald! Through such processes, shared reality in decision-making groups presumably plays a key role in groupthink (Janis, 1972) and other group biases such as preference for commonly known ("shared") information (Stasser & Titus, 1985; see Echterhoff & Schmalbach, 2018).

Another serious downside from motivated

cognition is that the content of the shared reality can itself be socially disruptive and destructive. For example, members of one race, ethnicity, or religion can share hatred for the members of a different race, ethnicity, or religion and share the belief that they should die, leading to pogroms. Members of one group can discriminate against the members of a different group with shared-reality justifications, such as believing that members of the other group are inferior to them and don't deserve equal treatment.

A final serious downside from motivated cognition is that the shared reality is treated as the whole truth and nothing but the truth, despite existing evidence to the contrary and/or the ambiguity of information upon which the shared reality is based. Unlike cases in which the shared reality is wrong, the shared reality might be simply incomplete or limited. Greater truth could be obtained from being open to new information. But the shared reality has produced cognitive closure—seizing and freezing (Dugas & Kruglanski, 2018). People only want to communicate with like-minded others (Jost, van der Linden, Panagopoulos, & Hardin, 2018).

The large-scale growth of online communication and the exploding availability of Internet devices (smartphones) allow users to choose and live in their own epistemic "bubbles." This phenomenon jeopardizes the ability of different groups to establish overarching shared realities. This fraying of our social fabric is one of the chief problems of our time.

ACKNOWLEDGMENTS

The preparation of this chapter was facilitated by an Anneliese Maier Research Award from the Alexander von Humboldt Foundation, awarded to E. Tory Higgins upon nomination by Gerald Echterhoff, and by a research grant awarded to Gerald Echterhoff by the German Research Foundation (DFG EC 317/10-1) for his project in the Research Group "Constructing Scenarios of the Past" (FOR2812).

REFERENCES

Andersen, S. M., & Chen, S. (2002). The relational self: An interpersonal social-cognitive theory. *Psychological Review, 109,* 619–645.

Andersen, S. M., & Przybylinski, E. (2018). Shared reality in interpersonal relationships. *Current Opinion in Psychology, 23,* 42–46.

Asch, S. E. (1951). Effects of group pressure upon the modification and distortion of judgments. In H. S. Guetzkow (Ed.), *Groups, leadership and men* (pp. 177–190). Pittsburgh, PA: Carnegie Press.

Asch, S. E. (1956). Studies of independence and conformity: I. A minority of one against a unanimous majority. *Psychological Monographs: General and Applied, 70*(9), 1–70.

Axelrod, R. (1984). *The evolution of cooperation.* New York: Basic Books.

Baron, R. S., Vandello, J., & Brunsman, B. (1996). The forgotten variable in conformity research: Impact of task importance on social influence. *Journal of Personality and Social Psychology, 71,* 915–927.

Baron-Cohen, S. (1995). The eye direction detector (EDD) and the shared attention mechanism (SAM): Two cases for evolutionary psychology. In C. Moore & P. J. Dunham (Eds.), *Joint attention: Its origins and role in development* (pp. 41–59). Hillsdale, NJ: Erlbaum.

Baumeister, R. F., & Leary, M. R. (1995). The need to belong: Desire for interpersonal attachments as a fundamental human motivation. *Psychological Bulletin, 117,* 497–529.

Brewer, M. B. (1997). On the social origins of human nature. In C. McGarty & S. A. Haslam (Eds.), *The message of social psychology* (pp. 54–62). Oxford, UK: Blackwell.

Brewer, M. B. (1999). The psychology of prejudice: Ingroup love and outgroup hate? *Journal of Social Issues, 55*(3), 429–444.

Brickman, P. (1978). Is it real? In J. H. Harvey, W. Ickes, & R. F. Kidd (Eds.), *New directions in attribution research* (Vol. 2, pp. 5–34). Hillsdale, NJ: Erlbaum.

Butterworth, G., & Jarrett, N. (1991). What minds have in common is space: Spatial mechanisms serving joint visual attention in infancy. *British Journal of Developmental Psychology, 9,* 55–72.

Campbell, D. T. (1983). Two distinct routes beyond kin selection to ultrasociality: Implications for the humanities and social sciences. In D. Bridgeman (Ed.), *The nature of prosocial development: Theories and strategies* (pp. 11–41). New York: Academic Press.

Chiu, C. Y., Krauss, R. M., & Lau, I. Y.-M. (1998). Some cognitive consequences of communication. In S. R. Fussell & R. Kreuz (Eds.), *Social and cognitive approaches to interpersonal communication* (pp. 259–278). Hillsdale, NJ: Erlbaum.

Clark, H. H. (2003). Pointing and placing. In S. Kita (Ed.), *Pointing: Where language, culture, and cognition meet* (pp. 243–268). Hillsdale, NJ: Erlbaum.

Clark, H. H., & Marshall, C. E. (1981). Definite reference and mutual knowledge. In A. K. Joshi, B. Webber, & I. Sag (Eds.), *Elements of discourse understanding* (pp. 10–63). Cambridge, UK: Cambridge University Press.

Conley, T. D., Rabinowitz, J. L., & Matsick, J. L. (2016). US ethnic minorities' attitudes towards Whites: The role of shared reality theory in intergroup relations. *European Journal of Social Psychology, 46,* 13–25.

Cooley, C. H. (1964). *Human nature and the social order.* New York: Schocken Books. (Original work published 1902)

Csibra, G., & Volein, A. (2008). Infants can infer the presence of hidden objects from referential gaze information. *British Journal of Developmental Psychology, 26,* 1–11.

Deutsch, M., & Gerard, H. B. (1955). A study of normative and informational social influences upon individual judgment. *Journal of Abnormal and Social Psychology, 51,* 629–636.

Dugas, M., & Kruglanski, A. W. (2018). Shared reality as collective closure. *Current Opinion in Psychology, 23,* 72–76.

Echterhoff, G. (2010). Shared reality: Antecedents, processes, and consequences. *Social Cognition, 28,* 273–276.

Echterhoff, G., & Higgins, E. T. (2017). Creating shared reality in interpersonal and intergroup communication: The role of epistemic processes and their interplay. *European Review of Social Psychology, 28,* 175–226.

Echterhoff, G., & Higgins, E. T. (2018a). Editorial: Shared reality. *Current Opinion in Psychology, 23,* vii–xi.

Echterhoff, G., & Higgins, E. T. (2018b). Shared reality: Construct and mechanisms. *Current Opinion in Psychology, 23,* iv–vii.

Echterhoff, G., Higgins, E. T., & Groll, S. (2005). Audience-tuning effects on memory: The role of shared reality. *Journal of Personality and Social Psychology, 89,* 257–276.

Echterhoff, G., Higgins, E. T., Kopietz, R., & Groll, S. (2008). How communication goals determine when audience tuning biases memory. *Journal of Experimental Psychology: General, 137,* 3–21.

Echterhoff, G., Higgins, E. T., & Levine, J. M. (2009). Shared reality: Experiencing commonality with others' inner states about the world. *Perspectives on Psychological Science, 4,* 496–521.

Echterhoff, G., & Hirst, W. (2009). Social influence on memory. *Social Psychology, 40,* 106–110.

Echterhoff, G., Kopietz, R., & Higgins, E. T. (2013). Adjusting shared reality: Communicators' memory changes as their connection with their audience changes. *Social Cognition, 31,* 162–186.

Echterhoff, G., Kopietz, R., & Higgins, E. T. (2017). Shared reality in intergroup communication: Increasing the epistemic authority of an out-group audience. *Journal of Experimental Psychology: General, 146,* 806–825.

Echterhoff, G., Lang, S., Krämer, N., & Higgins, E. T. (2009). Audience-tuning effects on communicators' memory: The role of audience status in sharing reality. *Social Psychology, 40,* 150–163.

Echterhoff, G., & Schmalbach, B. (2018). How shared reality is created in interpersonal communication. *Current Opinion in Psychology, 23,* 57–61.

Eich, E. E., & Macauley, D. (2000). Fundamental factors in mood-dependent memory. In J. P. Forgas (Ed.), *Feeling and thinking: The role of affect in social cognition* (pp. 109–130). New York: Cambridge University Press.

Erb, H.-P., & Bohner, G. (2010). Consensus as the key: Towards parsimony in explaining minority and majority influence. In R. Martin & M. Hewstone (Eds.), *Minority influence and innovation: Antecedents, processes and consequences* (pp. 79–103). Hove, UK: Psychology Press.

Festinger, L. (1950). Informal social communication. *Psychological Review, 57,* 271–282.

Frith, C. D. (2007). *Making up the mind: How the brain creates our mental world.* Malden, MA: Blackwell.

Harari, Y. N. (2015). *Sapiens: A brief history of humankind.* New York: Harper-Collins.

Hardin, C. D., & Conley, T. D. (2001). A relational approach to cognition: Shared experience and relationship affirmation in social cognition. In G. B. Moskowitz (Ed.), *Cognitive social psychology: The Princeton Symposium on the legacy and future of social cognition* (pp. 3–17). Mahwah, NJ: Erlbaum.

Hardin, C. D., & Higgins, E. T. (1996). Shared reality: How social verification makes the subjective objective. In R. M. Sorrentino & E. T. Higgins (Eds.), *Handbook of motivation and cognition: The interpersonal context* (Vol. 3, pp. 28–84). New York: Guilford Press.

Harris, P. L. (2012). *Trusting what you're told: how children learn from others.* Cambridge, MA: Harvard University Press.

Harris, S. (2005). *The end of faith: Religion, terror and the future of reason.* New York: Norton.

Hatfield, E., Cacioppo, J. T., & Rapson, R. L. (1994). *Emotion contagion.* Cambridge, UK: Cambridge University Press.

Hausmann, L. R. M., Levine, J. M., & Higgins, E. T. (2008). Communication and group perception: Extending the "saying is believing" effect. *Group Processes and Intergroup Relations, 11,* 539–554.

Heider, F. (1958). *The psychology of interpersonal relations.* New York: Wiley.

Heiphetz, L. (2018). The development and importance of shared reality in the domains of opinion, morality, and religion. *Current Opinion in Psychology, 23,* 1–5.

Heleven, E., & Van Overwalle, F. (2018). The neural basis of representing others' inner states. *Current Opinion in Psychology, 23,* 98–103.

Henrich, J. (2016). *The secret of our success: How culture is driving human evolution, domesticating our species, and making us smarter.* Princeton, NJ: Princeton University Press.

Henrich, N., & Henrich, J. (2007). *Why humans cooperate.* Oxford, UK: Oxford University Press.

Higgins, E. T. (1992). Achieving "shared reality" in the communication game: A social action that creates meaning. *Journal of Language and Social Psychology, 11,* 107–131.

Higgins, E. T. (1996a). Knowledge activation: Accessibility, applicability, and salience. In E. T. Higgins & A. W. Kruglanski (Eds.), *Social psychology: Handbook of basic principles* (pp. 133–168). New York: Guilford Press.

Higgins, E. T. (1996b). Shared reality in the self-system: The social nature of self-regulation. In W. Stroebe & M. Hewstone (Eds.), *European review of social psychology* (Vol. 7, pp. 1–29). Chichester, UK: Wiley.

Higgins, E. T. (1998). The aboutness principle: A pervasive influence on human inference. *Social Cognition, 16,* 173–198.

Higgins, E. T. (1999). "Saying is believing" effects: When sharing reality about something biases knowledge and evaluations. In L. L. Thompson, J. M. Levine, & D. M. Messick (Eds.), *Shared cognition in organizations: The management of knowledge* (pp. 33–49). Mahwah, NJ: Erlbaum.

Higgins, E. T. (2011). Sharing inner states: A defining feature of human motivation. In G. R. Semin & G. Echterhoff (Eds.), *Grounding sociality: Neurons, minds, and culture* (pp. 149–173). New York: Psychology Press.

Higgins, E. T. (2012). *Beyond pleasure and pain: How motivation works.* New York: Oxford University Press.

Higgins, E. T. (2016). Shared-reality development in childhood. *Perspectives on Psychological Science, 11,* 466–495.

Higgins, E. T. (2019). *Shared reality: What makes us strong . . . and tears us apart.* New York: Oxford University Press.

Higgins, E. T., Echterhoff, G., Crespillo, R., & Kopietz, R. (2007). Effects of communication on social knowledge: Sharing reality with individual versus group audiences. *Japanese Psychological Research, 49,* 89–99.

Higgins, E. T., & Pittman, T. S. (2008). Motives of the human animal: Comprehending, managing, and sharing inner states. *Annual Review of Psychology, 59,* 361–385.

Higgins, E. T., & Rholes, W. S. (1978). "Saying is believing": Effects of message modification on memory and liking for the person described. *Journal of Experimental Social Psychology, 14,* 363–378.

Hogg, M. A., & Rinella, M. J. (2018). Social identities and shared realities. *Current Opinion in Psychology, 23,* 6–10.

Huneke, M., & Pinel, E. C. (2016). Fostering selflessness through I-sharing. *Journal of Experimental Social Psychology, 63,* 10–18.

Huntsinger, J. R., Sinclair, S., Kenrick, A. C., & Ray, C. (2016). Affiliative social tuning reduces the activation of prejudice. *Group Processes and Intergroup Relations, 19,* 217–235.

Janis, I. L. (1972). *Victims of groupthink.* Boston: Houghton Mifflin.

Johnson, M. K., & Raye, C. L. (1981). Reality monitoring. *Psychological Review, 88,* 67–85.

Johnston, A. M., Byrne, M., & Santos, L. R. (2018). What is unique about shared reality?: Insights from a new comparison species. *Current Opinion in Psychology, 23,* 30–33.

Jost, J. T., Ledgerwood, A., & Hardin, C. D. (2007). Shared reality, system verification, and the relational basis of ideological beliefs. *Social and Personality Psychology Compass, 2,* 171–186.

Jost, J. T., van der Linden, S., Panagopoulos, C., & Hardin, C. D. (2018). Ideological asymmetries in conformity, desire for shared reality, and the spread of misinformation. *Current Opinion in Psychology, 23,* 77–83.

Keysar, B., & Barr, D. J. (2002). Self-anchoring in conversation: Why language users do not do what they "should." In T. Gilovich, D. W. Griffin, & D. Kahneman (Eds.), *Heuristics and biases: The psychology of intuitive judgment* (pp. 150–166). Cambridge, UK: Cambridge University Press.

Keysers, C., & Gazzola, V. (2007). Integrating simulation and theory of mind: From self to social cognition. *Trends in Cognitive Sciences, 11,* 194–196.

Kopietz, R., Echterhoff, G., Niemeier, S., Hellmann, J. H., & Memon, A. (2009). Audience-congruent biases in eyewitness memory and judgment: Influences of a co-witness' liking of a suspect. *Social Psychology, 3,* 138–149.

Kopietz, R., Hellmann, J. H., Higgins, E. T., & Echterhoff, G. (2010). Shared-reality effects on memory: Communicating to fulfill epistemic needs. *Social Cognition, 28,* 353–378.

Kruglanski, A. W., Bélanger, J. J., Gelfand, M., Gunaratna, R., Hettiarachchi, M., Reinares, F., et al. (2013). Terrorism—A (self) love story: Redirecting the significance quest can end violence. *American Psychologist, 68,* 559–575.

Kruglanski, A. W., Fishbach, A., Woolley, K., Bélanger, J. J., Chernikova, M., Molinario, E., et al. (2018). A structural model of intrinsic motivation: On the psychology of means–ends fusion. *Psychological Review, 125,* 165–182.

Kruglanski, A., & Fishman, S. (2009). Psychological factors in terrorism and counterterrorism: Individual, group, and organizational levels of analysis. *Social Issues and Policy Review, 3,* 1–44.

Kruglanski, A. W., Orehek, E., Dechsne, M., & Pierro, A. (2010). Lay epistemic theory: The motivational, cognitive, and social aspects of knowledge formation. *Social and Personality Psychology Compass, 4,* 939–950.

Kruglanski, A. W., Raviv, A., Bar-Tal, D., Raviv, A., Sharvit, K., Ellis, S., Bar, R., et al. (2005). Says who?: Epistemic authority effects in social judgment. In M. P. Zanna (Ed.), *Advances in experimental social psychology* (Vol. 37, pp. 345–392). New York: Academic Press.

Leslie, A. M., Friedman, O., & German, T. P. (2004). Core mechanisms in "theory of mind." *Trends in Cognitive Sciences, 8,* 528–533.

Levine, J. M. (2018). Socially-shared cognition and consensus in small groups. *Current Opinion in Psychology, 23,* 52–56.

Lewin, K. (1947). Group decision and social change. In T. M. Newcomb & E. L. Hartley (Eds.), *Readings in social psychology* (pp. 330–344). New York: Holt.

Liszkowski, U. (2018). Emergence of shared reference and shared minds in infancy. *Current Opinion in Psychology, 23,* 26–29.

Liu, Z., & Slepian, M. L. (2018). Secrecy: Unshared realities. *Current Opinion in Psychology, 23,* 124–128.

Lun, J., Sinclair, S., Whitchurch, E. R., & Glenn, C. (2007). (Why) do I think what you think?: Epistemic social tuning and implicit prejudice. *Journal of Personality and Social Psychology, 93,* 957–972.

Malle, B. F. (1999). How people explain behavior: A new theoretical framework. *Personality and Social Psychology Review, 3,* 21–43.

Malle, B. F., & Hodges, S. D. (Eds.). (2005). *Other minds: How humans bridge the divide between self and other.* New York: Guilford Press.

Mannetti, L., Levine, J. M., Pierro, A., & Kruglanski, A. W. (2010). Group reaction to defection: The impact of shared reality. *Social Cognition, 28,* 447–464.

McAllister, D. J. (1995). Affect- and cognition-based trust as foundations for interpersonal cooperation in organizations. *Academy of Management Journal, 38,* 24–59.

McCann, C. D., & Higgins, E. T. (1992). Personal and contextual factors in communication: A review of the "communication game." In G. R. Semin & K. Fiedler (Eds.), *Language, interaction and social cognition* (pp. 144–171). London: SAGE.

Mead, G. H. (1934). *Mind, self, and society.* Chicago: University of Chicago Press.

Molenberghs, P., Johnson, H., Henry, J. D., & Mattingley, J. B. (2016). Understanding the minds of others: A neuroimaging meta-analysis. *Neuroscience and Biobehavioral Reviews, 65,* 276–291.

Moscovici, S. (1981). On social representations. In J. P. Forgas (Ed.), *Social cognition: Perspectives on everyday understanding* (pp. 181–209). London: Academic Press.

Murray, S. L., Lamarche, V., & Seery, M. D. (2018). Romantic relationships as shared reality defense. *Current Opinion in Psychology, 23,* 34–37.

Newcomb, T. M. (1959). Individual systems of orientation. In S. Koch (Ed.), *Psychology: A study of a science: Formulations of the person and the social context* (Vol. 3, pp. 384–422). New York: McGraw-Hill.

Newman, L. S., Higgins, E. T., & Vookles, J. (1992). Self-guide strength and emotional vulnerability: Birth order as a moderator of self–affect relations. *Personality and Social Psychology Bulletin, 18,* 402–411.

Nickerson, R. S. (2001). The projective way of knowing: A useful heuristic that sometimes misleads. *Current Directions in Psychological Science, 10,* 168–172.

Pierucci, S., Echterhoff, G., Marchal, C., & Klein, O. (2014). Creating shared reality about ambiguous sexual harassment: The role of stimulus ambiguity in audience-tuning effects on memory. *Journal of Applied Research in Memory and Cognition, 3,* 300–306.

Pierucci, S., Klein, O., & Carnaghi, A. (2013). You are the one I want to communicate with!: Relational motives driving audience-tuning effects on memory. *Social Psychology, 44,* 16–25.

Pinel, E. C. (2018). Existential isolation and I-sharing: Interpersonal and intergroup implications. *Current Opinion in Psychology, 23,* 84–87.

Pinel, E. C., Long, A. E., Landau, M. J., Alexander, K., & Pyszczynski, T. (2006). Seeing I to I: A pathway to interpersonal connectedness. *Journal of Personality and Social Psychology, 90,* 243–257.

Pryor, J., & Day, J. (1988). Interpretations of sexual harassment—an attributional analysis. *Sex Roles, 18*(7–8), 405–417.

Reznik, I., & Andersen, S. M. (2007). Agitation and despair in relation to parents: Activating emotional suffering in transference. *European Journal of Personality, 21,* 281–301.

Rossignac-Milon, M., Bolger, N., Zee, K. S., Boothby, E., & Higgins, E. T. (in press). Merged minds:

Generalized shared reality in dyadic relationships. *Journal of Personality and Social Psychology*.

Rossignac-Milon, M., & Higgins, E. T. (2018a). Beyond intrapersonal cognitive consistency: Shared reality and the interpersonal motivation for truth. *Psychological Inquiry, 29,* 86–93.

Rossignac-Milon, M., & Higgins, E. T. (2018b). Epistemic companions: Shared reality development in close relationships. *Current Opinion in Psychology, 23,* 66–71.

Schachter, S. (1959). *The psychology of affiliation: Experimental studies of the sources of gregariousness.* Stanford, CA: Stanford University Press.

Semin, G. R. (2007). Grounding communication: Synchrony. In A. W. Kruglanski & E. T. Higgins (Eds.), *Social psychology: Handbook of basic principles* (2nd ed., pp. 630–649). New York: Guilford Press.

Shah, J. (2003). The motivational looking glass: How significant others implicitly affect goal appraisals. *Journal of Personality and Social Psychology, 85,* 424–439.

Shepherd, S. V. (2010). Following gaze: Gaze-following behavior as a window into social cognition. *Frontiers in Integrative Neuroscience, 4,* 5.

Sherif, M. (1935). A study of some social factors in perception. *Archives of Psychology, 187,* 60.

Sherif, M. (1936). *The psychology of social norms.* New York: Harper & Brothers.

Shteynberg, G. (2015). Shared attention. *Perspectives on Psychological Science, 10,* 579–590.

Shteynberg, G. (2018). A collective perspective: Shared attention and the mind. *Current Opinion in Psychology, 23,* 93–97.

Sinclair, S., Lowery, B. S., Hardin, C. D., & Colangelo, A. (2005). Social tuning of automatic racial attitudes: The role of affiliative motivation. *Journal of Personality and Social Psychology, 89,* 583–592.

Sinclair, S., & Lun, J. (2010). Social tuning of ethnic attitudes. In B. Mesquita, L. Feldman Barrett, & E. R. Smith (Eds.), *The mind in context* (pp. 214–230). New York: Guilford Press.

Skorinko, J., Lun, J., Sinclair, S., Marotta, S. A., Calanchini, J., & Paris, M. H. (2015). Reducing prejudice across cultures via social tuning. *Social Psychological and Personality Science, 6,* 363–372.

Skorinko, J., & Sinclair, S. (2018). Shared reality through social tuning of implicit prejudice. *Current Opinion in Psychology, 23,* 109–112.

Slotter, E. B., Emery, L. F., & Luchies, L. B. (2014). Me after you: Partner influence and individual effort predict rejection of self-aspects and self-concept clarity after relationship dissolution.

Personality and Social Psychology Bulletin, 40, 831–844.

Smith, E. R., & Semin, G. R. (2004). Socially situated cognition: Cognition in its social context. In M. P. Zanna (Ed.), *Advances in experimental social psychology* (Vol. 36, pp. 53–115). San Diego, CA: Academic Press.

Sokolowski, K., Schmalt, H.-D., Langens, T., & Puca, R. (2000). Assessing achievement, affiliation, and power motives all at once: The Multi-Motive Grid (MMG). *Journal of Personality Assessment, 74,* 126–145.

Stasser, G., & Titus, W. (1985). Pooling of unshared information in group decision making: Biased information sampling during discussion. *Journal of Personality and Social Psychology, 48*(6), 1467–1478.

Stern, C., & Ondish, P. (2018). Political aspects of shared reality. *Current Opinion in Psychology, 23,* 11–14.

Sullivan, H. S. (1953). *The interpersonal theory of psychiatry.* New York: Norton.

Thompson, L., & Fine, G. A. (1999). Socially shared cognition, affect, and behavior: A review and integration. *Personality and Social Psychology Review, 3,* 278–302.

Tomasello, M. (2008). *Origins of human communication.* Cambridge, MA: MIT Press.

Tomasello, M. (2009). *Why we cooperate.* Cambridge, MA: MIT Press.

Tomasello, M. (2014a). *A natural history of human thinking.* Cambridge, MA: Harvard University Press.

Tomasello, M. (2014b). The ultra-social animal. *European Journal of Social Psychology, 44,* 187–194.

Tomasello, M., Melis, A. P., Tennie, C., Wyman, E., & Herrmann, E. (2012). Two key steps in the evolution of human cooperation. *Current Anthropology, 53*(6), 673–692.

Turner, J. C., & Oakes, P. J. (1997). The socially structured mind. In C. McGarty & S. A. Haslam (Eds.), *The message of social psychology: Perspectives on mind in society* (pp. 355–373). Cambridge, MA: Blackwell.

Wilder, D. A. (1990). Some determinants of the persuasive power of in-groups and out-groups: Organization of information and attribution of independence. *Journal of Personality and Social Psychology, 59,* 1202–1213.

Williams, K. D. (2009). Ostracism: A temporal need-threat model. *Advances in Experimental Social Psychology, 41,* 275–314.

Wyer, R. S., & Srull, T. K. (1989). *Memory and cognition in its social context.* Hillsdale, NJ: Erlbaum.

CHAPTER 11

Goal Transactivity

Eli J. Finkel
Gráinne M. Fitzsimons

Make no little plans. They have no magic to stir men's blood.
—DANIEL H. BURNHAM

As an aimless young man in the 1860s, Daniel H. Burnham failed his college entrance exams. "I went to Harvard for examination," he later recalled, "with two men not as well prepared as I; both passed easily, and I flunked having sat through two or three examinations without being able to write a word." He also failed his exam for Yale. He found employment in Chicago as a salesman, but quit after 4 months. After a brief period of introspection, he wrote to his mother, at age 23, that he had found his passion: "I shall try to become the greatest architect in the city or country. Nothing less will be near the mark I have set for myself, and I am not afraid but that I can become so." He even mapped out a rough strategy: "There needs but one thing. A determined and persistent effort" (in Hines, 2009, p. 12).

But despite Burnham's considerable self-efficacy and goal commitment, he remained unmoored. Not long after sending that letter, he went to Nevada in search of silver. While there, he ran for political office. Echoing his academic endeavors in the East, his pursuit of financial and political success in the West ended in failure. Chastened, he returned to Chicago

in 1872 and, with his father's help, procured an entry-level position in the architectural office of Carter, Drake and Wight, one of the firms working to rebuild the city following the great fire of 1871. Under the tutelage of Peter Wight, Burnham rediscovered his passion for architecture. More importantly, he met the young John Root, with whom he would ultimately build the most influential architectural firm of the late 1800s.

Burnham had long been desperate to earn the respect of the intellectual elite, so he was pleased when Harvard and Yale awarded him honorary degrees in the 1890s. By then, he had achieved—at least to his own satisfaction—his goal of becoming "the greatest architect in the city or country." But although the young Burnham was correct that "a determined and persistent effort" was essential in pursuit of such goals, he was incorrect in assuming that nothing else would be required. Indeed, the story of his success may be less about determination than about collaboration. And although his circumstances are unique, the broader truth that human achievement is inextricably bound up in social relationships is not.

Reconceptualizing the Unit of Analysis for Research on Goal Pursuit

In contrast to the dominant theories of self-regulation and goal pursuit in social psychology, transactive goal dynamics theory (TGD theory) conceptualizes the unit of analysis for "self"-regulation as the social group rather than the individual (Fitzsimons, Finkel, & vanDellen, 2015). The basic principle underlying TGD theory is *goal transactivity*: that the interdependence of goal setting, pursuit, and outcomes among members of meaningful social units (romantic partners, family members, friends, coworkers, teammates, etc.) is typically so strong that it ceases to make sense to consider the group members as independent self-regulating entities. Each individual is a subcomponent of a broader self-regulating system. As elaborated below, reconceptualizing the unit of analysis as the social group rather than the individual has profound consequences for the theories and research methods we use to understand how people set, pursue, and achieve goals.

Consider some empirical examples that underscore the importance of adopting a relational level of analysis. The conscientiousness level of an employee's spouse is positively linked to the employee's likelihood of promotion, even after controlling for his or her own conscientiousness level (Solomon & Jackson, 2014). Employees' productivity is greater to the extent that their coach's motivational orientation matches their own (Sue-Chan, Wood, & Latham, 2012). At-risk students' mathematics performance is stronger when they are taught by an instructor who teaches with high rather than low energy (Klusmann, Richter, & Lüdtke, 2016). Young adolescents with diabetes exhibit better metabolic control to the extent that their parents are more involved in monitoring their blood glucose levels (Anderson, Ho, Brackett, Findelstein, & Laffel, 1997). Mainstream theories and research methods from the self-regulation literature likely would miss these sorts of effects, treating them as part of the error term.

In expanding the unit of analysis for goal dynamics from the individual to the social unit, TGD theory owes a major debt to John Thibaut and Harold Kelley's (1959) interdependence theory (also see Kelley et al., 2003; Kelley &

Thibaut, 1978). "Humans are enmeshed in the fabric of their social milieu," observe Caryl Rusbult and Paul Van Lange (1996, p. 564) in their chapter on the nature of human interdependence in *Social Psychology: Handbook of Basic Principles*. "Accordingly," they continue,

> it is surprising that many theories of social psychological processes present the individual social agent as their theoretical centerpiece, largely ignoring the interpersonal circumstances encompassing the individual's preferences, thoughts, and actions. Social psychological explanations focusing on the individual are likely to be as limited as explanations of cellular processes focusing on a single cell—such explanations may tell us a good deal about the cell under consideration, yet fail to discern the broader meaning of its structure and functioning. (p. 564)

This insight—that frameworks seeking to understanding human tendencies at the level of the individual neglect not only vast swaths of explainable variance but also many of the most exciting research questions—serves as a major source of inspiration for the development of TGD theory.

Historical Perspective

Social psychological research on self-control and self-regulation has been remarkably influential since the 1960s. Consider, for example, the seminal studies that Walter Mischel (1974) conducted on preschoolers in the 1960s and 1970s. Across an ingenious research program, Mischel and his collaborators confronted young children with a dilemma. The children sat, alone, at a table with a marshmallow on it, weighing whether to eat the marshmallow now or to wait an unknown duration for the experimenter to return with a second marshmallow as a reward for their patience. Children who waited longer for a second marshmallow—who were better at delaying gratification—grew into teenagers who performed better academically and, eventually, into adults with stronger social relationships (Mischel, 2014).[1]

This particular research paradigm was unique, but the tendency to build theories and research paradigms that isolate the individual was not. This tendency is a manifestation of the highly individualistic *Zeitgeist* of social psychological research on goal setting, pursuit, and achievement before the 21st century. Collectively, the achievements of this *Zeitgeist* are monumental, but, in our view, they have also left a less fortunate legacy, one that has gone largely unnoticed in the interim half-century: The marshmallow studies contributed to a vision of goal pursuit that is strongly individualistic and, consequently, contributed to the development of a subfield of social psychology that is replete with theories and empirical paradigms oriented toward understanding goal setting, pursuit, and outcomes as largely individual-level phenomena. Hence the dominance of the terms *self*-regulation and *self*-control when referring to this subfield, which probably should be called something more general, perhaps *goal dynamics*.

With these observations in mind, it is useful to consider another example—beyond conscientious spouses, motivationally aligned coaches, high-energy teachers, and glucose-monitoring parents—of the fundamental role that relationship partners play in each other's goal outcomes. This example is, in our view, crucial in helping us understand when children actually eat marshmallows in the real world: Among overweight or obese children enrolled in a parent–child treatment program, the tendency to lose weight was stronger to the extent that their parent also lost weight, largely because their tendency to eat healthier food was linked to their parent's tendency to do so (Best et al., 2016). Related evidence comes from a study demonstrating that preadolescent children eat more sweets when their mother is experiencing greater-than-usual difficulty coping with stress (Mason et al., 2019). It seems that children eat more healthfully, and overweight and obese children lose more weight, to the extent that their parents purchase and serve healthy food and currently possess the psychological resources to promote healthful eating habits in the family. This parental tendency is precisely the sort of variable that gets shunted into the error term when our theories of goal dynamics treat relationship processes as noise to be eliminated rather than as signal to be investigated.

When we study goal dynamics by isolating participants in laboratory rooms or computer cubicles, we have indeed created a well-controlled empirical situation. But, frequently, we have done so at the expense of studying the variables and processes that are especially influential in determining the behavior we seek to understand (e.g., eating behavior).

The Dominance of Individual–Level Perspectives in the Social Psychology of Self-Regulation

To be sure, research on self-regulation has flourished in recent decades, producing an abundance of influential theoretical principles. For example, people are especially likely to enjoy goal success when they set clear goals and clear plans for pursuing them (Gollwitzer, 1999); feel confident that they can achieve their goals (Bandura, 1977); closely monitor the effectiveness of their pursuit and make adjustments as needed (Carver & Scheier, 1982); pursue important goals when their self-regulatory resources are intact rather than depleted (Baumeister & Heatherton, 1996); believe that goal-relevant abilities are malleable rather than fixed (Dweck & Leggett, 1988); deliberately distract themselves from temptations (Mischel, Shoda, & Rodriguez, 1989); automatically, when encountering a temptation, think about the goal that would be violated if they succumbed to the temptation (Fishbach, Friedman, & Kruglanski, 2003); and pursue goals with means that match their preferred self-regulatory orientation, such as when a gain-oriented person adopts an eager means of pursuit or a loss-oriented person adopts a vigilant means of pursuit (Higgins, 2000). This list is far from exhaustive, but it points to both the immense intellectual ferment in the science of goal pursuit and the strong tendency to treat the individual goal-pursuer as the unit of analysis. Such tendencies are echoed in the related literatures in personality psychology (Roberts, Lejuez, Krueger, Richards, & Hill, 2014) and social neuroscience (Wagner & Heatherton, 2016).[2]

To the extent that evidence continues to demonstrate the robustness and importance of these individual-level principles, they remain necessary components of any comprehensive theory of goal dynamics. But from the perspective of TGD theory, they are insufficient; they must be incorporated into a broader theoretical framework that also accounts for the social processes relevant to the setting, pursuit, and achievement of goals. Here, social psychology and its kindred disciplines come up short. For example, the most recent edition of the highly influential *Handbook of Self-Regulation* (Vohs & Baumeister, 2016) includes a chapter on TGD theory (Finkel, Fitzsimons, & vanDellen, 2016), but none of the other chapters from social psychologists is fundamentally social. Existing theories sometimes do explore how individual-level self-regulatory processes influence social outcomes (e.g., aggression), but, by and large, the relational focus is incidental to the basic causal mechanism under investigation. Before the arrival of TGD theory in 2015, there existed no social psychological theory of goal dynamics that incorporated social processes into its core principles.[3]

Toward the Conceptualization of a Shared Psyche

In a sense, the tendency of social psychologists to treat social processes as incidental rather than central to goal dynamics is bizarre. After all, such scholars have done major work underscoring the porous boundaries between *self* and *other*. Research in relationship science, for example, suggest that the self-concept gets expanded to incorporate aspects of close relationship partners (Agnew, Van Lange, Rusbult, & Langston, 1998; Aron, Aron, Tudor, & Nelson, 1991). Findings at the intersection of social psychology and judgment/decision making suggest that members of social units can, beyond any individual-level effects, strategically reason about problems and delegate decisions in ways that bolster collective goal achievement (Grossman & Kross, 2014; Polman & Vohs, 2016). Social psychological scholarship on management and organizations suggests that groups vary in their collective intelligence, independent of each member's individual intelligence; group performance depends on both bottom-up compositional features such as members' skills and top-down interaction features such as inclusive communication norms (Woolley, Aggarwal, & Malone, 2016).

Of particular relevance to this chapter is social psychologist Daniel Wegner's construct of *transactive memory* (Wegner, 1987; Wegner, Erber, & Raymond, 1991). According to Wegner, members of interdependent social units (romantic partners, team members, etc.) develop a shared memory pool—literally, a shared mind—that allows individuals to understand which members are likely to remember which information and to allocate, often implicitly, the responsibility for remembering information in accord with that understanding. Although research on transactive memory (e.g., Austin, 2003; Hollingshead, 1998; Liang, Moreland, & Argote, 1995) does not engage deeply with many of the topics that are essential to building a model of goal dynamics, the idea that individual minds serve as subparts of a social memory system was a second major source of inspiration for the development of TGD theory.

And generalizing the idea to the goal domain affords novel perspectives on goal-relevant constructs such as skills and resources (vanDellen & Baker, 2011). For example, one individual's skills or resources can influence another's goal setting, pursuit, and outcomes, such as when a husband's expertise regarding dieting and exercise may be sufficient for both himself and his wife to enjoy a healthy lifestyle. Or multiple individuals' skills or resources can combine in ways that bolster or undermine goal setting, pursuit, and outcomes, such as when employees perform better when embedded in a work team with others whose dispositional approach to goal pursuit—a tendency to set aside time for critical evaluation versus sustain forward movement—differs from their own (Pierro, Presaghi, Higgins, Klein, & Kruglanski, 2012). Topics such as these become increasingly central once we have reconceptualized the unit of analysis for goal pursuit to be the social group rather than the individual.

The next two sections make up the bulk of the chapter. First, in the section on transactive density, we present a social framework for conceptualizing goal setting and pursuit, develop a typology of goals emerging from that framework, and conceptualize goal outcomes (or achievement) within it. Next, in the section on transactive goal dynamics theory, we discuss the theory's six tenets and briefly review the empirical literature relevant to each of them.

Transactive Density

Transactivity density refers the level of interdependence among group members vis-à-vis goal setting, pursuit, and outcomes—the extent to which group members' goal systems are intertwined. Density assessments can extend to various goal properties (value, efficacy, standards), and to the effort one exerts and the means one employs in pursuit of the goal (Finkel et al., 2016). However, we simplify the discussion here to consider binary (present vs. absent) assessments of goal setting, pursuit, and outcomes for each group member with regard to the self and the other members. All of the ideas generalize to larger groups, but we focus primarily on the dyadic case.

A Factorial Framework
for Goal Setting and Goal Pursuit:
Setting × Target × Pursuit

We begin by setting aside goal outcomes to focus on goal setting and goal pursuit. TGD theory does so by considering three questions:

1. Who sets the goal?
2. Who is the target of the goal (i.e., toward whose outcomes is the goal oriented)?
3. Who pursues that goal?

In Figure 11.1, we represent these three questions in terms of a 2 (goal setting) × 2 (goal target) × 2 (goal pursuit) framework, which we consider from the perspective of our architects Daniel Burnham and John Root. The left panel encompasses goals that Burnham sets, and right panel encompasses the goals that Root sets—regardless of whether a given goal targets the outcomes of Burnham, Root, or both, and regardless of whether the goal is pursued by Burnham, Root, both, or neither. The left column in each panel encompasses goals for which Burnham is the target, and the right column in each panel encompasses goals for which Root is the target—regardless of whether a given goal is set by Burnham, Root, or both, and regardless of whether the goal is pursued by Burnham, Root, both, or neither. The top row in each panel encompasses goals for which Burnham is the pursuer, and the bottom row in each panel encompasses goals for which Root is the pur-

suer—regardless of whether a given goal is set by Burnham, Root, or both, and regardless of whether a given goal targets the outcomes of Burnham, Root, or both.

Our reading of the self-regulation literature is that the vast majority of research fits within Cell 1 (Burnham sets a goal for himself and pursues it alone) or Cell 8 (Root sets a goal for himself and pursues it alone). The major theoretical principles in the self-regulation literature tend to ignore instances in which, for example, one person sets a goal for his or her partner ("I want my partner to be nicer to me"), one person sets a goal for himself that is pursued by a relationship partner ("I want to lose weight, so my partner stops stocking the pantry with Oreos"), or both people set a goal for both of them that is pursued by one of them ("My wife and I want to save enough money for a trip to Iceland, so she cuts back on golfing expenses"). Although such cases pervade everyday life, they are largely absent from theories and empirical paradigms in the self-regulation literature.

A Structural Typology of Goals:
A TGD Theory Perspective

Our *Psychological Review* article (Fitzsimons et al., 2015, especially Table 1) provides a detailed discussion of the different types of goals that emerge from the typology depicted in Figure 11.1. It identifies seven prototypical types of goals—nested within three categories (one person's goals, parallel goals, and shared goals)—that emerge from adopting a TGD theory perspective. We provide an abbreviated discussion here.

One Person's Goals

The simplest category of goal types encompasses goals set by one person, and TGD theory identifies three major subcategories in this space. *Self-oriented goals* are those that a given person sets for him- or herself, such as when Burnham sets a goal to hone his drawing skills (Cell 1, Cell 3, or both). *Partner-oriented goals* are those that a given person sets for his or her partner, such as when Burnham sets a goal for Root to win an architectural award (Cell 2, Cell 4, or both). *System-oriented goals* (or, in the dyadic case, "dyad-oriented goals") are those that a given person

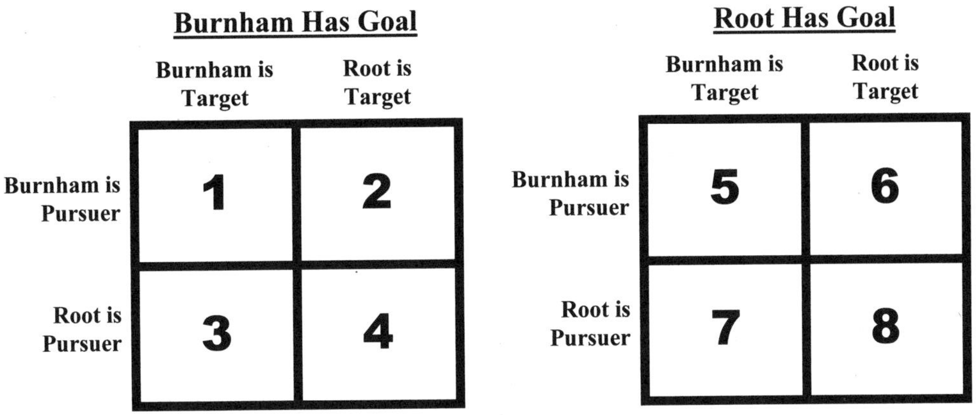

Burnham Has Goal

	Burnham is Target	Root is Target
Burnham is Pursuer	1	2
Root is Pursuer	3	4

Root Has Goal

	Burnham is Target	Root is Target
Burnham is Pursuer	5	6
Root is Pursuer	7	8

FIGURE 11.1. The three-way structure of goal setting and pursuit in TGD systems: who possesses the goal (left vs. right side of figure) × who is the target of the goal (left vs. right column) × who pursues the goal (top vs. bottom row). Adapted with permission from Fitzsimons et al. (2015).

sets for both (or all) members of the transactive system, such as when Burnham sets a goal for "Burnham and Root" to become the preeminent architectural firm of its time (Cells 1 and 2, Cells 3 and 4, or both of these pairs of cells).

As is clear from the previous paragraph's parenthetical information about which cells in Figure 11.1 are relevant in each case, this discussion of goal types is orthogonal to a consideration of who pursues a given goal. Burnham's goal to hone his drawing skills might be pursued by him practicing at home after his kids are asleep (Cell 1), by Root purchasing higher-quality supplies for the office (Cell 3), or by Root tutoring Burnham on a new technique (Cells 1 and 3). Burnham's goal for Root to win an architectural award might be pursued by Burnham writing a nomination letter (Cell 2), by Root schmoozing members of the award committee (Cell 4), or by the two of them hosting the committee members for a guided tour of their firm (Cells 2 and 4). Burnham's goal for "Burnham and Root" to become the preeminent architectural firm might be pursued by him doubling the number of draftsmen in the firm and procuring enough business to keep them busy (Cells 1 and 2), by Root working an extra 10 hours per week to bolster the firm's reputation for finishing buildings on time (Cells 3 and 4), or by the two of them working together to create a novel vision for the corporate skyscraper (Cells 1, 2, 3, and 4).

Parallel Goals

The second category of goal types encompasses goals set by both people for separate targets, and TGD theory identifies two major subcategories in this space. *Parallel self-oriented goals* are those simultaneously set by both people for themselves but not for the partner, such as when both Burnham and Root set a goal to lose weight (Cell 1, Cell 3, or both—and Cell 6, Cell 8, or both). *Parallel partner-oriented goals* are those simultaneously set by both people for the partner but not for themselves, such as when both Burnham and Root set a goal for the other person to bring more adventure into his life (Cell 2, Cell 4, or both—and Cell 5, Cell 7, or both).

With regard to pursuit, Burnham and Root's parallel self-oriented goal to lose weight might be pursued by Burnham ridding the office of unhealthy snacks (Cells 1 and 6), by Root ordering leaner lunches for the two of them (Cells 3 and 8), or by the two of them holding their daily state-of-the-firm meeting while running outside rather than while seated in Burnham's office (Cells 1, 3, 6, and 8). Burnham and Root's parallel partner-oriented goal to have the other person experience more adventure might be pursued by Burnham getting a group of their shared friends together for a hiking trip in the Rocky Mountains (Cells 2 and 5), by Root signing them up for a 19th-century version of *The*

Amazing Race (Cells 4 and 7), or by the two of them starting a *Fight Club*–style bare-knuckle boxing club (Cells 2, 4, 5, and 7).

Shared Goals

The third category of goal types encompasses goals set by both people for the same target (rather than for a different target, as with parallel goals), and TGD theory identifies two major subcategories in this space. *Shared target-oriented goals* are those simultaneously set by both people for one partner or the other, such as when both Burnham and Root want Root to recover from a case of pneumonia (Cell 2, Cell 4, or both—and Cell 6, Cell 8, or both). *Shared dyad-oriented goals* (or, more generally, shared system-oriented goals) are those simultaneously set by both people for both of them, such as when both Burnham and Root set the goal to procure the commission for the World Fair (Cells 1 and 2, Cells 3 and 4, or both of these pairs of cells—and Cells 5 and 6, Cells 7 and 8, or both of these pairs of cells).

With regard to pursuit, Burnham and Root's shared target-oriented goal for Root to recover from a case of pneumonia might be pursued by Burnham coordinating Root's medical care (Cells 2 and 6), by Root forcing himself to drink plenty of fluids (Cells 4 and 8), or by both of them engaging in these pursuits (Cells 2, 4, 6, and 8). Burnham and Root's shared system-oriented goal to procure the commission for the World Fair might be pursued by Burnham using his political skills to close the deal (Cells 1, 2, 5, and 6), by Root wowing the selection committee with a particularly innovative design (Cells 3, 4, 7, and 8), or by the two of them working together to build a scale model of their proposal (Cells 1, 2, 3, 4, 5, 6, 7, and 8).

Goal Outcomes in Transactive Systems

Beyond goal setting and goal pursuit, transactive density also encompasses *goal outcomes*—the extent to which progress is made regarding the goals set by members of the transactive system. Indeed, a primary goal of TGD theory is to discern the circumstances under which people achieve good or bad goal outcomes. In addition, the extent to which goal outcomes are good or bad reverberates throughout the transactive

system, influencing subsequent goal setting, pursuit, and outcomes (Finkel et al., 2016). For example, our romantic partner's success after setting the goal to lose weight might make us more likely to set that goal for ourselves (Lockwood & Kunda, 1997). Such success might also make our partner more likely to set that goal for us, even creating a detailed spreadsheet for us that incorporates daily caloric intake and an exercise regimen for the next 3 months.

Transactive Goal Dynamics Theory

With the transactive density construct as the foundation, we started wondering circa 2012 what it might look like to develop a theory of goal dynamics (a theory of "self-regulation") that was deeply, inextricably social. This task was different from the ones we had previously pursued at the intersection of self-regulation and close relationships, which involved identifying specific research questions of a magnitude that could be tested in a single empirical article—questions such as the following:

1. Does thinking about a significant other associated with a given goal increase one's exertions in pursuit of that goal (Fitzsimons & Bargh, 2003)?
2. Do inefficient social interactions undermine one's goal performance on subsequent tasks (Finkel et al., 2006)?
3. Does thinking about how helpful a romantic partner is in the pursuit of one's goal undermine one's own effort exertion (Fitzsimons & Finkel, 2011)?
4. Does having low power in a relationship increase the tendency to prioritize one's partner's goals over one's own (Laurin et al., 2016)?

We remain excited about questions of this magnitude, but, by 2012, we had come to believe that an exclusive focus on such questions would not allow for the development of a truly social theory of goal setting, pursuit, and achievement.

Our first effort along these lines appear in our "Transactive Goal Dynamics" article (Fitzsimons et al., 2015). In combination with Figure 11.2, the ensuing sections provide an

overview of TGD theory, along with brief discussions of the state of the empirical evidence
relevant to each of the theory's tenets. In several cases, including those summarized in the
note underneath Figure 11.2, this discussion
represents a slightly revised, updated version
of the theory presented in Fitzsimons and colleagues (2015).

Tenet 1: Relationships Vary in Their Level of Transactive Density

Some relationships exhibit greater transactive
density than others, and the level of transactive
density within a given relationship varies across
time and circumstance.[4] Figure 11.3 provides a
stylized illustration of this idea by considering

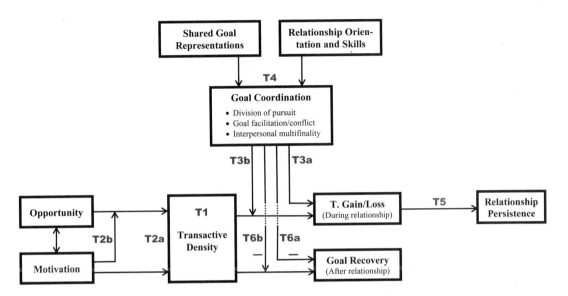

FIGURE 11.2. An overview of TGD theory. The Tenet 1 (T1) box captures the density of the transactive
system's goal setting, pursuit, and outcomes. Tenet 2 captures the hypotheses that opportunity and motivation are the key antecedents of transactive density (T2a), and that motivation moderates the effect of
opportunity on transactive density (T2b). Tenet 3 captures the hypotheses that effective goal coordination
both predicts transactive gain rather than loss ("T. Gain/Loss"; T3a) and makes the effect of transactive
density on transactive gain rather than loss more positive (T3b). Tenet 4 (T4) captures the hypotheses that
shared goal representations and relationship orientation and skills are the key antecedents of goal coordination. Tenet 5 (T5) captures the hypotheses that transactive gain rather than loss predicts relationship
persistence. Tenet 6 captures the hypotheses that when considering outcomes following relationship dissolution, effective goal coordination when the relationship was intact both predicts transactive loss rather
than gain (T6a) and makes the effect of transactive density when the relationship was intact on transactive
loss rather than gain more positive (T6b). This figure is adapted with permission from Fitzsimons et al.
(2015), with four notable changes. First, this figure adds an arrow representing the moderational effect of
motivation on the association between ability and transactive density, which required splitting the initial
Tenet 2 into two tenets; T2a was the original tenet, and T2b captures the new moderational hypothesis.
Second, this figure adds an arrow representing the main effect of goal coordination on transactive gain/
loss, which required splitting the initial Tenet 3 into two tenets; T3a captures this new main-effect hypothesis, whereas T3b was the original tenet. Third, in parallel manner, this figure adds an arrow representing the main effect of goal coordination on transactive goal recovery, which required splitting the initial Tenet 6 into two tenets; T6a captures this new main-effect hypothesis, whereas T6b was the original
tenet. And fourth, for conceptual simplicity, this figure splits shared goal representations and relationship
orientation/skills into separate boxes, a change underscoring that these are two distinct constructs that
can independently influence goal coordination.

the transactive density characterizing Burnham and Root's relationship in 1872, shortly after they first met (left panel), and that in 1890, after they had built their firm into a juggernaut (right panel).

In 1873, they launched their firm into the teeth of a major recession. But soon, their luck improved. Both were skilled architects, but Root was the more innovative of the two. Burnham was the better salesman and organizational mastermind; Root was the deeper intellectual. Root developed a revolutionary system for building foundations—a "floating raft system" involving interlocked steel beams—which made it possible for Chicago to become the center of innovation for tall buildings despite its marshy soil. The system made it possible for Burnham and Root to build the Montauk Building in 1882—a structure that many consider the first skyscraper. Throughout the decade, the firm built a number of monumental buildings, including many that continue to awe observers today.

"The Chicago skyscraper, soon exported elsewhere" observes the Burnham biographer Thomas Hines (2009, p. 69), "became the new cathedral, the votive symbol, of turn-of-the-century American culture—an architectural offering created of and for the time, that unified the worlds of science, of commerce, and of art." By 1890, Burnham and Root were among the hardest-working architects in the world, and pretty much everything each man did influenced the other. The magnitude of their goal-related interdependence was clear to observers all along, but it became especially obvious when Root succumbed to pneumonia in 1891, at the age of 41, a topic we consider when discussing Tenet 6 below. For now, the central point is that transactive density is an essential measure of interdependence, one that varies substantially from one relationship to the next and within a relationship over time. Understanding the causes and consequences of this interdependence is the primary purpose of TGD theory.

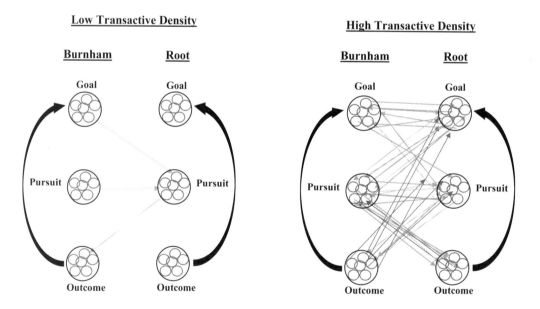

FIGURE 11.3. A depiction of transactive density. The left panel depicts a stylized representation of Daniel Burnham and John Root's goal-related interdependence in 1872, when they first became acquainted at the architectural firm of Carter, Drake and Wight. The right panel depicts a stylized representation of their goal-related interdependence in 1890, when their own architectural firm was at peak productivity. In both panels, the solid arrows represent effects from Burnham to Root, dashed arrows represent effects from Root to Burnham, and thicker lines represent stronger links. Adapted with permission from Fitzsimons et al. (2015).

Tenet 2: Opportunity and Motivation Exhibit Main and Interactive Effects on Transactive Density

Tenet 2 addresses the circumstances under which a transactive system is likely to exhibit lower versus higher levels of transactive density. According to Tenet 2a, a system exhibits higher levels of density to the extent that (1) circumstances afford the *opportunity* for interdependence, such as when management assigns two employees to work together on a project; and (2) the group members *desire* deeper rather than shallower interdependence, such as when the two employees ask management to assign them to shared projects again in the future. In other words, the cross-partner interdependence of the goals that members set, pursue, and achieve is likely to grow over time to the extent that external forces have pushed them to interact in meaningful ways more frequently (opportunity) and the partners want to interact in such ways (motivation).

Opportunity and motivation do not constitute transactive density in and of themselves; they set the stage for density to emerge over time. Management might assign several employees to work together on a project, which will increase the transactive density of the employees on average. But, as represented in Tenet 2b, the extent to which any two employees in this work team become interdependent will vary according to how much they are motivated to increase their goal-related interdependence—not only regarding the assigned project but perhaps also regarding other work-related goals (e.g., seeking feedback from each other on independent work) and non-work-related goals (e.g., getting the two families together for holiday festivities).

Burnham and Root obviously never could have become "Burnham and Root" had their paths not crossed. It was to their mutual good fortune that Burnham's father was able to persuade Peter Wight to hire his ne'er-do-well son into an architecture firm that happened to employ Root. Because they worked in the same firm, Burnham's and Root's goal systems inevitably intersected, creating a modest, necessary level of interdependence. When the two men discovered how much they loved working together, they founded their own firm, a setup that afforded the opportunity for them to be-

come deeply interdependent across many goals, including those linked to their reputations, their financial well-being, the enjoyment of their work, and so on.

Research provides compelling clues about what makes people seek more versus less density with a potential partner. For example, teams of individuals who are assigned to work together come to exhibit especially high levels of density to the extent that the members hold egalitarian values (Wageman & Gordon, 2005). Individuals tend to reduce their density with people who are highly competitive (Van Lange & Visser, 1999). People with low self-control are especially likely to pursue greater density with a partner who has high self-control (Shea, Davisson, & Fitzsimons, 2013).

Motivation also influences transactive density by altering transactive structure. Neither the number of people in a transactive system nor the nature of transactive density among them is necessarily fixed. Some groups are receptive to adding new members who become incorporated into a more complex web of goal-related interdependence, whereas other groups are less so. One intriguing case from our own discipline is Daniel Kahneman and Amos Tversky, who, according to Michael Lewis's (2016) *The Undoing Project,* exerted effort during their peak period of collaborative genius to keep others out of their transactive system of two.

Tenet 3: Goal Coordination Predicts Transactive Gain (vs. Loss) and Moderates the Effect of Transactive Density on Transactive Gain (vs. Loss)

In Tenet 3, we start investigating the consequences of transactive density, especially in terms the circumstances under which it promotes rather than undermines system-level goal outcomes. Specifically, this tenet introduces the construct of goal coordination, which both promotes system-level goal outcomes (Tenet 3a) and moderates the effect of density on such outcomes (Tenet 3b). Specifically, the effect of density on system-level goal outcomes becomes increasingly positive as goal coordination gets better but increasingly negative as goal coordination gets worse.[5]

The terms *transactive gain* and *transactive loss* capture the extent to which involvement in this relationship—in this transactive system—increases or decreases the members' collective goal outcomes. Researchers can adopt one or both of two benchmarks for such comparisons: the goal outcomes the members would have experienced (1) on their own (e.g., Burnham founding his own architecture firm) or (2) in a different transactive system (i.e., Burnham founding an architecture firm with somebody other than Root). Whichever benchmark researchers use, they can conceptualize transactive gain or loss in terms of the extent to which the whole is greater or less than the sum of its parts vis-à-vis goal achievement.

Goal coordination refers to the alignment and integration of goal pursuit across the array of goals in the transactive system, including the prioritization of more important over less important goals. Not surprisingly, research supports the hypothesis that transactive systems characterized by stronger coordination tend to exhibit better goal outcomes (Tenet 3a). Adolescents with type 1 diabetes tend to cope better with their medical condition to the extent that they enjoy collaborating with their mother to manage it (Berg, Schindler, & Maharajh, 2008). Elderly individuals with type 2 diabetes tend to falter more regarding their diet to the extent that their spouse tempt them with forbidden foods (Henry, Rook, Stephens, & Franks, 2013). People involved in new dating relationships make more progress on a given goal to the extent that it aligns with their partner's goals (Gere & Impett, 2018).

In accord with Tenet 3b is research demonstrating that transactive density and goal coordination interact to predict goal outcomes. Teams with a very high proportion of talented individuals tend to perform better than teams with a lower proportion of talented individuals when success is largely determined by the performance of individuals (e.g., in baseball)—but the performance of these highly talented teams suffers when success is largely determined by coordinated performance (e.g., in basketball), in part because status conflicts undermine team coordination (Swaab, Schaerer, Anicich, Ronay, & Galinsky, 2014). In other words, greater transactive density (basketball rather than baseball) predicts transactive gain when the team has a blend of elite and nonelite play-

ers, but it predicts transactive loss when the team has a particularly high proportion of elite players, apparently because goal coordination, such as who sets the pick and who shoots the ball, is problematic in the latter case. Analogously, adolescents who perceive that their family makes frequent demands on them tend to exhibit potentially harmful immunological activation (cytokine production in response to bacterial stimulation), but only if the family is close (Levine, Hoffer, & Chen, 2017). In other words, greater transactive density (close rather than nonclose familial context) predicts transactive gain when the demands are infrequent, but it predicts transactive loss when demands are frequent, apparently because goal coordination (alignment of goal-relevant behaviors) is problematic in the latter case.

Such studies provide intriguing support for Tenet 3b's transactive density × goal coordination interaction effect (task interdependence × status conflicts; family closeness × frequency of demands), but they offer few clues about the forms that goal coordination can take. TGD theory identifies three such forms: division of pursuit, transactive facilitation/conflict, and interpersonal multifinality.

Division of Pursuit

The first form involves the division of goal pursuit across members of the transactive system. To the extent that such division leverages the strengths and preferences of the members rather than focusing on, say, which member happened to set a given goal, the system enjoys greater transactive gain (or less transactive loss). One of the primary reasons why Burnham and Root enjoyed so much success is that they had complementary skills and specialized their efforts accordingly. Burnham was particularly interested in serving as a chief executive and in developing broad-brushstroke visions for the buildings, whereas Root was especially interested in the artistic components of architecture and in developing a philosophy linked to it. Because they were able to play to their respective strengths—and because they were able to integrate this division of labor with the opportunities afforded to them by industrial advances and the architectural demands in Chicago following the 1871 fire—they were able to achieve much more together than they could have achieved separately or with a less complementary partner.

Goal Facilitation/Conflict

The second form involves the extent to which one member's goal pursuit facilitates or interferes with other members' goal pursuit. If Burnham insisted on holding business meetings near the drafting area, he would have interfered with the quiet concentration required for Root to maximize his creativity and productivity. If Root had been uninterested in giving philosophical lectures, which enhanced the reputation of the firm, Burnham would have found it more difficult to procure major commissions. Rather than enduring such goal conflict, the gears that turned as the two of them pursued goals generally aligned, with the salutary consequence that each person's pursuit facilitated that of the other.

Interpersonal Multifinality

The third form differs from the first two in that it involves the system-level consequences of one person's pursuit. Here, we build on the goal systems theory construct of multifinality (Kruglanski et al., 2002), an individual-level variable capturing the extent to which the pursuit of a given means (e.g., walking the dog) serves multiple goals (e.g., caring for the dog, getting exercise, and enjoying the fresh air). Interpersonal multifinality captures the extent to which an individual's pursuit of a given goal serves multiple goals in the transactive system. Root's expertise in helping to design the stockyard magnate John B. Sherman's house in the firm's first major commission not only bolstered the shared goals of making money and enhancing the firm's reputation but also helped Burnham's personal life by impressing Sherman's daughter Margaret, whom Burnham ultimately married.

The Orthogonality of Transactive Density and Goal Coordination

TGD theory conceptualizes transactive density and goal coordination as independent constructs. A given transactive system, such as a married couple, might possess high versus low density; independently, it might possess strong versus weak coordination. Empirically speaking, density and coordination may be positively correlated because, all else being equal, people are likely to increase density over time when coordination is strong, and to decrease density over time when it is weak. But this idea represents a testable hypothesis rather than a feature of the theory itself. The theory conceptualizes density and coordination as constructs that can, and often do, vary independently.

Tenet 4: Shared Goal Representations and Relationship Orientation and Skills Predict Goal Coordination

Given how crucial goal coordination is in determining whether transactive density makes the whole better or worse than the sum of its parts, it is important to understand what helps members of transactive systems coordinate more successfully. TGD theory identifies two major factors that bolster goal coordination: (1) shared goal representations and relationship orientation and (2) skills.

Shared Goal Representations

A widespread, albeit weakly supported (Tidwell, Eastwick, & Finkel, 2013), belief among scholars and laypersons alike is that similarity—in terms of psychological attributes such as personality, attitudes, and values—is linked to greater interpersonal attraction and relationship quality. TGD theory focuses not on qualities that people have in common (e.g., both partners are conscientious), but rather on the goals and the preferred patterns of pursuit that people share *for specific targets* within their transactive system: Who should achieve what outcomes? Who should do what in pursuit of those outcomes? How should they do it? To the extent that the members of a transactive system align in answering such questions, their goal coordination is likely to be better. In particular, they will find it easier to divide pursuit sensibly, to enjoy more transactive facilitation and less transactive conflict, and to engage in more behaviors characterized by strong interpersonal multifinality.

Many studies illustrate the importance of shared goal representations. For example, people who make concrete exercise plans with a significant other pursue their exercise goals more effectively, and lose more weight, than do people who make concrete exercise plans for themselves or people who ask a significant other to help them exercise more but without making concrete plans (Prestwich et al., 2012). The concrete social plans appear to be especially effective because they include shared representations of both the targeted goal (that partner *A* will exercise more) and the means of pursuit. Older spouses with a larger proportion of shared target-oriented or shared dyad-oriented goals tend to experience greater psychological well-being, in part because these shared goal representations are linked to greater enjoyment of daily collaboration (Schindler, Berg, Butler, Fortenberry, & Wiebe, 2010). The main effect of shared goal representations is especially robust in couples who collaborate together more frequently—a reasonable indicator of transactive density—which is consistent with the moderational path implied by the intersection of Tenet 4 and Tenet 3b.

Relationship Orientation and Skills

Possessing shared goal representations is a major predictor of effective goal coordination, but it is far from the whole story. Dedication to the well-being of the relationship, along with the social skills required to facilitate it, is also essential (Feeney & Collins, 2015). People who feel highly committed to a relationship are especially willing to deviate from their self-interested preferences (narrowly defined) in order to benefit their partner and the relationship (Van Lange et al., 1997). In doing so, they are more likely than their less committed counterparts to prioritize overall goal achievement within the transactive system rather than simply prioritizing achievement of their own goals. According to TGD theory, such individuals are especially likely to seek out opportunities for efficient division of pursuit, transactive goal facilitation, and interpersonal multifinality.

Of course, adopting a relationship orientation of this sort is no guarantee that one's efforts will be effective. The odds of success are higher to the degree that individuals are skilled and attentive—that they can accurately perceive each other's goals and preferred means and can behave in ways that align with them. Consider so-

cial support. People differ in the sort of support they typically like to receive (e.g., emotional vs. instrumental), in the sort of support that is especially relevant in a given situation (e.g., information vs. money), in the relational dynamics they experience with a given support partner (e.g., an easygoing relationship vs. one on which one feels excessively dependent), and so forth—not to mention complex interactions among such variables. As such, a transactive system characterized by strong goal coordination is unlikely to be one in which members use cookie-cutter means of supporting one another's pursuit goals; rather, it is one in which goal-pursuit efforts are sensitively tailored to members' idiosyncratic needs, dispositions, and preferences (Finkel, Larson, Carswell, & Hui, 2014; also see Clark & Lemay, 2010; Reis, 2007).

Abundant research demonstrates the importance of providing such tailored, responsive support. Individuals talking to their romantic partner about their goal-related challenges tend to feel more deeply understood to the extent that their partner is generally more skilled at understanding other people's feelings (Leuchtmann et al., 2018). The long-term trajectories of physical functioning among individuals with osteoarthritis are better to the extent that their spouse calibrate support to align with their pain-related needs on a given day, dialing the level of support up or down to match their current pain level (Wilson, Martire, & Sliwinski, 2017).

But tailoring support is challenging, as any given approach can have downsides. For example, parents' direct academic support is linked not only to stronger mastery goals for their adolescent children but also to greater test anxiety (Song, Bong, Lee, & Kim, 2015). HIV-positive individuals who feel confident in their primary romantic partner's dedication to the relationship tend to enjoy strong medication-relevant self-efficacy regardless of how much medication-relevant support the partner provides, but HIV-positive individuals who feel uncertain of their romantic partner's dedication exhibit less self-efficacy to the extent that their partner provides more medication-relevant support, perhaps as a result of dissonance associated with being dependent on somebody who is unreliable (VanderDrift, Ioerger, Mitzel, & Vanable, 2017). Individuals with sleep apnea adhere better to their medical regimen when their spouse makes them feel supported for adherence, but worse when their spouse pressures them about it (Baron et al., 2011).

Tenet 5: System–Level Goal Achievement Predicts Relationship Quality and Persistence

As we have seen, TGD theory predicts that goal coordination, which is predicted by shared goal representations and relationship orientation and skills (Tenet 4), promotes transactive gain (vs. loss) through both a main effect (Tenet 3a) and an interaction effect with transactive density (Tenet 3b). According to Tenet 5, greater transactive gain in turn predicts higher relationship quality, including (in voluntary relationships) longer relationship persistence. No longitudinal research has examined the hypothesized link between transactive gain and relationship persistence, but several studies have demonstrated that greater *partner instrumentality*—a relationship partner's greater assistance with the achievement of one's goals—is linked to higher relationship quality (Fitzsimons & Shah, 2008; Orehek, Forest, & Wingrove, 2018). For example, individuals who experience their romantic partner as particularly instrumental during their moment-to-moment goal pursuit throughout a given week exhibit an increase in relationship satisfaction across that week (Hofmann, Finkel, & Fitzsimons, 2015). Individuals also exhibit elevated state-level relationship quality at moments during which they experience their partner as more instrumental than usual, an effect that is especially strong when individuals are fatigued or stressed—presumably because these are circumstances under which people benefit the most from their partner's instrumentality (Larson, Finkel, Fitzsimons, & Hofmann, 2018).

Tenet 6: Predissolution Goal Coordination Predicts Worse Goal Recovery and Negatively Moderates the Effect of Predissolution Transactive Density on Goal Recovery

Tenet 6 is, in a sense, the inverse of Tenet 3: Whereas Tenet 3 points to the positive main and interactive effects of goal coordination on

members' combined goal outcomes while the transactive system is intact (e.g., while two individuals are dating), Tenet 6 points to the negative main and interactive effects of goal coordination on members' combined goal outcomes after the transactive system has been dissolved (e.g., following a breakup). To the extent that goal coordination was strong while the system was intact, the members are likely to experience poorer goal-related outcomes following dissolution (Tenet 6a), especially to the extent that transactive density was high (Tenet 6b).

Although no research to date offers precise tests of these hypotheses, the available evidence is consistent with them. For example, when elite scientists die at the apex of their career, the publication rate of their collaborators declines sharply (Azoulay, Fons-Rosen, & Zivin, 2015), presumably in part because these collaborators had developed skill sets that facilitated coordination with the elite scientist but may be less effective independent of him or her. Similar results emerge when inventors die prematurely—their co-inventors' earnings and citation-weighted patents decline sharply (Jaravel, Petkova, & Bell, 2016), presumably for similar reasons. When a romantic relationship remains intact, individuals tend to make more goal progress to the extent that their partner is highly instrumental regarding those goals—but when the relationship has dissolved, individuals tend to make less progress to the extent that their partners had been highly instrumental while the relationship was ongoing (Gomillion, Murray, & Lamarche, 2015).

It is no small feat to disentangle the dense, messy web of goal-related interdependence characterizing systems with high transactive density. Recall that members of such systems function less as individual self-regulating entities than as subcomponents of a multiperson self-regulating system (see, again, the right panel of Figure 11.3). In successful systems—those characterized by strong goal coordination—members' skills improve in certain domains and atrophy in others (as a result of effective division of pursuit), they find their goal pursuit easier than it otherwise would be (as a result of strong goal facilitation), and they even find some of their goals achieved without them having to exert any effort at all (as a result of frequent interpersonal multifinality). When the system dissolves—due to a romantic breakup, a spousal death, or an organizational restructuring, for example—it can be difficult for members to disentangle their goal-related interdependence to develop an adapted set of goal-related mechanisms that yield strong goal-related outcomes.

Consider an example: Even though romantic couples often make decisions about which partner will have greater responsibility for financial matters on the basis of factors unrelated to skills in this domain (e.g., amount of responsibility in other domains), the person who adopts this role tends to become increasingly financially literate over time, while the partner does not (Ward & Lynch, 2017; also see Wegner et al., 1991). If the relationship dissolves, the person who did not become increasingly financially literate must confront a world in which he or she cannot rely on the erstwhile partner to compensate for that limitation.

Some of these consequences are visible when we consider Burnham's rather mixed architectural output following Root's abrupt death in 1891. This output is best exemplified by considering how Burnham managed the Chicago World's Fair, which took place in 1893. Burnham and Root were awarded the commission several years earlier, and the two of them had made some initial plans, seeking to create a small-scale version of an ideal city. After Root died, Burnham supervised an all-star team to create a hugely successful social and cultural event, one canonized anew in Erik Larson's (2004) *The Devil in the White City*. But in the eyes of some architectural critics—most stridently Burnham's contemporary Louis Sullivan (1924), the principal mentor of Frank Lloyd Wright—the Fair represented a giant step backward for the cause of architectural innovation. The source of the criticism is that Burnham, with Root dead and the pressure of producing a world-class event on a tight time line and with insufficient funding, turned away from innovation in favor of neoclassical designs. And although Burnham collaborated on some nice buildings in the two decades between Root's death and his own, he never approached the level of architectural creativity that he had achieved with Root in the 1880s.

Sullivan argued that Burnham's inability to recapture the magic of Burnham and Root resulted from Burnham's inherent lack of skill, but the biographer Thomas Hines (2009, p. 71) disagrees: "The worst and later work of D. H. Burnham and Company was not the 'real Burnham' finally exposed after Root no longer lived to cover up and carry on. It was a different Burnham, with both negative and positive manifestations, a Burnham changed not so much by Root's death as by his partner's life and by their close association of eighteen years." Hines continues, "With Root as a kind of intellectual 'authority,' Burnham had felt secure to combine his vision and his practicality in a large, aggressive way without fear of ultimate academic, artistic, or intellectual 'error.' His failure after Root's death to find the same kind of lasting human authority forced him, for the most part, into a gradual dependence upon 'the book,' upon the abstract academic authority of the 'classics.'" In this sense, Burnham is like the rest of us—if we are lucky enough to find ourselves in a transactive system characterized by strong transactive density and efficient goal coordination, we will probably struggle to maximize our goal success if the system dissolves.

Discussion

TGD theory represents a major departure from all major social psychological theories of goal dynamics in adopting the foundational assumption that goal setting, pursuit, and outcomes are fundamentally embedded within social units. It introduces the basic principle of goal transactivity, reconceptualizing the unit of analyses for goal dynamics, conceptualizing individuals as subcomponents of a self-regulating social group (Tenet 1). It then investigates both the causes (Tenet 2) and the consequences (Tenets 3–5) of transactive density for the social unit, including the implications of the unit's transactive density for its members following its dissolution (Tenet 6).

An Inextricably Social Species

As significant as TGD theory's departure is from mainstream theorizing in the social psychology of goal dynamics—of *self*-regulation and *self*-control—it aligns entirely with diverse perspectives that treat the social group as the unit of analysis for understanding various phenomena, including Thibaut and Kelley's (1959) interdependence theory and Wegner's (1987) work on transactive memory. "There is no such thing as a baby," observes the child psychiatrist Donald Woods Winnicott (1958, p. 99), meaning that it is virtually impossible to make sense of infants' experiences and development without accounting for their relationship and social interactions with their primary caregiver. "The smallest indivisible human unit is two people, not one; one is a fiction," says the playwright Tony Kushner. "From such nets of souls societies, the social world, human life springs."

Such perspectives are more than stylized abstractions. According to the Nobel Prize-winning physicist Neils Bohr (1934, p. 37), "Subatomic particles [are] definable and observable only through their interaction with other systems." The relationship scientist Ellen Berscheid (1999) argues that a similar truth applies to the human experience—it is largely defined in terms of interaction with other people. In *Reality Is Not What It Seems* (2018, p. 256), the physicist Carlo Rovelli underscores this idea by interpreting the pre-Socratic Greek philosopher Democritus's observations of humanity as follows: "The nature of man is not his internal structure but the network of personal, familial, and social interactions within which he exists."

None of this is to question the value of theories or research methods that conceptualize goal dynamics as individual-level phenomena. Such perspectives have proven to be immensely generative and surely will remain so. But, from the perspective of TGD theory, they neglect vast swaths of explanatory territory. To the extent that individual-level perspectives become increasingly embedded within a broader, social framework, they will account for a much greater proportion of the variance in explaining how people set, pursue, and achieve goals, conquering new territory at the intersection of the individual and the group levels of analysis.

A Glance to the Future

All perspectives that take human sociality seriously are complex, and TGD Theory is no exception. Indeed, the present discussion has simplified reality in major ways. The story becomes much more complicated as group size increases to three or more (Fitzsimons, Sackett, & Finkel, 2016). As just one example, parallel target-oriented goals in dyadic systems refer to cases in which both partners hold the same goal, but only for the other person, such as when both spouses want the partner to be kinder but believe that the self is already kind enough. But what about a work team with five members? Now a parallel target-oriented goal refers to cases in which multiple members of the team—two, three, four, or all five of them—hold the same goal but for a different teammate or teammates (if it were for the same teammate, it would be a shared goal). Perhaps Alice wants Betty to give the presentation, but Betty wants Charlie to do it, and Charlie thinks that Dwayne and Evan should do it together. Such phenomena are complex, but they are also important and worthy of empirical investigation.

The story gets even more complex when we appreciate that social units do not exist in isolation. All of us are embedded within multiple transactive systems—say, a marriage, a cycling club, a work team, and a church board—and the goal transactivity within any of them reverberates throughout all of them. Recall that Burnham and Root's first major commission was for the John B. Sherman house. They were able to procure this commission in part because Sherman's protégé, George Chambers, was Root's friend. Stated otherwise, Burnham had the opportunity to sign his first major deal because Chambers happened to be involved in one transactive system with Root and in another with Sherman.

Speaking of Sherman, Burnham's marriage to his daughter, Margaret, yielded a new transactive system that aligned symbiotically with the one Burnham had already developed with Root. "With the success of the Sherman commission and the influence of the Sherman family with important Chicago socialites and business magnates," observes Hines (2009, p. 21), "the young firm's 'starving time' would quickly end. New clients led to social invitations to attend parties and join clubs, which led, in turn, to more clients. . . . Daniel and Margaret rose socially as Burnham and Root rose professionally, the movement of both inevitably and inextricably entwined." Given widespread concerns about work–life balance, it seems that such smooth alignment across an individual's transactive systems can be difficult to achieve.

Conclusion

In the end, Burnham did make big plans, which did indeed have the magic to stir people's blood. But, as with the rest of us, the goals he set, the nature of his goal pursuit, and the extent of his achievement were not the result of one individual toiling away in isolation. They were, in the deepest, most fundamental sense, socially embedded. Burnham deserves credit for his titanic contributions to architecture, as does Root. But considering either man's contributions independently of the other's—and independently of both men's broader network of social relationships—represents a seriously oversimplified version of the truth. Such a simplification cannot, in the end, come close to explaining how they accomplished what they did.

NOTES

1. As we were revising this chapter, a conceptual replication attempt revealed additional evidence that the marshmallow test predicts long-term outcomes, although the effects were smaller in magnitude than in the initial research, emerged on fewer of the dependent variables, and were largely explained by differences in socioeconomic status (Watts, Duncan, & Quan, 2018). Debate about the magnitude and explanation of the *delay of gratification* effect is ongoing (Doebel, Michaelson, & Munakata, 2020).

2. As illustrated here, many of the seminal papers investigating self-regulation—virtually all of them treating goal setting, pursuit, and achievement as predominantly individual-level phenomena—were coauthored rather than sole-authored, which raises questions about the extent to which the processes elucidated in those papers would be sufficient to explain how the authors were able to achieve the goal of writing those very papers!

3. Perhaps surprisingly, developmental and health psychologists have done more than social psychologists to incorporate social dynamics into theories of goal pursuit, albeit typically constraining their theorizing to specific relationships (e.g.,

parent–child), process (e.g., social support), or behavioral domains (e.g., smoking).

4. This characterization of Tenet 1 is slightly different from the characterization in the *Psychological Review* article, in which the tenet reads as follows: "Relationship partners tend to form a shared system of goal pursuit" (Fitzsimons et al., 2015, p. 651). The revised text we employ here focuses on the *extent* of transactive density rather than merely on its presence or absence, and it recognizes that the level of transactive density in a given relationship fluctuates over time.

5. In participant samples characterized by consistently high levels of density, such as most serious dating or marital relationships, the main effect of goal coordination (Tenet 3a) is likely to be much stronger than the transactive density × goal coordination interaction effect (Tenet 3b).

REFERENCES

Agnew, C. R., Van Lange, P. A., Rusbult, C. E., & Langston, C. A. (1998). Cognitive interdependence: Commitment and the mental representation of close relationships. *Journal of Personality and Social Psychology, 74*(4), 939–954.

Anderson, B., Ho, J., Brackett, J., Finkelstein, D., & Laffel, L. (1997). Parental involvement in metabolic control in young adolescents with insulin-dependent diabetes mellitus. *Journal of Pediatrics, 130*, 257–265.

Aron, A., Aron, E. N., Tudor, M., & Nelson, G. (1991). Close relationships as including other in the self. *Journal of Personality and Social Psychology, 60*, 241–253.

Austin, J. R. (2003). Transactive memory in organizational groups: The effects of content, consensus, specialization, and accuracy on group performance. *Journal of Applied Psychology, 88*, 866–878.

Azoulay, P., Fons-Rosen, C., & Zivin, J. S. G. (2015). *Does science advance one funeral at a time?* (No. w21788). Cambridge, MA: National Bureau of Economic Research.

Bandura, A. (1977). Self-efficacy: Toward a unifying theory of behavioral change. *Psychological Review, 84*, 191–215.

Baron, K. G., Smith, T. W., Berg, C. A., Czajkowski, L. A., Gunn, H., & Jones, C. R. (2011). Spousal involvement in CPAP adherence among patients with obstructive sleep apnea. *Sleep and Breathing, 15*(3), 525–534.

Baumeister, R. F., & Heatherton, T. F. (1996). Self-regulation failure: An overview. *Psychological Inquiry, 7*(1), 1–15.

Berg, C. A., Schindler, I., & Maharajh, S. (2008). Adolescents' and mothers' perceptions of the cognitive and relational functions of collaboration and adjustment in dealing with type 1 diabetes. *Journal of Family Psychology, 22*(6), 865–874.

Berscheid, E. (1999). The greening of relationship science. *American Psychologist, 54,* 260–266.

Best, J. R., Goldschmidt, A. B., Mockus-Valenzuela, D. S., Stein, R. I., Epstein, L. H., & Wilfley, D. E. (2016). Shared weight and dietary changes in parent–child dyads following family-based obesity treatment. *Health Psychology, 35*(1), 92–95.

Bohr, N. (1934). *Atomic physics and the description of nature.* Cambridge, UK: Cambridge University Press.

Carver, C. S., & Scheier, M. F. (1982). Control theory: A useful conceptual framework for personality–social, clinical, and health psychology. *Psychological Bulletin, 92*(1), 111–135.

Clark, M. S., & Lemay, E. P. (2010). Close relationships. In S. T. Fiske, D. T. Gilbert, & L. Gardner (Eds.), *Handbook of social psychology* (Vol. 2, 5th ed., pp. 898–940). Hoboken, NJ: Wiley.

Doebel, S., Michaelson, L. E., & Munakata, Y. (2020). Good things come to those who wait: Delaying gratification likely does matter for later achievement (a commentary on Watts, Duncan, & Quan, 2018). *Psychological Science, 31,* 97–99.

Dweck, C. S., & Leggett, E. L. (1988). A social-cognitive approach to motivation and personality. *Psychological Review, 95,* 256–273.

Feeney, B. C., & Collins, N. L. (2015). A new look at social support: A theoretical perspective on thriving through relationships. *Personality and Social Psychology Review, 19,* 113–147.

Finkel, E. J., Campbell, W. K., Brunell, A. B., Dalton, A. N., & Scarbeck, S. J., & Chartrand, T. L. (2006). High-maintenance interaction: Inefficient social coordination impairs self-regulation. *Journal of Personality and Social Psychology, 91,* 456–475.

Finkel, E. J., & Fitzsimons, G. M., & vanDellen, M. R. (2016). Self-regulation as a transactive process: Reconceptualizing the unit of analysis for goal setting, pursuit, and outcomes. In K. D. Vohs & R. F. Baumeister (Eds.), *Handbook of self-regulation: Research, theory, and applications* (3rd ed., pp. 264–282). New York: Guilford Press.

Finkel, E. J., Larson, G. M., Carswell, K. L., & Hui, C. M. (2014). Marriage at the summit: Response to the commentaries. *Psychological Inquiry, 25,* 120–145.

Fishbach, A., Friedman, R. S., & Kruglanski, A. W. (2003). Leading us not into temptation: Momentary allurements elicit overriding goal activation. *Journal of Personality and Social Psychology, 84,* 296–309.

Fitzsimons, G. M., & Bargh, J. A. (2003). Thinking of you: Nonconscious pursuit of interpersonal goals associated with relationship partners. *Journal of Personality and Social Psychology, 84*(1), 148–164.

Fitzsimons, G. M., & Finkel, E. J. (2011). Outsourcing self-regulation. *Psychological Science, 22*(3), 369–375.

Fitzsimons, G. M., Finkel, E. J., & vanDellen, M. R. (2015). Transactive goal dynamics. *Psychological Review, 122*(4), 648–673.

Fitzsimons, G. M., Sackett, E., & Finkel, E. J. (2016). Transactive goal dynamics theory: A relational goals perspective on work teams and leadership. *Research on Organizational Behavior, 36,* 135–155.

Fitzsimons, G. M., & Shah, J. Y. (2008). How goal instrumentality shapes relationship evaluations. *Journal of Personality and Social Psychology, 95*(2), 319–337.

Gere, J., & Impett, E. A. (2018). Shifting priorities: Effects of partners' goal conflict on goal adjustment processes and relationship quality in developing romantic relationships. *Journal of Social and Personal Relationships, 35,* 793–810.

Gollwitzer, P. M. (1999). Implementation intentions: Strong effects of simple plans. *American Psychologist, 54,* 493–503.

Gomillion, S., Murray, S. L., & Lamarche, V. M. (2015). Losing the wind beneath your wings: The prospective influence of romantic breakup on goal progress. *Social Psychological and Personality Science, 6*(5), 513–520.

Grossmann, I., & Kross, E. (2014). Exploring Solomon's Paradox: Self-distancing eliminates the self-other asymmetry in wise reasoning about close relationships in younger and older adults. *Psychological Science, 25*(8), 1571–1580.

Henry, S. L., Rook, K. S., Stephens, M. A., & Franks, M. M. (2013). Spousal undermining of older diabetic patients' disease management. *Journal of Health Psychology, 18*(12), 1550–1561.

Higgins, E. (2000). Making a good decision: Value from fit. *American Psychologist, 55,* 1217–1230.

Hines, T. S. (2009). *Burnham of Chicago: Architect and planner* (2nd ed.). Chicago: University of Chicago Press.

Hofmann, W., Finkel, E. J., & Fitzsimons, G. M. (2015). Close relationships and self-regulation: How relationship satisfaction facilitates momentary goal pursuit. *Journal of Personality and Social Psychology, 109*(3), 434–452.

Hollingshead, A. B. (1998). Communication, learning, and retrieval in transactive memory systems. *Journal of Experimental Social Psychology, 34,* 423–442.

Jaravel, X., Petkova, N., & Bell, A. (2016). *Team-specific capital and innovation.* Unpublished manuscript, Stanford University, Stanford, CA.

Kelley, H. H., Holmes, J. G., Kerr, N. L., Reis, H. T., Rusbult, C. E., & Van Lange, P. A. M. (2003). *An atlas of interpersonal situations.* New York: Cambridge.

Kelley, H. H., & Thibaut, J. W. (1978). *Interpersonal relations: A theory of interdependence.* New York: Wiley.

Klusmann, U., Richter, D., & Lüdtke, O. (2016). Teachers' emotional exhaustion is negatively related to students' achievement: Evidence from a large-scale assessment study. *Journal of Educational Psychology, 108*(8), 1193–1203.

Kruglanski, A. W., Shah, J. Y., Fishbach, A., Friedman, R., Chun, W. Y., & Sleeth-Keppler, D. (2002). A theory of goal systems. In M. P. Zanna (Ed.), *Advances in experimental social psychology* (Vol. 34, pp. 311–378). New York: Academic Press.

Larson, E. (2004). *The devil in the white city: Murder, magic, and madness at the fair that changed America.* Visalia, CA: Vintage.

Larson, G. M., Finkel, E. J., Fitzsimons, G. M., & Hofmann, W. (2018). *When happiness is conditional: Compromised self-regulatory resources, partner instrumentality, and relationship satisfaction.* Unpublished manuscript, Northwestern University, Evanston, IL.

Laurin, K., Fitzsimons, G. M., Finkel, E. J., Carswell, K. L., vanDellen, M. R., Hofmann, W., et al. (2016). Power and the pursuit of a partner's goals. *Journal of Personality and Social Psychology, 110*(6), 840–868.

Leuchtmann, L., Zemp, M., Milek, A., Nussbeck, F. W., Brandstätter, V., & Bodenmann, G. (2018). Role of clarity of other's feelings for dyadic coping. *Personal Relationships, 25,* 38–49.

Levine, C. S., Hoffer, L. C., & Chen, E. (2017). Moderators of the relationship between frequent family demands and inflammation among adolescents. *Health Psychology, 36*(5), 493–501.

Lewis, M. (2016). *The undoing project: A friendship that changed our minds.* New York: Norton.

Liang, D., Moreland, R., & Argote, L. (1995). Group versus individual training and group performance: The mediating factor of transactive memory. *Personality and Social Psychology Bulletin, 21,* 384–393.

Lockwood, P., & Kunda, Z. (1997). Superstars and me: Predicting the impact of role models on the self. *Journal of Personality and Social Psychology, 73*(1), 91–103.

Mason, T. B., O'Connor, S. G., Schembre, S. M., Huh, J., Chu, D., & Dunton, G. F. (2019). Momentary affect, stress coping, and food intake in mother–child dyads. *Health Psychology, 38,* 238–247.

Mischel, W. (1974). Processes in delay of gratification. In L. Berkowitz (Ed.), *Advances in experimental social psychology* (Vol. 7, pp. 249–292). New York: Academic Press.

Mischel, W. (2014). *The marshmallow test: Understanding self-control and how to master it.* New York: Random House.

Mischel, W., Shoda, Y., & Rodriguez, M. I. (1989). Delay of gratification in children. *Science, 244,* 933–938.

Orehek, E., Forest, A. L., & Wingrove, S. (2018). People as means to multiple goals: Implications for interpersonal relationships. *Personality and Social Psychology Bulletin, 44*(10), 1487–1501.

Pierro, A., Presaghi, F., Higgins, E. T., Klein, K. M., & Kruglanski, A. W. (2012). Frogs and ponds: A multilevel analysis of the regulatory mode complementarity hypothesis. *Personality and Social Psychology Bulletin, 38*(2), 269–279.

Polman, E., & Vohs, K. D. (2016). Decision fatigue, choosing for others, and self-construal. *Social Psychological and Personality Science, 7*(5), 471–478.

Prestwich, A., Conner, M. T., Lawton, R. J., Ward, J. K., Ayres, K., & McEachan, R. R. (2012). Randomized controlled trial of collaborative implementation intentions targeting working adults' physical activity. *Health Psychology, 31*(4), 486–495.

Reis, H. T. (2007). Steps toward the ripening of relationship science. *Personal Relationships, 14,* 1–23.

Roberts, B. W., Lejuez, C., Krueger, R. F., Richards, J. M., & Hill, P. L. (2014). What is conscientiousness and how can it be assessed? *Developmental Psychology, 50*(5), 1315–1330.

Rovelli, C. (2018). *Reality is not what it seems: The journey to quantum gravity.* New York: Penguin.

Rusbult, C. E., & Van Lange, P. A. M. (1996). Interdependence processes. In E. T. Higgins & A. Kruglanski (Eds.), *Social psychology: Handbook of basic principles* (pp. 564–596). New York: Guilford Press.

Schindler, I., Berg, C. A., Butler, J. M., Fortenberry, K. T., & Wiebe, D. J. (2010). Late-midlife and older couples' shared possible selves and psychological well-being during times of illness: The role of collaborative problem solving. *Journals of Gerontology B: Psychological Sciences and Social Sciences, 65*(4), 416–424.

Shea, C. T., Davisson, E. K., & Fitzsimons, G. M. (2013). Riding other people's coattails: Individuals with low self-control value self-control in other people. *Psychological Science, 24*(6), 1031–1036.

Solomon, B. C., & Jackson, J. J. (2014). The long reach of one's spouse: Spouses' personality influences occupational success. *Psychological Science, 25*(12), 2189–2198.

Song, J., Bong, M., Lee, K., & Kim, S. I. (2015). Longitudinal investigation into the role of perceived social support in adolescents' academic motivation and achievement. *Journal of Educational Psychology, 107*(3), 821–841.

Sue-Chan, C., Wood, R. E., & Latham, G. P. (2012). Effect of a coach's regulatory focus and an individual's implicit person theory on individual performance. *Journal of Management, 38*(3), 809–835.

Sullivan, L. (1924). *The autobiography of an idea.* New York: Press of the American Institute of Architects.

Swaab, R. I., Schaerer, M., Anicich, E. M., Ronay, R., & Galinsky, A. D. (2014). The too-much-talent effect: Team interdependence determines when more talent is too much or not enough. *Psychological Science, 25*(8), 1581–1591.

Thibaut, J. W., & Kelley, H. H. (1959). *The social psychology of groups.* New York: Wiley.

Tidwell, N. D., Eastwick, P. W., & Finkel, E. J. (2013). Perceived, not actual, similarity predicts initial attraction in a live romantic context: Evidence from the speed-dating paradigm. *Personal Relationships, 20,* 199–215.

Van Lange, P. A., Rusbult, C. E., Drigotas, S. M., Arriaga, X. B., Witcher, B. S., & Cox, C. L. (1997). Willingness to sacrifice in close relationships. *Journal of Personality and Social Psychology, 72,* 1373–1395.

Van Lange, P. A., & Visser, K. (1999). Locomotion in social dilemmas: How people adapt to cooperative, tit-for-tat, and noncooperative partners. *Journal of Personality and Social Psychology, 77*(4), 762–773.

vanDellen, M. R., & Baker, E. (2011). Implicit delegation of responsibility: Joint self-control in close relationships. *Social Psychological and Personality Science, 2*(3), 277–283.

VanderDrift, L. E., Ioerger, M., Mitzel, L. D., & Vanable, P. A. (2017). Partner support, willingness to sacrifice, and HIV medication self-efficacy. *AIDS and Behavior, 21*(8), 2519–2525.

Vohs, K. D., & Baumeister, R. F. (Eds.). (2016). *Handbook of self-regulation: Research, theory, and applications* (3rd ed.). New York: Guilford Press.

Wageman, R., & Gordon, F. M. (2005). As the twig is bent: How group values shape emergent task interdependence in groups. *Organization Science, 16*(6), 687–700.

Wagner, D. D., & Heatherton, T. F. (2016). The cognitive neuroscience of self-regulatory failure. In K. D. Vohs & R. F. Baumeister (Eds.), *Handbook of self-regulation: Research, theory, and applications* (3rd ed., pp. 111–130). New York: Guilford Press.

Ward, A. F., & Lynch, J. G. (2017). *On a need-to-know basis: How the distribution of responsibility between couples shapes financial literacy and financial outcomes.* Unpublished manuscript, University of Texas–Austin, Austin, TX.

Watts, T. W., Duncan, G. J., & Quan, H. (2018). Revisiting the marshmallow test: A conceptual replication investigating links between early delay of gratification and later outcomes. *Psychological Science, 29,* 1159–1177.

Wegner, D. M. (1987). Transactive memory: A contemporary analysis of the group mind. In B. Mullen & G. R. Goethals (Eds.), *Theories of group behavior* (pp. 185–208). New York: Springer Science + Business Media.

Wegner, D. M., Erber, R., & Raymond, P. (1991). Transactive memory in close relationships. *Journal of Personality and Social Psychology, 61,* 923–929.

Wilson, S. J., Martire, L. M., & Sliwinski, M. J. (2017). Daily spousal responsiveness predicts longer-term trajectories of patients' physical function. *Psychological Science, 28*(6), 786–797.

Winnicott, D. W. (1958). *Collected papers: Through paediatrics to psycho-analysis.* London: Tavistock.

Woolley, A. W., Aggarwal, I., & Malone, T. W. (2016). Collective intelligence and group performance. *Current Directions in Psychological Science, 24*(6), 420–424.

CHAPTER 12

Major Principles of Attachment Theory
Overview, Hypotheses, and Research Ideas

Jeffry A. Simpson
W. Steven Rholes
Jami Eller
Ramona L. Paetzold

During the past five decades, few theories in psychology have generated as much interest, research, and debate as attachment theory (Bowlby, 1969/1982, 1973, 1980, 1988) and its recent extensions (see Cassidy & Shaver, 2016). Attachment theory is an extensive, inclusive theory of personality and social development "from the cradle to the grave" (Bowlby, 1979, p. 129). Being a lifespan theory, it is relevant to several areas in psychology, including developmental, personality, social, cognitive, neuroscience, and clinical.

Because attachment theory covers the entire life course, it has several fundamental principles and core hypotheses, most of which address how and why people think, feel, and behave in particular ways within relationships at different points of their lives. Given the focus of this volume, our primary goal in this chapter is to provide a brief, representative overview of the key principles and central hypotheses that underlie attachment theory, both as originally articulated by Bowlby and his contemporaries (e.g., Ainsworth, Blehar, Waters, & Wall, 1978) and as expanded upon in recent theory and research (Cassidy & Shaver, 2016).

Attachment theory has two major components: (1) a *normative component,* which ex-plains modal (species-typical) attachment processes and patterns of behavior in humans, and (2) an *individual-difference component,* which explains individual deviations from modal processes and behavioral patterns. Most of the major principles and hypotheses we discuss in this chapter are normative ones, but we also highlight principles associated with well-established individual differences in attachment patterns (in children) and attachment orientations (in adults), including how they are related to a host of personal and relational processes and outcomes.

We began our work on this chapter by surveying the theoretical and empirical literature on attachment processes across the lifespan and generated an initial list of potential principles and hypotheses. We then asked several leading attachment scholars working in different areas of psychology (e.g., clinical, developmental, personality, social) to indicate what they thought were the most important principles/hypotheses.[1] Informed by this information, we next identified what we believe are nine of the most important, foundational principles and hypotheses that serve as the foundation of attachment theory (see Table 12.1, which serves as a guide to the following discussion).

TABLE 12.1. Major Attachment Principles and Hypotheses

Principle A: Attachment theory is an evolutionary, biologically based theory explaining a predisposition to engage in proximity to important others for safety and survival.

1. All human infants, and certain other species, engage in this behavior (universality hypothesis) as a means of meeting basic physical and emotional needs.

2. The relationship state of engaging in proximity with an important caregiver who can meet basic safety and survival needs is referred to as an attachment.

3. Close others who meet the attachment needs of an individual are attachment figures.

Principle B: The attachment system coexists with other innate behavioral systems, such as the caregiving system, the sexuality system, and the exploration system.

1. All of these systems are important and interrelated.

2. However, the attachment behavioral system comes to the forefront (is dominant) during times of distress, fear, loss, pain, or separation (threat activation hypothesis), motivating proximity seeking to attachment figures.

Principle C: The connection between the attachment and caregiving systems determines whether infants form attachments that are secure or insecure.

1. Attachment-relevant behavior develops largely in response to the quality of early caregiving, such that high-quality and consistent early caregiving—particularly during times of distress—leads to attachment security (sensitivity hypothesis).

2. Early inconsistent, rejecting, or absent caregiving by attachment figures during times of distress leads to attachment insecurity.

Principle D: There are three major functions of attachment relationships—to promote proximity seeking, provide a safe haven, and offer a secure base—all of which facilitate self-regulation and emotion regulation.

1. Proximity seeking promotes safety and survival of the individual, through either greater physical closeness to an attachment figure or internalized feelings of closeness to an attachment figure (felt security).

2. A safe haven helps the individual regulate emotions during times of actual or perceived distress/threat.

3. A secure base allows the individual to explore the world and develop greater autonomy, growth, and competence, eventually resulting in better self-regulation and psychological development.

Principle E: Attachment figures, and types of attachments to them (secure vs. insecure), shape internal working models (mental representations) of the self and others.

1. Internal working models consist of preverbal and verbal memories, which shape cognitions, perceptions, emotions, attitudes, and behaviors toward the self, others, and the world more generally.

2. In infants and young children, the organization of attachment behavior (e.g., expressing distress, seeking comfort, being soothed by comforting) varies based on prior caregiving experiences with attachment figures (e.g., parents or other caregivers). Children are classified as secure, ambivalent (anxious), avoidant, or disorganized based on their responses to their attachment figures. These responses are viewed as adaptive given the specific nature of the child's caregiving environment.

3. Over time, internal working models become more elaborate and important, eventually developing into adult attachment orientations, which include anxiety, avoidance, and disorganization (with low scores on these dimensions representing greater security).

Principle F: The attachment system is relevant from "the cradle to the grave."

1. Internal working models based on an individual's entire attachment history with various caregivers guide cognitions, perceptions, emotions, attitudes, and behaviors across the individual's entire life.

2. Attachment orientations in adulthood are relatively stable within people across time and context; they are "trait-like," particularly attachment security (stability hypothesis).

3. However, attachment orientations can change in response to attachment-relevant events/contexts (e.g., therapy, experiences that sharply contradict existing internal working models) (change hypothesis).

(continued)

TABLE 12.1. *(continued)*

Principle G: Attachment security is an inner resource that can facilitate resilience (broaden-and-build hypothesis), whereas attachment insecurity is a vulnerability often associated with poorer life outcomes.

1. Mental health outcomes

2. Interpersonal difficulties

Principle H: Individuals have specific reactions when they are separated from or lose their attachment figures.

1. They experience three stages of grief: protest, despair, and detachment.

2. Each of these responses serves an adaptive purpose.

Principle I: The attachment system, although universal, is culturally dependent and promotes culturally specific forms of adaptation and development.

1. In some cultures, most individuals develop secure attachments, because they are exposed to sensitive and appropriate caregiving by their attachment figures/caregivers (normativity and sensitivity hypotheses), especially in plentiful, nonthreatening environments.

2. In other cultures, relatively more individuals develop insecure attachments, because they are exposed to less sensitive and inappropriate caregiving by their attachment figures/caregivers, especially in less plentiful, more threatening environments.

Major Principles

We now discuss each principle and the key hypotheses associated with it, present representative research relevant to each principle/hypothesis, and identify a few important, unanswered questions relevant to each principle.

Principle A: Attachment Theory Is an Evolutionary, Biologically Based Theory

According to Bowlby (1969/1982, 1973, 1980, 1988), the attachment system evolved and is deeply ingrained in our nature because it solved one of the greatest adaptive challenges our ancestors faced—how to improve the chances of survival during childhood in ancestral environments. Inspired by Darwin (1859, 1872), Bowlby (1969/1982) believed that the "attachment system" was genetically wired into our species through directional selection. At its core, the attachment system is designed to detect and respond to potential threats when they arise. The system has three central features: (1) monitoring/appraising potentially threatening events, which activate (turn on) the attachment system, (2) monitoring/appraising the availability and responsiveness of another person who can provide protection/comfort in response to the threat, and (3) monitoring/appraising the likeli-

hood that seeking proximity to this person can (or will) be achieved (Bowlby, 1973; Mikulincer & Shaver, 2003).

Bowlby believed that all human infants—as well as young offspring in many other species—engage in behaviors that reflect the operation of the attachment system, most notably when they are either acutely or chronically ill, stressed, fatigued, or threatened. This is termed the *universality hypothesis*. Bowlby further claimed that the state of seeking and maintaining proximity with a person who can meet one's basic safety and survival needs involves being attached to that person, and that people who meet attachment needs become "attachment figures."

Bowlby also highlighted the important role that care and nurturance assume in the survival, growth, and thriving of all individuals, including in nonthreatening situations. He claimed that good caregivers tend to provide "a secure base from which a child or an adolescent can make sorties into the outside world and to which he [*sic*] can return knowing for sure that he will be welcomed when he gets there, nourished physically and emotionally, comforted if distressed, reassured if frightened" (1988, p. 11). This type of care and nurturance, which Bowlby believed was governed primarily by the parenting behavioral system in nonthreatening situations, allows individuals to develop many of the skills, attributes, and abilities necessary for competent functioning in other life domains, such as learning new tasks, developing self-confidence, and establishing warm, communal relationships with other people.

Several gaps in our understanding of these issues remain. For example, we need to know more about how attachment relationships are formed across time, particularly among adults and their romantic partners. We also need to know more about how children and adults develop and manage relationships with multiple attachment figures, including the conditions under which they turn to and use specific attachment figures for specific needs or purposes (e.g., for comfort, reassurance, support, information, advice). Finally, regarding the universality hypothesis, we need to know more about the conditions under which attachment relationships may develop in early deviant environments.

Principle B: The Attachment System Coexists with Other Behavioral Systems

The attachment system is one of several biologically based behavioral systems, each of which affects and interacts with the others to impact what a person does in a specific situation. In children, for example, the other primary behavioral systems include the *exploration system* (which can activate when the attachment system is inactive, permitting the learning of new information and skills relevant to survival and social development), the *social system* (which also can activate when the attachment system is quiescent, allowing individuals to reap the benefits of forging personal ties with different people), and the *caregiving system* (which operates in tandem with the attachment system to provide care and protection, particularly when an offspring or partner's attachment system is activated; Cassidy, 2016). In adulthood, other biologically based behavioral systems become relevant, especially the *sexual/mating system,* which evolved to promote reproductive fitness (Birnbaum, 2016).

According to Bowlby (1969/1982, 1973, 1980), and as supported by considerable research with children (e.g., Marvin, Britner, & Russell, 2016) and adults (e.g., Mikulincer & Shaver, 2016; Simpson & Rholes, 2012), the attachment system dominates attention and guides behavior (relative to the other behavioral systems) when children and adults feel threatened, distressed, fatigued, or fearful, especially in response to potential, impending, or actual loss or separation of their attachment figures. This is known as the *threat activation hypothesis,* which makes attachment theory unique compared to other theories of personality and social development. The primary evolved function of threat activation is to motivate "at-risk" individuals to seek closer physical and/or psychological proximity to their attachment figures. As threatening events and distress terminate or abate, the attachment system becomes deactivated and attachment-relevant behavior (e.g., seeking proximity) subsides, permitting other behavioral systems once again to become activated by relevant motives and environmental cues.

Our knowledge regarding how these behavioral systems operate in relation to one another is still limited. What we currently know is that the attachment system becomes activated and tends to suppress the operation of many other systems (e.g., exploration, mating/sexuality) when individuals feel threatened. The attachment system, however, most likely plays an important role in triggering and/or facilitating the operation of other systems, especially the caregiving system (in adult–child and adult–adult attachment relationships) and the mating/sexuality system (in adult–adult attachment relationships). In adults, for instance, attachment processes probably facilitate the emotional bonds necessary to keep parents together long enough to raise their children, which may have been necessary for survival in ancestral environments (Fletcher, Simpson, Campbell, & Overall, 2015; Zeifman & Hazan, 2016).

Principle C: The Attachment System and the Caregiving System Are Interrelated

This principle involves the special connection between the attachment and caregiving behavioral systems, which largely determines whether infants and adults form secure or insecure attachment patterns with their attachment figures. Although most children and adults become attached to their caregivers/attachment figures, not all individuals become securely attached (Bowlby, 1956). According to attachment theory, the types of bonds that children and adults form depend on the type, quantity, and quality of caregiving they have received from prior caregivers/attachment figures.

Bowlby's (1944) observations of maladjusted youth led him to conjecture that disruptions in the early caregiver–child relationship often generate certain predispositions that affect a person's later life outcomes. Children, for example, can detect whether and the degree to which their caregivers are sensitive, responsive, and attentive to their needs, particularly when they are upset. According to the *sensitivity hypothesis,* attachment-relevant behavior develops primarily in response to the type and quality of early care received, with higher-quality and more consistent early care usually resulting in attachment security, and with lower-quality and/or more inconsistent care generating attachment insecurity.

The sensitivity hypothesis has been supported by meta-analytic evidence (e.g., De Wolff & van IJzendoorn, 1997) and holds true across several different cultures and social contexts, affirming Bowlby's original claims (see Mesman, van IJzendoorn, & Sagi-Schwartz, 2016). Although the exact behaviors that constitute sensitive care vary somewhat from culture to culture, the function and outcome of these behaviors is the same cross-culturally. Sensitive care, however, does not always take the same form or have the same impact on all children within the same culture (Fearon & Belsky, 2016). Variability exists due to the specific needs, motives, and dispositions of each child, which may affect what the optimal form of caregiving may be.

Inspired by Bowlby, Mary Ainsworth (1967) conducted the first series of naturalistic behavioral observations by examining how different caregiving behaviors were associated with different attachment-related motivations. Based on these observations, she and colleagues developed the Strange Situation procedure to evaluate young children's patterns of attachment with their mothers (Ainsworth et al., 1978). The Strange Situation consists of two brief separations and reunions during which the caregiver and a stranger enter and leave the room, while the child's reactions to these events are observed and coded. The absence of an at-tachment figure, coupled with the presence of a stranger, should be alarming to children in the age range (12–18 months) for which the Strange Situation was developed.

Four behavioral patterns are witnessed in the Strange Situation (Ainsworth et al., 1978). Secure (Type B) infants explore and are comfortable with the stranger when their caregiver is present, become upset when the caregiver leaves, and are rather easily and quickly calmed when the caregiver returns to the room. Anxious–avoidant (Type A) infants typically do not explore the room (regardless of the caregiver's or the stranger's presence or absence) and display minimal visible affective changes when their caregiver leaves or reenters the room. Anxious–ambivalent (Type C) infants are often distressed before separation from their caregiver, become even more upset when their caregiver leaves the room, and often fail to calm down when their caregiver returns. Disorganized (Type D) infants exhibit strange, inconsistent, and sometimes bizarre behaviors in the Strange Situation, which can include signs of fear, odd movements, freezing, or other unusual reactions when they are separated from or reunited with their caregiver (see Main & Hesse, 1990).

Each of these attachment patterns has distinct caregiving origins (Ainsworth et al., 1978). Secure attachment typically develops when children receive consistent, warm, and responsive care from their caregivers. Anxious–avoidant attachment usually develops when children receive rejecting and/or absent care from their caregivers. Anxious–ambivalent attachment often develops when children receive inconsistent or mixed care from their caregivers. And disorganized attachment develops when children are exposed to frightening, strange, or unusual parenting often associated with abuse or their caregiver's clinical disorders (Lyons-Ruth & Jacobvitz, 2016). These latter three forms of attachment represent types of attachment insecurity.

A number of unanswered questions still exist. For example, how are the caregiving and attachment systems interrelated? Some research suggests they may operate in a bidirectional fashion to one another (Fearon & Belsky, 2016), but further research is needed to determine the exact nature of this bidirectional association.

Additionally, under what circumstances might attachment insecurity be more functional or adaptive than attachment security? One possibility is that the behavioral tendencies that define insecurity might be more adaptive in harsh or unpredictable environments in which resources are either limited or highly variable, other people cannot be trusted, and watching out for one's best interests is necessary (Szepsenwol & Simpson, 2019). Our knowledge of the unique ways in which avoidance, anxiety, and disorganization might be adaptive in specific environments and social situations is negligible. Furthermore, precisely how does security protect or buffer people when separations from their attachment figures occur, and what are the long-term effects on health, well-being, and social functioning? Although some researchers are beginning to address this important issue (e.g., Sbarra & Coan, 2017), our understanding remains limited.

Principle D: Attachment Relationships Serve Three Functions—Proximity Seeking, Safe Haven, and Secure Base

The need to feel safe and secure is one of the most fundamental human needs (Bowlby, 1969/1982). Indeed, both children and adults need to feel safe, with some amount of "felt security" (Sroufe & Waters, 1977) before they can engage in and benefit from other important life tasks such as exploring, playing, and affiliating with others. Individuals who are effective attachment figures typically foster these outcomes by providing and facilitating three essential functions, especially when their children or partners feel distressed: remaining open to proximity seeking, providing a safe and comforting haven from threats and stressors, and providing a secure base from which their partners can reengage with the world.

The first function, seeking proximity to one's attachment figure, promotes safety and protection, a tendency that most likely enhanced the survival of children and perhaps adults during evolutionary history (Bowlby, 1969/1982). Proximity seeking is achieved by establishing closer physical contact with one's attachment figure or via internalized perceptions of greater contact/closeness to him or her, both of which begin the process of increasing the sense of felt security. According to attachment theorists (e.g., Bowlby, 1969/1982; Mikulincer & Shaver, 2003), proximity seeking is the primary default strategy of the attachment behavioral system, and most people—including adults—resist unnecessary or prolonged separations from their primary attachment figures (Fraley & Shaver, 1998).

In young children, proximity seeking manifests in attempts to gain closer physical proximity to one's primary caregiver(s). Children do this with signaling behaviors (e.g., distressed facial expressions), aversive behaviors (e.g., crying), approach behaviors (e.g., moving toward the caregiver), or contact maintenance behaviors (e.g., clinging to the caregiver). Most adults also seek closer contact with their attachment figures (typically their romantic partners), particularly when their attachment system is activated (Collins & Feeney, 2004). However, the way in which adults seek proximity differs from that of children, particularly when threat/stress is at lower levels. Adult proximity seeking typically involves direct forms of verbal communication in which the distressed adult's specific needs, concerns, or desires are expressed to their attachment figures (Feeney & Woodhouse, 2016).

Once proximity has been achieved, the safe haven function becomes relevant. Attachment figures who provide a safe haven help their distressed partners down-regulate to assuage their negative emotions and thoughts. Attachment figures who effectively enact the safe haven function support their partners by allowing them to return to and remain in the relationship in order to receive comfort, reassurance, and assistance until their distress attenuates (Bowlby, 1988; Collins & Feeney, 2000). They accomplish this by providing the specific type and amount of support their partners actually need, taking into account the current situation, their partners' goals, wishes, concerns, and the need to express their feelings, after which they adjust their caregiving behaviors accordingly (Bowlby, 1988). Less sensitive and less responsive attachment figures, on the other hand, neglect, fail to understand, or are either overinvolved or out of synchrony with their distressed partners' actual needs (Kunce & Shaver, 1994). The net result of effective safe haven behavior is the further restoration of felt security (Feeney & Collins, 2014).

Unlike that for young children, an adult's safe haven behavior can involve mental representations of his or her supportive attachment figure. Studies in which threat is experimentally induced have revealed that these manipulations automatically trigger mental representations of romantic partners who serve the safe haven function. When this happens, adults report less negative affect, even though their romantic partners (attachment figures) are not physically present (e.g., Mikulincer, Gillath, & Shaver, 2002).

After distressed partners have been soothed, the third function—providing a secure base—helps calmed partners to reengage once again in other life tasks. A secure base promotes autonomy, growth, and competence, eventually resulting in better self-regulation, greater well-being, and positive psychosocial development (Feeney & Woodhouse, 2016). Attachment figures who effectively serve as a secure base for their partners remain available, do not interfere with their partners' explorations, and actively encourage such explorations (Bowlby, 1988; Feeney & Thrush, 2010). Those who are ineffective do not notice or disregard their partners' goals, needs, and feelings, intrude on their partners' explorations, discourage and impede them, and tend to be unsupportive or unhelpful.

In young children, secure base behaviors include looking back or "checking in" to ensure their caregiver's presence as they explore their surroundings. As children age, they start venturing farther from their attachment figures, particularly those who provide a solid, secure base. In adults, secure base behavior involves attachment figures providing support for partners' important needs, plans, and goals, and responding in a timely, responsive, and sensitive manner when partners embark on new or challenging life tasks (Waters & Cummings, 2000). In general, more effective proximity-seeking, safe haven, and secure base behaviors tend to be enacted by attachment figures and distressed partners (both children and adults) who are securely rather than insecurely attached (Feeney & Woodhouse, 2016).

At present, a few basic questions remain unanswered. For example, how are proximity-seeking, safe haven, and secure base functions "transferred" from parents (or early attachment figures) to adult romantic partners? To what extent do the behaviors of one's parents or early attachment figures impact this process, and to what extent do the novel characteristics of adult attachment figures override these earlier experiences (see Zeifman & Hazan, 2016)? Moreover, how does the attachment security of the distressed person or his or her attachment figure facilitate better, more effective exploration and the accomplishment of other important life tasks in adulthood? These questions need to be answered.

Principle E: Attachment Figures, and the Type of Attachment to Them, Shape Internal Working Models

Bowlby (1969/1982, p. 81) introduced the concept of "internal working models" to describe a mental representational system that is dynamic, allowing individuals to conduct "small-scale experiments within the head" in order to understand and predict behavior, particularly that of their attachment figures. *Internal working models* are aggregate representations of a person's entire life history of attachment-relevant experiences (Sroufe, Egeland, Carlson, & Collins, 2005). They capture preverbal and early language experiences, along with conscious and unconscious attitudes, emotions, cognitions, beliefs, and expectations (Collins, Guichard, Ford, & Feeney, 2004). In essence, working models encapsulate an individual's attachment-related thoughts about, feelings toward, and experiences with their attachment figures.

No systematic theory of internal working models exists in Bowlby's writings (Bretherton & Munholland, 2016), but he posited several things that had to be true for working models to fulfill some basic functions in attachment relationships. Bowlby theorized the following functions, among others: Working models (1) store, manipulate, and update information to help individuals decide how to react and behave in specific situations (Bowlby, 1988); (2) facilitate appraisals of others, oneself, and the world more broadly (Bowlby, 1969/1982); (3) identify attachment figures and form expectations about their availability and responsiveness (Bowlby, 1988); (4) allow for conscious and unconscious applications of stored information in attachment-related situations (Bowlby, 1969/1982); and (5) provide a means of internalization, such that the working model becomes part of one's self-concept and identity (Bowlby, 1988).

According to Bowlby (1969/1982; 1973), working models have two parts: (1) a model of the self and (2) a model of specific attachment figures and attachment figures in general. These have both evaluative and internal structural components. The models of self and specific attachment figure(s) or attachment figures in general can be positive or negative. Each of these models can also be either internally consistent or incoherent, and individuals may have more than one working model of the same person (Bowlby, 1980). When they exist, multiple models typically consist of a simple, rudimentary model developed in infancy or early childhood and a later model that is more fully articulated, more sophisticated, and often more accessible to conscious awareness. Bowlby believed that both working models were important because they guided behavior, thought, perceptions, and emotions. He conjectured that in some situations, earlier, more primitive models could be more influential than later ones (Bowlby, 1980).

A major question about working models is how internally consistent they tend to be. Models of the self and other (i.e.., the attachment figure) can be incongruent, especially if the attachment figure's behavior is inconsistent or unpredictable. Models may also be incongruent if their basic components—what individuals experience, what they are told by attachment figures, and what they learn from other people—are inconsistent with one another. For example, Bowlby (1973) wrote that a child might be labeled a "bad child" by his or her mother based on behavior of which the mother disapproved. However, the child might also be told that the mother loves the child dearly, despite his or her badness. From this, the child might learn that he or she is bad, but not so bad as to be unlovable. The behavior of this "loving" mother, however, might actually be quite unloving, resulting in the storage of inconsistent information between the mother's words and the child's actual experiences with her. Bowlby also believed that many young children find it

difficult to dismiss or ignore what their attachment figures tell them. Thus, in cases like these, young children, because they have more limited cognitive abilities than adults, may find themselves with irreconcilable information, resulting in highly incongruent working models. Bowlby hypothesized that such children often develop uneasy, unstable compromises in an attempt to reconcile such conflicting information. Finally, working models can also be incoherent because attachment figures teach their children not to think independently. For example, parents may teach their children that they cannot view their parents' actions objectively, but simply must accept what their parents say about themselves (Bowlby, 1973). Incongruent models make the world less predictable and less explainable, making decisions about how to behave within relationships more difficult, sometimes even contributing to clinical disorders (Liotti, 1992). For example, multiple images of attachment figures can make it difficult to decide how to behave in their presence. As another example, dissociation is associated with contradictions within the self system.

Working models underlie attachment patterns in children. As children develop into adolescents and adults, these attachment patterns are replaced by attachment orientations. There are two primary adult attachment orientations: anxiety and avoidance. The adult attachment literature has covered them extensively, particularly in conjunction with relationship conflict, caregiving and support, relationship satisfaction, emotion regulation, stress, and depression (e.g., Mikulincer & Shaver, 2016). A third attachment orientation, disorganized attachment, is less understood and is just beginning to be studied (Paetzold, Rholes, & Kohn, 2015). It is important to note that attachment orientations reflect habitual patterns of behavior, preferences, goals, fears, and so forth, that one brings to relationships. Although attachment orientations are a reflection of working models, they should not be confused with them, even though they are often discussed somewhat interchangeably in some of the attachment literature. An understanding of working models is essential to a broader understanding of the attachment system. The precise workings and structure of working models have not been examined directly. Fraley (2007), however, has begun to lay the groundwork for a theory of how working models typically operate. Using a connectionist approach, Fraley suggests that working models operate across different interpersonal and social contexts that also allow for within-person variability across time. This approach provides clues regarding how and why multiple representations of attachment figures exist and may shift from being relationship-specific to more general (global) in nature. This approach also explains why working models tend to be rather stable over time but can also change in response to changing environments (see Principle F below). One strength of this approach is that early experiences tend to have a "privileged status" in the working model memory system, even if they recur rarely over time, which is in line with Bowlby's (1980) initial assumptions.

Other strengths of this approach include notions that (1) mental representations are based on an individual's own learning systems; (2) no a priori notions are needed about how general representations are constructed from relationship-specific ones because general (global) models emerge from a set of repeated, specific experiences; (3) behaviors can be contingently inconsistent over time, depending on context, which indicates that working models are more than merely a set of "if–then" scripts (as has commonly been believed; Mikulincer & Shaver, 2016); and (4) the organization of working models is based on characteristics of the relationship partner rather than his or her relationship status. If, for example, a new relationship partner resembles an individual's mother, working model organization may be based on the shared characteristics of mother and partner instead of the category "relationship partner" (Fraley, 2007).

Several important issues still need to be investigated, and the connectionist approach offers insights to address them. These include determining how working models differ from general schemas or sets of scripts, how new information is incorporated over time and how much weight is given to particular experiences, how working models tend to transform from early infancy and childhood into adulthood, and how close the information that organizes working models must be to actual attachment experiences in order to influence working models.

Principle F: The Attachment System Is Operative from "the Cradle to the Grave"

Bowlby (1979, p. 129) believed that attachment processes are relevant from "the cradle to the grave." There are several things this phrase could mean. One is that early attachment experiences have enduring effects. Another is that proximity seeking and other attachment behaviors are just as relevant to older people as they are to infants, children, and younger adults because the attachment system continues to operate similarly throughout life. Yet another is that working models and attachment orientations, once formed, remain relatively constant across the lifespan. The issue of temporal stability is particularly relevant to attachment theory because the theory maintains that although change in working models and attachment orientations is possible, it is the exception rather than the rule (Bowlby, 1980).

According to the theory, attachment orientations and working models should be relatively constant and stable over time (the stability hypothesis). Consistent with this view, studies of adult romantic attachment reveal that attachment orientations show fairly high test–retest correlations (e.g., .60–.80 over varying lengths of time; Stern et al., 2018). Correlations by themselves, however, do not provide the best evidence for or against stability. There are two possible ways in which change in attachment orientations can occur. One possibility is known as the revisionist model, and the other is the prototype model. According to the revisionist model, environmental changes (e.g., the development of a new relationship or the demise of an old one) affect and sometimes change working models and attachment orientations, often gradually over time. In test–retest studies, the longer the period between tests, the more opportunity for environmental events to influence attachment orientations. Thus, there should be less similarity (i.e., a lower correlation) between testing sessions. The prototype model, in contrast, suggests there is an unchanging attachment prototype underlying attachment orientations that limits the amount of change that can occur. If so, test–retest correlations should remain at similar levels across time, no matter how long the intervals between testing. Current empirical evidence favors the prototype model

(Fraley, Vicray, Brumbaugh, & Roisman, 2011; Jones et al., 2018), which implies that, absent a change in the underlying prototype, changes in attachment orientations are likely to be superficial or temporary, and they will eventually revert to prototypical levels.

Although prototypes limit change, they do not eliminate it. Bowlby (1973) proposed that change in attachment orientations occurs slowly and rather arduously (*the change hypothesis*). He stated:

> In general when new information clashes with established [working] models . . . an old model may be replaced by a new one. Nevertheless, much evidence suggests that we undertake such replacements only very reluctantly. . . . To dismantle a model which has played and is still playing a major part in our daily life and to replace it with a new one is a slow and arduous task. (Bowlby, 1973, pp. 230–231)

There are several reasons why replacement tends to be uncommon, slow, and difficult. One source of resistance to change is the tendency for new information to be accepted if it is consistent with existing perspectives and rejected if it is not (Lord, Ross, & Lepper, 1979). Another is the tendency to appraise new information in ways that make it seem consistent with old information, which also limits change. An additional relevant factor is that, with time, information processing becomes automated and less subject to conscious inspection, decreasing the likelihood that new information will be reflected upon and its inconsistency with old information will be noticed. Also relevant is Bowlby's (1980) notion that some attachment figures tell their children that they cannot view them (the parents) objectively, but must accept the parents as they present themselves (Bowlby, 1980, p. 56). When parents successfully do this, it is difficult for individuals to unlearn what they were taught and reflect on their attachment history and working models objectively.

Simpson, Rholes, Campbell, and Wilson (2003) tested Bowlby's idea that clashes between incoming information and information stored in working models may produce changes in working models. For example, when a highly avoidant person perceives that he or she is providing emotional support to the partner—a behavior that is incongruent with an avoidant attachment orientation—does the inconsistency between support giving and the cardinal features of avoidance weaken the avoidant working model, resulting in lower levels of avoidance? Simpson and colleagues found that, consistent with Bowlby's hypothesis, clashes between new, incoming information and old information stored in working models predicted changes in attachment orientations across a chronically stressful life event (the transition to parenthood).

Several other researchers have tested whether interpersonal and psychotherapeutic experiences motivate change. Kirkpatrick and Davis (1994), for example, found that the experience of divorce increased attachment insecurity, and that entry into a new relationship was associated with the growth of security (i.e., decreased avoidance). In a longitudinal study, Fraley, Roisman, Booth-LaForce, Owen, and Holland (2013) found that receiving nurturing maternal care and having a close childhood friendship increased security. In another longitudinal study, Chopik, Moors, and Edelstein (2014) documented that having a nurturing mother is associated with greater security across time. Conceptualizing psychopathology as a vulnerability factor for instability in adult attachment orientations, Davila, Burge, and Hammen (1997) found that psychopathology is related to larger changes in attachment orientations.

While informative, this literature has limitations. First, most studies reveal that positive relationship events are associated with increases in security, and vice versa. However, they have not sufficiently addressed how, why, or when this occurs. Questions of mediation and moderation have not received the attention they deserve. Second, past work has not examined the full lifespan of the changes that have been observed. Are changes deep and permanent, or are they superficial, eventually returning to baseline values over time? The evidence supporting the prototype model suggests that they may often be superficial.

Principle G: Attachment Security Is an Inner Resource That Facilitates Resilience; Attachment Insecurity Is a Vulnerability Associated with Poorer Outcomes

According to Bowlby, attachment security in early life prepares people to cope better with trauma by allowing them to be more resilient (*the competence hypothesis*; Bowlby, 1980; van IJzendoorn, 1990). Attachment insecurity, on the other hand, leads individuals to cope with the world's unpredictability by either "shrinking from it or by doing battle with it" (Bowlby, 1973, p. 208). Thus, Bowlby viewed attachment insecurity as a vulnerability or risk factor for poorer life outcomes, including depression (1980), anxiety disorders (1973), and agoraphobia (which he viewed as an extension of separation anxiety; Bowlby, 1973).

In recent years, resilience has come to be viewed through the *"broaden-and-build" hypothesis* (Fredrickson, 2001), based on the notion that positive emotions, which provide emotional stability in times of stress, allow for a broadening of internal resources (e.g., skills, flexibility in coping) and an increased ability to use external resources via strong social connections (Sroufe et al., 2005). Frederickson's (2001) upward spiral model of the broaden-and-build hypothesis for resilience is bidirectional, allowing for the development of inner resources that permit reappraisal of past experiences, which can generate even greater resilience over time. Sroufe (2016) has tied Frederickson's ideas to attachment security, based on the notion that secure people are better able to recuperate from stress, cope with adversity, regulate negative emotions, rely on the support of others, and use adversity as an opportunity for personal growth. Additionally, highly secure individuals have positive views of themselves and others, along with greater positivity, which helps them be more hopeful and optimistic (Berant, Mikulincer, & Florian, 2001).

A considerable amount of research has verified Bowlby's belief that attachment insecurity is associated with poorer life outcomes, including both internalizing and externalizing behaviors. Social and clinical psychologists have examined psychopathologies such as depression, social anxiety disorder, generalized anxiety disorder, posttraumatic stress disorder (PTSD), eating disorders, agoraphobia, borderline personality disorder, and dissociation, as well as general reactions to stress, to determine their linkages to attachment orientations. More recently, psychosis and obsessive–compulsive disorders also have been shown to be related to

attachment insecurity. Additionally, externalizing symptomatology, such as substance abuse and antisocial behaviors, have been linked to attachment insecurity (see Ein-Dor & Doron, 2016).

Most studies examining poor life outcomes and attachment insecurity are correlational and conducted on community samples. Conradi, Kamphuis, and de Jonge (2018) conducted one study that is noteworthy for its longitudinal design (7 years) and use of clinically diagnosed participants. They found that higher levels of attachment anxiety and avoidance were associated with higher severity of depression and lower perceptions of being symptom-free. Other studies reveal a positive association with attachment anxiety, but equivocal results for avoidance, perhaps due to the absence of important moderators. Similarly, anxiety disorders have been linked to attachment anxiety, but the connection for avoidance is less clear. Agoraphobia has been associated with anxiety in adulthood, as has borderline personality disorder in both community and clinical samples. Recent connections have also been established between attachment insecurity and coping with stress, dissociation, and schizophrenia (e.g., Fillo, Simpson, Rholes, & Kohn, 2015; Paetzold, Rholes, & Andrus, 2017).

Despite all this research, several issues still need to be explored. First, appropriate moderators of the connection between attachment orientations and poorer life outcomes are needed. This could help to resolve the equivocal findings for attachment avoidance. Second, understanding the mechanisms that link attachment insecurity to poorer life outcomes is important. For example, Kwon, Lee, and Kwon (2017) have shown that excessive reassurance seeking mediates the relation between anxiety and depression. Others (e.g., Shaver, Schachner, & Mikulincer, 2005) argue that excessive reassurance seeking is part of the anxiety construct itself. A distinct and viable mediating construct could be emotion dysregulation, which mediates the relation between attachment anxiety/avoidance and depression/generalized anxiety disorder (Marganska, Gallagher, & Miranda, 2013).

Finally, nearly all the data on resilience and vulnerability is correlational and cross-sectional. Longitudinal studies are needed to identify causal, explanatory pathways connecting security to resilience or vulnerability to insecurity. These models should include the possibility of bidirectional relationships in line with the broaden-and-build hypothesis.

Principle H: Individuals Experience a Specific Sequence of Reactions When Separated from or When They Lose Their Attachment Figures

Across many, if not all, human cultures (Rosenblatt, 2008) and myriad species (Archer, 1999), young, vulnerable children (as well as most adults) experience a series of reactions after being separated from their caregivers/attachment figures (Bowlby, 1980). Immediately following separation, young children (and especially adults) become disoriented and experience "numbness," which often is quickly followed by intense protest as individuals search for their missing caregiver/attachment figure. Bowlby conjectured that numbness alerts and directs an individual's attention to the caregiver's/attachment figure's absence. Following this, a period of protest during the initial phases of caregiver absence is a good strategy to promote survival (Archer, 1999), especially for young offspring in species that have developmentally immature, highly dependent young. In many instances, intense protest draws caregivers back to their young children who, during evolutionary history, would have been susceptible to injury or predation if left unattended.

If persistent protest fails to retrieve the caregiver/attachment figure, most young children and many adults enter a state of despair, during which their activity diminishes and they fall silent. From an evolutionary standpoint, despondency is a good second strategy to promote survival, especially in young, vulnerable children, because excessive movement could result in accident or injury, and loud, prolonged protests might draw predators. If protest fails to bring back the caregiver, the next best survival strategy is to disengage from actions that might increase the risk of self-inflicted harm or predation.

Over time, most young children and many adults who do not reunite with their caregivers/attachment figures experience a final stage—detachment/reorganization. During this phase,

individuals gradually begin to resume normal activities without their caregiver/attachment figure, resume exploring the environment, and become more self-reliant. According to Bowlby (1980), the function of detachment/reorganization is to come to terms with the loss, which facilitates the forging of new affectional bonds with subsequent caregivers/attachment figures. From the standpoint of evolution, detachment/reorganization helps individuals to reformulate representations of themselves and their lost caregiver/attachment figure, which helps them establish new attachment bonds with partners who can provide the attention, protection, and resources needed for survival (in children) and reproduction (in adults). Bowlby believed that these reactions to separation not only evolved via natural selection primarily to promote the survival of young, vulnerable children (see also Cassidy, 2016), but they also characterize adults who experience prolonged or permanent separations from their romantic partners (Parkes, 2006).

Bowlby (1980) did not view these stages as occurring in a rigid or fixed sequence. People can and do move between different stages, or they may experience a mixture of two stages within short periods of time (e.g., vacillating between protest and despair), depending on their attachment orientations and the circumstances of their separation or loss. Bowlby's key contribution was to identify the evolutionary functions and psychological experiences associated with each stage of the general grief/bereavement process (Fraley & Shaver, 2016).

It is also important to note that numbing (and the disorientation associated with it) is often more prolonged in adults than in young children. Protest and despair also tend to be expressed differently in children versus adults, and the process of detachment/reorganization is different due to the greater cognitive and inferential abilities of adults compared to young children.

Contrary to some claims, Bowlby (1980) believed that individuals retain attachment bonds with their former figures, even when they detach from them (Fraley & Shaver, 2016). During the detachment process, most people—especially older children and adults—reorganize their working models of their lost attachment figures by integrating their former partner's memory and continued psychological presence into their own revised identity, plans, and life story (Bowlby, 1980; Fraley & Shaver, 2016). Detachment, therefore, does not involve completely severing psychological ties to departed or deceased attachment figures.

A growing body of research has revealed that anxiously attached adults are more likely to experience prolonged or chronic grief/mourning following the loss of their romantic partners, as indexed by greater depression, anxiety, and prolonged grief symptoms. Some highly avoidant adults are inclined to experience the absence of grief/mourning and significantly less emotional disruption, whereas other highly avoidant adults experience greater dysfunction and more chronic problems in the aftermath of loss. Secure adults, who tend to be more well regulated, exhibit more normal patterns of grief/mourning (i.e., strong emotional distress early in the process, followed by gradual recovery), and they adjust better across time (Fraley & Shaver, 2016).

When individuals fail to move through and "resolve" the stages of grief, they may experience pathological mourning. Ten to 15% of people have such severe grief reactions (Bonanno, 2004), but most are resilient following major interpersonal losses (Fraley & Shaver, 2016; Parkes, 2006). Some highly avoidant people may not experience the stages of grief in the way that other people do because they may not form strong attachment bonds with their romantic partners, which means that their typically subdued reactions may not be pathological.

In summary, this attachment principle is pivotal because it is not only a hallmark feature of the attachment behavioral system, but it also ushers in the formation of new attachment bonds, both completing and restarting a cycle in which the other attachment principles once again become relevant. Several important questions, however, still need to be addressed. For example, little is known about detachment/reorganization, including how this process works, how long it takes to complete, whether cultural differences affect its expression, and how "detached" or "reorganized" children and adults must be to start forming strong, enduring attachment bonds with new attachment figures.

Principle I: The Attachment System Is Universal, Yet Also Culturally Dependent

The attachment system, which ostensibly evolved and should be universal, is affected by cultural events, norms, rules, and practices that can result in culturally specific forms of adaptation and social development. To date, the majority of attachment research in developmental psychology has focused on attachment processes and patterns in young children, primarily in Western cultures. While there is a growing body of attachment research on individuals raised in various non-Western cultures (see Mesman et al., 2016), we are just beginning to learn about them.

Most cross-cultural attachment research has examined four central attachment hypotheses: the *universality hypothesis* (when given an opportunity, virtually all infants become attached to one or more caregivers), the *normativity hypothesis* (most infants develop secure attachments, especially in stable, nonthreatening environments), the *sensitivity hypothesis* (attachment security is shaped by the quality of caregiving, particularly sensitivity and contingent responsiveness), and the *competence hypothesis* (secure attachment typically leads to more positive developmental outcomes).

Reviewing studies conducted in different cultures in Africa, East Asia, Latin America, and the Middle East, Mesman and colleagues (2016) conclude there is strong cross-cultural support for three of these hypotheses. Specifically, in virtually all of these cultures, almost all nonneurophysiologically impaired infants become attached to one or more caregivers, the majority of infants form secure attachments in nonthreatening environments, and attachment security is strongly tied to sensitive, responsive caregiving provided by attachment figures. There currently is less evidence bearing on the competence hypothesis because it has been tested less frequently. The available evidence, however, suggests there also may be a connection between early attachment security and more adaptive functioning later in life (e.g., Aviezer, Sagi, & van IJzendoorn, 2002; Gini, Oppenheim, & Sagi-Schwartz, 2007).

Additionally, there is a reasonable amount of variation both within and between cultures with respect to these outcomes. This is particularly true of outcomes associated with the sensitivity hypothesis. For example, young children raised in Japan, Indonesia, Israel, and several African cultures are somewhat more likely to develop anxious attachment patterns than young children raised in most Western cultures, where rates of the avoidance pattern tend to be slightly higher (Grossmann, Grossmann, Spangler, Suess, & Unzner, 1985; van IJzendoorn & Sagi-Schwartz, 2008). These cultural differences may be partly attributable to different parenting goals, expectations, and practices enacted in these cultures. In many non-Western cultures, parents strive to instill a sense of interdependence with and connections to others, whereas parents in many Western cultures place greater emphasis on fostering independence and autonomy in their children (Rothbaum, Weisz, Pott, Miyake, & Morelli, 2000).

What is most striking, however, is how similar the base rates of different attachment patterns tend to be across diverse cultures that have different practices. One likely reason for this is that distinctive parenting behaviors may serve similar or identical functions across different cultures (Bornstein, Cote, Haynes, Suwalsky, & Bakeman, 2012). Moreover, the amount of sensitive, responsive caregiving tends to be fairly similar across most (but not all) cultures, despite the fact it is expressed somewhat differently (e.g., Kartner, Keller, & Yovsi, 2010). When deviations from common base rates in attachment patterns are found, they can usually be explained by the unique parenting practices enacted within a specific culture.

In cultures in which there tend to be fewer stressors and more resources, relatively more children should be securely attached because they are more inclined to receive sensitive, responsive caregiving from their caregivers (Belsky, Steinberg, & Draper, 1991). Conversely, in cultures in which there is greater stress and fewer resources, relatively more children should be insecurely attached because they are more likely to receive poorer caregiving. Indeed, cross-cultural research on socioeconomically disadvantaged groups confirms that insecure attachment patterns are significantly more common among such groups (Mesman et al., 2016). This is another instance of the potential "adaptive value" of insecure working models

and behavioral tendencies within harsh or unpredictable environments, in which trusting and depending on others who may be less trustworthy or undependable could result in poorer long-term outcomes, including well-being (Main, 1990; Simpson & Belsky, 2016).

Cultures also differ in the norms and roles ascribed to different caregivers. Multiple caregivers or *alloparents* (e.g., aunts, uncles, grandparents) are common in many Asian and African cultures, most of which grant specific roles and responsibilities to each caregiver (Mesman et al., 2016). Children in these cultures frequently form attachment relationships with different caregivers but typically have a primary attachment figure to whom they turn, especially when distressed.

Less is known about how culture impacts attachment process and orientations in adults. Some research has addressed whether living in a collectivistic versus individualistic culture affects how individuals tend to fare, based on their attachment orientation. Collectivistic cultures emphasize the well-being of the group and maintaining social harmony, which generates strong adherence to group norms and making sacrifices for the good of the group (Hofstede, 1984). Individualistic cultures place greater importance on the independence and autonomy of each person in the group, which results in greater freedom to make decisions based on one's personal goals and preferences. Thus, people who have an avoidant orientation in a collectivistic culture should find themselves in a difficult position because their personal orientation (to be independent) should be at odds with the norms of their culture (to be interdependent). In a study comparing people in three cultures, Friedman and colleagues (2010) found that people who are avoidantly attached to their romantic partners experienced greater conflict, perceived less support and investment from their partners, and had poorer relationship satisfaction if they lived in Hong Kong (a collectivistic culture) than in the United States (an individualistic culture). In Mexico, which is an autonomous-relatedness culture between Hong Kong and the United States, avoidance was more strongly associated with lower relationship satisfaction, less perceived partner support, and greater relationship conflict than in the United States.

Several pressing cross-cultural questions remain unanswered. For instance, how are basic attachment processes, such as the ways in which attachment bonds form, are maintained, and dissolve, expressed in different cultures? What kinds of interpersonal experiences produce stability or change in people's attachment orientations across the lifespan in different cultures? And how do important, culturally specific norms and practices shape or alter the normative attachment processes discussed in the chapter?

Conclusion

In this chapter, we have reviewed the major key principles that have defined attachment theory and guided prior research. While doing so, we have highlighted some of the most central hypotheses, postulates, and ideas associated with each key principle. Additionally, we have proposed several novel and potentially fruitful directions in which future work on attachment processes might head. Our hope is that coverage of these essential features of attachment theory will help to spawn the next generation of research applying one of psychology's grandest and most powerful lifespan approaches to personality and social development from the cradle to the grave.

NOTE

1. We thank Ximena Arriaga, Mary Dozier, Judy Feeney, Chris Fraley, Omri Gillath, Sue Johnson, Gery Karantzas, Geoff MacDonald, Mario Mikulincer, Nikola Overall, Paula Pietromonaco, Glenn Roisman, and Alan Sroufe for their comments on key principles underlying attachment theory. Their expert insights and general consensus played an important role in the development of this chapter.

REFERENCES

Ainsworth, M. D. S. (1967). *Infancy in Uganda: Infant care and the growth of attachment.* Baltimore: Johns Hopkins University Press.

Ainsworth, M. D. S., Blehar, M., Waters, E., & Wall, S. (1978). *Patterns of attachment: A psychological study of the Strange Situation.* Hillsdale, NJ: Erlbaum.

Archer, J. (1999). *The nature of grief: The evolution and psychology of reactions to loss.* New York: Routledge.

Aviezer, O., Sagi, A., & van IJzendoorn, M. H. (2002). Collective sleeping for kibbutz children: An experiment in nature predestined to fail. *Family Process, 41,* 435–454.

Belsky, J., Steinberg, L., & Draper, P. (1991). Childhood experience, interpersonal development, and reproductive strategy: An evolutionary theory of socialization. *Child Development, 62,* 647–670.

Berant, E., Mikulincer, M., & Florian, V. (2001). Attachment style and mental health: A 1-year follow-up study of mothers of infants with congenital heart disease. *Personality and Social Psychology Bulletin, 27,* 956–968.

Birnbaum, G. E. (2016). Attachment and sexual mating: The joint operation of separate motivational systems. In J. Cassidy & P. R. Shaver (Eds.), *Handbook of attachment: Theory, research, and clinical applications* (3rd ed., pp. 464–483). New York: Guilford Press.

Bonanno, G. (2004). Loss, trauma, and human resilience: Have we underestimated the human capacity to thrive after extremely aversive events? *American Psychologist, 59,* 20–28.

Bornstein, M. H., Cote, L. R., Haynes, O. M., Suwalsky, J. T. D., & Bakeman, R. (2012). Modalities of infant–mother interaction in Japanese, Japanese American immigrant, and European American dyads. *Child Development, 83,* 2073–2088.

Bowlby, J. (1944). Forty-four juvenile thieves: Their characters and home life. *International Journal of Psycho-Analysis, 25,* 19–52, 107–127.

Bowlby, J. (1956). The growth of the independence in the young child. *Royal Society of Health Journal, 76,* 587–591.

Bowlby, J. (1973). *Attachment and loss: Vol. 2. Separation: Anxiety and anger.* New York: Basic Books.

Bowlby, J. (1979). *The making and breaking of affectional bonds.* London: Tavistock.

Bowlby, J. (1980). *Attachment and loss: Vol. 3. Loss: Sadness and depression.* New York: Basic Books.

Bowlby, J. (1982). *Attachment and loss: Vol. 1. Attachment* (2nd ed.). New York: Basic Books. (Original work published 1969)

Bowlby, J. (1988). *A secure base: Clinical applications of attachment theory.* London: Routledge.

Bretherton, I., & Munholland, K. A. (2016). The internal working model construct in light of contemporary neuroimaging research. In J. Cassidy & P. R. Shaver (Eds.), *Handbook of attachment: Theory, research, and clinical applications* (3rd ed., pp. 63–88). New York: Guilford Press.

Cassidy, J. (2016). The nature of the child's ties. In J. Cassidy & P. R. Shaver (Eds.), *Handbook of attachment: Theory, research, and clinical applications* (3rd ed., pp. 3–24). New York: Guilford Press.

Cassidy, J., & Shaver, P. R. (Eds.). (2016). *Handbook of attachment: Theory, research, and clinical applications* (3rd ed.). New York: Guilford Press.

Chopik, W. J., Moors, A. C., & Edelstein, R. S. (2014). Maternal nurturance predicts decreases in attachment avoidance in emerging adulthood. *Journal of Research in Personality, 53,* 47–53.

Collins, N. L., & Feeney, B. C. (2000). A safe haven: An attachment theory perspective on support seeking and caregiving in intimate relationships. *Journal of Personality and Social Psychology, 78,* 1053–1073.

Collins, N. L., & Feeney, B. C. (2004). Working models of attachment shape perceptions of social support: Evidence from experimental and observational studies. *Journal of Personality and Social Psychology, 87,* 363–383.

Collins, N. L., Guichard, A. C., Ford, M. B., & Feeney, B. C. (2004). Working models of attachment: New developments and emerging themes. In W. S. Rholes & J. A. Simpson (Eds.), *Adult attachment: Theory, research and clinical implications* (pp. 196–239). New York: Guilford Press.

Conradi, H. J., Kamphuis, J. H., & de Jonge, P. (2018). Adult attachment predicts the seven-year course of recurrent depression in primary care. *Journal of Affective Disorders, 225,* 160–166.

Darwin, C. (1859). *The origin of species by means of natural selection: Or, the preservation of favored races in the struggle for life.* London: John Murray.

Darwin, C. (1872). *The expression of the emotions in man and animals.* London: John Murray.

Davila, J., Burge, D., & Hammen, C. (1997). Why does attachment style change? *Journal of Personality and Social Psychology, 73,* 826–838.

De Wolff, M., & van IJzendoorn, M. H. (1997). Sensitivity and attachment: A meta-analysis on parental antecedents of infant attachment. *Child Development, 68,* 571–591.

Ein-Dor, T., & Doron, G. (2016). Extending the transdiagnostic model of attachment and psychopathology. *Frontiers in Psychology, 7,* 1–6.

Fearon, R. M. P., & Belsky, J. (2016). Precursors of attachment security. In J. Cassidy & P. R. Shaver (Eds.), *Handbook of attachment: Theory, research, and clinical applications* (3rd ed., pp. 291–313). New York: Guilford Press.

Feeney, B. C., & Collins, N. L. (2014). A theoretical perspective on the importance of social connections for thriving. In M. Mikulincer & P. R. Shaver (Eds.), *Mechanisms of social connection: From brain to group* (pp. 291–314). Washington, DC: American Psychological Association.

Feeney, B. C., & Thrush, R. L. (2010). Relationship influences on exploration in adulthood: The characteristics and function of a secure base. *Journal of Personality and Social Psychology, 98,* 57–76.

Feeney, B. C., & Woodhouse, S. S. (2016). Caregiving. In J. Cassidy & P. R. Shaver (Eds.), *Handbook of attachment: Theory, research, and clinical applications* (3rd ed., pp. 827–851). New York: Guilford Press.

Fillo, J., Simpson, J. A., Rholes, W. S., & Kohn, J. L. (2015). Dads doing diapers: Individual and relational outcomes associated with the division of childcare across the transition to parenthood. *Journal of Personality and Social Psychology, 108,* 298–316.

Fletcher, G. J. O., Simpson, J. A., Campbell, L., & Overall, N. C. (2015). Pair-bonding, romantic love, and evolution: The curious case of *Homo sapiens. Perspectives on Psychological Science, 10,* 20–36.

Fraley, R. C. (2007). A connectionist approach to the organization and continuity of working models of attachment. *Journal of Personality, 75,* 1157–1180.

Fraley, R. C., Roisman, G. I., Booth-LaForce, C., Owen, M. T., & Holland, A. S. (2013). Interpersonal and genetic origins of adult attachment styles: A longitudinal study from infancy to early adulthood. *Journal of Personality and Social Psychology, 104,* 817–838.

Fraley, R. C., & Shaver, P. R. (1998). Airport separations: A naturalistic study of adult attachment dynamics in separating couples. *Journal of Personality and Social Psychology, 75,* 1198–1212.

Fraley, R. C., & Shaver, P. R. (2016). Attachment, loss, and grief: Bowlby's views, new developments, and current controversies. In J. Cassidy & P. R. Shaver (Eds.), *Handbook of attachment: Theory, research, and clinical applications* (3rd ed., pp. 40–62). New York: Guilford Press.

Fraley, R. C., Vicray, A. M., Brumbaugh, C. C., & Roisman, G. I. (2011). Patterns of stability in adult attachment: An empirical test of two models of continuity and change. *Journal of Personality and Social Psychology, 101,* 974–992.

Fredrickson, B. L. (2001). The role of positive emotions in positive psychology: The broaden-and-build theory of positive emotions. *American Psychologist, 56,* 218–226.

Friedman, M., Rholes, W. S., Simpson, J. A., Bond, M. H., Diaz-Loving, R., & Chan, C. (2010). Attachment avoidance and the cultural fit hypothesis: A cross-cultural investigation. *Personal Relationships, 17,* 107–126.

Gini, M., Oppenheim, D., & Sagi-Schwartz, A. (2007). Negotiation styles in mother–child narrative co-constructions in middle childhood: Associations with early attachment. *International Journal of Behavioral Development, 31,* 149–160.

Grossmann, K., Grossmann, K. E., Spangler, G., Suess, G., & Unzner, L. (1985). Maternal sensitivity and newborns' orientation responses as related to quality of attachment in northern Germany. *Monographs of the Society for Research in Child Development, 50*(1–2, Serial No. 209), 233–257.

Hofstede, G. (1984). *Culture's consequences: International differences in work-related values.* Newbury Park, CA: SAGE.

Jones, J. D., Fraley, R. C., Ehrlich, K. B., Stern, J. A., Lejuez, D. W., Shaver, P. R., & Cassidy, J. (2018). Stability of attachment style in adolescence: An empirical test of alternative developmental processes. *Child Development, 89,* 871–880.

Kartner, J., Keller, H., & Yovsi, R. D. (2010). Mother–infant interaction during the first 3 months: The emergence of culture-specific contingency patterns. *Child Development, 81,* 540–554.

Kirkpatrick, L. A., & Davis, K. E. (1994). Attachment style, gender, and relationship stability: A longitudinal analysis. *Journal of Personality and Social Psychology, 66,* 502–512.

Kunce, L. J., & Shaver, P. R. (1994). An attachment-theoretical approach to caregiving in romantic relationships. In K. Bartholomew & D. Perlman (Eds.), *Advances in personal relationships* (Vol. 5, pp. 205–237). London: Jessica Kingsley.

Kwon, H., Lee, J. S., & Kwon, J. H. (2017). Interpersonal mediating mechanism underlying insecure attachment and depression in people with major depressive disorder. *Journal of Social and Clinical Psychology, 36,* 64–86.

Liotti, G. (1992). Disorganized/disoriented attachment in the etiology of the dissociative disorders. *Dissociation: Progress in the Dissociative Disorders, 5,* 196–204.

Lord, C., Ross, L., & Lepper, M. (1979). Biased assimilation and attitude polarization: The effect of prior theories on subsequently considered evidence. *Journal of Personality and Social Psychology, 37,* 2098–2109.

Lyons-Ruth, K., & Jacobvitz, D. (2016). Attachment disorganization from infancy to adulthood: Neurobiological correlates, parenting contexts, and pathways to disorder. In J. Cassidy & P. R. Shaver (Eds.), *Handbook of attachment: Theory, research, and clinical applications* (3rd ed., pp. 667–695). New York: Guilford Press.

Main, M. (1990). Cross-cultural studies of attachment organization: Recent studies, changing methodologies, and the concept of conditional strategies. *Human Development, 33,* 48–61.

Main, M., & Hesse, E. (1990). Parents' unresolved traumatic experiences are related to infant disorganized attachment status: Is frightened and/or frightening parental behavior the linking mechanism? In M. T. Greenberg, D. Cicchetti, & E. M. Cummings (Eds.), *Attachment in the preschool years: Theory, research, and intervention* (Vol. 1, pp. 161–182). Chicago: University of Chicago Press.

Marganska, A., Gallagher, M., & Miranda, R. (2013). Adult attachment, emotion dysregulation, and symptoms of depression and generalized anxiety disorder. *American Journal of Orthopsychiatry, 83,* 131–141.

Marvin, R. S., Britner, P. A., & Russell, B. S. (2016). Normative development: The ontogeny of attachment in childhood. In J. Cassidy & P. R. Shaver (Eds.), *Handbook of attachment: Theory, research, and clinical applications* (3rd ed., pp. 273–290). New York: Guilford Press.

Mesman, J., van IJzendoorn, M. H., & Sagi-Schwartz, A. (2016). Cross-cultural patterns of attachment. In J. Cassidy & P. R. Shaver (Eds.), *Handbook of attachment: Theory, research, and clinical applications* (3rd ed., pp. 852–877). New York: Guilford Press.

Mikulincer, M., Gillath, O., & Shaver, P. R. (2002). Activation of the attachment system in adulthood: Threat-related primes increase the accessibility of mental representations of attachment figures. *Journal of Personality and Social Psychology, 83,* 881–895.

Mikulincer, M., & Shaver, P. R. (2003). The attachment behavioral system in adulthood: Activation, psychodynamics, and interpersonal processes. In M. P. Zanna (Ed.), *Advances in experimental social psychology* (Vol. 35, pp. 53–152). New York: Academic Press.

Mikulincer, M., & Shaver, P. R. (2016). *Attachment in adulthood* (2nd ed.). New York: Guilford Press.

Paetzold, R. L., Rholes, W. S., & Andrus, J. L. (2017). A Bayesian analysis of the link between disorganized attachment and dissociative symptoms. *Personality and Individual Differences, 107,* 17–22.

Paetzold, R. L., Rholes, W. S., & Kohn, J. L. (2015). Disorganized attachment in adulthood: Theory, measurement, and implications for romantic relationships. *Review of General Psychology, 19,* 146–156.

Parkes, C. M. (2006). *Love and loss: The roots of grief and its complications.* New York: Taylor & Francis.

Rosenblatt, P. C. (2008). Grief across cultures: A review and research agenda. In M. S. Stroebe, R. O. Hansson, H. Schut, & W. Stroebe (Eds.), *Handbook of bereavement research and practice: Advances in theory and intervention* (pp. 207–222). Washington, DC: American Psychological Association.

Rothbaum, F., Weisz, J., Pott, M., Miyake, K., & Morelli, G. (2000). Attachment and culture: Security in the United States and Japan. *American Psychologist, 55,* 1093–1104.

Sbarra, D. A., & Coan, J. A. (2017). Divorce and health: Good data in need of better theory. *Current Opinion in Psychology, 13,* 91–95.

Shaver, P. R., Schachner, D. A., & Mikulincer, M. (2005). Attachment style, excessive reassurance seeking, relationship processes, and depression. *Personality and Social Psychology Bulletin, 31,* 343–359.

Simpson, J. A., & Belsky, J. (2016). Attachment theory within a modern evolutionary framework. In J. Cassidy & P. R. Shaver (Eds.), *Handbook of attachment: Theory, research, and clinical applications* (3rd ed., pp. 91–116). New York: Guilford Press.

Simpson, J. A., & Rholes, W. S. (2012). Adult attachment orientations, stress, and romantic relationships. In P. Devine & A. Plant (Eds.), *Advances in experimental social psychology* (Vol. 45, pp. 279–328). San Diego, CA: Academic Press.

Simpson, J. A., Rholes, W. S., Campbell, L., & Wilson, C. L. (2003). Changes in attachment orientations across the transition to parenthood. *Journal of Experimental Social Psychology, 39,* 317–331.

Sroufe, L. A. (2016). The place of attachment in development. In J. Cassidy & P. R. Shaver (Eds.), *Handbook of attachment: Theory, research, and clinical applications* (3rd ed., pp. 997–1011). New York: Guilford Press.

Sroufe, L. A., Egeland, B., Carlson, E., & Collins, W. A. (2005). *The development of the person: The Minnesota Study of Risk and Adaptation from Birth to Adulthood.* New York: Guilford Press.

Sroufe, L. A., & Waters, E. (1977). Attachment as an organizational construct. *Child Development, 48,* 1184–1199.

Stern, J. A., Fraley, R. C., Jones, J. D., Gross, J. T., Shaver, P. R., & Cassidy, J. (2018). Developmental processes across the first two years of parenthood: Stability and change in adult attachment style. *Developmental Psychology, 54,* 975–988.

Szepsenwol, O., & Simpson, J. A. (2019). Attachment within life history theory: An evolutionary perspective of individual differences in attachment. *Current Opinion in Psychology, 25,* 65–70.

van IJzendoorn, M. H. (1990). Developments in cross-cultural research on attachment: Some methodological notes. *Human Development, 33,* 3–9.

van IJzendoorn, M. H., & Sagi-Schwartz, A. (2008). Cross-cultural patterns of attachment: Universal and contextual dimensions. In J. Cassidy & P. R. Shaver (Eds.), *Handbook of attachment: Theory, research, and clinical applications* (2nd ed., pp. 880–905). New York: Guilford Press.

Waters, E., & Cummings, E. M. (2000). A secure base from which to explore close relationships. *Child Development, 71,* 164–172.

Zeifman, D. M., & Hazan, C. (2016). Pair bonds as attachments: Mounting evidence in support of Bowlby's hypothesis. In J. Cassidy & P. R. Shaver (Eds.), *Handbook of attachment: Theory, research, and clinical applications* (3rd ed., pp. 416–434). New York: Guilford Press.

CHAPTER 13

Relational Motives

Harry T. Reis

Few aphorisms are as timeworn as "humans are social animals." Yet packed into this undeniable truth is an abundance of assumptions, propositions, and questions that have preoccupied philosophers, political and religious leaders, novelists, poets, and scientists for centuries. In the past 100 or so years, a scholarly discipline has emerged that accepts this assertion as a starting point and uses empirical methods to better understand its roots, mechanisms, and implications. That discipline is, of course, social psychology, the subject matter of this volume (for historical reviews, see Jahoda, 2007; Kruglanski & Stroebe, 2012; Reis, 2019).

Although the social world influences our behavior in many and diverse ways, in this chapter I posit more precisely as fundamental the ongoing relationships in which most human activity is carried out (Reis, Collins, & Berscheid, 2000). From birth to the end of life, our associations with other people, especially significant others, profoundly affect our thoughts, feelings, activities, and well-being. In spite of this reality, and perhaps ironically, theories in social psychology do not always account for the relationship context of behavior. In this chapter, I offer a framework for such an accounting. This framework begins with the idea that human behavior often depends on who else is involved in a situation, and how one's relationship with that person (or those persons) influences our perceptions, preferences, and actions. These latter attributes, in turn, depend on people's motives with respect to their interaction partners. For this reason, a full understanding of relational motives is essential to most, if not all, theoretical models of the impact of situational factors on human behavior.

To illustrate, consider the following simple example: How might Paul decide which new car to buy? As a young man, if he seeks to impress his friends about his dashing personality, Paul might prefer a sleek Mazda Miata, but if his desired image is more along the lines of a New Age consciousness, he might instead opt for a Tesla Model 3. Later in life, as a parent of young children, when he needs a vehicle that can transport himself, his partner, and his five children, Paul might choose a commodious SUV. Still later in life, when Paul and his partner are saving for retirement, he might favor a well-preserved, preowned Toyota Camry. Or, if Paul wishes to staunchly assert his individualism, he might ignore all relational and practical considerations and instead purchase the Mustang convertible he has coveted since childhood. In each of these instances, Paul's choice follows from his situation-specific, relationship-relevant goals.

In this chapter I review general theories and specific examples describing the influence of relationship motives on social behavior. The chapter begins with a brief explanation of why relational motives matter for a full understanding human behavior, emphasizing the role of interdependence. This is followed by an overview of a general conceptual framework for specifying and integrating the various relational motives that existing research has identified. Next, I review several prominent relational motives from the literature, namely, those motives that apply to close dyadic relationships, such as romantic and family relationships, and friendship. The chapter concludes with my brief commentary on the prospects of this framework for enhancing the depth and usefulness of social psychological theories.

Interdependence: Why Relational Motives Matter Broadly

Evolutionary psychologists have often asserted that sociality embodies humankind's key adaptive advantage. For example, Berscheid (2003, p. 37) observed, "*Homo sapiens* is an extraordinarily tough animal to have survived on planet Earth for as long as it has. Our ancestors survived, and . . . we survive today, only with the aid of other humans." Buss and Kenrick (1998) summarized much of the work underlying this assertion by describing the adaptive benefits that, throughout evolutionary history, accrued to those individuals who could most effectively interact with others as they went about the central activities contributing to survival and reproduction. In their view, these benefits fostered the development of human neural architecture and regulatory systems designed to be social: that is, brains innately geared to deal with the problems and concerns inherent in living, working, and reproducing interdependently with others (Principle 1 in Table 13.1).

Nowhere is this idea explored more clearly than in interdependence theory (Kelley et al., 2003; Kelley & Thibaut, 1978; Rusbult & Van Lange, 1996; Thibaut & Kelley, 1959). Interdependence theory is based on the premise that in nearly all circumstances, the outcomes we obtain depend not solely on our individual actions but rather on the manner in which we coordinate those actions with the actions of others. This coordination depends on a process called *transformation of motivation*—namely, the way that people adjust their personal preferences to account for the preferences of interaction partners, as well as the requirements of the situation.

Figure 13.1 illustrates this process. Any interdependent situation—that is, any situation that calls for coordinated action between two persons—affords various potential behavioral options, each of which would yield certain outcomes for the individuals involved. When partners' personal preferences differ, some sort of reconciliation is needed. For example, suppose Deb and Sheila favor seeing different movies on their date night. To resolve their conflicting preferences, Deb might doggedly insist that they see her personal favorite, or defer to Sheila's wish, or advocate that they separately

TABLE 13.1. Four Key Principles Relevant to the Operation and Impact of Relational Motives

Principle 1: The human brain evolved to provide us with an extensive set of mechanisms for dealing with the problems and concerns inherent in living, working, and reproducing interdependently with others.

Principle 2: Success in carrying out many important tasks depends on the ability to efficiently and satisfyingly coordinate one's own actions with the actions of others implicated in the same task.

Principle 3: Relational motives—what each partner in an interdependent situation wishes to accomplish in that circumstance, at that moment in time, with regard to relevant partners—determine people's behavioral choices from among the various potential alternative behaviors afforded by a particular situation.

Principle 4: Differing adaptive mechanisms are most relevant to different types of relationships, and as such need to be understood in the context of the relationship domains in which they most often apply.

attend their own first choices. She might even suggest that they go bowling instead. The ultimate resolution among these alternatives—that is, the transformation of a personal preference into behavior that involves both partners—depends on each of their relational motives.[1] *Relational motives* refer to what the individual wishes to accomplish in that circumstance, at that moment in time, with that partner, construed broadly to include both personal and relational outcomes. In other words, the choice of a particular action from the various behavioral alternatives afforded in a given situation reflects each person's most salient relational motives. A key insight of interdependence theory is that these motives pertain to not only the choice of a movie but also the relational message conveyed by the process of resolving differing preferences: for example, asserting dominance in the relationship, striving to please one's partner, or eschewing conflict. In other words, transformations demonstrate partners' motives toward each other—how each partner in an interdependent situation prioritizes his or her own, relative to his or her partner's, preferences.

Extensive literatures support the general idea that the success of interdependent dyads and teams depends on their ability to transform discrepant personal preferences in a manner that fulfills two basic criteria: efficiently facilitating productive behavior while, at the same time, satisfying the needs (to a reasonable degree) of the persons involved (e.g., Steiner, 1972) (Principle 2 in Table 13.1). Of particular relevance in this chapter is the idea of *transactive goal dynamics* (Fitzsimons, Finkel, & vanDellen, 2015), which stipulates that in a close relationship, repeated instances of interdependence lead individuals to become a single regulatory system, such that both partners' goals and their pursuit of those goals become shared and indivisible. Transactive goal dynamics are evident in many common relationship phenomena. For example, couples generally pursue shared goals as a single entity, such as in having children, taking vacations, planning for retirement, and buying a house together. They may also internalize each other's more personal goals by "including the other in the self" (Aron, Aron, Tudor, & Nelson, 1991), so that a partner's goals acquire all

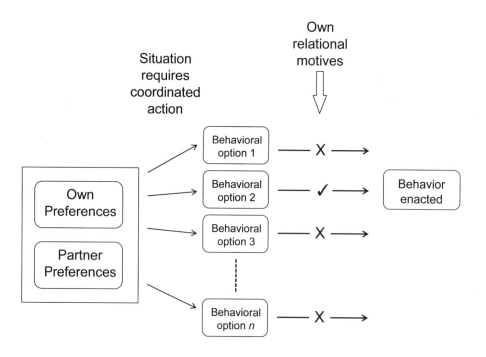

FIGURE 13.1. How motives drive behavioral choices.

or most of the valence and drive of one's own goals. Moreover, in such dyads, each partner's goal pursuit often involves assistance from the other, such as when partners are instrumental or emotionally supportive for accomplishing personal goals (cf., Orehek & Forest, 2016; Rusbult, Finkel, & Kumashiro, 2009), or when they share encoding, storage, and retrieval of knowledge, presumably to maximize efficiency and expertise (called *transactive memory*; Wegner, 1986). Importantly, in these examples, goal pursuit is properly conceptualized in interdependent terms, as Principle 2 articulates, because each party's actions differ from what either of them might have done alone, and both experience joy or disappointment, respectively, when the goal is fulfilled or unrealized.

The process of adopting shared perspectives on personal goals is fundamental to the concept of shared reality. Early in life, young children infer, then accept the goals and standards that their caregivers have for them, a process that Freud called *internalization* (Higgins, 2016). Such internalized self-guides are an early manifestation of shared reality, which Rossignac-Millon and Higgins (2018) describe as fundamental to establishing close adult relationships that satisfy epistemic needs to "make sense of the world together" (p. 66)—that is, to develop a vision of life and circumstances that encourages coordinated action, mutuality of affect (Rimé, 2009), and, ultimately, a shared sense of identity. Although I focus in this chapter on dyadic relationships, it bears noting that principles underlying the adoption and impact of shared reality apply broadly across many domains of social life, including work, politics, religion, and communities (Echterhoff & Higgins, 2018). Relational motives, in this larger sense, influence behavior in most life contexts.

Relational motives are those motives that affect our choices in interdependent situations and, as such, they are critical to coordinated goal pursuit (Principle 3 in Table 13.1). For example, in support situations, instrumentality presumes a partner's motive to be helpful. If a partner were instead motivated to undermine one's goal pursuit, the likelihood of success would be diminished, or at least progress would be impaired. In the conceptual language of interdependence theory, and as shown in Figure 13.1, situations offer

opportunities for partners to interact in various ways, but they do not mandate which of the situationally relevant options the partner will (or should) choose. Thus, for example, if Ron needs assistance editing his dissertation, his roommate Steve might decide to provide that help or, alternatively, he might opt not to help. Steve's choice depends in large part on his motives toward Ron, that is, whether he is motivated to be altruistic or unkind. Analogously, cooperative motives may lead classmates to help each other master a difficult assignment, whereas competitive motives might induce them to ignore their peers' predicament. In this way, then, relational motives help determine how partners respond to the interdependent situations in which they find themselves. It is important to recognize that many of the most influential motives activated in interdependent situations are relational motives, as I detail later in this chapter—motives that refer to the outcomes and individual wishes to achieve with respect to the other person(s) involved in that situation.

Because many of the phenomena studied in social psychology—and, for that matter, more generally, in the behavioral sciences—involve interdependence to some degree, relational motives have greater significance than is generally acknowledged. Reis and colleagues (2000) theorized that human behavior is pervasively affected by the relationship context in which those behaviors occur, and they exemplified this principle in the literatures on emotion, social cognition, and health (although it also applies diffusely in many other areas; see Clark, Lemay, & Reis, 2020; Reis, 2008). If so, the concept of relational motives, which in social psychology textbooks has traditionally been confined to a discrete chapter, may have considerably broader relevance throughout the field. In other words, whom one is with or thinking about, and one's motives toward him or her, may affect the operation of countless social psychological processes. I return to this idea in the concluding section of this chapter.

A Hierarchical Framework for Conceptualizing Relational Motives

Existing models describe relational motives with varying levels of specificity, which can engender conceptual confusion. To provide some clarity, this chapter adopts an organizational scheme suggested by Elliot's (1997, 2006; Elliot & Fryer, 2008) hierarchical model of motivation. At the highest level, this framework proposes the existence of particular *adaptive mechanisms* that regulate social behavior. These mechanisms, which appear in both human and nonhuman animals, albeit in somewhat different forms, play a fundamental role in shaping evolutionarily significant social behaviors.[2] Beginning an analysis of human relational motives at this level acknowledges the origin of certain motives in behaviors that had adaptive significance well before the human species emerged (Buss & Kenrick, 1998). More importantly, it highlights the critical role of social interaction in carrying out these important species-general tasks, as noted in Principle 2. To be more explicit: Specific social behaviors helped earlier organisms solve adaptive problems related to survival and reproduction, and these behaviors are precursors to the more complex relational manifestations that modern-day humans exhibit (Buss & Kenrick, 1998; Cosmides & Tooby, 1992; Eastwick, 2009). For example, many attributes of adult attachment relationships derive from simpler behaviors that are evident in other mammalian species (Bowlby, 1969/1982). Of course, these earlier-evolved mechanisms could not have been mediated by the kinds of higher mental processes that constitute existing theoretical models of human relational motives; rather, they should be considered rudimentary building blocks elaborated and extended through humans' more advanced cognitive and affective processes. Beginning at this level of analysis also provides important clues to the neurobiological mechanisms that underlie human relational behavior (Beckes & Coan, 2013; Bugental, 2000).

At the middle level of explanation, the hierarchical model describes valenced tendencies, or *motives,* that orient and energize people toward particular, relatively general, end states. They derive from higher-level adaptive mechanisms in the sense that they represent specific processes by which individuals strive to fulfill adaptive imperatives, but, at the same time, they are directed at (and explained by, as mediators) more distinct cognitive and affective processes. For example, the motive to be appreciated and accepted by relationship partners might be considered as a somewhat more specialized and complex representation of what happens when people seek to satisfy proximity needs (inasmuch as when one feels appreciated and accepted, one can anticipate adequate levels of proximity when sought). These midlevel mechanisms are characterized as motives both here and in the literature because they describe relatively abstract and common tendencies that activate behavior targeted at achieving a desired outcome. But because motives refer to relatively abstract processes, they are imprecise about particular actions and particular end states; this is instead the conceptual function of *goals* (Elliot, 1997, 2006; Elliot & Fryer, 2008). Goals articulate explicit behaviors that are intended to fulfill general motives. Diverse goals can fulfill a given motive (*equifinality*), and a given goal may sometimes accomplish different motives, a construct sometimes referred to as *multifinality* (Kruglanski et al., 2013). (For example, the goal of having sex with a popular other can fulfill intimacy motives or, alternatively, a motive to be perceived by peers as having high mate value.) For that reason, although the constructs of goals and motives are clearly intertwined, and often simultaneously activated, when examining any particular goal, it is also important to ask with what motive (or motives) it is associated.

Table 13.2 lists several relational motives that have received substantial attention in the literature. The list is organized around three adaptive mechanisms that contribute to mammalian social connections, grouped according to the types of human relationships in which these mechanisms are most commonly expressed. The idea behind these groupings borrows from Bugental's (2000) seminal descriptions of the algorithms of social life. Bugental argues that human adaptation to the recurrent problems of social life led, through inheritance and learning, to the development of *algorithms* (i.e., internalized regulatory systems that help individuals respond to these problems) that are expressed in specific types of relationships. These algorithms are instantiated by a network of innate neurohormonal mechanisms, which, through developmental experience, incorporate learned modifications and elaborations, allowing individuals a great deal of flexibility in their behavioral response to situational demands. Different algorithms have been designed to address different adaptive problems, and as such pertain to different types of relationships, or domains (Principle 4 in Table 13.1). For present purposes, Table 13.2 is intended to highlight how these algorithms give rise to particular relational motives, thereby providing individuals with a suite of regulatory systems that, when needed, activate and direct behavior. Like any motives, they can function automatically, outside of awareness, or under more deliberate, conscious control.

I have chosen to emphasize the three relational domains listed in the leftmost column of Table 13.2 because of their popularity in the literature.[3] *Communal caregiving* refers to relationships in which partners are concerned about each other's well-being, often, though not exclusively, mutually. As I describe later, communal caregiving motives likely evolved out of the adaptive benefits of maintaining one's own and significant others' safety and security, through proximity to and bonding between caregivers and care recipients. with caregivers. *Peer belonging* pertains to the connections people form with less-close others, usually in groups and social networks. This category has been referred to in earlier models in terms of exchange (Clark & Aragon, 2013), equality matching (Fiske, 1992), reciprocity (Bugental, 2000), bonding with acquaintances in social groups (Abrams & Hogg, 2006), and weak ties (Fingerman, 2009). I use the more generic label here to emphasize what is common among these definitions and

TABLE 13.2. A Hierarchical Model of Relational Motives

Relationship domains and their central adaptive mechanisms	Representative relational motives	Potential situation-specific goals
Communal caregiving relationships Protection and caring by concerned partners fosters individual survival and well-being	Attachment security Safe haven Secure base Prorelationship motives (commitment and trust) Responsiveness Giving and garnering care and support	Minimize conflict about potential relationship threats. Stay in regular contact with my partner. Protect my partner/children from harm. Do something special to please my partner. Pay no attention to alternative romantic partners. Reveal normatively private information about myself to my partner. Try to find a mutually agreeable solution to an important disagreement with my partner. Ask my partner for help with a personal problem.
Peer belonging relationships Social affiliation facilitates cooperative strategies for addressing challenges; provides access to reproductive opportunities.	Belonging Self-presentation Ostracism Cooperation Fairness	Join a club. Wear a shirt from my favorite sports team. Cultivate friendship network. Follow old friends on social media. Tell friends about personal accomplishments. Try to be a good team player. Don't cheat in business transactions and monitor others' possible cheating.
Mating Identify reproductive opportunities; bond with and retain high-value reproductive partners.	Sexual desire Passionate and companionate love Mate retention and mate poaching Pair-bonding	Flirt with a desired partner. Subscribe to an online dating service. Make arrangements for a romantic weekend with one's partner. Interfere with potential rivals' access to one's partner.

also to highlight a link with the adaptive task of using social connection to facilitate coordinated, jointly beneficial activity with peers. The final category, *mating,* refers to the evident adaptive significance of finding, bonding with, and retaining access to reproductive partners.

It is worth reiterating that each of these domains describes a type of relationship: an ongoing association between individuals (or the groups to which they belong) who repeatedly find themselves in interdependent situations (Kelley, 1983). *Interdependent situations,* as discussed earlier, occur when people modify their behavior to account for the necessity of coordinating their own and others' actions in order to accomplish life tasks. Because over evolutionary time humans lived in groups with relatively stable membership of well-acquainted individuals (Caporael, 1997), these associations typically met the requirements of a relationship: Each person's behavior exerted causal effects on the other's behavior, frequently, influentially, and diversely, over time (Kelley, 1983). The motives that drive people's behavior in these interdependent situations are therefore intrinsically *relational* motives: They reflect not only the instrumental demands of the immediate circumstances but also their knowledge about one another from shared history, their expectations about future interaction, and the long-term socioaffective outcomes that each kind of interaction might be expected to produce (Principle 3). In other words, the goals that drive behavior often have more to do with the social context than with the task at hand. This is why successful relationships are a major predictor of well-being and performance in most activities at all stages of the life cycle (e.g., Hartup & Stevens, 1997).

Table 13.2 lists several key relational motives representing each domain, as well as specific goals that are distinctive to each domain, as suggested by Principle 4.[4] These examples are intended to be illustrative rather than prescriptive; that is, I make no claim that the list is exhaustive or that the entries are ideal illustrations. Rather, the examples have been chosen because of their prominence in the literature, and as such, are informative about the range and impact of relational motives in human behavior. Another key idea that readers might

keep in mind is that a given relationship may embody more than one adaptive function. In other words, these domains are not mutually exclusive: Any or all may apply to a particular relationship, as occurs, for example, when mating partners comfort each other in distressing circumstances, or when neighbors inquire about each other's health. Furthermore, a given relational motive may contribute to more than one domain, especially when fulfillment of those motives yields similar outcomes. For example, belongingness motives apply to both the communal and peer group domains because, in both instances, motive satisfaction yields similar affective outcomes (Hirsch & Clark, 2019). Indeed, people's flexibility in applying these relational motives across different relationships might be considered an indication of our species' versatility in adapting to the complexity of social roles and interactions.

Relational Motives Relevant to Communal Caregiving Relationships

In communal caregiving relationships, people are concerned with their partners' welfare (Clark & Aragon, 2013). The prototype of a communal caregiving relationship is the bond between parents and their children, in which caregiving is typically one-sided (i.e., from parent to child). In adulthood, communal caregiving relationships tend to be more mutual, with each partner giving and expecting care from the other.[5] Thus, these motives focus on providing assistance or kindness when a need exists or when it might be beneficial; for example, helping partners deal with problems, offering them useful resources, and promoting their happiness (Crocker & Canevello, 2008). Likewise, in adult communal caregiving relationships, people are motivated to rely on their partners to facilitate their own health and well-being. Because these benefits accrue most commonly in ongoing relationships, communal caregiving motives are often manifested in behaviors that strengthen the relationship; in essence, the welfare of the relationship becomes a goal in and of itself, intrinsic to, and in some cases, indistinguishable from the well-being of the partners as individuals. Although communal concern is typically described in terms of alleviating a partner's distress, it is important to recognize that these motives can have either a prevention focus (e.g., preventing or resolving problems) or a promotion focus (e.g., supporting a partner's growth and development or contributing to his or her happiness; cf. Higgins, 1998).

Various terms are used in the literature to describe relationships in which communal caregiving motives are expressed, for example, *communal, communal sharing, intimate, close,* and *attachment relationships.* Although certain particulars distinguish these examples from one another, they share a common interest in the provision and expectation of mutual concern and caregiving.

Attachment

The central insight of attachment theory is the adaptive significance of proximity: Young individuals (including both humans and nonhumans) who stayed physically proximate to a protective adult were more likely to survive than those without such protection (Bowlby, 1969/1982). In the most elementary sense, then, achieving an acceptable degree of proximity, especially in threatening or dangerous circumstances, is the fundamental, underlying attachment motive for both infants and their caregivers. In Bowlby's terminology, proximity represents the "set goal" of the attachment behavioral system. When current circumstances satisfy the individual's set goal, he or she feels safe and secure, and can pursue growth, learning, and exploration. When the set goal is not satisfied, however, a set of innate mechanisms is activated to restore proximity or, alternatively, to defensively adapt to its absence. These defensive strategies represent the individual's effort to modify normative proximity-seeking tendencies, either through *hypervigilance*—exaggerated attempts to recruit protection from the caregiver or others—or *deactivation*—dampening of the proximity-seeking drive and its attendant distress (Shaver & Mikulincer, 2002; Simpson, Rholes, Eller, & Paetzold, Chapter 12, this volume).

Attachment-related motives become active in situations in which the individual feels threatened and seeks protection from caregivers—in other words, when an interdependent situation exists in which the effectiveness of an individual's behavioral options depends on a caregiver's response. More generally, in human adult relationships, the basic attachment motive can be described in terms of the desire to achieve and maintain a stable sense of personal security. In most adults, this motive is considerably more varied and complex than the simple act of seeking proximity to caregivers. For one thing, normal developmental processes foster the internalization of early experience, so that baseline levels of felt security, as well as individual differences in responding when attachment needs are activated, become relatively stable characteristics of the individual—so-called "internal working models of attachment" (Fraley, 2002). For another, with maturation, people become better able to reestablish their set goal of proximity through more diverse behavioral channels, such as verbal interaction, that need not require the caregiver's actual physical presence (e.g., mentally accessing representations of an attachment figure or communicating electronically). A third reason is that, in adulthood, attachment relationships become less one-sided than they are during infancy, with the same individuals commonly serving as both security-seeker and caregiver (although not necessarily at the same time; Hazan & Shaver, 1994).

Two particular components of attachment motives have been emphasized in research. The first, *safe haven,* refers to the heightened desire for contact with attachment figures in the face of threat. Thus, for example, research has shown that adults actively seek out attachment figures when stress occurs (e.g., Collins & Feeney, 2000) and that mental accessibility of representations of attachment figures increases following subliminal activation of the attachment system (e.g., Mikulincer, Gillath, & Shaver, 2002). The second, *secure base,* describes the use of attachment relationships as a reliable base or resource from which individuals can safely and confidently explore other, nonattachment-related goals. For example, priming with a secure attachment relationship increases people's openness to a variety of exploratory activities (Luke, Sedikides, & Carnelley, 2012) and their creative problem solving (Mikulincer, Shaver, & Rom, 2011). Also, responsive support from a secure-base figure has been shown to facilitate goal striving, personal growth, and exploratory behavior (e.g., Feeney, 2004; Feeney & Thrush,

2010).[6] These and many other similar studies point to the motivational significance of attachment relationships across a broad spectrum of human activities (for elaboration, see Simpson et al., Chapter 12, this volume).

Commitment and Trust

Commitment is one way to distinguish single-time social interactions from ongoing relationships, inasmuch as the latter involve expectations about ongoing interactions and interdependence. Rusbult and colleagues proposed that partners become committed to their relationships—that is, they form expectations that the relationship will continue into the future—to the extent that they depend on those relationships for satisfying important needs and obtaining desired rewards (Rusbult, Martz, & Agnew, 1998; Rusbult, Olsen, Davis, & Hannon, 2001; Rusbult & Van Lange, 1996). Nevertheless, although people establish committed relationships because of the anticipated rewards, commitment also entails inherent risk: the possibility of exploitation by a partner as well as the cost of forgoing potentially greater rewards from alternative relationships. Prorelationship behaviors—behaviors that make a relationship more satisfying—help minimize these risks, and these follow directly from commitment (Rusbult et al., 2001).

Commitment per se is not a motive; rather, it describes an intention to persist in a relationship over time. But in order to maximize the probability that one's commitment will pay off, committed partners do two things: They strive to maintain and enhance their own level of reward within the relationship ("It is better than any other relationship I could find right now") and they attend to their partners' level of reward (to forestall the partner being tempted by alternatives). This is not just a matter of instrumental calculus, however. One reason is that committed partners are more likely to see things in terms of "we" rather than "you and me" (Agnew, Van Lange, Rusbult, & Langston, 1998), essentially incorporating the partner's perspectives and identity with one's own (Aron et al., 1991). For another, commitment fosters shared reality, which may fulfill epistemic needs more effectively than individualized perspectives do (Rossignac-Millon & Higgins, 2018). Rusbult's

conception of maximizing own and partner's benefits, therefore, should be thought of in the broadest sense possible, encompassing both tangible and highly subjective outcomes.

Partners benefit from each other's commitment because committed partners are motivated to think and act in ways that will support their commitment (Murray & Holmes, 2011)—that is, they adopt *prorelationship motives* (Rusbult et al., 2001). These motives include both approach (promoting desired goals) and avoidance (preventing nondesired goals) examples (Gable & Strachman, 2008), and are manifested in behavioral or psychological outcomes. With regard to the former, for example, committed partners are more willing to sacrifice for their partners' well-being (Van Lange et al., 1997) and are more likely to respond constructively when their partners misbehave (Rusbult, Verette, Whitney, Slovik, & Lipkus, 1991). As for the latter, committed partners tend to perceive their partners more positively than those partners see themselves (so-called *positive illusions*; Murray, Holmes, & Griffin, 1996), believe that their relationships are superior to other people's relationships (Reis, Caprariello, & Velickovic, 2011; Rusbult, Van Lange, Wildschut, Yovetich, & Verette, 2000), and devalue potential alternative partners (Lydon & Karremans, 2015). In each of these examples, a prorelationship motive helps people choose between behavioral or psychological options that will support or undermine continuity of their relationship. Conversely, prorelationship motives are less likely to be influential when commitment wanes; they may even, in the case of very low levels of commitment, undermine relationship stability.

Trust, which Rempel, Holmes, and Zanna (1985, p. 96) define as "feelings of confidence and security in the caring response of the partner and the strength of the relationship," is a key part of this process. In their influential risk regulation model, Murray, Holmes, and Collins (2006) posed the following question: When interdependent partners have conflicting preferences or goals, how should they choose between doing what is best (or safest) for the self and what is best for the relationship (or partner)? This commonplace dilemma pits autonomy—acting according to personal priorities—against the relational benefits and risks of sacrifice. Trust encourages the latter, relationship-promoting option: By engendering faith in the partner's beneficence toward oneself, as well as in the durability of the relationship, trust justifies setting aside self-interest in order to invest in the relationship.[7] In the absence of trust, however, self-interest represents a safer, more self-protective choice, by minimizing the possibility of harm or loss. Murray and Holmes (2011, p. 103) explain how trust helps partners to commit confidently, making the relationship "a valued end in and of itself," and thereby strengthening it. In this way, trust is an important source of prorelationship motives.

Responsiveness

The paradigmatic interaction sequence for describing intimate interaction consists of one partner's self-disclosure and the other's responsive listening (Reis & Shaver's [1988] *intimacy process* model). When opportunities for self-disclosing revelations and responsive listening arise—for example, when two people find themselves talking about potentially self-revealing matters—relational motives help determine whether each will follow through, that is, whether the discloser will open up or hold back, and whether the listener will respond encouragingly or dismissively. It follows, then, that trust has particular importance for self-disclosure and responsiveness. Self-disclosure creates risk and vulnerability, so that, much as described in the previous section, beliefs about a partner's trustworthiness will prompt openness (e.g., Larzelere & Huston, 1980; Wheeless & Grotz, 1977). Similar logic applies to being a responsive listener because engaged listening requires openness to the discloser, as well as to the likelihood of reciprocally self-disclosing.

Reis and Shaver (1988) decompose the interaction sequence that engenders perceptions of a partner's responsiveness into three elements that each may also be considered a relational motive, in the sense that it orients and energizes people toward intimate interactions. These are *understanding* (believing that the partner "gets the facts right" about oneself), *validation* (attaining a partner's respect and appreciation), and *caring* (believing that the partner is interested in one's well-being). Existing research documents the motivational significance of each component.

For example, people strive for others to understand their view of the world (i.e., to establish shared reality; Higgins & Pittman, 2008), they prefer partners who understand them over partners who like them (Swann, 1990), and they tend to overattribute understanding to their partners in committed relationships (Reis, Lemay, & Finkenauer, 2017). Validation is a key drive underlying several well-known social cognitive processes, such as social comparison (Wood, 1989) and self-enhancement (Sedikides & Strube, 1997), both of which are influential in close-relationship contexts. Caring, or support, is described in the next section.

Interaction sequences such as those described by the intimacy process model are distinctive because they unfold successfully only when both partners' motives are well coordinated; that is, a self-discloser's motive to establish intimacy is fulfilled only when his or her partner is also motivated to be a responsive listener; likewise, responsive listening is unlikely to have much impact if the speaker is not revealing something meaningful about him- or herself. Interdependence theory refers to situations such as these as coordination problems because interacting persons must first identify, then carry out behavior that meshes effectively with the partner's behavior, rather than simply implementing their own preferred actions (Kelley et al., 2003). In ongoing relationships, partners are likely to have an extensive bank of information about each other's preferences, abilities, and goals, which makes close relationships a particularly fertile area for studying the influence of motives on coordination.

Giving and Garnering Care

The provision of help, care, and support in close relationships is a paramount and much-studied process. In the prototypical case, called *communal relationships* (Clark & Aragon, 2013; Clark & Mills, 1979), people expect their partners to be noncontingently helpful when a need occurs, and, in turn, they expect to provide assistance to those partners when their need arises. Thus, in the language of Figure 13.1, one partner's need creates an opportunity for the other to help; whether or not partners choose to do so depends on their communal motives. Communal motives (akin to Crocker & Canevello's [2008] concept of compassionate goals) are defined by people's concern about another person's well-being and their intent to support that person. People sometimes do render help outside of a communal relationship (e.g., in exchange relationships), but in these instances, their helping is governed by motives related to exchange norms and feelings of indebtedness rather than by caregiving motives. This section focuses on the latter.

Much research has established the benefits of caregiving for human health and well-being (for a review, see Robles, Slatcher, Trombello, & McGinn, 2014). In communal relationships, support is motivated by the caregiver's desire to meet the care recipient's need along at least three dimensions: (1) the degree of need; (2) the costliness of help to the provider, in terms of time, money, and effort; and (3) the *communal strength* of the relationship. This last factor refers to the degree of responsibility felt by the provider for the recipient and varies from one relationship to another. Clark and Aragon (2013) rank-order normative levels of communal strength as follows (from most to least): children, spouse, best friend, friend, neighbor, and stranger. The greater the communal strength of a relationship, the stronger the caregiver's motive to provide care in response to the partner's need. Presumably, because communal relationships are typically mutual and reciprocal, the strength of the motive to solicit help from communal partners follows a similar rank ordering (excluding nonadult children).

Within the social support literature, there is debate about the extent to which the actual receipt of support, as opposed to its perceived availability, is beneficial; that is, some studies indicate that support receipt is associated with worse outcomes (e.g., Bolger, Zuckerman, & Kessler, 2000; Rafaeli & Gleason, 2009), perhaps because the support transaction highlights the recipient's inability to deal with the stressful circumstances on his or her own. However, even when support receipt is associated with heightened individual distress, it tends to foster more favorable relationship outcomes (e.g., Gleason, Iida, Shrout, & Bolger, 2008)—likely implying the recipient's gratitude for the caregiver's support, regardless of its outcome. This finding illustrates the relational significance of caregiving motives—that is, caregiving is a

relationally significant act whose meaning and impact extend beyond the specifics of whatever concrete help is provided.

Relational Motives Relevant to Peer Relationships

By far the largest portion of the relationship science literature investigates nominally communal relationships: romantic partners, families, and close friends. But noncommunal peer relationships also matter. Throughout evolutionary times, peer relationships have played an important role in human activity and adaptation. Much as they do today, humans lived and worked in small cooperative groups whose shared activity facilitated key tasks such as resource acquisition, protection from predators, contending with enemies and environmental threats, socializing offspring, and enacting social structures and rituals. Success in these tasks offered distinct adaptive advantages, leading to the evolution of a suite of physiological mechanisms designed to regulate peer-belonging processes such as affiliation and cooperation (Bugental, 2000)—for example, social rejection and ostracism typically trigger autonomic responses that are thought to underlie coping with situational demands (e.g., Mendes, Major, McCoy, & Blascovich, 2008). Peer belonging situations differ from the caregiving situations described earlier because they do not centrally concern a caregiver's provision of help or protection; rather, they focus on interacting with peers to achieve mutually beneficial solutions to shared problems. As a consequence, a different set of relational motives is implicated.

Belonging

The often-heralded need to belong describes "a pervasive drive to form and maintain at least a minimum of lasting, positive, and significant interpersonal relationships" (Baumeister & Leary, 1995, p. 497). This motive has been proposed as a direct precursor to such fundamental human behaviors as the tendency to affiliate with others, to form groups, to bond with family, to experience a variety of negative emotions (particularly, but not exclusively, loneliness) and to suffer ill-health and even a heightened risk of premature mortality when isolated (Holt-Lunstad, Smith, Baker, Harris, & Stephenson, 2015), and to ostracize norm-breakers (Baumeister & Leary, 1995; Cacioppo & Patrick, 2008; Williams, 2007). That these tendencies are well established in all known human societies, in very young children, and, for that matter, in many mammalian species, strongly suggests deep roots in human neural architecture.

Diverse evidence supports the idea that belongingness is a relational motive—that is, a motive that impels people to pursue and maintain social connections. For one, when people feel insufficiently connected with others, a state commonly called *loneliness*, they often seek out social contact (Shaver, Furman, & Buhrmester, 1985). Similarly, experimental studies have demonstrated that social exclusion prompts heightened interest in forming bonds with new partners (Maner, DeWall, Baumeister, & Schaller, 2007). This finding is consistent with research on ostracism, or exclusion from a group or social network, which has been shown to have deleterious effects on self-esteem, self-regulation, and emotional well-being (Williams, 2007), even when the ostracizing group is offensive (Gonsalkorale & Williams, 2007). On the other hand, substantial evidence indicates that when belongingness needs are satiated, people are less inclined to pursue new connections (see review by Leary & Baumeister, 2000). Also relevant is research showing that people are reluctant to break existing bonds, especially when those bonds are long-standing and even when those relationships have been unsatisfying or abusive (Herbert, Silver, & Ellard, 1991), and they experience distress, which is often profound, when close relationships are ruptured, such as through bereavement (Stroebe, Schut, & Stroebe, 2007) or divorce (Amato & Hohmann-Marriott, 2007). Finally, extensive research indicates that much of people's cognitive and emotional processing is tailored specifically toward perceiving, interpreting, and regulating belonging circumstances, implying that these systems evolved to help people manage the vicissitudes of social life (see Reis et al., 2000, for a review).

Self-presentation can be understood as an expression of belongingness motives. Self-presentation can be strategic, in the sense of delib-erate, or nonstrategic, in the sense of motives to enhance one's reputation that operate largely outside of awareness. In either instance, when people attempt to convey desirable images of themselves, they seek esteem in the eyes of others, presumably because the more valued attributes one possesses, the greater one's relational value and likelihood of acceptance by others (Hirsch & Clark, 2019). People have evolved to be concerned about and promote their reputations (e.g., to avoid being excluded, which undermines survival and reproduction; Maner & Kenrick, 2010). As a result, people often strive to highlight socially valued attributes in their public personae. Such social approbation may emphasize any of numerous dimensions—for example, attractiveness, social skill, athletic or intellectual ability, status or social standing, wealth, or personal connections with famous others ("basking in reflected glory").

The benefits of successful impression management may also extend to self-perception. In one experiment, participants instructed to present themselves to an interviewer in a self-enhancing manner subsequently reported higher self-esteem (Jones, Rhodewalt, Berglas, & Skelton, 1981). In other research, self-esteem was most closely tied to those traits that were most likely to garner others' acceptance (Anthony, Holmes, & Wood, 2007). These findings support *sociometer theory,* which proposes that self-esteem provides an internal monitor of one's perceived relational value—whether one can anticipate being accepted or rejected by others (Leary & Baumeister, 2000). A related theory posits that self-regard also acts as a hierometer, tracking perceived social status, which serves a similar functional purpose in monitoring anticipated levels of liking and acceptance (Mahadevan, Gregg, & Sedikides, 2019). These theories, and the empirical studies that support them, imply that belongingness motives may help to account for the vast array of social psychological phenomena that have been linked to self-esteem maintenance and enhancement, and status acquisition and management.

Cooperation

The motive to cooperate becomes relevant in situations in which people must choose between maximizing joint outcomes with an interaction partner—that is, selecting behavioral options in which both partners come out ahead, even if this entails lesser outcomes for oneself—or prioritizing one's own relative gain over that of the partner. When either of two affects is salient—fear that a partner will exploit one by not reciprocating cooperation, and greed, or the desire to take selfish advantage of a partner's cooperation (Van Lange & Rusbult, 2012)—the tendency to cooperate diminishes. Thus, acting on cooperative motives depends on one's intentions regarding the self relative to a partner, as well as one's inferences about the partner's likely behavior. As such, it seems self-evident that relationship variables will play an influential role in determining whether cooperative motives predominate, and extensive research has supported this conjecture. Trust, in particular, is strongly associated with cooperative behavior (see Dawes, 1980, for a review).

Which situational variables strengthen people's motivation to act cooperatively? Expecting frequent and continued interaction is one well-documented influence, probably because people anticipate better, or perhaps more predictable, future outcomes from a cooperative than from a noncooperative relationship (e.g., Heide & Miner, 1992). Emphasizing common fate, a prototypical feature of ongoing relationships, also increases cooperation (Van Lange & Joireman, 2008), as does positive affect toward interaction partners, as shown, for example, in research on empathy (Batson & Ahmad, 2001),[8] respect (De Cremer, 2002), and liking (Tedeschi, 1974). The last of these factors is particularly germane to intergroup cooperation, in which friendship and attraction have been shown to be important (Johnson, Johnson, & Maruyama, 1983). General value orientations also may broadly affect a person's motivation to cooperate. In their seminal work, Messick and McClintock (1968) classified individuals as *prosocials* (i.e., people who tend to maximize joint outcomes), *individualists* (i.e., people who generally maximize their own outcomes), and *competitors* (i.e., people who prefer to maximize their own outcomes relative to others). Numerous studies have shown that, all other things being equal, prosocials are more likely to act cooperatively (for reviews, see Bogaert, Boone, & Declerck,

2008; Van Lange, 1999), likely reflecting their stronger motivation to cooperate.

Fairness

Societies establish social norms about the expected distribution of outcomes as a means of codifying favored patterns of interdependence: If interaction partners understand and agree upon the level of outcome that each party should expect, then interaction is more likely to proceed efficiently and harmoniously, with a minimum of conflict. A *fair* interaction, then, is one in which people believe that they and their partners have each received appropriate levels of whatever the relevant outcomes are. Although several specific principles have been proposed for defining just what level of outcomes is considered fair—most notably, equity (Walster, Walster, & Berscheid, 1978), equality, and need (Deutsch, 1985)—common to them is the underlying desire for fairness as a motivating force; that is, people seek to contribute and obtain the outcomes they believe they deserve; they wish for their partners to do similarly; and they react both emotionally, with anger (if underbenefited) or guilt (if overbenefited), and behaviorally, by seeking restitution, if they perceive that their outcomes are not commensurate with their entitlement.

This chapter construes fairness as a relational motive because of its relevance to *exchange relationships*—relationships in which partners benefit each other proportionally to comparable benefits received in the past or expected future benefits (Clark & Mills, 1979). Exchange relationships differ from communal relationships, discussed earlier, primarily in terms of the motive for benefiting a partner: in exchange relationships, rather than meeting a partner's need, the main goal is to achieve a fair exchange—for example, to pay employees a proper wage for their labor or to repay a neighbor for feeding one's cat during a vacation by doing the same for the neighbor during his or her vacation. Research has shown, for example, that compared to communally related partners, people in exchange relationships feel more liking for partners who allow their help to be reciprocated (Clark & Mills, 1979) and are more likely to feel exploited by a partner who does not repay a debt (Clark & Waddell, 1985).

Evolutionary psychologists explain the motivational significance of fairness through the principle of *reciprocal altruism*—the tendency of organisms to accept costs for helping others, when they anticipate later receiving help from those others. For reciprocal altruism to have adaptive value, the human mind had to incorporate mechanisms for detecting and punishing "cheaters"—individuals who fail to live up to the implied contract (Cosmides & Tooby, 1992)—as well as internalized drives to self-regulate situationally appropriate compliance. Fairness motives represent this latter drive. Of course, fairness motives are revealed in varied forms. Different circumstances implicate different norms (see, e.g., Fiske's [1992] four elementary forms of sociality, which describe four distinct forms, or principles, for regulating outcomes of social relationships). Beyond their concern about outcome fairness, people also value procedural justice—whether parties follow impartial procedures to resolve conflicting preferences (Brockner, 2010; Thibaut & Walker, 1975; Tyler, 2006). The idea of a fairness motive takes no position about which standard ought to be applied in which circumstance; rather, it speaks to people's motivation to comply with identifiable standards of fairness and thereby be entitled to their corresponding benefits. This suggests, of course, considerable flexibility in how the fairness motive is interpreted in particular circumstances.

Relational Motives Relevant to Mating

The adaptive significance of mating-relevant motives is unmistakable. Because mating is an intrinsically relational act, relational motives play a key role in determining how people behave when potential mating situations exist. Some of these motives apply to the sexual act itself (e.g., sexual desire), whereas others, more the focus in recent social-psychological research, pertain to the relationship (short-lived or ongoing) between reproductive partners. In this latter respect, because modern reproductive relationships usually also involve caregiving and belonging, mating-relevant motives may operate in tandem with motives from those domains. Nonetheless, in their origins and functions, mating-relevant motives apply to a narrower range of relationships than the other motives discussed in this chapter, perhaps explaining why, until recently, social psychologists have paid relatively little attention to sexual relationships. Even so, mating relationships represent for many people their most consequential and compelling relationships, suggesting a need for additional attention and research.

Sexual Desire

Functional analyses suggest that sexual activity can be instigated by a variety of motives. For example, Cooper, Shapiro, and Powers (1998) identified six motives that may lead people to engage in sex: self-enhancement (i.e., pleasure/enjoyment), intimacy, peer approval, partner approval, coping with stress, and self-affirmation. Among the more conspicuous motives for sexual behavior is *sexual desire,* defined by Birnbaum (2018, p. 102) as "the subjective experience of an inclination to engage in sexual activity with a specific individual." Theorists have long argued that *sexual desire* evolved to inspire actions that would pass on one's genes to the next generation (Birnbaum, 2018). Sexual desire is usually targeted toward a particular person, although sometimes with little or no implications about an ongoing relationship with that person (Diamond, 2013). In other cases, however, sexual desire plays a functionally significant role in the development of a relationship. To Birnbaum, sexual desire is a gatekeeper for relationship initiation, signaling oneself about the desirability of interaction with a potential partner and spurring behavioral displays that communicate that interest (e.g., flirting, warmth; Birnbaum, Mizrahi, & Reis, 2019). High levels of desire, accompanied by the rewarding sexual encounters that they may engender, can help partners overcome the doubts and insecurities that often characterize the transition from budding relationship to full-fledged romantic interdependence (Birnbaum, 2018).

Sexual desire typically declines as relationships mature, both because an instigator is no longer needed and because other processes, some of which were described earlier in this chapter, become more influential in relationship maintenance. The normative decline notwithstanding, recent evidence suggests that sexual desire may continue to motivate pleasurable contact and commitment in long-term relationships (Muise, Impett, Kogan, & Desmarais, 2013). When sexual desire fuels satisfying sexual interactions, it may buffer the adverse consequences of relationship insecurities (Little, McNulty, & Russell, 2010). On the other hand, for some, the absence of sexual desire can be a motivating concern, either for its own sake or because it may signify a loss of intimacy or of feeling loved (Augin & Heiman, 2004; Sprecher & Cate, 2004). In these instances, low sexual desire may prompt repair efforts (e.g., through self-help or couple therapy) or destabilize relationships (e.g., through infidelity or divorce).

Love

Among the varieties of love that characterize human relationships (Reis & Aron, 2008), two have received the most attention from researchers: *passionate love* (a state of intense longing for union with another person) and *companionate love* (feelings of mutual trust, respect, and affection for another person). The motivational significance of these two forms of love can be encapsulated in a phrase: Passionate love solves the attraction problem, whereas companionate love solves the commitment problem (adapted from Gonzaga, Keltner, Londahl, & Smith, 2001); that is, passionate love evolved to help people identify and pursue bonds with potential reproductive partners.[9] Companionate love, on the other hand, evolved to encourage and reinforce those bonds, once a relationship has been formed. Although passionate and companionate love tend to be correlated, especially in new relationships, research has generally characterized them in distinct motivational profiles.

Some researchers consider passionate love to be an emotion rather than a motive; however, several studies have established that the pattern of neural activation associated with passionate love more nearly resembles the latter than the former (e.g., Aron et al., 2005; specifically, passionate love activates dopamine-sensitive, reward-relevant regions of the brain). In Aron and Aron's *self-expansion theory* (Aron et al., 1991), passionate love motivates lovers to "include the other in the self," thereby expanding their resources, identity, and perspectives. Empirical evidence supports this hypothesis.

For example, in one study, committed couples who underwent a self-expansion exercise in the laboratory subsequently reported higher levels of passionate love (Aron, Norman, Aron, McKenna, & Heyman, 2000). Other motivationally significant manifestations of passionate love include heightened preoccupation with the beloved (Tennov, 1979), sometimes persistently so, even when unrequited (Baumeister, Wotman, & Stillwell, 1993), and a relatively high level of idealization of one's partner (Gunaydin & DeLong, 2015; White, Fishbein, & Rutstein, 1981; for a review, see Niehuis, Lee, Reifman, Swenson, & Hunsaker, 2011).

Companionate love, in contrast, is more closely linked to pair-bonding, discussed below. For present purposes, I note that because of its close conceptual linkage with communal caring, responsiveness, and trust, companionate motives may well depend on the same underlying processes and structures described earlier for those motives. This reasoning is consistent with the common observation that companionate love, and its associated goals, is more likely than passionate love to apply to nonromantic relationships.

Mate Retention and Mate Poaching

Traditionally, researchers have conceptualized mate retention largely in terms of relationship maintenance—doing what one can do to keep a partner happy and committed (Rusbult et al., 2001). Evolutionary theorizing has added another dimension to this literature: *mate guarding,* which refers to strategies enacted to restrict potential rivals' access to a partner. Motivationally, mate guarders have two main aims: blocking rivals from the possibility of sexual contact with one's partner and preserving one's own reproductive advantage (Buss, 1988). *Jealousy* often stimulates mate-guarding behavior: When people fear the loss of a valued romantic relationship due to the real or imagined presence of a competitor, they experience a range of emotions (e.g., hurt, anger, and fear; Guerrero, Trost, & Yoshimura, 2005) that typically elicit behavior intended to safeguard their own privileged access to the relationship. These behaviors can, of course, be constructive (e.g., voicing concerns in a nondefensive manner, attempting to please one's partner) or destructive (e.g., stalking, threatening violence). Jealousy is widely thought to have its evolved roots in mate guarding (Maner & Kenrick, 2010), although it also may motivate relationship-preserving efforts in nonromantic, nonreproductive relationships, such as those between close friends or siblings.

Mate guarding would not exist if sexual rivals posed no threat, implicating the complementary construct of *mate poaching.* Mate poaching, which is well documented among nonhuman animals, is also common among humans (Schmitt, 2004). Mate poaching is designed to attract a sexual partner who is already in a romantic relationship with someone else and can focus on the short-term (transient sexual encounters) or long-term (substituting a relationship with oneself for the existing relationship) (Schmitt & Buss, 2001). In either case, the underlying motive involves besting a sexual competitor by engaging the attention and favors of a valuable partner (i.e., one who has already achieved a mating relationship). The motive behind mate poaching differs from ordinary sexual desire by emphasizing its competitive aspect—poachers simultaneously seek to create opportunities for themselves while obstructing their competitors' prospects.

Pair–Bonding

Many theorists credit pair-bonding with a singularly significant role in human evolution. For example, Fletcher, Simpson, Campbell, and Overall (2015, p. 29) asserted that "romantic pair-bonding facilitated the evolution of the advanced levels of mind reading and social intelligence seen in modern humans," while Gavrilets (2012, p. 9923) similarly linked "the appearance of some of the unique human features to a major transition in life history strategy that transformed the social structure of early hominids from promiscuous groups to multimale/multifemale groups with strong pair-bonding." Chapais (2008) drew the same conclusion, subtitling his synthesis of primatological and anthropological work on human evolution, *How Pair-Bonding Gave Birth to Human Society.*

There can be little doubt about the importance of *pair-bonding,* the human tendency to join with another person in a stable, sexual, affect-laden, and highly interdependent relationship

around which many important life activities are organized. Neurobiological studies ascribe much of this tendency to the neuropeptides oxytocin and vasopression (Young & Wang, 2004). However, it is unclear whether, from a motivational standpoint, pair-bonding should be conceptualized as an independent motive with its own precursors and behavioral manifestations. Consider the alternative possibility that pair-bonding synthesizes in one relationship all of the relational motives described in this chapter; that is, in many societies, pair-bonds serve as an attachment relationship, fulfilling for most adults the major attachment functions of proximity maintenance, a safe haven, and a secure base (Hazan & Diamond, 2000), as well as nurturant support for the partner's interests (Rusbult et al., 2009). Pair-bonded relationships, at least when they live up to typical aspirations, involve relatively high levels of responsiveness, commitment, and trust, as well as the provision and receipt of care and support. Pair-bonds also provide a primary context for satisfying the need to belong (Leary & Baumeister, 2000), and they are usually cooperative, with an equitable balance of contributions and outcomes (Kluwer, 2009). Finally, sexual desire, love, and mate retention are obviously relevant in pair-bonded relationships. The point, then, is that pair-bonding, rather than representing a unique and specialized set of relational motives, may actually embody all of them, wrapped up and expressed in a single, multifaceted, and highly interdependent relationship.

From a pragmatic perspective, this speculation implies that pair-bonded relationships may epitomize human sociality in the sense of assimilating multiple motives, along with their associated goals, in a single relationship. Of course, this need not mean that pair-bonded relationships are the ideal, nor that they are invariably successful in satisfying these various motives. Indeed, the *suffocation model* proposed by Finkel, Hui, Carswell, and Larson (2014) suggests that this sort of many-sided agenda may beget an extensive list of desiderata that marriages will often struggle to meet. Nonetheless, this reasoning suggests that pair-bonded relationships may not differ qualitatively from other relationships, as is often assumed by both marital and evolutionary researchers. Rather, pair-bonded relationships may more straight-forwardly provide a vehicle for a more numerous and diverse set of relational motives, as well as, perhaps, stronger versions of them. Instead of studying pair-bonds as a discrete relationship category, then, it might be more fruitful to investigate how multiple motivated processes intertwine in this uniquely focal kind of relationship. Taking this idea one step further, the question then emerges whether the resulting entity (i.e., the pair-bonded relationships) is best understood as the simple sum of its constituent elements or as an organizational whole whose properties embody a more synthetic, Gestalt-like combination. Addressing this question will require novel research methods: Instead of focusing on single processes within a type of given relationship, it will be necessary to investigate the simultaneous operation of multiple processes within a single relationship.

Conclusion

This chapter offers an interdependence theory perspective on relational motives (Kelley et al., 2003). Building on four core principles (Table 13.1), its central premise is that motives supply the fuel behind behavioral choices. Social psychology is often identified as the science that investigates situational causes of behavior, but it is misleading to construe that definition as meaning that situations or their features cause behavior (as many social psychologists do). A more thoughtful analysis suggests that situations provide interacting parties with a variety of behavioral options, each of which would yield certain specifiable outcomes to the individuals involved. How people select among these available options depends on their motives: what the person wishes to accomplish in that circumstance, at that moment in time, with that partner (or partners). Conceptualized in this manner, motives are properly understood neither as individual differences nor as situational variables, but rather as the place these often-dichotomized entities come together: the person's attempt to attain desired ends out of what is possible.

The list of relational motives that affect human behavior is extensive, much more so than can be covered in a single chapter. The specific motives I decided to review in this chapter

are among the most studied examples, and they have the further advantage of illustrating how adaptive problems relevant to interdependence give rise to multiple, yet clearly connected motives. Other motives may eventually turn out to be as, or even more, important than these. I hope that this analysis encourages others to think about the ways in which humans evolved interdependent, and not just independent, solutions to important problems of living and reproducing, and in turn to describe the relational motives that regulate those behaviors.

Much existing research on motives is arelational, yet there is good reason to view relational motives as essential to any understanding of motivation. Many of the most influential theories of motivation treat behavior and its impellance as a property of individuals acting in pseudoisolation, their motives translated into behavior without consideration of the influence of, and on, relevant others. Yet many, if not most, of the tasks that people enact in everyday life concern relationships with others—initiating, monitoring, maintaining, enhancing, repairing, enjoying, remembering, suffering through, worrying about, and sometimes terminating relationships dominates our attention and activity from infancy through old age. Sometimes these activities concern relationship life itself, but more often, they focus on the myriad ways in which ordinary pursuits—tasks material to schooling, work, recreation, spirituality, or financial planning, for example—depend on coordinating our actions with others. In this sense, then, it might be said that relational motives are the most fundamental of motives, underlying nearly all meaningful human activity.

NOTES

1. It may also be influenced by general personality traits and social norms (Rusbult & Van Lange, 1996), but these are not our focus here.

2. To be clear, the mechanisms proposed here are not the same ones identified by Elliot, although his model also originates in adaptive considerations.

3. These categories are similar to Bugental's (2000) domains, although there are also important differences. Bugental also includes two group-oriented domains: hierarchical relations and coalitions

among groups. Research on these two domains appears elsewhere in this volume.

4. Of course, there are many situation-specific goals that would apply across all three domains. For example, taking an interaction partner's perspective or minimizing conflict is relevant in communal caregiving, peer belonging, and mating relationships.

5. There are, however, some notable examples of one-sided communal caregiving relationships in adulthood, such as those between patients and their health care providers or between elderly or handicapped individuals and their caregivers.

6. To be sure, other theoretical models (e.g., self-determination theory; Deci & Ryan, 2000) see exploration and mastery as intrinsic human goals rather than as secondary to attachment security. In these frameworks, communal relationships still play an important role in facilitating or discouraging these goal-directed behaviors.

7. Of course, this logic presumes that a successful relationship has long-term benefits for the self. The decision process outlined by Murray and Holmes (2011) describes the momentary considerations that partners face in deciding among behavioral options.

8. In this study and others, researchers could not distinguish between *altruistic*—other-benefiting—and *cooperative*—maximizing joint outcomes. Although this distinction has theoretical importance, in practice, altruistic and cooperative motives often are manifested similarly.

9. Researchers commonly differentiate passionate love and sexual desire, despite the fact that these constructs share key properties. The distinction reflects the fact that people often report experiencing passionate love in the absence of sexual desire, for example, with one's children, siblings, or a close friend. Similarly, people often experience lustful feelings without a passionate attraction, for example, in sexual fantasies or in one-time encounters. Presumably, the desire for union in nonsexual yet still intensely rewarding relationships exapted (took advantage of) the neural mechanisms underlying sexual attraction. This logic is supported by the conceptual similarity of passionate love in sexual and nonsexual relationships (Aron & Westbay, 1986).

REFERENCES

Abrams, D., & Hogg, M. A. (2006). *Social identifications: A social psychology of intergroup relations and group processes.* London: Routledge.

Agnew, C. R., Van Lange, P. A., Rusbult, C. E., & Langston, C. A. (1998). Cognitive interdependence: Commitment and the mental representation of close relationships. *Journal of Personality and Social Psychology, 74*(4), 939–954.

Amato, P. R., & Hohmann-Marriott, B. (2007). A comparison of high- and low-distress marriages that end in divorce. *Journal of Marriage and Family, 69*(3), 621–638.

Anthony, D. B., Holmes, J. G., & Wood, J. V. (2007). Social acceptance and self-esteem: Tuning the sociometer to interpersonal value. *Journal of Personality and Social Psychology, 92*(6), 1024–1039.

Aron, A., Aron, E. N., Tudor, M., & Nelson, G. (1991). Close relationships as including other in self. *Journal of Personality and Social Psychology, 60*, 241–253.

Aron, A., Fisher, H., Mashek, D. J., Strong, G., Li, H., & Brown, L. L. (2005). Reward, motivation, and emotion systems associated with early-stage intense romantic love. *Journal of Neurophysiology, 94*(1), 327–337.

Aron, A., Norman, C. C., Aron, E. N., McKenna, C., & Heyman, R. E. (2000). Couples' shared participation in novel and arousing activities and experienced relationship quality. *Journal of Personality and Social Psychology, 78*, 273–284.

Aron, A., & Westbay, L. (1996). Dimensions of the prototype of love. *Journal of Personality and Social Psychology, 70*(3), 535–551.

Augin, S., & Heiman, J. R. (2004). Sexual dysfunction from a relationship perspective. In J. H. Harvey, A. Wenzel, & S. Sprecher (Eds.), *The handbook of sexuality in close relationships* (pp. 477–517). Mahwah, NJ: Erlbaum.

Batson, C. D., & Ahmad, N. (2001). Empathy-induced altruism in a prisoner's dilemma: II. What if the target of empathy has defected? *European Journal of Social Psychology, 31*(1), 25–36.

Baumeister, R. F., & Leary, M. R. (1995). The need to belong: Desire for interpersonal attachments as a fundamental human motivation. *Psychological Bulletin, 117*, 497–529.

Baumeister, R. F., Wotman, S. R., & Stilwell, A. M. (1993). Unrequited love: On heartbreak, anger, guilt, scriptlessness, and humiliation. *Journal of Personality and Social Psychology, 64*, 377–394.

Beckes, L., & Coan, J. A. (2013). Toward an integrative neuroscience of relationships. In J. A. Simpson & L. Campbell (Eds.), *The Oxford handbook of close relationships* (pp. 685–710). New York: Oxford University Press.

Berscheid, E. (2003). The human's greatest strength: Other humans. In L. G. Aspinwall & U. M. Staudinger (Eds.), *A psychology of human strengths: Fundamental questions and future di-*

rections for a positive psychology (pp. 37–47). Washington, DC: American Psychological Association.

Birnbaum, G. E. (2018). The fragile spell of desire: A functional perspective on changes in sexual desire across relationship development. *Personality and Social Psychology Review, 22*(2), 101–127.

Birnbaum, G. E., Mizrahi, M., & Reis, H. T. (2019). Fueled by desire: Sexual activation facilitates the enactment of relationship-initiating behaviors. *Journal of Social and Personal Relationships, 36*(10), 3057–3074.

Bogaert, S., Boone, C., & Declerck, C. (2008). Social value orientation and cooperation in social dilemmas: A review and conceptual model. *British Journal of Social Psychology, 47*(3), 453–480.

Bolger, N., Zuckerman, A., & Kessler, R. C. (2000). Invisible support and adjustment to stress. *Journal of Personality and Social Psychology, 79,* 953–961.

Bowlby, J. (1982). *Attachment and loss: Vol. 1. Attachment* (2nd ed.). New York: Basic Books. (Original work published 1969)

Brockner, J. (2010). *A contemporary look at organizational justice: Multiplying insult times injury.* New York: Routledge.

Bugental, D. B. (2000). Acquisition of the algorithms of social life: A domain-based approach. *Psychological Bulletin, 126,* 187–219.

Buss, D. M. (1988). From vigilance to violence: Tactics of mate retention in American undergraduates. *Evolution and Human Behavior, 9*(5), 291–317.

Buss, D. M., & Kenrick, D. T. (1998). Evolutionary social psychology. In D. Gilbert & S. Fiske (Eds.), *The handbook of social psychology* (4th ed., Vol. 2, pp. 982–1026). Boston: McGraw-Hill.

Cacioppo, J. T., & Patrick, B. (2008). *Loneliness: Human nature and the need for social connection.* New York: Norton.

Caporael, L. (1997). The evolution of truly social cognition: The core configurations model. *Personality and Social Psychology Review, 1,* 276–298.

Chapais, B. (2008). *Primeval kinship: How pairbonding gave birth to human society.* Cambridge, MA: Harvard University Press.

Clark, M. S., & Aragon, O. (2013). Communal (and other) relationships: History, theory development, recent findings, and future directions. In J. A. Simpson & L. Campbell (Eds.), *The Oxford handbook of close relationships* (pp. 255–280). New York: Oxford University Press.

Clark, M. S., Lemay, E. P., & Reis, H. T. (2020). Other people as situations: Relational context shapes psychological phenomena. In J. F. Rauthmann, R. A. Sherman, & D. C. Funder (Eds.), *The Oxford handbook of psychological situations.* New York: Oxford University Press.

Clark, M. S., & Mills, J. (1979). Interpersonal attraction in exchange and communal relationships. *Journal of Personality and Social Psychology, 37,* 12–24.

Clark, M. S., & Waddell, B. (1985). Perceptions of exploitation in communal and exchange relationships. *Journal of Social and Personal Relationships, 2*(4), 403–418.

Collins, N., & Feeney, B. (2000). A safe haven: An attachment theory perspective on support seeking and caregiving in intimate relationships. *Journal of Personality and Social Psychology, 78,* 1053–1073.

Cooper, M. L., Shapiro, C. M., & Powers, A. M. (1998). Motivations for sex and risky sexual behavior among adolescents and young adults: A functional perspective. *Journal of Personality and Social Psychology, 75*(6), 1528–1558.

Cosmides, L., & Tooby, J. (1992). Cognitive adaptations for social exchange. In J. H. Barkow, L. Cosmides, & J. Tooby (Eds.), *The adapted mind: Evolutionary psychology and the generation of culture* (pp. 163–228). New York: Oxford University Press.

Crocker, J., & Canevello, A. (2008). Creating and undermining social support in communal relationships: The role of compassionate and self-image goals. *Journal of Personality and Social Psychology, 95*(3), 555–575.

Dawes, R. M. (1980). Social dilemmas. *Annual Review of Psychology, 31,* 169–193.

De Cremer, D. (2002). Respect and cooperation in social dilemmas: The importance of feeling included. *Personality and Social Psychology Bulletin, 28*(10), 1335–1341.

Deci, E. L., & Ryan, R. M. (2000). The "what" and "why" of goal pursuits: Human needs and the self-determination of behavior. *Psychological Inquiry, 11*(4), 227–268.

Deutsch, M. (1985). *Distributive justice.* New Haven, CT: Yale University Press.

Diamond, L. M. (2013). Sexuality in relationships. In J. Simpson & L. Campbell (Eds.), *Handbook of close relationships* (pp. 589–614). New York: Oxford University Press.

Eastwick, P. W. (2009). Beyond the Pleistocene: Using phylogeny and constraint to inform the evolutionary psychology of human mating. *Psychological Bulletin, 135*(5), 794–821.

Echterhoff, G., & Higgins, E. T. (2018). Shared reality: Construct and mechanisms. *Current Opinion in Psychology, 23,* iv–vii.

Elliot, A. J. (1997). Integrating the classic and contemporary approaches to achievement motivation:

A hierarchical model of approach and avoidance achievement motivation. In M. Maehr & P. Pintrich (Eds.), *Advances in motivation and achievement* (Vol. 10, pp. 143–179). Greenwich, CT: JAI Press.

Elliot, A. J. (2006). The hierarchical model of approach–avoidance motivation. *Motivation and Emotion, 30,* 111–116.

Elliot, A. J., & Fryer, J. W. (2008). The goal construct in psychology. In J. Y. Shah & W. L. Gardner (Eds.), *Handbook of motivation science* (pp. 235–250). New York: Guilford Press.

Feeney, B. C. (2004). A secure base: Responsive support of goal strivings and exploration in adult intimate relationships. *Journal of Personality and Social Psychology, 87,* 631–648.

Feeney, B. C., & Thrush, R. L. (2010). Relationship influences on exploration in adulthood: The characteristics and function of a secure base. *Journal of Personality and Social Psychology, 98,* 57–76.

Fingerman, K. L. (2009). Consequential strangers and peripheral ties: The importance of unimportant relationships. *Journal of Family Theory and Review, 1*(2), 69–86.

Finkel, E. J., Hui, C. M., Carswell, K. L., & Larson, G. M. (2014). The suffocation of marriage: Climbing Mount Maslow without enough oxygen. *Psychological Inquiry, 25*(1), 1–41.

Fiske, A. P. (1992). The four elementary forms of sociality: Framework for a unified theory of social relations. *Psychological Review, 99,* 689–723.

Fitzsimons, G. M., Finkel, E. J., & vanDellen, M. R. (2015). Transactive goal dynamics. *Psychological Review, 122*(4), 648–673.

Fletcher, G. J., Simpson, J. A., Campbell, L., & Overall, N. C. (2015). Pair-bonding, romantic love, and evolution: The curious case of *Homo sapiens. Perspectives on Psychological Science, 10*(1), 20–36.

Fraley, R. C. (2002). Attachment stability from infancy to adulthood: Meta-analysis and dynamic modeling of developmental mechanisms. *Personality and Social Psychology Review, 6*(2), 123–151.

Gable, S. L., & Strachman, A. (2008). Approaching social rewards and avoiding social punishments. In J. Y. Shah & W. L. Gardner (Eds.), *Handbook of motivation science* (pp. 561–575). New York: Guilford Press.

Gavrilets, S. (2012). Human origins and the transition from promiscuity to pair-bonding. *Proceedings of the National Academy of Sciences of the USA, 109*(25), 9923–9928.

Gleason, M. E. J., Iida, M., Shrout, P. E., & Bolger, N. (2008). Receiving support as a mixed blessing: Evidence for dual effects of support on psychological outcomes. *Journal of Personality and Social Psychology, 94,* 824–838.

Gonsalkorale, K., & Williams, K. D. (2007). The KKK won't let me play: Ostracism even by a despised outgroup hurts. *European Journal of Social Psychology, 37*(6), 1176–1186.

Gonzaga, G. C., Keltner, D., Londahl, E. A., & Smith, M. D. (2001). Love and the commitment problem in romantic relations and friendship. *Journal of Personality and Social Psychology, 81*(2), 247–262.

Guerrero, L. K., Trost, M. R., & Yoshimura, S. M. (2005). Romantic jealousy: Emotions and communicative responses. *Personal Relationships, 12*(2), 233–252.

Gunaydin, G., & DeLong, J. E. (2015). Reverse correlating love: Highly passionate women idealize their partner's facial appearance. *PLOS ONE, 10*(3), e0121094.

Hartup, W. W., & Stevens, N. (1997). Friendships and adaptation in the life course. *Psychological Bulletin, 121,* 355–370.

Hazan, C., & Diamond, L. M. (2000). The place of attachment in human mating. *Review of General Psychology, 4,* 186–204.

Hazan, C., & Shaver, P. R. (1994). Attachment as an organizational framework for research on close relationships. *Psychological Inquiry, 5,* 1–22.

Heide, J. B., & Miner, A. S. (1992). The shadow of the future: Effects of anticipated interaction and frequency of contact on buyer–seller cooperation. *Academy of Management Journal, 35*(2), 265–291.

Herbert, T. B., Silver, R. C., & Ellard, J. H. (1991). Coping with an abusive relationship: I. How and why do women stay? *Journal of Marriage and the Family, 53,* 311–325.

Higgins, E. T. (1998). Promotion and prevention: Regulatory focus as a motivational principle. In M. P. Zanna (Ed.), *Advances in experimental social psychology* (Vol. 30, pp. 1–46). New York: Academic Press.

Higgins, E. T. (2016). Shared-reality development in childhood. *Perspectives on Psychological Science, 11,* 466–495.

Higgins, E. T., & Pittman, T. S. (2008). Motives of the human animal: Comprehending, managing, and sharing inner states. *Annual Review of Psychology, 59,* 361–385.

Hirsch, J., & Clark, M. S. (2019). Paths to belonging we should study together. *Perspectives on Psychological Science, 14*(2), 238–255.

Holt-Lunstad, J., Smith, T. B., Baker, M., Harris, T., & Stephenson, D. (2015). Loneliness and social isolation as risk factors for mortality: A meta-analytic review. *Perspectives on Psychological Science, 10*(2), 227–237.

Jahoda, G. (2007). *A history of social psychology: From the Eighteenth-Century Enlightenment to the Second World War.* New York: Cambridge University Press.

Johnson, D. W., Johnson, R. T., & Maruyama, G. (1983). Interdependence and interpersonal attraction among heterogeneous and homogeneous individuals: A theoretical formulation and a meta-analysis of the research. *Review of Educational Research, 53*(1), 5–54.

Jones, E. E., Rhodewalt, F., Berglas, S., & Skelton, J. A. (1981). Effects of strategic self-presentation on subsequent self-esteem. *Journal of Personality and Social Psychology, 41*(3), 407–421.

Kelley, H. H. (1983). Analyzing close relationships. In H. H. Kelley, E. Berscheid, A. Christensen, J. H. Harvey, T. L. Huston, G. Levinger, et al. (Eds.), *Close relationships* (pp. 20–67). New York: Freeman.

Kelley, H. H., Holmes, J. G., Kerr, N., Reis, H. T., Rusbult, C. E., & Van Lange, P. A. M. (2003). *An atlas of interpersonal situations.* New York: Cambridge University Press.

Kelley, H. H., & Thibaut, J. W. (1978). *Interpersonal relations: A theory of interdependence.* New York: Wiley.

Kluwer, E. (2009). Fairness in personal relationships. In H. T. Reis & S. Sprecher (Eds.), *Encyclopedia of human relationships* (Vol. 2, pp. 588–591). Thousand Oaks, CA: SAGE.

Kruglanski, A. W., Köpetz, C., Bélanger, J. J., Chun, W. Y., Orehek, E., & Fishbach, A. (2013). Features of multifinality. *Personality and Social Psychology Review, 17*(1), 22–39.

Kruglanski, A. W., & Stroebe, W. (Eds.). (2012). *Handbook of the history of social psychology.* New York: Psychology Press.

Larzelere, R. E., & Huston, T. L. (1980). The Dyadic Trust Scale: Toward understanding interpersonal trust in close relationships. *Journal of Marriage and the Family, 42,* 595–604.

Leary, M. R., & Baumeister, R. F. (2000). The nature and function of self-esteem: Sociometer theory. In M. P. Zanna (Ed.), *Advances in experimental social psychology* (Vol. 32, pp. 1–62). San Diego, CA: Academic Press.

Little, K. C., McNulty, J. K., & Russell, V. M. (2010). Sex buffers intimates against the negative implications of attachment insecurity. *Personality and Social Psychology Bulletin, 36*(4), 484–498.

Luke, M. A., Sedikides, C., & Carnelley, K. (2012). Your love lifts me higher!: The energizing quality of secure relationships. *Personality and Social Psychology Bulletin, 38*(6), 721–733.

Lydon, J., & Karremans, J. C. (2015). Relationship regulation in the face of eye candy: A motivated cognition framework for understanding responses to attractive alternatives. *Current Opinion in Psychology, 1,* 76–80.

Mahadevan, N., Gregg, A. P., & Sedikides, C. (2019). Is self-regard a sociometer or a hierometer?: Self-esteem tracks status and inclusion, narcissism tracks status. *Journal of Personality and Social Psychology, 116*(3), 444–466.

Maner, J. K., DeWall, C. N., Baumeister, R. F., & Schaller, M. (2007). Does social exclusion motivate interpersonal reconnection?: Resolving the "porcupine problem." *Journal of Personality and Social Psychology, 92,* 42–55.

Maner, J. K., & Kenrick, D. T. (2010). Evolutionary social psychology. In R. F. Baumeister & E. J. Finkel (Eds.), *Advanced social psychology* (pp. 613–653). New York: Oxford University Press.

Mendes, W. B., Major, B., McCoy, S., & Blascovich, J. (2008). How attributional ambiguity shapes physiological and emotional responses to social rejection and acceptance. *Journal of Personality and Social Psychology, 94*(2), 278–291.

Messick, D. M., & McClintock, C. G. (1968). Motivational bases of choice in experimental games. *Journal of Experimental Social Psychology, 4*(1), 1–25.

Mikulincer, M., Gillath, O., & Shaver, P. R. (2002). Activation of the attachment system in adulthood: Threat-related primes increase the accessibility of mental representations of attachment figures. *Journal of Personality and Social Psychology, 83*(4), 881–895.

Mikulincer, M., Shaver, P. R., & Rom, E. (2011). The effects of implicit and explicit security priming on creative problem solving. *Cognition and Emotion, 25*(3), 519–531.

Muise, A., Impett, E. A., Kogan, A., & Desmarais, S. (2013). Keeping the spark alive: Being motivated to meet a partner's sexual needs sustains sexual desire in long-term romantic relationships. *Social Psychological and Personality Science, 4*(3), 267–273.

Murray, S. L., & Holmes, J. G. (2011). *Interdependent minds.* New York: Guilford Press.

Murray, S. L., Holmes, J. G., & Collins, N. L. (2006). Optimizing assurance: The risk regulation system in relationships. *Psychological Bulletin, 132,* 641–666.

Murray, S. L., Holmes, J. G., & Griffin, D. (1996). The benefits of positive illusions: Idealization and the construction of satisfaction in close relationships. *Journal of Personality and Social Psychology, 70,* 79–98.

Niehuis, S., Lee, K. H., Reifman, A., Swenson, A., & Hunsaker, S. (2011). Idealization and disillusionment in intimate relationships: A review of theory, method, and research. *Journal of Family Theory and Review, 3*(4), 273–302.

Orehek, E., & Forest, A. L. (2016). When people serve as means to goals: Implications of a motivational account of close relationships. *Current Directions in Psychological Science, 25*(2), 79–84.

Rafaeli, E., & Gleason, M. E. J. (2009). Skilled support within intimate relationships. *Journal of Family Theory and Review, 1,* 20–37.

Reis, H. T. (2008). Reinvigorating the concept of situation in social psychology. *Personality and Social Psychology Review, 12,* 311–329.

Reis, H. T. (2019). A brief history of social psychology. In R. F. Baumeister & E. J. Finkel (Eds.), *Advanced social psychology: The state of the science* (2nd ed., pp. 9–38). New York: Oxford University Press.

Reis, H. T., & Aron, A. (2008). Love: What is it, why does it matter, and how does it operate? *Perspectives on Psychological Science, 3,* 80–86.

Reis, H. T., Caprariello, P. A., & Velikcovic, M. (2011). The relationship superiority effect is moderated by the relationship context. *Journal of Experimental Social Psychology, 47,* 481–484.

Reis, H. T., Collins, W. A., & Berscheid, E. (2000). The relationship context of human behavior and development. *Psychological Bulletin, 126,* 844–872.

Reis, H. T., Lemay, E. P., & Finkenauer, C. (2017). Toward understanding understanding: The importance of feeling understood in relationships. *Social and Personality Psychology Compass, 11,* e12308.

Reis, H. T., & Shaver, P. R. (1988). Intimacy as an interpersonal process. In S. Duck (Ed.), *Handbook of personal relationships* (pp. 367–389). Chichester, UK: Wiley.

Rempel, J. K., Holmes, J. G., & Zanna, M. P. (1985). Trust in close relationships. *Journal of Personality and Social Psychology, 49*(1), 95–112.

Rimé, B. (2009). Emotion elicits the social sharing of emotion: Theory and empirical review. *Emotion Review, 1*(1), 60–85.

Robles, T. F., Slatcher, R. B., Trombello, J. M., & McGinn, M. M. (2014). Marital quality and health: A meta-analytic review. *Psychological Bulletin, 140*(1), 140–187.

Rossignac-Milon, M., & Higgins, E. T. (2018). Epistemic companions: Shared reality development in close relationships. *Current Opinion in Psychology, 23,* 66–71.

Rusbult, C. E., Finkel, E. J., & Kumashiro, M. (2009). The Michelangelo phenomenon. *Current Directions in Psychological Science, 18,* 305–309.

Rusbult, C. E., Martz, J. M., & Agnew, C. R. (1998). The investment model scale: Measuring commitment level, satisfaction level, quality of alternatives, and investment size. *Personal Relationships, 5,* 357–391.

Rusbult, C. E., Olsen, N., Davis, J. L., & Hannon, P. A. (2001). Commitment and relationship maintenance mechanisms. In J. H. Harvey & A. Wenzel (Eds.), *Close romantic relationships: Maintenance and enhancement* (pp. 87–113). Mahwah, NJ: Erlbaum.

Rusbult, C. E., & Van Lange, P. A. M. (1996). Interdependence processes. In E. T. Higgins & A. Kruglanski (Eds.), *Social psychology: Handbook of basic mechanisms and processes* (pp. 564–596). New York: Guilford Press.

Rusbult, C. E., Van Lange, P. A. M., Wildschut, T., Yovetich, N. A., & Verette, J. (2000). Perceived superiority in close relationships: Why it exists and persists. *Journal of Personality and Social Psychology, 79,* 521–545.

Rusbult, C. E., Verette, J., Whitney, G. A., Slovik, L. F., & Lipkus, I. (1991). Accommodation processes in close relationships: Theory and preliminary empirical evidence. *Journal of Personality and Social Psychology, 60,* 53–78.

Schmitt, D. P. (2004). Patterns and universals of mate poaching across 53 nations: The effects of sex, culture, and personality on romantically attracting another person's partner. *Journal of Personality and Social Psychology, 86*(4), 560–584.

Schmitt, D. P., & Buss, D. M. (2001). Human mate poaching: Tactics and temptations for infiltrating existing mateships. *Journal of Personality and Social Psychology, 80*(6), 894–917.

Sedikides, C., & Strube, M. J. (1997). Self evaluation: To thine own self be good, to thine own self be sure, to thine own self be true, and to thine own self be better. In M. P. Zanna (Ed.), *Advances in experimental social psychology* (Vol. 29, pp. 209–269). San Diego, CA: Academic Press.

Shaver, P. R., Furman, W., & Buhrmester, D. (1985). Aspects of a life transition: Network changes, social skills and loneliness. In S. W. Duck & D. Perlman (Eds.), *Understanding personal relationships* (pp. 193–219). London: SAGE.

Shaver, P. R., & Mikulincer, M. (2002). Attachment-related psychodynamics. *Attachment and Human Development, 4,* 133–161.

Sprecher, S., & Cate, R. (2004). Sexual satisfaction and sexual expression as predictors of relationship satisfaction and stability. In J. H. Harvey, A. Wenzel, & S. Sprecher (Eds.), *Handbook of sexuality in close relationships* (pp. 235–256). Mahwah, NJ: Erlbaum.

Steiner, I. D. (1972). *Group process and productivity.* New York: Academic Press.

Stroebe, M., Schut, H., & Stroebe, W. (2007). Health

outcomes of bereavement. *Lancet, 370*(9603), 1960–1973.

Swann, W. B., Jr. (1990). To be adored or to be known: The interplay of self-enhancement and self-verification. In R. Sorrentino & E. T. Higgins (Eds.), *Handbook of motivation and cognition* (Vol. 2, pp. 408–448). New York: Guilford Press.

Tedeschi, J. T. (1974). Attributions, liking, and power. In T. L. Huston (Ed.), *Foundations of interpersonal attraction* (pp. 193–215). New York: Academic Press.

Tennov, D. (1979). *Love and limerence: The experience of being in love.* New York: Stein & Day.

Thibaut, J. W., & Kelley, H. H. (1959). *The social psychology of groups.* New York: Wiley.

Thibaut, J. W., & Walker, L. (1975). *Procedural justice: A psychological analysis.* Hillsdale, NJ: Erlbaum.

Tyler, T. (2006). *Why people obey the law.* Princeton, NJ: Princeton University Press.

Van Lange, P. A. M. (1999). The pursuit of joint outcomes and equality in outcomes: An integrative model of social value orientation. *Journal of Personality and Social Psychology, 77*(2), 337–349.

Van Lange, P. A. M., & Joireman, J. A. (2008). How we can promote behavior that serves all of us in the future. *Social Issues and Policy Review, 2*(1), 127–157.

Van Lange, P. A. M., & Rusbult, C. E. (2012). Interdependence theory. In P. A. M. Van Lange, A.

W. Kruglanski, & E. T. Higgins (Eds.), *Handbook of theories of social psychology* (Vol. 2, pp. 251–272). Thousand Oaks, CA: SAGE.

Van Lange, P. A. M., Rusbult, C. E., Drigotas, S. M., Arriaga, X. B., Witcher, B. S., & Cox, C. L. (1997). Willingness to sacrifice in close relationships. *Journal of Personality and Social Psychology, 72*(6), 1373–1395.

Walster, E., Walster, G. W., & Berscheid, E. (1978). *Equity: Theory and research.* Boston: Allyn & Bacon.

Wegner, D. M. (1986). Transactive memory: A contemporary analysis of the group mind. In B. Mullen & G. R. Goethals (Eds.), *Theories of group behavior* (pp. 185–208). New York: Springer-Verlag.

Wheeless, L. R., & Grotz, J. (1977). The measurement of trust and its relationship to self-disclosure. *Human Communication Research, 3*(3), 250–257.

White, G. L., Fishbein, S., & Rutstein, J. (1981). Passionate love and the misattribution of arousal. *Journal of Personality and Social Psychology, 41,* 56–62.

Williams, K. D. (2007). Ostracism. *Annual Review of Psychology, 58,* 425–452.

Wood, J. V. (1989). Theory and research concerning social comparisons of personal attributes. *Psychological Bulletin, 106,* 231–248.

Young, L. J., & Wang, Z. (2004). The neurobiology of pair bonding. *Nature Neuroscience, 7*(10), 1048–1054.

INTRAGROUP LEVEL

CHAPTER 14

Indirect Reciprocity, Gossip, and Reputation–Based Cooperation

Daniel Balliet
Junhui Wu
Paul A. M. Van Lange

Humans not only live incredibly social lives, but they also live incredibly prosocial lives. Biologists and social scientists have long marveled at the human ability to join together in efforts to produce public goods that could not be achieved by any single person alone. The ability for humans to cooperate, that is, to engage in behaviors that benefit others (sometimes even at a cost to oneself), underlies some of the most notable human accomplishments. Yet cooperation can sometimes be very challenging for individuals in a group (or between groups) because some situations can contain a conflict of interest, such that it is in each individual's immediate self-interest to free ride and take advantage of others' cooperation (i.e., social dilemmas; De Dreu, 2010; Fehr, Fischbacher, & Gächter, 2002; Van Lange, Rockenbach, & Yamagishi, 2014).

For decades theorists and researchers have attempted to understand why humans cooperate in social dilemmas (Dawes, 1980; Komorita & Parks, 1995; Pruitt & Kimmel, 1977; Van Lange, Balliet, Parks, & Van Vugt, 2014). One of the most long-standing traditions has been from a biological perspective. According to Darwinian theory of evolution, a species cannot evolve to be cooperative unless there are survival and reproductive benefits from cooperation, and cooperative traits must compete with noncooperative alternatives, which can result in potentially greater fitness benefits if social interactions are modeled as a social dilemma (see Rand & Nowak, 2013). This problem of cooperation has attracted some of the greatest minds across a number of scientific disciplines in the biological and social sciences.

Since the 1960s, many theories have been proposed to explain why humans evolved to cooperate. Hamilton (1964) formalized the idea that cooperating with kin can increase the replication of one's own genes by increasing the chance of survival and reproduction of others who share one's genes (i.e., inclusive fitness). This was followed by Trivers's (1971) model that people may cooperate with others from whom they expect future cooperation (i.e., direct reciprocity). With direct reciprocity, actors receive (sometimes delayed) benefits directly from the individual they helped. Several additional candidate models have been forwarded in more recent years, including costly signaling (Gintis, Smith, & Bowles, 2001), generalized reciprocity (Pfeiffer, Rutte, Killingback, Taborsky, & Bonhoeffer, 2005), and gene–culture coevolution (Richerson et al., 2016).

In this chapter, we draw attention to a model of how humans evolved to cooperate (and also avoid interactions with noncooperators)—reputation-based indirect reciprocity—and this model carries rich potential for understanding some basic cognitive and motivational processes underlying social behavior. Indirect reciprocity involves two events: (1) An actor extends a benefit (or not) to a recipient and (2) a third party obtains knowledge of the actor's behavior and decides to cooperate (or not) with the actor at some point in the future (Alexander, 1987/2017; Boyd & Richerson, 1989; Nowak & Sigmund, 1998b). An essential element for indirect reciprocity to occur is that a third party directly observes the interaction between the actor and the recipient or learns about the actor's behavior through communication, such as gossip. Direct and indirect reciprocity vary in how an actor acquires benefits from his or her own cooperation. *Direct reciprocity* occurs when the recipient of the benefit of a cooperative action returns a benefit to the cooperative actor. *Indirect reciprocity,* on the other hand, occurs when anyone, except for the recipient of the benefit of a cooperative action, delivers a benefit to the cooperative actor. Direct and indirect reciprocity can also involve responding to others' noncooperative actions by imposing either direct or indirect costs on the noncooperative actor, respectively. In this chapter, we focus on indirect reciprocity and reputation-based cooperation. Indirect reciprocity could be a unique evolutionary pathway to human cooperation, although a few examples suggest that indirect reciprocity can also occur in other species, such as cleaner fish (Bshary & Grutter, 2006) and song sparrows (Akçay, Reed, Campbell, Templeton, & Beecher, 2010). Regardless, the capacity for language has enabled humans to exploit this route to cooperation in large groups of genetically unrelated individuals (Dunbar, 2004).

Although much of the theoretical work on indirect reciprocity emerged from the biological sciences, the topic of indirect reciprocity is now widely studied by a growing number of scientists across numerous disciplines, including behavioral economics and psychology. They have studied (1) the influence of indirect reciprocity on cooperation in the lab and field, (2) environmental conditions that facilitate indirect reciprocity, and (3) the proximate psychological processes that underlie this human ability. Our purpose in this chapter is to integrate biological, economic, and psychological research on how indirect reciprocity facilitates cooperation. In doing so, we use models in evolutionary biology to generate insights about how humans have evolved to engage in reputation-based indirect reciprocity and discuss ideas and research about the proximate psychological mechanisms operating to make this form of cooperation possible.

Evolutionary Dynamics, Direct Reciprocity, and Indirect Reciprocity

With the exception of species that reproduce incredibly fast (e.g., fruit flies), we cannot observe how the process of evolution selects for the adaptive design of a species. Because it can be exceedingly difficult, or even impossible, to study the process by which evolution shapes organisms, scientists have resorted to creating their own "organisms" (i.e., agents) in computer programs. Agent-based modeling is an approach used to study how evolutionary dynamics can select for certain behavioral strategies in a population of agents. This method has become incredibly popular over the last few decades and has yielded several valuable insights about how evolution could have shaped human social behavior (Nowak, 2006).

The models always begin with a population of agents that have preprogrammed behavioral strategies (e.g., always cooperate, always defect, tit for tat, and win–stay, lose–shift), and then these agents interact with each other over a lifespan in a situation that contains specified outcomes. The outcome is the number of offspring an agent produces in a lifetime, and offspring always have a higher chance to inherit the behavioral strategy of their parents. In the context of the study of cooperation, agents are most often specified to interact in a prisoner's dilemma (PD; or some variant of the PD, see Figure 14.1). In the PD, each person can decide to deliver a benefit (b) to the other at some cost (c) to him- or herself. When the benefit to the other is greater than the cost to oneself ($b > c$), then both can obtain better outcomes if each person decides to extend a benefit to the other. However, in this type of situation, the best outcome for each person can be obtained by not paying the cost to deliver a benefit to the other, and nonetheless receive a benefit delivered by the partner. Thus, cooperation in the PD is mutually beneficial, but it is always vulnerable to exploitation and free riding by noncooperators. A corpus of literature has formed around understanding the behavioral strategies that can successfully maintain cooperation in a species and are robust to invasion by noncooperators (for reviews, see Nowak, 2006; Rand & Nowak, 2013; West, Griffin, & Gardner, 2007).

These models have generated support and insights about behavioral strategies of direct reciprocity in a population characterized by repeated encounters. Early modeling work demonstrated that the simple rule of tit for tat (i.e., cooperate first, then follow one's partner's previous behavior) outperformed many other more complex strategies (Axelrod, 1984). Subsequent modeling work discovered another strategy that outcompeted tit for tat—win–stay, lose–shift (i.e., cooperate only if both players had the same behavior on the previous round; Nowak & Sigmund, 1993). Yet these strategies can make costly errors in environments where people sometimes intend to cooperate but end up defecting. In these environments, a more for-giving tit-for-tat strategy (i.e., cooperates once again after a partner defects, but then defects after a partner's second defection; tit for two tats; Wu & Axelrod, 1995) is more successful. Also, adding some generosity to the tit-for-tat strategy can be effective in "noisy" environments in which it is not always certain that an intended choice results in actual choice (Kollock, 1993). Indeed, changing parameters of the environment itself (e.g., the situation is noisy or not) or the social environment (i.e., the strategies followed by others) can affect which strategy is most successful. Thus, modeling work can benefit from attempting to make plausible assumptions about the ancestral conditions in which humans evolved to cooperate (Tooby & Cosmides, 1996).

The modeling work reported here provides us insights about how evolution may have shaped certain strategies of cooperation that could acquire direct benefits, and still prevent a population from being invaded and exploited by defectors. The models can be used to generate hypotheses about different adaptions humans could have developed to regulate their cooperation to acquire direct benefits (see Delton, Krasnow, Cosmides, & Tooby, 2011), such as cheater detection (Cosmides, Barrett, & Tooby,

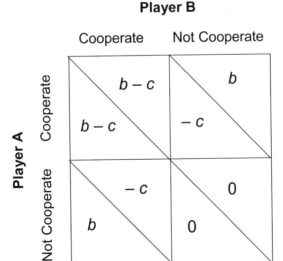

FIGURE 14.1. The interdependence structure of a prisoner's dilemma. Cooperation means delivering a benefit (b) to one's partner at a cost (c) to oneself ($b > c$).

2010), revenge and forgiveness (McCullough, Kurzban, & Tabak, 2013), gratitude (Ma, Tunney, & Ferguson, 2017), generosity (Van Lange, Ouwerkerk, & Tazelaar, 2002), and inferences about future interactions (Delton et al., 2011).

Similarly, agent-based models have also provided insights about how evolution may have shaped the way humans engage in indirect reciprocity and its role in the maintenance of large-scale cooperation. Nowak and Sigmund (1998a, 1998b) found that indirect reciprocity can evolve if agents have knowledge about how their partners have behaved toward others in previous interactions (i.e., image score), then condition their behavior on their partners' past behavior. In this modeling work, in each round of interactions between agents, agents were randomly assigned to be a donor or a receiver. The donor could decide to pay a small cost to provide the receiver with a larger benefit. Each donor would receive a positive point for each helping behavior and a negative point for each failure to help. Cooperation evolved when agents assigned as donors conditioned their decisions to help based on the recipients' image score (i.e., only help if the recipient has a positive image score). Since this initial work, a number of models have further examined how different environments and decision rules can affect the evolution of cooperation via indirect reciprocity (e.g., Ohtsuki & Iwasa, 2006).

The modeling research described here serves two complementary goals. First, modeling behavioral strategies of indirect reciprocity can help us understand how humans evolved to cooperate. Second, the modeling work can be used to develop and test hypotheses about how evolution could have modified the design of an organism to cooperate to acquire direct and indirect benefits. Modeling evolutionary dynamics can be viewed as a way to develop theories and generate new predictions that can be tested using behavioral experiments—and this is where the modeling becomes most relevant for psychologists.

An initial step in testing predictions from an agent-based model is conducting behavioral experiments to observe whether human behavior varies according to how the models predict (for a list of predictions generated by specific agent-based models of indirect reciprocity, see Table 14.1). For example, empirical researchers could design lab experiments to examine whether the possibility of punishing defectors, with the decision to punish affecting one's reputation, is especially effective at promoting cooperation in larger groups (e.g., groups of eight vs. groups of four; dos Santos & Wedekind, 2015).

A further step would be unpacking the abilities that could have evolved to promote these types of behavior—and this is often an entirely different enterprise in applying evolution to understanding human behavior, often referred to as an *adaptationist approach* or *evolutionary psychology* (Tooby & Cosmides, 1992). The agent-based models provide insights about the evolutionary success of certain behavioral strategies, but the models are agnostic about the actual psychological mechanisms that could have evolved through the process of evolution to promote such behaviors. Importantly, evolution does not select for organisms to engage in a specific behavior. Instead, the outputs of the evolutionary process are psychological mechanisms that process input from the environment and produce behavior. Interestingly, there has been much more agent-based modeling work on the role of indirect reciprocity on cooperation compared to an adaptationist approach. Much of what comes next is a discussion of the possible psychological mechanisms that could be operating to enable indirect reciprocity to promote large-scale cooperation. Yet prior to discussing the proximate psychology of indirect reciprocity, we take a moment to consider recent work that has documented the phenomenon that people actually engage in indirect reciprocity in their daily lives and in controlled lab environments.

Indirect Reciprocity in the Field

Agent-based modeling of the evolution of indirect reciprocity suggests that humans could have adaptations that regulate their cooperative behavior in a way that is structured according to indirect reciprocity. One of the first steps in a program of research on this topic is to document that humans in fact do behave in ways that look like indirect reciprocity, and a number of recent field studies give us insights in this matter.

TABLE 14.1. Examples of Testable Hypotheses about Human Behavior Derived from Agent-Based Modeling on Indirect Reciprocity

Study	Model description	Hypotheses
dos Santos & Wedekind (2015)	Computer simulations tested two reputation systems (reputation based on cooperative and noncooperative actions and reputation based on punitive and nonpunitive actions) in a public goods game involving groups of unrelated individuals.	Compared to reputation systems based on cooperation, reputation systems based on punishment (1) are more likely to lead to the evolution of cooperation in larger groups, (2) more effectively sustains cooperation within larger groups, and (3) are more robust to errors in reputation assessment.
Leimar & Hammerstein (2001)	Simulations tested how cooperation evolves through two indirect reciprocity strategies (i.e., image scoring and standing strategy).	(1) Image scoring strategies enhance cooperation only when the cost of cooperation is small. (2) Standing strategy outperforms image scoring even when there are errors in perception.
Roberts (2008)	Evolutionary simulations compared indirect reciprocity strategies (i.e., image scoring and simple standing) with direct reciprocity strategies in large groups with less repeated interactions and in small groups with more repeated interactions.	(1) As probability of repeated interactions increases, indirect reciprocity through image scoring becomes less stable in promoting cooperation than direct reciprocity by experience scoring. (2) Indirect reciprocity through standing strategy is as stable as direct reciprocity in promoting cooperation when individuals have repeated interactions with few partners.
Sasaki, Okada, & Nakai (2017)	An evolutionary analysis compared a simple "staying" norm with other prevailing social norms that discriminate the good and the bad.	Staying is most effective in establishing cooperation than other social norms that rely on constant monitoring and unconditional assessment (i.e., scoring, simple-standing, stern-judging, and shunning).[a]
Giardini, Paolucci, Villatoro, & Conte (2014)	An agent-based simulation assessed how cooperation rates change when agents can punish others or know others' reputation and then defect with free riders or refuse to interact with them.	(1) Both punishment and reputation-based partner selection are effective in maintaining cooperation. (2) Cooperation decreases when people defect after learning about free riders' reputations. (3) A combination of punishment and reputation-based partner selection leads to higher cooperation rates.
Giardini & Vilone (2016)	An agent-based model tested the conditions under which gossip and ostracism might enhance cooperation in groups of different sizes by addressing the effects of quantity and quality of gossip, network structure, and errors in gossip transmission.	(1) Cooperation is more likely to thrive in larger groups when the amount of gossip exchanged is abundant. (2) Inclusion errors (i.e., one's negative reputation is understood as positive) in gossip transmission are more detrimental to cooperation than exclusion errors (i.e., one's positive reputation is understood as negative).

[a]Staying = the reputation of a person who gives help stays the same as in the last assessment if the recipient has a bad reputation; scoring (or image scoring) = people lose reputations anytime they fail to help someone in need; simple standing (or standing strategy) = reputation declines when one fails to help someone with a good reputation; stern judging = people lose reputations when they help someone with a bad reputation or fail to help a person with a good reputation; shunning = people gain a good reputation only when they help someone with a good reputation; otherwise they lose a good reputation.

In a field study with 2,413 residents, researchers collaborated with a utility company to examine participation in a program to prevent blackouts during high electricity demand (Yoeli, Hoffman, Rand, & Nowak, 2013). They found that participation rate was tripled when residents' identities were observable (vs. concealed) on the sign-up sheet, and this positive effect of observability was four times larger than that of monetary reward. More importantly, observability had a larger effect for homeowners (vs. temporary renters) and people living in apartments (vs. houses), as they tend to have longer-term relationships with neighbors. In this study, we clearly see that people are more cooperative when their behavior is observable, and so can affect their reputation within their social network.

Similarly, van Apeldoorn and Schram (2016) examined indirect reciprocity in a field experiment utilizing an online platform in which people can ask and offer services to each other for free. They created new member profiles that vary in serving history (i.e., "serving" or "neutral" profile), then sent out service requests to worldwide members. People were more likely to reward a service request from someone who had previously offered services to others. Another natural field experiment conducted in a hair salon revealed that customers tended to offer more tips to hairdressers who were collecting donations to a charity, compared to doing nothing (Khadjavi, 2016). These studies support the idea that people are more cooperative with others who have a cooperative reputation.

In fact, people are strongly influenced by information about others' reputations, even more so than information about their similarity with others. Abrahao, Parigi, Gupta, and Cook (2017) conducted a large-scale online experiment with 8,906 users of Airbnb playing an interpersonal investment game. In this game, the users had to make trust decisions toward potential receivers whose profiles varied in distance (i.e., the extent to which the receiver matched the demographic attributes of participants across four categories) and two reputation features (i.e., the average ratings and the number of reviews on Airbnb). The users had 100 credits that they could keep or invest in the receivers they chose. Any amount invested was tripled and the re-

ceiver could then decide to return some amount to users. The authors found that people tend to trust receivers with a better reputation even though they are dissimilar, and this was further confirmed when analyzing real-world data of 1 million actual hospitality interactions among users of Airbnb.

Taken together, these field studies show that indirect reciprocity promotes cooperation in contexts outside of the laboratory. Specifically, this work documents that people are willing to (1) behave in ways that maintain a positive and cooperative reputation and (2) condition their cooperation on their partners' reputations.

Indirect Reciprocity in the Lab

Several experiments using economic games as a paradigm to study cooperation have demonstrated that people do engage in indirect reciprocity. Wedekind and Milinski (2000) conducted a behavioral experiment with a design similar to previous modeling work (i.e., Nowak & Sigmund, 1998b). In this study, participants interacted with each other in several rounds, and in each round they were selected to interact with a different person as a donor or a receiver. The donor decided whether to give 2 Swiss Francs to a receiver who would then earn four Swiss Francs. In each round, participants (assigned a pseudonym) could see the previous decisions made by their partners. The study revealed that people were more likely to give money to another person who had given money to others in the past.

Similar experiments have revealed that people are more likely to help others who have a positive reputation (Engelmann & Fischbacher, 2009; Seinen & Schram, 2006; Stanca, 2009). When people can build a reputation in a group based on their helping behavior, then groups display higher levels of cooperation (Milinski, Semmann, & Krambeck, 2002). Furthermore, when people can gossip about each other during interactions in a repeated public goods game (i.e., a multiperson PD), then people become more cooperative, compared to when gossip is not allowed (Feinberg, Willer, & Schultz, 2014; Wu, Balliet, & Van Lange, 2015).

Of course, people may strategically build reputations to achieve higher earnings (e.g., only help others when being observed), and economists have been interested in empirically distinguishing such strategic behaviors aimed at maximizing self-interest from a motivation to extend benefits to others who have a cooperative reputation. To accomplish this, Engelmann and Fischbacher (2009) had participants interact in an 80-trial helping game involving a donor and a receiver. Participants were randomly assigned to be a donor or a receiver in each trial, and had a public or private score for the first or last 40 trials (i.e., public scores displayed past behaviors to current partners, and this information was not provided to current partners in the private score condition). This design allowed participants to interact with others who had private or public scores. Importantly, they found that people with a private score were still willing to help others with a higher positive public score. Thus, participants with a private score had no strategic incentives to condition their cooperation toward people with a cooperative reputation, so it is unlikely that a motivation to maximize own outcomes was directing these behaviors. The authors take this as evidence that people have a social preference to help others who have a helpful and cooperative reputation.

Lab studies have also examined how effective and efficient indirect reciprocity can be at promoting cooperation. This question becomes especially relevant when one compares gossip (i.e., reputation sharing) with another mechanism that can support cooperation: the possibility to punish others' past behavior. A prior study revealed that gossip is more effective and efficient than punishment (Wu, Balliet, & Van Lange, 2016a). Although punishment can be an effective means to promoting cooperation, punishment is costly to enact and can result in retaliation. Gossip, on the other hand, may be less costly to enact and involves less exposure to the costs of retaliation. There can be reputational costs in gossip, but this is not always true (Feinberg, Cheng, & Willer, 2012).

The agent-based models suggest that indirect reciprocity is a possible route through which evolutionary processes shape human cooperation, and now we see that both lab and field experiments have documented that people do engage in indirect reciprocity. However, documenting the existence, effectiveness, and efficiency of indirect reciprocity does not provide an explanation for this behavioral phenomenon. Moreover, agent-based models and economic models do not specify the cognitive and motivational processes that produce behaviors in a system of indirect reciprocity. Currently, there is a need to develop theories about the proximate psychological mechanisms that could be operating to produce these forms of behavior.

An Evolutionary Psychology Approach

Agent-based models suggest that humans could have evolved to cooperate in a system of indirect reciprocity, so an evolutionary psychology approach can be applied to hypothesize about the proximate psychological mechanisms that could have evolved to produce these behaviors. Evolutionary psychology aims to understand how different cognitive and motivational mechanisms of the human mind have evolved to function and produce behavior. Prior to applying this perspective, we need to understand a few key concepts (for several reviews, see Confer et al., 2010; Cosmides & Tooby, 2013; for comparisons of this perspective to other approaches in the social sciences, see Tooby & Cosmides, 1992, 2015).

An evolutionary psychology approach is an adaptationist research program, in that researchers test hypotheses about some adaptive designs of an organism that promote a functional output. An *adaptation* has four properties: (1) It is a system of reliably developing properties of a species, (2) it is incorporated into the design of an organism, (3) it is coordinated with the structure of the environment, and (4) it causes a functional outcome (at least increases the probability of a functional outcome within the environment that it evolved; see Tooby & Cosmides, 2015). Adaptations must solve a problem necessary for the reproduction of an organism and can be understood as the output of the evolutionary process. Thus, an evolutionary psychology research program is largely about understanding the adaptations that underlie and explain variability in human behavior.

To understand any single adaptation, researchers need to generate hypotheses about the *environment of evolutionary adaptedness (EEA)*. The EEA "for a given adaptation is the statistical composite of the enduring selection pressures or cause-and-effect relationships that pushed the alleles underlying an adaptation systematically upward in frequency until they became species-typical or reached a frequency-dependent equilibrium" (Tooby & Cosmides, 2015, p. 25). Each adaptation would have a corresponding specialized EEA with which the adaptation is coordinated to promote a behavior that enhanced survival and reproductive success within those environmental conditions. The EEA is not a specific time or place, but it contains the reliably recurring environmental challenges and opportunities that gave rise to the adaptation. Thus, an evolutionary psychology program of research generally tests hypotheses about an adaptive psychological mechanism that enables a specific behavior, and uses knowledge and assumptions about the EEA to generate hypotheses about how the adaptation (i.e., proximate psychological mechanism) might work to produce the behavior. Furthermore, this approach can be used to forward hypotheses about how an adaptation that evolved to function for one purpose can be exapted and applied to a different purpose (Andrews, Gangestad, & Matthews, 2002; Buss, Haselton, Shackelford, Bleske, & Wakefield, 1998). The distinction between adaptations and exaptations may be especially important in understanding the emergence of indirect reciprocity, and how the phylogenetically older psychological mechanisms that evolved for direct reciprocity could be exapted to enable indirect reciprocity.

In the following sections, we break down a system of indirect reciprocity into its most simple elements—three persons in a social network. We discuss specific potential adaptive challenges and opportunities in the EEA for each person in this network and hypothesize about possible adaptations that motivate fitness-enhancing behaviors to resolve those adaptive problems.

Emergence of Indirect Reciprocity in the EEA

Humans lived in small hunter–gatherer groups prior to the advent of agriculture, and it is thought that many human adaptations for co-

operation have arisen from reliably recurring opportunities and challenges before and during this period. Research comparing humans to chimps and bonobos suggests that a common ancestor may have already possessed some key adaptations for cooperation, such as for direct reciprocity—to help others who are helpful to you, and not help those who did not help you (De Waal, 2008; Jaeggi, Stevens, & Van Schaik, 2010; Warneken & Tomasello, 2006). Adaptations for direct reciprocity could have provided the foundation for indirect reciprocity to emerge in human societies.

Direct reciprocity can be an effective strategy to maintain cooperation in small groups in which people will interact with each other in the future, can observe everyone's behavior, and share a history with each interaction partner. However, direct reciprocity may face difficulties in sustaining cooperation in larger groups, or at least indirect reciprocity would enable people to more effectively avoid costly interactions with noncooperators (even during the first encounter), and to capture even greater benefits from cooperation by netting not only direct but also indirect benefits in larger groups. Furthermore, language was likely a key ability that amplified the benefits of indirect reciprocity. Language enabled people to communicate their own social interaction experiences with many others, and this information could be used as an input to learn about others' past behavior, to update reputations, and to condition cooperation (Dunbar, 2004). Thus, as human groups expanded in size, this increased the frequency of people having valuable first-encounter interactions and decreased the ability to directly observe all possible interaction partners. These changes in the social ecology, along with an enhanced ability for language, were key conditions that amplified the indirect benefits of cooperation and paved the way for indirect reciprocity, thereby enabling natural selection to shape psychological mechanisms functionally specialized for this structure of social interactions.

How did indirect reciprocity become a major force shaping human social behavior? One critical action in a system of indirect reciprocity involves one person cooperating or not with another person, and this would have been occurring deep into our ancestral past, and beyond a common ancestor we share with the other great apes. Therefore, it is possible that indirect reciprocity takes hold when people learn about others' reputation and condition their behavior toward others based on that reputation (as opposed to previous direct experience or benefits). As mentioned earlier, humans likely had adaptations for direct reciprocity, and these preexisting psychological mechanisms could have been exapted to acquire input from others' experiences shared via language. Language enabled people to communicate their experiences with many others, and if people conditioned their cooperation toward the actor based on this input, then this enabled opportunities for people to behave in ways to affect their reputations and receive indirect benefits. This perspective predicts that at least some adaptations for direct reciprocity, such as abilities for cheater detection and welfare tradeoffs (Cosmides, 1989; Cosmides & Tooby, 1992; Sznycer, Delton, Robertson, Cosmides, & Tooby, 2019), could use language as input to condition cooperation and partner selection.

Once humans were able to share information with each other, then use that information to condition their cooperation, this form of structured interactions would have enabled natural selection to operate on functionally specialized abilities to (1) condition behavior to acquire indirect benefits, (2) share information to acquire direct benefits (since gossip has value to interaction partners), and (3) evaluate gossip and use it to select cooperative partners and condition cooperation. An important line of future research may consider understanding what adaptations for direct reciprocity have been exapted for indirect reciprocity and which, if any, adaptations are unique to indirect reciprocity. This line of research will need to clearly delineate the different adaptive challenges of a system of indirect reciprocity. Figure 14.2 displays the essential components of a system of indirect reciprocity and identifies distinct adaptive challenges that can occur for different persons within the network. Next, we discuss the different adaptive problems, some hypothesized solutions, and relevant research on these topics.

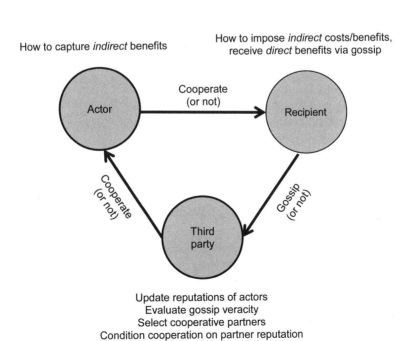

FIGURE 14.2. Indirect reciprocity and adaptive problems faced by the actor, recipient, and third party.

Managing a Cooperative Reputation (the Actor)

In a system of indirect reciprocity, cooperative people can capture indirect benefits from others and avoid ostracism in social interactions, and this can offset the cost of cooperation. Thus, conditioning cooperation in ways to acquire these benefits and avoid these costs could be a reliably recurring adaptive challenge. A generalized learning system would have difficulty in solving this problem because indirect benefits can be incredibly challenging to anticipate, and the rewards of one's cooperative behavior can occur a long distance in time from the actual cooperative behaviors. In fact, to anticipate these indirect benefits, people would need to understand that the recipient would evaluate their behavior positively, remember their behavior, share that information with others—and especially others with whom the actor would meet and interact in the future, that the recipients of the gossip would use that information to form an evaluation of the actor, that the recipients of gossip would meet them in the future and condition their behavior on that information, and that the benefit received from that future interaction would be larger than the cost of the present cooperation. Previous research suggests that people find this difficult to do, even when they obtain very explicit information about how their actions affect the recipient, that the recipient will communicate with a third person, and that the third person has a chance to select them as a partner (and to possibly reward them with a larger benefit). For example, Wu, Balliet, and Van Lange (2015b) conducted three studies in which participants knew (or not) that a recipient of their generous behavior could gossip about their behavior to a third person, and that this third person could use that information to condition his or her own behavior toward them in a future interaction. Although participants were more cooperative when they knew their behavior would be gossiped about, this increase in cooperation was not explained by the participants' expectation that the third person would be kind to them in a future interaction. Perhaps the problem of identifying opportunities to cooperate to acquire indirect benefits is better solved by a functionally specialized ability to use *cues* in social interactions that would identify situa-

tions in which people could often acquire greater indirect benefits for their cooperation.

Social network structures can provide some insights about situations that may result in greater indirect benefits. Recent work has revealed that several characteristics are reliably recurring in social networks in large-scale modern societies, as well in small-scale hunter–gatherer societies (Apicella, Marlowe, Fowler, & Christakis, 2012; Hamilton, Milne, Walker, Burger, & Brown, 2007; Hill et al., 2011; Mc-Glohon, Akoglu, & Faloutsos, 2011; Porter, Mucha, Newman, & Warmbrand, 2005). Two of these social network properties are that (1) social networks are "small" and (2) some people are better connected than others. Specifically, in most social networks, it takes very few connections to travel from one node to another, so gossip and reputational information can easily spread widely throughout a social network. Furthermore, the number of network connections any single individual has in a social network is unevenly distributed, with some people having more network connections than others. If these properties of social networks did indeed covary with the probability of actions translating into indirect benefits, then it might be possible that natural selection would favor an ability to condition cooperation on the social network properties of an interaction partner (or any observer of one's behavior).

In order for this to be possible, there would need to be cues that reliably covary across social interactions that could be used to indicate which situations are more likely to translate into indirect benefits. Cues that a person is either connected to one's social network or that the person is well connected within one's social network could both indicate opportunities for indirect benefits (Wu et al., 2016c). Previous research indicates that people extended greater cooperation and generosity to a person who could communicate to a future interaction partner (Wu et al., 2015), and that people were more generous toward others who could communicate with a greater number of their possible future interaction partners (Wu et al., 2016c). Thus, initial evidence provides support for the idea that cues that covary with network properties may be used to condition cooperation to acquire indirect benefits. Similarly, Yamagishi, Jin, and Kiyonari (1999) suggested that people use group membership as a cue of a shared social network, and that cooperation with ingroup members is a strategy to acquire indirect benefits.

Another possible cue for indirect benefits is observability. Observers may select or avoid an actor based on the observed behavior, and observers may also gossip about what they have witnessed. Prior research indicates that reducing anonymity tends to increase cooperation (Andreoni & Petrie, 2004; Wang et al., 2017), and researchers have argued that this effect may be due to reputational concerns (e.g., Sparks & Barclay, 2013). Watching eyes, such as a pair of eyes on a computer screen when people are making decisions, have been found to enhance generosity and cooperation (Haley & Fessler, 2005). Recent meta-analyses, however, have either found no effect of eye cues (Northover, Pedersen, Cohen, & Andrews, 2017) or discovered only a few situations in which the effect may be found. For example, eye cues only increase the probability of giving but not the overall level of generosity (Nettle et al., 2013), only increase cooperation after brief exposure (Sparks & Barclay, 2013), and the eyes need to be open and attentive (Manesi, Van Lange, & Pollet, 2016). Furthermore, it may be that observability affects cooperation via a different process than reputation. For example, the presence of others may serve as a cue of being mutually dependent on another person (Balliet, Tybur, & Van Lange, 2017). Observability is certainly a central issue in indirect reciprocity that may have enabled a simple form of indirect reciprocity prior to the existence of language and sharing gossip about others. Future research can attempt to better understand how anonymity and observability influence behaviors that are aimed at reputation management, while controlling and accounting for alternative explanations.

Two interrelated issues for future research on reputation management are (1) how to manage several dimensions of reputation and (2) how the social ecology shapes the strategies people use to manage their reputation. Modeling and experimental research on cooperation has tended to focus on how people can form cooperative reputations, but reputations can be multifaceted and track many other traits and characteristics of people (e.g., dominance, competence, and

mate value). Recent work in our lab had people describe their daily-life events about which they either shared or received gossip (Dores Cruz et al., 2018). We found that the gossip people reported in their daily lives covers a broad range of personal characteristics that fall into the six broad dimensions of personality (i.e., Honesty–Humility, Emotionality, Extroversion, Agreeableness, Conscientiousness, Openness to Experience) and the major dimensions of social perception (i.e., warmth, competence, dominance, and morality). One adaptive challenge in managing one's reputation is to understand how a behavior would be evaluated along each of these dimensions, as well as what characteristics would be of value to future interaction partners. Moreover, little is understood about how reputation management strategies vary across social ecologies. One possibility is that variation across societies in the opportunity costs of forming new relationships (Thomson et al., 2018) relates to how much people will invest in a cooperative reputation and which traits people attempt to communicate to others.

Gossip and Reputation Sharing (the Recipient)

People engage in actions that directly affect others' outcomes, and these actions can spark recipient evaluations and behaviors in response to these actions and outcomes—a topic that has been widely studied as moral evaluations, judgment, and behavior (e.g., Skowronski & Carlston, 1987). From an evolutionary perspective, humans may have evolved strategies in social interactions to increase the chance of future benefits and reduce potential future costs. These strategies would function to shape others' behavior that can affect one's outcomes. One strategy is to directly reciprocate benefits and costs. For example, when an individual is mistreated, he or she may experience anger, which mobilizes direct confrontation that can function to adjust the transgressors' actions in future encounters (e.g., become more cooperative; Sell, Tooby, & Cosmides, 2009). An alternative strategy is to share information with others who will confer benefits and impose costs on the actor. For example, a person who is exploited in an interaction can share this experience with a third party, who then may decide against selecting the actor as a future cooperative partner. Here we focus on the adaptive challenges of when and how to share information about others' behavior (e.g., gossip).

Human communication via language greatly expands the human capacity to obtain knowledge about others in their social networks. People often talk about other people, and this is pervasive across small- and large-scale societies (see Dunbar, 2004). Previous theory has suggested that humans may use language strategically to communicate information about others, and especially absent third parties. For example, people who have been treated poorly by another could directly aggress against that person or impose harm on him or her, but this is a strategy that is exposed to the costs of retaliation. Instead, people could share information about that person's past behavior with others in the absence of the actor, and the recipients of that information could then impose costs on the actor (i.e., indirect aggression; Archer & Coyne, 2005) or avoid the person in the future. Humans may have a functionally specialized ability to share information about others in ways that increase the likelihood that benefits and costs occur to others because the behavior

could indirectly enhance an individual's reproductive fitness by further enhancing the fitness of a cooperative ally or reducing the fitness of a previously uncooperative exchange partner (Molho, Tybur, Van Lange, & Balliet, 2020).

Talking about others, especially in their absence, is known as gossip. Unfortunately, gossip has not received extensive research attention, perhaps because it has been widely viewed as a trivial social behavior of little consequence. Thus, when and how people gossip about others is an understudied topic of research, and this is unfortunate given that theory of indirect reciprocity provides a functional account of gossip in regulating social relationships and that people around the world engage in this behavior.

Research over the past few decades has approached and defined gossip in many different ways (for an overview of definitions, see Table 14.2). Common themes across these definitions are that gossip involves communicating information about an absent third party (or at least the third party is not knowledgeable of the information exchanged). Other approaches have emphasized that the communicated information must contain some evaluative content (e.g., Foster, 2004) and that the communication must be

TABLE 14.2. Definitions of Gossip

Reference	Definition of *gossip*
Dunbar (2004)	"conversation about social and personal topics" (p. 109)
Feinberg, Cheng, & Willer (2012)	"sharing of evaluative information about an absent third party" (p. 25)
Fine & Rosnow (1978)	"a topical assertion about personal qualities or behavior, usually but not necessarily formulated on the basis of hearsay, that is deemed trivial or nonessential within the immediate social context" (p. 161)
Fonseca & Peters (2017)	"the class of speech that transmits information about the behaviors and attributes of third parties" (p. 254)
Foster (2004)	"the exchange of personal information (positive or negative) in an evaluative way (positive or negative) about absent third parties" (p. 83)
Hess & Hagen (2006)	"personal conversations about reputation-relevant behavior" (p. 339)
Noon & Delbridge (1993)	"the process of informally communicating value-laden information about members of a social setting" (p. 25)
Piazza & Bering (2008)	"the mechanism by which social information (derived from direct experience) gets transmitted to absent third parties" (p. 172)
Wittek & Wielers (1998)	"the provision of information by one person (ego) to another person (alter) about an absent third person (tertius)" (p. 189)

informal (Noon & Delbridge, 1993). Yet previous theory of indirect reciprocity does not specify that the information communicated needs to be evaluative; it could simply be factual, and neither should it have to be informal. In fact, formal evaluations, such as an employer giving an evaluation of an employee, is an institutionalization of gossip—organizations understand the functional benefits of gossip in terms of selecting and retaining cooperative allies. We take the perspective that gossip is the sharing of information about a third party who is not knowledgeable about the information exchange. Such gossip does not need to be evaluative; it can be simply factual and can be either formal or informal.

There are several adaptive problems of gossip, such as when, how, and with whom to gossip to impose costs or benefits on an actor. First, people may gossip in ways that amplify the benefits and costs to the actor. People may strategically share gossip with others who will have future interactions with the target of gossip, and thus may be especially likely to share gossip with ingroup members or people who are connected to their social network. People may share gossip in a way that communicates attributes (e.g., competence, trustworthiness) of the target that would make him or her especially (un)desirable as a cooperation partner to others. People could have an ability to understand when to share facts versus evaluations, and when to exaggerate certain evaluations of the target.

Second, people may use gossip as a resource in exchange for other direct benefits from the recipients of gossip. From the perspective of indirect reciprocity, gossip can be a valuable resource that enables others to select mutually beneficial, cooperative allies and avoid costly encounters with noncooperators. Thus, people should be willing to reciprocate the benefits received from gossip. Indeed, previous work has indicated that exchanging gossip can enhance trust, reciprocity, and social bonding (Peters, Jetten, Radova, & Austin, 2017). Furthermore, sharing highly negative gossip about others could make the gossiper even more vulnerable and, indeed, people tend to share negative gossip only when they trust the recipient (Ellwardt, Wittek, & Wielers, 2012; Grosser, Lopez-Kidwell, & Labianca, 2010). An interesting possibility is that

sharing negative gossip could especially help to further build trust and bonding between individuals.

Third, people may gossip in ways that reduce the likelihood of exposure and retaliation from the target of gossip. How would people avoid the cost of retaliation for being exposed for gossiping? People should be sensitive to the qualities of the relationship between the recipient and the target of gossip. In particular, people may be less likely to share negative gossip about targets who are genetically related to the recipient or close to the recipient. Moreover, certain qualities of the recipient may increase the chance of detection, such as the person being well connected within a social network, untrustworthy, or highly dominant. In addition, certain qualities of the target, such as how well connected the target is in his or her social network, and his or her prestige and standing within the group, may also increase the chance of detection.

Reputation Updating, Partner Selection, and Conditional Cooperation (Third Party)

Previous modeling work has clearly displayed that sharing information about others' behavior in a social network can promote the evolution of cooperation, and we recognize at least three adaptive problems for the recipients of gossip (i.e., third parties): (1) how to update an actor's reputation based on new information, (2) how to use reputation to select and avoid partners, and (3) how to use others' reputations to condition their own cooperation.

Reputation has been discussed and defined in many ways across different literatures (for some prominent definitions, see Table 14.3). Across these definitions, there are some key similarities and differences. Reputation can be thought to involve information that is shared about a person among multiple people. The information is usually about some attribute of the person, and possibly a corresponding evaluation of that attribute. Many scholars theorize that reputation exists at a collective level of analysis and refers to a shared belief and evaluation of a person (Anderson & Shirako, 2008; Emler, 1990). However, most research also acknowledges that an individual's evaluation of another's actions can contribute to shaping that person's reputation in the mind of the individual, and if shared with others, then the individual's evaluation contributes to the collectively shared evaluation of that person. Reputation is meaningfully tied to social status, prestige, and one's standing in a social group (Tedeschi & Melburg, 1984). Indeed, future research can more clearly delineate the uniqueness of reputation beyond these existing constructs and situate reputation in the nomological net of existing constructs in psychology.

One adaptive problem is how to form a reputation of the actor based on his or her actions toward the recipient. The actor's reputation would ideally enable the third party to avoid being exploited by a noncooperator and facilitate selecting cooperative partners for mutually beneficial exchange. Initial models of indirect reciprocity tested a simple rule of assessing reputation called *image scoring* (Nowak & Sigmund, 1998b). To assess an image score, people just kept track of whether someone was cooperative (+1) or noncooperative (–1) with others in prior interactions, then cooperate with others having a positive image score. However, this reputation-updating strategy may be too simple and actually punishes a person who defects (i.e., refuses to cooperate) with another person having a negative image score. An additional strategy that has been modeled in previous work is called *standing strategy* (i.e., assigning a negative reputation only to someone who fails to cooperate with a cooperator; see Yamamoto, Okada, Uchida, & Sasaki, 2017). Although this strategy places greater demands on memory to update reputational scores, the standing strategy does not impose punishment on people who do not cooperate with others who have been uncooperative in the past, and thus can distinguish between justified and unjustified noncooperators.

Some prior research has tested whether humans use image scoring or standing strategy to update reputations. Milinski, Semmann, Bakker, and Krambeck (2001) conducted an experiment to observe how people behave toward others who cooperate, or not, with a noncooperative person. They found that participants who did not cooperate with a noncooperative person were defected on in subsequent interactions. This was taken as evidence that the

people did not take into account the interaction partner's reputation but used a simpler updating rule based on an actors' behavior (cooperate or not). In contrast, Bolton, Katok, and Ockenfels (2005) found that while providing information about a partner's past behavior (i.e., image scoring) increased cooperation, there was an even higher increase in cooperation when participants were provided with second-order information (i.e., the partner's previous partner's past action), which suggests that standing strategy exists. Thus, it is still uncertain whether people follow a more complicated reputation-updating rule like a standing strategy. It has been argued that image scoring is a simpler heuristic that avoids the problem of recursive reasoning, for example, that a person should know his or her partner's (say, person A) previous behavior toward person B, person B's previous actions toward person C, person C's actions toward person D, person D's actions toward person E, and so on. If any single interaction is missing, then a person cannot adequately use a standing strategy to update the reputation of a partner, so this could result in an image scoring heuristic as a useful, though imperfect, shortcut. That said, an evolved ability to update reputational information may circumvent these problems by only searching and using input from first-order and second-order information, and not attempt to secure all the information about the history of interactions (which is likely an insurmountable computational problem). Future research is necessary to better understand how humans update reputations.

People may also spread false information about others. There can be possible benefits to an individual to manipulate gossip to derogate competitors and enhance one's relative standing in a social network (Barkow, 1992; Emler, 1990). Moreover, gossip can also contain errors that occur during communication (Hess & Hagen, 2006). In order for indirect reciprocity to promote cooperation, people need to be able to accurately assess others' reputations. Thus, one adaptive problem is assessing the veracity of gossip. Hess and Hagen conducted several experiments to test cues of gossip veracity and found that people perceive gossip to be more accurate (1) when they receive the same information from multiple independent sources

TABLE 14.3. Definitions of Reputation

Reference	Definition of reputation
Anderson & Shirako (2008)	"the set of beliefs, perceptions, and evaluations a community forms about one of its members" (p. 320)
Emler (1990)	"that set of judgments a community makes about the personal qualities of one of its members" (p. 171)
Milinski (2016)	"the current standing the person has gained from previous investments or refusal of investments in helping others" (p. 1)
Stiff & Van Vugt (2008)	"socially shared information about a potential interaction partner" (p. 156)
Whitmeyer (2000)	"an attribute attached to actors (or perhaps objects) that signals that they are more or less likely to be desirable for some sort of interaction than those without the attribute" (p. 189)
Wu, Balliet, & Van Lange (2016b)	"a set of collective beliefs, perceptions, or evaluative judgments about someone among members within a community" (p. 351)

and (2) when there is no detectable conflict or competition between the gossiper and the target of gossip. Thus, it seems that people use cues that enable them to assess the accuracy of gossip, and this could be an adaptation that enabled more accurate updating of others' reputations and better selection of cooperative partners.

Innovative Directions for Future Research

Social Learning, Reputation, and Indirect Reciprocity

Societies and groups can have social norms of cooperation, that is, a shared set of beliefs that people should cooperate, and that noncooperation will result in negative evaluations, punishment, and ostracism from group members (Fehr & Fischbacher, 2004). Learning social norms and the punishment of counternormative behavior may account for why people choose to cooperate with others who are cooperative and choose to defect with or ostracize noncooperators. From this perspective, people copy, mimic, and learn the common (and successful) behaviors they observe from ingroup members (Henrich & Boyd, 2001)—and can be biased to especially learn from prestigious group members (Chudek, Heller, Birch, & Henrich, 2012). This approach offers hypotheses about when people will choose to cooperate, and the motivations

they have for cooperating, that differ from reputation-based indirect reciprocity.

For example, when people are part of a group that contains a majority of noncooperative members, a social norm perspective would predict that people would learn to defect. However, what would happen in this situation when a group member interacts with a newcomer to the group who has a cooperative reputation? To examine this issue, Romano and Balliet (2017) assigned participants to a group in which other group members were always noncooperative or cooperative with a newcomer to the group. They also manipulated whether the newcomer was always cooperative or not in previous interactions. A social norm learning approach predicts that people should follow the majority group member behavior, but this research found that people condition their behavior on their partner's past (and expected future) behavior (i.e., their partner's reputation). Moreover, when people did conform to their group members' behavior (i.e., behaving as though conforming to a social norm), they reported doing so because they were concerned about their reputation in the group. Thus, people were conforming to group member behavior in order to avoid being negatively evaluated by ingroup members. These findings suggest that the psychological mechanisms of indirect reciprocity may have greater influence on decisions to cooperate than the psychological mechanisms underlying the learning of social norms. Future research can further test the contrasting predictions of theories about social norms and indirect reciprocity, with a focus on distinguishing the psychological mechanisms that are hypothesized to underlie each of these phenomena.

One line of inquiry can test to what extent a general learning ability can account for how people cooperate to acquire indirect benefits. For example, humans could have a general learning ability that identifies when their behavior can translate into good or bad reputational outcomes, and so indirect benefits and costs. However, reputational consequences of one's current actions often occur in the distant future, and this presents a challenge for leaning about how one can adjust his or her behavior to maintain a cooperative reputation. Instead, humans may have decision rules or heuristics that help them solve exactly this problem. People may use cues that are reliably associated with indirect costs and benefits, then condition their behavior on these cues. Future research can contrast a reinforcement learning account of reputation management, with an alternative account of functionally specialized decision rules that rely on cues that can be associated with indirect benefits.

Indirect Reciprocity from a Developmental Perspective

As we discussed earlier, humans may have evolved abilities that enable reputation-based indirect reciprocity, and this proposition has inspired several researchers to examine when these abilities emerge through development. Field research making observations at a school playground has documented that 5- to 6-year-old children are more likely to receive help after having previously helped another child (Kato-Shimizu, Onishi, Kanazawa, & Hinobayashi, 2013). Such notable field observations present immense challenges in ruling out alternative interpretations, such as direct reciprocity and the effects of the history of the relationships between the children.

However, lab research has also documented that young children display indirect reciprocity. Olson and Spelk (2008) presented 3½-year-olds a puppet story with a protagonist who had to decide how to divide resources among other puppets. The participants learned that one of the other puppets had previously helped other puppets, while another puppet decided against helping someone in the past. They found that the children recommended that the protagonist give more to the puppet that had previously been helpful, compared to the puppet that did not help previously, suggesting that children at this age engage in indirect reciprocity. Similarly, Kenward and Dahl (2011) found that 4½-year-olds, but not 3-year-olds, would decide to give more resources to a puppet that had previously helped another puppet, compared to a puppet that was a hindrance to another puppet. Importantly, across both studies, children only distributed resources as would be expected according to indirect reciprocity when they were forced to decide how to distribute unequal resources (e.g., three cookies between two persons). However, when they could divide the resources equally (e.g., two cookies between two persons), they preferred dividing the resources equally between helpers and nonhelpers. Such field and lab studies suggest that children at a young age, and potentially even 3 years old, are motivated to give more benefits to others whom they observed to be helpful to others in previous occasions.

Interestingly, the cognitive and motivational mechanisms of indirect reciprocity may emerge even earlier in development. Previous research has found that even 10-month-old infants seem to expect third parties to behave positively toward someone who has behaved in an egalitarian way in a previous interaction, compared to someone who behaved unfairly (Meristo & Surian, 2013). There is a need for future research along these lines on the development of specific cognitive and motivational abilities that underlie indirect reciprocity.

Do Reputations Transcend Group Boundaries?

Social networks often contain clusters of individuals who have strong ties to each other, and these clusters can be considered groups. Yamagishi and colleagues (1999) have claimed that reputational benefits of cooperation may be contained within groups. According to a bounded generalized reciprocity perspective, groups contain a system of reputation-based indirect reciprocity, and humans have evolved a decision heuristic to be more cooperative with ingroup members than with outgroup members, in order to enhance their cooperative reputation and to avoid being ostracized from the group. Previous research using minimal group paradigm has supported this claim through the observation that ingroup favoritism in cooperation only occurs when people have common knowledge of each other's group membership (Balliet, Wu, & De Dreu, 2014; Yamagishi et al., 1999). When participants have unilateral knowledge of group membership (i.e., participants knew their partners' group membership, but also learned that their partners did not know their own group membership), they could not gain reputational benefits–costs from their behavior, and so they did not discriminate in cooperation between ingroup and outgroup members. A recent meta-analysis of the literature on ingroup favoritism indeed found that people only cooperated more with ingroup than with outgroup members when there was common knowledge, but this ingroup favoritism completely disappeared in the unilateral knowledge condition (Balliet et al., 2014). This work is complemented by research showing that 5-year-old children invest in a positive reputation with ingroup, but not outgroup, members (Engelmann, Over, Herrmann, & Tomasello, 2013).

Theory and research suggest that reputational benefits of cooperation are contained within groups, or at least that people have a reputation management strategy that is conditional on group membership. However, research supporting this view has mostly relied on the common knowledge paradigm to manipulate whether actions can have reputational consequences. Other research using different methodologies has resulted in the conclusion that people care about their reputation when interacting with both ingroup *and* outgroup members (Romano, Balliet, & Wu, 2017; Semmann, Krambeck, & Milinski, 2005). Romano, Balliet, and Wu (2017) conducted five studies in which they manipulated both partner group membership (using minimal and natural groups) and cues of reputation (e.g., anonymity, gossip) via several methods, and found that reputation promoted

cooperation during interactions with both ingroup and outgroup members. Additionally, a large-scale study across 17 societies attempted to replicate the previous work by Yamagishi and colleagues (1999) testing how common/unilateral knowledge affected ingroup favoritism in cooperation (Romano, Balliet, Yamagishi, & Liu, 2017). This study manipulated partner nationality (own country vs. one of 16 other countries) and common (vs. unilateral) knowledge of partner group membership, and found that these two factors did not interact to predict cooperation as would be expected by the bounded generalized reciprocity theory. However, common knowledge (and also reputational benefits) promoted cooperation with both ingroup and outgroup members.

It is unclear why these studies result in inconsistent findings, and there is a need for future work to closely examine how reputation and reputational benefits can generalize across groups. This issue can inform why people might discriminate in favor of their ingroup, which can not only result in benefits for the ingroup but also provoke conflict between groups (De Dreu, & Balliet, & Halevy, 2014). Furthermore, if reputation transcends group boundaries, then it may be wielded as a tool to reduce intergroup discrimination.

Individual Differences in Reputation Management

Although reputation-based indirect reciprocity could result in universal human adaptations, there may be individual differences in how these mechanisms would operate to produce behavior. For example, people may not display similar levels of concern for their reputations, and they may not invariably cooperate in response to cues that their behavior can lead to indirect benefits. Some personality traits (e.g., social value orientation, prevention focus, and chronic public self-awareness) are likely to account for potential variation in reputation management.

There exist stable individual differences in the weighting of own and others' outcomes during interdependent decision-making tasks, with some people (e.g., proselfs) only valuing their own welfare, and other people (e.g., prosocials) displaying a positive valuation of both self and others' outcomes (Van Lange, 1999; Van Lange, Otten, De Bruin, & Joireman, 1997). While prosocials tend to be generally more cooperative than proselfs in both economic games and real-world situations (Balliet, Parks, & Joireman, 2009; Van Lange, Schippers, & Balliet, 2011), proselfs have been found to be strategically more cooperative in situations with cues that their behavior can lead to potential future indirect benefits (e.g., the presence of third-party observers or potential for gossip), compared to an anonymous situation (Feinberg, Willer, Stellar, & Kellner, 2012; Simpson & Willer, 2008; Wu et al., 2015; Wu, Balliet, & Van Lange, 2016c). Thus, proself individuals can be more strongly influenced to cooperate when their reputations are at stake.

Individuals differences in *prevention focus*— one's general tendency to minimize negative outcomes and prevent losses (Higgins, 1998)— can also shape strategies of reputation management. Some initial evidence reveals that prevention-focused individuals tend to generally show greater concern for their reputations (Cavazza, Guidetti, & Pagliaro, 2015) and also donate more money when they are exposed to subtle cues of watching eyes (Pfattheicher, 2015). In addition, people with a strong chronic public self-awareness also tend to be behave more prosocially in response to cues of being watched (Pfattheicher & Keller, 2015). While some previous research has been done on individual differences in gossip (Nevo, Nevo, & Derech-Zehavi, 1993), very little research has examined individual differences in the context of indirect reciprocity, and several candidate traits include Honesty–Humility, Dark Triad, Forgivingness, and Revengefulness (see Thielmann, Spadaro, & Balliet, 2020).

Conclusions

Humans possess a remarkable ability to coordinate and cooperate to produce public goods. Biologists and psychologists believe that this ability has its roots in the phylogeny of our species. Indeed, natural selection can favor cooperative strategies that result in direct *and* indirect benefits of cooperation. Thus, indirect

reciprocity may have shaped human abilities to evaluate others' behavior (e.g., person perception, moral judgment) and to engage in certain social behaviors (e.g., reputation and impression management, partner selection, and conditional cooperation) to acquire these benefits. In this chapter, we have discussed several fitness-relevant adaptive problems (e.g., capturing indirect benefits, strategically sharing gossip, and selecting cooperative partners and avoiding exploitation by free riders) that can occur when social interactions are structured according to indirect reciprocity. Specifying these adaptive problems can be useful in generating hypotheses about how the mind might work to solve these problems, and we proposed several possibilities, many of which require future research and empirical scrutiny.

Several agent-based models discussed in this chapter support the idea that indirect reciprocity could have influenced the evolution of human cooperation. And here we reported an abundance of evidence, from both the field and lab, that people engage in behaviors that can be recognized as indirect reciprocity. We believe the most exciting next steps on this topic involve identifying the proximate psychological processes underlying these behaviors. In this regard, bridging evolutionary models of indirect reciprocity and social psychology should be exceptionally useful in generating hypotheses to test in behavioral experiments. Specifically, psychologists can use these evolutionary models of ultimate mechanisms as inspiration to develop and test hypotheses about the proximal cognitive and motivational processes that underlie the human ability for indirect reciprocity. Another topic may focus on the broader circumstances that may limit or facilitate the workings of indirect reciprocity. For example, it is unclear whether people cooperate to secure a good reputation among outgroup members. Such issues could illuminate and extend classic topics in social psychology, such as stereotyping, discrimination, and impression formation. We predict that the next decade will witness a cascade of work on gossip, reputation, and reputation-based cooperation, thereby increasing our understanding about how humans evolved to become such a cooperative species.

REFERENCES

Abrahao, B., Parigi, P., Gupta, A., & Cook, K. S. (2017). Reputation offsets trust judgments based on social biases among Airbnb users. *Proceedings of the National Academy of Sciences of the USA, 114,* 9848–9853.

Akçay, Ç., Reed, V. A., Campbell, S. E., Templeton, C. N., & Beecher, M. D. (2010). Indirect reciprocity: Song sparrows distrust aggressive neighbours based on eavesdropping. *Animal Behaviour, 80,* 1041–1047.

Alexander, R. (2017). *The biology of moral systems.* New York: Routledge. (Original work published 1987)

Anderson, C., & Shirako, A. (2008). Are individuals' reputations related to their history of behavior? *Journal of Personality and Social Psychology, 94,* 320–333.

Andreoni, J., & Petrie, R. (2004). Public goods experiments without confidentiality: A glimpse into fund-raising. *Journal of Public Economics, 88,* 1605–1623.

Andrews, P. W., Gangestad, S. W., & Matthews, D. (2002). Adaptationism—how to carry out an exaptationist program. *Behavioral and Brain Sciences, 25,* 489–504.

Apicella, C. L., Marlowe, F. W., Fowler, J. H., & Christakis, N. A. (2012). Social networks and cooperation in hunter–gatherers. *Nature, 481,* 497–501.

Archer, J., & Coyne, S. M. (2005). An integrated review of indirect, relational, and social aggression. *Personality and Social Psychology Review, 9,* 212–230.

Axelrod, R. (1984). *The evolution of cooperation.* New York: Basic Books.

Balliet, D., Parks, C., & Joireman, J. (2009). Social value orientation and cooperation in social dilemmas: A meta-analysis. *Group Processes and Intergroup Relations, 12,* 533–547.

Balliet, D., Tybur, J. M., & Van Lange, P. A. M. (2017). Functional interdependence theory: An evolutionary account of social situations. *Personality and Social Psychology Review, 21,* 361–388.

Balliet, D., Wu, J., & De Dreu, C. K. W. (2014). Ingroup favoritism in cooperation: A meta-analysis. *Psychological Bulletin, 140,* 1556–1581.

Barkow, J. H. (1992). Beneath new culture is old psychology: Gossip and social stratification. In J. H. Barkow, L. Cosmides, & J. Tooby (Eds.), *The adapted mind: Evolutionary psychology and the generation of culture* (pp. 627–637). New York: Oxford University Press.

Bolton, G. E., Katok, E., & Ockenfels, A. (2005). Cooperation among strangers with limited information about reputation. *Journal of Public Economics, 89,* 1457–1468.

Boyd, R., & Richerson, P. J. (1989). The evolution of indirect reciprocity. *Social Networks, 11,* 213–236.

Bshary, R., & Grutter, A. S. (2006). Image scoring and cooperation in a cleaner fish mutualism. *Nature, 441,* 975–978.

Buss, D. M., Haselton, M. G., Shackelford, T. K., Bleske, A. L., & Wakefield, J. C. (1998). Adaptations, exaptations, and spandrels. *American Psychologist, 53,* 533–548.

Cavazza, N., Guidetti, M., & Pagliaro, S. (2015). Who cares for reputation?: Individual differences and concern for reputation. *Current Psychology, 34,* 164–176.

Chudek, M., Heller, S., Birch, S., & Henrich, J. (2012). Prestige-biased cultural learning: Bystander's differential attention to potential models influences children's learning. *Evolution and Human Behavior, 33,* 46–56.

Confer, J. C., Easton, J. A., Fleischman, D. S., Goetz, C. D., Lewis, D. M., Perilloux, C., et al. (2010). Evolutionary psychology: Controversies, questions, prospects, and limitations. *American Psychologist, 65,* 110–126.

Cosmides, L. (1989). The logic of social exchange: Has natural selection shaped how humans reason?: Studies with the Wason selection task. *Cognition, 31,* 187–276.

Cosmides, L., Barrett, H. C., & Tooby, J. (2010). Adaptive specializations, social exchange, and the evolution of human intelligence. *Proceedings of the National Academy of Sciences of the USA, 107,* 9007–9014.

Cosmides, L., & Tooby, J. (1992). Cognitive adaptations for social exchange. In J. H. Barkow, L. Cosmides, & J. Tooby (Eds.), *The adapted mind: Evolutionary psychology and the generation of culture* (pp. 163–228). Oxford, UK: Oxford University Press.

Cosmides, L., & Tooby, J. (2013). Evolutionary psychology: New perspectives on cognition and motivation. *Annual Review of Psychology, 64,* 201–229.

Dawes, R. M. (1980). Social dilemmas. *Annual Review of Psychology, 31,* 169–193.

De Dreu, C. K. W. (2010). Social conflict: The emergence and consequences of struggle and negotiation. In S. T. Fiske, D. T. Gilbert, & L. Gardner (Eds.), *Handbook of social psychology* (pp. 983–1023). New York: Wiley.

De Dreu, C. K. W., Balliet, D. P., & Halevy, N. (2014). Parochial cooperation in humans: Forms and functions of self-sacrifice in intergroup conflict. In A. Elliot (Ed.), *Advances in motivational science* (Vol. 1, pp. 1–48). New York: Elsevier.

De Waal, F. B. (2008). Putting the altruism back into altruism: The evolution of empathy. *Annual Review of Psychology, 59,* 279–300.

Delton, A. W., Krasnow, M. M., Cosmides, L., & Tooby, J. (2011). Evolution of direct reciprocity under uncertainty can explain human generosity in one-shot encounters. *Proceedings of the National Academy of Sciences of the USA, 108,* 13335–13340.

Dores Cruz, T., Thielmann, I., Balliet, D., Righetti, F., Beersma, B., Molho, C., et al. (2020). Gossip in daily life [Raw data], VU Amsterdam.

dos Santos, M., & Wedekind, C. (2015). Reputation based on punishment rather than generosity allows for evolution of cooperation in sizable groups. *Evolution and Human Behavior, 36,* 59–64.

Dunbar, R. I. M. (2004). Gossip in evolutionary perspective. *Review of General Psychology, 8,* 100–110.

Ellwardt, L., Wittek, R., & Wielers, R. (2012). Talking about the boss effects of generalized and interpersonal trust on workplace gossip. *Group and Organization Management, 37,* 521–549.

Emler, N. (1990). A social psychology of reputation. *European Review of Social Psychology, 1,* 171–193.

Engelmann, D., & Fischbacher, U. (2009). Indirect reciprocity and strategic reputation building in an experimental helping game. *Games and Economic Behavior, 67,* 399–407.

Engelmann, J. M., Over, H., Herrmann, E., & Tomasello, M. (2013). Young children care more about their reputation with ingroup members and potential reciprocators. *Developmental Science, 16,* 952–958.

Fehr, E., & Fischbacher, U. (2004). Social norms and human cooperation. *Trends in Cognitive Sciences, 8,* 185–190.

Fehr, E., Fischbacher, U., & Gächter, S. (2002). Strong reciprocity, human cooperation, and the enforcement of social norms. *Human Nature, 13,* 1–25.

Feinberg, M., Cheng, J. T., & Willer, R. (2012). Gossip as an effective and low-cost form of punishment. *Behavioral and Brain Sciences, 35,* 25.

Feinberg, M., Willer, R., & Schultz, M. (2014). Gossip and ostracism promote cooperation in groups. *Psychological Science, 25,* 656–664.

Feinberg, M., Willer, R., Stellar, J., & Keltner, D. (2012). The virtues of gossip: Reputational information sharing as prosocial behavior. *Journal of Personality and Social Psychology, 102,* 1015–1030.

Fine, G. A., & Rosnow, R. L. (1978). Gossip, gossipers, gossiping. *Personality and Social Psychology Bulletin, 4,* 161–168.

Fonseca, M. A., & Peters, K. (2017). Will any gossip do?: Gossip does not need to be perfectly accurate to promote trust. *Games and Economic Behavior, 107,* 253–281.

Foster, E. K. (2004). Research on gossip: Taxonomy, methods, and future directions. *Review of General Psychology, 8,* 78–99.

Giardini, F., Paolucci, M., Villatoro, D., & Conte, R. (2014). Punishment and gossip: Sustaining cooperation in a public goods game. In B. Kamiński & Grzegorz Koloch (Eds.), *Advances in social simulation* (pp. 107–118). Berlin, Germany: Springer.

Giardini, F., & Vilone, D. (2016). Evolution of gossip-based indirect reciprocity on a bipartite network. *Scientific Reports, 6,* Article No. 37931.

Gintis, H., Smith, E. A., & Bowles, S. (2001). Costly signaling and cooperation. *Journal of Theoretical Biology, 213,* 103–119.

Grosser, T. J., Lopez-Kidwell, V., & Labianca, G. (2010). A social network analysis of positive and negative gossip in organizational life. *Group and Organization Management, 35,* 177–212.

Haley, K. J., & Fessler, D. M. (2005). Nobody's watching?: Subtle cues affect generosity in an anonymous economic game. *Evolution and Human Behavior, 26,* 245–256.

Hamilton, M. J., Milne, B. T., Walker, R. S., Burger, O., & Brown, J. H. (2007). The complex structure of hunter–gatherer social networks. *Proceedings of the Royal Society of London B: Biological Sciences, 274,* 2195–2203.

Hamilton, W. D. (1964). The genetical evolution of social behaviour II. *Journal of Theoretical Biology, 7,* 17–52.

Henrich, J., & Boyd, R. (2001). Why people punish defectors: Weak conformist transmission can stabilize costly enforcement of norms in cooperative dilemmas. *Journal of Theoretical Biology, 208,* 79–89.

Hess, N. H., & Hagen, E. H. (2006). Psychological adaptations for assessing gossip veracity. *Human Nature, 17,* 337–354.

Higgins, E. T. (1998). Promotion and prevention: Regulatory focus as a motivational principle. *Advances in Experimental Social Psychology, 30,* 1–46.

Hill, K. R., Walker, R. S., Božičević, M., Eder, J., Headland, T., Hewlett, B., et al. (2011). Co-residence patterns in hunter–gatherer societies show unique human social structure. *Science, 331,* 1286–1289.

Jaeggi, A. V., Stevens, J. M., & Van Schaik, C. P. (2010). Tolerant food sharing and reciprocity is precluded by despotism among bonobos but not chimpanzees. *American Journal of Physical Anthropology, 143,* 41–51.

Kato-Shimizu, M., Onishi, K., Kanazawa, T., & Hinobayashi, T. (2013). Preschool children's behavioral tendency toward social indirect reciprocity. *PLOS ONE, 8*, e70915.

Kenward, B., & Dahl, M. (2011). Preschoolers distribute scarce resources according to the moral valence of recipients' previous actions. *Developmental Psychology, 47*, 1054–1064.

Khadjavi, M. (2016). Indirect reciprocity and charitable giving—evidence from a field experiment. *Management Science, 63*, 3708–3717.

Kollock, P. (1993). An eye for an eye leaves everyone blind: Cooperation and accounting systems. *American Sociological Review, 58*, 768–786.

Komorita, S. S., & Parks, C. D. (1995). Interpersonal relations: Mixed-motive interaction. *Annual Review of Psychology, 46*, 183–207.

Leimar, O., & Hammerstein, P. (2001). Evolution of cooperation through indirect reciprocity. *Proceedings of the Royal Society of London B: Biological Sciences, 268*, 745–753.

Ma, L. K., Tunney, R. J., & Ferguson, E. (2017). Does gratitude enhance prosociality?: A meta-analytic review. *Psychological Bulletin, 143*, 601–635.

Manesi, Z., Van Lange, P. A. M., & Pollet, T. (2016). Eyes wide open: Only eyes that pay attention promote prosocial behavior. *Evolutionary Psychology, 14*, 1–15.

McCullough, M. E., Kurzban, R., & Tabak, B. A. (2013). Putting revenge and forgiveness in an evolutionary context. *Behavioral and Brain Sciences, 36*, 41–58.

McGlohon, M., Akoglu, L., & Faloutsos, C. (2011). Statistical properties of social networks. In C. C. Aggarwal (Ed.), *Social network data analytics* (pp. 17–42). New York: Springer.

Meristo, M., & Surian, L. (2013). Do infants detect indirect reciprocity? *Cognition, 129*, 102–113.

Milinski, M. (2016). Reputation, a universal currency for human social interactions. *Philosophical Transactions of the Royal Society of London B: Biological Sciences, 371*, 20150100.

Milinski, M., Semmann, D., Bakker, T. C., & Krambeck, H. J. (2001). Cooperation through indirect reciprocity: Image scoring or standing strategy? *Proceedings of the Royal Society of London B: Biological Sciences, 268*, 2495–2501.

Milinski, M., Semmann, D., & Krambeck, H. J. (2002). Reputation helps solve the "tragedy of the commons." *Nature, 415*, 424–426.

Molho, C., Tybur, J. M., Van Lange, P. A. M., & Balliet, D. (2020). *Direct and indirect punishment in daily life.* Manuscript under review.

Nettle, D., Harper, Z., Kidson, A., Stone, R., Penton-Voak, I. S., & Bateson, M. (2013). The watching eyes effect in the Dictator Game: It's not how much you give, it's being seen to give something. *Evolution and Human Behavior, 34*, 35–40.

Nevo, O., Nevo, B., & Derech-Zehavi, A. (1993). The development of the tendency to gossip questionnaire: Construct and concurrent validation for a sample of Israeli college students. *Educational and Psychological Measurement, 53*, 973–981.

Noon, M., & Delbridge, R. (1993). News from behind my hand: Gossip in organizations. *Organization Studies, 14*, 23–36.

Northover, S. B., Pedersen, W. C., Cohen, A. B., & Andrews, P. W. (2017). Artificial surveillance cues do not increase generosity: Two meta-analyses. *Evolution and Human Behavior, 38*, 144–153.

Nowak, M. A. (2006). Five rules for the evolution of cooperation. *Science, 314*, 1560–1563.

Nowak, M., & Sigmund, K. (1993). A strategy of win–stay, lose–shift that outperforms tit-for-tat in the Prisoner's Dilemma Game. *Nature, 364*, 56–58.

Nowak, M. A., & Sigmund, K. (1998a). The dynamics of indirect reciprocity. *Journal of Theoretical Biology, 194*, 561–574.

Nowak, M. A., & Sigmund, K. (1998b). Evolution of indirect reciprocity by image scoring. *Nature, 393*, 573–577.

Ohtsuki, H., & Iwasa, Y. (2006). The leading eight: Social norms that can maintain cooperation by indirect reciprocity. *Journal of Theoretical Biology, 239*, 435–444.

Olson, K. R., & Spelke, E. S. (2008). Foundations of cooperation in young children. *Cognition, 108*, 222–231.

Peters, K., Jetten, J., Radova, D., & Austin, K. (2017). Gossiping about deviance: Evidence that deviance spurs the gossip that builds bonds. *Psychological Science, 28*, 1610–1619.

Pfattheicher, S. (2015). A regulatory focus perspective on reputational concerns: The impact of prevention-focused self-regulation. *Motivation and Emotion, 39*, 932–942.

Pfattheicher, S., & Keller, J. (2015). The watching eyes phenomenon: The role of a sense of being seen and public self-awareness. *European Journal of Social Psychology, 45*, 560–566.

Pfeiffer, T., Rutte, C., Killingback, T., Taborsky, M., & Bonhoeffer, S. (2005). Evolution of cooperation by generalized reciprocity. *Proceedings of the Royal Society of London B: Biological Sciences, 272*, 1115–1120.

Piazza, J., & Bering, J. M. (2008). Concerns about reputation via gossip promote generous allocations in an economic game. *Evolution and Human Behavior, 29*, 172–178.

Porter, M. A., Mucha, P. J., Newman, M. E., & Warmbrand, C. M. (2005). A network analysis of committees in the US House of Representatives. *Proceedings of the National Academy of Sciences of the USA, 102,* 7057–7062.

Pruitt, D. G., & Kimmel, M. J. (1977). Twenty years of experimental gaming: Critique, synthesis, and suggestions for the future. *Annual Review of Psychology, 28,* 363–392.

Rand, D. G., & Nowak, M. A. (2013). Human cooperation. *Trends in Cognitive Sciences, 17,* 413–425.

Richerson, P., Baldini, R., Bell, A., Demps, K., Frost, K., Hillis, V., et al. (2016). Cultural group selection plays an essential role in explaining human cooperation: A sketch of the evidence. *Behavioral and Brain Sciences, 39,* e30.

Roberts, G. (2008). Evolution of direct and indirect reciprocity. *Proceedings of the Royal Society of London B: Biological Sciences, 275,* 173–179.

Romano, A., & Balliet, D. (2017). Reciprocity outperforms conformity to promote cooperation. *Psychological Science, 28,* 1490–1502.

Romano, A., Balliet, D., & Wu, J. (2017). Unbounded indirect reciprocity: Is reputation-based cooperation bounded by group membership? *Journal of Experimental Social Psychology, 71,* 59–67.

Romano, A., Balliet, D., Yamagishi, T., & Liu, J. H. (2017). Parochial trust and cooperation across 17 societies. *Proceedings of the National Academy of Sciences of the USA, 114,* 12702–12707.

Sasaki, T., Okada, I., & Nakai, Y. (2017). The evolution of conditional moral assessment in indirect reciprocity. *Scientific Reports, 7,* Article No. 41870.

Seinen, I., & Schram, A. (2006). Social status and group norms: Indirect reciprocity in a repeated helping experiment. *European Economic Review, 50,* 581–602.

Sell, A., Tooby, J., & Cosmides, L. (2009). Formidability and the logic of human anger. *Proceedings of the National Academy of Sciences of the USA, 106,* 15073–15078.

Semmann, D., Krambeck, H. J., & Milinski, M. (2005). Reputation is valuable within and outside one's own social group. *Behavioral Ecology and Sociobiology, 57,* 611–616.

Simpson, B., & Willer, R. (2008). Altruism and indirect reciprocity: The interaction of person and situation in prosocial behavior. *Social Psychology Quarterly, 71,* 37–52.

Skowronski, J. J., & Carlston, D. E. (1987). Social judgment and social memory: The role of cue diagnosticity in negativity, positivity, and extremity biases. *Journal of Personality and Social Psychology, 52,* 689–699.

Sparks, A., & Barclay, P. (2013). Eye images increase generosity, but not for long: The limited effect of a false cue. *Evolution and Human Behavior, 34,* 317–322.

Stanca, L. (2009). Measuring indirect reciprocity: Whose back do we scratch? *Journal of Economic Psychology, 30,* 190–202.

Stiff, C., & Van Vugt, M. (2008). The power of reputations: The role of third party information in the admission of new group members. *Group Dynamics: Theory, Research, and Practice, 12,* 155–166.

Sznycer, D., Delton, A. W., Robertson, T. E., Cosmides, L., & Tooby, J. (2019). The ecological rationality of helping others: Potential helpers integrate cues of recipients' need and willingness to sacrifice. *Evolution and Human Behavior, 40,* 34–45.

Tedeschi, J. T., & Melburg, V. (1984). Impression management and influence in the organization. In S. B. Bacharach & E. J. Lawler (Eds.), *Research in the sociology of organizations* (Vol. 3, pp. 31–58). Greenwich, CT: JAI.

Thielmann, I., Spadaro, G., & Balliet, D. (2020). Personality and prosocial behavior: A theoretical framework and meta-analysis. *Psychological Bulletin, 146*(1), 30–90.

Thomson, R., Yuki, M., Talhelm, T., Schug, J., Kito, M., Ayanian, A. H., et al. (2018). Relational mobility predicts social behaviors in 39 countries and is tied to historical farming and threat. *Proceedings of the National Academy of Sciences of the USA, 115,* 7521–7526.

Tooby, J., & Cosmides, L. (1992). The psychological foundations of culture. In J. H. Barkow, L. Cosmides, & J. Tooby (Eds.), *The adapted mind: Evolutionary psychology and the generation of culture* (pp. 19–136). New York: Oxford University Press.

Tooby, J., & Cosmides, L. (1996). Friendship and the banker's paradox: Other pathways to the evolution of adaptations for altruism. In W. G. Runciman, J. M. Smith, & R. I. M. Dunbar (Eds.), *Proceedings of the British Academy: Vol. 88. Evolution of social behaviour patterns in primates and man* (pp. 119–143). New York: Oxford University Press.

Tooby, J., & Cosmides, L. (2015). The theoretical foundations of evolutionary psychology. In D. M. Buss (Ed.), *The handbook of evolutionary psychology: Vol. 1. Foundations* (2nd ed., pp. 3–87). Hoboken, NJ: Wiley.

Trivers, R. L. (1971). The evolution of reciprocal altruism. *Quarterly Review of Biology, 46,* 35–57.

Van Apeldoorn, J., & Schram, A. (2016). Indirect reciprocity: A field experiment. *PLOS ONE, 11,* e0152076.

Van Lange, P. A. M. (1999). The pursuit of joint outcomes and equality in outcomes: An integrative model of social value orientation. *Journal of Personality and Social Psychology, 77,* 337–349.

Van Lange, P. A. M., Balliet, D., Parks, C. D., & Van Vugt, M. (2014). *Social dilemmas: The psychology of human cooperation.* New York: Oxford University Press.

Van Lange, P. A. M., Otten, W., De Bruin, E. M. N., & Joireman, J. A. (1997). Development of prosocial, individualistic, and competitive orientations: Theory and preliminary evidence. *Journal of Personality and Social Psychology, 73,* 733–746.

Van Lange, P. A. M., Ouwerkerk, J. W., & Tazelaar, M. J. A. (2002). How to overcome the detrimental effects of noise in social interaction: The benefits of generosity. *Journal of Personality and Social Psychology, 82,* 768–780.

Van Lange, P. A. M., Rockenbach, B., & Yamagishi, T. (2014). *Reward and punishment in social dilemmas.* New York: Oxford University Press.

Van Lange, P. A. M., Schippers, M., & Balliet, D. (2011). Who volunteers in psychology experiments?: An empirical review of prosocial motivation in volunteering. *Personality and Individual Differences, 51,* 284–297.

Wang, Z., Jusup, M., Wang, R. W., Shi, L., Iwasa, Y., Moreno, Y., et al. (2017). Onymity promotes cooperation in social dilemma experiments. *Science Advances, 3,* e1601444.

Warneken, F., & Tomasello, M. (2006). Altruistic helping in human infants and young chimpanzees. *Science, 311,* 1301–1303.

Wedekind, C., & Milinski, M. (2000). Cooperation through image scoring in humans. *Science, 288,* 850–852.

West, S. A., Griffin, A. S., & Gardner, A. (2007). Evolutionary explanations for cooperation. *Current Biology, 17,* R661–R672.

Whitmeyer, J. M. (2000). Effects of positive reputation systems. *Social Science Research, 29,* 188–207.

Wittek, R., & Wielers, R. (1998). Gossip in organizations. *Computational and Mathematical Organization Theory, 4,* 189–204.

Wu, J., & Axelrod, R. (1995). How to cope with noise in the iterated prisoner's dilemma. *Journal of Conflict Resolution, 39,* 183–189.

Wu, J., Balliet, D., & Van Lange, P. A. M. (2015). When does gossip promote generosity?: Indirect reciprocity under the shadow of the future. *Social Psychological and Personality Science, 6,* 923–930.

Wu, J., Balliet, D., & Van Lange, P. A. M. (2016a). Gossip versus punishment: The efficiency of reputation to promote and maintain cooperation. *Scientific Reports, 6,* Article No. 23919.

Wu, J., Balliet, D., & Van Lange, P. A. M. (2016b). Reputation, gossip, and human cooperation. *Social and Personality Psychology Compass, 10,* 350–364.

Wu, J., Balliet, D., & Van Lange, P. A. M. (2016c). Reputation management: Why and how gossip enhances generosity. *Evolution and Human Behavior, 37,* 193–201.

Yamagishi, T., Jin, N., & Kiyonari, T. (1999). Bounded generalized reciprocity: Ingroup boasting and ingroup favoritism. *Advances in Group Processes, 16,* 161–197.

Yamamoto, H., Okada, I., Uchida, S., & Sasaki, T. (2017). A norm knockout method on indirect reciprocity to reveal indispensable norms. *Scientific Reports, 7,* Article No. 44146.

Yoeli, E., Hoffman, M., Rand, D. G., & Nowak, M. A. (2013). Powering up with indirect reciprocity in a large-scale field experiment. *Proceedings of the National Academy of Sciences of the USA, 110,* 10424–10429.

CHAPTER 15

Aggression, Violence, and Revenge

C. Nathan DeWall
David S. Chester

Humans flourish despite their aggressive urges. They pause when angered, work when frustrated, and turn the other cheek when provoked. Amid boiling blood and the desire to get even, people often keep their aggressive urges in check. But sometimes they don't, lashing out at their provocateurs or even innocent victims. In this chapter we seek to explain why aggressive urges sometimes translate into aggressive actions.

The chapter is organized into six sections. First, we offer detailed definitions of aggression, violence, and revenge. The definitions differentiate the three types of actions and also describe their different forms and functions. Second, we discuss the development of aggression over time and across the lifespan. We review evidence about massive historical shifts in aggression and violence, along with how the risk for aggression ebbs and flows across an individual's lifespan. Third, we provide a chronological review of social psychology's dominant theories of aggression: *frustration–aggression theory; cognitive neoassociation theory; social learning theory; excitation transfer theory; social, cognitive, and information-processing theory;* the *general aggression model;* and I³ *(I-cubed) meta-theory.* Fourth, we offer a compre-

hensive review of neural, genetic, and hormonal factors that can increase or decrease aggression. Specifically, we focus on the role of various neural networks, approaches to the study of genetics, and the additive and interactive effects of various hormones on aggression. Sixth, we briefly review some of the most common causes of aggression. These six sections represent the basic principles and conceptualizations of aggression.

What Are Aggression, Violence, and Revenge?

Aggression is any action intended to harm another person who is motivated to avoid the harm (Anderson & Bushman, 2002; Baron & Richardson, 1994; Bushman & Huesmann, 2010). This definition has three components. First, aggression is an action—it is as easy to observe as any other behavior. Aggression is neither an emotion nor a cognition. Drivers or sports fans may feel angry or think hostile thoughts, but unless they put those feelings and thoughts into action, they are not behaving aggressively. You must *do* something in order for your actions to satisfy this definition of aggression. Punching, kicking, biting, throwing objects, or threatening people with a weapon are examples of aggressive actions.

Second, aggression occurs on purpose rather than accidentally, and it is intended to harm someone. Imagine walking down the hall with a box of books and seeing a colleague whom you dislike. Knowing your colleague likes to ski, you intentionally drop the books on his foot, causing him physical pain that prevents him from attending a planned skiing vacation. Now imagine taking the same actions toward a cherished colleague, with the exception that you accidentally (rather than intentionally) drop the books. You still caused your colleague physical pain and hijacked his ability to enjoy a skiing vacation, only your action was not aggressive because you didn't intend to do it.

Third, aggressive actions must harm victims who are motivated to avoid the harm. Most people do not relish opportunities for being harmed, but some people do. For example, masochistic sex involves people willingly being spanked, choked, slapped, or otherwise physically dominated by others. Although masochistic sexual activities involve experiencing intentional harm, its participants are not considered victims of aggression because they were motivated to approach the harm rather than avoid it.

Violence is a more extreme version of aggression. Specifically, *violence* is an action intended to cause extreme physical injury to another person who is motivated to avoid the extreme physical injury. For example, an aggressive act may involve punching someone, whereas a violent act may involve shooting or stabbing someone. The U.S. Federal Bureau of Investigation (FBI) identifies four crimes as meeting the definition of violence: homicide, aggravated assault, forcible rape, and robbery. Criminologists often separate violent from nonviolent crime according to the likelihood that the victim requires medical attention. Social psychologists set a lower bar for actions to meet the definition of violence. As long as someone intends to cause a victim extreme physical injury, social psychologists consider the action violent.

People use different approaches to act aggressively. That is, aggression takes different forms. Aggression is often expressed physically, such as by hitting, stabbing, or choking. But people also express their aggression ver-

bally by yelling, screaming, swearing, or calling people unkind or humiliating names. Sometimes people direct their aggression toward innocent victims rather than the source of their anger or provocation. For example, after being publicly humiliated by one's boss at the office, a worker may decide not to retaliate against her boss because doing so would result in her getting fired. Instead, she returns to her apartment and kicks her dog. Drawing on Freudian notions of displacement, psychologists call this *displaced aggression* because the woman substitutes a new target (her dog) for the aggressive action because harming the original target (her boss) is deemed dangerous or unacceptable (Marcus-Newhall, Pedersen, Carlson, & Miller, 2000; Reijntjes et al., 2013; Scott, DiLillo, Maldonado, & Watkins, 2015). Sometimes people displace their aggression, but the third-party victim isn't completely innocent. For example, a woman who is humiliated by her boss returns home and kicks her dog because the dog chewed up her favorite photos. Psychologists call this *triggered displaced aggression* because people displace their aggression toward a third-party target that committed an offense that triggered an aggressive urge (Pedersen, Gonzales, & Miller, 2000). Numerous factors increase the likelihood of triggered displaced aggression, including rumination, alcohol intoxication, and the salience of the triggering event (Bushman, Bonacci, Pedersen, Vasquez, & Miller, 2005; Denson et al., 2008; Denson, Spanovic, et al., 2011; Vasquez et al., 2013).

People express aggression directly or indirectly. The key difference between these two forms of aggression is the presence or absence of the victim. In *direct* aggression, the victim is always present, such as when a husband punches his wife in the face. In indirect aggression, the victim is not present. For example, a husband may destroy his wife's car while she is at work. The same distinction holds for verbal aggression, in which a husband's aggression can be direct (e.g., calling his wife fat or ugly) or indirect (e.g., telling lies about his wife to her friends, family, and coworkers). Men tend to use direct aggression more than women do, whereas women more often use indirect aggression (e.g., Björkqvist, Lagerspetz, & Kaukiainen, 1992; Lagerspetz, Björkqvist, & Peltonen, 1988).

Different motivations drive people to act aggressively. *Reactive aggression* refers to aggression that is motivated by "hot," negative emotional states such as anger or frustration. *Proactive* aggression is motivated by a desire to achieve a specific goal, such as obtaining money, status, or power. Whereas reactive aggression is often an impulsive reaction to provocation, *proactive aggression* relies less on emotion and is instead a "cool," premeditated action. Although some researchers have demonstrated distinctions between reactive and proactive aggression (e.g., Merk, Orobio de Castro, Koops, & Matthys, 2005; Miller & Lynam, 2006), the two motivations often correlate highly with each other (e.g., Vize, Miller, & Lynam, 2018). Other researchers have argued that it is difficult to identify aggressive acts that do not involve both reactive and proactive components at some level (Bushman & Anderson, 2001). For example, a man might feel angry when he learns that his girlfriend has left him for another man. The jilted man's anger might motivate him to get revenge on his ex-girlfriend, leading him to form a plot to kill her and her new boyfriend. Such was the case with Charles Victor Thompson, who was sentenced to death for killing his ex-girlfriend, Denise Hayslip, and her new boyfriend, Darren Cain (McNamara, 2005). Were Thompson's violent aggressions motivated by his anger? Or were Thompson's actions the result of his premeditated goal to get revenge? Probably both motivations drove Thompson's actions. According to Anderson and Huesmann (2003), a potentially more useful approach to understanding the motives underlying aggression may result from asking three questions:

1. How much is the primary and the ultimate aim to harm the victim rather than benefit the perpetrator?
2. How much negative affect is present?
3. How much did the perpetrator consider the consequences of taking the aggressive or violent action?

Revenge is a subtype of aggression and violence. People who seek revenge aim to intentionally harm someone who is both motivated to avoid the harm and previously inflicted harm or committed some other act that violated norms

for appropriate behavior (Carlsmith & Darley, 2008; Frijda, 1994; McCullough, Bellah, Kilpatrick, & Johnson, 2001). Although people may seek revenge to improve their mood (e.g., Chester & DeWall, 2017), other theorists have argued that revenge evolved more broadly as a means for helping organisms solve survival and reproductive goals (McCullough, Kurzban, & Tabak, 2013).

Summary

The first principle is that aggression, violence, and revenge are actions. To engage in aggression, violence, or revenge is to carry out an action intentionally to harm someone who is motivated to avoid the harm. Simply feeling or thinking about aggression, violence, or revenge is not enough. You must *do* something in order to enact aggression, violence, or revenge. The main difference between the three concepts depends on the action's severity to the victim (aggression vs. violence) and whether the victim previously transgressed toward the perpetrator (aggression and violence vs. revenge).

Development of Aggression

Over Human History

Do we live in a safe historical period? If you turn on the television, surf the Internet, or read newspapers, you might conclude that it is a dangerous period in human history. Terrorist bombings, gang violence, and school shootings seem widespread. Yet according to several sources of data, the world has never experienced such low levels of aggression and violence.

Understanding historical shifts in aggression are difficult because of changing definitions of aggression. At certain points in time and in certain locations, people may have used different definitions of aggression. To bypass this problem, it is useful to focus on a single behavior that is unambiguously aggressive: homicide. It is also valuable to examine both long-term and short-term historical trends in the same aggression behavior.

Archaeologists have examined sites from around the world to estimate the percentage of people who died due to homicide. As shown in Figure 15.1, death due to homicide varied con-

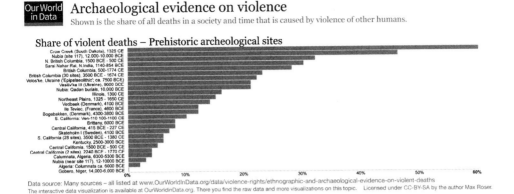

FIGURE 15.1. Archaeological evidence on the percentage of deaths in a society due to violence. From Our World in Data. Licensed under Creative Commons 4.0.

siderably between different groups. But overall, the rate of homicide was at least 1 in 10 people. As culture progressed over time, homicide rates decreased. For example, consider Western European homicide rates beginning in the year 1300 (Figure 15.2). Beginning in the year 1300, about 47 in 100,000 people from the Netherlands and Belgium died due to homicide. Over time, Western European homicide rates plummeted. In 2016, the homicide rate in the Neth-

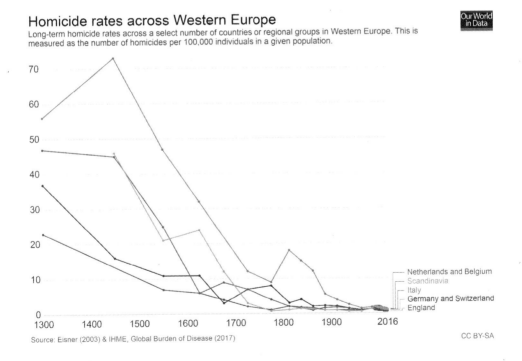

FIGURE 15.2. Homicide rates in Western Europe, 1300–2016. From Our World in Data. Licensed under Creative Commons 4.0.

erlands and Belgium was 1.1 in 100,000 people. Reductions in homicides over long periods of time are also observed in many other countries (Pinker, 2011, 2018).

Aggression researchers have also examined changes in homicide rates over much smaller periods of time, searching for changes across decades rather than centuries. With some exceptions, most countries have demonstrated dramatic drops in homicide rates over the past 40 years. For example, between the 1980 and 2016, the homicide rate in the United States decreased from 10.2 per 100,000 to 5.3 per 100,000, respectively (FBI, 2017; U.S. Bureau of the Census, 2011). In other words, Americans today, compared with those before 1980, are half as likely to die from homicide. These findings add to a growing body of evidence suggesting a shift toward greater personal safety in society.

Despite the promising nature of these historical downward trends, many people each year continue to experience physical and psychological harm due to others' aggressive and violent actions. Aggression research continues to be a worthwhile scientific enterprise. By understanding aggression's causes and consequences, it becomes more possible for researchers and policymakers to understand how to prevent it.

Over the Lifespan

Aggression is not evenly distributed across the lifespan. Certain ages increase or decrease the likelihood that people will engage in aggressive behavior. When are people most likely to act aggressively? Between ages 1 and 3 (e.g., Côté, Vaillancourt, LeBlanc, Nagin, & Tremblay, 2006; Miner & Clarke-Steward, 2008; Tremblay et al., 2004). During this development stage, about 1 in 4 social interactions between children involve aggression (Tremblay, 2000). Although these aggressive actions often do not cause severe physical injuries, they can cause emotional distress and undermine the quality of children's relationships. Three factors help explain why young children act with such frequent aggression. First, children do not begin to learn to inhibit their aggression until after age 3. Second, children struggle to simulate other children's mental states because of an underdeveloped theory of mind (Premack & Woodruff, 1978; Rubio-Fernández & Geurtz, 2013). With-

out a fully functioning capacity to understand and simulate how their actions might affect others, children are less likely to restrain their actions that cause others harm. Third, young children are egocentric, focusing primarily on their self-centered thoughts and desires. Such an egocentric mindset can help explain the genesis of many aggression interactions between young children, which often begin when one child takes another child's possession or refuses to share his or her own possessions with others.

The next most aggressive point in the lifespan occurs between late adolescence and early adulthood. For example, rape or sexual assault, robbery, and aggravated assault peaks between ages 18 and 34 (U.S. Department of Justice, 2018). Homicide shows a similar developmental pattern, with the highest rates between ages 15 and 49 (see Figure 15.3).

Summary

The second basic principle is that aggressive propensity changes over time and across the lifespan. Although human biology has remained relatively unchanged over the past several thousand years, human culture has changed dramatically. Cultural progress gives people better options for resolving conflict than aggression or violence. As a result, historical data show dramatic reductions in aggression and violence over time. Aggression peaks very early in life, before people develop the ability to overcome their aggressive urges. Adolescence and early adulthood are the main periods in which people engage in violence because of their increased size and shifting motivations for sexual, status, and power.

Theoretical Foundations of Aggression

Frustration–Aggression Theory

In 1939, social psychologists made their first major theoretical foray into understanding aggression. In that year, John Dollard, Leonard Doob, Neal Miller, O. H. Mowrer, and Robert Sears (1939) published their seminal volume, *Frustration and Aggression*. The initial formulation of frustration–aggression theory asserted that frustration is a necessary and sufficient cause of aggression. Frustration occurs when an organism encounters an obstacle to an ex-

Homicide rate by age (per 100,000), World

Homicide rates measured per 100,000 individuals across various age categories. Also shown is the total death rate across all ages (not age-standardized) and the age-standardized death rate. Age-standardization assumes a constant population age & structure to allow for comparisons between countries and with time without the effects of a changing age distribution within a population (e.g. aging).

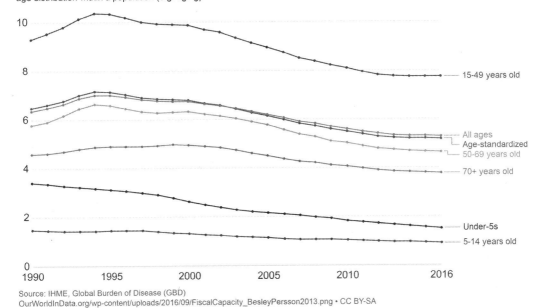

Source: IHME, Global Burden of Disease (GBD)
OurWorldInData.org/wp-content/uploads/2016/09/FiscalCapacity_BesleyPersson2013.png • CC BY-SA

FIGURE 15.3. Homicide rates across the lifespan, 1990–2016. From Our World in Data. Licensed under Creative Commons 4.0.

pected goal. Therefore, if an organism became frustrated, that organism was guaranteed to behave aggressively. If an organism encountered a stimulus thought to increase frustration but did not behave aggressively, then the stimulus was not frustrating.

In this way, frustration–aggression theory was a product of its historical era, owing largely to the influence of philosophy on the advent of psychology theorizing (James, 1890). Unfortunately, this theoretical rigidity posed problems in terms of making frustration–aggression theory falsifiable (Popper, 1959). As a result, future iterations of frustration–aggression theory were modified to account for the possibility that frustration may not always increase aggression (Miller, 1941). However, these reformulations continued to argue that if an organism acted aggressively, it was always due to increased frustration (Zillman, 1979). Hence, frustration–aggression theory no longer claimed that

frustration was a sufficient cause of aggression, but it continued to assert that frustration was a necessary cause of aggression.

Cognitive Neoassociation Theory

Cognitive neoassociation (CNA) theory grew out of frustration–aggression theory (Berkowitz, 1989, 2012). Unlike frustration–aggression theory, CNA theory was heavily influenced by the cognitive revolution and emerging work on discrete emotions (anger and fear vs. general frustration). Specifically, CNA theory asserts that people behave aggressively because they encounter unpleasant situational cues that automatically activate cognitive associations with either fight or flight responses. When cognitive associations with fight responses become activated, people tend to experience anger. In contrast, cognitive associations with flight responses often lead people to experience fear. These emotions and the fight or flight responses they influence become stored in memory, awaiting activation if people encounter a similar unpleasant situational cue. Thus, CNA theory goes beyond frustration–aggression theory by emphasizing the importance of cognition in driving aggression, the difference between anger and fear in fight-or-flight responses, and how those emotional responses mediate the relationship between the activation of the cognitive association and the behavioral response.

For example, imagine rushing to a restaurant after work to celebrate your best friend's birthday. On the way, you accidently bump into a pedestrian on the sidewalk. The pedestrian immediately pushes you and yells, "Watch where you're walking, idiot!" The push hurt your shoulder and you felt embarrassed. Onlookers watch you, wondering whether you'll retaliate. That's when you see the pedestrian walk toward you with clenched fists. Suddenly, he lunges at you, yelling, "Now I'm really going to make you hurt." According to CNA theory, you would be prone to behave aggressively in this scenario for at least three reasons. First, you would be exposed to a situational cue that is unpleasant and automatically activates cognitive associations with a fight response. Knowing that the other person had caused you pain and intended to continue to harm you, the automatic association would be to defend yourself rather than let yourself be harmed again. Second, the automatic activation of cognitive associations with a fight response would likely cause you to experience anger, which is associated with aggression and other approach-relevant behaviors. Third, the activation of cognitive associations with fighting, the activation of anger, and your initial aggressive response may perpetuate an escalating cycle of aggression, in which your aggressive responses increase over several iterations of hitting, name-calling, or other aggressive acts. The risk for aggression would be lower if the pedestrian you bumped acted kindly and said, "No problem. I know it was an accident and you look like you're in a hurry. Have a good night." Hence, you would still experience an unpleasant event because it might hurt to bump into someone, but this experience would not activate the same cognitive associations linked with fight responses, anger, and aggressive action.

Social Learning Theory

Social learning theory was formulated in the wake of the learning revolution that dominated psychological science in the early to mid-20th century. Operant conditioning and classical conditioning can help explain why humans and nonhuman animals behave aggressively. *Positive reinforcement* increases children's aggression, whereas *negative reinforcement* decreases their aggression (Cowan & Walters, 1963; Lovaas, 1961; Patterson, Littman, & Bricker, 1967). Children also show signs of stimulus discrimination and generalization, in which they learn to associate certain situations (but not others) with aggression and apply their learning history to new situations (Eron, 1987; Eron, Walder, & Lefkowitz, 1971; Sears, Whiting, Nowlis, & Sears, 1953). Using operant conditioning, most mice quickly learn to associate aggression with reward and later remain aggressive even when doing so earns them punishment (Golden et al., 2017).

Albert Bandura (1977) argued that social learning through observation, imitation, and modeling can help explain aggression. In some of the most classic psychological studies, children observed an adult hitting and yelling at a "Bobo" doll—an inflated toy doll that gets up after being knocked down (Bandura, Ross, & Ross, 1961, 1963). To evoke frustration, children played with toys, had the toys removed, and were then told that they could play with the other toys, including the Bobo doll. Compared with children who observed an adult interacting peacefully with the Bobo doll, those who observed an aggressive adult were more likely to act aggressively toward the Bobo doll. Social learning theory has been used to help explain numerous aggressive acts, including media violence effects and the greater likelihood for children whose parents spank them to act actively during adulthood (Bartholow & Anderson, 2002; Gershoff & Grogan-Kaylor, 2016).

Excitation Transfer Theory

Why might riding an exercise bike increase people's propensity to behave aggressively? According to excitation transfer theory (Zillmann, 1979, 1988), arousal from one event leaves a residue that affects subsequent events. Because arousal is a basic component of emotion common to many events (Russell & Barrett, 1999; Wundt, 1897), it is easy to transfer excitation from one experience to another because it does not need to fit each context. Within the context of aggression, initial arousal that is transferred to another person or situation can cause people to misattribute feelings of anger to the second experience, thereby increasing their likelihood for aggression. In a famous test of excitation transfer theory, participants completed an initial nonaggressive task designed to increase their arousal (i.e., riding an exercise bike) or to leave their arousal levels unchanged (i.e., threading discs onto a wire; Zillmann & Bryant, 1974). Next, participants were given an opportunity to transfer their high or normal levels of arousal to a second situation, namely, an annoying or mild-mannered confederate. Consistent with excitation transfer theory, the most aggressive participants were those who initially experienced high levels of arousal and transferred it to an annoying confederate. Subsequent work showed that given positive environmental situations, excitation transfer theory can also be used to help explain prosocial behavior (Mueller, Donnerstein, & Hallam, 1983; Van Assche et al., 2017).

Social, Cognitive, and Information-Processing Theory

Psychology's cognitive revolution seeped into aggression theorizing by encouraging researchers to understand how memory, perceptions, and attributions influence people's predisposition to act aggressively. Two theoretical perspectives have dominated cognitive information-processing models of aggression. The first perspective emphasizes the importance of normative beliefs about aggression that develop through observation and the formation of behavioral scripts (Huesmann, 1982, 1988, 1998; Huesmann & Eron, 1984). *Scripts* develop from previously acted or observed behaviors that people retrieve from memory to help them navigate situations with the appropriate role in the script. Scripts help explain why children who observe others behave aggressively become predisposed to act aggressively (Huesmann et al., 2017). By retrieving their observed behavioral history from memory, people assume a role in a script, in

which aggression is a normative response (i.e., walk down the street, someone frustrates you, express your anger verbally, act aggressively if the other person escalates the conflict).

The second theoretical perspective emphasizes the importance of attributions that increase the likelihood of aggression (Dodge, 1980, 1986, 1993; Dodge & Frame, 1982; Fite, Goodnight, Bates, Dodge, & Pettit, 2008). *Attributions* refer to how people explain the causes others' actions. According to this perspective, people who have a *hostile attribution bias* show a heightened propensity toward aggression because they tend to explain the causes for others' neutral actions as hostile. Meta-analytic findings support the link between hostile attribution bias and aggression (Bushman, 2016; Yeager, Miu, Powers, & Dweck, 2013)

The General Aggression Model

The general aggression model (GAM; Anderson & Bushman, 2002; DeWall, Anderson, & Bushman, 2011; see Figure 15.4) synthesizes perspectives from multiple aggression theories into a parsimonious, unified metatheoretical framework. The GAM incorporates social, cognitive, developmental, personality, and biological processes that occur over the short- and long-term, and that inform judgment and decision-making processes. In contrast to rigid, essentialist theories of aggression (e.g., frustration–aggression theory), the GAM offers a flexible approach to understanding aggression because it takes a knowledge structure approach. *Knowledge structures* represent people's perceptions, expectations, knowledge, and beliefs about other people, the environment, outcomes, and options for how to behave in response to different events. According to the GAM, the development of knowledge structures influences the likelihood of aggression by affecting psychological processes at every stage of the so-called "social cognitive stream" (attention, memory, judgments and attributions, and behavioral decision making; Maner et al., 2003).

The GAM includes three basic components: inputs, internal states, and outcomes of appraisal and decision-making processes. Inputs can originate from the person (e.g., trait physical aggressiveness) or the situation (e.g., provocation). Internal states include emotion, cognitive,

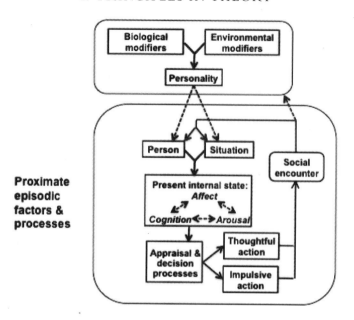

FIGURE 15.4. The GAM (Anderson & Bushman, 2002; DeWall, Anderson, & Bushman, 2011).

arousal, or neural activity. Within the appraisal and decision-making process, internal states can increase or decrease the probability that people will engage in impulsive or thoughtful actions. The GAM also includes a feedback loop that can help explain how and why violence can escalate or deescalate over multiple social interactions (Anderson, Buckley, & Carnagey, 2008).

Crucially, the GAM makes no value judgment on aggression, focusing instead on whether the action fulfills proximal (changing one's current emotional or cognitive state) or ultimate (solving an adaptive problem related to survival and reproduction) goals. For example, socially rejected people may behave aggressively as part of a proximal emotion regulation goal of improving their mood (Chester & DeWall, 2017). Social rejection may also motivate people to engage in aggression because doing so can help them achieve the ultimate goal of earning the attention and respect of desirable mates (Kavanagh, Robins, & Ellis, 2010).

I^3 (I–Cubed) Meta–Theory

I-cubed meta-theory also integrates across many theoretical perspectives, arguing that ag-

gression is determined by a combination of im-pellance, instigation, and inhibition (hence, the three i's in I-cubed meta-theory; Denson, DeWall, & Finkel, 2012; Finkel & Eckhardt, 2013; Finkel & Hall, 2018; Finkel et al., 2012). Impellance encompasses the effects of situational or stable factors that increase the likelihood that (or the intensity with which) the individual will enact the afforded behavior when encountering that target object in that context. An "afforded" behavior refers to the target-object-directed behavioral options that the target object furnishes the individual. For example, the presence of a firearm affords a violent response more than the absence of a firearm because these violent behaviors are behavioral options that accompany firearms. Indeed, Americans who have access to firearms are twice as likely to die from homicide and three times as likely to die by suicide compared to Americans who have no access to firearms (Center for Injury Research and Prevention, 2018). Instigation encompasses the effects of exposure to a particular target object in a particular context that normatively affords a certain behavior. For example, being flagrantly insulted affords a strong aggressive response (Anderson & Bushman, 2002). Inhibition encompasses the effects of situational or stable factors that increase the likelihood that (or the intensity with which) people will override the effects of impellance and instigation on behavior, thereby reducing the likelihood or the intensity of the behavior. Alcohol intoxication often increases aggression by reducing inhibition (Giancola, 2004). Compared to people with weak executive control, for example, people with strong executive control can override their aggressive urges (DeWall, Baumeister, Stillman, & Gailliot, 2007; Finkel et al., 2012).

According to *I*-cubed meta-theory, predicting the likelihood of aggression and violence requires defining impelling, instigating, and inhibiting processes that explain how these behaviors work in a given domain. Using theoretical and statistical principles of moderation, researchers can identify the conditions under which aggression is most likely to occur, what the *I*-cubed meta-theory describes as the "perfect storm theory": high impellance, high instigation, and low inhibition. For example, perfect storm theory would predict the highest probability of aggression when a firearm is present (vs. absent), when someone has been insulted (vs. praised), and when the person is experiencing alcohol intoxication (vs. sobriety).

Summary

The third principal is that social psychological theorizing on aggression has grown increasingly complex. Early theories emphasized a single emotion and a single aggressive act (frustration–aggression theory). In contrast, today's dominant meta-theories highlight interactive models that involve multiple moderating and mediating factors underlying a dynamic feedback loop of aggressive actions (the GAM and *I*-cubed meta-theory).

Genes, the Brain, and Hormones

Genes

Heritability

To what extent is aggression genetically inherited from our ancestors versus learned from our environments? Such genetic heritability estimates can be obtained from studies that compare monozygotic to dizygotic twins or ad-

opted to biological children who shared similar developmental environments. These investigations have yielded heritability estimates of 50–80% for human aggressiveness (e.g., Burt, 2009; Ferguson, 2010; Porsch et al., 2016; Tuvblad & Baker, 2011). This robust influence of genetics is largely stable across developmental stages (Van Beijsterveldt, Bartels, Hudziak, & Boomsma, 2003) and may even gradually become stronger as individuals advance into adolescence and adulthood (Burt, 2009). Although genetic effects on aggression may change, individual differences in aggression itself are quite stable over time, and genetic forces largely explain this stability over the developmental time span (Van Beijsterveldt et al., 2003).

Candidate Genes

A host of candidate genetic polymorphisms have been linked to aggression, including (yet certainly not limited to) the oxytocin receptor (*OXTR*; Malik, Zai, Abu, Nowrouzi, & Beitchman, 2012), catechol-*O*-methyltransferase (*COMT*; Rujescu, Giegling, Gietl, Hartmann, & Möller, 2003), serotonin transfer promoter variant (*5-HTTLPR*; Sukonick et al., 2001), arginine vasopressin receptor (*AVPR1A*; Vogel et al., 2012), and dopamine transporter (*DAT1*; Guo, Roettger, & Shih, 2007) and receptor (*DRD2*; Chester, DeWall, et al., 2016) genes (for a more comprehensive review see Fernàndez-Castillo & Cormand, 2016; Pavlov, Chistiakov, & Chekhonin, 2012). Most notable among these monoaminergic candidate genes that are associated with aggression is the monoamine oxidase A (*MAO-A*) gene, often referred to as "the warrior gene" (Chester et al., 2015). Despite the massive literature linking these candidate genetic polymorphisms to aggression, candidate gene findings are increasingly questioned due to a growing number of failures to replicate (e.g., Albaugh et al., 2010; Byrd & Manuck, 2014; Sakai et al., 2006; Young et al., 2006; for a meta-analytic estimate, see Ioannidis, Ntzani, Trikalinos, & Contopoulos-Ioannidis, 2001). As a complex social behavior, it is unlikely that a single candidate gene can reliably predict aggression. To alleviate these issues, new approaches model interactive effects between such candidate genes with the social environment.

Candidate Gene-by-Environment Interactions

Candidate gene-by-environment (cG × E) approaches examine the interactive effects of candidate genetic polymorphisms and environmental factors in predicting aggressive behavior (for a review, see Moffitt, 2005). For instance, the effect of low-functioning *MAO-A* genotype on aggression is magnified by childhood maltreatment (Kim-Cohen et al., 2006). The cG × E approach is undergirded by the proposal that certain genetic polymorphisms may render some individuals either more vulnerable to detrimental environmental inputs or simply sensitive to their developmental environments, which would magnify aggression in adverse conditions and buffer against it in improved conditions (Belsky et al., 2009). Much like the candidate gene studies, cG × E interaction studies have been plagued by failures to replicate (Duncan & Keller, 2011; Eaves & Verhulst, 2014).

Genomics

Unlike the candidate gene approach, the genome-wide association study (GWAS) approach examines the association between all genetic polymorphisms across the entire genome and aggression. Several initial GWASs failed to find any genomewide correlates of aggression, though this was likely due to smaller sample sizes ($N = 1,800$: Brevik et al., 2016; $N = 4,816$: Tielbeek et al., 2012). Subsequent GWASs using larger samples have observed several polymorphisms associated with aggression, mostly localized on chromosome 2 (Dick et al., 2011; Pappa et al., 2016). Future research will determine the reliability of these findings.

Epigenetics

Epigenetics research demonstrates that the environment plays a critical role in whether genetic polymorphisms are expressed. Through epigenetic mechanisms such as methylation, the environment can amend genotypes, altering their phenotypic expression. For example, exposure to violence is reliably linked to the erosion of telomeres, the protective terminals of chromosomes that prevent the deterioration of genetic information held within (Shalev et al., 2013). Thus, aggression can change the human genotype via epigenetic mechanisms, which may increase the likelihood for aggression.

The Brain

The neuroscience of aggression has arisen in the hopes of identifying the brain functions and structures that give rise to aggression. Various neural regions, subregions, and minute nuclei do not function in isolation, but instead serve as constituents of larger circuits or networks of brain regions. We articulate six distinct and overlapping brain networks that play established roles in aggressive behavior: the cingulo-insular pain network, the default mode network, the cingulo-opercular control network, the fronto-amygdalar threat network, the fronto-parietal executive network, and the fronto-striatal reward network (Figure 15.5).

Cingulo-Insular Pain Network

Pain reliably increases aggression (Berkowitz, 1988; Berkowitz, Cochran, & Embree, 1981). Experiences of pain are represented in the somatosensory cortices, posterior insula, dorsal anterior cingulate cortex (DACC), anterior insula, the periaqueductal gray and dorsomedial thalamus (Lieberman & Eisenberger, 2015; Price, 2000; Rainville, Duncan, Price, Carrier, & Bushnell, 1997). Neuroimaging studies indicate a reliable association between recruitment of the cingulo-insular network during socially painful experiences and subsequent aggression. The DACC and anterior insula are reliably recruited during negative social feedback (e.g., insults), and subsequent retaliatory aggression is linked to greater DACC and anterior insula activity during such aggression (Dambacher et al., 2014; Denson, Pedersen, Ronquillo, & Nandy, 2009; Krämer, Jansma, Tempelmann, & Münte, 2007). DACC activity during social rejection was associated with greater aggression toward the sources of rejection, though only among individuals who were unable to regulate this socially painful experience (Chester et al., 2014). Individuals with borderline personality disorder, a form of psychopathology characterized by reactive aggression, exhibit a magnified anterior insula response to insulting social feedback (Peters, Chester, Walsh, DeWall, & Baer, 2018). This ability of social pain to pro-

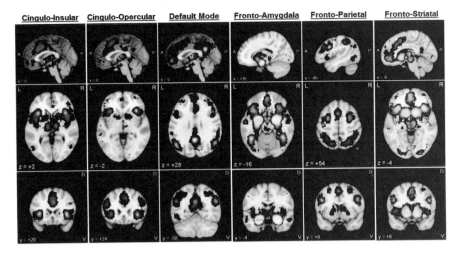

| Cingulo-Insular | Cingulo-Opercular | Default Mode | Fronto-Amygdala | Fronto-Parietal | Fronto-Striatal |

FIGURE 15.5. Brain networks implicated in human aggression, as seen from the side (top row), above/below (middle row), and front/back (bottom row). Meta-analytic maps created via Neurosynth (Yarkoni, Poldrack, Nichols, Van Essen, & Wager, 2011) using as keywords the search terms *pain, cognitive control, default mode, threat, fronto-parietal,* and *reward,* from left to right.

mote aggression exists not just in humans. Mice that were reared in social isolation exhibit both hyperactivity in the ACC and greater aggressive behavior (Toth et al., 2012). Across these sources of evidence, it is clear that pain does give rise to aggression and that the cingulo-insular affective pain network is a likely substrate of this effect.

Cingulo-Opercular Control Network

The cingulo-opercular control network consists of the midcingulate cortex and overlying supplemental motor area, as well as the bilateral ventrolateral prefrontal cortex (VLPFC), which aids attentional and behavioral control (Dosenbach et al., 2007; Hampshire, Chamberlain, Monti, Duncan, & Owen, 2010; Zhang & Li, 2012). Deficits in the cingulo-opercular control network produce deficits in self-control and increase aggression. A meta-analysis of 43 neuroimaging studies revealed that aggression was substantially associated with functional and structural impairments of the orbital aspect of the right VLPFC (Yang & Raine, 2009). Excessive recruitment of the VLPFC aspect of this network may also increase aggression. For example, individuals who exhibited greater VLPFC recruitment during an instance of social rejection were subsequently

more aggressive toward their rejecters (Chester, Lynam, Milich, & DeWall, 2018). Thus, deficient or exaggerated activation in this network can increase aggression.

Default Mode Network

The default mode network is activated when individuals are at rest and not processing any specific tasks or stimuli, and broadly comprises dorsal and ventral aspects of medial PFC (DMPFC/VMPFC), posterior cingulate cortex (PCC), and bilateral temporoparietal junction (TPJ; Buckner, Andrews-Hanna, & Schacter, 2008). This network strongly overlaps with the mentalizing network, which subserves theory-of-mind and cognitive empathy processes of social cognition (Schilbach, Eickhoff, Rotarska-Jagiela, Fink, & Vogeley, 2008). Aggression, as a necessarily social behavior, has profound roots in altered function and structure of the default mode network and the social cognitive processes it subserves.

The default mode network includes almost the entire MPFC, extending from its more dorsal aspects in Brodmann's area 9 to its ventral terminus above the orbitofrontal cortex in Brodmann's area 10 (Buckner et al., 2008). This dorsal–ventral gradient of the MPFC corresponds to a social cognitive gradient as well. During interpersonal judgments and perception, the tendency to distinguish others from the self tracks with this dorsal–ventral gradient (Denny, Kober, Wager, & Ochsner, 2012). More specifically, DMPFC recruitment reflects "other" and VMPFC recruitment reflects "self" (Denny et al., 2012). Aggressive individuals tend to show a dorsal bias in MPFC recruitment during interpersonal interactions that may reflect a chronic "othering" of social targets. For instance, participants who had previously perpetrated violence against an intimate partner exhibited a bias towards recruitment of the DMPFC versus the VMPFC during provocation from a stranger (Chester & DeWall, 2019). DMPFC activity during opportunities to retaliate against a provocateur are linked with greater aggressive acts during this time (Lotze, Veit, Anders, & Birbaumer, 2007). This DMPFC bias may also reflect a ruminative process, as the DMPFC is recruited during rumination about provocations and predicts tendencies to displace provocation-related aggression onto innocent others (Denson et al., 2009). Such neural biases may even help explain why alcohol increases aggression. Alcohol, compared to placebo, increased both aggressive behavior and DMPFC activation during such aggression (Denson, Blundell, Schofield, Schira, & Krämer, 2018).

The default mode network is not just the MPFC, however, and the most promising investigations are those that seek to characterize how aggression arises from network-level disruptions. As just such as example, young adult males with conduct disorder exhibited reduced connectivity within the default mode network regions (Zhou et al., 2016). This functional discoordination may extend to brain structures, as violent offenders demonstrated reduced white-matter integrity in the tract that anatomically connects the central hubs of the default mode network (Sethi et al., 2015). Individuals with functionally cohesive and structurally intact default mode networks may be less aggressive, but the mechanisms underlying this association remain unclear.

Fronto-Amygdalar Threat Network

The fronto-amygdalar threat network includes the amygdala, which is intimately involved in aggression. The amygdala encodes the motivational salience of stimuli (i.e., "Is this stimulus relevant to my current goals?"; Cunningham & Brosch, 2012). Because organisms are motivated to avoid threats, most research on the amygdala has focused on its relation to threat. Animal models of aggression emphasized a "RAGE system" that centered on the amygdala and served to mitigate threats in the environment through aggression (Panksepp & Zellner, 2004). In humans, this amygdalar network is more articulated and has remarkably pronounced connections with the DLPFC, VLPFC, and VMPFC, which largely serve to regulate and tune amygdalar responses to evocative stimuli (Kim et al., 2011; Wager, Davidson, Hughes, Lindquist, & Ochsner, 2008).

Dysfunction of this fronto-amygdalar network can increase the likelihood of aggression. Hyperactivation of the amygdala may then bias the perception of stimuli toward being perceived as threats, motivating individuals to respond to such threats with aggression (Coccaro, McCloskey, Fitzgerald, & Phan, 2007). Violent offenders also exhibited reduced connectivity between the amygdala and VMPFC after engaging in an anger rumination task, as compared to healthy controls (Siep et al., 2018). Such dysregulated amygdalar responses may occur even in the absence of external stimuli. Indeed, combat veterans with impulsive aggression exhibited reduced functional connectivity between the amygdala and lateral PFC at rest, as compared to nonaggressive combat veterans (Varkevisser, Gladwin, Heesink, van Honk, & Geuze, 2017).

Fronto-Parietal Executive Network

The front-parietal executive network consists of the bilateral dorsolateral PFC (DLPFC) and superior parietal lobe. This network facilitates executive functioning processes such as working memory, attention allocation, and inhibition (Niendam et al., 2012). Deficits in executive functioning cause increases in aggression, likely due to an inability to inhibit such inappropriate behavior and attentional biases towards provocative stimuli (Giancola, 2000). As such, dysfunctional fronto-parietal networks promote aggressive acts and effective recruitment of this network is likely to suppress aggression (Achterberg et al., 2018; Denson, O'Dean, Blake, & Beames, 2018; Klimecki, Sander, & Vuilleumier, 2018). Aggressive and violent individuals from clinical and forensic populations show functional and structural deficits in the DLPFC (Yang & Raine, 2009). As with the cingulo-opercular network, when dysfunction reigns in the neural substrates of self-regulation, aggression is increased.

Fronto-Striatal Reward Network

The fronto-striatal reward network extends from subcortical nuclei such as the ventral tegmentum, ventral pallidum, and ventral striatum into the medial aspects of VMPFC (Berridge & Kringelbach, 2015). The ventral striatum largely serves to promote the subjective experience of reward (i.e., positive affect in anticipation or receipt of an appetitive outcome; Berridge, 2003). The VMPFC serves, in part, to adaptively tune the reward response of the striatum based on motivational and situational factors (Haber & Knutson, 2010). Although this circuit has long been examined within the context of substance abuse and external rewards, recent evidence points to its relation to appetitive aggression (Chester, 2017; Chester, Lynam, Milich, & DeWall, 2017).

Aggressive individuals have a larger ventral striatum than their less aggressive counterparts (Ducharme et al., 2011; Van Donkelaar et al., 2018). Greater ventral striatum activation is associated with more aggression in response to provocation and social rejection (Chester & DeWall, 2016, 2018; Chester, Lynam, Milich, & DeWall, 2018). This striatal–aggression effect is greatest when functional coupling between the ventral striatum and the VLPFC is reduced (Buades-Rotger, Brunnlieb, Münte, Heldmann, & Krämer, 2016; Chester & DeWall, 2016). Stimulating dopaminergic neurons in the ventral striatum increases aggression in mice (Ferrari, Van Erp, Tornatzky, & Miczek, 2003; Van Erp & Miczek, 2000). It is thus clear that aggression is linked to a functional and structural neural imbalance in the fronto-striatal reward circuit, in which the reward-eliciting ventral striatum is hyperexpressed, and the regulatory PFC is hypoexpressed.

Murine Hypothalamic Aggression Circuit

Animal models of aggression allow for neurological specificity that are currently unobtainable in the six human neural circuits described earlier. Using mouse models of aggressive attack behavior, neuroscientists have clearly articulated a mechanistic model that centers on the hypothalamus. Stimulation of the ventrolateral subdivision of the ventromedial hypothalamus (VMHvl) causes mice to engage in both proactive and reactive aggression, whereas inhibiting this region with pharmacological agents reduces such behavior (Lin et al., 2011). Activity in this "hypothalamic attack area" then begins a cascade of neural co-activations that ultimately elicit the aggressive response and serves as the neural hub of the aggression network (Miczek, Takahashi, Gobrogge, Hwa, & de Almeida, 2015). Given the monumental neuroanatomical differences between humans and rodents, it remains uncertain how conserved this aggression circuit remains in our species. Findings such as the observation that hypothalamic activity during retaliatory aggression is observed in humans and linked to psychopathic and aggressive traits (Veit et al., 2010) suggest that these hypothalamic circuits observed in mice remain at play in human aggression.

Hormones

Cortisol

The body responds to stressors in many ways. Perhaps one of the most robust responses to stress is the release of the hormone cortisol, which mobilizes the body's autonomic nervous system to adaptively respond to threats (Snoek, Van Goozen, Matthys, Buitelaar, & Van Engeland, 2004). Alterations in cortisol levels are reliably linked to aggression. Over 2 years, adolescent boys' onset and persistence of aggressive behavior both were associated with lower overall cortisol levels (McBurnett, Lahey, Rathouz, & Loeber, 2000). This association holds for females as well, with adolescent females with conduct disorder exhibiting lower baseline cortisol levels than controls (Pajer, Gardner, Rubin, Perel, & Neal, 2001). Lower baseline cortisol levels also predict greater aggression when soccer fans watched their favorite team lose a match (Van der Meij et al., 2015). Beyond the semistatic cortisol baseline, aggressive individuals also exhibited a blunted cortisol response to acute stressors (Fairchild et al., 2008). These findings suggest that aggressive individuals exhibit an abnormal stress response, which is characterized by a low baseline level of autonomic stress activity coupled with a diminished cortisol reactivity to acute stressors. These findings suggest that individuals who are most likely to engage in arousing, aggressive actions are those who have relatively low levels of cortisol at baseline and in response to acute stressors. Yet cortisol alone is not enough to provide an endocrine basis for aggression. Testosterone and its relative ratio with cortisol plays an impactful and dynamic role in predisposing people to act aggressively (Montoya, Terburg, Bos, & Van Honk, 2012).

Testosterone

Perhaps the most popular of the biological correlates of aggression is the hormone testosterone. Colloquially it is linked with a masculine, brutish tendency to impulsively harm others. Testosterone is responsible for profound developmental changes in both men and women and has pronounced psychological effects. Chief among testosterone's influences on human thought, feeling, and behavior is the increased tendency for status seeking (Hamilton, Carré, Mehta, Olmstead, & Whitaker, 2015). Testosterone drives individuals, especially males, to seek dominance over others and a higher place in the social hierarchy (Mazur & Booth, 1998).

This role of testosterone in promoting status-seeking behaviors may explain the often-fraught literature on the testosterone–aggression link. Although both baseline testosterone levels and testosterone reactivity to interpersonal challenges are associated with greater aggression, this effect is quite modest in size and context-dependent (Archer, 2006; Archer, Graham-Kevan, & Davies, 2005; Book, Starzyk, & Quinsey, 2001). The testosterone–aggression link is most likely an interactive effect, not a simple main effect. Aggression is one of many strategies people use to achieve social status (the central motivation of testosterone). Sometimes an aggressive act can secure a more dominant role in the hierarchy, yet in some contexts and for some types of people, an aggressive act would

result in a severe loss of status in the local pecking order. As such, testosterone should only be associated with aggression when the social situation suggests that aggression is a viable route to gaining higher status.

Another explanation for the modest size and fickle nature of the testosterone–aggression link is that this effect depends on the individual's other hormone levels. Testosterone does not increase aggression for everyone, but it has pronounced effects in men who are relatively high in dominant and impulsive personality traits (Carré et al., 2017). The interaction between testosterone and cortisol is particularly crucial, with aggression being most reliably linked to a ratio of high testosterone to low levels of cortisol (Carré & Mehta, 2011). Though this interaction is specific to physical and overt forms of aggression and is not observed among relational and subtle forms of aggression (Popma et al., 2007). These findings suggest that testosterone does not share a simple one-to-one relationship with aggression but instead depends on the status-seeking context and the ratio of this hormone to others such as cortisol.

Aggression must ultimately be enacted by neural circuits that control behavior, which raises the question: On what neural mechanisms does testosterone operate to increase aggression? Testosterone appears to exert its aggression-enhancing abilities by blunting the regulatory influence of the VMPFC (Mehta & Beer, 2010). This is sensible given the established influence of testosterone on dysregulating the fronto-striatal reward network by blunting VMPFC activity while simultaneously magnifying ventral striatum reactivity (de Macks et al., 2011).

Ovarian Hormones: Estradiol and Progesterone

Whereas testosterone is considered a "masculinizing" hormone, the ovarian hormones estradiol and progesterone are considered "feminizing" hormones. Estradiol, an estrogen hormone, and progesterone, both regulate physiological states of females, such as menstrual and reproductive cycles. As with testosterone, these hormones also impact psychological states across the estrous and menstrual cycle (e.g., negative affect, self-regulation; Eisenlohr-Moul, DeWall, Girdler, & Segerstrom, 2015). Research on the roles of these hormones in human aggression is sparse. Estradiol baseline levels were negatively associated with self-reported dominance in anxious females (Ziomkiewicz, Wichary, Gomula, & Pawlowski, 2015). During the luteal phase of the menstrual cycle, aggressive females had lower levels of progesterone than their nonaggressive counterparts (Ziomkiewicz et al., 2012). These negative associations between aggression and ovarian hormone levels fit with the larger functions of these steroid hormones, which serve to regulate emotions and cognition (Eisenlohr-Moul et al., 2015) and motivate individuals to form, maintain, and repair social bonds (Maner, Miller, Schmidt, & Eckel, 2010).

Neuropeptide Hormones: Oxytocin and Vasopressin

Two peptide hormones that have profound implications for human social functioning are oxytocin and vasopressin. Unlike other hormones, these are constrained to the central nervous system and have acute effects. Like the ovarian hormones, oxytocin and vasopressin are known to promote social motivations, such as caretaking (Campbell, 2008). Caretaking can assume the form of aggression, in the context of parental, defensive aggression toward perceived threats to offspring. Both oxytocin and vasopressin are critical motivators of such parental aggression (Bosch & Neumann, 2010; Campbell, 2008). Neuroimaging evidence suggests that oxytocin is able to motivate such parental aggression by suppressing the fear response and up-regulating the parasympathetic branch of the autonomic nervous system (Bosch & Neumann, 2010; Huber, Veinante, & Stoop, 2005). In this way, these neuropeptides allow parents to face down indomitable threats and protect their young.

Humans no longer simply live in kin groups that share a genetic ancestry. In modern society we occupy larger, more diverse groups. The role of oxytocin (but not vasopressin) appears to have scaled with this development in modern group dynamics, in that the functions that once served to protect offspring may now apply to unrelated group members (De Dreu, 2012). Nasal administrations of oxytocin elicited a protective response toward vulnerable ingroup members and a noncooperative response toward outgroup members in the context of an intergroup competition, compared to placebo (De Dreu, Shalvi, Greer, Van Kleef, & Handgraaf, 2012). Such parochial and parental aggression are the likely consequences of the neuropeptides oxytocin and vasopressin.

Summary

The third principle is that genetic, neural, and hormonal factors play a large role in predicting aggression. Aggressiveness is highly heritable, and genetic mutations can also increase the likelihood that people will respond to environmental cues with aggression. We reviewed six brain networks—the cingulo-insular pain network, the default mode network, the cingulo-opercular control network, the fronto-amygdalar threat network, the fronto-parietal executive network, and the fronto-striatal reward network—that directly influence aggression. Low levels of the hormones cortisol and estradiol and high levels of testosterone, estradiol, and vasopressin tend to increase aggression, but their influence differs according to the target of aggression. It is impossible to gain a comprehensive understanding of aggression without considering the powerful role of genes, the brain, and hormones.

Dispositional Aggressiveness

Trait Aggression

Some individuals tend to be more aggressive than others. These individual differences in aggression are often consistent over time and across situations (Huesmann & Eron, 1984). Although the biological processes we covered in the previous section account for a great degree of this variance, psychological constructs are clearly involved as well. *Trait aggression* is a construct invoked to articulate these between-person individual differences in aggressive tendencies. Self-report measures of trait aggression have revealed the existence of four subfacets of trait aggression: trait physical aggression, trait verbal aggression, trait anger, and trait hostility (Buss & Perry, 1992). These subfacets reflect behavioral (i.e., trait physical and verbal aggression), emotional (i.e., trait anger), and cognitive (i.e., trait hostility) aspects of being dispositionally aggressive. Although some critics argue that aggression is not a personality trait and should only be viewed as a behavioral outcome (Paulhus, Curtis, & Jones, 2018), the trait aggression framework has been a remarkably generative approach to understanding why some people tend to be more prone to harming others.

Personality Predictors of Aggression

Numerous personality traits correlate with aggressive behavior. To bring parsimony to this literature, we look to broader frameworks of personality. The five-factor model is the most accepted theoretical structure of personality (McCrae & Costa, 1987). Within this framework, aggression has been investigated in relation to the "Big Five" trait clusters: Agreeableness, Conscientiousness, Extraversion, Neuroticism, and Openness to Experience. Meta-analyses have revealed that Agreeableness is the single, most reliable personality correlate of aggression and explains the most variance in this outcome (Hyatt, Zeichner, & Miller, 2019; Jones, Miller, & Lynam, 2011; Vize et al., 2018). More specifically, low Agreeableness (i.e., antagonism) is associated with greater aggressiveness. Antagonistic individuals are characterized by antisocial traits (e.g., arrogance, callousness, combativeness, distrust, immorality; Lynam & Miller, 2019). Antagonism thus represents a promising avenue for future work on the personality bases of aggression.

Summary

The fifth principle is that individuals tend to differ in how aggressive they are across situations and time. Such variability can be productively viewed from the trait aggression framework and is best predicted by antagonistic personality traits.

Environmental Causes of Aggression, Violence, and Revenge

Provocation/Rejection

Humans have a fundamental motivation to form and maintain positive relationships (Baumeister & Leary, 1995). Provocation and social rejection strike at the core of this need to belong, causing people to react aggressively. Anderson and Bushman (2002) declared provocation as "perhaps the most important single cause of aggression" (p. 37). Provocations can range from simple annoyances to outright insults. Social rejection can also take various forms (e.g., being left out of a ball-tossing game, being voted out of a group activity, or being told that another person refused to work with you). Despite the variety of these provocation and rejection manipulations, all tend to increase aggression (Berkowitz, 1993; Bushman & Baumeister, 1998; DeWall, Twenge, Gitter, & Baumeister, 2009; Gaertner, Iuzzini, & O'Mara, 2008; Twenge, Baumeister, Tice, & Stucke, 2001; Warburton, Smith, & Cairns, 2006). Some individual-difference factors known to increase aggression do so most reliably in the presence of provocation, such as gender and narcissism (Bettencourt, Talley, Benjamin, & Valentine, 2006; Rasmussen, 2016). Thus, threats to positive and inclusive relationships often increase aggression.

Alcohol

Alcohol is a psychoactive drug that affects numerous cognitive, emotional, and behavioral outcomes. Alcohol consumption is a major predictor of aggression, with up to 95% of violent crime on college campuses involving the use of alcohol (National Council on Alcoholism and Drug Dependence, 2015). Alcohol affects the central nervous system through the gamma-aminobutyric acid $(GABA_A)$ receptor, which governs the brain's primary inhibitory neurotransmitters (Lobo & Harris, 2008). Hence, alcohol exerts its effect on aggression primarily by reducing inhibition (Denson, Blundell, et al., 2018; Giancola, 2004).

Why is alcohol a social cause of aggression? There are two main reasons. First, alcohol is a socially consumed drug. Most people consume alcohol with others rather than alone, especially when drinking to intoxication (Johnston, O'Malley, Bachman, & Schulenberg, 2006). Second, alcohol intoxication enhances social bonding, increasing people's propensity to make new friends (Sayette et al., 2012). Therefore, alcohol consumption often occurs with others and drives people to form social bonds. In that way, alcohol is a social cause of aggression because alcohol increases the chances that intoxicated people—who have reduced inhibitory abilities—will be surrounded by others when an aggressive urge is stimulated and in need of being overridden.

Aggressive Cues

Aggressive cues refer to any object or piece of information that relates to performing aggressive acts. The prototypical aggressive cue is a weapon. In one classic study, participants exposed to a weapon behaved more aggressively toward an annoying confederate than did those who were exposed to a tennis racket (Berkowitz & LePage, 1967). This so-called "weapons effect" has been replicated numerous times, with researchers showing that merely presenting participants with weapons-related words is enough to spark aggressive thoughts and actions (Anderson, Benjamin, & Bartholow, 1998). Compared with people who had a tennis racket in the front passenger seat, people who drove a car with a weapon in the front passenger seat behaved more aggressively (Bushman, Kerwin, Whitlock, & Weisenberger, 2017). A meta-analysis of 78 studies with nearly 8,000 participants suggested a reliable, small- to medium-size effect of the presence of weapon-related stimuli on aggressive thoughts and actions (Benjamin, Kepes, & Bushman, 2017).

Experience with aggressive cues matters. For example, when shown hunting rifles and assault weapons, nonhunters show increased aggression (Bartholow, Anderson, Carnagey, & Benjamin, 2005). However, hunters, whose experience caused them to encode hunting rifles as tools more than weapons, only displayed greater aggression after exposure to assault weapons. These findings help explain factors that interact with the presence of aggressive cues to predispose people to act aggressively.

Violent Media

Social psychologists studying aggression have spent decades examining whether viewing violent media predicts aggressive thoughts, feelings, and actions. With adolescents consuming entertainment media at least 9 hours per day (Common Sense Media, 2015), understanding whether exposure to violent media themes continues to be of importance. Numerous studies have demonstrated a positive association between violent media use and aggressive outcomes, including aggressive behavior (see Anderson et al., 2010, for a meta-analytic review). Experimental and longitudinal studies have likewise produced valid and reliable evidence that violent media use predicts greater aggression, including evidence from Western and Eastern countries (Anderson et al., 2017). A 2015 American Psychological Association Task Force on Violent Media concluded that "research demonstrates a consistent relation between violent video game use and increases in aggressive behavior, aggressive cognitions, and aggressive affect, and decreases in prosocial behavior, empathy, and sensitivity to aggression" (p. 11).

Skeptics question the robustness of these effects, noting a potential bias to publish only studies with statistically significant results (Hilgard, Engelhardt, & Rouder, 2017). Others wonder how to reconcile surging sales and consumption of violent video games with dramatic declines in societal violence (Ferguson, 2015). Such debates will continue to unfold as researchers continue to examine how, when, and why violent media affects aggressive outcomes.

Cultural Norms

Norms are standards for behavior that communicate to people how members of a group ought to behave. In the context of aggression, norms have waxed and waned in terms of cultural approval for different forms and functions of aggression. As noted earlier, norms have shifted considerably over the past several centuries in terms of perceived appropriateness of aggression, with fewer and fewer people perpetrating murder each year (e.g., Pinker, 2011, 2018). Cultural norms condoning other forms of aggression have also decreased over time. For example, in 1962, the popular U.S. group The Crystals released the song, "He Hit Me (And It Felt Like a Kiss)," in which a female sang about how her male romantic partner was justified in abusing her because she had engaged in infidelity. Three decades later, the U.S. group Hole played the same song, with lead singer Courtney Love denouncing its theme, saying, "This is a really sick song." Norms have shifted regarding other forms of aggression. In 1970, corporal punishment in school was legal in 49 of 50 U.S. states. By 2018, it was legal in only 19 of 50 U.S. states (Gershoff & Font, 2016; Straus, Douglas, & Medeiros, 2013).

In which U.S. states does most corporal punishment in school occur? States marked by a culture of honor, namely, those in the Southern U.S. culture of honor theory proposes that retaliation is expected when people perceive threats to their personal reputation or status, property, or personal relationships (Cohen, Nisbett, Bowdle, & Schwarz, 1996). Rather than retreating, a culture of honor endorses aggressive action when doing so restores a feeling of safety and security to one's personal reputation and immediate environment. Investigations using correlational, epidemiological, experimental, and computer simulation methodologies have supported culture of honor theory's predictions related to aggression between strangers and intimate partners (Brown, 2016; Cohen et al., 1996; Nowak, Gelfand, Borkowski, Cohen, & Hernandez, 2015). A meta-analysis of 69 effect sizes from more than 5 million individuals revealed a small-to-medium overall effect size of culture of honor on aggression (Enjaian & DeWall, 2018).

Environmental Features (e.g., Temperature, Noise)

Social psychologists study the effect of the environmental situation on individual and group behavior. Because aggression is a highly social behavior—aggressive acts require at least two people—social psychologists have spent most of their time examining intricacies of the dyad or group that can increase or decrease aggression. But other environmental factors also impact aggression, such as temperature, noise, and odors.

Temperature has received the most theoretical and empirical attention as a predictor of aggression and violence. Epidemiological studies have shown that hotter temperatures predict various indicators of aggression and violence, including violent crime (Anderson, 1989; Anderson & Anderson, 1996; Krenzer & Splan, 2018). Experiments have also shown a consistent causal relationship between higher temperatures and greater levels of aggression (e.g., Anderson, Anderson, & Deuser, 1996; Baron &

Bell, 1976). Some researchers have argued that increasing average ambient temperatures and lower seasonal variability may increase aggression by impacting time orientation and self-control (Van Lange, Rinderu, & Bushman, 2017).

Less attention has focused on other environmental features that can influence aggression, such as noise. In rats and humans, experiments have demonstrated a causal relationship between unpleasant noise and greater aggression (Geen, 1978; Sheard, Astrachan, & Davis, 1975). The effect of unpleasant noise on aggression is especially pronounced following provocation (Donnerstein & Wilson, 1976).

Poor Self-Control

Nearly 30 years ago, criminologists Travis Gottfredson and Travis Hirschi proposed a general theory of crime (Gottfredson & Hirschi, 1990). After combing through hundreds of studies, they identified what they argued are the two best predictors of crime (including aggressive and violent crime): opportunity and poor self-control. Meta-analytic evidence supports the general theory of crime, leading Pratt and Cullen (2000) to assert that poor self-control is one of the "strongest known correlates of crime" (p. 952).

Self-control refers to the motivation and ability to override an unwanted urge in order to remain in line with standards for acceptable behavior (Baumeister, 1998; Inzlicht, Schmeichel, & Macrae, 2014). Social psychologists have compiled a large body of evidence that poor self-control contributes to aggression between strangers and intimate partners. Some evidence linking poor self-control to greater aggression draws on the theoretical perspective that people have a limited motivation and ability to exert self-control (Baumeister, Bratslavsky, Muraven, & Tice, 1998; Muraven & Baumeister, 2000). Several studies have shown that when people use self-control, they become more aggressive on subsequent occasions when provoked (Denson, Pedersen, Friese, Hahm, & Roberts, 2011; DeWall et al., 2007; Watkins, DiLillo, Hoffman, & Templin, 2015). Low levels of glucose, which have been linked to impulsive decision making (Orquin & Kurzban, 2016), also predict higher intimate partner violence inclinations (Bushman, DeWall, Pond,

& Hanus, 2014). The implication is that depleting limited self-control energy undermines people's ability and motivation to override their aggressive urges.

Although self-control ability and motivation fluctuate over time, some people tend to have chronically high and low levels of self-control. Using cross-sectional and longitudinal designs, numerous studies indicate that poor trait self-control is associated with greater aggression toward strangers and romantic partners (Moffitt et al., 2011; Pulkkinen, Lyyra, & Kokko, 2011; Quigley et al., 2018). These findings conceptually replicate the laboratory evidence linking lower self-control to greater aggression.

Some skepticism exists regarding the reliability of experimental manipulations designed to deplete people of their limited self-control energy (e.g., Hagger et al., 2016). Others have shown that individual and cultural implicit theories of self-control can nullify and reverse typical undesirable effects that accompany prior self-control exertion (Job, Dweck, & Walton, 2010; Savani & Job, 2017). These critiques, extensions, and identification of boundary conditions will sharpen future research that seeks to understand the reliability and validity of the association between poor self-control and aggression.

Childhood Exposure to Adversity

Few factors predispose people toward adolescent and adult aggression more than childhood exposure to adversity, such as sexual abuse, physical abuse, urbanicity, migration, and problematic alcohol and cannabis use (Mitjans et al., 2018). Each childhood adversity risk factor often predicts greater adolescent and adult aggression, especially in the presence of biological (e.g., genetic; Caspi et al., 2002; Weder et al., 2009) or other social risk factors (e.g., provocation; McDermott, Tingley, Cowden, Frazzetto, & Johnson, 2009). But the accumulation of these risk factors dramatically increases the odds of future aggression, with estimates of between a five- and tenfold increase in the likelihood of a violent criminal conviction (Mitjans et al., 2018). To maximize the reliability of research in this area, future research will benefit from taking a cumulative approach to understanding the role of childhood exposure to adversity and adolescent and adult aggression.

Summary

The sixth principle is that environmental factors are the leash that restrains or enhances aggression. Our environment inundates us with experiences that can increase our aggression, such as provocation, violent media, aggressive cues (e.g., weapons). When the environment or alcohol saps our self-control and inhibition, we become more likely to behave aggressively. Exposure to norms that encourage aggression and experiences of childhood adversity dramatically increase the potential for aggressiveness. Social factors can keep our aggressive inclinations at bay, such as when we receive praise rather than provocation. But social factors can also unleash our aggressive traits, increasing our propensity to perpetrate aggression.

Concluding Remarks

Aggression intrigues and befuddles social psychologists, policymakers, and laypersons. Most societies admonish their citizens to refrain from aggression, regardless of the strength of their aggressive urge. Yet sometimes people do act aggressively, intentionally harming others who are motivated to avoid the harm. In extreme cases, aggression escalates to violence, causing victims severe physical injury or death. This chapter defined aggression, violence, and revenge; reviewed the development of aggression over time and across the lifespan; summarized dominant social psychological theories of aggression; discussed neural, genetic, and hormonal factors that help explain why people do and do not behave aggressively; examined the individual differences in aggression and their bases in personality; and surveyed common causes of aggression. Given the vastness of the aggression literature, this chapter has only scratched the surface of the intricacies regarding the causes and consequences of aggression. We hope this chapter offers a glimpse into a scientifically and humanly significant research topic that will help explain why people behave aggressively and how to prevent it.

REFERENCES

Achterberg, M., Van Duijvenvoorde, A. C., van der Meulen, M., Bakermans-Kranenburg, M. J., & Crone, E. A. (2018). Heritability of aggression following social evaluation in middle childhood: An fMRI study. *Human Brain Mapping, 39*(7), 2828–2841.

Albaugh, M. D., Harder, V. S., Althoff, R. R., Rettew, D. C., Ehli, E. A., Lengyel-Nelson, T., et al. (2010). COMT Val158Met genotype as a risk factor for problem behaviors in youth. *Journal of the American Academy of Child and Adolescent Psychiatry, 49*, 841–849.

Anderson, C. A. (1989). Temperature and aggression: Ubiquitous effects of heat on the occurrence of human violence. *Psychological Bulletin, 106*, 74–96.

Anderson, C. A., & Anderson, K. B. (1996). Violent crime rate studies in philosophical context: A destructive testing approach to heat and southern culture of violence effects. *Journal of Personality and Social Psychology, 70*, 740–756.

Anderson, C. A., Anderson, K. B., & Deuser, W. E. (1996). Examining an affective aggression framework: Weapon and temperature effects on aggressive thoughts, affect, and attitudes. *Personality and Social Psychology Bulletin, 22*, 366–376.

Anderson, C. A., Benjamin, A. J., & Bartholow, B. D. (1998). Does the gun pull the trigger?: Automatic priming effects of weapon pictures and weapon names. *Psychological Science, 9*, 308–314.

Anderson, C. A., Buckley, K. E., & Carnagey, N. L. (2008). Creating your own hostile environment: A laboratory examination of trait aggression and the violence escalation cycle. *Personality and Social Psychology Bulletin, 34*, 462–473.

Anderson, C. A., & Bushman, B. J. (2002). Human aggression. *Annual Review of Psychology, 53*, 27–51.

Anderson, C. A., & Huesmann, L. R. (2003). Human aggression: A social-cognitive view. In M. A. Hogg & J. Cooper (Eds.), *Handbook of social psychology* (pp. 296–323). London: SAGE.

Anderson, C. A., Shibuya, A., Ihori, N., Swing, E. L., Bushman, B. J., Sakamoto, A., et al. (2010). Violent video game effects on aggression, empathy, and prosocial behavior in Eastern and Western countries. *Psychological Bulletin, 136*, 151–173.

Anderson, C. A., Suzuki, K., Swing, E. L., Groves, C. L., Gentile, D. A., Prot, S., et al. (2017). Media violence and other aggression risk factors in seven nations. *Personality and Social Psychology Bulletin, 43*, 986–998.

American Psychological Association Task Force on Violent Media. (2015). *Technical report on the review of the violent video game literature.* Washington, DC: American Psychological Association.

Archer, J. (2006). Testosterone and human aggression: An evaluation of the challenge hypothesis. *Neuroscience and Biobehavioral Reviews, 30*(3), 319–345.

Archer, J., Graham-Kevan, N., & Davies, M. (2005). Testosterone and aggression: A reanalysis of Book, Starzyk, and Quinsey's (2001) study. *Aggression and Violent Behavior, 10*(2), 241–261.

Bandura, A. (1977). *Social learning theory.* New York: Prentice Hall.

Bandura, A., Ross, D., & Ross, S. A. (1961). Transmission of aggression through imitation of aggressive models. *Journal of Abnormal and Social Psychology, 63*, 575–582.

Bandura, A., Ross, D., & Ross, S. A. (1963). Vicarious reinforcement and imitative learning. *Journal of Abnormal and Social Psychology, 67*, 601–607.

Baron, R. A., & Bell, P. A. (1976). Aggression and heat: The influence of ambient temperature, negative affect, and a cooling drink on physical aggression. *Journal of Personality and Social Psychology, 33*, 245–255.

Baron, R. A., & Richardson, D. R. (1994). *Human aggression* (2nd ed.). New York: Plenum Press.

Bartholow, B. D., & Anderson, C. A. (2002). Effects of violent video games on aggressive behavior: Potential sex differences. *Journal of Experimental Social Psychology, 38*, 283–290.

Bartholow, B. D., Anderson, C. A., Carnagey, N. L., & Benjamin, A. J. (2005). Interactive effects of life experience and situational cues on aggression: The weapons priming effect in hunters and nonhunters. *Journal of Experimental Social Psychology, 41*, 48–60.

Baumeister, R. F. (1998). The self. In D. T. Gilbert, S. T. Fiske, & G. Lindzey (Eds.), *Handbook of social psychology* (4th ed., pp. 680–740). New York: McGraw-Hill.

Baumeister, R. F., Bratslavsky, E., Muraven, M., & Tice, D. M. (1998). Ego depletion: Is the active self a limited resource? *Journal of Personality and Social Psychology, 74*, 1252–1265.

Baumeister, R. F., & Leary, M. R. (1995). The need to belong: Desire for interpersonal attachments as a fundamental human motivation. *Psychological Bulletin, 117*, 497–529.

Belsky, J., Jonassaint, C., Pluess, M., Stanton, M., Brummett, B., & Williams, R. (2009). Vulnerability genes or plasticity genes? *Molecular Psychiatry, 14*, 746–754.

Benjamin, A. J., Kepes, S., & Bushman, B. J. (2017). Effects of weapons on aggressive thoughts, angry feelings, hostile appraisals, and aggressive behavior: A meta-analytic review of the weapons effect literature. *Personality and Social Psychology Review, 22*, 347–377.

Berkowitz, L. (1988). Frustrations, appraisals, and aversively stimulated aggression. *Aggressive Behavior, 14*, 3–11.

Berkowitz, L. (1989). Frustration–aggression hypothesis: Examination and reformulation. *Psychological Bulletin, 106*, 59–73.

Berkowitz, L. (1993). *Aggression: Its causes, consequences, and control.* New York: McGraw-Hill.

Berkowitz, L. (2012). A cognitive–neoassociation theory of aggression. In P. A. M. Van Lange, A. W. Kruglanski, & E. T. Higgins (Eds.), *Handbook of theories of social psychology* (pp. 99–117). Thousand Oaks, CA: SAGE.

Berkowitz, L., Cochran, S. T., & Embree, M. C. (1981). Physical pain and the goal of aversively stimulated aggression. *Journal of Personality and Social Psychology, 40*, 687–700.

Berkowitz, L., & LePage, A. (1967). Weapons as aggression-eliciting stimuli. *Journal of Personality and Social Psychology, 7*, 202–207.

Berridge, K. C., & Kringelbach, M. L. (2015). Pleasure systems in the brain. *Neuron, 86*, 646–664.

Bettencourt, B. A., Talley, A., Benjamin, A. J., & Valentine, J. (2006). Personality and aggressive behavior under provoking and neutral conditions: A meta-analytic review. *Psychological Bulletin, 132*, 751–777.

Björkqvist, K., Lagerspetz, K. M. J., & Kaukiainen, A. (1992). Do girls manipulate and boys fight?: Developmental trends in regard to direct and indirect aggression. *Aggressive Behavior, 18*(2), 117–127.

Book, A. S., Starzyk, K. B., & Quinsey, V. L. (2001). The relationship between testosterone and aggression: A meta-analysis. *Aggression and Violent Behavior, 6*(6), 579–599.

Bosch, O. J., & Neumann, I. D. (2010). Vasopressin released within the central amygdala promotes maternal aggression. *European Journal of Neuroscience, 31*(5), 883–891.

Brevik, E. J., van Donkelaar, M. M., Weber, H., Sánchez-Mora, C., Jacob, C., Rivero, O., et al. (2016). Genome-wide analyses of aggressiveness in attention-deficit hyperactivity disorder. *American Journal of Medical Genetics B: Neuropsychiatric Genetics, 171*(5), 733–747.

Brown, R. P. (2016): *Honor bound: How a cultural ideal has shaped the American psyche.* New York: Oxford University Press.

Buades-Rotger, M., Brunnlieb, C., Münte, T. F., Heldmann, M., & Krämer, U. M. (2016). Winning is not enough: Ventral striatum connectivity during physical aggression. *Brain Imaging and Behavior, 10*(1), 105–114.

Buckner, R. L., Andrews-Hanna, J. R., & Schacter, D. L. (2008). The brain's default network. *Annals of the New York Academy of Sciences, 1124*(1), 1–38.

Burt, S. A. (2009). Are there meaningful etiological differences within antisocial behavior?: Results of a meta-analysis. *Clinical Psychology Review, 29*(2), 163–178.

Bushman, B. J. (2016). Violent media and hostile appraisals: A meta-analytic review. *Aggressive Behavior, 42*, 605–613.

Bushman, B. J., & Anderson, C. A. (2001). Is it time to pull the plug on the hostile versus instrumental aggression dichotomy? *Psychological Review, 108*, 273–279.

Bushman, B. J., & Baumeister, R. F. (1998). Threatened egotism, narcissism, self-esteem, and direct and displaced aggression: Does self-love or self-hate lead to violence? *Journal of Personality and Social Psychology, 75*, 219–229.

Bushman, B. J., Bonacci, A. M., Pedersen, W. C., Vasquez, E. A., & Miller, N. (2005). Chewing on it can chew you up: Effects of rumination on triggered displaced aggression. *Journal of Personality and Social Psychology, 88*, 969–983.

Bushman, B. J., DeWall, C. N., Pond, R. S., & Hanus, M. D. (2014). Low glucose relates to greater aggression in married couples. *Proceedings of the National Academy of Sciences of the USA, 111*, 6254–6257.

Bushman, B. J., & Huesmann, L. R. (2010). Aggression. In S. T. Fiske, D. T. Gilbert, & G. Lindzey (Eds.), *Handbook of social psychology* (Vol. 2, 5th ed., pp. 833–863). Hoboken, NJ: Wiley.

Bushman, B. J., Kerwin, T., Whitlock, T., & Weisenberger, J. M. (2017). The weapons effect on wheels: Motorists drive more aggressively when there is a gun in the vehicle. *Journal of Experimental Social Psychology, 73*, 82–85.

Buss, A. H., & Perry, M. (1992). The aggression questionnaire. *Journal of Personality and Social Psychology, 63*, 452–459.

Byrd, A. L., & Manuck, S. B. (2014). MAOA, childhood maltreatment, and antisocial behavior: Meta-analysis of a gene–environment interaction. *Biological Psychiatry, 75*(1), 9–17.

Campbell, A. (2008). Attachment, aggression and affiliation: The role of oxytocin in female social behavior. *Biological Psychology, 77*(1), 1–10.

Carlsmith, K. M., & Darley, J. M. (2008). Psychological aspects of retributive justice. *Advances in Experimental Social Psychology, 41*, 193–236.

Carré, J. M., Geniole, S. N., Ortiz, T. L., Bird, B. M., Videto, A., & Bonin, P. L. (2017). Exogenous testosterone rapidly increases aggressive behavior in dominant and impulsive men. *Biological Psychiatry, 82*(4), 249–256.

Carré, J. M., & Mehta, P. H. (2011). Importance of considering testosterone–cortisol interactions in predicting human aggression and dominance. *Aggressive Behavior, 37*(6), 489–491.

Caspi, A., McClay, J., Moffitt, T. E., Mill, J., Martin, J., Craig, I. W., et al. (2002). Role of genotype in the cycle of violence in maltreated children. *Science, 297,* 851–854.

Center for Injury Research and Prevention. (2018). Gun violence: Facts and statistics. Retrieved from *https://injury.research.chop.edu/violence-prevention-initiative/types-violence-involving-youth/gun-violence/gun-violence-facts-and#.W4AXls5Kjcs.*

Chester, D. S. (2017). The role of positive affect in aggression. *Current Directions in Psychological Science, 26*(4), 366–370.

Chester, D. S., & DeWall, C. N. (2016). The pleasure of revenge: Retaliatory aggression arises from a neural imbalance toward reward. *Social Cognitive and Affective Neuroscience, 11*(7), 1173–1182.

Chester, D. S., & DeWall, C. N. (2017). Combating the sting of rejection with the pleasure of revenge: A new look at how emotion shapes aggression. *Journal of Personality and Social Psychology, 112,* 413–430.

Chester, D. S., & DeWall, C. N. (2018). Aggression is associated with greater subsequent alcohol consumption: Shared neural basis in the ventral striatum. *Aggressive Behavior, 44*(3), 285–293.

Chester, D. S., & DeWall, C. N. (2019). Intimate partner violence perpetration corresponds to a dorsal-ventral gradient in medial PFC reactivity to interpersonal provocation. *Social Neuroscience, 14*(2), 173–182.

Chester, D. S., DeWall, C. N., Derefinko, K. J., Estus, S., Lynam, D. R., Peters, J. R., et al. (2016). Looking for reward in all the wrong places: Dopamine receptor gene polymorphisms indirectly affect aggression through sensation-seeking. *Social Neuroscience, 11*(5), 487–494.

Chester, D. S., DeWall, C. N., Derefinko, K. J., Estus, S., Peters, J. R., Lynam, D. R., et al. (2015). Monoamine oxidase A (MAOA) genotype predicts greater aggression through impulsive reactivity to negative affect. *Behavioural Brain Research, 283,* 97–101.

Chester, D. S., Eisenberger, N. I., Pond, R. S., Jr., Richman, S. B., Bushman, B. J., & DeWall, C. N. (2014). The interactive effect of social pain and executive functioning on aggression: An fMRI experiment. *Social Cognitive and Affective Neuroscience, 9*(5), 699–704.

Chester, D. S., Lynam, D. R., Milich, R., & DeWall, C. N. (2017). Physical aggressiveness and gray matter deficits in ventromedial prefrontal cortex. *Cortex, 97,* 17–22.

Chester, D. S., Lynam, D. R., Milich, R., & DeWall, C. N. (2018). Neural mechanisms of the rejection–aggression link. *Social Cognitive and Affective Neuroscience, 13*(5), 501–512.

Coccaro, E. F., Fitzgerald, D. A., Lee, R., McCloskey, M., & Phan, K. L. (2016). Frontolimbic morphometric abnormalities in intermittent explosive disorder and aggression. *Biological Psychiatry: Cognitive Neuroscience and Neuroimaging, 1*(1), 32–38.

Cohen, D., Nisbett, R. E., Bowdle, B. F., & Schwarz, N. (1996). Insult, aggression, and the Southern Culture of Honor: An "experimental ethnography." *Journal of Personality and Social Psychology, 70,* 945–960.

Common Sense Media. (2015). Common sense census: Media use by tweens and teens. Retrieved from *www.commonsensemedia.org/research/the-common-sense-census-media-use-by-tweens-and-teens.*

Côté, S., Vaillancourt, T., LeBlanc, J., Nagin, D. W., & Tremblay, R. E. (2006). The development of physical aggression from toddlerhood to preadolescence: A nation wide longitudinal study of Canadian children. *Journal of Abnormal Child Psychology, 34*(1), 71–85.

Cowan, P. A., & Walters, R. A. (1963). Studies of reinforcement of aggression: I. Effects of scheduling. *Child Development, 34,* 543–551.

Cunningham, W. A., & Brosch, T. (2012). Motivational salience: Amygdala tuning from traits, needs, values, and goals. *Current Directions in Psychological Science, 21*(1), 54–59.

Dambacher, F., Sack, A. T., Lobbestael, J., Arntz, A., Brugman, S., & Schuhmann, T. (2014). Out of control: Evidence for anterior insula involvement in motor impulsivity and reactive aggression. *Social Cognitive and Affective Neuroscience, 10*(4), 508–516.

De Dreu, C. K. (2012). Oxytocin modulates cooperation within and competition between groups: An integrative review and research agenda. *Hormones and Behavior, 61*(3), 419–428.

De Dreu, C. K., Shalvi, S., Greer, L. L., Van Kleef, G. A., & Handgraaf, M. J. (2012). Oxytocin motivates non-cooperation in intergroup conflict to protect vulnerable in-group members. *PLOS ONE, 7*(11), e46751.

de Macks, Z. A. O., Moor, B. G., Overgaauw, S., Güroğlu, B., Dahl, R. E., & Crone, E. A. (2011). Testosterone levels correspond with increased ventral striatum activation in response to monetary rewards in adolescents. *Developmental Cognitive Neuroscience, 1*(4), 506–516.

Denny, B. T., Kober, H., Wager, T. D., & Ochsner, K. N. (2012). A meta-analysis of functional neuroimaging studies of self- and other judgments reveals a spatial gradient for mentalizing in medial prefrontal cortex. *Journal of Cognitive Neuroscience, 24*(8), 1742–1752.

Denson, T. F., Aviles, F. E., Pollock, V. E., Earleywine, M., Vasquez, E. A., & Miller, N. (2008). The effects of alcohol and the salience of aggressive cues on triggered displaced aggression. *Aggressive Behavior, 34,* 25–33.

Denson, T. F., Blundell, K. A., Schofield, T. P., Schira, M. M., & Krämer, U. M. (2018). The neural correlates of alcohol-related aggression. *Cognitive, Affective, and Behavioral Neuroscience, 18*(2), 203–215.

Denson, T. F., DeWall, C. N., & Finkel, E. J. (2012). Self-control and aggression. *Current Directions in Psychological Science, 21*(1), 20–25.

Denson, T. F., O'Dean, S. M., Blake, K. R., & Beames, J. R. (2018). Aggression in women: Behavior, brain, and hormones. *Frontiers in Behavioral Neuroscience, 12,* Article 81.

Denson, T. F., Pedersen, W. C., Friese, M., Hahm, A., & Roberts, L. (2011). Understanding impulsive aggression: Angry rumination and reduced self-control capacity are mechanisms underlying the provocation–aggression relationship. *Personality and Social Psychology, 37,* 850–862.

Denson, T. F., Pedersen, W. C., Ronquillo, J., & Nandy, A. S. (2009). The angry brain: Neural correlates of anger, angry rumination, and aggressive personality. *Journal of Cognitive Neuroscience, 21,* 734–744.

Denson, T. F., Spanovic, M., Aviles, F. E., Pollock, V. E., Earleywine, M., & Miller, N. (2011). The effects of acute alcohol intoxication and self-focused rumination on triggered displaced aggression. *Journal of Aggression, Maltreatment, and Trauma, 20,* 128–147.

DeWall, C. N., Anderson, C. A., & Bushman, B. J. (2011). The general aggression model: Theoretical extensions to violence. *Psychology of Violence, 1,* 245–258.

DeWall, C. N., Baumeister, R. F., Stillman, T. F., & Gailliot, M. T. (2007). Violence restrained: Effects of self-regulation and its depletion on aggression. *Journal of Experimental Social Psychology, 43,* 62–76.

DeWall, C. N., Twenge, J. M., Gitter, S. A., & Baumeister, R. F. (2009). It's the thought that counts: The role of hostile cognition in shaping aggressive responses to social exclusion. *Journal of Personality and Social Psychology, 96,* 45–59.

Dick, D. M., Aliev, F., Krueger, R. F., Edwards, A., Agrawal, A., Lynskey, M., et al. (2011). Genome-wide association study of conduct disorder symptomatology. *Molecular Psychiatry, 16*(8), 800–808.

Dodge, K. A. (1980). Social cognition and children's aggressive behavior. *Child Development, 51,* 620–635.

Dodge, K. A. (1986). A social information processing model of social competence in children. In M. Perlmutter (Ed.), *The Minnesota Symposium on Child Psychology* (Vol. 18, pp. 77–125). Hillsdale, NJ: Erlbaum.

Dodge, K. A. (1993). Social-cognitive mechanisms in the development of conduct disorder and depression. *Annual Review of Psychology, 44,* 559–584.

Dodge, K. A., & Frame, C. L. (1982). Social cognitive biases and deficits in aggressive boys. *Child Development, 53,* 620–635.

Dollard, J., Doob, L., Miller, N., Mowrer, O., & Sears, R. (1939). *Frustration and aggression.* New Haven, CT: Yale University Press.

Donnerstein, E., & Wilson, D. W. (1976). Effects of noise and perceived control on ongoing and subsequent aggressive behavior. *Journal of Personality and Social Psychology, 34,* 774–781.

Dosenbach, N. U., Fair, D. A., Miezin, F. M., Cohen, A. L., Wenger, K. K., Dosenbach, R. A., et al. (2007). Distinct brain networks for adaptive and stable task control in humans. *Proceedings of the National Academy of Sciences of the USA, 104*(26), 11073–11078.

Ducharme, S., Hudziak, J. J., Botteron, K. N., Ganjavi, H., Lepage, C., Collins, D. L., et al. (2011). Right anterior cingulate cortical thickness and bilateral striatal volume correlate with child behavior checklist aggressive behavior scores in healthy children. *Biological Psychiatry, 70*(3), 283–290.

Duncan, L. E., & Keller, M. C. (2011). A critical review of the first 10 years of candidate gene-by-environment interaction research in psychiatry. *American Journal of Psychiatry, 168*(10), 1041–1049.

Eaves, L., & Verhulst, B. (2014). Problems and pitfalls in testing for G × E and epistasis in candidate gene studies of human behavior. *Behavior Genetics, 44*(6), 578–590.

Eisenlohr-Moul, T. A., DeWall, C. N., Girdler, S. S., & Segerstrom, S. C. (2015). Ovarian hormones and borderline personality disorder features: Preliminary evidence for interactive effects of estradiol and progesterone. *Biological Psychology, 109,* 37–52.

Enjaian, B. S., & DeWall, C. N. (2018). *Does a culture of honor impact aggression, mental health, anger, and shame?: A meta-analytic review of the literature.* Manuscript submitted for publication.

Eron, L. D. (1987). The development of aggressive behavior from the perspective of a developing behaviorist. *American Psychologist, 42,* 435–442.

Eron, L. D., Walder, L. O., & Lefkowitz, M. M.

(1971). *The learning of aggression in children.* Boston: Little, Brown.

Fairchild, G., van Goozen, S. H., Stollery, S. J., Brown, J., Gardiner, J., Herbert, J., et al. (2008). Cortisol diurnal rhythm and stress reactivity in male adolescents with early-onset or adolescence-onset conduct disorder. *Biological Psychiatry, 64*(7), 599–606.

Federal Bureau of Investigation. (2017). 2016 crime in the United States. Retrieved from *https://ucr.fbi.gov/crime-in-the-u.s/2016/crime-in-the-u.s.-2016/topic-pages/murder.*

Ferguson, C. J. (2010). Genetic contributions to antisocial personality and behavior: A meta-analytic review from an evolutionary perspective. *Journal of Social Psychology, 150*(2), 160–180.

Ferguson, C. J. (2015). Do angry birds make for angry children?: A meta-analysis of video game influences on children's and adolescents' aggression, mental health, prosocial behavior, and academic performance. *Perspectives on Psychological Science, 10,* 646–666.

Fernàndez-Castillo, N., & Cormand, B. (2016). Aggressive behavior in humans: Genes and pathways identified through association studies. *American Journal of Medical Genetics B: Neuropsychiatric Genetics, 171*(5), 676–696.

Ferrari, P. F., Van Erp, A. M. M., Tornatzky, W., & Miczek, K. A. (2003). Accumbal dopamine and serotonin in anticipation of the next aggressive episode in rats. *European Journal of Neuroscience, 17*(2), 371–378.

Finkel, E. J., DeWall, C. N., Slotter, E. B., McNulty, J. K., Pond, R. S., & Atkins, D. C. (2012). Using I^3 theory to clarify when dispositional aggressiveness predicts intimate partner violence. *Journal of Personality and Social Psychology, 102,* 533–549.

Finkel, E. J., & Eckhardt, C. I. (2013). Intimate partner violence. In J. A. Simpson & L. Campbell (Eds.), *The Oxford handbook of close relationships* (pp. 452–474). New York: Oxford University Press.

Finkel, E. J., & Hall, A. N. (2018). The I^3 model: A metatheoretical framework for understanding aggression. *Current Opinion in Psychology, 19,* 125–130.

Fite, J. E., Goodnight, J. A., Bates, J. E., Dodge, K. A., & Pettit, G. S. (2008). Adolescent aggression and social cognition in the context of personality: Impulsivity as a moderator of predictions from social information processing. *Aggressive Behavior, 34,* 511–520.

Frijda, N. H. (1994). The lex talionis: On vengeance. In S. H. M. van Goozen, N. E. Van de Poll, & J. A. Sargeant (Eds.), *Emotions: Essays on emotion theory* (pp. 263–289). Mahwah, NJ: Erlbaum.

Gaertner, L., Iuzzini, J., & O'Mara, E. M. (2008). When rejection by one fosters aggression against many: Multiple-victim aggression as a consequence of social rejection and perceived groupness. *Journal of Experimental Social Psychology, 44,* 958–970.

Geen, R. G. (1978). Effects of attack and uncontrollable noise on aggression. *Journal of Research in Personality, 12,* 15–29.

Gershoff, E. T., & Font, S. A. (2016). Corporal punishment in U.S. public schools: Prevalence, disparities in use, and status in state and federal policy. *Social Policy Report, 30,* 1–25.

Gershoff, E. T., & Grogan-Kaylor, A. (2016). Spanking and child outcomes: Old controversies and new meta-analyses. *Journal of Family Psychology, 30,* 453–469.

Giancola, P. R. (2000). Executive functioning: A conceptual framework for alcohol-related aggression. *Experimental and Clinical Psychopharmacology, 8*(4), 576–597.

Giancola, P. R. (2004) Executive functioning and alcohol-related aggression. *Journal of Abnormal Psychology, 113,* 541–555.

Golden, S. A., Heins, C., Venniro, M., Caprioli, D., Zhang, M., Epstein, D. H., et al. (2017). Compulsive addiction-like aggressive behavior in mice. *Biological Psychiatry, 82,* 239–248.

Gottfredson, M. R., & Hirschi, T. (1990). *A general theory of crime.* Stanford, CA: Stanford University Press.

Guo, G., Roettger, M. E., & Shih, J. C. (2007). Contributions of the DAT1 and DRD2 genes to serious and violent delinquency among adolescents and young adults. *Human Genetics, 121*(1), 125–136.

Haber, S. N., & Knutson, B. (2010). The reward circuit: Linking primate anatomy and human imaging. *Neuropsychopharmacology, 35*(1), 4–26.

Hagger, M. S., Chatzisarantis, N. L. D., Alberts, H., Anggono, C. O., Batailler, C., Birt, A. R., et al. (2016). A multilab preregistered replication of the ego-depletion effect. *Perspectives on Psychological Science, 11,* 546–573.

Hamilton, L. D., Carré, J. M., Mehta, P. H., Olmstead, N., & Whitaker, J. D. (2015). Social neuroendocrinology of status: A review and future directions. *Adaptive Human Behavior and Physiology, 1*(2), 202–230.

Hampshire, A., Chamberlain, S. R., Monti, M. M., Duncan, J., & Owen, A. M. (2010). The role of the right inferior frontal gyrus: Inhibition and attentional control. *NeuroImage, 50*(3), 1313–1319.

Hilgard, J., Engelhardt, C. R., & Rouder, J. N. (2017). Overstated evidence for short-term effects of violent games on affect and behavior: A reanalysis of Anderson et al. (2010). *Psychological Bulletin, 143,* 757–774.

Huber, D., Veinante, P., & Stoop, R. (2005). Vasopressin and oxytocin excite distinct neuronal populations in the central amygdala. *Science, 308,* 245–248.

Huesmann, L. R. (1982). Television violence and aggressive behavior. In D. Pearl, L. Bouthilet, & J. Lazar (Eds.), *Television and behavior: Ten years of scientific progress and implications for the eighties: Vol. 2. Technical reviews* (pp. 126–137). Washington, DC: U.S. Government Printing Office.

Huesmann, L. R. (1988). An information processing model for the development of aggression. *Aggressive Behavior, 14,* 13–24.

Huesmann, L. R. (1998). The role of social information processing and cognitive schema in the acquisition and maintenance of habitual aggressive behavior. In R. G. Geen & E. Donnerstein (Eds.), *Human aggression: Theories, research, and implications for policy* (pp. 73–109). New York: Academic Press.

Huesmann, L. R., Dubow, E. F., Boxer, P., Landau, S. F., Gvirsman, S. D., & Shikaki, K. (2017). Children's exposure to violent political conflict stimulates aggression at peers by increasing emotional distress, aggressive script rehearsal, and normative beliefs favoring aggression. *Development and Psychopathology, 29,* 39–50.

Huesmann, L. R., & Eron, L. D. (1984). Cognitive processes and the persistence of aggressive behavior. *Aggressive Behavior, 10,* 243–251.

Hyatt, C. S., Zeichner, A., & Miller, J. D. (2019). Laboratory aggression and personality traits: A meta-analytic review. *Psychology of Violence, 9*(6), 675–689.

Inzlicht, M., Schmeichel, B. J., & Macrae, C. N. (2014). Why self-control seems (but may not be) limited. *Trends in Cognitive Sciences, 18,* 127–133.

Ioannidis, J. P., Ntzani, E. E., Trikalinos, T. A., & Contopoulos-Ioannidis, D. G. (2001). Replication validity of genetic association studies. *Nature Genetics, 29*(3), 306–309.

James, W. (1890). *The principles of psychology.* New York: Holt.

Job, V., Dweck, C. S., & Walton, G. M. (2010). Ego depletion—is it all in your head?: Implicit theories about willpower affect self-regulation. *Psychological Science, 21,* 1686–1693.

Johnston, L. D., O'Malley, P. M., Bachman, J. G., & Schulenberg, J. E. (2006). *Monitoring the future: National results on adolescent drug use: Overview of key findings, 2005.* Bethesda, MD: National Institutes of Health, U.S. Department of Health and Human Services.

Jones, S. E., Miller, J. D., & Lynam, D. R. (2011). Personality, antisocial behavior, and aggression: A meta-analytic review. *Journal of Criminal Justice, 39,* 329–337.

Kavanagh, P. S., Robins, S. C., & Ellis, B. J. (2010). The mating sociometer: A regulatory mechanism for mating aspirations. *Journal of Personality and Social Psychology, 99,* 120–132.

Kim, M. J., Loucks, R. A., Palmer, A. L., Brown, A. C., Solomon, K. M., Marchante, A. N., et al. (2011). The structural and functional connectivity of the amygdala: From normal emotion to pathological anxiety. *Behavioural Brain Research, 223*(2), 403–410.

Kim-Cohen, J., Caspi, A., Taylor, A., Williams, B., Newcombe, R., Craig, I. W., et al. (2006). MAOA, maltreatment, and gene–environment interaction predicting children's mental health: New evidence and a meta-analysis. *Molecular Psychiatry, 11*(10), 903–913.

Klimecki, O. M., Sander, D., & Vuilleumier, P. (2018). Distinct brain areas involved in anger versus punishment during social interactions. *Scientific Reports, 8*(1), Article No. 10556.

Krämer, U. M., Jansma, H., Tempelmann, C., & Münte, T. F. (2007). Tit-for-tat: The neural basis of reactive aggression. *NeuroImage, 38*(1), 203–211.

Krenzer, W. L. D., & Splan, E. D. (2018). Evaluating the heat-aggression hypothesis: The role of temporal and social factors in predicting baseball related aggression. *Aggressive Behavior, 44,* 83–88.

Lagerspetz, K. M., Björkqvist, K., & Peltonen, T. (1988). Is indirect aggression typical of females?: Gender differences in aggressiveness in 11- to 12-year-old children. *Aggressive Behavior, 14,* 403–414.

Lieberman, M. D., & Eisenberger, N. I. (2015). The dorsal anterior cingulate cortex is selective for pain: Results from large-scale reverse inference. *Proceedings of the National Academy of Sciences of the USA, 112*(49), 15250–15255.

Lin, D., Boyle, M. P., Dollar, P., Lee, H., Lein, E. S., Perona, P., et al. (2011). Functional identification of an aggression locus in the mouse hypothalamus. *Nature, 470*(7333), 221–226.

Lobo, I. A., & Harris, R. A. (2008). GABA(A) receptors and alcohol. *Pharmacology, Biochemistry, and Behavior, 90,* 90–94.

Lotze, M., Veit, R., Anders, S., & Birbaumer, N. (2007). Evidence for a different role of the ventral and dorsal medial prefrontal cortex for social reactive aggression: An interactive fMRI study. *NeuroImage, 34*(1), 470–478.

Lovaas, O. I. (1961). Interaction between verbal and non-verbal behavior. *Child Development, 32,* 329–336.

Lynam, D. R., & Miller, J. D. (2019). The basic trait of antagonism: An unfortunately underappreciated construct. *Journal of Research in Personality, 81,* 118–126.

Malik, A. I., Zai, C. C., Abu, Z., Nowrouzi, B., & Beitchman, J. H. (2012). The role of oxytocin and oxytocin receptor gene variants in childhood-onset aggression. *Genes, Brain and Behavior, 11*(5), 545–551.

Maner, J. K., Kenrick, D. T., Becker, D. V., Delton, A. W., Hofer, B., Wilbur, C. J., et al. (2003). Sexually selective cognition: Beauty captures the mind of the beholder. *Journal of Personality and Social Psychology, 85,* 1107–1120.

Maner, J. K., Miller, S. L., Schmidt, N. B., & Eckel, L. A. (2010). The endocrinology of exclusion: Rejection elicits motivationally tuned changes in progesterone. *Psychological Science, 21,* 581–588.

Marcus-Newhall, A., Pedersen, W. C., Carlson, M., & Miller, N. (2000). Displaced aggression is alive and well: A meta-analytic review. *Journal of Personality and Social Psychology, 78,* 670–689.

Mazur, A., & Booth, A. (1998). Testosterone and dominance in men. *Behavioral and Brain Sciences, 21*(3), 353–363.

McBurnett, K., Lahey, B. B., Rathouz, P. J., & Loeber, R. (2000). Low salivary cortisol and persistent aggression in boys referred for disruptive behavior. *Archives of General Psychiatry, 57*(1), 38–43.

McCrae, R. R., & Costa, P. (1987). Validation of the five factor model of personality across instruments and observers. *Journal of Personality and Social Psychology, 52,* 81–90.

McCullough, M. E., Bellah, C. G., Kilpatrick, S. D., & Johnson, J. L. (2001). Vengefulness: Relationships with forgiveness, rumination, well-being, and the Big Five. *Personality and Social Psychology Bulletin, 27,* 601–610.

McCullough, M. E., Kurzban, R., & Tabak, B. A. (2013). Cognitive systems for revenge and forgiveness. *Behavior and Brain Sciences, 36,* 1–58.

McDermott, R., Tingley, D., Cowden, J., Frazzetto, G., & Johnson, D. D. P. (2009). Monoamine oxidase A gene (MAOA) predicts behavioral aggression following provocation. *Proceedings of the National Academy of Sciences of the USA, 106,* 2118–2123.

McNamara, M. (2005). Death row escapee caught. Retrieved from *www.cbsnews.com/news/death-row-escapee-caught.*

Mehta, P. H., & Beer, J. (2010). Neural mechanisms of the testosterone–aggression relation: The role of orbitofrontal cortex. *Journal of Cognitive Neuroscience, 22*(10), 2357–2368.

Merk, W., Orobio de Castro, B., Koops, W., & Matthys, W. (2005). The distinction between reactive and proactive aggression: Utility for theory, diagnosis, and treatment? *European Journal of Developmental Psychology, 2,* 197–220.

Miczek, K. A., Takahashi, A., Gobrogge, K. L., Hwa, L. S., & de Almeida, R. M. (2015). Escalated aggression in animal models: Shedding new light on mesocorticolimbic circuits. *Current Opinion in Behavioral Sciences, 3,* 90–95.

Miller, J. D., & Lynam, D. R. (2006). Reactive and proactive aggression: Similarities and differences. *Personality and Individual Differences, 41,* 1469–1480.

Miller, N. (1941). The frustration–aggression hypothesis. *Psychological Review, 48,* 337–342.

Miner, J. L., & Clarke-Steward, K. A. (2008). Trajectories of externalizing behavior from age 2 to age 9: Relations with gender, temperament, ethnicity, parenting, and rater. *Developmental Psychology, 44*(3), 771–786.

Mitjans, M., Seidel, J., Begemann, M., Bockhop, F., Moya-Higueras, J., Bansal, V., et al. (2019). Violent aggression predicted by multiple pre-adult environmental hits. *Molecular Psychiatry, 24*(10), 1549–1574.

Moffitt, T. E. (2005). The new look of behavioral genetics in developmental psychopathology: Gene–environment interplay in antisocial behaviors. *Psychological Bulletin, 131*(4), 533–554.

Moffitt, T. E., Arseneault, L., Belsky, D., Dickson, N., Hancox, R. J., Harrington, H., et al. (2011). A gradient of childhood self-control predicts health, wealth, and public safety. *Proceedings of the National Academy of Sciences of the USA, 108,* 2693–2698.

Montoya, E. R., Terburg, D., Bos, P. A., & Van Honk, J. (2012). Testosterone, cortisol, and serotonin as key regulators of social aggression: A review and theoretical perspective. *Motivation and Emotion, 36*(1), 65–73.

Mueller, C. W., Donnerstein, E., & Hallam, J. (1983). Violent films and prosocial behavior. *Personality and Social Psychology Bulletin, 9,* 83–89.

Muraven, M., & Baumeister, R. F. (2000). Self-regulation and depletion of limited resources: Does self-control resemble a muscle? *Psychological Bulletin, 126,* 247–259.

National Council on Alcoholism and Drug Dependence. (2015). Alcohol, drugs and crime. Retrieved from *www.ncadd.org/about-addiction/alcohol-drugs-and-crime.*

Niendam, T. A., Laird, A. R., Ray, K. L., Dean, Y. M., Glahn, D. C., & Carter, C. S. (2012). Meta-analytic evidence for a superordinate cognitive control network subserving diverse executive functions. *Cognitive, Affective, and Behavioral Neuroscience, 12*(2), 241–268.

Nowak, A., Gelfand, M. J., Borkowski, W., Cohen, D., & Hernandez, I. (2015). The evolutionary basis of honor cultures. *Psychological Science, 27*, 12–24.

Orquin, J. L., & Kurzban, R. (2016). A meta-analysis of blood glucose effects on human decision making. *Psychological Bulletin, 142*, 546–567.

Pajer, K., Gardner, W., Rubin, R. T., Perel, J., & Neal, S. (2001). Decreased cortisol levels in adolescent girls with conduct disorder. *Archives of General Psychiatry, 58*(3), 297–302.

Panksepp, J., & Zellner, M. R. (2004). Towards a neurobiologically based unified theory of aggression. *Revue Internationale de Psychologie Sociale, 17*, 37–62.

Pappa, I., St Pourcain, B., Benke, K., Cavadino, A., Hakulinen, C., Nivard, M. G., et al. (2016). A genome-wide approach to children's aggressive behavior: The EAGLE consortium. *American Journal of Medical Genetics B: Neuropsychiatric Genetics, 171*(5), 562–572.

Patterson, G. R., Littman, R. A., & Bricker, W. (1967). Assertive behavior in children: A step toward a theory of aggression. *Monographs of the Society for Research in Child Development, 32*, 1–43.

Paulhus, D. L., Curtis, S. R., & Jones, D. N. (2018). Aggression as a trait: The Dark Tetrad alternative. *Current Opinion in Psychology, 19*, 88–92.

Pavlov, K. A., Chistiakov, D. A., & Chekhonin, V. P. (2012). Genetic determinants of aggression and impulsivity in humans. *Journal of Applied Genetics, 53*(1), 61–82.

Pedersen, W. C., Gonzales, C., & Miller, N. (2000). The moderating effect of trivial triggering provocation on displaced aggression. *Journal of Personality and Social Psychology, 78*, 913–927.

Peters, J. R., Chester, D. S., Walsh, E. C., DeWall, C. N., & Baer, R. A. (2018). The rewarding nature of provocation-focused rumination in women with borderline personality disorder: A preliminary fMRI investigation. *Borderline Personality Disorder and Emotion Dysregulation, 5*, 1.

Pinker, S. (2011). *The better angels of our nature.* New York: Viking.

Pinker, S. (2018). *Enlightenment now: The case for reason, science, humanism, and progress.* New York: Viking.

Popma, A., Vermeiren, R., Geluk, C. A., Rinne, T., van den Brink, W., Knol, D. L., et al. (2007). Cortisol moderates the relationship between testosterone and aggression in delinquent male adolescents. *Biological Psychiatry, 61*(3), 405–411.

Popper, K. R. (1959). *The logic of scientific discovery.* Abingdon-on-Thames, UK: Routledge.

Porsch, R. M., Middeldorp, C. M., Cherny, S. S., Krapohl, E., Van Beijsterveldt, C. E., Loukola, A., et al. (2016). Longitudinal heritability of childhood aggression. *American Journal of Medical Genetics Part B: Neuropsychiatric Genetics, 171*(5), 697–707.

Pratt, T. C., & & Cullen, F. T. (2000). The empirical status of Gottfredson and Hirschi's general theory of crime: A meta-analysis. *Criminology, 38*, 931–964.

Premack, D., & Woodruff, G. (1978). Does the chimpanzee have a theory of mind? *Behavioral and Brain Sciences, 1*(4), 515–526.

Price, D. D. (2000). Psychological and neural mechanisms of the affective dimension of pain. *Science, 288*, 1769–1772.

Pulkkinen, L., Lyyra, A.-L., & Kokko, K. (2011). Is social capital a mediator between self-control and psychological and social functioning across 34 years? *International Journal of Behavioral Development, 35*, 475–481.

Quigley, B. M., Levitt, A., Derrick, J. L., Testa, M., Houston, R. J., & Leonard, K. E. (2018). Alcohol, self-regulation and partner physical aggression: Actor–partner effects over a three-year time frame. *Frontiers in Behavioral Neuroscience, 12*, Article ID 130.

Rainville, P., Duncan, G. H., Price, D. D., Carrier, B., & Bushnell, M. C. (1997). Pain affect encoded in human anterior cingulate but not somatosensory cortex. *Science, 277*, 968–971.

Rasmussen, K. (2016). Entitled vengeance: A meta-analysis relating narcissism to provoked aggression. *Aggressive Behavior, 42*, 362–379.

Reijntjes, A., Thomaes, S., Kamphuis, J. H., Bushman, B. J., Reitz, E., & Telch, M. J. (2013). Youths' displaced aggression against in- and out-group peers: An experimental examination. *Journal of Experimental Child Psychology, 115*, 180–187.

Rubio-Fernández, P., & Geurts, B. (2013). How to pass the false-belief task before your fourth birthday. *Psychological Science, 24*, 27–33.

Rujescu, D., Giegling, I., Gietl, A., Hartmann, A. M., & Möller, H. J. (2003). A functional single nucleotide polymorphism (V158M) in the COMT gene is associated with aggressive personality traits. *Biological Psychiatry, 54*(1), 34–39.

Russell, J. A., & Barrett, L. F. (1999). Core affect, prototypical emotional episodes, and other things called "emotion": Dissecting the elephant. *Journal of Personality and Social Psychology, 76*, 805–819.

Sakai, J. T., Young, S. E., Stallings, M. C., Timberlake, D., Smolen, A., Stetler, G. L., et al. (2006). Case–control and within-family tests for an association between conduct disorder and 5HTTLPR.

American Journal of Medical Genetics B: Neuropsychiatric Genetics, 141(8), 825–832.

Savani, K., & Job, V. (2017). Reverse ego-depletion: Acts of self-control can improve subsequent performance in Indian cultural contexts. *Journal of Personality and Social Psychology, 113,* 589–607.

Sayette, M. A., Creswell, K. G., Dimoff, J. D., Fairbairn, C. E., Cohn, J. F., Heckman, B. W., et al. (2012). Alcohol and group formation: A multimodel investigation of the effects of alcohol on emotion and social bonding. *Psychological Science, 23,* 869–878.

Schilbach, L., Eickhoff, S. B., Rotarska-Jagiela, A., Fink, G. R., & Vogeley, K. (2008). Minds at rest?: Social cognition as the default mode of cognizing and its putative relationship to the "default system" of the brain. *Consciousness and Cognition, 17*(2), 457–467.

Scott, J. P., DiLillo, D., Maldonado, R. C., & Watkins, L. E. (2015). Negative urgency and emotion regulation strategy use: Associations with displaced aggression. *Aggressive Behavior, 41,* 502–512.

Sears, R. R., Whiting, J. W. M., Nowlis, V., & Sears, P. S. (1953). Some child-rearing antecedents of aggression and dependency in young children. *Genetic Psychology Monographs, 47*(2), 135–236.

Sethi, A., Gregory, S., Dell'Acqua, F., Thomas, E. P., Simmons, A., Murphy, D. G., et al. (2015). Emotional detachment in psychopathy: Involvement of dorsal default-mode connections. *Cortex, 62,* 11–19.

Shalev, I., Moffitt, T. E., Sugden, K., Williams, B., Houts, R. M., Danese, A., et al. (2013). Exposure to violence during childhood is associated with telomere erosion from 5 to 10 years of age: A longitudinal study. *Molecular Psychiatry, 18*(5), 576–581.

Sheard, M. H., Astrachan, D. I., & Davis, M. (1975). Effect of noise on shock-elicited aggression in rats. *Nature, 257,* 43–44.

Siep, N., Tonnaer, F., van de Ven, V., Arntz, A., Raine, A., & Cima, M. (2019). Anger provocation increases limbic and decreases medial prefrontal cortex connectivity with the left amygdala in reactive aggressive violent offenders. *Brain Imaging and Behavior, 13*(5), 1311–1323.

Snoek, H., Van Goozen, S. H., Matthys, W., Buitelaar, J. K., & Van Engeland, H. (2004). Stress responsivity in children with externalizing behavior disorders. *Development and Psychopathology, 16*(2), 389–406.

Straus, M. A., Douglas, E. M., & Medeiros, R. A. (2013). *The primordial violence: Spanking children, psychological development, violence, and crime.* New York: Routledge.

Sukonick, D. L., Pollock, B. G., Sweet, R. A., Mulsant, B. H., Rosen, J., Klunk, W. E., et al. (2001). The 5-HTTPR S/L polymorphism and aggressive behavior in Alzheimer disease. *Archives of Neurology, 58*(9), 1425–1428.

Tielbeek, J. J., Medland, S. E., Benyamin, B., Byrne, E. M., Heath, A. C., Madden, P. A., et al. (2012). Unraveling the genetic etiology of adult antisocial behavior: A genome-wide association study. *PLOS ONE, 7*(10), e45086.

Toth, M., Tulogdi, A., Biro, L., Soros, P., Mikics, E., & Haller, J. (2012). The neural background of hyper-emotional aggression induced by post-weaning social isolation. *Behavioural Brain Research, 233*(1), 120–129.

Tremblay, R. E. (2000). The development of aggressive behavior during childhood: What have we learned in the past century. *International Journal of Behavioral Development, 24,* 129–141.

Tremblay, R. E., Nagin, D. S., Seguin, J. R., Zoccolillo, M., Zelazo, P., Boivin, M., et al. (2004). Physical aggression during early childhood: Trajectories and predictors. *Pediatrics, 114*(1), e43–e50.

Tuvblad, C., & Baker, L. A. (2011). Human aggression across the lifespan: Genetic propensities and environmental moderators. *Advances in Genetics, 75,* 171–214.

Twenge, J. M., Baumeister, R. F., Tice, D. M., & Stucke, T. S. (2001). If you can't join them, beat them: Effects of social exclusion on aggressive behavior. *Journal of Personality and Social Psychology, 81,* 1058–1069.

U.S. Bureau of the Census. (2011). Section 5: Law enforcement, courts, and prisons. Retrieved from *www.census.gov/prod/2011pubs/12statab/law.pdf.*

U.S. Department of Justice. (2018). Criminal victimization, 2015 (National Crime Victimization Survey). Retrieved from *www.bjs.gov/content/pub/pdf/cv15.pdf250180.*

Van Assche, J., Van Hiel, A., Stadeus, J., Bushman, B. J., De Cremer, D., & Roets, A. (2017). When the heat is on: The effect of temperature on voter behavior in presidential elections. *Frontiers in Psychology, 8,* 929.

Van Beijsterveldt, C. E. M., Bartels, M., Hudziak, J. J., & Boomsma, D. I. (2003). Causes of stability of aggression from early childhood to adolescence: A longitudinal genetic analysis in Dutch twins. *Behavior Genetics, 33*(5), 591–605.

Van der Meij, L., Klauke, F., Moore, H. L., Ludwig, Y. S., Almela, M., van Lange, P. A. M. (2015). Football fan aggression: The importance of low basal cortisol and a fair referee. *PLOS ONE, 10,* e0120103.

Van Donkelaar, M. M., Hoogman, M., Pappa, I., Tiemeier, H., Buitelaar, J. K., Franke, B., et al.

(2018). Pleiotropic contribution of MECOM and AVPR1A to aggression and subcortical brain volumes. *Frontiers in Behavioral Neuroscience, 12,* 61.

Van Erp, A. M., & Miczek, K. A. (2000). Aggressive behavior, increased accumbal dopamine, and decreased cortical serotonin in rats. *Journal of Neuroscience, 20*(24), 9320–9325.

Van Lange, P. A. M., Rinderu, M. I., & Bushman, B. J. (2017). Aggression and violence around the world: A model of climate, aggression, and self-control in humans (CLASH). *Behavioral and Brain Sciences, 40,* 1–63.

Varkevisser, T., Gladwin, T. E., Heesink, L., van Honk, J., & Geuze, E. (2017). Resting-state functional connectivity in combat veterans suffering from impulsive aggression. *Social Cognitive and Affective Neuroscience, 12*(12), 1881–1889.

Vasquez, E. A., Pedersen, W. C., Bushman, B. J., Kelley, N. J., Demeestere, P., & Miller, N. (2013). Lashing out after stewing over public insults: The effects of public provocation, provocation intensity, and rumination on triggered displaced aggression. *Aggressive Behavior, 39,* 13–29.

Veit, R., Lotze, M., Sewing, S., Missenhardt, H., Gaber, T., & Birbaumer, N. (2010). Aberrant social and cerebral responding in a competitive reaction time paradigm in criminal psychopaths. *NeuroImage, 49*(4), 3365–3372.

Vize, C. E., Miller, J. D., & Lynam, D. R. (2018). FFM facets and their relations with different forms of antisocial behavior: An expanded meta-analysis. *Journal of Criminal Justice, 57,* 67–75.

Vogel, F., Wagner, S., Baskaya, Ö., Leuenberger, B., Mobascher, A., Dahmen, N., et al. (2012). Variable number of tandem repeat polymorphisms of the arginine vasopressin receptor 1A gene and impulsive aggression in patients with borderline personality disorder. *Psychiatric Genetics, 22*(2), 105–106.

Wager, T. D., Davidson, M. L., Hughes, B. L., Lindquist, M. A., & Ochsner, K. N. (2008). Prefrontal–subcortical pathways mediating successful emotion regulation. *Neuron, 59*(6), 1037–1050.

Warburton, W. A., Williams, K. D., & Cairns, D. R. (2006). When ostracism leads to aggression: The moderating effects of control deprivation. *Journal of Experimental Social Psychology, 42,* 213–220.

Watkins, L. E., DiLillo, D., Hoffman, L., & Templin, J. (2015). Do self-control depletion and negative emotion contribute to intimate partner aggression?: A lab-based study. *Psychology of Violence, 5,* 35–45.

Weder, N., Yang, B. Z., Douglas-Palumbri, H.,

Massey, J., Krystal, J. H., Gelernter, J., et al. (2009). *MAOA* genotype, maltreatment, and aggressive behavior: The changing impact of genotype at varying levels of trauma. *Biological Psychiatry, 65,* 417–424.

Wundt, W. (1897). *Outlines of psychology.* St. Clair Shores, MI: Scholarly Press.

Yang, Y., & Raine, A. (2009). Prefrontal structural and functional brain imaging findings in antisocial, violent, and psychopathic individuals: A meta-analysis. *Psychiatry Research: Neuroimaging, 174*(2), 81–88.

Yarkoni, T., Poldrack, R. A., Nichols, T. E., Van Essen, D. C., & Wager, T. D. (2011). Large-scale automated synthesis of human functional neuroimaging data. *Nature Methods, 8*(8), 665–670.

Yeager, D. S., Miu, A. S., Powers, J., & Dweck, C. S. (2013). Implicit theories of personality and attributions of hostile intent: A meta-analysis, an experiment, and a longitudinal intervention. *Child Development, 84,* 1651–1667.

Young, S. E., Smolen, A., Hewitt, J. K., Haberstick, B. C., Stallings, M. C., Corley, R. P., et al. (2006). Interaction between MAO-A genotype and maltreatment in the risk for conduct disorder: Failure to confirm in adolescent patients. *American Journal of Psychiatry, 163*(6), 1019–1025.

Zhang, S., & Li, C. S. R. (2012). Functional networks for cognitive control in a stop signal task: Independent component analysis. *Human Brain Mapping, 33,* 89–104.

Zhou, J., Yao, N., Fairchild, G., Cao, X., Zhang, Y., Xiang, Y. T., et al. (2016). Disrupted default mode network connectivity in male adolescents with conduct disorder. *Brain Imaging and Behavior, 10,* 995–1003.

Zillmann, D. (1979). *Hostility and aggression.* Hillsdale, NJ: Erlbaum.

Zillmann, D. (1988). Cognitive–excitation interdependencies in aggressive behavior. *Aggressive Behavior, 14,* 51–64.

Zillmann, D., & Bryant, J. (1974). Effect of residual excitation on the emotional response to provocation and delayed aggressive behavior. *Journal of Personality and Social Psychology, 30,* 782–791.

Ziomkiewicz, A., Pawlowski, B., Ellison, P. T., Lipson, S. F., Thune, I., & Jasienska, G. (2012). Higher luteal progesterone is associated with low levels of premenstrual aggressive behavior and fatigue. *Biological Psychology, 91,* 376–382.

Ziomkiewicz, A., Wichary, S., Gomula, A., & Pawlowski, B. (2015). Trait anxiety moderates the association between estradiol and dominance in women. *Physiology and Behavior, 143,* 97–103.

CHAPTER 16

Cultural Systems

Attunement, Tension, and Lewinian Social Psychology

Dov Cohen
Xi Liu
Faith Shin

Seen from one perspective, cultural psychology is an *enfant terrible,* its chief organizing principle being to upend other principles established by different branches of psychology. For example: People have an incessant drive to self-enhance, so much so that the tendency seems evolutionarily baked into our genes. Maybe not; in East Asia, tendencies toward self-criticism seem at least as strong (Heine, Lehman, Markus, & Kitayama, 1999). People make the fundamental attribution error, explaining behavior in terms of dispositions rather than situations. However, this seems truer in the West than in East or South Asia (Nisbett, 2004). Expressing anger is a risk factor for poor health. Letting people choose for themselves is the best motivator. Cognitive ability is mostly a matter of genes, not environment. Responses to these three assertions might be "Not in Japan," "True for individualists," and "The reverse seems true among the poor in the United States," respectively (Iyengar & Lepper, 1999; Miyamoto, Yoo, & Wilken, 2019; Tucker-Drob & Bates, 2016).

From another perspective, however, cultural psychology is less psychology's *enfant terrible* and more like psychology's zealous missionary, taking some of social, cognitive, biological, and developmental psychology's most abstract grounding principles (about attunement to the social world, bounded rationality, brain plasticity, subjective construal, and self-selection of social niches) into places they had not gone before; that is, it brings a psychological lens to problems that are usually left to other disciplines (anthropology, sociology), and it can illuminate cultural phenomena that would otherwise seem puzzling.

This chapter covers some of the basic principles animating cultural psychology—some of the psychological ideas that it brings on its mission. It also explores some "exceptions" to those big ideas and how they may be understood in terms of the overall system. Cultural psychology's principles and assumptions might be seen as deriving from "big ideas" in psychology such as (1) homeostasis as achieved by top-down and bottom-up regulation as people become attuned to their environment, (2) bounded rationality and heuristics guiding human thinking, (3) the importance of construal and the subjective nature of perception and understanding, and (4) emergent properties of groups.

From a cultural psychology perspective, these principles—explained below—might be described in terms of (1) the attunement of people to their culture through mechanisms going from the neuropsychological to the interpersonal to the macrosocial; (2) cultures as quasi-rational, functional—or at least nonawful—adaptations to the environment; (3) the importance of different cultural construals and different cultural logics organizing behavior, thus giving rise to both the multifinality and equifinality of cultural systems; and (4) continuities and disjunctions between the individual and the collective.

These four principles of cultural psychology very much involve systems thinking: how systems emerge, how constituent elements cohere and fit together, how they self-regulate and respond to their environment—and how they occasionally go awry, producing results that no one necessarily wanted. Of course, cultural psychologists are primarily biased toward seeing people as well socialized and attuned to their environment. They are biased to view cultures as systems that work, as functional adaptations to ecological and social challenges. This is in part because alternatives to these biased assumptions are so unpalatable. (People are primarily disattuned to their culture or misfit for their environments? Cultural systems develop as dysfunctional or as random responses to challenges?).

However, as will be seen, assumptions of attunement and functionality are indeed *assumptions*. Interesting phenomena may be missed by psychologists' tendencies to see people as well socialized and (boundedly) rational and by psychologists' penchant for thinking in terms of positive feedback loops between the person and environment. Later in this chapter, we focus on disattunement, negative feedback loops, misperceptions, countercurrents, and consequences neither wanted nor forseen. These are not ephemera to ignore. Rather, in considering them, we harken back to classic social psychology in the Lewinian tradition. One of the metaprinciples underlying Lewinian social psychology was that of the "tension system" (Lewin, 1948/1997). Individuals and groups always exist as, and exist in, a field of forces, some of which impel, others of which restrain, and all of which are interdependent elements of the life space. Cultures, too, may be conceived of as "tension systems" (Ross & Nisbett, 1991). Forces of attunement, functionality, and posi-

tive feedback exist in tension with forces that push for disharmony, irrationality, and counternormative behavior. The interdependent push and pull of such forces—the tensions, breaks, and opportunities they create—are all part of understanding cultural systems, as summarized in Table 16.1.

Homeostasis and Attunement

We begin with basic assumptions of attunement and functionality: We consider how individuals become attuned to their social environment and, in a subsequent section, we examine how cultures become functional adaptations to their ecologies and the natural or material world (Table 16.1, points 1–3). These sections resonate well with psychology's general conceptions of bodies, minds, persons, and (occasionally) groups as homeostatic systems, achieving equilibrium in their environments through both bottom-up and top-down processes.

Cultural psychology's emphasis on people's attunement to the social world also embraces processes occurring at many different levels. This attunement most famously takes the form of shaping self-schemas (Markus & Kitayama, 1991). However, the principle of attunement goes further "down" in an *intra*personal sense to an individual's more basic cognitive and perceptual habits and his or her biological or neuronal processes. Attunement processes also go further "up" in an *inter*personal sense by sensitizing individuals to the various affordances in social situations and through the establishment of institutions and norms, the creation of collective products, and the construction of the built environment.

For example, the most well-established distinction within cultural psychology is that whereas some cultures are more collectivistic (emphasizing group goals, distinctions between ingroup and outgroup, and the social conferral of worth), others are more individualistic (emphasizing personal goals, autonomy, and the sovereignty of the individual).

What follows from these different individualistic versus collectivistic social systems? Early work concentrated on the formation of self-schemas, with collectivistic societies shaping interde-

TABLE 16.1. Summary Points: Attunement and Tension

Thinking about cultures involves thinking in terms of systems. Systems thinking is involved in (1) how people become attuned to their culture through mechanisms going from the biological to the interpersonal to the macrosocial; (2) how cultural patterns arise in response to ecological and economic environments; and (3) how different cultural logics organize behavior in different societies, resulting in equifinality and multifinality. The overarching meta-principle of the culture-as-a-tension system (Lewin, 1948/1997; Ross & Nisbett, 1991) also involves systems thinking, requiring us to think about opposing forces that keep each other in balance and about negative feedback loops (as well as positive ones).

1. Early work focused on the self (independent vs. interdependent) and attunement to the cultural environment. Subsequent work has gone both "down" (examining basic cognitive, perceptual, and neuropsychological processes) as well as "up" (examining interpersonal situations, collective products, and macrosocial structures) to study attunement.

2. Causal processes are theorized to run both bottom-up and top-down. Successful attunement seems to predict psychological and physical well-being.

3. Cultural patterns also arise in response to ecologies and economies (as noted in the examples of collectivistic syndromes and honor syndromes).

4. Cultural psychologists usually assume that cultural patterns are functional adaptations. This is not necessarily so. Patterns may be maladaptive, outlive their usefulness, or confer benefits on the few at the expense of the many.

5. Cultural patterns exhibit both equifinality and multifinality. Different cultural logics can lead societies with similar starting points to different outcomes (multifinality), and they can lead societies with different starting points to similar outcomes (equifinality). In the realm of ideology, equifinality can be seen with welfare states emerging from both the political left and right, and multifinality can be seen with individualistic nations developing as either welfare states (Scandinavia) or laissez-faire (the United States).

6. The premises and rules organizing various cultures do not follow a single, universal cultural logic. Cultural logics differ and need only be psycho-logically plausible rather than "rational." A logic that both creates anxiety (like the Calvinist doctrine of predestination) and provides a way to assuage it (the Protestant work ethic) can be quite motivating.

7. Psychologists also must pay attention to the forces that lead to disattunement between people and environments, as well as to negative feedback loops.

8. Such forces include (a) payoff structures that allow counternormative strategies to succeed and (b) heavy-handed pressures that undermine the values they are designed to inculcate (through crowding-out or overjustification effects).

9. Pluralistic ignorance also leads to misalignment between public behaviors and private beliefs, producing both conservative lag and then rapid change when pluralistic ignorance is broken.

10. Unintended change also occurs when value-expressive behavior is pursued without regard to consequences and leads to its own demise (as in the case of Protestant asceticism, as well as stigmatization of debt).

Forces and counterforces operate interdependently within a cultural system and are parts of individuals' life spaces.

pendent self-schemas and individualistic societies shaping independent self-schemas (Markus & Kitayama, 1991; Triandis, 1989). Independent self-schemas emphasized a self that was expressive, authentic, agentic, and consistent across times and situations. Interdependent self-schemas emphasized a self defined by its position with respect to other people or a hierarchy, saw groups and relationships as the source of agency, and believed people behaved appropriately when they adjusted to (or at least considered) social circumstances (Keller, 2019; Markus & Hamedani, 2019). Conceptions of the self, however, were only a piece of the puzzle as researchers explored how these social orientations had consequences for basic cognitive processes.

Going Down: Intrapersonal Consequences of Social Orientation

Classic early work on social orientation and cognitive style by Witkin and Goodenough (1981) showed that those living in more collectivistic settings developed a "field dependent" (vs. "field independent") cognitive style. For example, they showed that those from collectivistic backgrounds differed on tasks involving orienting lines with respect to a surrounding frame or perceiving figures in an embedded figures task. Later work by Nisbett (2004) and colleagues greatly expanded on this point by discussing how individualistic cultures create cognitive habits and practices that comprise an "analytic" thinking style, whereas collectivistic cultures create cognitive habits and practices comprising a "holistic" thinking style. A more analytic style would focus on central objects rather than context; categorize objects based on rules; rely heavily on formal, deductive logic to discern truth; abhor contradiction; and believe that change (if it occurred) would be linear. Conversely, a more holistic style would emphasize contexts and focus on the relations between objects; rely on practical experience more than logic; understand contradiction as natural in a world that could be seen from multiple different perspectives; and believe that change is constant and likely to be circular or cyclical rather than linear (Norenzayan, Choi, & Peng, 2007).

Cognitive habits learned in the *social* world— for example, in interdependent cultures, being aware of all the actors in a setting; paying attention to relationships; understanding behavior as a function of the situation rather than enduring dispositions of the person; realizing that different people have different perspectives and that there is likely to be some truth in each; emphasizing harmony over confrontation and outright argument; understanding that the social world is complicated, that things change, and fortunes can reverse—become cognitive habits that guide how one reasons about the world in general (Masuda, Russell, Li, & Lee, 2019; Nisbett, 2004).

Nisbett and colleagues' work relied heavily on East–West distinctions, but the same holistic versus analytic distinction seemed to occur in differences between collectivistic working-class versus individualistic middle-class participants; collectivistic Eastern Europeans versus more individualistic Western Europeans; collectivistic southern Chinese versus relatively more individualistic northern Chinese; and collectivistic farmers versus individualistic herders in neighboring areas of Turkey's Black Sea region (Nisbett, 2019; Talhelm & Oishi, 2019).

The causal process could also be demonstrated in microcosm in the lab. Giving experimental participants individualistic primes (e.g., by having them unscramble sentences with words such as *I, me, mine*) made them more analytic on cognitive tasks, whereas giving participants collectivist primes (unscrambling sentences with words such as *we, us, ours*) made them more holistic on such tasks (Oyserman & Lee, 2007).

Like a fair amount of research in cognitive psychology, this work subsequently became neuroscientific. Researchers began to uncover how deep these habits of the heart and mind went. *Cultural neuroscience,* a term first introduced in 2007, boomed in the next decade (Kitayama, Varnum, & Salvador, 2019). From a methodological perspective, such research was important because it helped establish that cultural differences were "real," in the sense of not being simply a product of biases in self-report. For example, researchers used heightened neural responses (P2 and N400) to show that Asians were more likely to attend to negative self-relevant information and find positive self-descriptions semantically incongruent, whereas Anglo Americans were more likely to attend to positive self-relevant information and find negative self-descriptions incongruous. Furthermore, because such studies allowed researchers to examine fast, less conscious processing, it allowed them to explore cognitive processes that participants themselves could not introspect about, or might not want to report, even if they could. For example, P2 and N400 responses occur 200 and 400 milliseconds poststimulus, respectively; and on a cognitive task in which participants could earn money for either themselves or a friend, differences in error-related negativity (ERN) show up almost concurrent with the error. In this latter case, ERN was greater when earning for the self rather than a friend among Anglo participants, but not among Asian participants—a difference that occurred despite

Anglos and Asians reporting similar levels of friendship closeness.

Additionally, because behavior is much more constrained and influenced by situational demands than mental life is, neuroscience studies could tap into differences that might not appear if one was simply observing a participant's action in a particular experimental setting. Experience changes the brain. Frequent responses lead to a process of long-term potentiation, as "neurons that fire together, wire together." Thus, over time, repeated experience in a culture can carve response channels in the brain—hence, neuroscience studies might provide a "natural history" of long-term socialization in a particular cultural milieu.

Kitayama and colleagues (2019) argued that cultural neuroscience helps demonstrate how deep culture goes in shaping biology. Such findings reinforce contemporary trends in neuroscience emphasizing brain plasticity. Furthermore, they point to a domain in which cultural psychology may have its greatest export value (Cohen & Kitayama, 2019). The assumptions of universality in neuroscientific work are generally quite strong: Scan any 15 brains of sophomores at, say, Yale and learn about the "human" brain. However, cultural researchers have, for example, shown that the region of the brain heavily involved in processing information about the self (among Westerners) may actually be seen as the region of the brain processing information about the self, mom, the spouse, and the kids among Chinese participants. Or they have shown that different regions of the brain are activated in certain language, face processing, and executive function tasks, and that regions mature more quickly or more slowly depending on culture and socioeconomic status (Hackman, Farah, & Meaney, 2010; LeWinn, Sheridan, Keyes, Hamilton, & McLaughlin, 2017).

This cognitive and neuroscience work thus "drilled down" to some "basic" levels of thought, perception, and biology. It is surely true that biology shapes culture in the sense of evolution shaping adaptations and providing a menu of responses that can be evoked by different cultural environments and circumstances (see Tooby & Cosmides, 1992). Additionally, over long periods of time, cognitive adaptations

and genes coevolve (as in the spread of lactose-tolerance genes in dairy-farming regions, alcohol-processing genes in places where fermented rice products are produced, and sickle-cell genes among slash-and-burn agriculturalists whose practices leave the standing water in which malarial mosquitos breed; Mesoudi, 2019). Over much shorter time scales, such as an individual life, culture also shapes "basic" cognitive or perceptual habits and the biology of the brain (Kitayama et al., 2019).

Moving Up: Attunement in Interpersonal Processes

Attunement happens as people interact with the world, with people of different cultures being exposed to different situations and becoming differentially sensitive to the rewards and pitfalls in their environment. For example, when Japanese and U.S. participants were asked to recall situations in which they had influenced others or adjusted to them, Japanese respondents recalled more adjustment situations, whereas U.S. respondents recalled more influence situations. Moreover, such adjustment situations made Japanese feel especially close to others, whereas influence situations made Americans feel particularly self-efficacious, suggesting that each group became sensitized to the culturally sanctioned rewards of these situations (Morling, Kitayama, & Miyamoto, 2002). Savani, Morris, Naidu, Kumar, and Berlia (2011) also showed that prototypical "influence" situations were different in India and the United States. When Indian respondents were asked to recall recent situations of interpersonal influence, respondents recalled situations in which others tried to influence the respondent to behave in ways that would benefit the respondent. U.S. respondents recalled situations in which the influencer tried to influence the respondent in ways benefiting the *influencer*. In a laboratory setting, Savani and colleagues showed that exposure to such prototypical situations might cause people to learn different default responses to others' attempts at influencing them. Thus, all persons exposed to prototypical Indian situations grew more open to influence by others in subsequent situations (regardless of whether these subsequent situations were generated by Indians or Americans). Conversely, all persons exposed to prototypical American situations grew less open to influence by others (again, regardless of who generated the subsequent situations).

Everyday Situations:
Construal and Social Identity

Work by Savani, Markus, and Conner (2008) also showed how culture shapes the opportunities people see in the environment. Middle-class Americans seem to have fetishized choice as a means of displaying autonomy and engaging in self-expression. This seems not to be true among either working-class or middle-class Indians. In one lab study, participants walked through a stream of a dozen (rather trivial) behaviors in which they could sit in one of two cubicles in the waiting room, use one of two colored pens filling out a form, help themselves to candy in a bowl or not, and so on. When asked to recall the "choices" they had made in the past few minutes, Americans recalled six choices, whereas Indians recalled three. The Americans were seeing or remembering opportunities for choice and self-expression that their Indian counterparts did not.

Everyday behaviors can also get coded by people in terms of their cultural identities, which becomes important for facilitating or inhibiting certain types of behaviors. As Black students in Detroit schools code studying as something that *we as Black people* do, the students study more (Oyserman, 2015). As obsessing over calories becomes something that those middle-class White people do, non-White participants may eat less healthily (Oyserman, Fryberg, & Yoder, 2007). As academic strategies become something that *we as first-generation college students* might use, college kids from working-class backgrounds may use them more (Stephens, Hamedani, & Destin, 2014). Hence, actions may take on a cultural meaning, and engaging in or refraining from those actions may further shape a person's cultural identity.

Thus, at the interpersonal level, people's selves and default response tendencies get shaped by the different situations to which they are exposed; moreover, people of different cultures see different opportunities in these situations; they become sensitized to different culturally sanctioned rewards and punishments in their environments; and they invest actions and responses with a higher-level meaning as either congruent or incongruent with their cultural identities. All these tendencies help bring people, the situations they encounter, and the affordances they perceive into resonance with cultural ideals.

Macrosocial Mechanisms

At a more macro level, the collective products, policies, and institutions that people build also create alignment. Language is a collective product par excellence. Kashima and Kashima (1998) argued that languages allowing speakers to drop pronouns (e.g., Spanish) draw attention away from actors and toward contexts, and pronoun drop is correlated with indicators of collectivism (see also Abdurazokzoda & Davis, 2015). Languages that are more "agentive" may lead to less charitable attributions for bad actions. For example, people assign more blame when a woman (accidentally) "overturns a table" than when she jumps back and "the table overturns," and such agentive descriptions are more common in English than in Spanish or Japanese (Fausey, Long, Inamori, & Boroditsky, 2010).

Cultures that stress independence produce artwork that more often concentrates attention on a central individual, whereas cultures stressing interdependence produce artwork with greater attention to context and background (Masuda et al., 2019). Additionally, interdependent cultures focus on relations between objects and produce built environments (cityscapes) that are more visually complex and overlapping. In turn, exposure to such cityscapes seems to facilitate more holistic thinking (Miyamoto, Nisbett, & Masuda, 2006).

Cultures emphasizing honor make different laws, social policies, media representations, and institutional standards about what a "reasonable person" (or a reasonable nation) should do when threatened (Cohen, 1996; Cohen & Nisbett, 1997). Thus, in the honor culture of the U.S. South (vs. non-South), newspapers are more likely to portray honor-related crimes sympathetically, institutions are less likely to discriminate against job applicants who have killed in defense of their honor, state laws are more permissive with respect to handguns and more likely to allow persons to stand their ground and kill rather than retreat, and federal legislators from the region are more likely to vote hawkishly on foreign policy. Folktales, advertisements, children's books, proverbs, and songs also create public representations of ideal motivations and emotions (Han & Shavitt, 1994; Kim and Markus, 1999; Snibbe & Markus, 2005; Tsai & Clobert, 2019). They show what happiness looks like (with greater exuberance and wider smiles in U.S. vs. Taiwanese picture books), what should motivate us (with more emphasis on ingroup benefits in Korean vs. U.S. magazine ads), and tell us whether we should either control our destiny or adjust to it (with greater emphasis on accepting reality in country music songs preferred by working-class Americans vs. greater emphasis on exerting control in rock songs preferred by middle-class Americans).

Alignment and Contentment

All of these features potentially bring people and situations into alignment with a cultural ideal, going "down" to the level of cognitions, perceptions, and biology, and going "up" to the level of interpersonal situations, collective products, and institutional standards. The various levels of phenomena are thought to come into alignment through processes that are hypothesized to be causally bidirectional (running down from macrosocial structures to interpersonal situations to selves to cognitions to perceptions to brains and running bottom-up in the reverse direction). It should be noted that this causal theorizing often runs ahead of the actual data that have been produced in this relatively young field (Cohen & Kitayama, 2007, 2019). Furthermore, a number of methodological issues complicate inferences about causality and statistical analysis (e.g., "Galton's problem" or the nonindependence of observations) when there actually are relevant data (Cohen, 2007, 2019). However, imperfect and incomplete data do exist for some phenomena, and they are generally congruent with the basic theoretical sketch of attunement between persons (genes, brains, percepts, cognitions) and their environment (interpersonal situations, group affiliation, collective products, and institutions), even if the causal processes leading to attunement are not always well understood.

Finally, the extent to which a person's self and emotions are attuned to cultural norms predicts an individual's well-being. For example, the more similar a person's emotional profile is to those of others in the culture, the higher well-being he or she reports in relevant domains (Mesquita, De Leersnyder & Jasini, 2019). In terms of physiological markers of health, negative emotions related to sadness and anxiety predict inflammation among Americans (as indicated by an interleukin-6 biomarker). But in Japan, where such negative emotions are not considered so problematic, they did not predict inflammation (Miyamoto et al., 2019). Neuroticism may predict better health (less inflammation, better cardiovascular functioning) in Japan, but not in the United States (Kitayama et al., 2019). As with other lines of research, more work is needed on the "benefits-of-cultural-fit" hypothesis (see Fulmer et al., 2010). However, initial data suggest that consequences of attunement and disattunement are a promising area for future research.

Adaptations to Ecology and Economy

The social environment is not the only environment cultural psychologists study. There is a long history within cross-cultural psychology of studying cultures as adaptations to the ecology and physical environment. Some environments are more bountiful than others. For example, lands with domesticable plants and animals got a head start in civilization building (Diamond, 1997). Agriculture made possible sedentary living (rather than nomadic or semi-nomadic hunting and gathering). The surpluses that agriculture generated made possible higher population densities and specialization of labor. This led to both technological advancement and the eventual growth of an administrative state, along with the empire building on which such states often embark.

Other theories have stressed water. Access to navigable waterways gives a place a leg up on developing trade. Trade creates wealth and brings with it the exchange of technology and ideas (Ridley, 2010).

Climates that are threatening and require long-term planning may lead to norms requiring group coordination and self-control (Gelfand et al., 2011; Van Lange, Rinderu, & Bushman, 2017). Climate also figures into Diamond's explanation of why Eurasian cultures have dominated the globe. The Eurasian continent primarily runs East–West. Africa and the Americas primarily run North-South. This means that farmers and their agriculture could easily spread across Eurasia because the continent has relatively similar climate across its width. Continents that ran North–South, however, did not have this advantage (see also Van de Vliert & Van Lange, 2019, on "latitudinal psychology").

The type of farming and landscape also seems to be important in shaping people's orientation toward the group, propensity to cooperate, or tendencies toward self-sufficiency. As one example, Talhelm and Oishi (2019) argued that rice growing and wheat growing make very different demands on farmers. Traditional rice farming often relied on irrigation systems that required farmers to cooperate with one another. Wheat, on the other hand, relies on rain, which "falls whether families cooperate or not" (p. 123). As a consequence, people from wheat-farming regions are more individualistic and analytic (vs. holistic) in their thinking styles.

The bases of production may shape norms for economic and interpersonal behavior more broadly. Two experimental games often used by economists are the dictator game and the ultimatum game. In dictator games, one participant is given a pot of money and told to split it in any way that he or she chooses with the other person in the study. In the ultimatum game, the offerer proposes the split, and if the recipient accepts, the deal goes through; if not, both parties get nothing. When economists teamed up with anthropologists and ran these games in small-scale societies all over the planet, they found a great range of responses (Henrich et al., 2005). However, there were two general patterns: In societies in which economic production depends on people working in teams (e.g., whale hunting among the Lamalera in Indonesia), offers were more generous. And in cultures in which there was greater integration with markets (measured in one study by the percent of an average family's calories that were bought instead of self-produced), offers were also greater. Even if they may not necessarily generate norms of benevolence, the smooth running of markets demands

trust; thus, markets seem to inculcate an abstract sense of fair play with strangers (but see Winking & Mizer, 2013).

The outliers are also notable. In two cultures, the Au and Gnau of Papua New Guinea, offers were often "hyperfair" (over 50% of the pot)— and they were routinely rejected. These were gift-giving cultures in which people were extremely reluctant to take gifts from others that might put them under a heavy obligation later. At the other extreme were the Machiguenga of Peru. Average offers were routinely 20% of the pot—and they were accepted. This tribe might seem the epitome of the "rational person" ideal of economists, but what is notable about this tribe was the self-sufficiency of the family as an economic unit; among the Machiguenga, there were almost no economic relationships outside the family. Offerers took the lion's share of the pot and offered only small amounts to offerees. Offerees, having no expectations that others would share, accepted it.

Economies and ecologies that make people vulnerable to predation create a need for self-sufficiency in another sense; that is, in places where people are subject to predation *and there is no adequate law enforcement to protect them,* self-help justice becomes an imperative. Crop farmers may have to deal with animals eating their crops, but they do not need to worry much about human predators coming to harvest their fields and steal their yields. On the other hand, pastoralists, who have their herds graze in open spaces, do have to worry about human predators. Their wealth has high per-unit value and legs that can walk. Thus, their livelihood can be literally rustled away from them instantly. Where the state cannot provide adequate protection—and many pastoral regions are remote, often sparsely populated, or mountainous and hence difficult to effectively police—people must depend on themselves for protection. As a backcountry North Carolina proverb put it, "Every man should be sheriff on his own hearth" (Fischer, 1989).

In such a world of self-help justice, cultures of honor develop. Being in an inherently vulnerable position, persons cultivate a reputation for toughness to ward off potential predators (Cohen & Nisbett, 1994; Daly & Wilson, 1998; Uskul, Cross, Gunsoy, & Gul, 2019). Insults, affronts, and "minor" threats become probes for who can do what to whom. And a person who establishes that he or she will not be walked over on small matters establishes that he or she will not be walked over on big matters either. Thus, males become prickly about their honor and are ready to use violence against those who would insult, threaten, or intimidate them. Such honor cultures have been independently invented the world over, as among pastoralists in the frontier U.S. South, the Mediterranean and Near East, the borderlands of Afghanistan and Pakistan, the steppes of Asia, and so on (Brown, 2016; Nisbett & Cohen, 1996).

Herding cultures in arid or mountainous regions are, however, just special cases of the more general rule that cultures of self-help justice emerge in places where the state cannot or will not go. Such regions need not be geographically remote. Inner cities of the United States are in urban areas with high population density. Yet the police cannot or will not go there. There is a saying: "Call for the police. Call for an ambulance. Call for a pizza. See which gets there first." In areas where the pizza wins, people have to rely on themselves for protection. Prisons, too, have honor cultures because while its residents are effectively cordoned off from society at large, there may be little effective law enforcement by the prison's officials within its walls. Finally, criminal organizations that deal in contraband also cannot go to the police if threatened or stolen from; thus, they, too, often create their own honor culture. As Pitt-Rivers (1968, p. 510) remarked, "Whenever the authority of law is questioned or ignored, the code of honor reemerges . . . as among aristocracies and criminal underworlds, school boy and street corner societies, open frontiers and the closed communities where reigns 'The Honorable Society,' as the mafia calls itself."

Thus, cultures are often responses to ecological and economic systems. The ecology often shapes how we approach the fundamental duties of life—earning a living, keeping one's family safe, withstanding climactic and environmental threats—and so gives rise to certain types of economic relations, social organization, and state administration. The ecology, social structures, and people's individual psychologies thus come to be adjusted to one another.

Issues of Functionality, Multifinality, and Equifinality

The previous statement about mutual adjustment deserves some pushback and clarification (Table 16.1, points 4–6). First, to say that cultures are often *responses* to ecology and economy is *not* to say that they are *optimal or* even *functional* responses to the environment. Second, to say that ecology, social structures, and individual psyches are adjusted to one another is not to say that causality always runs from ecology to social structure to psyche. Causality likely runs in both directions. These two points are related and are in turn related to larger points about equifinality and multifinality in cultural systems.

As noted in our opening remarks, the first point about cultures being functional adaptations is often one of cultural psychology's hidden *assumptions*. The assumption is often a sensible place to *start* rather than alternatives such as "culture is a dysfunctional response to the environment" or "culture is a random response to the environment." However, it is an assumption nonetheless, and it is easy to fall into Pangloss's fallacy that cultures are optimally functional adaptations, or functional adaptations, or even adaptations at all.

Those who study evolution argue that many human adaptations date to an early ancestral environment. They are not adaptations to contemporary circumstances. Thus, our ancestors craved sugar, salt, and fat because those tastes signaled nutrients that were important but relatively rare. We still have such cravings, but contemporary Americans are surrounded by cheap and abundant cheeseburgers, Pepsi, and fried foods. What was a functional adaptation in the past may not be adaptive in current circumstances.

Whereas cultural evolution can move much faster than biological evolution (and can therefore potentially adapt more quickly to the current situation), cultural features may also be adapted to *historical* circumstances rather than contemporary ones. This is reflected in instances of cultural lag, the outsize influence of a region's initial settlers (Fischer, 1989), and equilibria that are difficult to escape. Some cultural equilibria are difficult to escape because there are institutions and interest groups with a major stake in the status quo. Others may be difficult to escape because there are coordination problems—for example, who will be the first to cooperate rather than defect, to stop using violence, or to promulgate a new norm when everyone else is defecting, using violence, or punishing those who do not follow the old norm?

Norms and patterns of behavior that were once functional may not be functional now. They may not even have been functional in the past. Edgerton (1992), for example, has attacked the view that we should assume that cultural patterns are adaptive or rational. The benefits of any given cultural norm may be distributed quite unevenly, in some cases benefiting a minority of the population: men but not women; older adults over the young, or vice versa; Whites rather than non-Whites; colonists rather than the colonized; leaders rather than the rank and file; the wealthy rather than the poor, and so on. All we can say, Edgerton argues, is that a given cultural pattern was able to preserve itself and resist being replaced. Psychologists—because of disciplinary biases that do not seem to focus on societal power structures and resultant inequalities—sometimes mistake what is functional for some to be functional for most, and mistake acquiescence or conformity for consensus and endorsement.

Even when there is not a question of vested interests, structural power, or sticky equilibria, cultural solutions to problems are rarely optimal. They may be "good enough," but even "good enough" may not be very good in some absolute sense. Individuals or individuals banding together as groups or institutions decide how they will use their environment: how much they will explore versus exploit, how they will act toward neighboring tribes, how much they will embrace tradition versus novelty, how much they will consume versus invest, and so on. Persons and peoples may differ in their choices. And a little luck sometimes helps—or hurts (as in the "curse of oil," in which oil-rich countries tend to rely too much on petroleum exports rather than build up and diversify their economies).

Two groups may begin in similar ecologies, but human choice, chance, and small differences in initial conditions may drive them in different directions (Cohen, 2001). Many systems—

especially those with humans at the center of them—exhibit the principle of multifinality, a multiplicity of different outcomes. This is not to say that cultures do not respond to ecologies. They do. But their responses need not be optimal, fair, rational, or even functional—even if people could agree on what those terms mean.

Equifinality and Multifinality in Psycho-Logic

Cultures do not just illustrate multifinality. They also illustrate equifinality—as in the case of honor cultures developing within inner cities, the deserts of the Middle East, institutions such as prisons, and among warrior classes from ancient civilizations to outlaws, samurai, medieval knights, and modern military. The logic of self-help justice emerges in these disparate environments.

However, equifinality and multifinality occur not simply in response to environments. They also occur in the realm of ideas. In many domains, cultural logics differ: Starting at similar premises, cultures may arrive at vastly different conclusions; and beginning with different premises, cultures may arrive at similar end points (for other applications of equifinality and multifinality principles in psychology, see, e.g., Cicchetti & Rogosch, 1996; Kruglanski, Chernikova, Babush, Dugas, & Schumpe, 2015).

The premises and rules that organize a culture do not follow a single universal logic (Cohen, 2001, 2019; Leung & Cohen, 2011). They can differ, and they follow a psycho-logic that can sometimes lead to nonobvious places. As an example, on paper, the doctrine of predestination would seem like an inauspicious principle for creating a thriving society. This doctrine—that G-d had decided in advance who would be saved and who would not be, that the vast majority were damned to hell, and that there was nothing persons could do to alter their fate—would presumably breed hopelessness and passivity. But economically, it had, according to Max Weber, the opposite effect. Because the Elect would sometimes be given success in this life, worried Calvinists tried to assuage anxieties about their own damnation and depravity by working hard in their "calling." In the process, they gained wealth and developed an ethic of diligence, thrift, and rationality (the "Protestant" work ethic) that kick-started economic growth in Europe after the Reformation, according to Weber (1905). (For experimental evidence about depravity anxieties getting sublimated into productive activity among contemporary Protestants, see Cohen, Kim, & Hudson, 2014; Kim & Cohen, 2017).

In fact, the turn in subjective psycho-logic that converted the hopelessness of predestination to the diligent activity of the Protestant work ethic may be seen as a special case of classic Protestant psycho-logic. Traditional Protestant theology holds that good deeds do *not* lead to salvation. It is the reverse; that is, salvation (through either faith alone or through grace) leads to good deeds. The "reward" (salvation) precedes the behavior. Few economic theories of rationality would plausibly generate a theology with incentives like that. However, if culture both *effectively creates anxiety* (about depravity and Hell) and *provides the means for assuaging those anxieties* (faith, work, signs of Election, and salvation), it can motivate behavior as well as any operant principle developed in a Skinner box can (Kim, Zeppenfeld, & Cohen, 2013; also see Sullivan, 2013). Powerful human motivators such as anxiety, reciprocity and feelings of indebtedness, fear, and the search for meaning can make many seemingly unworkable, implausible cultural logics become psycho-logically compelling (Pye, 2000; Weber, 1905). (Obviously, there is also equifinality here: Plenty of cultures have managed to coax good behavior and hard work out of people without holding to Protestant theology.)

As another example of the way different cultural logics can lead to equifinality and multifinality, consider also different cultural understandings of "freedom" and how this affects the contemporary politics of redistribution. The American construal of freedom is primarily about liberty, a freedom from constraints imposed by institutions, especially the state. In the "triangle drama" (Berggren & Trägårdh, 2011) between the individual, the family, and the state, Americans traditionally view the individual and family as allied against the coercive power of the state. Americans' "rugged individualism" is associated with conservative, free-market, competitive, and antiredistributionist ideologies.

Other countries are also individualistic, but their construal of freedom and what limits it are different. In Scandinavia, the "triangle drama" is played out, with the state and the individual allied against the family. Thus, the Swedish welfare state emerges to break the bonds of dependency within the family. Berggren and Trägårdh (2011) argue for a "Swedish theory of love," in which true love exists only between equals. "One can discern," they write (pp. 14–15),

> an overarching ambition in the Nordic countries not to socialize the economy but to liberate the individual citizen from all forms of subordination and dependency within the family and in civil society: the poor from charity, the workers from their employers, wives from their husbands, children from parents—and vice versa when the parents become elderly. In practice, the primacy of individual autonomy has been institutionalized through a plethora of laws and policies affecting Nordics in matters minute and mundane as well as large and dramatic. Interdependency within the family has been minimized through individual taxation of spouses, family law reforms have revoked obligations to support elderly parents, more or less universal day care makes it possible for women to work, student loans without means tests in relation to the incomes of parents or spouse give young adults a large degree of autonomy in relation to their families. . . .
>
> This legislation has made the Nordic countries into the least family-dependent and most individualized societies on [earth]. To be sure, the family remains a central social institution . . . but it too is infused with the same moral logic stressing autonomy and equality. The ideal family is made up of adults who work and are not financially dependent on the other, and children who are encouraged to be as independent as early as possible.

According to eminent Swedish anthropologist Ake Daun, Swedes do their utmost to avoid dependency relationships and being a burden. They offer to *buy* cigarettes from coworkers and may bring their own sheets when sleeping over at another's house (Daun, 1991). This individualistic Swedish quest for autonomy and horror of dependency animates the welfare state. The individualistic American thirst for liberty animates the opposite sort of policies.

In yet other countries, the triangle drama played out differently. In Germany, the welfare state has historically been a product of the right.

The state and family comprise the central alliance, "with a much smaller role of either U.S.-style individual rights or a Nordic emphasis on individual autonomy" (Berggren & Trägårdh, 2011, p. 21). In Germany, the

> welfare state has largely been the result of efforts by *conservative* regimes from Bismarck through Hitler and Adenauer to Kohl. . . . In the German case, notions like solidarity and equality are secondary to the high levels of health, education, and social peace thought to be essential lubricants for the economic machine. . . . [This] partly accounts for the [contrast between the] egalitarian, anti-elitist, and individualist thrust of Swedish welfare-state policies and the much more traditional, elitist, and pro-family character of corresponding German policies. (Trägårdh, 1990, p. 575)

As Bismarck reportedly remarked, it is much easier to control a person with a pension than someone without one. Similar principles seemed to be at work in other places that became what historian Murray Rothbard (1978, p. 22) called "welfare–warfare states." Citing examples from Japan between 1937 and 1950 and elsewhere, Kasza (2006, p. 53) argued that "long mass wars stand among the primary causes of the welfare state." Under this right-wing model, the state maintains order and provides for the needs of citizens, who in turn owe their fealty to the state and its jingoistic pursuits.

On the left, the Swedish welfare state tries to break the bonds of family dependency. On the right, the welfare–warfare state tries to create familial-like bonds between citizens and the Motherland, Fatherland, or Volk. Thus, individualism (of the liberty-loving sort in the United States and of the autonomous, egalitarian sort in Scandinavia) illustrates a principle of multifinality, being consonant with conservative, free-market, rugged individualism in one case and a social-democratic welfare state in the other. Equifinality is illustrated in the way the welfare state can be a product of either the left or right, especially the militarist right.

Disjunctions and Negative Feedback Loops

We began this chapter with (1) a discussion of people's attunement to their social environ-

ment and proceeded to (2) a discussion of cultural patterns as responses to the physical environment. The previous section pushed back against the usual assumption that such cultural responses were functional and rational, noting that these responses were not necessarily functional, might be ill-suited to current circumstances, and could be governed by different and potentially contradictory cultural logics.

The assertion in the first part of the chapter—that people are attuned to their social environments—also deserves some clarification and pushback. Again, attunement is a reasonable starting assumption because alternative starting assumptions—that people respond randomly to their environments or are disattuned to their environments—seem problematic. However, believing that there is perfect attunement or anything close to it is unrealistic, and there are several principles that suggest a lack of attunement is not simply "error" and that provide clues as to where to expect discrepancies. Classical Lewinian social psychology conceived of individuals and groups as tension systems. Cultures also exist in a state of tension, with forces aligning and opposing each other in an interdependent fashion. The notion of "tension systems" is an important *meta-principle*. The next sections describe some of the forces creating such tensions: Whereas positive feedback loops produce "more and more of the same," (1) negative feedback loops create tensions that hold systems in equilibrium; (2) multiple niches allow for variability and counternormative strategic behavior; (3) forces that become too heavy-handed can undermine internalization and lead to "crowding out" of the desired behavior; (4) mistaken perceptions and pluralistic ignorance can produce cultural lag as public behaviors and private beliefs fall out of alignment; and (5) value-expressive actions that are pursued without regard to consequences can sometimes contain the seeds of their own undoing (Table 16.1, points 7–10).

Multiple Niches

The basic notion that there are multiple niches within any cultural system is a powerful idea. Different niches exist because payoff structures often make it profitable to engage in a strategy different than that of the majority. In a world of honest people, a certain number of dishonest people will be able to prosper, until "too many" people behave dishonestly and a crackdown occurs. In a world of defectors, cooperators who can find each other can band together and succeed (Axelrod, 1984). In a world of sellers, it will pay to be a buyer; and in a world of buyers, it will pay to be a seller. Exactly where there will be an equilibrium—between hawks and doves, honest people and dishonest people, cooperators and defectors, alphas and betas, buyers and sellers, honorables and dishonorables—will depend on the payoff structures for the various agents, agents' frequencies in the population, the probabilities of their meeting up, and the likelihood of repeat encounters (Cohen et al., 2020; Cohen, Shin, & Liu, 2019; Smith, 1982). But there likely will not be just one strategy that is the best in all settings or configurations of the population.

Moreover, payoff structures that are stable have a way of returning a system to equilibrium, regardless of the motivations of people within the system. For example, suppose a system is in equilibrium—meaning that no one can gain by unilaterally changing strategies—when there are 85 honest people and 15 cheaters. Suppose further that the honest people comprise 50 "truly" honest people who would be honest no matter what and 35 people who are honest because it is the most beneficial policy given what everyone else is doing. As Cooter (1996, p. 961) notes, if we suppose one of the cheaters "gets religion" and decides to become truly honest, then the system will shift to disequilibrium with 86 honest people and 14 cheaters. It will then become more profitable to cheat, so one of the 35 people who had been honest out of expediency will now cheat out of expediency, returning the system to an 85–15 equilibrium. There are more "truly" honest people in the system, but there is no overall increase in honest behavior. Only changing the payoff structure—or eliminating all expedient actors—will shift the equilibrium in this scenario.

Overjustification or "Crowding Out"

Institutional structures and social forces that apply too much pressure to produce a behavior can crowd out intrinsic motivation for that behavior. At the micro level, psychologists know

this from the overjustification effect (Deci, Koestner, & Ryan 1999; Lepper, Greene, & Nisbett, 1973). Threatened external sanctions that are too severe can make forbidden fruit look all the more tasty, and external rewards that are too salient can turn even playful activity into work. The principle holds for all sorts of social behaviors, coloring attributions for our own actions and those for others' actions.

Yamagishi refers to Japan as a heavy monitoring and sanctioning society, more so than the United States. In experimental games, however, in the absence of a sanctioning system, Japanese participants cooperate less and are more likely to opt out of the interaction if they can do so (Yamagishi, 1988a, 1988b). This is potentially because heavy sanctioning has crowded out cooperation, by undermining participants' internal motivation to cooperate (Houser, Xiao, McCabe, & Smith, 2008; Tenbrunsel & Messick, 1999). Or it could also be that participants' reluctance to trust is driven by their fear that *others'* behavior is only held in line through sanctioning (Mulder, Van Dijk, De Cremer, & Wilke, 2006). The severe punishments that normally follow noncooperation in everyday life make people discount others' internal motivation to cooperate, so they become wary of how others will behave when sanctions are absent.

Outside the lab, money rewards have the potential to crowd out civic virtue, as monetary fines can become "prices," turning questions of conscience into considerations of costs and benefits. Under a cost–benefit frame, people are psychologically permitted to purchase the right to act in ways that they might otherwise consider inappropriate. Thus, out of courtesy, Israeli parents might not want to inconvenience a day care worker by being late to pick up their children, but if a $3 fine is introduced for doing so, the $3 may be construed as a price for an extra hour of care—and a bargain at that. After the daycares implemented the fine, parents' tardiness went up (Gneezy & Rustichini, 2000). Or out of a sense of civic virtue and a belief that citizens should share national burdens, Swiss citizens might agree to have a nuclear waste repository in their community. But if they are offered $4,000 for having the repository, that amount is either a bribe or a price, and who would risk the health of their family for that? Offering the money reduced Swiss citizens' willingness to accept the nuclear dump (Frey, Oberholzer-Gee, & Eichenberger, 1996). Money (and other salient rewards and punishments) can change how people construe choices and acts.

In general, societies want to use rewards and punishments to signal what is good behavior and incentivize it (Fiorillo, 2011). And with the right level of incentives they can "crowd in" good behavior, influencing more people to behave in ways that they may then internalize (Cameron, Banko, & Pierce, 2001). However, it is a delicate balance, and a too-heavy hand may change attributions and construals, undermining the trust and internalization of values it is trying to promote (Aronson & Carlsmith, 1963; Bohnet, Frey, & Huck, 2001).

Both the "crowding out" principle and the principle of stable payoff structures creating multiple niches illustrate *negative* feedback loops: Pressures in one direction lead to pressures in the other direction, bringing the system back to a "quasi-stationary" equilibrium (see also Lewin, 1948/1997). For the most part, cultural psychologists have stressed processes that implied *positive* feedback loops, as changes produce vicious or virtuous circles. However, as Boulding (1986) noted, positive feedback loops are uncommon in nature because they often lead systems to break. Having cultural psychologists think in terms of negative feedback loops that keep a system regulated or in a state of tension/balance is a useful complement to the usual way of thinking (Cohen, Shin, & Lawless, 2020).

Public Knowledge and Pluralistic Ignorance

Another phenomenon that reflects disattunement is pluralistic ignorance, and it often (though not always) preserves the status quo. People generally express opinions and act in ways that they think others will approve of (Chiu & Hong, 2019; Higgins, 1992). Dissenting opinions are held privately and may not be acted upon. Because our perceptions of what others believe come from observations of their public behavior, it is possible that people are all conforming to a public norm that none of them actually privately believe. Classic examples from Schanck (1932) showed that people's beliefs about alcohol and minor vices were not as severe as their public behavior implied; contemporary examples include students' beliefs about alcohol and casual sex that are not as lenient as their public behavior implies (Lambert, Kahn, & Apple, 2003; Miller & Prentice, 1994).

Public knowledge—knowledge that everyone knows and everyone recognizes as universally known—provides a coordinating point for people's behavior. Thus, as Miller and Prentice (1994) note, a collective norm continues to be upheld, even though it may be in disagreement with people's private beliefs. This is one explanation for "cultural lag." Conversely, it is also one reason why some cultural shifts may be extremely rapid: Once pluralistic ignorance is broken, the dominoes begin to fall. Kuran (1995) gives examples of how quickly formal systems were dismantled with respect to caste in India, apartheid in South Africa, and communism in the former Soviet bloc. It is not that people's attitudes changed so quickly. The private attitudes had likely already changed. It was just that people now realized their neighbors also shared their opposition to the status quo and were ready to act on it, if others would as well. When citizens of the former Soviet bloc spoke out—and when resistance by their governments proved much more timid than was supposed—change came quickly. As a banner said when the communist regime in Czechoslovakia suddenly crumbled, "Poland—10 years, Hungary—10 months, East Germany—10 weeks, Czechoslovakia—10 days" (Kuran, 1995, p. 274). Recent shifts in American life concerning gay marriage, gender categories, and sexual harassment likely followed this dynamic, at least in part, as well. People's conservative attitudes had likely softened considerably in private prior to the public norms undergoing their rapid shift.

Processes of Change

An additional factor that leads to at least temporary disharmony among cultural elements involves processes of change. Writing about the "unanticipated consequences" of purposeful "social action," Merton (1936) outlined several reasons why cultures change in unforeseen (and hence, unintended) ways. There is ignorance and error, of course. But perhaps more interesting is another class of cases: those in which actions are pursued for their value-expressive functions, without regard to consequences. In this class, Merton gives the example of the Protestant work ethic's (partial) undoing, in which "active asceticism paradoxically leads to its own decline through the accumulation of wealth and possessions entailed by decreased consumption and intense productive activity" (p. 903). The realization of values leads to its own demise, or as John Wesley (1786/1901, p. 130) put it, "For the Methodists in every place grow diligent and frugal; consequently, they increase in goods. Hence, they proportionately increase in pride, in anger, in the desire of the flesh. . . . So, although the form of religion remains, the spirit is swiftly vanishing away." (One should not overstate the decline of the Protestant ethic, however; see, e.g., Cohen et al., 2014; Uhlmann & Sanchez-Burks, 2014.)

Relatedly, we might also consider the case of Protestantism and attitudes toward debt and credit. As a gross oversimplification, historically Catholicism stigmatized lenders, forbidding usury because loans were supposed to be an act of charity. Protestantism—beginning primarily with Calvin—shifted stigma from the lender to the debtor. Debtors who could not repay might be stigmatized everywhere, but Protestantism went further: "By the beginning of the nineteenth century evangelical Protestants [considered] borrowing as sinful [per se], even when the debt was serviced and repaid" on time (Friedman, 2014, p. 50). In England, paying in cash was consider morally correct (Graeber, 2014).

From this, one might expect that there would be very low levels of debt in Protestant countries today. However, the reverse is true. Because of cultural attitudes stigmatizing borrowing, Protestant countries established rules, institutions, and practices favoring lenders (Djankov, McLiesh, & Shleifer, 2007; La Porta, Lipez-De-Silanes, Shleifer, & Vishny, 1997). This greater protection for lenders meant that lenders were more willing to extend credit. With cheaper and more abundant credit, people borrowed more money, and it is now households in the Protestant rather than Catholic countries of Europe that show high levels of indebtedness today (Cohen et al., 2019, 2020; Cohen & Shin, 2020).

Both the cases of Protestants' declining asceticism and their increasing debt provide examples in which a cultural push in one direction led to stronger countervailing pressures in the other direction. This resembles the negative feedback loops described earlier, but in this case, the opposing push does not create balance that keeps the cultural system in stasis. Instead it creates change.

Conclusion: Attunement, Disattunement, and the Meta-Principle of the Lewinian Tradition

In summary, the overarching picture for cultural psychologists involves the attunement of people to their cultural settings. People become sensitized to the rewards and punishments in their cultural environment in ways that studies (including neuroscience studies) help us identify. They develop selves and cognitive and perceptual styles in accord with dominant cultural ideals. They construe and construct situations highlighting dominant cultural themes. And they create collective representations, institutions, and macro-social structures in accordance with such values. A cultural mosaic is created as elements come together to establish a coherent pattern, according to a particular cultural logic (Cohen, 2015, 2019). People and environments become attuned, as processes bring biological, perceptual, cognitive, self-related, interpersonal, and macrosocial elements into rough alignment in some sort of functioning system that is boundedly rational—or at least able to persist over time.

However, one would commit the error of adopting the "oversocialized conception of [people]" (Wrong, 1961) to focus too much on congruity and attunement, and neglect the multiple niches within a culture, the existence of subgroups, the payoffs from using counternormative strategies, the heavy-handedness of forces that can undermine the internalization of values, the fallibility of interpersonal perception and possibility of pluralistic ignorance, and the pursuit of value-expressive behavior without regard to consequences, potentially leading to its own undoing. And add to this the existence of human irrationality, malice, nearsightedness, and the downright stubbornness of people who temperamentally cannot or just do not want to fit the mold.

Forces of attunement and disattunement co-exist. And this is where one of the "meta-principles" from social psychology might be most applicable. In the Lewinian tradition, individual psyches as well as groups are conceived of as systems in a state of tension. Cultural systems can be conceived of this way as well (Ross & Nisbett, 1991).

Forces and counterforces operate interdependently within a cultural system, and they exert influence on the psychology of the individual. And here culture and Lewinian social psychology merge. As Cartwright (in Lewin, 1948/1997) observed,

Many of Lewin's contributions to the understanding of human behavior consisted of showing that a wider and wider realm of determinants must be treated as part of a single, interdependent field and that phenomena traditionally parceled out to separate "disciplines" must be treated in a single coherent system of constructs. In the last few months of his life, he was coming to recast considerably his conception of motivation to emphasize "need" less and to stress more such determinants as group membership, personal ability, economic and political resources, social channels, and other influences usually omitted from psychological theories of motivation. (p. 162)

The forces cultural psychologists study—the varied meanings people bring to events, the different cultural logics with which they reason, the situational affordances and institutional constraints they confront, and the larger ecological, social, and economic environments they inhabit—are all crucial parts of the Lewinian life space.

REFERENCES

Abdurazokzoda, F., & Davis, L. (2015). Language, culture and institutions. Retrieved from *https://ssrn.com/abstract=2366649*.

Aronson, E., & Carlsmith, J. M. (1963). Effect of the severity of threat on the devaluation of forbidden behavior. *Journal of Abnormal and Social Psychology, 66*(6), 584–588.

Axelrod, R. (1984). *The evolution of cooperation.* New York: Basic Books.

Berggren, H., & Trägård, L. (2011). Social trust and radical individualism. In A. Partanen (Ed.), *The Nordic way* (pp. 12–27). Stockholm, Sweden: Global Utmaning.

Bohnet, I., Frey, B. S., & Huck, S. (2001). More order with less law. *American Political Science Review, 95*(1), 131–144.

Boulding, K. (1986). System breaks and positive feedback as sources of catastrophe. In A. Diekman & P. Miller (Eds.), *Paradoxical effects of social behavior (*pp. 47–54). Heidelberg, Germany: Physica-Verlag.

Brown, R. P. (2016). *Honor bound.* New York: Oxford University Press.

Cameron, J., Banko, K. M., & Pierce, W. D. (2001). Pervasive negative effects of rewards on intrinsic motivation. *The Behavior Analyst, 24*(1), 1–44.

Chiu, C.-Y., & Hong, Y-Y. (2019). Culture and creativity/innovation. In D. Cohen & S. Kitayama (Eds.), *Handbook of cultural psychology* (2nd ed., pp. 699–720). New York: Guilford Press.

Cicchetti, D., & Rogosch, F. (1996). Equifinality and multifinality in developmental psychopathology. *Development and Psychopathology, 8,* 597–600.

Cohen, D. (1996). Law, social policy, and violence. *Journal of Personality and Social Psychology, 70*(5), 961–978.

Cohen, D. (2001). Cultural variation. *Psychological Bulletin, 127*(4), 451–471.

Cohen, D. (2007). Methods in cultural psychology. In S. Kitayama & D. Cohen (Eds.), *Handbook of cultural psychology* (pp. 196–236). New York: Guilford Press.

Cohen, D. (2015). Cultural psychology. In M. Mikulincer & P. R. Shaver (Eds.), *APA handbook of personality and social psychology* (pp. 415–456). Washington, DC: American Psychological Association.

Cohen, D. (2019). Methods in cultural psychology. In D. Cohen & S. Kitayama (Eds.), *Handbook of cultural psychology* (2nd ed., pp. 163–206). New York: Guilford Press.

Cohen, D., Hernandez, I., Gruschow, K., Nowak, A., Gelfand, M., & Borkowski, W. (2020). *The importance of being unearnest: Opportunists and the making of culture.* Unpublished manuscript, University of Illinois.

Cohen, D., Kim, E., & Hudson, N. W. (2014). Religion, the forbidden, and sublimation. *Current Directions in Psychological Science, 23*(3), 208–214.

Cohen, D., & Kitayama, S. (2007). Cultural psychology: This stanza and the next. In S. Kitayama & D. Cohen (Eds.), *Handbook of cultural psychology* (pp. 847–851). New York: Guilford Press.

Cohen, D., & Kitayama, S. (2019). Young and still developing. In D. Cohen & S. Kitayama (Eds.), *Handbook of cultural psychology* (2nd ed., pp. 1–10). New York: Guilford Press.

Cohen, D., & Nisbett, R. E. (1994). Self-protection

and the culture of honor. *Personality and Social Psychology Bulletin, 20*(5), 551–567.

Cohen, D., & Nisbett, R. E. (1997). Field experiments examining the culture of honor. *Personality and Social Psychology Bulletin, 23*(11), 1188–1199.

Cohen, D., & Shin, F. (2020). Institutional inversion and the connection between collective attitudes and behavior. *Current Opinion in Psychology, 32,* 133–137.

Cohen, D., Shin, F., & Lawless, R. M. (2020). *Attitudes, behavior, and institutional inversion: The case of debt.* Unpublished manuscript, University of Illinois.

Cohen, D., Shin, F., & Liu, X. (2019). Cultural psychology of money. In D. Cohen & S. Kitayama (Eds.), *Handbook of cultural psychology* (2nd ed., pp. 599–629). New York: Guilford Press.

Cooter, R. (1996). Normative failure theory of law. *Cornell Law Review, 82,* 947–979.

Daly, M., & Wilson, M. (1988). *Homicide.* New York: Aldine DeGruyter.

Daun, Å. (1991). Individualism and collectivity among Swedes. *Ethnos, 56*(3–4), 165–172.

Deci, E. L., Koestner, R., & Ryan, R. M. (1999). A meta-analytic review of experiments examining the effects of extrinsic rewards on intrinsic motivation. *Psychological Bulletin, 125*(6), 627–668.

Diamond, J. (1997). *Guns, germs and steel.* New York: Norton.

Djankov, S., McLiesh, C., & Shleifer, A. (2007). Private credit in 129 countries. *Journal of Financial Economics, 84*(2), 299–329.

Edgerton, R. (1992). *Sick societies.* New York: Free Press.

Fausey, C. M., Long, B. L., Inamori, A., & Boroditsky, L. (2010). Constructing agency. *Frontiers in Psychology, 1,* 162.

Fiorillo, D. (2011). Do monetary rewards crowd out the intrinsic motivation of volunteers? *Annals of Public and Cooperative Economics, 82*(2), 139–165.

Fischer, D. H. (1989). *Albion's seed.* New York: Oxford University Press.

Frey, B. S., Oberholzer-Gee, F., & Eichenberger, R. (1996). The old lady visits your backyard. *Journal of Political Economy, 104*(6), 1297–1313.

Friedman, B. M. (2014). The pathology of Europe's debt. *New York Review of Books, 61*(15), 50–51.

Fulmer, C. A., Gelfand, M. J., Kruglanski, A. W., Kim-Prieto, C., Diener, E., Pierro, A., et al. (2010). On "feeling right" in cultural contexts: How person–culture match affects self-esteem and subjective well-being. *Psychological Science, 21*(11), 1563–1569.

Gelfand, M. J., Raver, J. L., Nishii, L., Leslie, L. M., Lun, J., Lim, B. C., et al. (2011). Differences between tight and loose cultures. *Science, 332*(6033), 1100–1104.

Gneezy, U., & Rustichini, A. (2000). A fine is a price. *Journal of Legal Studies, 29*(1), 1–17.

Graeber, D. (2014). *Debt.* New York: Melville House.

Hackman, D. A., Farah, M. J., & Meaney, M. J. (2010). Socioeconomic status and the brain. *Nature Reviews Neuroscience, 11*(9), 651–659.

Han, S. P., & Shavitt, S. (1994). Persuasion and culture. *Journal of Experimental Social Psychology, 30*(4), 326–350.

Heine, S. J., Lehman, D. R., Markus, H. R., & Kitayama, S. (1999). Is there a universal need for positive self-regard? *Psychological Review, 106*(4), 766–794.

Henrich, J., Boyd, R., Bowles, S., Camerer, C., Fehr, E., Gintis, H., et al. (2005). "Economic man" in cross-cultural perspective. *Behavioral and Brain Sciences, 28*(6), 795–815.

Higgins, E. T. (1992). Achieving "shared reality" in the communication game. *Journal of Language and Social Psychology, 11*(3), 107–131.

Houser, D., Xiao, E., McCabe, K., & Smith, V. (2008). When punishment fails. *Games and Economic Behavior, 62*(2), 509–532.

Iyengar, S. S., & Lepper, M. R. (1999). Rethinking the value of choice. *Journal of Personality and Social Psychology, 76*(3), 349–366.

Kashima, E. S., & Kashima, Y. (1998). Culture and language. *Journal of Cross-Cultural Psychology, 29*(3), 461–486.

Kasza, G. J. (2006). *One world of welfare.* Ithaca, NY: Cornell University Press.

Keller, H. (2019). Culture and development. In D. Cohen & S. Kitayama (Eds.), *Handbook of cultural psychology* (2nd ed., pp. 397–423). New York: Guilford Press.

Kim, E., & Cohen, D. (2017). Roads more and less traveled. *Journal of Personality and Social Psychology, 112*(6), 901–925.

Kim, E., Zeppenfeld, V., & Cohen, D. (2013). Sublimation, culture, and creativity. *Journal of Personality and Social Psychology, 105*(4), 639–666.

Kim, H., & Markus, H. R. (1999). Deviance or uniqueness, harmony or conformity? *Journal of Personality and Social Psychology, 77*(4), 785–800.

Kitayama, S., Varnum, M. E. W., & Salvador, C. E. (2019). Cultural neuroscience. In D. Cohen & S. Kitayama (Eds.), *Handbook of cultural psychology* (2nd ed., pp. 79–118). New York: Guilford Press.

Kruglanski, A. W., Chernikova, M., Babush, M., Dugas, M., & Schumpe, B. (2015). The architecture of goal systems. *Advances in Motivation Science, 2,* 69–98.

Kuran, T. (1995). *Private truths, public lies.* Cambridge, MA: Harvard University Press.

La Porta, R., Lopez-De-Silanes, L., Shleifer, A., & Vishny, R. (1997). Legal determinants of external finance. *Journal of Finance, 52*(3), 1131–1150.

Lambert, T. A., Kahn, A. S., & Apple, K. J. (2003). Pluralistic ignorance and hooking up. *Journal of Sex Research, 40*(2), 129–133.

Lepper, M., Greene, D., & Nisbett, R. (1973). Undermining children's intrinsic interest with extrinsic reward. *Journal of Personality and Social Psychology, 28,* 129–137.

Leung, A. K. Y., & Cohen, D. (2011). Within- and between-culture variation. *Journal of Personality and Social Psychology, 100*(3), 507–526.

Lewin, K. (1997). *Resolving social conflicts and field theory in social science.* Washington, DC: American Psychological Association. (Original work published 1948)

LeWinn, K. Z., Sheridan, M. A., Keyes, K. M., Hamilton, A., & McLaughlin, K. A. (2017). Sample composition alters associations between age and brain structure. *Nature Communications, 8,* 874.

Markus, H. R., & Hamedani, M. G. (2019). People are culturally shaped shapers. In D. Cohen & S. Kitayama (Eds.), *Handbook of cultural psychology* (2nd ed., pp. 11–52). New York: Guilford Press.

Markus, H. R., & Kitayama, S. (1991). Culture and the self. *Psychological Review, 98*(2), 224–253.

Masuda, T., Russell, M., Li, L., & Lee, H. (2019). Cognition and perception. In D. Cohen & S. Kitayama (Eds.), *Handbook of cultural psychology* (2nd ed., pp. 222–243). New York: Guilford Press.

Merton, R. K. (1936). The unanticipated consequences of purposive social action. *American Sociological Review, 1*(6), 894–904.

Mesoudi, A. (2019). Cultural evolution and cultural psychology. In D. Cohen & S. Kitayama (Eds.), *Handbook of cultural psychology* (2nd ed., pp. 144–162). New York: Guilford Press.

Mesquita, B., DeLeersnyder, J., & Jasini, A. (2019). The cultural psychology of acculturation. In D. Cohen & S. Kitayama (Eds.), *Handbook of cultural psychology* (2nd ed., pp. 502–535). New York: Guilford Press.

Miller, D. T., & Prentice, D. A. (1994). Collective errors and errors about the collective. *Personality and Social Psychology Bulletin, 20*(5), 541–550.

Miyamoto, Y., Nisbett, R. E., & Masuda, T. (2006). Culture and the physical environment. *Psychological Science, 17*(2), 113–119.

Miyamoto, Y., Yoo, J., & Wilken, B. (2019). Well-being and health. In D. Cohen & S. Kitayama (Eds.), *Handbook of cultural psychology* (2nd ed., pp. 319–342). New York: Guilford Press.

Morling, B., Kitayama, S., & Miyamoto, Y. (2002). Cultural practices emphasize influence in the United States and adjustment in Japan. *Personality and Social Psychology Bulletin, 28*(3), 311–323.

Mulder, L. B., Van Dijk, E., De Cremer, D., & Wilke, H. A. (2006). Undermining trust and cooperation. *Journal of Experimental Social Psychology, 42*(2), 147–162.

Nisbett, R. (2004). *The geography of thought.* New York: Free Press.

Nisbett, R. E. (2019). Culture and intelligence. In D. Cohen & S. Kitayama (Eds.), *Handbook of cultural psychology* (2nd ed., pp. 207–221). New York: Guilford Press.

Nisbett, R. E., & Cohen, D. (1996). *Culture of honor.* Boulder, CO: Westview.

Norenzayan, A., Choi, I., & Peng, K. (2007). Perception and cognition. In S. Kitayama & D. Cohen (Eds.), *Handbook of cultural psychology* (pp. 569–594). New York: Guilford Press.

Oyserman, D. (2015). *Pathways to success through identity-based motivation.* New York: Oxford University Press.

Oyserman, D., Fryberg, S. A., & Yoder, N. (2007). Identity-based motivation and health. *Journal of Personality and Social Psychology, 93*(6), 1011–1027.

Oyserman, D., & Lee, S. W. S. (2007). Priming "culture." In S. Kitayama & D. Cohen (Eds.), *Handbook of cultural psychology* (pp. 255–279). New York: Guilford Press.

Pitt-Rivers, J. (1968). Honor. In D. Sills (Ed.), *International encyclopedia of the social sciences* (pp. 509–510). New York: Macmillan.

Pye, L. (2000). Asian values. In L. Harrison & S. Huntington (Eds.), *Culture matters* (pp. 244–255). New York: Basic Books.

Ridley, M. (2010). *The rational optimist.* New York: Harper.

Ross, L., & Nisbett, R. E. (1991). *The person and the situation.* New York: McGraw-Hill.

Rothbard, M. N. (1978). *For a new liberty: The libertarian manifesto.* Auburn, AL: Ludwig von Mises Institute.

Savani, K., Markus, H. R., & Conner, A. L. (2008). Let your preference be your guide? *Journal of Personality and Social Psychology, 95*(4), 861–876.

Savani, K., Morris, M. W., Naidu, N. V. R., Kumar, S., & Berlia, N. V. (2011). Cultural conditioning. *Journal of Personality and Social Psychology, 100,* 84–102.

Schanck, R. (1932). A study of community and its groups and institutions conceived of as behaviors of individuals. *Psychological Monographs, 43,* 1–133.

Smith, J. (1982). *Evolution and the theory of games.* Cambridge, UK: Cambridge University Press.

Snibbe, A. C., & Markus, H. R. (2005) "You can't always get what you want." *Journal of Personality and Social Psychology, 88,* 703–720.

Stephens, N. M., Hamedani, M. G., & Destin, M. (2014). Closing the social-class achievement gap. *Psychological Science, 25*(4), 943–953.

Sullivan, D. (2013). From guilt-oriented to uncertainty-oriented culture. *Journal of Theoretical and Philosophical Psychology, 33,* 107–124.

Talhelm, T., & Oishi, S. (2019). Culture and ecology. In D. Cohen & S. Kitayama (Eds.), *Handbook of cultural psychology* (2nd ed., pp. 119–143). New York: Guilford Press.

Tenbrunsel, A. E., & Messick, D. M. (1999). Sanctioning systems, decision frames, and cooperation. *Administrative Science Quarterly, 44*(4), 684–707.

Tooby, J., & Cosmides, L. (1992). The psychological foundations of culture. In J. Barkow, L. Cosmides, & J. Tooby (Eds.), *The adapted mind* (pp. 19–136). New York: Oxford University Press.

Trägårdh, L. (1990). Swedish model or Swedish culture? *Critical Review, 4*(4), 569–590.

Triandis, H. (1989). *Culture and social behavior.* New York: McGraw-Hill.

Tsai, J., & Clobert, M. (2019). Cultural influences on emotion. In D. Cohen & S. Kitayama (Eds.), *Handbook of cultural psychology* (2nd ed., pp. 292–318). New York: Guilford Press.

Tucker-Drob, E. M., & Bates, T. C. (2016). Large cross-national differences in gene × socioeconomic status interaction on intelligence. *Psychological Science, 27*(2), 138–149.

Uhlmann, E. L., & Sanchez-Burks, J. (2014). The implicit legacy of American Protestantism. *Journal of Cross-Cultural Psychology, 45*(6), 992–1006.

Uskul, A., Cross, S., Gunsoy, C., & Gul, P. (2019). Cultures of honor. In D. Cohen & S. Kitayama (Eds.), *Handbook of cultural psychology* (2nd ed., pp. 793–821). New York: Guilford Press.

Van de Vliert, E., & Van Lange, P. A. (2019). Latitudinal psychology: An ecological perspective on creativity, aggression, happiness, and beyond. *Perspectives on Psychological Science, 14*(5), 860–884.

Van Lange, P. A., Rinderu, M. I., & Bushman, B. J. (2017). Aggression and violence around the world: A model of CLimate, Aggression, and Self-control in Humans (CLASH). *Behavioral and Brain Sciences, 40,* 1–58.

Weber, M. (1905). *The Protestant ethic and the "spirit" of capitalism.* New York: Penguin.

Wesley, J. (1901). *Selections from the writings of the Rev. John Wesley.* New York: Eaton & Mains. (Original work published 1786)

Winking, J., & Mizer, N. (2013). Natural-field dictator game shows no altruistic giving. *Evolution and Human Behavior, 34*(4), 288–293.

Witkin, H. A., & Goodenough, D. R. (1981). Cognitive styles. *Psychological Issues, 51,* 1–141.

Wrong, D. H. (1961). The oversocialized conception of man in modern sociology. *American Sociological Review, 26,* 183–193.

Yamagishi, T. (1988a). Exit from the group as an individualistic solution to the free rider problem in the United States and Japan. *Journal of Experimental Social Psychology, 24,* 530–542.

Yamagishi, T. (1988b). The provision of a sanctioning system in the United States and Japan. *Social Psychology Quarterly, 51,* 265–271.

CHAPTER 17

Social Ostracism

Theoretical Foundations and Basic Principles

Andrew H. Hales
Kipling D. Williams

If we were to nominate a set of core principles for the field of social psychology as a whole, the ancient dictum that *humans are social animals* would be high on the list. As far back as 1890, in the classic *Principles of Psychology*, William James wrote, "No more fiendish punishment could be devised, were such a thing physically possible, than that one should be turned loose in society and remain absolutely unnoticed by all the members thereof" (p. 293).

This principle is so basic that the now rigorously documented facts that social exclusion is painful and that individuals will go to great lengths to avoid it, were unstated premises in the work of many early theorists. Why would people conform to absurd norms, obey unconscionable orders, or justify irrational behaviors were it not for at least some ultimate concern about maintaining their social standing? James implied as much when, elaborating on his earlier statement, he quoted Locke in describing the characteristic of humans that would later be examined by social ostracism researchers, saying there is not "one in ten thousand who is stiff and insensible enough to bear up under the constant dislike and condemnation of his own club" (p. 295).

In recent decades, the *social animal* dictum has transitioned from an unarticulated assumption to an active subfield of social psychology working to answer the question, *What happens when the social animal is not permitted to be social?* In this chapter we aim to distill the main lessons from this area of research. We describe social ostracism as a scientific concept, review its modern theoretical foundation, and outline seven principles that are central to its understanding. Our aim is to provide an overview of these broad principles. Our review of the research is not exhaustive and instead focuses on the most essential foundations (for a more thorough treatment of the topics addressed, see Williams, 2007, 2009; Williams & Nida, 2017). The principles are summarized in Table 17.1.

What Is Social Ostracism?

Social ostracism is defined as ignoring and excluding by individuals or groups (Williams, 2009). When people hear the word *ostracism*, they often think of its most extreme instantiation: complete and unambiguous shunning carried out by an entire community. While this is

TABLE 17.1. Basic Principles of Social Ostracism

1. Ostracism is more than fully isolating shunning.

2. Ostracism is detected quickly and crudely.

3. Ostracism threatens belonging, self-esteem, control, and meaningful existence.

4. Ostracism threatens certainty.

5. Ostracism motivates restoration of basic needs.

6. Recovery from ostracism is typical but not inevitable.

7. Ostracism is applied nonrandomly.

certainly a form that ostracism can take, the definition is broader and allows the construct to refer to a wide band of experiences. For example, an individual may be ignored and excluded by some, but not all, members of a community. Or an individual may be ignored and excluded by all members of a community, but only partially so, through social contact that is *reduced* but not *eliminated.* Ignoring and excluding may take forms that are relatively extreme (i.e., pretending not to hear someone when they speak), to relatively subtle (i.e., terse or delayed verbal responses, or decreased eye contact). This is the first principle of social ostracism, and the only one to refer to its scope, rather than its substance.

Principle 1: Ostracism Is More Than Fully Isolating Shunning

To appreciate the significance of this principle, it is important to notice that scientific disciplines sometimes face a tension between defining a construct too narrowly (and thereby failing to capture all its facets), and defining a construct too broadly (and thereby diluting its meaning; Haslam, 2016). The definition of ostracism intentionally tilts toward breadth. This allows researchers to ask questions about different variants of ostracism, ultimately producing a rich theoretical understanding.

As an example, consider a case in which an individual at a social event believes that he or she was snubbed by another, who, in reality, did not notice the individual amid the commotion. Are we to say that this event is not ostracism because it was not intended? It is easy to picture how, in groups, a person may be ignored and excluded

by others, quite unintentionally, for example when these others are simply more interested in attending to different people, rather than *not* wanting to attend to the target. If the definition of ostracism were *intentionally excluding and ignoring,* then these events would not be of interest to an ostracism researcher. Moreover, if ostracism is, by definition, intentional, it would be impossible to ask the question, *Is ostracism more hurtful when it is believed to be intentional?*—which would cause researchers to forego interesting theoretical avenues.

Of course, distinctions can and should be made between different variants of ostracism. The original model of ostracism (Williams, 1997) outlined four dimensions on which it can vary: quantity (from partial to complete), visibility (i.e., whether the target is physically removed from the sources vs. ignored while in their presence), motive (e.g., punishment, obliviousness), and causal certainty (from ambiguous to obvious). Some of these types of ostracism are more severe and consequential than others. Hales (2018) coarsely identified *severe* ostracism as instances that are complete, believed to be motivated by dislike, from close others, and lasting an appreciable amount of time. Alternatively, *mundane* ostracism refers to instances that are partial, believed to be motivated by circumstance, from strangers, and short-lived. In terms of the distinction between *physical* and *social* ostracism, physical ostracism may hurt more because one is literally isolated from others. Alternatively, social ostracism may hurt more because one must watch others carry on as if one is not present. What is clear is that some forms of ostracism are more extreme than others. Does ostracism hurt, even in its mundane forms? We answer this question below, but for now simply note that it is a question that would be unaskable if the concept of ostracism were restricted to its extreme forms.

Although ostracism is highly variable in forms that it can take, there are commonalities that apply across all forms. The temporal need–threat model of ostracism (Williams, 2009) provides a generative framework for understanding the basic principles of social ostracism. As a theory, much of its value derives from the fact that it abstracts from the particular forms that ostracism can take to more general principles and also generates novel predictions, allowing greater progress in understanding the phenomenon (Van Lange, 2013). In the next section, we present the seven remaining principles of social ostracism, drawing on insights from this model as we explain each in turn.

The Temporal Need–Threat Model of Social Ostracism

According to the temporal need–threat model (Williams, 2009), when someone is ostracized, his or her experience unfolds dynamically in three sequential stages. First, in the *reflexive stage,* the target detects ostracism and experiences immediate pain, negative affect, and threat to four basic human needs: belonging, self-esteem, control, and meaningful existence. Second, in the *reflective stage,* the target appraises the situation and engages a variety of strategies that are motivated to restore basic need satisfaction. Some strategies are more effective than others, and are driven by situational availability and individual differences in coping. Finally, if the ostracism is prolonged, the individual enters the third, *resignation stage* of ostracism. In this stage, if the individual is unable to restore the satisfaction of the four basic needs, he or she succumbs to chronic feelings of alienation, unworthiness, helplessness, and depression.

Principle 2: Ostracism Is Detected Quickly and Crudely

A primary tenet of the temporal need–threat model is that ostracism is detected quickly and

crudely (in the reflexive stage), and produces immediate negative affect, pain, and threat to basic needs. Humans are in fact social animals and depend on one another to meet the challenges of survival. From an evolutionary perspective, then, ostracism represents a serious threat to one's ultimate fitness (Buss, 1990; Kerr & Levine, 2008; Spoor & Williams, 2007; Wesselmann, Nairne, & Williams, 2012). Ancestral humans who were oblivious to early signs of social ostracism would have had a serious survival and reproductive disadvantage compared to those who were sensitively tuned and thus able to make necessary adjustments to their behavior to either prevent further ostracism from an existing group or seek new affiliations. Moreover, the immediate costs of overdetecting ostracism when it is not actually occurring are relatively minor (i.e., redirecting cognitive and motivational resources toward one's social standing), in comparison to the costs of failing to notice when one truly is being ostracized (i.e., forfeiting the benefits of social life). Based on this perspective, it is reasonable to expect people to be highly sensitive to even minimal forms of ostracism.

Indeed, research confirms that this is the case. Social psychologists have a variety of experimental procedures to induce substantial threats to one's belonging. For example, in the *life-alone* paradigm, people are led to believe, based on personality tests, that they are likely to live a life filled with few social connections (Twenge, Baumeister, Tice, & Stucke, 2001). In the *reliving* paradigm, they vividly recall an actual experience of being ostracized (Pickett, Gardner, & Knowles, 2004). Or, in the *get-acquainted* paradigm, they are led to believe that a group of peers opted not to interact with them (Twenge et al., 2001). Not surprisingly, these paradigms reliably induce a variety of negative outcomes.

More surprisingly, however, are findings from the Cyberball paradigm, which was designed to induce an insubstantial threat to one's belonging. In Cyberball, people are led to believe that they are playing an online ball-tossing game with two strangers connected via the Internet, and depicted with minimalistic avatars (Williams, Cheung, & Choi, 2000; Williams & Jarvis, 2006). In a typical inclusion condition, participants are thrown the ball fairly. In a typical ostracism condition, they receive a few throws at the beginning of the game (demonstrating that the game functions properly), but then receive no more throws.

Logically, ostracism in Cyberball should not be distressing; participants have no prior connection to the players in the game and never expect to meet them in the future. The game lasts only a few minutes. The other players know nothing about the participant, so the treatment cannot reflect some perceived personality defect, and it has no implications for future connections. Also, any effects of the game cannot be due to believing that one has failed to complete the task at hand; participants are instructed that the purpose of the game is to practice their mental visualization skills, and that it does not matter who receives the ball, so long as they are picturing the scene in their mind.

Nevertheless, Cyberball strongly induces negative affect, pain, and threat to basic psychological needs, with differences between control and ostracism conditions often exceeding a standard deviation (e.g., Hartgerink, van Beest, Wicherts, & Williams, 2015; Williams et al., 2000).

The detection mechanism appears to be crude and inexact as well. Not only is the impact of this (and other) ostracism inductions strong, but it is also surprisingly robust to variations that rationally ought to neutralize its effect. Consider, for example, one's ingroup–outgroup relation to the other players in the game. Based on decades of social identity research and theory (Tajfel & Turner, 1986) people should experience worse outcomes when ostracized by members of their ingroup compared to members of a group to which they did not belong in the first place. In fact, based on the principle of *positive distinctiveness* (Turner, 1975), one might even expect favorable psychological outcomes when one is ostracized by an outgroup. Yet Cyberball's immediate impact is strong, even when the other players are members of a group with which participants would never consider affiliating: the Klu Klux Klan (Fayant, Muller, Hartgerink, & Lantian, 2014; Gonsalkorale & Williams, 2007).

Beyond group membership, other situational factors that one would expect to render ostracism harmless have failed to do so. Cyberball-induced ostracism has been shown to hurt, even when it is financially beneficial to be excluded (van Beest & Williams, 2006), and even when being thrown the ball represents symbolic death (van Beest, Williams, & van Dijk, 2011). It also hurts when participants are made aware that the other players are operated by the computer (Zadro, Williams, & Richardson, 2004). It appears then that whatever minimal anthropomorphism humans bestow on computers (Epley, Waytz, & Caciopppo, 2007) is sufficient for ostracism to be substantially painful, even when it comes from sources that only *appear* vaguely human (i.e., the figures in the game), even though people are cognitively aware it is not human.

Similar outcomes are observed when people are exposed to subtle nonverbal cues of exclusion, such as reduced eye-contact (Böckler, Hömke, & Sebanz, 2014; Wesselmann, Cardoso, Slater, & Williams, 2012; Wirth, Sacco, Hugenberg, & Williams, 2010), prolonged conversational pauses (Koudenburg, Postmes, & Gordijn, 2011), cell phone use during a face-to-face interaction (Hales, Dvir, Wesselmann, Kruger, & Finkenauer, 2018; Roberts & David, 2016), and sexually objectifying eye gaze (Dvir, Kelly, & Williams, 2018).

Beyond nonverbal cues, subtle verbal cues have also been documented to produce the same outcomes as ostracism. For example, women who read descriptions of job advertisements that use gender-exclusive pronouns (e.g., "We usually know a good employee when we see him") report threatened basic psychological needs and less interest in the job (Stout & Dasgupta, 2011). Similarly, unfamiliar abbreviations and references to popular culture that one has never heard of (i.e., unfamiliar celebrities), can also threaten basic needs (Hales & Williams, 2018; Iannone, Kelly, & Williams, 2018). Finally, people need not be the direct target of ostracism to experience its effects. *Vicarious ostracism* is a robust phenomenon that has been observed across a range of circumstances (Claypool, Trujillo, Bernstein, & Young, 2020; Giesen & Echterhoff, 2018; Wesselmann, Williams, & Hales, 2013). For example, viewing a movie clip depicting ostracism can threaten one's own basic needs (Coyne, Nelson, Robinson, & Gundersen, 2011).

Extreme sensitivity to cues of potential ostracism is further corroborated by neuroimaging research. Ostracism, induced with Cyberball, has been found to produce patterns of brain activation that are similar to those caused by physical pain (Eisenberger, Lieberman, & Williams, 2003), and this activation can be mitigated with the antithesis of ostracism: a supportive partner (Eisenberger et al., 2011; Karremans, Heslenfeld, van Dillen, & Van Lange, 2011).

Principle 3: Ostracism Threatens Belonging, Self-Esteem, Control, and Meaningful Existence

According to the need–threat model, ostracism threatens four fundamental needs. Ostracism is not necessary to threaten these needs; plenty of other experiences can cause people to feel variously outcast, unworthy, helpless, or invisible. However, ostracism does appear to be sufficient to threaten these needs, and do so simultaneously. A heated argument or a physical altercation may cause a person to feel like an outsider or to question his or her worth. But at least in these contexts the person still has some amount of control over the social environment, and at least the other person is acknowledging him or her. Ostracism is unique in its capacity to threaten all four needs simultaneously.

We conceptualize the term *need* broadly. Beyond obvious physical necessities, we consider something a psychological need not only if failure to satisfy it threatens survival (as has been argued of the need to belong; Baumeister & Leary, 1995), but also if it significantly interferes with one's growth, thriving, or ultimate life satisfaction or well-being (a distinction made by Pittman & Zeigler, 2007).

Furthermore, it should be noted that the needs outlined below are themselves broadly construed. This breadth is an asset for theories that postulate these needs and allows for regularities to be documented and predictions to be made. But a consequence of this breadth is that the needs overlap at the boundaries, and what may appear to one theorist as a threat to one need may appear to another theorist as a threat to a different need. This is part of the scientifically healthy tension between parsimony of explanation versus comprehensiveness of explanation. But for our purposes, a motive constitutes a

need if substantial scientific literature attests to the harms that can be realized when it is not met. For context, Pittman and Zeigler (2007) reviewed six broad theories of human needs. The theories range from postulating between three to five needs, and each tends to overlap with the four needs reviewed below with some reasonable adjustments. In other words, there may not literally be exactly four needs, but this summary of needs is not unreasonable, and it has proved useful in advancing the study of ostracism.

Belonging

Ostracism is a clear signal that one does not belong. Baumeister and Leary's (1995) theory of the need to belong emphasizes its central role in survival and reproductive fitness, and how failure to satisfy this need produces depression, anxiety, and stress, as well as physical illness. For example, lonely individuals show indications of greater stress and poorer heart health (Hawkley, Burleson, Berntson, & Cacioppo, 2003). Belongingness is also implicated in social identity theories prominent in social psychology (Tajfel & Turner, 1986).

Self-Esteem

Ostracism usually occurs for a reason (see Principle 7, below), and that reason is often opaque to the target given that ostracism can occur without any explicit notice or explanation. The target may ruminate about possible reasons and wonder whether he or she is engaged in some taboo behavior or has violated some important norm. Or the target may wonder if he or she has some stable trait that has caused others to cut him or her off. These reasons may or may not be the actual reasons for the ostracism, but in either case, targets of ostracism are likely to have some awareness of these antecedents; thus, ostracism threatens their belief that they are good people (or valued by others, as in the sociometer account of self-esteem; Leary & Baumeister, 2000). One possible reason why ostracism may be especially threatening to self-esteem is that the ambiguity inherent in ostracism allows people to ruminate and generate far more reasons for the ostracism than are actually relevant, and by merely contemplating these reasons—regardless of their accuracy—these individuals confront negative aspects of the self (Williams, 2009). Whereas there is disagreement about the ultimate theoretical origins of self-esteem, its importance for psychological well-being is uncontroversial (Leary & Baumeister, 2000; Pyszczynski, Greenberg, Solomon, & Arndt, 2004).

Control

Ordinary conflicts involve an exchange; partners may attempt to persuade, argue, coerce, or even attack one another. Ostracism, in contrast, represents a one-sided behavior in which one party disregards the other. In such a situation, the target's behavior bears no effect on his or her social environment, and the person becomes helpless to cause any influence on what is happening. The sense that one can control outcomes in one's environment plays an important role in maintaining mental health (Seligman, 1975; Wortman & Brehm, 1975).

Meaningful Existence

Finally, ostracism can induce the sense that one's existence is meaningless. It has been argued that ostracism is a metaphor for death, giving people a glimpse into what the world would be like if they did not exist (Case & Williams, 2004). Inversely, it has also been suggested that *death* is a useful metaphor for ostracism—one that might lead to new hypotheses and insights (Hales, 2018). Research suggests that ostracism could activate the concept of death, making more accessible words that are related to it (Steele, Kidd, & Castano, 2015), and also that social exclusion can induce a sense of meaninglessness (Stillman et al., 2009). Theorists have argued that our belief in the meaningfulness of our own existence is critical to our functioning (e.g., Greenberg, Pyszczynski, & Solomon, 1986; Heine, Proulx, & Vohs, 2006). Also, ostracism very likely damages people's sense of a shared reality with others—a factor that enables people to translate subjective experiences into more objective beliefs (Hardin & Higgins, 1996), and thereby imbues them with meaning. In the absence of this shared reality, meaning becomes all the more difficult to achieve.

Principle 4: Ostracism Threatens Certainty

In addition to the four basic needs outlined in earlier formulations of the temporal need–threat model, emerging evidence has pointed toward a fifth need that is also reliably threatened by ostracism: the need for certainty, or, framed more naturally, the need to avoid or reduce uncertainty when it arises. People are generally motivated to achieve coherent and predictable understandings of both themselves (Festinger, 1954; van den Bos, 2009) and the world around them (Kruglanksi, 1990; Heine et al., 2006). As with other needs (e.g., the need to belong; Leary, Kelly, Cottrell, & Schreindorfer, 2013), people can vary in their motivation to resolve uncertainty (Webster & Kruglanski, 1994), and this has important consequences for how people relate to others and identify with groups (Hogg, 2007). Uncertainty about one's environment can even cause people to expose themselves to painful experiences just to know what produces them (Hsee & Ruan, 2016), and a growing body research show that waiting to receive uncertain news is a distinctly aversive experience (Sweeny, 2018). It appears that people need to have not only some amount of leverage over the social environment but also some ability to understand the past with confidence, and predict the future with accuracy.

Ostracism is an inherently ambiguous experience. Unlike other forms of interpersonal conflict, ostracism can be thought of as a nonbehavior; that is, it is characterized by the actions targets refrain from enacting rather than behaviors they positively enact (Williams, 1997). For example, ostracism may manifest as an invitation *not* extended, a question that is *not* answered, or eye contact that is *not* returned. This is a recipe for tremendous uncertainty (Chen, Law, & Williams, 2010).

More specifically, ostracism can induce uncertainty in at least three different ways (Williams, Hales, & Michels, 2019). First, targets may be uncertain about whether they are even being ostracized to begin with (or at least whether the source *intended* to ignore/exclude the target or was merely oblivious to the target; Williams, 1997). In theory this ambiguity could serve as a protective force, allowing people to avoid the uncomfortable possibility that they are not welcome (e.g., Crocker & Major, 1989). However, in practice, people may find the uncertainty aversive. Second, targets may be uncertain about the reasons why they are being ostracized. Correlational research indicates that people who can report a clear reason for *why* they were ostracized report less severe outcomes (Sommer, Williams, Ciarocco, & Baumeister, 2001). Finally, ostracism can cause people to feel uncertain about aspects of their own selves. Group memberships and affiliations provide important information about one's identity and prototypes from which individuals can extrapolate how they ought to act (Hogg, 2007). When ostracism communicates that these affiliations cannot be relied on, individuals may be left wondering who they are and how they should behave.

Recent investigations have provided support for the notion that ostracism can induce feelings of uncertainty about the self. When participants are given information that they are highly *peripheral* group members (i.e., that their personality more closely resembles that of the typical outgroup member than the typical ingroup member) they report greater levels of uncertainty about themselves, endorsing statements such as "I wonder what kind of person I really am" (Hohman, Gaffney, & Hogg, 2017). Additionally, when participants are directly ostracized by a group in Cyberball, they also report greater uncertainty about their actions, and also their identity (Hales & Williams, 2018). The observation that ostracism has the power to induce self-uncertainty has caused researchers to ask whether it might also leave people open to more extreme groups and movements that are clearer on their stances—a possibility that we discuss below.

Principle 5: Ostracism Motivates Restoration of Basic Needs

If ostracism threatens basic needs, then it follows that people will display behavioral and motivational signs that promote refortification of the basic needs. Three broad classes of behaviors have been documented in response to ostracism: affiliative, retaliatory, and retractive (Ren, Hales, & Williams, 2017).

Following ostracism, people appear to be sensitively tuned to social information (i.e., information that is relevant to helping restore the threatened needs). For example, they display improved memory for social information (Gardner, Pickett, & Brewer, 2000), improved ability to discriminate between sincere smiles and insincere smiles (Bernstein, Young, Brown, Sacco, & Claypool, 2008), and greater attending to information about specific individuals (Claypool & Bernstein, 2014).

This heighten social sensitivity also manifests behaviorally, with ostracism causing people to seek out social connections (Maner, DeWall, Baumeister, & Schaller, 2007), and output more effort in group tasks (Williams & Sommer, 1997). Ostracism has also been documented to leave people more open to the three major forms of social influence: conformity (Williams et al., 2000), compliance (Carter-Sowell, Chen, & Williams, 2008), and obedience (Riva, Williams, Torstrick, & Montali, 2014).

This ostracism-induced tendency to behave in socially mindful ways appears to be adaptive and is likely a healthy response in many circumstances. However, growing research shows that ostracism has the potential to leave people susceptible to recruitment into extreme or unsavory groups (Knapton, 2014; Wesselmann & Williams, 2010). For example, following ostracism, college participants reported a greater willingness to attend a meeting for a group that advocated using extreme methods to accomplish its goals (e.g., blockading campus, and disrupting classes), and also greater openness to the idea of gang membership (Hales & Williams, 2018). Similarly, ostracism-induced threat to the need for control has been found to produce increased endorsement of violence (Pfundmair, 2018). Moreover, ostracism may cause a preference for extreme groups over moderate groups because they have a cluster of properties that are well suited to address the threatened needs. Extreme groups tend to comprise members that are highly identified and similar (i.e., "entitative"; Campbell, 1958; Hogg, 2014), making them a strong source of belonging (provided one is able to gain membership). They also tend to stake out strong and certain positions, offering a sense of perceived superiority and purpose/meaning (Toner, Leary, Asher, & Jongman-Sereno, 2013), which should promote self-esteem. Finally, to promote their goals, extreme groups are often willing to engage in a wider range of actions, promoting a sense of control. Because many of these actions are also provocative in nature, it should be especially appealing to ostracized individuals, who are motivated to be noticed.

In contrast to the (generally) prosocial responses to ostracism, abundant research has also documented the potential for ostracism to cause people to behave aggressively toward both the sources of the ostracism (e.g., Twenge et al., 2001), and third-party others (e.g., Aydin, Fischer, & Frey, 2010; for a review, see Ren, Wesselmann, & Williams, 2018). These aggressive behaviors appear to be effective in helping people feel better following rejection (Chester & DeWall, 2017), plausibly as a result of exercising some degree of control over the environment (Warburton, Williams, & Cairns, 2006).

The affiliative and aggressive responses are, of course, at odds. It is not always clear what factors motivate people to express one set of behaviors versus another; however, at least two key moderators have been identified. First, the specific needs that are most salient following ostracism likely influence whether people aggress. When people are particularly motivated to restore belonging and self-esteem, they should behave more prosocially, but when they are motivated to restore control and meaningful existence, they should behave more aggressively (Williams, 2009). There may be times when it is more important to be noticed than to be liked. Experimental evidence for this type of process was demonstrated with the need for control: Ostracism was shown to provoke significantly less aggression when individuals were randomly assigned to a condition in which they were able to exert control over specific aspects of their environment (Warburton et al., 2006). Second, it appears that ostracism is more likely to provoke aggression when people sense that they do not have any chance of being reincluded (DeWall & Richman, 2011; Smart Richman & Leary, 2009; Twenge et al., 2007). The mirror image of this process has also been shown: People tend to be less reliant on stereotypes, and instead rely on individuating information in an apparent push to reconnect with others (as it is necessary to attend to *individual* characteristics in order to identify which candidates are potential sources of connection). However, this only occurs for individuals who belong to groups that the person would even entertain affiliating with in the first place (i.e., not avowed racists; Claypool & Bernstein, 2014). An additional possible reason for the discrepant responses documented in the literature is that studies very often measure either only prosocial responding *or* aggressive responding, but not both. When both options are available, participants may choose the one that is most impactful, whether that be prosocial or antisocial (Schade, Domachowska, Mitchell, & Williams, 2014).

Finally, a third general response to ostracism that has received less empirical attention is the tendency to withdraw. Following ostracism, rather than continue to risk the prospect of further painful exclusion, when given the opportunity, people can seek solitude to recover privately—a tendency that is especially strong among people who are more introverted even prior to the ostracism (Ren, Wesselmann, & Williams, 2016).

Principle 6: Recovery from Ostracism Is Typical but Not Inevitable

The reflective stage begins just moments after ostracism occurs. As the name suggests, the *reflexive* stage is brief and should be measured in seconds. People immediately begin the process of recovering their basic psychological needs. The speed with which this recovery occurs has been shown to depend on both individual differences (e.g., Zadro, Boland, & Richardson, 2006), and situational factors (e.g., Ren, Wesselmann, & Williams, 2013; Wirth & Williams, 2009). In the next section we outline different processes in which people engage to enable this process, but for now, just note that a cluster of behaviors has been found to effectively promote recovery, including distraction (Wesselmann, Ren, Swim, & Williams, 2013), mindfulness (Molet, Macquet, Lefebvre, & Williams, 2013), and prayer (Hales, Wesselmann, & Williams, 2016).

While people quickly recover their basic needs after a single episode of ostracism, it is reasonable to ask what happens when ostracism occurs not in a single episode but is sustained over longer periods of days, months, or even years. According to the temporal need-threat model, such chronic ostracism will have serious consequences for mental health and well-being, especially if people are not able to fortify their basic needs (Williams, 2009). It is theorized that persistent threat to the four needs will eventually give way to alienation, worthlessness, learned helplessness, and depression.

Empirically studying the resignation stage is logistically and ethically more difficult than the earlier stages of ostracism; however, existing work largely supports the conclusion that chronic ostracism produces these negative effects. First, qualitative interviews have provided a rich source of information about the phenomenological experience of prolonged ostracism. Targets report distress, with some even claiming that they would prefer physical abuse to ostracism (Williams & Zadro, 2001). Second, correlational research shows that people who are socially excluded for 3 or more months experience greater levels of alienation, worthlessness, hopelessness, and depression compared to not only to healthy control participants but also people experiencing chronic *physical* pain (Riva, Montali, Wirth, Curioni, & Williams, 2017). These outcomes did not occur after a single instance of ostracism, suggesting that it is the accumulated impact of ostracism over time than produces these effects in the resignation stage, rather than merely a momentary reaction.

Principle 7: Ostracism Is Applied Nonrandomly

For the final principle, we shift our attention from the experience of being a target of ostracism to the dynamics that produce ostracism in the first place. While most ostracism research has focused on the experience of targets, there is growing interest in the experience of sources (e.g., Zadro & Gonsalkorale, 2014), precipitating causes of ostracism (e.g., Hales, Kassner, Graziano, & Williams, 2016), and behaviors in which sources engage to minimize the sting of ostracism in those instances when it is necessary (e.g., Freedman, Williams, & Beer, 2016).

Ostracism is clearly a painful experience; however, it occurs surprisingly frequently, with daily diary studies showing that people tend to experience it about once per day (Nezlek, Wesselmann, Wheeler, & Williams, 2012). While people tend to underestimate the pain caused by social exclusion (Nordgren, Banas, & McDonald, 2011), they also negatively morally

judge others who use ostracism for apparently arbitrary reasons (Rudert, Sutter, Corrodi, & Greifeneder, 2018). It follows that people will not be especially inclined to ostracize others in the absence of good reasons.

People use ostracism for a variety of reasons, such as punishing others, observing social norms (i.e., not including a waiter in a conversation), and even sheer obliviousness (Williams, 1997). Additionally, research shows that people are especially likely to ostracize targets who are disagreeable because they are less trustworthy (Hales et al., 2016), targets who are less conscientious (and therefore less able to effectively contribute to groups; Rudert, Keller, Hales, Walker, & Greifeneder, 2019), and targets who directly interfere with group progress (e.g., Schachter; 1951; Wesselmann, Wirth, Pryor, Reeder, & Williams, 2013). The prospect of ostracism has been shown to increase cooperation within groups (Feinberg, Willer, & Schultz, 2014). While ostracism is a painful experience for targets, overall, it does appear to have at least some adaptive functions within groups (Hales, Ren, & Williams, 2017; Schachter, 1951).

Conclusion

There is little doubt that humans are indeed social animals. Decades of ostracism research have now shown that this expression is truer than initially realized. The principles presented in this chapter are well established. As ostracism research continues, we expand our understanding of processes currently at the frontier of ostracism theory, such as the long-term consequences, and the antecedents that cause sources to choose to use ostracism. For now, it is safe to conclude that ostracism is a painful experience—the prospect of which helps to account for much of humans' social behavior.

REFERENCES

Aydin, N., Fischer, P., & Frey, D. (2010). Turning to God in the face of ostracism: Effects of social exclusion on religiousness. *Personality and Social Psychology Bulletin, 36,* 742–753.

Baumeister, R. F., & Leary, M. R. (1995). The need to belong: Desire for interpersonal attachments as a fundamental human motivation. *Psychological Bulletin, 117,* 497–529.

Bernstein, M. J., Young, S. G., Brown, C. M., Sacco, D. F., & Claypool, H. M. (2008). Adaptive responses to social exclusion: Social rejection improves detection of real and fake smiles. *Psychological Science, 19,* 981–983.

Böckler, A., Hömke, P., & Sebanz, N. (2014). Invisible man: Exclusion from shared attention affects gaze behavior and self-reports. *Social Psychological and Personality Science, 5,* 140–148.

Buss, D. M. (1990). The evolution of anxiety and social exclusion. *Journal of Social and Clinical Psychology, 9,* 196–201.

Campbell, D. T. (1958). Common fate, similarity, and other indices of the status of aggregates of persons as social entities. *Behavioral Science, 3,* 14–25.

Carter-Sowell, A. R., Chen, Z., & Williams, K. D. (2008). Ostracism increases social susceptibility. *Social Influence, 3,* 143–153.

Case, T. I., & Williams, K. D. (2004). Ostracism: A metaphor for death. In J. Greenberg, S. L. Koole, & T. Pyszczynski (Eds.), *Handbook of experimental existential psychology* (pp. 336–351). New York: Guilford Press.

Chen, Z., Law, A. T., & Williams, K. D. (2010). The uncertainty surrounding ostracism: Threat amplifier or protector? In R. M. Arkin, K. C. Oleson, & P. J. Carroll (Eds.), *Handbook of the uncertain self* (pp. 291–302). New York: Psychology Press.

Chester, D. S., & DeWall, C. N. (2017). Combating the sting of rejection with the pleasure of revenge: A new look at how emotion shapes aggression. *Journal of Personality and Social Psychology, 112,* 413–430.

Claypool, H. M., & Bernstein, M. J. (2014). Social exclusion and stereotyping: Why and when exclusion fosters individuation of others. *Journal of Personality and Social Psychology, 106,* 571–589.

Claypool, H. M., Trujillo, A., Bernstein, M. J., & Young, S. (2020). Experiencing vicarious rejection in the wake of the 2016 presidential election. *Group Processes and Intergroup Relations, 23,* 163–178.

Coyne, S. M., Nelson, D. A., Robinson, S. L., & Gundersen, N. C. (2011). Is viewing ostracism on television distressing? *Journal of Social Psychology, 151,* 213–217.

Crocker, J., & Major, B. (1989). Social stigma and self-esteem: The self-protective properties of stigma. *Psychological Review, 96,* 608–630.

DeWall, C. N., & Richman, S. B. (2011). Social exclusion and the desire to reconnect. *Social and Personality Psychology Compass, 5,* 919–932.

Dvir, M., Kelly, J. R., & Williams, K. D. (2018, April). *Is sexual objectification a form of ostracism?* Research talk presented at the Society for Industrial and Organizational Psychology Annual Conference, Chicago, IL.

Eisenberger, N. I., Lieberman, M. D., & Williams, K. D. (2003). Does rejection hurt?: An fMRI study of social exclusion. *Science, 302,* 290–292.

Eisenberger, N. I., Master, S. L., Inagaki, T. K., Tayler, S. E., Shirinyan, D. S., Lieberman, M. D., et al. (2011). Attachment figures activate a safety signal-related neural region and reduce pain experience. *Proceedings of the National Academy of Sciences of the USA, 108,* 11721–11726.

Epley, N., Waytz, A., & Cacioppo, J. T. (2007). On seeing human: A three factor theory of anthropomorphism. *Psychological Review, 114,* 864–886.

Fayant, M. P., Muller, D., Hartgerink, C. H. J., & Lantian, A. (2014). Is ostracism by a despised outgroup really hurtful?: A replication and extension of Gonsalkorale and Williams (2007). *Social Psychology, 45,* 489–494.

Feinberg, M., Willer, R., & Schultz, M. (2014). Gossip and ostracism promote cooperation in groups. *Psychological Science, 25,* 656–664.

Festinger, L. (1954). A theory of social comparison processes. *Human Relations, 7,* 117–140.

Freedman, G., Williams, K. D., & Beer, J. S. (2016). Softening the blow of social exclusion: The responsive theory of social exclusion. *Frontiers in Psychology, 7,* 1570.

Gardner, W. L., Pickett, C. L., & Brewer, M. B. (2000). Social exclusion and selective memory: How the need to belong influences memory for social events. *Personality and Social Psychology Bulletin, 26,* 486–496.

Giesen, A., & Echterhoff, G. (2018). Do I really feel your pain?: Comparing the effects of observed and personal ostracism. *Personality and Social Psychology Bulletin, 44,* 550–561.

Gonsalkorale, K., & Williams, K. D. (2007). The KKK won't let me play: Ostracism even by a despised outgroup hurts. *European Journal of Social Psychology, 37,* 1176–1186.

Greenberg, J., Pyszczinski, T., & Solomon, S. (1986). The causes and consequences of the need for self-esteem: A terror management theory. In R. F. Baumeister (Ed.), *Public and private self* (pp. 189–212). New York: Springer.

Hales, A. H. (2018). Death as a metaphor for ostracism: Social invincibility, autopsy, necromancy, and resurrection. *Mortality, 23,* 366–380.

Hales, A. H., Dvir, M., Wesselmann, E. D., Kruger, D., & Finkenauer, C. (2018). Cellphone-induced ostracism threatens basic needs. *Journal of Social Psychology, 158,* 460–473.

Hales, A. H., Kassner, M. P., Williams, K. D., & Graziano, W. G. (2016). Disagreeableness as a cause and consequence of ostracism. *Personality and Social Psychology Bulletin, 42,* 782–797.

Hales, A. H., Ren, D., & Williams, K. D. (2017). Protect, correct, and eject: Ostracism as a social influence tool. In S. J. Harkins, J. M. Burger, & K. D. Williams (Eds.), *The Oxford handbook of social influence* (pp. 205–217). New York: Oxford University Press.

Hales, A. H., Wesselmann, E. D., & Williams, K. D. (2016). Prayer, self-affirmation, and distraction improve recovery from short-term ostracism. *Journal of Experimental Social Psychology, 64,* 8–20.

Hales, A. H., & Williams, K. D. (2018). Marginalized individuals and extremism: The role of ostracism in openness to extreme groups. *Journal of Social Issues, 74,* 75–92.

Hardin, C. D., & Higgins, E. T. (1996). Shared reality: How social verification makes the subjective objective. In R. M. Sorrentino & E. T. Higgins (Eds.), *Handbook of motivation and cognition: Vol. 3. The interpersonal context* (pp. 28–84). New York: Guilford Press.

Hartgerink, C. J., van Beest, I., Wicherts, J. M., & Williams, K. D. (2015). The ordinal effects of ostracism: A meta-analysis of 120 Cyberball studies. *PLOS ONE, 10*(5), e0127002.

Haslam, N. (2016). Concept creep: Psychology's expanding concepts of harm and pathology. *Psychological Inquiry, 27,* 1–17.

Hawkley, L. C., Burleson, M. H., Berntson, G. G., & Cacioppo, J. T. (2003). Loneliness in everyday life: Cardiovascular activity, psychosocial context, and health behaviors. *Journal of Personality and Social Psychology, 85,* 105–120.

Heine, S. J., Proulx, T., & Vohs, K. D. (2006). The meaning maintenance model: On the coherence of social motivations. *Personality and Social Psychology Review, 10,* 88–110.

Hogg, M. A. (2007). Uncertainty-identity theory. In M. P. Zanna (Ed.), *Advances in experimental social psychology* (Vol. 39, pp. 69–126). New York: Academic Press.

Hogg, M. A. (2014). From uncertainty to extremism: Social categorization and identity processes. *Current Directions in Psychological Science, 23,* 338–342.

Hohman, Z. P., Gaffney, A. M., & Hogg, M. A. (2017). Who am I if I am not like my group?: Self-uncertainty and feeling peripheral in a group. *Journal of Experimental Social Psychology, 72,* 125–132.

Hsee, C. K., & Ruan, B. (2016). The Pandora effect: The power and peril of curiosity. *Psychological Science, 27,* 659–666.

Iannone, N. E., Kelly, J. R., & Williams, K. D. (2018). "Who's that?": The negative consequences of being out of the loop on pop culture. *Psychology of Popular Media Culture, 7,* 113–129.

James, W. (1890). *Principles of psychology* (Vol. 1). New York: Dover.

Karremans, J. C., Heslenfeld, D. J., van Dillen, L. F., & Van Lange, P. A. M. (2011). Secure attachment partners attenuate neural responses to social exclusion: An fMRI investigation. *International Journal of Psychophysiology, 81,* 44–50.

Kerr, N. L., & Levine, J. M. (2008). The detection of social exclusion: Evolution and beyond. *Group Dynamics: Theory, Research, and Practice, 12,* 39–52.

Knapton, M. K. (2014). The recruitment and radicalization of Western citizens: Does ostracism have a role in homegrown terrorism? *Journal of European Psychology Students, 5,* 38–48.

Koudenburg, N., Postmes, T., & Gordijn, E. H. (2011). Disrupting the flow: How brief silences in group conversations affect social needs. *Journal of Experimental Social Psychology, 47,* 512–515.

Kruglanski, A. W. (1990). Lay epistemic theory in social-cognitive psychology. *Psychological Inquiry, 1,* 181–197.

Leary, M. R., & Baumeister, R. F. (2000). The nature and function of self-esteem: Sociometer theory. *Advances in Experimental Social Psychology, 32,* 1–62.

Leary, M. R., Kelly, K. M., Cottrell, C. A., & Schreindorfer, L. S. (2013). Construct validity of the Need to Belong Scale: Mapping the nomological network. *Journal of Personality Assessment, 95,* 610–624.

Maner, J. K., DeWall, C. N., Baumeister, R. F., & Schaller, M. (2007). Does social exclusion motivate interpersonal reconnection?: Resolving the "porcupine problem." *Journal of Personality and Social Psychology, 92,* 42–55.

Molet, M., Macquet, B., Lefebvre, O., & Williams, K. D. (2013). A focused attention intervention for coping with ostracism. *Consciousness and Cognition, 22,* 1262–1270.

Nezlek, J. B., Wesselmann, E. D., Wheeler, L., & Williams, K. D. (2012). Ostracism in everyday life. *Group Dynamics: Theory, Research, and Practice, 16,* 91–104.

Nordgren, L. F., Banas, K., & MacDonald, G. (2011). Empathy gaps for social pain: Why people underestimate the pain of social suffering. *Journal of Personality and Social Psychology, 100,* 120–128.

Pfundmair, M. (2018). Ostracism promotes a terroristic mindset. *Behavioral Sciences of Terrorism and Political Aggression, 4,* 1–15.

Pickett, C. L., Gardner, W. L., & Knowles, M. (2004). Getting a cue: The need to belong and enhanced sensitivity to social cues. *Personality and Social Psychology Bulletin, 30,* 1095–1107.

Pittman, T. S., & Zeigler, K. R. (2007). Basic human needs. In A. W. Kruglanski & E. T. Higgins (Eds.), *Social psychology: Handbook of basic principles* (pp. 473–489). New York: Guilford Press.

Pyszczynski, T., Greenberg, J., Solomon, S., & Arnd, J. (2004). Why do people need self-esteem?: A theoretical and empirical review. *Psychological Bulletin, 130,* 435–468.

Ren, D., Hales, A. H., & Williams, K. D. (2017). Ostracism: Being ignored and excluded. In K. D. Williams & S. A. Nida (Eds.), *Handbook of ostracism, exclusion, and rejection* (pp. 10–28). New York: Routledge.

Ren, D., Wesselmann, E. D., & Williams, K. D. (2013). Interdependent self-construal moderates coping with (but not the initial pain of) ostracism. *Asian Journal of Social Psychology, 16,* 320–326.

Ren, D., Wesselmann, E. D., & Williams, K. D. (2016). Evidence for another response to ostracism: Solitude seeking. *Social Psychology and Personality Science, 7,* 204–212.

Ren, D., Wesselmann, E. D., & Williams, K. D. (2018). Hurt people hurt people: Ostracism and aggression. *Current Opinion in Psychology, 19,* 34–38.

Riva, P., Montali, L., Wirth, J. H., Curioni, S., & Williams, K. D. (2017). Chronic social exclusion and evidence for the resignation stage: An empirical investigation. *Journal of Social and Personal Relationships, 34,* 541–564.

Riva, P., Williams, K. D., Torstrick, A. M., & Montali, L. (2014). Orders to shoot (a camera): Effects of ostracism on obedience. *Journal of Social Psychology, 154,* 208–216.

Roberts, J. A., & David, M. E. (2016). My life has become a major distraction from my cell phone: Partner phubbing and relationship satisfaction among romantic couples. *Computers and Human Behavior, 54,* 134–141.

Rudert, S. C., Keller, M. D., Hales, A. H., Walker, M., & Greifeneder, R. (2019). Who gets ostracized?: A personality perspective on risk and protective factors of social ostracism. *Journal of Personal and Social Psychology.* [Epub ahead of print]

Rudert, S. C., Sutter, D., Corrodi, V. C., & Greifeneder, R. (2018). Who's to blame?: Dissimilarity as a cue in moral judgments of observed ostracism episodes. *Journal of Personality and Social Psychology, 115,* 31–53.

Schachter, S. (1951). Deviation, rejection and communication. *Journal of Abnormal and Social Psychology, 46,* 190–207.

Schade, H., Domachowska, I., Mitchell, A., & Williams, K. D. (2014, July). *Help or hurt, I just want to matter: Desire for impact guides post-ostracism behavior.* Paper presented at the annual conference of the European Association for Social Psychology, Amsterdam, the Netherlands.

Seligman, M. E. P. (1975). *Helplessness: On depression, development, and death.* San Francisco: Freeman.

Smart Richman, L., & Leary, M. (2009). Reactions to discrimination, stigmatization, ostracism, and other forms of interpersonal rejection: A multimotive model. *Psychological Review, 116,* 365–383.

Sommer, K. L., Williams, K. D., Ciarocco, N. J., & Baumeister, R. F. (2001). Explorations into the intrapsychic and interpersonal consequences of social ostracism. *Basic and Applied Social Psychology, 23,* 227–245.

Spoor, J., & Williams, K. D. (2007). The evolution of an ostracism detection system. In J. P. Forgas, M. Haselton, & W. von Hippel (Eds.), *The evolution of the social mind: Evolutionary psychology and social cognition* (pp. 279–292). New York: Psychology Press.

Steele, C., Kidd, D. C., & Castano, E. (2015). On social death: Ostracism and the accessibility of death thoughts. *Death Studies, 39,* 19–23.

Stillman, T. F., Baumeister, R. B., Lambert, N. M., Crescioni, W. A., DeWall, N. C., & Fincham, F. D. (2009). Alone and without purpose: Life loses meaning following exclusion. *Journal of Experimental Social Psychology, 45,* 686–694.

Stout, J. G., & Dasgupta, N. (2011). When he doesn't mean you: Gender-exclusive language as ostracism. *Personality and Social Psychology Bulletin, 37,* 757–769.

Sweeny, K. (2018). On the experience of awaiting uncertain news. *Current Directions in Psychological Science, 27,* 281–285.

Tajfel, H., & Turner, J. C. (1986). The social identity theory of intergroup behavior. In S. Worchel & W. Austin (Eds.), *Psychology of intergroup relations* (pp. 7–24). Chicago: Nelson-Hall.

Toner, K., Leary, M. R., Asher, M. W., & Jongman-Sereno, K. P. (2013). Feeling superior is a bipartisan issue: Extremity (not direction) of political views predicts perceived belief superiority. *Psychological Science, 24,* 2454–2462.

Turner, J. C. (1975). Social comparison and social identity: Some prospects for intergroup behavior. *European Journal of Social Psychology, 5,* 5–34.

Twenge, J. M., Baumeister, R. F., Tice, D. M., & Stucke, T. S. (2001). If you can't join them, beat them: Effects of social exclusion on aggressive behavior. *Journal of Personality and Social Psychology, 81,* 1058–1069.

Twenge, J. M., Zhang, L., Catanese, K. R., Dolan-Pascoe, B., Lyche, L. F., & Baumeister, R. F. (2007). Replenishing connectedness: Reminders of social activity reduce aggression after social exclusion. *British Journal of Social Psychology, 46,* 205–224.

Van Beest, I., & Williams, K. D. (2006). When inclusion costs and ostracism pays, ostracism still hurts. *Journal of Personality and Social Psychology, 91,* 918–928.

Van Beest, I., Williams, K. D., & Van Dijk, E. (2011). Cyberbomb: Effects of being ostracized from a death game. *Group Processes and Intergroup Relations, 14,* 581–596.

van den Bos, K. (2009). Making sense of life: The existential self trying to deal with personal uncertainty. *Psychological Inquiry, 20,* 197–217.

Van Lange, P. A. M. (2013). What we should expect from theories in social psychology: Truth, abstraction, progress, and applicability as standards (TAPAS). *Personality and Social Psychology Review, 17,* 40–55.

Warburton, W. A., Williams, K. D., & Cairns, D. R. (2006). When ostracism leads to aggression: The moderating effects of control deprivation. *Journal of Experimental Social Psychology, 42,* 213–220.

Webster, D. M., & Kruglanski, A. W. (1994). Individual differences in need for cognitive closure. *Journal of Personality and Social Psychology, 67,* 1049–1062.

Wesselmann, E. D., Cardoso, F. D., Slater, S., & Williams, K. D. (2012). To be looked at as though air: Civil attention matters. *Psychological Science, 23,* 166–168.

Wesselmann, E. D., Nairne, J. S., & Williams, K. D. (2012). An evolutionary social psychological approach to studying the effects of ostracism. *Journal of Social, Evolutionary, and Cultural Psychology, 6,* 308–327.

Wesselmann, E. D., Ren, D., Swim, E., & Williams, K. D. (2013). Rumination hinders recovery from ostracism. *International Journal of Developmental Science, 7,* 33–39.

Wesselmann, E. D., & Williams, K. D. (2010). The potential balm of religion and spirituality for recovering from ostracism. *Journal of Management, Spirituality and Religion, 7,* 31–49.

Wesselmann, E. D., Williams, K. D., & Hales, A. H. (2013). Vicarious ostracism. *Frontiers in Human Neuroscience, 7,* 153.

Wesselmann, E. D., Wirth, J. H., Pryor, J. B., Reeder, G. D., & Williams, K. D. (2012). When do we ostracize? *Social Psychological and Personality Science, 4(1),* 108–115.

Williams, K. D. (1997). Social ostracism. In R. Kowalski (Ed.), *Aversive interpersonal behaviors* (pp. 133–170). New York: Plenum Press.

Williams, K. D. (2007). Ostracism. *Annual Review of Psychology, 58,* 425–452.

Williams, K. D. (2009). Ostracism: Effects of being excluded and ignored. In M. P. Zanna (Ed.), *Advances in experimental social psychology* (Vol. 41, pp. 275–314). New York: Academic Press.

Williams, K. D., Cheung, C. T., & Choi, W. (2000). Cyberostracism: Effects of being ignored over the Internet. *Journal of Personality and Social Psychology, 79,* 748–762.

Williams, K. D., Hales, A. H., & Michels, C. (2019). Social ostracism as a factor motivating interest in extreme groups. In S. C. Rudert, R. Greifeneder, & K. D. Williams (Eds.), *Current directions in ostracism, social exclusion and rejection research* (pp. 18–31). Oxford, UK: Routledge.

Williams, K. D., & Jarvis, B. (2006). Cyberball: A program for use in research on ostracism and interpersonal acceptance. *Behavior Research Methods, Instruments, and Computers, 38,* 174–180.

Williams, K. D., & Nida, S. A. (Eds.). (2017). *Frontiers handbook of ostracism, exclusion, and rejection.* New York: Psychology Press.

Williams, K. D., & Sommer, K. L. (1997). Social ostracism by coworkers: Does rejection lead to loafing or compensation? *Personality and Social Psychology Bulletin, 23,* 693–706.

Williams, K. D., & Zadro, L. (2001). Ostracism: On being ignored, excluded, and rejected. In M. R. Leary (Ed.), *Interpersonal rejection* (pp. 21–53). New York: Oxford University Press.

Wirth, J. H., Sacco, D. F., Hugenberg, K., & Williams, K. D. (2010). Eye gaze as relational evaluation: Averted eye gaze leads to feelings of ostracism and relational devaluation. *Personality and Social Psychology Bulletin, 36,* 869–882.

Wirth, J. H., & Williams, K. D. (2009). "They don't like our kind": Consequences of being ostracized while possessing a group membership. *Group Processes and Intergroup Relations, 12,* 111–127.

Wortman, C. B., & Brehm, J. W. (1975). Responses to uncontrollable outcomes: An integration of reactance theory and the learned helplessness model. In L. Berkowitz (Ed.), *Advances in experimental social psychology* (Vol. 8, pp. 277–336). San Diego, CA: Academic Press.

Zadro, L., Boland, C., & Richardson, R. (2006). How long does it last?: The persistence of the effects of ostracism in the socially anxious. *Journal of Experimental Social Psychology, 42,* 692–697.

Zadro, L., & Gonsalkorale, K. (2014). Sources of ostracism: The nature and consequences of excluding and ignoring others. *Current Directions in Psychological Science, 23,* 93–97.

Zadro, L., Williams, K. D., & Richardson, R. (2004). How low can you go?: Ostracism by a computer is sufficient to lower self-reported levels of belonging, control, self-esteem, and meaningful existence. *Journal of Experimental Social Psychology, 40,* 560–567.

CHAPTER 18

The Social Power of Emotions

Emerging Principles of the Social Functions and Effects of Emotional Expression

Gerben A. van Kleef

Scholarly interest in emotions dates back to the dawn of recorded civilization. Questions about the (dys)functionality of emotions infused the writings of Greek philosophers such as Plato and Aristotle, sparked the advent of the Stoics, and divided influential thinkers such as Descartes, Hume, Kant, and Nietzsche. Later, inquiries into the nature and purpose of emotions propelled the development of the scientific field of psychology (see James, 1884). Classic work on emotions in psychology revolved around the basic questions of where emotions come from and how they influence our thinking and action (Frijda, 1986; Lazarus, 1991). Over the past decades, this traditional focus has been complemented by a renascent conceptualization of emotions as regulators of social life (Keltner & Haidt, 1999; Parkinson, Fischer, & Manstead, 2005; Van Kleef, 2009), which finds its origins in Darwin's (1872) seminal work *The Expression of the Emotions in Man and Animals*. By now, a rich literature exists on the interpersonal functions and effects of emotions. These interpersonal functions and effects of emotions are the topic of this chapter.

What is meant by the word *emotion*? Formal definitions are elusive, but there is reasonable agreement about a number of key elements of emotions. Specifically, emotions arise as a result of an individual's conscious or unconscious evaluation or *appraisal* of some event as positively or negatively relevant to a particular concern or goal (Frijda, 1986; Lazarus, 1991); they involve specific patterns of phenomenological experience (Scherer & Tannenbaum, 1986), physiological reactions (Levenson, Ekman, & Friesen, 1990), and expressions (Ekman, 1993); and they are accompanied by a sense of action readiness (Frijda, 1986), in that they prepare the body and the mind for behavioral responses aimed at dealing with the circumstances that elicited the emotion.

Emotions differ from moods in that they are directed toward a specific stimulus—be it a person, an object, or an event; moods lack such object-directedness (Parrott, 2001). Emotions are also typically more differentiated and of shorter duration, whereas moods tend to be more enduring and pervasive, if generally of lower intensity (Frijda, 1994). Furthermore, in contrast to diffuse moods, "discrete" emotions are associated with distinct patterns of subjective experience, physiology, expression, and action (Ekman, 1993; Levenson et al., 1990; Roseman, Wiest, & Swartz, 1994; Scherer & Tannenbaum, 1986). Emotions and moods are generally seen as belonging to the overarching category of *affect,* which denotes subjective feeling states that can range from specific and acute emotions (e.g., happiness, anger) to diffuse moods (e.g., cheerfulness, depression) to "sentiments" (e.g., likes and dislikes; Frijda, 1994). I use these terms accordingly in this chapter.

The chapter unfolds as follows. I begin by discussing prevailing theoretical perspectives on the social functions and effects of emotions. Using an evolutionary lens, I develop the idea that emotions have evolved, at least in part, because of the functions they fulfil in coordinating social interaction. Against this theoretical backdrop, I identify seven basic principles of the social effects of emotions, which I support and illustrate with theoretical arguments, as well as empirical findings. I conclude by offering an integrative summary and suggesting new directions for future research.

The Social Functions of Emotions: An Interpersonal Perspective

Inspired by Darwin's (1872) early thinking, scholars have increasingly embraced the notion that emotions are functional in that they help organisms adapt to ever-changing environments. Classic theorizing and research revolved around the individual-level functionality of emotions (Lazarus, 1991), emphasizing the role of emotions in channeling attention (Farb, Chapman, & Anderson, 2013), supporting physiological adaptation to environmental changes (Levenson et al., 1990), and preparing body and mind for adaptive action (Frijda, 1986). Although these traditional approaches offer a useful lens for understanding many intraindividual processes, they are ill-suited to explain fundamental *social* questions about emotion. Why can our emotions be perceived by others from our facial expressions, bodily postures, and vocal tone? Why do we often feel the urge to communicate our emotional experiences to other people? And how do such intentional or unintentional emotional expressions influence others? Addressing these questions requires a radically different, interpersonal perspective on emotion. Such a perspective is provided by emotions as social information (EASI) theory (Van Kleef, 2009, 2016).

EASI theory offers a comprehensive framework for understanding the interpersonal dynamics of emotions. The theory is rooted in social functional approaches to emotion, which acknowledge that emotions influence not only those who experience them but also those who perceive their expressions (Keltner & Haidt, 1999; Parkinson et al., 2005; Van Kleef, 2009). The fact that emotions tend to be expressed in one way or another—whether verbally or nonverbally, mildly or intensely, knowingly or unknowingly, deliberately or inadvertently— implies that one person's emotions may become known to others via such expressions. By attending to the emotions of others, people may glean useful information about how others appraise the situation they are in and how they feel about it (Van Kleef, 2016). Moreover, emotional expressions can provide insight into how individuals (wish to) relate to one another, which helps address problems of commitment and cooperation that are central to human ultrasociality (Frank, 1988). For instance, expressions of love and compassion signal relational commitment (Gonzaga, Keltner, Londahl, & Smith, 2001). Displays of embarrassment and shame appease dominant individuals and signal submissiveness (Keltner & Buswell, 1997). Expressions of pride regulate social hierarchies by signaling status (Lange & Crusius, 2015; Shariff & Tracy, 2009). Displays of anger serve to identify and rectify social problems and clarify boundaries for acceptable behavior (Averill, 1982; Fischer & Roseman, 2007). Expressions of guilt signal interpersonal concern (Baumeister, Stillwell, & Heatherton, 1994) and social sensitivity (Van Kleef, De Dreu, & Manstead, 2006). In other words, emotional expressions can help individuals find adaptive ways of relating to one another.

It seems plausible that emotional expressions have been selected for over the course of evolution because of not only their intrapersonal functions (e.g., wrinkling the nose in disgust might prevent potential contaminants from entering the lungs), but also the functions they fulfil in enabling coordinated action (e.g., the resultant display of disgust might signal the presence of potential contaminants to others). As an ultrasocial species, humans accomplish many tasks relevant to survival and reproduction (e.g., provision and distribution of resources, raising of offspring, protection against predators) in highly coordinated, close-proximity, face-to-face relationships and groups (Caporael, 1997). As group sizes increased over the course of evolution (Dunbar, 2004), a critical challenge in human adaptation became to navigate the myriad relationships involved in social life.

In the early stages of group life, our hominoid ancestors likely communicated without formal language. Given that the emotional systems of the human brain (e.g., the amygdala and other parts of the limbic system) evolved much earlier than the centers that are responsible for language and speech (which are located in the cortex), it stands to reason that emotional expressions and other nonverbal behaviors constituted the primary communication devices in preliterate times. In the absence of formal language, observable nonverbal behaviors—including facial, vocal, and postural expressions of emotion—provided useful clues to other people's motives and intentions (Fridlund, 1994), making such expressions especially vital for social coordination, survival, and reproduction (Dunbar, 2004; Tooby & Cosmides, 1990). Emotional expressiveness and the ability to decode the emotional displays of others may have assisted our ancestors in dealing with the complex social problems that were posed by the emergence of group life (Boone & Buck, 2003).

With later evolution came humans' unique mastery of language, which added an additional layer of sophistication to emotional expression (Oatley, 2004). Rather than supplanting the critical functions of nonverbal expressions, language has provided humans with complementary ways of expressing their emotions and navigating increasingly complex social realities. Although there are certainly situations in which it may be advantageous to hide one's emotions, the ability to express one's emotions to others in appropriate ways, whether nonverbally or verbally, still is key to well-adjusted social relations and general life success. For instance, children who more effectively convey distress to their caregivers are more likely to be nurtured, and parents who are better attuned to their children's suffering are more likely to intervene when needed, thereby increasing the likelihood of their offsprings' survival. Individuals

who display anger at appropriate times and in the appropriate manner are more likely to ward off enemies and to defend their interests, just as challengers who are better attuned to signs of anger in their counterparts are more likely to avoid potential lethal combat (Fridlund, 1994). People who express happiness in the right circumstances may develop better social networks, receive more social support, and lead more successful social lives (Lopes, Salovey, Côté, & Beers, 2005). In short, appropriate use of and responses to emotional expressions are vital to successful social adaptation, and these benefits derive in large part from the evolved social-signaling functions of emotional expressions.

At the heart of the various coordination problems posed by human social interdependence (see Rusbult & Van Lange, 2003) lies the challenge of inferring other people's states of mind. In many situations, people have limited insight into each other's feelings, goals, needs, desires, and intentions, which poses a significant challenge to adaptive social interaction. If one does not know what goes on in other people's minds, it is difficult to relate to them, anticipate their behavior, and determine an appropriate course of action. EASI theory postulates that individuals gain insight into each other's states of mind through their own relatively automatic affective reactions to others' emotional expressions and/ or via more deliberate inferential processing of the meaning and implications of others' emotional expressions (Van Kleef, 2009)—two fundamental notions to which I return below.

Theorizing about the social functions of emotions has sparked a fast-growing body of empirical work on the interpersonal consequences of emotional expressions. Moving beyond the traditional questions of where our emotions come from and how they influence our own thinking and behavior, work at the interpersonal level of analysis has begun to illuminate how one person's emotional expressions influence the feelings, thoughts, and actions of other individuals (for reviews, see Elfenbein, 2007; Niedenthal & Brauer, 2012; Van Kleef, 2016). This literature has now reached a stage where it is possible to formulate a number of basic principles that capture the social functions and effects of emotional expressions. These principles are summarized in Table 18.1.

TABLE 18.1. Basic Principles of the Social Functions and Effects of Emotional Expressions

Principle 1: The rudimentary mechanisms underlying the social-signaling functions of emotional expressions exhibit continuity across cultures, across stages of development, and across related species.

Principle 2: The social effects of emotional expressions are functionally equivalent across expressive modalities (i.e., face, voice, body, words, symbols).

Principle 3: The social functionality of an emotional expression hinges on successful encoding by the expresser and successful decoding by the perceiver.

Principle 4: Emotional expressions elicit affective reactions in observers, which have downstream consequences for cognition and behavior.

Principle 5: Emotional expressions elicit inferential processes in observers, which have downstream consequences for cognition and behavior.

Principle 6: The relative influence of inferential processes in shaping responses to emotional expressions increases to the degree that the observer engages in thorough information processing, whereas the influence of affective reactions increases to the degree that information processing is reduced.

Principle 7: The relative influence of affective reactions in shaping observers' responses to others' emotional expressions increases to the degree that observers perceive the emotional expressions as inappropriate, whereas the influence of inferential processes increases to the degree that emotional expressions are perceived as appropriate.

Theoretical Underpinning and Empirical Illustration of Basic Principles

The basic principles listed in Table 18.1 jointly capture robust patterns in the empirical science of the social dynamics of emotional expressions. They describe the continuity of the basic mechanisms underlying the social effects of emotions across cultures, stages of development, and primate species (Principle 1); the functional equivalence of the social effects of emotional expressions across expressive modalities (Principle 2); the critical importance of successful encoding and decoding of emotional expressions (Principle 3); the affective (Principle 4) and inferential (Principle 5) processes that emotional expressions may trigger in observers; and the moderating role of observers' information processing (Principle 6) and the perceived appropriateness of the emotional expression (Principle 7) in shaping the relative potency of affective and inferential processes in guiding observers' behavioral responses to others' emotional expressions. In conjunction with the theoretical arguments outlined here, these principles reflect the current state of the science with regard to the interpersonal effects of emotional expressions.

Continuity of the Rudimentary Mechanisms of Emotional Communication

EASI theory maintains that emotional expressions have evolved in part because of their critical role in coordinating social interaction, and that over evolutionary history they have become hardwired systems of communication (Van Kleef, 2016). The areas in the brain that are responsible for generating and processing emotions are evolutionarily old. Rudimentary emotional processes that facilitate communication are therefore likely to have evolved before early humans started to migrate across the globe and develop unique cultural practices and modes of communication. If so, there should be appreciable overlap in the ways in which humans across cultures express their emotions and perceive others' emotional expressions. In other words, one would expect to see a degree of *cross-cultural continuity* in patterns of emotional communication. Furthermore, if patterns of emotional communication have been selected for over the course of evolutionary history due to their functionality in coordinating social exchange, one would expect to see evidence of emotional communication in infants. Although the finesses of emotional communication are developed and perfected across the lifespan through learning and socialization, the evolutionary argument implies that rudimentary building blocks enabling such emotional communication are present at birth, suggesting a degree of *ontological continuity*. Finally, given that brain regions involved in emotional processes are evolutionarily older than *Homo sapiens*, one may expect to see evidence of basic emotional communication in related species that branched off from the same evolutionary ancestors as humans, which would suggest a degree of *phylogenetic continuity*. I summarize evidence for these three interrelated tenets in turn.

Cross-Cultural Continuity

The question of universality versus cultural specificity of emotional communication is among the most contentious issues in affective science. Some have argued that displays of basic emotions are well recognized across cultures that have had little or no exposure to one another, pointing to universals in emotional expression and recognition (e.g., Ekman et al., 1987). Others have claimed, in contrast, that emotional expressions are shaped by cultural norms and socialization (e.g., Lutz & White, 1986). After decades of fierce debate, a growing group of scholars nowadays take an intermediate position, suggesting that the facial expression and recognition of emotions is characterized by a combination of fundamental universals and cultural dialects (e.g., Elfenbein & Ambady, 2003; Scherer & Wallbott, 1994). Recent work indicates, furthermore, that members of different cultural groups may vary in the degree to which they perceive one specific emotion or a combination of related emotions in a particular facial expression, although they tend to agree about the "primary" emotion that is conveyed by a particular expression (Fang, Sauter, & Van Kleef, 2018). In other words, despite variation across cultures in specific patterns of emotion perception, there is considerable consistency in the broader patterns of basic emotion perception. This is also true for the recognition and interpretation of vocal expressions of emotion, with evidence showing that vocalizations of "basic" emotions (e.g., anger, disgust, fear, joy, sadness) are recognized cross-culturally, whereas the recognition of "nonbasic" emotion

vocalizations (e.g., triumph, relief, sensual pleasure) is more culture-specific (Sauter, Eisner, Ekman, & Scott, 2010).

In short, cross-cultural studies of emotion expression and emotion recognition tend to reveal a combination of commonalities and differences in emotional patterns across cultures. Although scholars differ in the degree to which they interpret these mixed patterns as evidence for universality or cultural specificity, it seems fair to conclude that basic emotions such as joy/happiness, sadness, fear, anger, and disgust tend to be well recognized across cultural boundaries. Moreover, patterns of subjective experience (e.g., duration, intensity), physiological symptoms (e.g., arousal, temperature), and expressive tendencies (e.g., approach motivation; verbal, nonverbal, and paralinguistic expression) associated with these basic emotions are similar across cultures (Scherer & Wallbott, 1994). Such evidence is consistent with the possibility that basic emotional expressions have a biological basis that is shared by humans across cultures.

Ontogenetic Continuity

If emotional expressions have been selected for over the course of evolution because they afford adaptive benefits, one would expect the rudimentary mechanisms underlying this functionality to be observable early in the lifespan. Indeed, research shows that 4-month-old infants can already discriminate between facial expressions of emotions such as happiness and fear (Nelson, 1987). By 14 months of age, human babies understand that others' emotional expressions are directed at particular objects (Repacholi, 1998), and by age 18 months, they recognize that such emotional signals contain information about the expresser's desires vis-à-vis those objects (Repacholi & Gopnik, 1997). In other words, well before children can communicate using word-based language, they already have the ability to use others' emotional expressions as a source of information.

The potential adaptive value of this ability is illustrated by research on "social referencing" in infants. Classic studies on social referencing utilized a visual cliff, which consists of a glass-covered table that is divided into two halves: a shallow side under which a patterned surface is placed immediately beneath the glass plate, and a deep side under which a similar surface is visible at some distance below the glass (see, e.g., Sorce, Emde, Campos, & Klinnert, 1985). The critical manipulation in classic studies such as these involves a caregiver showing certain emotional expressions (e.g., happiness or fear) at the opposite side of the cliff. In one of the studies reported by Sorce and colleagues, none of the babies crossed the visual cliff when their caregiver looked fearful, whereas 74% of the babies crossed the cliff when the caregiver looked happy. Presumably the caregiver's emotional display signals that the environment is safe (happiness) or unsafe (fear), which informs the infant's behavior.

Later studies showed that human infants understand the referential content of others' emotional expressions and use this understanding to draw inferences about the expresser's preferences. In an illustrative study by Repacholi (1998), 14-month-old babies saw an adult open two boxes and show a facial display of happiness or disgust, depending on the content of the boxes. The infants were subsequently more likely to select the box that had elicited a happy expression from the adult than the box that had elicited a disgusted expression. In short, in keeping with the assumption that emotional expressions have been selected for because they facilitate social coordination, basic capabilities that are fundamental to social communication through emotional expressions can already be observed in infants.

Phylogenetic Continuity

Guided by Darwin's (1872) assumption of phylogenetic continuity of the emotion system—the idea that basic features of the emotion process are comparable across related species—a considerable body of research has documented similarities between human and nonhuman emotional expressions (Redican, 1982). Many human facial expressions appear to be rooted in ancestral primate communicative displays that are believed to serve a critical role in sustaining cooperative societies (Parr, Waller, & Fugate, 2005). Indeed, as in humans, basic patterns that support the functionality of emotional expressions can be observed in nonhuman primates living in social constellations. Various primate

species possess the ability to express and recognize basic emotions such as fear, anger, joy, and disgust (Parr, Hopkins, & de Waal, 1998). Moreover, apes, as well as certain types of monkeys, are capable of using other individuals' emotional expressions to gain information about these individuals' desires and to anticipate their behavior (Buttelmann, Call, & Tomasello, 2009), which helps them coordinate their mutual actions and solve (social) problems (de Waal, 2009). Early studies revealed that rhesus monkeys use the emotional expressions of their conspecifics to inform their own behavior (e.g., Mirsky, Miller, & Murphy, 1958). In some of these studies, monkeys witnessing expressions of fear in another monkey that anticipated an electrical shock quickly learned to switch a lever that eliminated the shock. Apparently, the monkeys used the emotional expression of the distressed individual to develop an understanding of what was happening and to determine what action was needed.

More recent work points to the remarkably sophisticated emotional understanding of chimpanzees, bonobos, gorillas, and orangutans. In one experiment, Buttelmann and colleagues (2009) found that apes used the experimenter's expressions of happiness versus disgust to inform their choices in a decision task. In this study, the experimenter reacted emotionally upon viewing the contents of two boxes, which were unknown to the subjects. The apes were subsequently more likely to pick the box to which the experimenter had reacted with a happy expression than the box to which the experimenter had reacted with an expression of disgust. These findings suggest that the apes inferred from the experimenter's emotional expressions how the experimenter felt about the contents of the various containers, which helped them decide which container to pick for themselves. Besides demonstrating that apes have the ability to use others' emotional expressions to inform their own behavior, these studies provide evidence for mutual recognition of emotional displays across species (also see Linnankoski, Laasko, & Leinonen, 1994, on the recognition of macaques' affective vocalizations by humans). Such findings suggest a degree of phylogenetic continuity in the expression of basic emotions, which is consistent with the possibility that basic emotional expressions have become hardwired over the course of evolution.

These three sets of evidence culminate in the first principle of the social functions and effects of emotional expressions:

> **Principle 1:** *The rudimentary mechanisms underlying the social-signaling functions of basic emotional expressions show considerable cross-cultural, ontogenetic, and phylogenetic continuity.*

Functional Equivalence of Emotions across Expressive Modalities

Building on the argument that emotions facilitate social interaction by providing relevant information to interaction partners, EASI theory posits that expressions of the same emotion that are emitted via different expressive modalities (i.e., in the face, through the voice, by means of bodily postures, with words, or via symbols [e.g., emoticons]) should in principle have comparable effects (Van Kleef, 2017). Obviously, the suitability of the various forms of emotional expression depends on the situation. For instance, facial expressions are likely to be generally more effective during face-to-face contact, vocal expressions during phone conversations, and verbal expressions during e-mail exchanges. Such obvious boundary conditions aside, however, EASI theory postulates that the social-signaling value of emotions is functionally equivalent across expressive modalities. The *magnitude* of the interpersonal effects of various forms of emotional expression may vary due to differences in the relative strength of expressions and the degree to which they are picked up by others, but the *direction* of the effects should be the same irrespective of the expressive channel, as long as the emotional expression is accurately perceived.

Research on the social effects of emotions has used a variety of procedures to manipulate emotional expressions, which makes it possible to evaluate the tenability of the functional equivalence hypothesis by comparing results across studies. Some studies relied on verbal expressions of emotion, which were often delivered in the context of (simulated) computer-mediated interactions (e.g., Adam, Shirako, & Maddux, 2010; Van Kleef, De Dreu, & Manstead, 2004a). Other studies used pictures of facial emotional expressions (e.g., Van Doorn, Heerdink, & Van Kleef, 2012) or film clips containing emotional expressions in face, voice, and/or posture (e.g., Hess & Blairy, 2001; Van Kleef et al., 2009). Still other studies utilized face-to-face paradigms, in which confederates were trained or naive participants were provoked to emit certain emotional expressions in interaction with another person (e.g., Barsade, 2002; Sinaceur & Tiedens, 2006; Sy, Côté, & Saavedra, 2005; Wang, Northcraft, & Van Kleef, 2012). Yet other research involved self-reports of emotions and/or perceptions or coding of emotional expressions as they arose in the context of ongoing social interactions (Averill, 1982; Fischer & Roseman, 2007). Finally, some reports contain a combination of studies that involved written emotion messages, emoticons, and pictures of facial displays; film clips containing facial, vocal, and postural expressions; and/or emotional expressions shown in face-to-face interaction (e.g., Heerdink, Van Kleef, Homan, & Fischer, 2013; Tiedens, 2001; Van Kleef, Van den Berg, & Heerdink, 2015).

Critically, all these different procedures have yielded highly consistent effects. For instance, in a persuasion context, expressions of happiness versus sadness had comparable effects on attitude formation and change regardless of whether the emotions were communicated in words, through facial expressions, or via a combination of facial, vocal, and postural cues (Van Kleef et al., 2015). Likewise, in a group decision-making setting, expressions of anger versus happiness had similar effects on conformity irrespective of whether the emotions were conveyed by means of words, emoticons, or a combination of facial, vocal, and bodily displays (Heerdink et al., 2013). When it comes to their interpersonal effects, it appears that different channels of emotional communication are functionally equivalent. This brings me to the second principle of the social dynamics of emotions:

> **Principle 2:** *The social-signaling function of emotional expressions is functionally equivalent across expressive modalities in*

that the direction (but not necessarily the magnitude) of the interpersonal effects of emotions is similar regardless of whether emotions are expressed in the face, through the voice, by means of bodily postures, and/or with words or symbols.

Encoding and Decoding of Emotions as Boundary Conditions of Social Functionality

A foundational assumption of EASI theory is that emotional expressions regulate social interaction. A general precondition for such functional effects is that the emotions a person experiences become known by others. This is not always the case. Felt emotions may not be expressed (e.g., because they are downregulated and suppressed; Gross, 1998), or the expressions may not be picked up by others. In other words, the social functions of emotions hinge on successful encoding (expression) and decoding (perception) of emotions.

Encoding: The Role of Emotional Expressivity

The first general precondition for any social effects of emotions to occur is that the emotion be expressed in one way or another, be it through facial expressions, tone of voice, bodily postures, written or spoken words, and/or use of symbols such as emoticons (cf. Principle 2). Even though people have a tendency to express the emotions they feel in one way or another, they do so in varying degrees. Emotional expressivity is guided in part by implicit or explicit norms and scripts that vary across situations (e.g., gender roles, organizational norms, cultural expectations; Ekman, 1993), an issue to which I return below in relation to the appropriateness of emotional expressions. In addition, emotional expressivity varies as a function of chronic individual differences (Kring, Smith, & Neale, 1994).

People who express their emotions in more outwardly visible ways logically provide more relevant information to others in their social environment than do individuals who suppress their emotional expressions. This implies that, *ceteris paribus*, people who interact with more emotionally expressive others should gain better insight into those others' needs, desires, goals, and intentions. Thus, people who interact with emotionally expressive others should be able to respond more appropriately to those others' needs and expectations, thereby contributing to smoother social interactions. In line with this argument, research has found that explicit instructions to suppress the expression of any felt emotions during face-to-face conversations increased stress, reduced rapport, and impeded friendship formation (Butler et al., 2003). Other work has linked parental emotional expressivity to children's socioemotional competence (Denham, Zoller, & Couchoud, 1994), social adjustment (Bronstein, Fitzgerald, Briones, Pieniadz, & D'Ari, 1993), and (particularly for positive emotions) the quality of parent–child relationships (Eisenberg, Cumberland, & Spinrad, 1998). In short, emotions can serve social communicative functions to the degree that they are expressed in observable ways.

Decoding: Emotional Intelligence and Emotion Perception Ability

The second general prerequisite for any social effects of emotions to occur is that the emotional expressions be perceived by one or more others. Although perhaps self-evident, this notion is important in relation to the presumed social functions of emotions. Theoretical perspectives on the social functions of emotions hinge on the assumption that people perceive one another's emotional states, yet individuals vary in their ability to accurately recognize and interpret others' emotional expressions. Besides various clinical conditions, such emotion perception ability is shaped by individual differences in *emotional intelligence,* "the ability to monitor one's own and others' feelings, to discriminate among them, and to use this information to guide one's thinking and action" (Salovey & Mayer, 1990, p. 189). Two aspects of emotional intelligence—perception and understanding— are particularly relevant to the decoding of emotional expressions.

Emotion perception ability involves the capacity to recognize emotions from others' facial, vocal, and postural expressions (Mayer, Salovey, & Caruso, 2004). Accurate perception of the emotions of other people is vital to adequate social responding. Indeed, studies have shown that the adequate decoding of emotional expressions is a significant predictor of relationship quality (Malouff, Schutte, & Thorsteinsson, 2014). Emotional understanding pertains to the comprehension and interpretation of one's own as well as others' emotions (Mayer et al., 2004). Understanding where other people's emotions come from, how they develop, and what their effects may be is equally vital to well-adjusted social relationships and general life success. For instance, research has shown that individuals who score higher on emotional understanding are more likely to emerge as leaders in groups (Côté, Lopes, Salovey, & Miners, 2010).

In summary, emotions can only be expected to bring about social consequences when they are both successfully encoded by the sender and successfully decoded by the receiver, as determined by the sender's expressive tendencies and the receiver's emotion perception and understanding. Thus, the expressive tendencies of the sender and the perceptive sensitivity of the receiver jointly determine the success of emotional communication. This points to a third principle of the social functions and effects of emotions:

Principle 3: *The informational value of emotions is more likely to be capitalized upon to the degree that emotions are (a) successfully encoded by the sender (as determined by the sender's emotional expressivity) and (b) successfully decoded by the receiver (as determined by the receiver's emotion perception and understanding abilities).*

Affective Processes Triggered in Observers by Others' Emotional Expressions

EASI theory postulates that emotional expressions can evoke in observers various types of affective reactions that may subsequently inform their behavior (Van Kleef, 2016). These affective reactions can take the form of *reciprocal* or *complementary* feeling states (Keltner & Haidt, 1999), as well as associated sentiments, such as likes or dislikes (Frijda, 1994). For instance, one person's displays of distress may evoke reciprocal feelings of distress and/ or complementary feelings of compassion in an observer (Batson, Fultz, & Schoenrade,

1987; Van Kleef et al., 2008), and these affective states may be accompanied by feelings of warmth and a desire to comfort the distressed person. Conversely, expressions of anger may inspire reciprocal anger and/or complementary fear in observers (Dimberg & Öhman, 1996), which may motivate fight versus flight responses, respectively. Affective reactions thus constitute a key mediating mechanism between the emotional expressions of one person and the (behavioral) responses of another.

The most extensively studied type of affective reaction to emotional expressions is *emotional contagion,* the tendency to "catch" other people's emotions (Hatfield, Cacioppo, & Rapson, 1994). So-called "primitive" emotional contagion occurs when individuals mimic others' nonverbal displays of emotion (e.g., facial, vocal, and postural expressions) and come to experience similar emotions via afferent feedback (i.e., physiological feedback from facial, vocal, and postural movements; Hatfield et al., 1994; Hawk, Fischer, & Van Kleef, 2012; Hess & Blairy, 2001; Neumann & Strack, 2000). Nonprimitive emotional contagion, in contrast, occurs via processes that do not require mimicry, such as classical conditioning and perspective taking (Hatfield et al., 1994). Although these nonprimitive forms of emotional contagion have received comparatively less research attention, there is accumulating evidence that emotional contagion can indeed occur even in the absence of face-to-face interaction and mimicry, for instance, through computer-mediated interaction (e.g., Cheshin, Rafaeli, & Bos, 2011; Friedman et al., 2004; Van Kleef et al., 2004a). As a result of these processes, individuals tend to catch others' emotions on a moment-to-moment basis, not only from their facial displays but also from vocal, postural, and verbal expressions. The resulting emotional similarity presumably facilitates reciprocal understanding, interpersonal rapport, and relationship building (Hatfield et al., 1994).

Besides the reciprocal emotional experiences that may come about via primitive or nonprimitive emotional contagion, emotional expressions can also arouse complementary emotional experiences in observers; that is, individuals may respond with particular patterns of emotional expressions and experiences that are different from those displayed by the expresser, yet match those expressions in terms of their meaning, function, and motivational implications. For instance, expressions of sadness and distress may elicit sympathy (Batson et al., 1987; Eisenberg, 2000) or compassion (Van Kleef et al., 2008) in observers, expressions of anger may elicit fear (Dimberg & Öhman, 1996), and expressions of disappointment may elicit guilt (Lelieveld, Van Dijk, Van Beest, & Van Kleef, 2013). Although research on complementary emotional reactions is relatively scarce, there is good evidence for the incidence and functionality of complementary emotional reactions.

For instance, building on the assumption that the intricate facial musculature of human and nonhuman primates has evolved to produce expressions that signal information about the expresser's emotional state and/or social intentions, Dimberg and Öhman (1996) argued that people should exhibit a tendency to spontaneously react with specific emotional responses to particular facial expressions to facilitate understanding, communication, and behavioral adjustment. Indeed, their research showed that angry faces evoke more fear in observers than happy faces—a finding that fits well with an evolutionary account of human emotional expression. People who are disposed to experience a certain degree of fear when confronted with others' expressions of anger may be more likely to avoid potentially dangerous encounters.

Another type of complementary emotional response that may be highly functional for social adaptation occurs when observers experience sympathy, concern, or compassion when confronted with the emotional suffering of another person (Batson et al., 1987). Several studies have shown that expressions of sadness, worry, and fear can elicit sympathetic emotions in observers, which in turn motivate supportive responses (e.g., Eisenberg et al., 1989). Such complementary emotional responses and concomitant behavioral tendencies can be highly functional for the quality of social relationships (Keltner & Haidt, 1999). For instance, research showed that strangers who were instructed to disclose episodes of emotional suffering felt more understood and appreciated, and expressed a greater desire to befriend their conversation partner, to the degree that the partner

showed more signs of compassion in response to their suffering (Van Kleef et al., 2008).

Finally, research in a variety of social psychological domains speaks to the idea that affective reactions mediate the effects of emotional expressions on observers' (behavioral) responses (e.g., Barsade, 2002; Friedman et al., 2004; Van Dijk, Van Kleef, Steinel, & Van Beest, 2008; Van Kleef et al., 2009). For instance, a seminal study by Barsade (2002) demonstrated that expressions of positive versus negative emotions by a confederate in a group decision-making task instilled similar emotions in the other group members, with contagion of positive emotions subsequently resulting in better group performance.

In summary, a person's affective reactions to the emotional expressions of another individual may afford insight into the expresser and the situation by facilitating the observer's understanding of the other's emotional state (Keltner & Haidt, 1999). Thus, individuals may gain information about other people by monitoring their own affective reactions to the emotions of others (Hatfield et al., 1994). Moreover, an observer's affective reactions to another person's emotional expressions may have downstream consequences for the observer's cognitions, attitudes, motivations, and actions vis-à-vis that person. This brings me to the fourth principle of the social functions and effects of emotions:

Principle 4: *Emotional expressions can elicit reciprocal and complementary affective reactions in observers, which in turn inform their behavior.*

Inferential Processes Triggered in Observers by Others' Emotional Expressions

EASI theory posits that observers can glean information from others' emotional expressions by drawing inferences about the antecedents, meaning, and implications of the emotion (Van Kleef, 2009). Because specific emotions arise in response to appraisals of specific situations (Frijda, 1986; Lazarus, 1991), observing a particular emotion in another person provides relatively differentiated information about how that person regards the situation. The implications of an emotional display vary as a function of the situation, but the basic informational value of discrete emotions generalizes across situations (Van Kleef, 2009). For instance, according to appraisal theories (e.g., Frijda, 1986; Smith, Haynes, Lazarus, & Pope, 1993), happiness arises when goals have been met (or good progress is being made toward attaining them) and expectations are positive; expressions of happiness therefore signal that the environment is appraised as favorable and benign. Anger arises when a person's goals are being frustrated and he or she blames someone else for it; expressions of anger therefore signal appraisals of goal blockage and other blame. Sadness arises when one faces irrevocable loss and experiences low coping potential; expressions of sadness therefore signal lack of control and helplessness. Guilt arises when a person feels that he or she has transgressed some social norm or moral imperative; expressions of guilt therefore signal that one is aware of (and possibly troubled by) one's misdemeanor (Van Kleef, De Dreu, & Manstead, 2010).

Because discrete emotions have such distinct appraisal patterns (Smith et al., 1993), they provide a wealth of information to observers (Hareli & Hess, 2010; Keltner & Haidt, 1999; Van Kleef, 2009). Besides informing observers about the expresser's appraisal of the situation (Manstead & Fischer, 2001), emotional expressions convey information about the expresser's current feelings (Ekman, 1993), his or her social intentions (Fridlund, 1994), and his or her orientation toward other people (Knutson, 1996). Individuals can therefore distill useful pieces of information from others' emotional expressions (Van Kleef, 2009). For instance, when one is the target of another's anger, one may infer that one did something wrong, and this inference may in turn inform one's behavior (e.g., apologizing, changing one's conduct). When confronted with another person's happiness, one may conclude that things are going well, which may lead one to stay the course. When confronted with another's sadness, one might infer that the other faces a loss and experiences low coping potential, which may lead one to offer help or consolation. And when one's partner shows guilt after a *faux pas*, one may infer that he or she cares about the relationship and is willing to make up for the transgression. In short, inferential processes

are a second key mediating mechanism between the emotional expressions of one person and the (behavioral) responses of another.

Numerous studies have documented the occurrence of such inferential processes, as well as their role in shaping responses to emotional expressions. Extending classic appraisal theories to the interpersonal domain, Scherer and Grandjean (2008) found that observers could reliably extract information from others' facial expressions about their emotions as well as their appraisals. Extending this basic notion to a social decision-making context, de Melo, Carnevale, Read, and Gratch (2014) found that participants interpreted a partner's expressions of happiness as a sign that a particular outcome was conducive to the expresser's goals, anger as a sign of goal obstruction and other blame, and regret as a sign of goal obstruction and self-blame. Such inferential processes can be functional, in that they help individuals make sense of ambiguous situations. A series of studies on the informational value of emotional expressions in ambiguous situations showed that expressions of regret fueled inferences that the expresser was responsible for an adverse situation, whereas expressions of anger fueled inferences that someone else was responsible (Van Doorn, Van Kleef, & Van der Pligt, 2015a).

People may also use others' emotional expressions to draw inferences about their dispositions. Knutson (1996) found in two experiments that perceivers inferred high degrees of dominance and affiliation from expressions of happiness, high degrees of dominance and low degrees of affiliation from expressions of anger and disgust, and low degrees of dominance from expressions of sadness and fear. Compatible findings were obtained in other research (e.g., Hareli & Hess, 2010; Hendriks & Vingerhoets, 2006). Recent work further revealed that inferences of traits such as dominance, affiliation, warmth, and competence are shaped more strongly by current emotional expressions than by preceding expressions (Fang, Van Kleef, & Sauter, 2018), suggesting that people flexibly update their inferences about others' dispositions in light of new emotional information.

Other research indicates that emotional expressions shape the construal of social situations in terms of cooperation versus competition. In a series of studies involving verbal as well as facial expressions, Van Doorn and colleagues (2012) demonstrated that a person's expressions of anger led participants to construe an anticipated interaction with that person as more competitive compared to expressions of happiness or disappointment, and to infer more cooperative intentions from expressions of happiness or disappointment compared to anger. Furthermore, more recent work indicated that people use emotional expressions to predict the trajectory of interactions between others (i.e., not involving themselves), with participants anticipating more cooperative interactions, greater interpersonal liking and trust, and less conflict when two people assigned to work together both showed happiness rather than sadness (Homan, Van Kleef, & Sanchez-Burks, 2016).

Finally, numerous studies indicate that the inferences people draw from others' emotional expressions influence their own behavior vis-à-vis those others. The nature of these behavioral effects logically depends heavily on the social context because different settings afford and require different types of behaviors. For instance, expressions of anger by a counterpart in the context of dyadic negotiation can trigger inferences of ambitious goals and toughness, which in turn motivate concession making when one is motivated to strike a deal (Sinaceur & Tiedens, 2006; Van Kleef et al., 2004b). Expressions of anger by group members in response to another member's deviant position in a group decision-making task can trigger inferences of impending exclusion from the group, which in turn motivate conformity among individuals who desire to remain in the group (Heerdink et al., 2013). Finally, expressions of anger by leaders in the context of a team task can elicit inferences of subpar performance (Sy et al., 2005), which in turn fuel greater effort when team members are motivated to think through the implications of the leader's anger (Van Kleef et al., 2009).

These theoretical considerations and empirical findings converge in the fifth principle of the social functions and effects of emotional expressions:

Principle 5: Emotional expressions can elicit inferential processes in observers pertaining to the expresser's appraisal of and orientation vis-à-vis the situation and the people involved, which in turn inform observers' behavior.

Processing the Meaning and Implications of Emotional Expressions

Building on the idea that emotional expressions provide information, EASI theory postulates that the interpersonal effects of emotional expressions depend on observers' information processing depth (Van Kleef, 2009). Classic dual-process models maintained that individuals assess situations and render judgments either by means of quick, effortless, and heuristic information processing or through more effortful, deliberate, and systematic processing (Chaiken & Trope, 1999; Petty & Cacioppo, 1986). More recent models departed from such categorical distinctions, conceptualizing shallow and deep information processing as points on a continuum rather than a dichotomy (Keren & Schul, 2009; Kruglanski & Gigerenzer, 2011). Thus, individuals may differ in the degree to which they are inclined to engage in shallow or deep processing. This notion has important implications for how individuals may process the emotional expressions of others. Affective reactions are more immediate than inferences, and they require less cognitive processing (Zajonc, 1980). This implies that affective reactions can occur even when individuals engage in relatively shallow information processing, as long as they register the emotional expression. Inferential processes, in contrast, require a greater degree of cognitive deliberation.

It follows that the predictive power of affective reactions relative to inferential processes should be greater to the degree that the observer of an emotional expression engages in shallower information processing. An observer in a relatively superficial information processing mode can still pick up the emotions of others because primitive emotional contagion is not mediated by conscious cognitive processes (Hatfield et al., 1994), and the resulting affective state may in turn influence the observer's cognition and behavior without the involvement of conscious computation (Forgas, 1995). The observer would be less likely to draw deliberate inferences from the other's emotional expressions, however, because this process requires conscious cognitive effort. By reverse logic, EASI theory posits that the relative predictive power of inferential processes increases to the extent that an observer engages in more thorough information processing (Van Kleef, 2009). This is not to say that affective reactions become irrelevant under conditions of deeper information processing; rather, the relative influence of affective reactions on an observer's (behavioral) responses decreases as the influence of inferential processes increases.

A pervasive insight in social cognition is that humans are "cognitive misers" who are motivated to employ their scarce mental resources as economically as possible (Fiske & Taylor, 1991). Given the abundance of social information people encounter on an everyday basis, and given that their cognitive resources are limited, people are inclined to navigate the social world by relying on mental shortcuts and heuristics (Tversky & Kahneman, 1974). Thorough information processing is effortful and cognitively taxing; therefore, individuals only engage in it when there is a good reason to do so and when the required cognitive resources can be mobilized. In other words, deep information processing requires both motivation and ability (Chaiken & Trope, 1999; Petty & Cacioppo, 1986).

Depth of information processing is influenced by an individual's epistemic motivation, that is, his or her willingness to expend effort to achieve a rich and accurate understanding of the world (Kruglanski, 1989). Individuals with higher epistemic motivation have a higher threshold of information sufficiency than individuals with lower epistemic motivation. As a consequence, people with higher epistemic motivation tend to engage in rather deliberate, systematic information search and processing before making judgments and decisions, whereas those with lower epistemic motivation are more likely to engage in shallower information processing (Kruglanski & Webster, 1996).

Epistemic motivation and associated perceptions of information sufficiency are partly rooted in personality. For instance, individuals with a higher need for cognition, lower need for cognitive closure, lower personal need for structure, and higher openness to experience have chronically higher epistemic motivation than their counterparts on the opposite poles of these scales, and as a result they engage in more deliberate information processing (De Dreu & Carnevale, 2003; Homan et al., 2008; Neuberg & Newsom, 1993; Van Kleef et al., 2009; Webster & Kruglanski, 1994). EASI theory posits that these individuals are more likely to reflect on other people's emotions, meaning that the effects of others' emotional expressions on their behavior are driven by deliberate inferential processes (as opposed to more automatic affective reactions) to a greater degree than is the case for individuals with lower levels of epistemic motivation (Van Kleef et al., 2010).

Epistemic motivation also varies as a function of the situation. For instance, epistemic motivation is increased when a task is perceived as attractive or personally involving, or when one is held accountable for one's judgments and decisions; conversely, epistemic motivation is undermined by factors such as mental fatigue and time pressure (for reviews, see De Dreu & Carnevale, 2003; Kruglanski & Webster, 1996). By influencing epistemic motivation, these factors influence the relative predictive strength of affective reactions and inferential processes, with inferential processes becoming progressively more influential as epistemic motivation increases (Van Kleef, 2016).

Besides motivation, a person's information processing depth logically depends on his or her ability to engage in effortful processing (Chaiken & Trope, 1999; Petty & Cacioppo, 1986). This ability is partly rooted in stable individual differences in general intelligence and working memory capacity (Conway et al., 2002). In addition, the ability to engage in systematic information processing is determined by momentary variations in (among other things) cognitive load and mental fatigue, which undermine people's processing capacity (Gilbert & Hixon, 1991). Under increasing cognitive load, working memory capacity is reduced (Engle, 2002). As a result, cognitive control and the ability to engage in systematic information processing are undermined (Lavie, Hirst, De Fockert, & Viding, 2004). Thus, individuals who are under high cognitive load should be less likely to engage in thorough processing of another person's emotional expressions, meaning that affective reactions to the other's emotions take on heightened importance in driving behavioral responses.

Support for the moderating role of information processing in shaping the relative potency of affective versus inferential processes in guiding behavioral responses to emotional expressions has begun to accumulate over the past decade. Evidence is provided by studies on the effects of emotional expressions in a variety of social settings (for a review, see Van Kleef, 2016). For instance, one study showed that team members with high epistemic motivation performed better under an angry rather than a happy leader because they inferred from the leader's anger that their previous performance was insufficient and they had to exert more effort; conversely, team members with low epistemic motivation performed better under a happy leader because they experienced positive emotions and developed a favorable impression of the leader, which helped them perform (Van Kleef et al., 2009). Studies have demonstrated such moderating effects of information processing as shaped by a variety of antecedents, ranging from dispositional characteristics, such as need for cognitive closure and personal need for structure, to situational factors, such as time pressure, cognitive load, power, and the security of one's position in a group (see Van Kleef, 2016).

These theoretical arguments and empirical findings bring me to the sixth basic principle of the social functions and effects of emotional expressions:

Principle 6: *The relative influence of inferential processes (as compared with affective reactions) in shaping responses to emotional expressions becomes greater to the degree that the observer of the emotional expression is motivated and able to engage in deep information processing; the relative influence of affective reactions increases to the degree that information processing motivation or ability is reduced.*

The Perceived Appropriateness of Emotional Expressions

EASI theory postulates that emotional expressions can contribute to effective social coordination and well-adjusted relationships to the degree that the expressions are aligned with the social context; conversely, misalignment of emotional expressions with the social context can disrupt social coordination and undermine the quality of social relationships. Emotional expressions that are misaligned with prevailing normative expectations in a particular social context may be perceived as inappropriate. EASI theory holds that such perceptions of inappropriateness influence the relative predictive strength of inferential processes and affective reactions triggered by others' emotional expressions (Van Kleef, 2016).

The relative potency of affective and inferential processes in shaping responses to emotional expressions shifts due to the influence of the perceived (in)appropriateness of the expressions on inferential as well as affective processes. Research on expectancy violations has established that even though unanticipated events can trigger increased information processing, negative affective reactions to expectancy violations tend to be primary (Bartholow, Fabiani, Gratton, & Bettencourt, 2001). Moreover, emotional displays that are perceived as inappropriate for the situation tend to evoke negative emotions in perceivers (Bucy, 2000), and these negative emotions may impede deeper processing of the emotional displays. Thus, to the degree that emotional expressions are perceived as more inappropriate within a particular social context, they are less likely to be processed deeply and more likely to trigger negative affective reactions.

Norms and expectations with regard to emotional expression vary across cultures (Matsumoto, 1990). Accordingly, the perceived appropriateness of a particular emotional expression is shaped by the cultural context within which the expression is exhibited. For example, in individualistic cultures, expressions of anger tend to be relatively acceptable, whereas in collectivistic cultures, such expressions are perceived as highly inappropriate because they pose a threat to group harmony (Kitayama, Mesquita, & Karasawa, 2006). Such "display rules" also vary across organizational cultures. For instance, some organizations have explicit guidelines regarding emotional expressions (e.g., service with a smile), whereas others do not. To the degree that individuals within a particular cultural context value positive emotional expressions, displays of negative emotions may be perceived as more inappropriate and may have detrimental consequences because they elicit negative affective reactions. Thus, even though the basic mechanisms involved in emotional communication are similar across cultures (see Principle 1), the degree to which these mechanisms are engaged is subject to cultural differences related to the normativity of particular patterns of emotional expression.

The perceived appropriateness of emotional expressions also depends on their intensity and authenticity. For instance, according to Geddes and Callister's (2007) dual-threshold model of anger, overly intense expressions of anger backfire because they are perceived as inappropriate, which elicits negative responses. Recent work indicates that overly intense expressions of happiness and sadness are also perceived as inappropriate and are therefore more likely to have unfavorable consequences (Cheshin, Amit, & Van Kleef, 2018). Furthermore, emotional expressions may be perceived as inappropriate when they appear inauthentic (Rafaeli & Sutton, 1989). Inauthentic emotional expressions may be perceived as dishonest, unethical, or manipulative attempts to influence the target (Côté, Hideg, & Van Kleef, 2013), which in turn elicits negative affective reactions.

Personality factors also influence to what extent emotional expressions are perceived as appropriate. For instance, some people have a strong desire for social harmony (e.g., individuals who score high on Agreeableness; McCrae & Costa, 1987), whereas others have less of such a desire. Individuals with a strong desire for social harmony are more likely to perceive expressions of anger as inappropriate and to respond negatively to such expressions because they may create hostility and conflict and thus undermine social harmony (Graziano, Jensen-Campbell, & Hair, 1996).

Finally, the perceived appropriateness of emotional expressions depends on characteristics of the people involved that are unrelated to personality, such as status. People tend to accept more from high-status others than from low-status others (Porath, Overbeck, & Pearson, 2008); therefore, expressions of anger from low-status others are more likely to arouse negative affective reactions than expressions of anger from high-status others. Accordingly, recent research has demonstrated that lower-ranking individuals are less likely to directly express their anger than higher-ranking individuals, while the former are more likely to express their anger indirectly, for instance by gossiping with others (Petkanopoulou, Rodriguez-Bailon, Willis, & Van Kleef, 2019).

In short, there is now considerable evidence that emotional expressions that are perceived as inappropriate arouse negative affective reactions in observers. As a result, affective reactions become progressively more predictive of behavioral responses to others' emotional expressions (and inferential processes become correspondingly less predictive) as the perceived inappropriateness of the expressions increases (e.g., Adam et al., 2010; Van Doorn, Van Kleef, & Van der Pligt, 2015b; Van Kleef & Côté, 2007).

These arguments and findings point to the seventh and final principle of the social functions and effects of emotional expressions:

Principle 7: *The relative influence of negative affective reactions (as compared with inferential processes) in shaping observers' responses to others' emotional expressions increases to the degree that observers perceive the emotional expressions as inappropriate rather than appropriate; the relative influence of inferential processes increases to the degree that emotional expressions are perceived as appropriate.*

Summary and Concluding Remarks

The past decades have seen a social revolution in the study of emotions. Moving beyond the questions of what triggers emotions and how they affect the self, researchers have begun to investigate the interpersonal dynamics of emotions. By now, an accumulated, rich body of theoretical ideas and empirical findings highlights the fundamentally social constitution of emotions. I have distilled seven basic principles from this literature that govern the social functions and effects of emotional expressions. These principles, and the theorizing and research that underlies them, paint an integrative picture of the inherently social nature of emotion.

Prompted by the emerging challenges of living in groups, our humanoid ancestors developed patterns of emotional expression that allowed them to address various coordination problems before the advent of formal language. These basic patterns of emotional expression show considerable continuity across cultures, stages of development, and primate species. Over the course of evolution, facial, vocal, and postural modes of emotional expression were complemented with language and symbols. The effectiveness of these different expressive modalities varies with situational demands and affordances, but the social effects of emotional expressions are functionally equivalent across expressive modalities.

Effective emotional communication requires successful emotional encoding (by the expresser) and emotional decoding (by the perceiver). When effectively conveyed, emotional expressions can elicit affective reactions and/or inferential processes in observers, both of which can have downstream behavioral consequences. The relative influence of these two processes depends on observers' information processing and the perceived appropriateness of the emotional expressions, with inferential processes becoming progressively more potent to the degree that observers are motivated and able to engage in thorough information processing and perceive the emotional expression as appropriate, and affective reactions becoming more potent to the degree that observers are less motivated and/or able to engage in thorough information processing or perceive the emotional expression as inappropriate.

Although the current state of the science provides rich insight in the social functions and effects of emotional expressions, our understanding is limited by an excessive focus in the literature on short-term effects of emotional expressions in relatively contrived (laboratory) settings. The prevailing paradigms allow for careful experimental control and therefore high internal validity, but it remains to be seen how the social dynamics of emotional expression evolve over time in real social situations, in which one person's response to another's emotional expression becomes a new emotional

stimulus in itself, sparking a spiral of mutual influence. Going forward, the critical challenge for this field will be to develop and adopt more sophisticated research methodologies and statistical procedures that will allow researchers to track reciprocal emotional influences between people over time. Such work promises to paint an even richer picture of the social nature of emotion, and to further attest to the fundamental role of emotional expressions in coordinating social life.

REFERENCES

Adam, H., Shirako, A., & Maddux, W. W. (2010). Cultural variance in the interpersonal effects of anger in negotiations. *Psychological Science, 21,* 882–889.

Averill, J. R. (1982). *Anger and aggression.* New York: Springer.

Barsade, S. G. (2002). The ripple effect: Emotional contagion and its influence on group behavior. *Administrative Science Quarterly, 47,* 644–675.

Bartholow, B. D., Fabiani, M., Gratton, G., & Bettencourt, B. A. (2001). A psychophysiological examination of cognitive processing of and affective responses to social expectancy violations. *Psychological Science, 12,* 197–204.

Batson, C. D., Fultz, J., & Schoenrade, P. A. (1987). Distress and empathy: Two qualitatively distinct vicarious emotions with different motivational consequences. *Journal of Personality, 55,* 19–39.

Baumeister, R. F., Stillwell, A. M., & Heatherton, T. F. (1994). Guilt: An interpersonal approach. *Psychological Bulletin, 115,* 243–267.

Boone, R. T., & Buck, R. (2003). Emotional expressivity and trustworthiness: The role of nonverbal behavior in the evolution of cooperation. *Journal of Nonverbal Behavior, 27,* 163–182.

Bronstein, P., Fitzgerald, M., Briones, M., Pieniadz, J., & D'Ari, A. (1993). Family emotional expressiveness as a predictor of early adolescent social and psychological adjustment. *Journal of Early Adolescence, 13,* 448–471.

Bucy, E. P. (2000). Emotional and evaluative consequences of inappropriate leader displays. *Communication Research, 27,* 194–226.

Butler, E. A., Egloff, B., Wilhelm, F. H., Smith, N. C., Erickson, E. A., & Gross, J. J. (2003). The social consequences of expressive suppression. *Emotion, 3,* 48–67.

Buttelmann, D., Call, J., & Tomasello, M. (2009). Do great apes use emotional expressions to infer desires? *Developmental Science, 12,* 688–698.

Caporael, L. R. (1997). The evolution of truly so-cial cognition: The core configurations model. *Personality and Social Psychology Review, 1,* 276–298.

Chaiken, S., & Trope, Y. (Eds.). (1999). *Dual-process theories in social psychology.* New York: Guilford Press.

Cheshin, A., Amit, A., & Van Kleef, G. A. (2018). The interpersonal effects of emotion intensity in customer service: Perceived appropriateness and authenticity of attendants' emotional displays shape customer trust and satisfaction. *Organizational Behavior and Human Decision Processes, 144,* 97–111.

Cheshin, A., Rafaeli, A., & Bos, N. (2011). Anger and happiness in virtual teams: Emotional influences of text and behavior on others' affect in the absence of non-verbal cues. *Organizational Behavior and Human Decision Processes, 116,* 2–16.

Conway, A. R., Cowan, N., Bunting, M. F., Therriault, D. J., & Minkoff, S. R. (2002). A latent variable analysis of working memory capacity, short-term memory capacity, processing speed, and general fluid intelligence. *Intelligence, 30,* 163–183.

Côté, S., Hideg, I., & Van Kleef, G. A. (2013). The consequences of faking anger in negotiations. *Journal of Experimental Social Psychology, 49,* 453–463.

Côté, S., Lopes, P. N., Salovey, P., & Miners, C. T. (2010). Emotional intelligence and leadership emergence in small groups. *Leadership Quarterly, 21,* 496–508.

Darwin, C. (1872). *The expression of the emotions in man and animals* (3rd ed.). London: HarperCollins.

De Dreu, C. K. W., & Carnevale, P. J. (2003). Motivational bases of information processing and strategy in conflict and negotiation. *Advances in Experimental Social Psychology, 35,* 235–291.

de Melo, C. M., Carnevale, P. J., Read, S. J., & Gratch, J. (2014). Reading people's minds from emotion expressions in interdependent decision making. *Journal of Personality and Social Psychology, 106,* 73–88.

de Waal, F. B. M. (2009). *The age of empathy: Nature's lessons for a kinder society.* New York: Harmony Books.

Denham, S. A., Zoller, D., & Couchoud, E. A. (1994). Socialization of preschoolers' emotion understanding. *Developmental Psychology, 30,* 928–936.

Dimberg, U., & Öhman, A. (1996). Behold the wrath: Psychophysiological responses to facial stimuli. *Motivation and Emotion, 20,* 149–182.

Dunbar, R. I. M. (2004). *The human story: A new history of mankind's evolution.* London: Faber.

Eisenberg, N., Cumberland, A., & Spinrad, T. L. (1998). Parental socialization of emotion. *Psychological Inquiry, 9,* 241–273.

Eisenberg, N., Fabes, R. A., Miller, P. A., Fultz, J., Mathy, R. M., Shell, R., et al. (1989). The relations of sympathy and personal distress to prosocial behavior: A multimethod study. *Journal of Personality and Social Psychology, 57,* 55–66.

Ekman, P. (1993). Facial expression and emotion. *American Psychologist, 48,* 384–392.

Ekman, P., Friesen, W. V., O'Sullivan, M., Chan, A., Diacoyanni-Tarlatzis, I., Heider, K., et al. (1987). Universals and cultural differences in the judgements of facial expressions of emotion. *Journal of Personality and Social Psychology, 53,* 712–717.

Elfenbein, H. A. (2007). Emotion in organizations: A review and theoretical integration. *Academy of Management Annals, 1,* 315–386.

Elfenbein, H. A., & Ambady, N. (2003). Universals and cultural differences in recognizing emotions. *Current Directions in Psychological Science, 12,* 159–164.

Engle, R. W. (2002). Working memory capacity as executive attention. *Current Directions in Psychological Science, 11,* 19–23.

Fang, X., Sauter, D. A., & Van Kleef, G. A. (2018). Seeing mixed emotions: The specificity of emotion perception from static and dynamic facial expressions across cultures. *Journal of Cross-Cultural Psychology, 49,* 130–148.

Fang, X., Van Kleef, G. A., & Sauter, D. A. (2018). Person perception from changing emotional expressions: Primacy, recency, or averaging effect? *Cognition and Emotion, 32,* 1597–1610.

Farb, N. A., Chapman, H. A., & Anderson, A. K. (2013). Emotions: Form follows function. *Current Opinion in Neurobiology, 23,* 393–398.

Fischer, A. H., & Roseman, I. J. (2007). Beat them or ban them: The characteristics and social functions of anger and contempt. *Journal of Personality and Social Psychology, 93,* 103–115.

Fiske, S. T., & Taylor, S. E. (1991). *Social cognition* (2nd ed.). New York: McGraw-Hill.

Forgas, J. P. (1995). Mood and judgment: The affect infusion model (AIM). *Psychological Bulletin, 117,* 39–66.

Frank, R. H. (1988). *Passions within reason: The strategic role of the emotions.* New York: Norton.

Fridlund, A. J. (1994). *Human facial expression: An evolutionary view.* San Diego, CA: Academic Press.

Friedman, R., Anderson, C., Brett, J., Olekalns, M., Goates, N., & Lisco, C. C. (2004). The positive and negative effects of anger on dispute resolution: Evidence from electronically mediated disputes. *Journal of Applied Psychology, 89,* 369–376.

Frijda, N. H. (1986). *The emotions.* Cambridge, UK: Cambridge University Press.

Frijda, N. H. (1994). Varieties of affect: Emotions and episodes, moods, and sentiments. In P. Ekman & R. J. Davidson (Eds.), *The nature of emotion: Fundamental questions* (pp. 59–67). New York: Oxford University Press.

Geddes, D., & Callister, R. R. (2007). Crossing the line(s): A dual threshold model of anger in organizations. *Academy of Management Review, 32,* 721–746.

Gilbert, D. T., & Hixon, J. G. (1991). The trouble of thinking: Activation and application of stereotypic beliefs. *Journal of Personality and Social Psychology, 60,* 509–517.

Gonzaga, G. C., Keltner, D., Londahl, E. A., & Smith, M. D. (2001). Love and the commitment problem in romantic relationships and friendship. *Journal of Personality and Social Psychology, 81,* 247–262.

Graziano, W. G., Jensen-Campbell, L. A., & Hair, E. C. (1996). Perceiving interpersonal conflict and reacting to it: The case for agreeableness. *Journal of Personality and Social Psychology, 70,* 820–835.

Gross, J. J. (1998). The emerging field of emotion regulation: An integrative review. *Review of General Psychology, 2,* 271–299.

Hareli, S., & Hess, U. (2010). What emotional reactions can tell us about the nature of others: An appraisal perspective on person perception. *Cognition and Emotion, 24,* 128–140.

Hatfield, E., Cacioppo, J. T., & Rapson, R. L. (1994). *Emotional contagion.* New York: Cambridge University Press.

Hawk, S. T., Fischer, A. H., & Van Kleef, G. A. (2012). Face the noise: Embodied responses to nonverbal vocalizations of discrete emotions. *Journal of Personality and Social Psychology, 102,* 796–814.

Heerdink, M. W., Van Kleef, G. A., Homan, A. C., & Fischer, A. H. (2013). On the social influence of emotions in groups: Interpersonal effects of anger and happiness on conformity versus deviance. *Journal of Personality and Social Psychology, 105,* 262–284.

Hendriks, M. C., & Vingerhoets, A. J. (2006). Social messages of crying faces: Their influence on anticipated person perception, emotions and behavioural responses. *Cognition and Emotion, 20,* 878–886.

Hess, U., & Blairy, S. (2001). Facial mimicry and emotional contagion to dynamic emotional facial expressions and their influence on decoding accuracy. *International Journal of Psychophysiology, 40,* 129–141.

Homan, A. C., Hollenbeck, J. R., Humphrey, S. E., van Knippenberg, D., Ilgen, D. R., & Van Kleef, G. A. (2008). Facing differences with an open mind: Openness to experience, salience of intragroup differences, and performance of diverse work groups. *Academy of Management Journal, 51,* 1204–1222.

Homan, A. C., Van Kleef, G. A., & Sanchez-Burks, J. (2016). Team members' emotional displays as indicators of team functioning. *Cognition and Emotion, 30,* 134–149.

James, W. (1884). What is an emotion? *Mind, 9,* 188–205.

Keltner, D., & Buswell, B. N. (1997). Embarrassment: Its distinct form and appeasement functions. *Psychological Bulletin, 122,* 250–270.

Keltner, D., & Haidt, J. (1999). Social functions of emotions at four levels of analysis. *Cognition and Emotion, 13,* 505–521.

Keren, G., & Schul, Y. (2009). Two is not always better than one: A critical evaluation of two-system theories. *Perspectives on Psychological Science, 4,* 533–550.

Kitayama, S., Mesquita, B., & Karasawa, M. (2006). Cultural affordances and emotional experience: Socially engaging and disengaging emotions in Japan and the United States. *Journal of Personality and Social Psychology, 91,* 890–903.

Knutson, B. (1996). Facial expressions of emotion influence interpersonal trait inferences. *Journal of Nonverbal Behavior, 20,* 165–182.

Kring, A. M., Smith, D. A., & Neale, J. M. (1994). Individual differences in dispositional expressiveness: Development and validation of the emotional expressivity scale. *Journal of Personality and Social Psychology, 66,* 934–949.

Kruglanski, A. W. (1989). *Lay epistemics and human knowledge: Cognitive and motivational bases.* New York: Plenum Press.

Kruglanski, A. W., & Gigerenzer, G. (2011). Intuitive and deliberate judgments are based on common principles. *Psychological Review, 118,* 97–109.

Kruglanski, A. W., & Webster, D. M. (1996). Motivated closing of the mind: "Seizing" and "freezing." *Psychological Review, 103,* 263–283.

Lange, J., & Crusius, J. (2015). The tango of two deadly sins: The social–functional relation of envy and pride. *Journal of Personality and Social Psychology, 109,* 453–472.

Lavie, N., Hirst, A., De Fockert, J. W., & Viding, E. (2004). Load theory of selective attention and cognitive control. *Journal of Experimental Psychology: General, 133,* 339–354.

Lazarus, R. S. (1991). *Emotion and adaptation*. New York: Oxford University Press.

Lelieveld, G.-J., Van Dijk, E., Van Beest, I., & Van Kleef, G. A. (2013). Does communicating disappointment in negotiations help or hurt?: Solving an apparent inconsistency in the social-functional approach to emotions. *Journal of Personality and Social Psychology, 105,* 605–620.

Levenson, R. W., Ekman, P., & Friesen, W. V. (1990). Voluntary facial action generates emotion-specific autonomic nervous system activity. *Psychophysiology, 27,* 363–384.

Linnankoski, I., Laasko, M. L., & Leinonen, L. (1994). Recognition of emotions in macaque vocalizations by children and adults. *Language and Communication, 14,* 183–192.

Lopes, P. N., Salovey, P., Côté, S., & Beers, M. (2005). Emotion regulation abilities and the quality of social interaction. *Emotion, 5,* 113–118.

Lutz, C., & White, G. M. (1986). The anthropology of emotions. *Annual Review of Anthropology, 15,* 405–436.

Malouff, J. M., Schutte, N. S., & Thorsteinsson, E. B. (2014). Trait emotional intelligence and romantic relationship satisfaction: A meta-analysis. *American Journal of Family Therapy, 42,* 53–66.

Manstead, A. S. R., & Fischer, A. H. (2001). Social appraisal: The social world as object of and influence on appraisal processes. In K. R. Scherer, A. Schorr, & T. Johnstone (Eds.), *Appraisal processes in emotion: Theory, research, application* (pp. 221–232). New York: Oxford University Press.

Matsumoto, D. (1990). Cultural similarities and differences in display rules. *Motivation and Emotion, 14,* 195–214.

Mayer, J. D., Salovey, J., & Caruso, D. R. (2004). Emotional intelligence: Theory, findings, and implications. *Psychological Inquiry, 15,* 197–215.

McCrae, R. R., & Costa, P. T., Jr. (1987). Validation of the five-factor model of personality across instruments and observers. *Journal of Personality and Social Psychology, 52,* 81–90.

Mirsky, I. A., Miller, R. E., & Murphy, J. V. (1958). The communication of affect in rhesus monkeys: I. An experimental method. *Journal of the American Psychoanalytic Association, 6,* 433–441.

Nelson, C. A. (1987). The recognition of facial expressions in the first two years of life: Mechanisms of development. *Child Development, 58,* 889–909.

Neuberg, S. L., & Newsom, J. T. (1993). Personal need for structure: Individual differences in the desire for simpler structure. *Journal of Personality and Social Psychology, 65,* 113–131.

Neumann, R., & Strack, F. (2000). "Mood contagion": The automatic transfer of mood between persons. *Journal of Personality and Social Psychology, 79,* 211–223.

Niedenthal, P. M., & Brauer, M. (2012). Social functionality of human emotion. *Annual Review of Psychology, 63,* 259–285.

Oatley, K. (2004). *Emotions: A brief history*. Malden, MA: Blackwell.

Parkinson, B., Fischer, A. H., & Manstead, A. S. R. (2005). *Emotion in social relations: Cultural, group, and interpersonal processes*. New York: Psychology Press.

Parr, L. A., Hopkins, W. D., & de Waal, F. B. M. (1998). The perception of facial expressions in chimpanzees, *Pan troglodytes*. *Evolution of Communication, 2,* 1–23.

Parr, L. A., Waller, B. M., & Fugate, J. (2005). Emotional communication in primates: Implications for neurobiology. *Current Opinion in Neurobiology, 15,* 716–720.

Parrott, W. G. (2001). Implications of dysfunctional emotions for understanding how emotions function. *Review of General Psychology, 5,* 180–186.

Petkanopoulou, K., Rodriguez-Bailon, R., Willis, G., & Van Kleef, G. A. (2019). Powerless people don't yell but tell: The effects of social power on direct and indirect expression of anger. *European Journal of Social Psychology, 49,* 533–547.

Petty, R. E., & Cacioppo, J. T. (1986). The elaboration likelihood model of persuasion. *Advances in Experimental Social Psychology, 19,* 123–205.

Porath, C. L., Overbeck, J. R., & Pearson, C. M. (2008). Picking up the gauntlet: How individuals respond to status challenges. *Journal of Applied Social Psychology, 38,* 1945–1980.

Rafaeli, A., & Sutton, R. I. (1989). The expression of emotion in organizational life. *Research in Organizational Behavior, 11,* 1–42.

Redican, W. K. (1982). An evolutionary perspective on human facial displays. In P. Ekman (Ed.), *Emotion in the human face* (2nd ed., pp. 212–280). Elmsford, NY: Pergamon Press.

Repacholi, B. M. (1998). Infants' use of attentional cues to identify the referent of another person's emotional expression. *Developmental Psychology, 34,* 1017–1025.

Repacholi, B. M., & Gopnik, A. (1997). Early reasoning about desires: Evidence from 14- and 18-month-olds. *Developmental Psychology, 33,* 12–21.

Roseman, I. J., Wiest, C., & Swartz, T. S. (1994). Phenomenology, behaviors, and goals differentiate discrete emotions. *Journal of Personality and Social Psychology, 67,* 206–221.

Rusbult, C. E., & Van Lange, P. A. (2003). Interdependence, interaction, and relationships. *Annual Review of Psychology, 54,* 351–375.

Salovey, P., & Mayer, J. D. (1990). Emotional intelligence. *Imagination, Cognition, and Personality, 9,* 185–211.

Sauter, D. A., Eisner, F., Ekman, P., & Scott, S. K. (2010). Cross-cultural recognition of basic emotions through nonverbal emotional vocalizations. *Proceedings of the National Academy of Sciences of the USA, 107,* 2408–2412.

Scherer, K., & Grandjean, D. (2008). Facial expressions allow inference of both emotions and their components. *Cognition and Emotion, 22,* 789–801.

Scherer, K. R., & Tannenbaum, P. H. (1986). Emotional experiences in everyday life: A survey approach. *Motivation and Emotion, 10,* 295–314.

Scherer, K. R., & Wallbott, H. G. (1994). Evidence for universality and cultural variation of differential emotion response patterning. *Journal of Personality and Social Psychology, 66,* 310–328.

Shariff, A. F., & Tracy, J. L. (2009). Knowing who's boss: Implicit perceptions of status from the nonverbal expression of pride. *Emotion, 9,* 631–639.

Sinaceur, M., & Tiedens, L. Z. (2006). Get mad and get more than even: When and why anger expression is effective in negotiations. *Journal of Experimental Social Psychology, 42,* 314–322.

Smith, C. A., Haynes, K. N., Lazarus, R. S., & Pope, L. K. (1993). In search of the "hot" cognitions: Attributions, appraisals, and their relation to emotion. *Journal of Personality and Social Psychology, 65,* 916–929.

Sorce, J. F., Emde, R. N., Campos, J., & Klinnert, M. D. (1985). Maternal emotional signaling: Its effect on the visual cliff behavior of 1 year olds. *Developmental Psychology, 21,* 195–200.

Sy, T., Côté, S., & Saavedra, R. (2005). The contagious leader: Impact of the leader's mood on the mood of group members, group affective tone, and group processes. *Journal of Applied Psychology, 90,* 295–305.

Tiedens, L. Z. (2001). Anger and advancement versus sadness and subjugation: The effect of negative emotion expressions on social status conferral. *Journal of Personality and Social Psychology, 80,* 86–94.

Tooby, J., & Cosmides, L. (1990). The past explains the present: Emotional adaptations and the structure of ancestral environments. *Ethology and Sociobiology, 11,* 375–424.

Tversky, A., & Kahneman, D. (1974). Judgment under uncertainty: Heuristics and biases. *Science, 185,* 1124–1131.

Van Dijk, E., Van Kleef, G. A., Steinel, W., & Van Beest, I. (2008). A social functional approach to emotions in bargaining: When communicating anger pays and when it backfires. *Journal of Personality and Social Psychology, 94,* 600–614.

Van Doorn, E. A., Heerdink, M. W., & Van Kleef, G. A. (2012). Emotion and the construal of social situations: Inferences of cooperation versus competition from expressions of anger, happiness, and disappointment. *Cognition and Emotion, 12,* 442–461.

Van Doorn, E. A., Van Kleef, G. A., & Van der Pligt, J. (2015a). Deriving meaning from others' emotions: Attribution, appraisal, and the use of emotions as social information. *Frontiers in Psychology, 6,* 1077.

Van Doorn, E. A., Van Kleef, G. A., & Van der Pligt, J. (2015b). How emotional expressions shape prosocial behavior: Interpersonal effects of anger and disappointment on compliance with requests. *Motivation and Emotion, 39,* 128–141.

Van Kleef, G. A. (2009). How emotions regulate social life: The emotions as social information (EASI) model. *Current Directions in Psychological Science, 18,* 184–188.

Van Kleef, G. A. (2016). *The interpersonal dynamics of emotion: Toward an integrative theory of emotions as social information.* Cambridge, UK: Cambridge University Press.

Van Kleef, G. A. (2017). The social effects of emotions are functionally equivalent across expressive modalities. *Psychological Inquiry, 28,* 211–216.

Van Kleef, G. A., & Côté, S. (2007). Expressing anger in conflict: When it helps and when it hurts. *Journal of Applied Psychology, 92,* 1557–1569.

Van Kleef, G. A., De Dreu, C. K. W., & Manstead, A. S. R. (2004a). The interpersonal effects of anger and happiness in negotiations. *Journal of Personality and Social Psychology, 86,* 57–76.

Van Kleef, G. A., De Dreu, C. K. W., & Manstead, A. S. R. (2004b). The interpersonal effects of emotions in negotiations: A motivated information processing approach. *Journal of Personality and Social Psychology, 87,* 510–528.

Van Kleef, G. A., De Dreu, C. K. W., & Manstead, A. S. R. (2006). Supplication and appeasement in conflict and negotiation: The interpersonal effects of disappointment, worry, guilt, and regret. *Journal of Personality and Social Psychology, 91,* 124–142.

Van Kleef, G. A., De Dreu, C. K. W., & Manstead, A. S. R. (2010). An interpersonal approach to emotion in social decision making: The emotions as social information model. *Advances in Experimental Social Psychology, 42,* 45–96.

Van Kleef, G. A., Homan, A. C., Beersma, B., Van Knippenberg, D., Van Knippenberg, B., & Damen, F. (2009). Searing sentiment or cold calculation?: The effects of leader emotional displays on team performance depend on follower epistemic motivation. *Academy of Management Journal, 52,* 562–580.

Van Kleef, G. A., Oveis, C., Van der Löwe, I., LuoKogan, A., Goetz, J., & Keltner, D. (2008). Power, distress, and compassion: Turning a blind eye to the suffering of others. *Psychological Science, 19,* 1315–1322.

Van Kleef, G. A., Van den Berg, H., & Heerdink, M. W. (2015). The persuasive power of emotions: Effects of emotional expressions on attitude formation and change. *Journal of Applied Psychology, 100,* 1124–1142.

Wang, L., Northcraft, G., & Van Kleef, G. A. (2012). Beyond negotiated outcomes: The hidden costs of anger expression in dyadic negotiation. *Organizational Behavior and Human Decision Processes, 119,* 54–63.

Webster, D. M., & Kruglanski, A. W. (1994). Individual differences in need for cognitive closure. *Journal of Personality and Social Psychology, 67,* 1049–1062.

Zajonc, R. B. (1980). Feeling and thinking: Preferences need no inferences. *American Psychologist, 35,* 151–175.

INTERGROUP LEVEL

CHAPTER 19

Intergroup Processes: Principles from an Evolutionary Perspective

David Pietraszewski

Groups are a daily part of our life. We may watch with horror a terrorist attack in some far-off land, done on behalf of one group against another. Or we may follow the trials and triumphs of our favorite political party or sports team every morning or evening. A world of only individual identities—in which there were no group identities—would be a strange and alien place.

Yet it is the things that are most familiar that are least understood. So it is with groups. One of the great surprises of 20th-century psychological research was that real, objective conflict is not necessary to elicit intergroup dynamics. For example, randomly assigning individuals to what could only be described loosely as belonging to the same group (on the basis of some experimental superficiality such as sharing an arbitrary judgment or button color) seemed to nevertheless produce the signature traces of *group-based favoritism*: the elicitation of more positive attitudes and giving directed toward members of the "ingroup" compared to the "outgroup" (Locksley, Ortiz, & Hepburn, 1980; Tajfel, 1970). A number of theories at the time required groups to be situated in real conflict with one another in order to elicit such effects (realistic conflict theory and its variants;

Campbell, 1965; Levine & Campbell, 1972). These and other results—from Sherif, Harvey, White, Hood, and Sherif's (1961) Robber's Cave studies to the Asch (1951) conformity study, to Tajfel's (1970) previously mentioned minimal group paradigm—suggested that the psychology of group relations was bringing more to the table than just reacting to the objective state of the world. Rather, there were motivations and values at play; groups were being created from nothing within the lab (Tajfel, 1982; Tajfel & Turner, 1979, 1986; Turner, Hogg, Oakes, Reicher, & Wetherell, 1987).

Where does this psychology come from? Can we understand it well enough to predict what it will do and describe how it works? These are fundamental questions that lie at the heart of social psychology. Indeed, part of coming to terms with the social, emotional, and physical wreckage of the Second World War involved studying the psychology of groups and group processes more seriously and in a more sustained way than it had before. Half a century later, the social psychology of groups is still a vibrant and ongoing enterprise, collecting ever more data and findings (e.g., Brown, 2000; Forsyth, 2014/2019; Macrae, Stangor, & Hewstone, 1996; Miller & Davidson-Podgorny, 1987; Sedikides, Schopler, & Insko, 1998; Tropp, 2012). Yet for all of this attention, it has been notoriously difficult to resolve these most pressing questions of why social groups exist in the first place, and how the psychology works at a precise level—that is, beyond a level that is a redescription of the phenomenon. For example, the following quotes are representative of the kinds of explanations and definitions of group phenomena that one can currently find in the literature:

"We tend to like members of our own ingroup."
"A group is two or more individuals who perceive themselves to be members of the same social category."
"A group exists when two or more people define themselves as members of it, and when its existence is recognized by at least one other."

The tension revealed by these quotes is the same tension that played out in theories of intergroup relations in the 20th century: that there is more to group psychology than just outward, objective circumstances. Yet, if we exclusively appeal to these internal states and motivations, we sometimes run the risk of becoming vacuous and tautological. For example, that we tend to like members of our ingroup cannot be used to explain why we tend to like members of our ingroup. And what is an ingroup besides the people we tend to like? Likewise, what are people perceiving when they perceive a social category? And what exactly is being recognized by at least one other? In other words, the psychological perception of a "group" becomes tautological if it becomes both the thing to be explained and the explanation. These issues remain unresolved (see, e.g., Allport, 1954/1958; Brown, 2000; Forsyth, 2014/2019; Lewin, 1948; McGrath, 1984; Shaw, 1981).

How, then, do we study these internal states and motivations? On most social psychological approaches, the phenomenon of groups and social identities is taken as the starting point of inquiry. Then one attempts to infer the underlying psychology that causes the phenomenon (e.g., Yzerbyt, Judd, & Corneille, 2004). This psychology is typically characterized as a process that the person uses—such as categoriza-

tion or perception (e.g., Brewer & Hewstone, 2004; Macrae & Bodenhausen, 2000), or as a value or motivation (e.g., Abrams & Hogg, 1999; Riek, Mania, & Gaertner, 2006), or both (e.g., Leonardelli & Toh, 2015). The body of knowledge produced by this approach is now vast. However, there are limits to how deeply and precisely we can understand the underlying psychology with any one approach. So, to go beyond our current body of knowledge, we will have to incorporate additional, complementary approaches to the study of groups and group relationships.

Here, we consider an evolutionary approach to intergroup relations, examine the underlying principles and worldview of this approach, and see how its use has led to a number of important insights and discoveries related to intergroup relations. Fundamentally, science should transform the way we think about everyday experiences. And a science of intergroup relations should transform the way we think about groups and their relations. We see how an evolutionary approach begins to move us in this direction.

The Principles and Worldview of an Evolutionary Approach

It is obvious that adopting an evolutionary approach involves incorporating Darwin's insight that differential reproductive success over multiple generations (i.e., natural selection) is what causes all manifestations of biological life. (For examples applied to sociality, see Axelrod, 1984; Axelrod & Hamilton, 1981; Gardner, 2009; Grafen, 2007; Hardy & Briffa, 2013; West, Griffin, & Gardner, 2007a, 2007b.) What is less obvious is how natural selection forces us to think differently about human psychology. In particular:

When adopting an evolutionary approach, human psychology is conceptualized as being composed exclusively of mechanisms.

Mechanisms are entities that are defined according to their function (Bechtel, 2008; Cosmides & Tooby, 1987). And a *function* is a particular goal or outcome. For example, the goal of the digestive system is to extract nutrients from food. So when adopting an evolutionary approach, the mind is conceptualized as being exclusively composed of mechanisms executing functions. Any intentional language (i.e., appealing to an internal thinker who has desires, thoughts, feelings, beliefs, and so on) is not allowed, but must rather be translated into this language of mechanisms (Smith & Winterhalder, 1992; Tooby & Cosmides, 1992, 2015).

This way of thinking is what the philosopher Dan Dennett (1987) has called adopting the *design stance,* which means that one is treating an entity (in this case, a person) as an artifact, and asking what functions or purposes are contained within it (in the same way we might ask what mechanisms-executing-functions exist within a car or a robot). Adopting the design stance contrasts with the typical approach to social psychology, the *intentional stance*—in which one views the mind as containing an agency that has thoughts, feelings, and beliefs, pursues desires, and so on. Fundamentally then, adopting the design stance is akin to treating humans as if they are robots designed by evolution. Such an approach may sound odd or alienating, but it is important because it allows us to constrain the way that we think about the mind in a useful way. In particular:

The mechanisms that make up the mind have to have evolved in response to those features of the world that were present over evolutionary time.

Mechanisms work by being sensitive to certain classes of inputs (i.e., all mechanisms can be described in terms of inputs and outputs; Cosmides & Tooby, 1987; Pietraszewski, 2020). For the mechanisms that make up the mind, these inputs are informational, and can be thought of as detecting a particular situation or circumstance based on cues (e.g., "Is there a face in front of me?"; "Am I sick?"). Because of the way evolution works, we can stipulate that mechanisms only exist because they are built by natural selection (the only other alternative is magic). This in turn means that mechanisms are *for* features of the environment that occur over evolutionary time. For example, we are allowed to assume that there is a mechanism in

the mind for identifying one's mother because identifying one's mother is a recurring feature of the world over evolutionary time. In contrast, we are not allowed to assume that there are mechanisms *for* dealing with evolutionary novelties such as electronic lighting, artificial sweeteners, automobiles, and so on.

We will see how identifying what a mechanism is for can have profound empirical implications. But for now, it is also important because of the next principle:

What mechanisms are for is differential reproductive success.

This means that mechanisms can only exist if they have some influence, however distally, on survival and reproduction. That is, we are forced to only postulate the existence of mechanisms that may help the body in which they resides to survive, reproduce, and invest in the next generation—all, on average, over evolutionary time. For example, we are not allowed to stipulate that there is a mechanism for identifying one's mother unless there is some reason why doing so would have some causal influence on survival and reproduction (and, in fact, there are several reasons why this would be so; e.g., Bowlby, 1969/1999; Lieberman, Tooby, & Cosmides, 2007).

A corollary of this principle comprises the fourth and final principle:

Emotions, intrinsic motivations, and values must all be translated into evolutionarily recurrent costs and benefits.

This means that we are not allowed to use internal subjective states as explanations for a phenomenon. For example, it may entirely reasonable on some approaches to explain why children run to their mothers by saying that it makes them feel better. But on an evolutionary account, we are not allowed to stop there. We must in turn ask, why does it make them feel better? And some causal account must be provided as to why proximity to a caregiver is positively valued (that an evolutionary approach requires such an account is the source of attachment theory and its subsequent findings;

Bowlby, 1969/1999; Cassidy & Shaver, 2002). Analogously, we are not allowed to explain why people eat sweets by appealing to the fact that sweets taste good. Rather, we must provide an account of causal interactions out the world over evolutionary time for why sweets taste good. Providing such a causal account sometimes simply provides a deeper causal explanation (e.g., that sweetness cued nutritional value over evolutionary time within a foraging ecology). But in many cases, it also provides unique insights and predictions (e.g., that sweetness perception activates subsequent digestion processes; that sweetness perception may not cue nutritional value for evolutionarily novel substances; that the body is designed to best digest the sugars present over evolutionary time, and so on; see also Scott-Phillips, Dickins, & West, 2011).

For the remainder of the chapter, we look at specific examples of how these principles have allowed researchers to generate novel, testable predictions about the psychological mechanisms responsible for producing various intergroup phenomena. In the process, we are starting to make headway into answering the pressing questions of why social groups exist in the first place, and how the psychology works at a (more) precise level.

The Psychological Mechanisms That May Be Responsible for Producing Racial Categorization

This first example demonstrates the value of thinking about the evolved function of psychological mechanisms. In particular, it shows the benefits of thinking about what features would in principle have been present in the world over evolutionary time. For decades, as soon as psychologists devised a way to study implicit social categorization, it was found that certain aspects (or dimensions) of people always elicited categorization in the minds of participants, even when these were not relevant to the social context. These were age, sex, and race (e.g., Hewstone, Hantzi, & Johnston, 1991; Stangor, Lynch, Duan, & Glass, 1992; Taylor, Fiske, Etcoff, & Ruderman, 1978). In contrast, most other aspects of people only became the basis of categorization when relevant to the situation at hand

(e.g., what they were wearing; Brewer, Weber, & Carini, 1995; Stangor et al., 1992; Weeks & Lupfer, 2004).

Subsequent work failed to find any experimental manipulation that could modify categorization by age, sex, or race—despite considerable efforts on the part of researchers to do so (Hamilton, Stroessner, & Driscoll, 1994; Messick & Mackie, 1989). For example, showing people discussing race relations versus some innocuous topic produced no difference in categorization by race (Brewer et al., 1995; Hewstone et al., 1991). Likewise, priming race, or priming a crosscutting dimension (e.g., sex) had no effect (e.g., Stangor et al., 1992).

Such results led researchers to construct taxonomies that would describe these results. Temporarily activated aspects became *momentarily accessible* dimensions. Those always used independent of context became *chronically accessible* dimensions (Blanz, 1999; Higgins, 1996; Oakes, 1987, 1994; Oakes, Turner, & Haslam, 1991). It was assumed then that all chronically accessible dimensions would behave in the same way across experimental contexts. And the goal of social categorization research became the enterprise of articulating how (e.g., one question was how chronically accessible categories would behave when crossed with one another; Midgal, Hewstone, & Mullen, 1998; Vescio, Hewstone, Crisp, & Rubin, 1999).

One nagging question that remained was why race, sex, and age were chronically activated dimensions of person perception. Previously, theorists had suggested that categorization occurs along inferentially rich dimensions (e.g., Rothbart & Taylor, 1992). But the details of *which* dimensions and *which* inferences had been left unspecified (Hamilton et al., 1994). While it was clear that race, sex, and age were important outside of the lab—and thus were activated when people stepped into the lab (e.g., Blanz, 1999; Oakes et al., 1991)—theories describing exactly why and for what purpose were not forthcoming.

Here, one can see both the benefits and the limits of a descriptive approach: We would never know about chronically accessible social categories without the approach. But it does not explain *why* chronic accessibility occurs. Asking such a why question is where an evolutionary approach becomes particularly useful because it provides a set of useful constraints for how to think about the purpose of mechanisms in the mind.

Thus, from an evolutionary perspective, these experimental results were not the end of the story, but rather, the beginning. Evolutionary psychologists began to consider what underlying information-processing mechanisms could be responsible for producing categorization by race, sex, and age (Cosmides, Tooby, & Kurzban, 2003: Kurzban, Tooby, & Cosmides, 2001; Pietraszewski, Cosmides, & Tooby, 2014). They deemed it possible that there could be mechanisms in the mind for sex and age. (*For* here means that age and sex differences would be a stable feature of the world over multiple generations of evolutionary time, and so could exert some influence on the structure of the mind's information processing. It does not mean that the stereotypes associated with age and sex are inevitable).

In contrast, a system for keeping track of race seemed less likely. Race is a social construct and does not correspond to ancestry from a global perspective; that is, the objective differences between people that we typically think of as belonging to a race reflect extremely recent physical adaptions to local climates, and these differences do not correlate globally with ancestry—which means that if you pluck any two people up at random from the earth and consider how similar they look to each other, this will not give you a very good idea about how recently-related they are (because different populations look similar to each other because they have been exposed to similar climates, rather than because they are more closely related; Feldman, Lewontin, & King, 2003; Graves, 2001).

More importantly, for there to be mechanisms in the mind *for* race would require that race be a stable feature of the environment over evolutionary time. But given the scale of ancestral travel, it would only be with modern transportation technology and high population densities that large-scale, systematic physical differences would be encountered among different populations of people. Thus, the kinds of physical differences that we think of as race would not likely have been present over evolutionary time. For example, recent estimates suggest that light

skin may have evolved only 7,000–10,000 years ago (Gibbons, 2007; Norton et al., 2007)—an eyeblink compared to the advent of anatomically modern (and psychologically modern) humans 200,000 years ago.

Thus, it seemed most likely that racial categorization would be caused by the operation of a mechanism with a different evolved function than for categorization by race per se. This way of thinking led to the hypothesis that racial categorization may be the product of mechanisms for detecting and keeping track of patterns of social affiliation out the world, or what has been called *coalitional psychology* (e.g., Harcourt & deWall, 1992).

Coalitional psychology may sound like group psychology, but it refers to something more specific: those multiagent dynamics that would have in principle have been (1) reliably present over evolutionary time and (2) had some influence, however distally, on survival and reproduction—meaning that we have to distinguish between *evolutionarily recurrent* and *evolutionarily novel* dynamics (because we are only allowed to posit mechanisms built *for* the former, but not for the latter). What are these dynamics? At the most basic and fundamental level, humans can either coordinate, cooperate, or compete with one another—and these relationships are found across all known cultures and times. Thus, at a fundamental level, the psychology of coalitions is the psychology that makes these kinds of relationships possible (constrained in its details according to the previously discussed evolutionary principles; for details of what this means in practice, see, e.g., Apicella & Silk, 2019; Pietraszewski, 2016a; West et al., 2007a).

How does coalitional psychology work? To put it plainly, in any social world, there will be relationships, and one fundamental challenge is then to be able to keep track of them as a way to predict others' behavior, and to guide one's own behavior (e.g., "Will this person help me or harm me?"). This means that coalitional psychology should "care" about patterns of coordination, cooperation, and competition, and take these as inputs (i.e., these patterns of interaction should be fundamental and most important). Also, it should keep track of who is in such a relationship with whom and use these representations to generate behavioral predictions, guide one's own behavior, and so on (Pietraszewski, 2013).

The notion that there should be mechanisms in the mind for executing these functions is highly plausible in an evolutionary approach: Both the aspect of the world (the social relationships) and the costs and benefits (predicting how people will behave) are highly plausible, unlike mechanisms for tracking race. The hypothesis, then, is that racial categorization occurs because of the operation of coalitional psychology operating in a modern environment: Participants grow up in a world in which particular physical features correlate with patterns of coordination, cooperation, and competition—such as how people treat one another, who interacts with whom, who lives near whom, and so on (Graves, 2001). Participants' coalitional psychologies pick up on these features as a way to predict how others will behave. And these are the physical features that we think of as race.

Because the function of coalitional psychology is to keep track of social relationships, and because social relationships can change, coalitional psychology should contain a particular set of design features (or attributes). In particular, it should not just be sensitive to cues that correlate with patterns of coordination, cooperation. It should also be adept at noticing changes in the validities of these cues. For example, suppose you have recently joined a gang and discover that people who dress in certain way tend to treat you in a particular way (that white hats are friendly, whereas red hats are foes). In such a world, hat color should become one of the things that you (or precisely, these mechanisms) keep track of when encountering a new person. Moreover, suppose that after some time (as happens in real gangs) the marker of gang membership changes. Now, how you tie your shoelaces (a real example) marks how others will treat you. This sort of switch in cue validities should be no problem for coalitional psychology: it should quickly pick up on the new cue (lace tying) and drop the now outdated one (hat color).

If coalitional psychology indeed underwrites racial categorization, then we can take the previous functional prediction and turn it into a testable prediction about the circumstances that should reduce or eliminate categorization by race: If participants were to see a social interaction in which race does not predict who is affiliated with whom (such that people of the same race belong to different groups and race does not correlate with group membership), then coalitional psychology should shift categorization away from race and onto the new patterns of group membership. Race in this case would be analogous to hat color—once relevant, but no longer.

In fact, this is exactly what has been found in an extensive series of studies (Pietraszewski, 2016b, 2018; Pietraszewski et al., 2014; Pietraszewski, Curry, Peterson, Cosmides, & Tooby, 2015). When participants are shown that race is uncorrelated with cooperation, competition, or coordination, categorization by race plummets to near zero. In contrast, the same manipulation has no effect on categorization by either age or sex.[1] That is, when race is crossed with social affiliation patterns, categorization goes down. However, when either sex or age is crossed with social affiliation patterns, there is no appreciable change in categorization. The selectivity of the reduction to race is important because it means that participants are not ignoring just any cross-cutting dimension. Rather, there seems to be something specific about the relationship between race and social affiliation patterns.

These results are important for a number of reasons. First, they imply that the reason the human mind categorizes people by their race is in order to predict their social affiliations (for converging evidence see, e.g., Bernstein, Young, & Hugenberg, 2007; Golkar & Olsson, 2017). Second, they show that the long-held assumption that all chronically accessible dimensions will behave in the same way across different contexts cannot be correct. In all cases, age, sex, and race were presented in the exact same experimental contexts. Yet race behaved very differently than the other two. This should not happen on many theories of social categorization. Third, these results also support the predictions of social dominance theory (Sidanius & Pratto, 1999), which posits that race is an arbitrary, fictive dimension of the social world, driven by social consensus rather than being a biological dimension such as age or sex. Social dominance theory is itself a product of integrating sociological, psychological, and evolutionary perspectives on intergroup relations.

Ecological Stereotypes about Race

The previously discussed work focuses on the initial process of categorization. But there is also a very large literature on the downstream consequences of categorization: the accumulation of stereotypes (information and evaluations related to these social categories; e.g., Blanz, 1999; Macrae et al., 1996). While vast and thorough, this literature has been largely descriptive. However, there is exciting new work addressing the underlying structure of stereotype content as well (Neuberg & Schaller, 2016; Neuberg & Sng, 2013; Sng, Williams, & Neuberg, 2017). This work grounds the stereotyping process in terms of underling functions that would have some cost–benefit logic over evolutionary time.

For example, one such project tests the hypothesis that racial stereotypes are driven by ecological stereotypes (Williams, Sng, & Neuberg, 2016). On this account, the psychological mechanisms responsible for making inferences about people based on their race are in fact only using race as a proxy for the home ecology of a person. The idea is that people who grow up and live within a harsh ecology—one that this unpredictable and low on resources—tend to adopt life strategies that are more impulsive and opportunistic compared to those ecologies that are less harsh. Because race (e.g., White vs. Black in North America) tends to correlate with the harshness of home ecology, race then becomes a basis of forming expectations about the kinds of life strategies that a person adopts. This is then argued to be the basis of the content of racial stereotypes. Indeed, a number of studies (e.g., Williams et al., 2016) now show that ecological information about a person can override racial information—that is, that ecological information trumps race when people are forming expectations about others.

For example, participants in one study were presented with target individuals who were depicted as either growing up in a poor, harsh, and unpredictable environment with few resources and prospects, or in a rich, comfortable, and predictable environment with an abundance of resources and prospects. The individuals were either White or Black. Participants were then asked to assess these individuals along a number of typically racialized stereotypes—evaluating how likely they would be sexually restricted, impulsive, given to opportunistic behavior, invested in their own education, and invested in their children. Results showed that the ecology the individual was from completely overrode any effects of the race of the individual on participants' judgments. That is, White targets from harsh environments were evaluated the same as Black targets from harsh environments. And Black targets from kind environments were evaluated the same as White targets from kind environments; that is, race seemed to be no longer driving judgments at all once the inferences that are typically filled in by race (in this case, ecology and life strategy) are provided by more direct cues.

Thus, in both this and the above categorization findings, the superficial category of race seems to be used as a proxy for some other underlying reason. And this reason seems to have little to do with race in and of itself. Rather, deeper, evolutionarily relevant dimensions of the social world are being tracked. As these results show, when we understand what these deeper dimensions are, we can modify how strongly race continues to be used.

The Minimal Group Paradigm and Bounded Generalized Reciprocity

This next example illustrates how one must translate emotions, intrinsic motivations, and values into evolutionarily recurrent costs and benefits. As mentioned in the introduction, one of the great surprises of 20th-century psychological research was that real, objective conflict was not necessary to elicit intergroup dynamics. For example, in Tajfel's minimal group paradigm, randomly assigning individuals to group membership seemed to nevertheless produce more positive attitudes and generosity to members of the "ingroup" and less to the "outgroup" (Locksley et al., 1980; Tajfel, 1970). This observation led to the creation of theories that appealed to the intrinsic value of social identities (some shared property or dimension within the immediate context), such as *social identity theory* and *self-categorization theory* (e.g., Tajfel & Turner, 1986; Turner et al., 1987).

However, from an evolutionary perspective, saying that people intrinsically value and respond to social identities (some mutually represented, shared feature) is the phenomenon to be explained. And the notion of why social identities matter in the lab should be explicable in terms of why they matter in the real world, and in the currency of costs and benefits over evolutionary time. In the real world over evolutionary time, one fundamental challenge is that people need to negotiate with one another to figure out with whom they want to coordinate and cooperate. They also have to figure out with whom others want to coordinate and cooperate. This requires solving the twin problems of (1) determining who will and who will not fall within the bounds of the relationship and (2) ensuring that everyone is coordinated about those bounds. That is, they must know that others know. These twin problems represent the coordination costs of creating a relationship. *Social identities* are solutions to these problems. They define the packets of coordination and cooperation, and provide common knowledge, thereby solving these coordination problems (see also Park & van Leeuwen, 2015; Smaldino, 2015, 2019).

From an evolutionary perspective, solving these problems is recurrent, with clear sets of costs and benefits over evolutionary time (Alexander, 1987). Thus, we are allowed to expect that there will be psychological mechanisms for solving these problems. One way forward, then, is to lay out the logic of how mechanisms would be expected to work if they can in fact actually solve them (this is called conducting an *evolutionary task analysis*; Pietraszewski, 2020; Tooby & Cosmides, 1992). We can then look at the minimal group paradigm findings through the lens of these likely-to-exist mechanisms.

On such an approach, the minimal group paradigm seems to provide a ready-made solution to a coordination problem. Thus, the situation may be framed as an opportunity to establish a mutually beneficial coordination or cooperation relationship. In other words, we should expect evolved mechanisms to take advantage of mutually represented similarities as an opportunity to probe for cooperative intent (Pietraszewski,

2013). Importantly, this means that the minimal group paradigm should not be driven by a blind, automatic response to the presence of possible social identities. Rather, the mind should be sophisticated and flexible, treating this situation as a testing of the waters—an initial proposal and chance to see if others also behave in the same way.

Indeed, the evolutionary scientist Toshio Yamagishi and colleagues showed that the minimal group effect is driven by participants who anticipate indirect reciprocity along the arbitrary dimension of similarity (Yamagishi, Jin, & Kiyonari, 1999; Yamagishi & Kiyonari, 2000; Yamagishi & Mifune, 2009). That is, if people are divided into X's and Y's, it is those participants who anticipate that other X's will give more to other X's that will also give more to other X's. This is true even if the particular X that they are giving to is not the X that gives to them (thus the "indirect" reciprocity; see Alexander, 1987). In other words, participants behaved in a particular way only when they expected that others would also behave in that same way (i.e., that everyone would coordinate).

What Yamagishi and colleagues found was that only a subset of participants allocated in a biased way to their minimal ingroup: those who anticipated this indirect reciprocity. Follow-up studies have more clearly established this expectation as the causal mechanism. For example, expecting an outgroup member to allocate to oneself greatly reduces or even eliminates the minimal group effect. Indeed, an extensive meta-analysis on decades of findings (Balliet, Wu, & De Dreu, 2014) found the following:

1. Individuals' expectations of indirect reciprocity explain much of the variance in ingroup versus outgroup favoritism.
2. Interdependence within the task substantially increases ingroup favoritism. That is, if the minimal ingroup can objectively provide more help, people cooperate with their minimal ingroup members more.
3. The assignment of common social identities (even without imposed interdependence in the task) is sufficient to elicit a small amount of ingroup bias. This is consistent with the interpretation of shared identities as an op-

portunity to signal intent to establish a relationship where none existed before.

4. The possibility of direct reciprocity between agents (rather than through social-identity-mediated indirect reciprocity) *decreases* ingroup favoritism. That is, if a participant is an *X* and knows that a *Y* can and will cooperate with them, there is much less ingroup favoritism.

5. Shared knowledge of group membership increases ingroup favoritism, whereas a lack of shared knowledge drastically reduces it—consistent with common knowledge being important.

6. Allocations directed toward ingroup members are higher than allocations to not only the outgroup but also to strangers. This suggests that indirect reciprocity does not require perceiving outsiders as threats or competitors (addressing the long-standing issue of whether ingroup love necessarily brings along with it outgroup hate; Brewer, 1999).

These findings suggest that the evolved mechanisms producing the minimal group effect are for dealing with coordination and cooperation opportunities. The way that these work is clearly not as simple as merely up-regulating positivity along any dimension of similarity (in contrast to the well-worn trope that "we tend to like similar others"). Rather, the mechanisms seem to be sensitive to real-time cues about how much a particular dimension of similarity is being used by others to behave discriminately. Or, if there are no such cues, the mechanism seems to probabilistically probe for receptivity in others.

As one would hope, these findings also hold outside of the lab. For example, Swiss army officers who had been randomly assigned to one of several different training platoons for 4 weeks were asked to make allocation and punishment decisions in a series of economic games (Goette, Huffman, & Meier, 2006). Consistent with the laboratory minimal group findings, the levels of cooperation within the games was higher among members of the same platoon compared to members of different platoons.

However, there was an interesting result found for punishment. When someone was directly exploited in the game, the participants would exploit them right back, regardless of their platoon membership. That is, participants were punishing anyone who hurt them within the game, regardless of their group membership. However, group membership became important again when coming to the aid of others. When a fellow platoon member was exploited, participants were more likely to punish that exploiter—that is, to provide third-party punishment—compared to when a nonplatoon member was being exploited.

This result is important because it shows that the cost–benefit calculus underlying the operation of these mechanisms is not simply attending to the payout structure of the game itself. Participants would be better off not performing third-party punishment within the strict confines of the game. However, out in the real world, in a real ecology, there can be conditions in which third-party punishment is favored, even from an evolutionary perspective. It is this issue we turn to next.

Acting on Behalf of the Group

The effect of platoon membership on third-party punishment brings up the issue of why mechanisms should care about how others are treated. For instance, why did the officers care enough to offer punishment themselves—even when it was not rational from the immediate perspective of the economic game? Again, on a nonevolutionary approach, we may simply say that people tend to care about fair treatment. (Although this does not explain why nonplatoon members were protected less, unless the notion is that fairness only matters for those similar to us. But then what determines which dimension of similarity will be important, and when?) However, on an evolutionary approach, we are not allowed to be satisfied with such an explanation.

Fundamentally, the structure (or function) of any evolved mechanism must be that it produces outcomes that would have led to the differential reproduction of that mechanism across multiple generations. In other words, the mechanism "cares" about its survival and reproduction into the next generation; it does not care about preserving the particular body that it finds at any one time indefinitely. (In fact, this is why we senesce; there is diminishing return for investing in the maintenance and upkeep of an individual body after that body invests in the next generation (Williams, 1957)— analogous to the consumer's dilemma of fixing an older piece of technology versus upgrading and buying new). This is important because it means that the level of selection—that is, the bookkeeping of what counts as "cost" or "benefit," or a "good" or "bad" outcome—is neither what happens to the individual, nor what happens to the groups to which that individual belongs, but rather to the existence of the mechanisms across individual bodies.[2]

But why is this important? On an ordinary approach to psychology, one might characterize how a person is behaving—rationally or irrationally, selfishly or generously, so on and so forth. But from an evolutionary perspective, these kinds of personal-attribute characterizations start to break down. That is, we cannot just think that natural selection will tend to produce selfish behavior, or that natural selection will tend to produce generous behavior because in both cases, the very notions of selfishness and generousness are based on intuitive (i.e., folk) standards of behavior, and these start to break down one we start to think from the mechanisms existing across bodies, cost–benefit perspective of natural selection.

For example, imagine two people stranded in a leaky rowboat in the middle of the ocean. Intuitively, it might seem rational or selfish to not help with either the rowing or the bailing, instead leaving it to one's boatmate. But if this were our policy, we would also sink into the ocean a few days later when our (understandably angry) boatmate collapses with exhaustion. As this example shows, we cannot just look at a single slice of time to determine what counts as a self-beneficial decision. Rather, we must consider the cumulative, lifetime effects of the decision policies—and it is exactly this kind of bookkeeping that natural selection uses when selecting between different mechanisms.

This principle of looking at longer-term effects has direct implications for the kinds of decisions we should expect to see, for example, produced by the mind's evolved mechanisms in cooperative interactions (e.g., Krasnow, Delton, Tooby, & Cosmides, 2013). And although this point may seem exceedingly simple, a large

amount of unnecessary confusion has been caused in the past by researchers misunderstanding this point (see West, Mouden, & Gardner, 2011).

The metaphor of individuals sitting in boats is also helpful for thinking about how evolved mechanisms should behave in the context of groups. If we extend the metaphor, boats are analogous to groups, and each individual will, within their lifetime, sit in many different boats, with different kinds (and numbers) of boatmates (e.g., some will be helpful, some exploitative, some healthy, some sick, and so on). The question then becomes, what kind of mechanism decision rules would be selected for given that each individual has to survive and thrive while existing in different groups/boats? One can't let one's boat sink, but within each boat, one can't be exploited by the other boatmates either (such that one gets sick or starves).

As this metaphor suggests, there will be times when the interest of all three entities—the mechanism sitting within the person, the person sitting within the boat, and the boat itself—all overlap, but in other cases, they may not. Returning to groups: In many cases, the interests of the mechanism and the individual will overlap with one another. And in some cases, the interests of the individual and the group as a whole overlap with one another (as we saw in the two boatmates example above). Thus, depending on the particular case, we can sometimes use a heuristic framework of thinking about what would be differentially beneficial to the group (i.e., what decision rules would keep the entire boat afloat?). And at other times, we can use what would be useful to the individual as a shorthand (e.g., one would want to ensure that one is not doing more work than others).

However, it is important to remember that these are shorthand heuristics. There will be cases where the interests of the mechanism and the group do not overlap. And, there will even be cases where the interests of the mechanism and the individual do not overlap (as we will see). In all of these cases, we are only allowed to expect that the interests of the mechanism will win out. That is, at the end of the day, what counts as a good decision rule is that the mechanisms within each individual have survived and thrived on average at least as well as, if not better than, alternative mechanisms within the entire population (where everyone else in the population is also sitting in a bunch of different groups or boats). The comparison is between everyone—not just between particular individuals in one particular boat, or just between all the individuals in one boat versus another. Thus, there is a strict and uniform criterion for what counts as a cost or a benefit—the survival of the mechanism compared to alternatives within the entire population. And the function of mechanisms (i.e., what the decision rules within mechanisms are built to produce) is to maximize the probability of benefits thus defined (for more details and other examples, see Axelrod, 1984; Axelrod & Hamilton, 1981; Barclay, 2013; Gardner, 2009; Grafen, 2007; Hardy & Briffa, 2013; West et al., 2007a, 2007b).

This way of thinking about costs and benefits provides us with a principled way to think about the kinds of outcomes that we should expect to see under different intergroup contexts and circumstances. For example, consider Figure 19.1, in which one agent, A, imposes a cost on B.

How should a mechanism residing in the starred third party evaluate A's attack on B (an attack that may either be social or physical, minor or major)? If mechanisms only care about harm, then it shouldn't matter why A did this to B; A's behavior should always be negatively evaluated and punished. However, if mechanisms function such that they "care" about themselves, then the reason why A hurt B should modify the evaluation and subsequent behavior produced.

For example, suppose B did something terrible to A just prior to this event. If we, the third party, did not also do something to A, then the mechanisms governing our perception and evaluation of that event should treat A's attack on B as a specific retaliation caused by B's previous action. That is, there is no basis for thinking that A will also attack us because we did not do anything to A. Thus, the mechanisms should not "care" about such an event.

In contrast, consider an alternative scenario in which A imposes a cost on B because B is perceived to be an instance of a category or social identity (e.g., in a gang). If we also belong to that same social identity, then this means that A would have also done the same to us. We just happened to be a little luckier today, and B less so. But tomorrow or the next day, we may not be so lucky. A (or another agent sharing A's stance toward our social identity) may do the same to us. In this case, mechanisms should treat this event as diagnosing a probabilistic future cost, and should produce outcomes in the world to re-

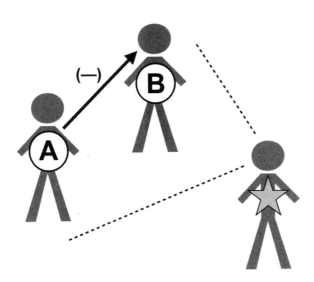

FIGURE 19.1. Two agents (A and B) considered from the perspective of a third (starred). A imposes a cost on B, denoted by arrow.

duce the probability of such future behaviors on the part of *A* or others (Pietraszewski, 2016a).

This is exactly what we see in the Swiss officers study. Officers see another officer of their same platoon being treated poorly by an officer of a different platoon. These officers (or precisely, the mechanism in the officers) infer that the poor treatment is based around platoon membership—an identity that they themselves share. Consequently, they may be treated the same way in the future. Consequently, there is a benefit to react against this event negatively, as seen in the study. Importantly, there is not a literal person inside the officer's mind or inside the mechanism thinking these things aloud. Rather, these context-sensitive contingencies are simply a result of the information-processing functions being executed.

This mechanism-level cost–benefit interpretation has been borne out in a number of studies. In particular, a substantial amount of converging evidence suggests that third-party punishment on behalf of fellow group members is mediated by inferences about how that observed behavior in turn predicts how the participant themselves will be treated (Delton & Krasnow, 2017).

The same result is also borne out in the real world. For example, there are different underlying cost–benefit dynamics to different kinds of intergroup conflict. Some conflicts, for example, are assessments of relative power and strength—scaled up versions of interpersonal posturing (Sell, 2011; Wrangham & Glowacki, 2012). In contrast, conflict with the explicit goal of incapacitation or lethality occurs under a much narrower set of circumstances. Studies of how soldiers behave in combat suggests that individual soldiers in most large-scale armies treat combat as ritualized assessments. Unless their rote training causes them to do otherwise, they often do not effectively kill enemy soldiers but rather posture toward them. It is only when direct known comrades are harmed that a desire for lethality is evoked (Grossman, 2009). These are exactly the kinds of situation-dependent contingencies that one would expect to see on this mechanism-level cost–benefit logic.

Indeed, the same underlying logic applies to decisions to join armies and fighting organizations in the first place. For example, in interviews with fighters, shared goals and experiences of conflict predict "fusion" or willingness to fight for real-world social identities (Whitehouse, McQuinn, Buhrmester, & Swann, 2014). That is, experiencing a social environment in which people "like me" are the targets of lethal aggression is what activates motivations to fight on behalf of that identity. Indeed, the same research group has shown in evolutionary models that sharing a fate or costs with others will produce concern about, and interest in fighting in, the conflict (Whitehouse et al., 2017).

Even something as apparently evolutionarily irrational as suicide on behalf of a group in fact behaves according to a similar logic (Blackwell, 2005, 2008). For example, most suicide bombers fall within a high-risk/high-reward social context in which they have few prospects; their friends, family, and so on, will gain much from their decision and the act itself is psychologically much more like going to combat rather than engaging in it—in that the destructive technology of the device removes the cues that would have over evolutionary time cued that the mechanisms within a mind that it was killing a large number of other people and that one was likely to die (such as in intimate physical combat). In other words, we can understand the technology used by those who send suicide bombers not just as a gruesome way to maximize death and destruction, but also a way to isolate the evolved mental mechanisms of the perpetrator from a decision to not follow through with their decision, as would more often be the case if such technologies were not used. (Indeed, the same logic applies to the training of soldiers; Grossman, 2009.)

This is not to say that mechanisms for dealing with life and death combat and raid situations (which are unfortunately evolutionarily recurrent situations; Wrangham & Glowacki, 2012) cannot at times produce decisions that lead toward death. Given that natural selection works across generations, and works on probabilities averaged across different individual bodies, something like an evolved decision rule that three-quarters of the time leads to death, but that one-quarter of the time leads to even higher benefits, could in principle be selected for within a population—which is a clear instance of mechanisms not "caring" about each particular body that they find themselves in (Tooby & Cosmides, 1988). Thus, even in such extreme cases of sacrifice on behalf of the group, mechanisms within the mind are not executing a dumb, inflexible allegiance to one's group or social identity—or even to one's own body. Rather, they are producing complex, context-dependent contingencies that follow an evolutionary, cost–benefit logic.

Groups and Morality

If all internal, subjective values must be translated into evolutionarily recurrent costs and benefits, why would evolved mechanisms be structured to care about a person with whom we have no relationship? Recall in Figure 19.1 that we shared a social identity with the victim. But what about the case when we do not? Consider A attacks B for no good reason. Even though we are not involved, mechanisms within us should "care" about such an unprovoked attack because this demonstrates that A is willing to impose costs on anyone, and anyone includes us. Consequently, we (or precisely, our mechanisms) should evaluate A's aggression negatively. In such a case, we may not respond as negatively in this case as when B shared a social identity with us, but we will still act more negatively than if A's attack was justified (Delton & Krasnow, 2017; DeScioli & Kurzban, 2009, 2013; Pietraszewski, 2016a).

And what of cases in which a group member or friend or ally does something morally wrong (where morally wrong means something that a disinterested third party would view negatively, for the above reason)? In this case, should the mechanisms take the side of the group member? In principle, while the answer may be "yes" under a range of circumstances, the answer may be "no" under others. In particular, the answer should be "no" when what was done by our group member would not be in our own long-term interest when weighed against the likely reaction from third parties. In such a situation, it would be ideal to cordon off the influence of the alliance and to side with the third parties. On particular theories, this is exactly why morality evolved: It is a set of information processing functions that allow us to forego the costs of siding with allies when they act in a way that runs against our own interests and the interests

of third parties (DeScioli & Kurzban, 2009, 2013). Thus, in this view, moral sentiments—the ability to take the side of what is right—are in fact a consequence of evolved information-processing mechanisms dealing with group dynamics over evolutionary time.

This view of moral sentiments suggests that morality is an important driver of social identities and a willingness to invest in causes. For example, moral outrage—the communication of what someone did to someone else—can serve as a coordination device for people to gang up against others (Tooby & Cosmides, 2010) and has been the tool of demagogues and tyrants throughout history (Lopez, 2019). Yet, at the same time, moral outrage is what drives the success of nonviolent resistance: If beatings, arrest, imprisonment, and torture occur in response to acts of nonviolent resistance, then we may view those committing this violence as unjust aggressors, and we will come to side with the victims for the reasons described above.

Flexibility in Relationships between "Ingroups" and "Outgroups"

An evolutionary perspective suggests that relationships between groups are not fixed or inevitable. Indeed, a mechanism that invariably produced antagonism toward outgroups would be ill-suited to handle the complex web of relationships that make up the real world (van den Berghe, 1999). Anthropologists who have looked beyond the walls of laboratory studies find a range of intergroup relationships between real-world groups (Barth, 1969; Brewer & Campbell, 1976; Hill et al., 2011; Moya & Boyd, 2015; Wertz & Moya, 2019). For example, groups defined by language differences are in some cases at odds with one another. But in other cases, they are a source of amicable trade and marriage prospects (Hill, 1978). Likewise, *ethnocentrism* (ingroup positivity) and *xenophobia* (outgroup negativity) do not correlate with each other across cultures and appear to have different determinants. In fact, groups with higher levels of xenophobia also tend to have higher levels of violence and conflict within their own group (Cashdan, 2001).

Furthermore, the relationships between groups do not seem to be capricious. Rather, it seems that people are evaluating the different groups in their environment in terms of what they might afford (Neuberg & Schaller, 2016), and these affordances in turn affect the nature of intergroup relationships. For example, in groups defined according to religion or ethnicity, one finds more generosity to outgroup strangers among individuals who lack local resources and who have some familiarity with members of the outgroup (Pisor & Gurven, 2016), suggesting that evolved mechanisms are searching for sources of mutually beneficial cooperation (a real-world analogue of the minimal group finding).

Expanding the "Us"

Finally, evolved mechanisms not only allow us to carve the social world into "us" versus "them," they also allow us to expand the "us." In particular, one important function of the mechanisms that evolved to deal with groups is to not only represent existing groups but to also generate new groups (Lopez, McDermott, & Petersen, 2001; Pietraszewski, 2020; Tooby & Cosmides, 2010). Expanding who belongs to the ingroup can in many cases be beneficial (for example, because of the benefits of trade and extended cooperation and foregoing the costs of conflict and dis-coordination). Thus, there is a cost–benefit logic for mechanisms to be structured such that they expand the "us" under the right circumstances—and to take the groupings handed to us from our parents, our society, and those around us with a grain of salt. Consequently, our capacity for seeing broader horizons of potential peace and prosperity is just as much a consequence of our evolved psychology as our capacity to fight against the tribe next door.

Looking Forward: Thinking Differently about Intergroup Relationships and How to Study Them

In summary, on an evolutionary approach,

- Human psychology is composed exclusively of mechanisms.
- These mechanisms are built around features present in the world over evolutionary time.

- What these mechanisms are for is *differential reproductive success* (the survival and reproduction of mechanisms, on average, as they exist across time and bodies in a population).
- Emotions, intrinsic motivations, and values must all be translated into evolutionarily recurrent costs and benefits.

We have seen how adopting these principles has allowed researchers to ask different kinds of questions and to generate new discoveries about social psychological phenomena (for additional reviews, see Kenrick, Maner, & Li, 2015; Neuberg & Schaller, 2016; Park & Hunt, 2018; Schaller, 2018; Schaller, Conway, & Peavy, 2010). However, we are still just in the very beginning phases of adopting this approach. And there is still much work to be done.

For example, we have yet to shift from accounting for known phenomena over to studying how evolved functions are actually carried out by mechanisms. An evolutionary approach to intergroup relations has thus far been largely occupied with explaining and understanding existing phenomena—such as racial categorization, discrimination and stereotyping, minimal group effects, and so on. However, in the process of investigating these phenomena, evolutionary researchers have been appealing to mechanisms whose function is execute basic functions—such as tracking patterns of cooperation and competition, predicting others' behaviors, probing for receptivity to coordination, and so on. But there is surprisingly little work into how these basic functions are actually carried out at the level of the mechanisms involved (i.e., at the level of what we have called *the design stance*).

For example, in the case of groups, we would expect to find the following functions within the mind:

- *Representation.* There should be mechanisms capable of representing and keeping track of patterns of coordination, cooperation, and competition. And because every agent will be engaged in many different relationships, each one will have to be assigned to multiple kinds of coordination, cooperation, and competition relationship representations.
- *Prediction and inference.* The point of tracking relationships is to anticipate specific be-

haviors and reactions. Thus, relationship representations are not static entities, but rather activate prediction and inference functions.

- *Motivation.* There must also be mechanisms for guiding and directing one's own motivations and behaviors. These are structured to navigate the costs and benefits presented by the social world and will be informed by the prior two functions.

We still know very little about these processes. And there are few explicit models of the kinds of representations and processes that could—even in principle—carry out these functions.

However, if we consider what these representations and processes might be, even in principle, then we can start to generate novel hypotheses about what we should expect to find within the mechanisms that make up mind. And at each step, one would use the principles listed above (for details of how to conduct such an analysis, see Tooby & Cosmides, 1992, pp. 73–74; for a recent example, see Pietraszewski, 2020). For example, one could ask what are the precise kinds of evolutionarily recurrent relationships that would need to be kept track of. (For recent examples of answers, see Balliet, Tybur, & van Lange, 2017; Pietraszewski, 2016a.) Likewise, one could ask what classes of behaviors and reactions from others would need to be predicted ahead of time, and what cues would likely be present in the environment—either over developmental or evolutionary time scales—that would afford making predictions about them. Asking these kinds of questions will provide us with unique insights as we continue to tackle the fundamental questions that lie at the heart of social psychology: Where does this psychology of groups come from? And can we understand it well enough to predict what it will do and describe how it works?

In sum, adopting an evolutionary approach will, in principle, allow us to resolve the long-standing tension (and discontinuity) between the outward, objective circumstances of group relationships and our subjective internal states and motivations surrounding them. On an evolutionary approach, our internal states and motivations were caused by the outward, objective circumstances of group relationships—but not of our current group relationships, but rather those that were reliability present over evo-

lutionary time. And these internal states and motivations are *for* producing mechanism-level differential reproductive success. Thus, the causal link between the external and internal nature of groups lies in our evolved history, a history that is being slowly uncovered.

ACKNOWLEDGMENTS

Mark Schaller, Oliver Sng, and Paul Van Lange kindly provided helpful feedback on previous versions of this chapter.

NOTES

1. Kurzban et al. (2001) are frequently cited as providing evidence of this hypothesis. However, in the fullness of time, we now know that there are a number of measurement and methodological issues with this paper, rendering it largely mute in terms of evidence (addressed in detail in Pietraszewski, 2019). However, even if that paper should no longer be considered a source of definitive evidence, it should still be considered (and cited as) the original source of this hypothesis.

2. A brief technical note: what replicates with fidelity are genes—the units of selection. But what *accumulates* over time, because of those genes, is the structure (or design) of mechanisms. So, when we talk about mechanisms "caring" about their survival and reproduction into the next generation, we are technically saying that the mechanism will be structured such that it causes the genes that have expressed that mechanism to differentially outcompete alternative variants of those genes over multiple generations. Or, to put it another way, we can use the shorthand of mechanisms caring about their survival and reproduction because this is more accurate than saying individuals care about their survival and reproduction. But we have to keep in mind that what is technically being preserved is the abstract structure (or design) of the mechanism, not the mechanism per se, and the bookkeeping is done according to what genes are selected to re-create this structure anew each generation.

REFERENCES

Abrams, D., & Hogg, M. A. (Eds.). (1999). *Social identity and social cognition.* Malden, MA: Blackwell.

Alexander, R. A. (1987). *The biology of moral systems.* New York: Routledge.

Allport, G. W. (1958). *The nature of prejudice*. New York: Doubleday Anchor. (Original work published 1954)

Apicella, C. L., & Silk, J. B. (2019). The evolution of human cooperation. *Current Biology, 29,* R447–R450.

Asch, S. (1951). Effects of group pressure upon the modification and distortion of judgement. In H. Guetzkow (Ed.), *Groups, leadership and men* (pp. 222–236). Pittsburgh, PA: Carnegie Press.

Axelrod, R. (1984). *The evolution of cooperation*. New York: Basic Books.

Axelrod, R., & Hamilton, W. D. (1981). The evolution of cooperation. *Science, 211,* 1390–1396.

Balliet, D., Tybur, J. M., & Van Lange, P. A. M. (2017). Functional interdependence theory: An evolutionary account of social situations. *Personality and Social Psychology Review, 21,* 361–388.

Balliet, D., Wu, J., & De Dreu, C. K. (2014). Ingroup favoritism in cooperation: A meta-analysis. *Psychological Bulletin, 140,* 1556–1581.

Barclay, P. (2013). Strategies for cooperation in biological markets, especially for humans. *Evolution and Human Behavior, 34,* 164–175.

Barth, F. (1969). *Ethnic groups and boundaries: The social organization of cultural difference*. Boston: Little, Brown.

Bechtel, W. (2008). *Mental mechanisms: Philosophical perspectives on cognitive neuroscience*. New York: Routledge.

Bernstein, M. J., Young, S. G., & Hungenberg, K. (2007). The cross-category effect: Mere social categorization is sufficient to elicit an own-group bias in face recognition. *Psychological Science, 18,* 342–345.

Blackwell, A. D. (2005). *Terrorism, heroism, and altruism: Kin selection and socio-religious cost–benefit scaling in Palestinian suicide attack*. Presented at the annual meeting of the Human Behavior and Evolution Society, Austin, TX.

Blackwell, A. D. (2008). *Middle-class martyrs: Modeling the inclusive fitness outcomes of Palestinian suicide attack*. Eugene: Anthropology Department, University of Oregon.

Blanz, M. (1999). Accessibility and fit as determinants of the salience of social categorizations. *European Journal of Social Psychology, 29,* 43–74.

Bowlby, J. (1999). *Attachment and Loss: Vol. 1. Attachment* (2nd ed.). New York: Basic Books. (Original work published 1969)

Brewer, M. B. (1999). The psychology of prejudice: Ingroup love or outgroup hate? *Journal of Social Issues, 55,* 429–444.

Brewer, M. B., & Campbell, D. T. (1976). *Ethnocentrism and intergroup attitudes: East African evidence*. New York: Wiley.

Brewer, M. B., & Hewstone, M. (Eds.). (2004). *Social cognition*. Malden, MA: Blackwell.

Brewer, M. B., Weber, J. G., & Carini, B. (1995). Person memory in intergroup contexts: Categorization versus individuation. *Journal of Personality and Social Psychology, 69,* 29–40.

Brown, R. (2000). *Group processes*. Malden, MA: Blackwell.

Campbell, D. T. (1965). Ethnocentric and other altruistic motives. In D. Levine (Ed.), *Nebraska Symposium on Motivation* (Vol. 13, pp. 283–311). Lincoln: University of Nebraska Press.

Cashdan, E. (2001). Ethnocentrism and xenophobia: A cross-cultural study. *Current Anthropology, 42,* 760–765.

Cassidy, J., & Shaver, P. R. (Eds.). (2002). *Handbook of attachment: Theory, research, and clinical applications*. New York: Guilford Press.

Cosmides, L., & Tooby, J. (1987). From evolution to behavior: Evolutionary psychology as the missing link. In J. Dupré (Ed.), *The latest on the best: Essays on evolution and optimality* (pp. 277–306). Cambridge, MA: MIT Press.

Cosmides, L., Tooby, J., & Kurzban, R. (2003). Perceptions of race. *Trends in Cognitive Science, 7,* 517–521.

Delton, A. W., & Krasnow, M. M. (2017). The psychology of deterrence explains why group membership matters for third-party punishment. *Evolution and Human Behavior, 38,* 734–743.

Dennett, D. (1987). *The intentional stance*. Cambridge, MA: MIT Press.

DeScioli, P., & Kurzban, R. (2009). Mysteries of morality. *Cognition, 112,* 281–299.

DeScioli, P., & Kurzban, R. (2013). A solution to the mysteries of morality. *Psychological Bulletin, 139,* 477–496.

Feldman, M. W., Lewontin, R. C., & King, M.-C. (2003). Race: A genetic melting pot. *Nature, 424,* 347.

Forsyth, D. R. (2019). *Group dynamics* (7th ed.). Boston: Cengage. (Original work published 2014)

Gardner, A. (2009). Adaptation as organism design. *Biology Letters, 5*(6), 861–864.

Gibbons, A. (2007). American Association of Physical Anthropologists meeting: European skin turned pale only recently, gene suggests. *Science, 316,* 364.

Goette, L., Huffman, D., & Meier, S. (2006). The impact of group membership on cooperation and norm enforcement: Evidence using random assignment to real social groups. *American Economic Review, 96,* 212–216.

Golkar, A., & Olsson, A. (2017). The interplay of social group biases in social threat learning. *Scientific Reports, 7,* Article No. 7685.

Grafen, A. (2007). The formal Darwinism project: A mid-term report. *Journal of Evolutionary Biology, 20,* 1243–1254.

Graves, J. L. (2001). *The emperor's new clothes: Biological theories of race at the millennium.* New Brunswick, NJ: Rutgers University Press.

Grossman, D. (2009). *On killing: The psychological cost of learning to kill in war and society.* New York: Back Bay.

Hamilton, D. L., Stroessner, S. J., & Driscoll, D. M. (1994). Social cognition and the study of stereotyping. In P. G. Devine, D. L. Hamilton, & T. M. Ostrom (Eds.), *Social cognition: Impact on social psychology* (pp. 291–346). San Diego, CA: Academic Press.

Harcourt, A. H., & deWall, F. B. M. (Eds.). (1992). *Coalitions and alliances in humans and other animals.* New York: Oxford University Press.

Hardy, I. C. W., & Briffa, M. (Eds.). (2013). *Animal contests.* Cambridge. UK: Cambridge University Press.

Hewstone, M., Hantzi, A., & Johnston, L. (1991). Social categorization and person memory: The pervasiveness of race as an organizing principle. *European Journal of Social Psychology, 21,* 517–528.

Higgins, E. T. (1996). Knowledge activation: Accessibility, applicability, and salience. In E. T. Higgins & A. W. Kruglanski (Eds.), *Social psychology: Handbook of basic principles* (pp. 133–168). New York: Guilford Press.

Hill, J. H. (1978). Language contact systems and human adaptations. *Journal of Anthropological Research, 43,* 1–26.

Hill, K. R., Walker, R. S., Božičević, M., Eder, J., Headland, T., Hewlett, B., et al. (2011). Co-residence patterns in hunter-gatherer societies show unique human social structure. *Science, 331,* 1286–1289.

Kenrick, D. T., Maner, J. T., & Li, N. P. (2015). Evolutionary social psychology. In D. M. Buss (Ed.), *The handbook of evolutionary psychology* (2nd ed., pp. 803–827). Hoboken, NJ: Wiley.

Krasnow, M. M., Delton, A. W., Tooby, J., & Cosmides, L. (2013). Meeting now suggests we will meet again: Implications for debates on the evolution of cooperation. *Scientific Reports, 3,* Article No. 1747.

Kurzban, R., Tooby, J., & Cosmides, L. (2001). Can race be erased?: Coalitional computation and social categorization. *Proceedings of the National Academy of Sciences of the USA, 98,* 15387–15392.

Leonardelli, G. J., & Toh, S. M. (2015). Social categorization in intergroup contexts: Three kinds of self-categorization. *Social and Personality Psychology Compass, 9,* 69–87.

Levine, R., & Campbell, D. (1972). *Ethnocentrism: Theories of conflict, ethnic attitudes, and group behavior.* New York: Wiley.

Lewin, K. (1948). *Resolving social conflict.* New York: Harper.

Lieberman, D., Tooby, J., & Cosmides, L. (2007). The architecture of human kin detection. *Nature, 445,* 727–731.

Locksley, A., Ortiz, V., & Hepburn, C. (1980). Social categorization and discriminatory behavior: Extinguishing the minimal intergroup discrimination effect. *Journal of Personality and Social Psychology, 39,* 773–783.

Lopez, A. C. (2019). Making "my" problem "our" problem: Warfare as collective action, and the role of leader manipulation. *Leadership Quarterly.* [Epub ahead of print]

Lopez, A. C., McDermott, R., & Petersen, M. B. (2011). States in mind: Evolution, coalitional psychology, and international politics. *International Security, 36,* 48–83.

Macrae, C. N., & Bodenhausen, G. V. (2000). Social cognition: Thinking categorically about others. *Annual Review of Psychology, 51,* 93–120.

Macrae, C. N., Stangor, C., & Hewstone, M. (Eds.). (1996). *Stereotypes and stereotyping.* New York: Guilford Press.

McGrath, J. E. (1984). *Groups: Interaction and performance.* Englewood Cliffs, NJ: Prentice Hall.

Messick, D. M., & Mackie, D. M. (1989). Intergroup relations. *Annual Review of Psychology, 40,* 45–81.

Migdal, M. J., Hewstone, M., & Mullen, B. (1998). The effects of crossed categorization on intergroup evaluations: A meta-analysis. *British Journal of Social Psychology, 37,* 303–324.

Miller, N., & Davidson-Podgorny, G. (1987). Theoretical models of intergroup relations and the use of cooperative teams as an intervention for desegregated settings. In C. Hendrick (Ed.), *Review of personality and social psychology: Vol. 9. Group processes and intergroup relations* (pp. 41–67). Thousand Oaks, CA: SAGE.

Moya, C., & Boyd, R. (2015). Different selection pressures give rise to distinct ethnic phenomena. *Human Nature, 26*(1), 1–27.

Neuberg, S. L., & Schaller, M. (2016). An evolutionary threat-management approach to prejudices. *Current Opinion in Psychology, 7,* 1–5.

Neuberg, S. L., & Sng, O. (2013). A life history theory of social perception: Stereotyping at the intersections of age, sex, ecology (and race). *Social Cognition, 31,* 696–711.

Norton, H. L., Kittles, R. A., Parra, E., McKeigue, P., Xianyun, M., Cheng, K., et al. (2007). Genetic evidence for the convergent evolution of light skin in Europeans and East Asians. *Molecular Biology and Evolution, 24,* 710–722.

Oakes, P. J. (1987). The salience of social categories. In J. Turner, M. A. Hogg, P. J. Oakes, S. D. Reicher, & M. S. Wetherell (Eds.), *Rediscovering the social group: A self-categorization theory* (pp. 117–141). Oxford, UK: Blackwell.

Oakes, P. J. (1994). The effects of fit versus novelty on the salience of social categories: A response to Biernat and Vescio (1993). *Journal of Experimental Social Psychology, 30,* 390–398.

Oakes, P. J., Turner, J. C., & Haslam, S. A. (1991). Perceiving people as group members: The role of fit in the salience of social categorizations. *British Journal of Social Psychology, 30,* 125–144.

Park, J. H., & Hunt, D. F. (2018). Evolutionary perspectives on the psychology of intergroup relations: Innate predispositions and cultural malleability. In C. L. Frisby & W. T. O'Donohue (Eds.), *Cultural competence in applied psychology* (pp. 269–280). Cham, Switzerland: Springer.

Park, J. H., & Van Leeuwen, F. (2015). Evolutionary perspectives on social identity. In V. Zeigler-Hill, L. Welling, & T. Shackelford (Eds.), *Evolutionary perspectives on social psychology* (pp. 115–125). New York: Springer.

Pietraszewski, D. (2013). What is group psychology?: Adaptations for mapping shared intentional stances. In M. Banaji & S. Gelman (Eds.), *Navigating the social world: What infants, children, and other species can teach us* (pp. 253–257). New York: Oxford University Press.

Pietraszewski, D. (2016a). How the mind sees coalitional and group conflict: The evolutionary invariances of *n*-person conflict dynamics. *Evolution and Human Behavior, 37,* 470–480.

Pietraszewski, D. (2016b). Priming race: Does the mind inhibit categorization by race at encoding or recall? *Social Psychological and Personality Science, 7,* 85–91.

Pietraszewski, D. (2018). A reanalysis of crossed-dimension "Who Said What?" paradigm studies, using a better error base-rate correction. *Evolution and Human Behavior, 39,* 479–489.

Pietraszewski, D. (2020). The evolution of leadership: Leadership and followership as a solution to the problem of creating and executing successful coordination and cooperation enterprises. *Leadership Quarterly, 31,* 101299

Pietraszewski, D., Cosmides, L., & Tooby, J. (2014). The content of our cooperation, not the color of our skin: An alliance detection system regulates categorization by coalition and race, but not sex. *PLOS ONE, 9*(2), e88534.

Pietraszewski, D., Curry, O., Peterson, M. B., Cosmides, L., & Tooby, J. (2015). Constituents of political cognition: Race, party politics, and the alliance detection system. *Cognition, 140,* 24–39.

Pisor, A. C., & Gurven, M. (2016). Risk buffering and resource access shape valuation of out-group strangers. *Scientific Reports, 6,* Article No. 30435.

Riek, B. M., Mania, E. W., & Gaertner, S. L. (2006). Intergroup threat and outgroup attitudes: A meta-analytic review. *Personality and Social Psychology Review, 10,* 336–353.

Rothbart, M., & Taylor, M. (1992). Category labels and social reality: Do we view social categories as natural kinds? In G. R. Semin & K. Fiedler (Eds.), *Language, interaction, and social cognition* (pp.11–36). London: SAGE.

Schaller, M. (2018). The parental care motivational system and why it matters (for everyone). *Current Directions in Psychological Science, 27*(5), 295–301.

Schaller, M., Conway, L. G., III, & Peavy, K. M. (2010). Evolutionary processes. In J. F. Dovidio, M. Hewstone, P. Glick, & V. M. Esses (Eds.), *Handbook of prejudice, stereotyping, and discrimination* (pp. 81–96). London: SAGE.

Scott-Phillips, T. C., Dickins, T. E., & West, S. A. (2011). Evolutionary theory and the ultimate-proximate distinction in the human behavioral sciences. *Perspectives in Psychological Science, 6,* 38–47.

Sedikides, C., Schopler, J., & Insko, C. A. (Eds.). (1998). *Intergroup cognition and intergroup behavior.* Mahwah, NJ: Erlbaum.

Sell, A. (2011). The recalibrational theory and violent anger. *Aggression and Violent Behavior, 16,* 381–389.

Shaw, M. E. (1981). *Group dynamics: The psychology of small group behavior* (3rd ed.). New York: McGraw-Hill.

Sherif, M., Harvey, O. J., White, B. J., Hood, W. R., & Sherif, C. (1961). *Intergroup conflict and cooperation: The robbers' cave experiment.* Norman: University of Oklahoma Press.

Sidanius, J., & Pratto, F. (1999). *Social dominance: An intergroup theory of social hierarchy and oppression.* New York: Cambridge University Press.

Smaldino, P. E. (2015). The evolution of the social self: Multidimensionality of social identity solves the coordination problems of a society. In A. C. Love & W. C. Wimsatt (Eds.), *Beyond the meme: Dynamical structures in cultural evolution.* Minneapolis: University of Minnesota Press.

Smaldino, P. E. (2019). Social identity and cooperation in cultural evolution. *Behavioural Processes, 161,* 108–116.

Smith, E. A., & Winterhalder, B. (1992). Natural selection and decision-making: Some fundamental principles. In E. A. Smith & B. Winterhalder (Eds.), *Evolutionary ecology and human behavior* (pp. 25–60). New York: de Gruyter.

Sng, O., Williams, K. E. G., & Neuberg, S. L. (2017). Evolutionary approaches to stereotyping and prejudice. In C. G. Sibley & F. K. Barlow (Eds.), *The Cambridge handbook of the psychology of prejudice* (pp. 21–46). New York: Cambridge University Press.

Stangor, C., Lynch, L., Duan, C., & Glass, B. (1992). Categorization of individuals on the basis of multiple social features. *Journal of Personality and Social Psychology, 62,* 207–218.

Tajfel, H. (1970). Experiments in intergroup discrimination. *Scientific American, 223,* 96–102.

Tajfel, H. (1982). Social psychology of intergroup relations. *Annual Review of Psychology, 33,* 1–39.

Tajfel, H., & Turner, J. C. (1979). An integrative theory of intergroup conflict. In W. G. Austin & S. Worchel (Eds.), *The social psychology of intergroup relations* (pp. 33–47). Monterey, CA: Brooks/Cole.

Tajfel, H., & Turner, J. C. (1986). The social identity theory of intergroup behavior. In S. Worchel & W. G. Austin (Eds.), *Psychology of intergroup relations* (pp. 7–24). Chicago: Nelson-Hall.

Taylor, S. E., Fiske, S. T., Etcoff, N. L., & Ruderman, A. J. (1978). Categorical and contextual bases of person memory and stereotyping. *Journal of Personality and Social Psychology, 36,* 778–793.

Tooby, J., & Cosmides, L. (1988). *The evolution of war and its cognitive foundations* (Institute for Evolutionary Studies Tech. Rep. No. 88-1). Palo Alto, CA: Institute for Evolutionary Studies.

Tooby, J., & Cosmides, L. (1992). The psychological foundations of culture. In J. Barkow, L. Cosmides, & J. Tooby (Eds.), *The adapted mind: Evolutionary psychology and the generation of culture* (pp. 19–136). New York: Oxford University Press.

Tooby, J., & Cosmides, L. (2010). Groups in mind: The coalitional roots of war and morality. In H. Høgh-Olesen (Ed.), *Human morality and sociality: Evolutionary and comparative perspectives* (pp. 91–234). New York: Palgrave Macmillan.

Tooby, J., & Cosmides, L. (2015). Conceptual foundations of evolutionary psychology. In D. M. Buss (Ed.), *The handbook of evolutionary psychology* (2nd ed., pp. 3–87). Hoboken, NJ: Wiley.

Tropp, L. R. (Ed.). (2012). *The Oxford handbook of intergroup conflict.* New York: Oxford University Press.

Turner, J. C., Hogg, M. A., Oakes, P. J., Reicher, S. D., & Wetherell, M. S. (1987). *Rediscovering the social group: A self-categorization theory.* Oxford, UK: Blackwell.

van den Berghe, P. (1999). Racism, ethnocentrism, and xenophobia: In our genes or in our memes? In K. Thienpont & R. Cliquet (Eds.), *In-group/out-group behaviour in modern societies: An evolutionary perspective* (pp. 21–36). Brussels, Belgium: NIDI CBGS.

Vescio, T. K., Hewstone, M., Crisp, R. J., & Rubin, M. (1999). Social categorization and social context: Is stereotype change a matter of information or meaning? In D. Abrams & M. A. Hogg (Eds.), *Social identity and social cognition* (pp. 111–140). Malden, MA: Blackwell.

Weeks, M., & Lupfer, M. B. (2004). Complicating race: The relationship between prejudice, race, and social class categorizations. *Personality and Social Psychology Bulletin, 30,* 972–984.

Wertz, A. E., & Moya, C. (2019). Pathways to cognitive design. *Behavioural Processes, 161,* 73–86.

West, S. A., Griffin, A. S., & Gardner, A. (2007a). Evolutionary explanations for cooperation. *Current Biology, 17,* R661–R672.

West, S. A., Griffin, A. S., & Gardner, A. (2007b). Social semantics: Altruism, cooperation, mutualism, strong reciprocity and group selection. *Journal of Evolutionary Biology, 20,* 415–432.

West, S. A., Mouden, C. E., & Gardner, A. (2011). Sixteen common misconceptions about the evolution of cooperation in humans. *Evolution and Human Behavior, 32,* 231–262.

Whitehouse, H., Jong, J., Buhrmester, M. D., Gómez, Á., Bastian, B., Kavanagh, C. M., et al. (2017). The evolution of extreme cooperation via shared dysphoric experiences. *Scientific Reports, 7,* Article No. 44292.

Whitehouse, H., McQuinn, B., Buhrmester, M., & Swann, W. B., Jr. (2014). Brothers in arms: Libyan revolutionaries bond like family. *Proceedings of the National Academy of Sciences of the USA, 111,* 1783–1785.

Williams, G. C. (1957). Pleiotropy, natural selection, and the evolution of senescence. *Evolution, 11,* 398–411.

Williams, K. E., Sng, O., & Neuberg, S. L. (2016). Ecology-driven stereotypes override race stereotypes. *Proceedings of the National Academy of Sciences of the USA, 113*(2), 310–315.

Wrangham, R. W., & Glowacki, L. (2012). Intergroup aggression in chimpanzees and war in nomadic hunter–gatherers. *Human Nature, 23,* 5–29.

Yamagishi, T., Jin, N., & Kiyonari, T. (1999). Bounded generalized reciprocity: In-group boasting and in-group favoritism. *Advances in Group Processes, 16,* 161–197.

Yamagishi, T., & Kiyonari, T. (2000). The group as the container of generalized reciprocity. *Social Psychological Quarterly, 63,* 116–132.

Yamagishi, T., & Mifune, N. (2009). Social exchange and solidarity: In-group love or out-group hate? *Evolution and Human Behavior, 30,* 229–237.

Yzerbyt, V., Judd, C. M., & Corneille, O. (Eds.). (2004). *The psychology of group perception: Perceived variability, entitativity, and essentialism.* New York: Psychology Press.

CHAPTER 20

The Stereotype Content Model
How We Make Sense of Individuals and Groups

Susan T. Fiske

Gandalf Nicolas

Xuechunzi Bai

Everyday encounters reveal a rich tapestry of national and religious origins. Now, more than ever, globalization and immigration, layered on past waves of migration, complicate simple ethnic images that people might once have used to make sense of each other. Starting with the basic stereotypes, science needs systematic principles to describe both the process of stereotyping and the content of stereotypes. Social psychologists have long studied stereotyping's cognitive processes (categorization, attention, inference, memory; starting with Allport, 1954, right up through Macrae & Bodenhausen, 2000).

More rarely, social psychologists have studied stereotype content. Starting with Katz and Braly (1933), periodic surveys at Princeton University have documented stereotypic traits describing 10 ethnic and national groups. Throughout the 20th century, Princeton students viewed Turkish people as cruel, Japanese as intelligent, Italians as artistic, and Americans as industrious (Bergsieker, Leslie, Constantine, & Fiske, 2012). But why do particular groups acquire their respective cultural images? Beyond describing the historical record, science needs theory to specify principles: What are the fundamental dimensions of stereotypes? And what are the antecedents that predict stereotype dimensions and consequences that follow? We describe in this chapter our lab's project for the last two decades.

We start with some prior work that—consciously or unconsciously—anticipated our model. Then, we describe in the first main section our two dimensions, conceptually and operationally, as well as their predictors, consequences, and dynamics. We review converging evidence from a variety of methods, case studies, levels of categories, and generality across cultures. We next describe competing models and our adversarial collaborations designed to understand the overlap and boundaries of each model. Finally, we close by considering limitations and future directions.

Prior Work

The stereotype content project all began with one of us (S. T. F.) agreeing to write a chapter for *The Handbook of Social Psychology* on bias: stereotyping, prejudice, and discrimination (Fiske, 1998). After addressing the history of the topic and mechanisms of bias, the literature's singular focus became obvious. Most of the work examined White-on-Black racism; less work examined sexism, anti-Semitism, and disability stigma; and a very few studies targeted other groups: Latinos, Asians, and homosexuals. Superficially, the array of groups seemed miscellaneous and begged the question of whether racism against Blacks would generalize to other target groups, given each one's distinctive history. Having a mind that prefers lumping to splitting, one searches for patterns among the differences.

Ingroup favoritism and outright derogation of some groups form an ingroup/outgroup dynamic already established by the social identity literature (Tajfel & Turner, 1986), so clearly some stereotypes will be all good or all bad. But many groups seem to have more mixed images—women, elderly adults, Jews, Asians. The possibility of ambivalence seemed to complete the description of stereotype content for all groups. Our lab had just identified ambivalent sexism (Glick & Fiske, 1996), whereby stereotypes of some women portray them as nice but not too bright, whereas other women appear stereotypically cold but competent. Based on this and on hunches about other groups, Fiske began exploring impressions of various groups as varying combinations of (dis)likeable and (not) respectworthy. To her chagrin, not all groups came across as ambivalent—high on one dimension but low on the other. But the dimensions themselves seemed to capture something useful.

Invited to a conference celebrating Allport, Fiske rediscovered Allport's 1954 description of compensatory contemporary stereotypes for Jewish people (hardworking and successful, but ambitious and overeager) and contemporary stereotypes for Black people (lazy and superstitious, but happy-go-lucky and musical). She presented preliminary data on (dis)liking and (dis)respecting different clusters of groups (Fiske, Xu, Cuddy, & Glick, 1999). At the same conference, much to our mutual surprise, Marilynn Brewer presented a model with some similar dimensions (Alexander, Brewer, & Herrmann, 1999). The hunt for shared principles was on.

In graduate school, Fiske had studied person perception, inspired by Solomon Asch's (1946) study of Gestalt impressions anchored in intelligence, efficiency, and skill—but contrasting

as warm or cold. Decades later, using multidimensional scaling, Rosenberg, Nelson, and Vivekananthan (1968) had generated independent dimensions of social good–bad and task good–bad. Still in graduate school, Fiske had used similar dimensions to code group interactions (Bales, 1950). Years later, the two seemingly universal dimensions were overdetermined. The lab started to gather data. The model resulted.

Dimensions of the Stereotype Content Model

The stereotype content model (SCM) has both conceptual rationale and operational evidence supporting the cognitive centrality and functional utility of two primary dimensions organizing social cognition about both groups and individuals.

Perceived Social Structure Explains Stereotypes' Two Main Dimensions

The SCM begins with perceivers interpreting social structure: Who is on my side (friend) and who is not (foe)? As interdependent social beings, we need to know others' intent and specific goals, whether cooperative or competitive, which predict how they will interact with us and our tribe. Perceived cooperative intent predicts expected warmth, which includes being both friendly and trustworthy. Warmth determines whom to trust, considering their motives to help or harm. Judging warmth can be subjective: Proving friendly intent and trust is difficult, and warmth judgments are more personal, less consensual, and less reliable than the other dimension (Kervyn, Fiske, & Yzerbyt, 2015; Koch et al., in press; Nicolas, Fiske, et al., 2020). As elusive as warmth is, the SCM treats it as primary.

The other structural dimension is status, which describes those who have the resources to act on their intent. Competence includes both capability and assertiveness. The status–competence association represents a widespread belief in meritocracy, that people's status reflects their talent. Of course, circumstances can determine status (or cooperation/competition), but perceivers tend to neglect situational causes.

Both inferences, cooperation → warmth and status → competence, reflect correspondence bias (Jones, 1990): People's behavior allegedly reflects their dispositions—underestimating the situation (Ross, 1977), especially in explaining negative outgroup behavior (Pettigrew, 1979). People observe the societal positions of various groups, their apparent intent and their status, then assume this reflects the content of their character. This is stereotypic logic because it paints the whole group (e.g., ethnicity) with the same brush (but no group is perfectly homogenous); it also fails to acknowledge that the group (e.g., immigrants) may be a biased sample (depending on who leaves and who stays). And the stereotypic inference confuses people's characteristics with their situations (e.g., who inhabits particular jobs and social status in a given era). Stereotypes, then, are accidents of history.

Operationalizing the Stereotypes

Many different labels describe the core dimensions of warmth and competence. The initial SCM (Fiske, Cuddy, Glick, & Xu, 2002) measured warmth as *friendly, well intentioned, trustworthy, warm, good-natured,* and *sincere.* Competence was operationally defined as *competent, confident, capable, efficient, intelligent,* and *skillful.* The traits came from Asch (1946), Rosenberg and colleagues (1968), Katz and Braly (1933), and our hunches. Luckily, warmth captured what would turn out to be both sociability and morality; competence items captured both capability and agency.

Specifically, in the standard procedure, preliminary participants first list social groups that come into their minds. Groups listed by at least 15% of participants are extracted for subsequent trait-rating tasks. Other participants then rate warmth- and competence-related traits for each of the social groups, using 5-point scales. The instructions specify rating on the basis of how the groups are viewed by the society. This seemed to avoid social desirability and to assess socially shared images. (We return to this point later.)

Over a series of studies with American students, nonstudents, and representative samples (Cuddy, Fiske, & Glick, 2007; Fiske et al., 2002), warmth and competence systematically differentiate diverse social groups, and many groups contain mixed stereotypes. For instance, older people and children are perceived as warm but incompetent; rich people and Asians are considered as not warm but competent; homeless and undocumented (Latino) immigrants are seen as neither warm nor competent; ingroups and reference groups (e.g., Whites, middle-class persons in the United States) are often evaluated as both warm and competent (see Figure 20.1).

In the interests of efficiency, subsequent studies (Cuddy, Fiske, & Glick, 2007; Cuddy et al., 2009; Fiske et al., 2002) narrowed down the trait options, using *friendly* and *warm* as the warmth dimension, *confident* and *competent* as the competence dimension. However, several researchers (e.g., Leach, Ellemers, & Barreto, 2007) propose the priority of morality (trustworthy and sincere) over sociability (friendly and warm) in the warmth dimension. Whereas sociability means cooperating and getting along with others, morality is more about a sense of right and wrong, or essential social values (see discussions in the next section on competing theories). Later studies (Kervyn et al., 2015) confirmed that sociability and morality items are operationally closely related, as indicated by high Cronbach's alphas, but are indeed useful subdimensions for a broader warmth definition. Therefore, refined warmth items include *warm, friendly, sincere, trustworthy,* and *well intentioned*; competence items include *competent, capable,* and *skilled,* but they would later be revised also.

As some critics (including Fiske) observed, another set of comparable but distinct dimensional traits are from the Osgood semantic differential of attitudes (SD; Osgood, Suci, & Tannenbaum, 1957). The semantic differential identifies evaluation (good–bad), potency (strong–weak), and activity (active–passive). One might wonder if the SD evaluation dimension corresponds to SCM warmth and SD potency/activity to SCM competence. (In perceiving people, potency and activity tend to combine into dynamism; Osgood et al., 1957.)

Psychometric analyses (Kervyn, Fiske, & Yzerbyt, 2013) found that the SD and SCM dimensions are neither orthogonal nor redundant, but rather align diagonally (see Figure 20.2). Specifically, evaluation runs from the low-competence/low-warmth quadrant (all bad) up

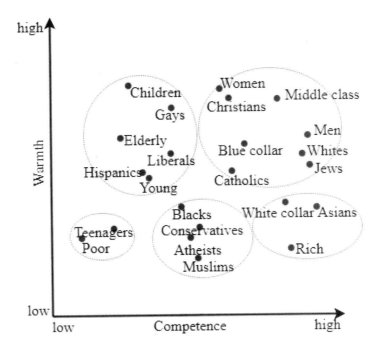

FIGURE 20.1. SCM cluster map. Warmth-by-competence map showing clusters of social groups in the United States. Drawn from data in Kervyn, Fiske, and Yzerbyt (2015).

to the high-competence/high-warmth quadrant (all good), whereas potency runs from the low-competence/high-warmth quadrant (no threat) to the high-competence/low-warmth quadrant (threat).

Operationalizing the Social Structural Predictors: Interdependence and Status

According to the SCM, social groups' perceived warmth and competence, respectively, result from their perceived competition/cooperation and relative socioeconomic status. Groups are perceived as more competent to the extent that they are perceived as powerful and high status, whereas groups are seen as warmer to the extent that they cooperate with others (Fiske et al., 2002). As noted, both reflect correspondence bias, such that people view even situationally determined behavior to reflect intrinsic characteristics.

In SCM studies that test the structure → stereotype prediction, participants rate the perceived status and competitiveness for each social group. Example questions for status include the following: How prestigious are the jobs generally held by members of this group? How economically successful are members of this group? Example items for competitiveness in early studies include only perceived realistic economic threat (e.g., If resources go to this group, to what extent does that take resources away from the rest of society?). Later studies (Kervyn et al., 2015) improved the measurement by adding perceived symbolic threat (e.g., the values and beliefs of this group are *not* compatible with the beliefs and values of most Americans).

Accumulated evidence reveals robust positive competence–status correlations (averaging Pearson's $r > .80$). Initial studies found consistent but smaller negative competitiveness–warmth correlations (averaging $r = -.30$) (Durante et al., 2013; Fiske, 2015). Refining the competition measures to include symbolic threat and using the full warmth scale (both sociability and morality) raised their correlation into the $-.70$'s (Kervyn et al., 2015); that is, con-

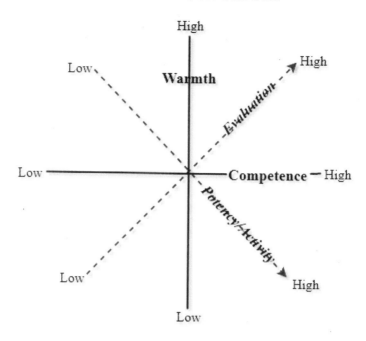

FIGURE 20.2. Comparing semantic differential and stereotype content model dimensions. SD appears as dashed lines and italic labels; SCM appears as solid lines and bold labels. See text and Kervyn et al. (2013).

necting social structural antecedents of status and competition with the warmth–competence space produces: high-status cooperative groups such as ingroups seem competent and warm; low-status cooperative groups such as children seem incompetent but warm; high-status competitive groups such as rich people seem competent but cold; low-status competitive groups such as undocumented immigrants seem incompetent and cold.

Operationalizing the Consequences: Stereotypes Predict Emotional Prejudices and Discriminatory Tendencies

The SCM proposes that the four warmth-by-competence stereotype combinations elicit four distinctive emotions of pity, envy, contempt, and admiration (Fiske et al., 2002; see Figure 20.3). In particular, competent and warm groups (e.g., citizens or middle-class persons) elicit pride and admiration, incompetent but warm groups (e.g., children, elders) elicit pity and sympathy, competent but cold groups (e.g., rich people, tech workers) elicit envy and jeal-

ousy, and incompetent and cold groups (e.g., homeless, drug addicts) elicit contempt and disgust. Various correlational and experimental studies have confirmed this stereotype–emotional prejudice hypothesis (Cuddy et al., 2007; Fiske et al., 2002).

The Behavior from Intergroup Affect and Stereotypes (BIAS) map extends the SCM by incorporating discriminatory tendencies (Cuddy et al., 2007). In this approach, the four combinations of warmth and competence, as well as corresponding distinctive emotions, elicit distinctive behavioral responses of active facilitation (e.g., helping, protecting), passive facilitation (e.g., associating, cooperating), passive harm (e.g., neglecting, demeaning), and active harm (e.g., fighting, attacking). (See Figure 20.3.)

Specifically: Admired, competent, and warm groups elicit both helping and associating, as with middle-class neighbors. Disgusting, incompetent, and cold groups elicit both attacking and neglecting, as when undocumented immigrants are mostly ignored but sometimes attacked. Envied, competent, but cold groups

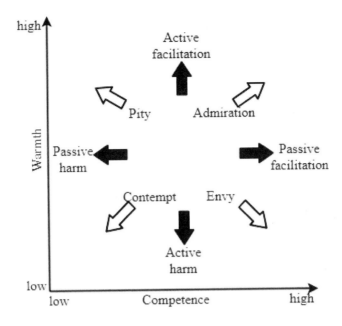

FIGURE 20.3. Emotions and behaviors predicted by the SCM and the BIAS map.

elicit mixed behaviors of associating and attacking, as when successful outsiders may have businesses that others use, but mobs may attack and loot the same businesses. Pitied, incompetent, but warm groups elicit mixed behaviors of helping and neglecting, as when society institutionalizes elders, simultaneously caretaking and isolating them.

Between stereotype contents and emotions, the emotions more strongly and directly predict behaviors (Cuddy et al., 2007). The predictive strength of emotions also appears in meta-analysis of emotional prejudices versus cognitive attitudes predicting discriminatory behavior (Talaska, Fiske, & Chaiken, 2008). Overall, in any case, perceived social structure predicts stereotypes, which in turn predict emotions, which proximally predict behavior.

Operationalizing Warmth–Competence Dynamics: Compensation Effect

To examine the internal dynamics of how the two dimensions of warmth and competence relate to each other, a series of experiments (Judd, James-Hawkins, Yzerbyt, & Kashima, 2005) asked participants to form impressions of two novel groups. The manipulated competence was

high for one group and low for another, while keeping warmth nondiagnostic or ambiguous. After reading vignettes about the behaviors of both groups, participants provided their impressions and rated the warmth and competence of both groups.

The manipulation tests three contradictory predictions. One possibility is a *halo effect*, whereby competent groups are perceived as both more competent and warmer, showing a positive relation between competence and warmth. Another possibility is the *compensation effect*, a trade-off, whereby competent groups are perceived as more competent but less warm, therefore establishing a negative, trade-off relation. Or warmth and competence might be completely *independent*, with null effects on each other. Results confirmed the compensation effect: The group portrayed by the experimental manipulation as higher on competence is judged even lower on warmth. The compensation effect also occurs in the reverse with a manipulation of warmth, such that participants judge the group higher on warmth as also lower on competence. The compensation effect serves motives for both justice and collective self-esteem because every group can claim a distinctive, good feature as its identity: These are the nice ones; those are the smart ones.

The compensation effects endure whether the targets are real groups (Yzerbyt, Kervyn, & Judd, 2008; Yzerbyt, Provost, & Corneille, 2005), artificial groups, or individuals (Judd et al., 2005), especially in comparative contexts, regardless of direct or indirect measurement (Kervyn, Yzerbyt, & Judd, 2011). More relevant here, the compensation effect holds only for the two core dimensions of warmth and competence, and not any other dimensions, such as healthiness (Holoien & Fiske, 2013; Yzerbyt et al., 2008). In comparative contexts, the higher-status group claims competence, which facilitates goal achievement; the lower-status group is ceded warmth, suggesting its members will cooperate with the hierarchy, but not helpful in societal goals that matter.

Furthermore, even in describing third parties, people likewise know to trade off warmth and competence in stereotypes. In the 20th century, as anti-bias norms developed, people describing societal groups began to omit whichever dimension was negative, preferring to accentuate the positive dimension; this stereotyping by omission still differentiates societal groups (Bergsieker et al., 2012). But the negative dimension is implied by omission: Trying to be tactful about a disrespected outgroup, one might say, "Well, they are really nice. . . . " Listeners do get the message and infer the omitted dimension (incompetence in this example) from its absence (Kervyn, Bergsieker, & Fiske, 2012).

Everyday self-presentation also illustrates. Such compensatory processes likewise influence people's impression management during interpersonal communication. People actively downplay one dimension to emphasize the other (Holoien & Fiske, 2013), playing dumb to be likable, or being mean to seem smart. Sexist women have long tried to appeal to sexist men, aiming to seem nicer by hiding their own competence. And in another domain, negative reviews that are more direct may seem smarter than negative feedback phrased in a nicer way.

This dynamic especially appears in cross-status interactions. Not wanting to seem arrogant and cold, a professor might use simpler vocabulary or slang ("getting down with the people") to connect with a lower-status service worker. Professors know they are seen as competent; high status in general confers an image of competence, but it does not confer warmth. Like the professor, to avoid being perceived as competent but cold, higher-status people downplay their own competence in order to appear warmer—while low-status people downplay their own warmth in order to appear more competent (Swencionis & Fiske, 2016). This reliable effect goes away when perceivers learn that their partner does not fit the status stereotypes, that status equals competence or that low-status equals warmth. This can create dysfunctional interactions, wherein the higher-status person wants to be liked and the lower-status person wants to be respected, so they have divergent goals for the encounter.

Cross-racial interaction also replicates these compensatory impression managements between high-status and low-status groups. Being generically lower status, racial minorities seek to be seen as competent more than Whites do, whereas generically higher-status Whites try to be seen as warm, more than racial minorities do (Bergsieker, Shelton, & Richeson, 2010). These interpersonal interaction studies fit interracial encounters in other settings. White liberals (who presumably care more about interracial relationships) similarly self-present to Black partners by downplaying their own competence, to seem warmer (Dupree & Fiske, 2019). Even Democratic Presidential candidates who are White show this competence downshift in speeches to minority audiences, compared with majority audiences; Republican candidates do not differentiate (but they give fewer such speeches).

Generality of the SCM

Going beyond the surveys asking about society's views, these studies of compensation, innuendo, and omission show the warmth–competence dimensions operating at a more personal level. As this section briefly overviews, other studies generalize the warmth and competence dimensions to situations that include individual reactions, interpersonal encounters, category subgroups, nonhuman intent-having entities, and cross-cultural variations.

Individual-Level Evidence

Adding to self-reports, neural activations and physiological responses provide converging individual-level evidence. Exposure to pictures of low-competence, low-warmth, disgusting groups (e.g., homeless people and those with addictions) can activate insula and amygdala, neural areas consistent with disgust emotions. Moreover, members of these low-low quadrant groups tend to be seen as less human, indicated by the absence of one typical neural signature for social cognition (activated medial prefrontal cortex [mPFC]). Questionnaire data corroborate these interpretations (Harris & Fiske, 2009).

Targeting high-status, competitive, enviable groups, such as the rich: People smile more in response to those groups' misfortunes, as measured by facial electromyography (EMG) on cheek muscle movements (Cikara & Fiske, 2012) and show pleasure indicated by neural reward regions' activation (Cikara, Botvinick, & Fiske, 2011; Cikara, Bruneau, & Saxe, 2011). Reward activation correlates with self-reports of harming the envied outgroup (Cikara et al., 2011).

Interpersonal Level

Borrowing principles of structural variables from group perception, individual interaction experiments examined how competition and status predict interpersonal perceptions (Russell & Fiske, 2008). Manipulating participants and their fictitious partners' structural relations created high- or low-status players in a cooperative or competitive game); participants evaluate the other players on warmth and competence. Competing targets are judged less warm than cooperating targets and high-status targets are judged more competent than low-status targets.

As previously described, studies of cross-status and cross-race interactions and their effects on warmth–competence dynamics also support the interpersonal level of the SCM.

Category Subgroups

Since the development of the SCM, prolific work has examined various subgroups of social groups. Subgroups reproduce the SCM space but offer nuanced differences. Initially, some derogated societal outgroups (Blacks, gay men)

appeared in neutral locations in the original SCM space (Fiske et al., 2002). However, Black subgroups of poor Blacks and Black professionals polarized into opposite corners, showing how they could cancel each other out in the general case (Cuddy et al., 2007). Similarly, although gay men in general initially appeared neutral in the warmth-by-competence space, subgroups spread out across the space, consistent with the subgroups averaging out to neutral in the aggregate (Clausell & Fiske, 2005).

Some subgroups predominantly fall into ambivalently high-competence/low-warmth or low-competence/high-warmth quadrants: This ambivalence represents many subgroups of immigrants (Lee & Fiske, 2006), gay men (Clausell & Fiske, 2005), men and women (Eckes, 2002), and older adults (Cuddy, Norton, & Fiske, 2005). However, subgroups of other overall groups fall into univalent quadrants, either high-high or low-low: Native Americans (Burkley, Durante, Fiske, Burkley, & Andrade, 2017), Black Americans (Fiske, Bergsieker, Russell, & Williams, 2009), lesbians (Brambilla, Carnaghi, & Ravenna, 2011), and rich people (Wu, Bai, & Fiske, 2018).

Multiple subgroup stereotypes potentially convey more varied and more precise information than a general category. For instance, research around the world shows a stable image of the rich being competent but cold, both as a group and as individuals (Durante, Tablante, & Fiske, 2017). Yet subgrouping studies (Wu et al., 2018) demonstrate that not all rich subgroups are envied, but only the stereotypical competent-but-cold rich (e.g., businessmen, lawyers). Warm and competent rich (e.g., doctors, entrepreneurs) are admired, while cold and incompetent rich (e.g., second generations of the rich, politicians) are resented. Deservingness and fairness may be involved (see below).

Similarly, Native American subgroups represent an assortment of polarized noble (e.g., wise elder) and ignoble (e.g., alcoholic) stereotypes that correspond, respectively, to distinctive emotions of admiration and contempt (Burkley et al., 2017). Likewise, immigrant subgroup analysis reveals that Americans perceive Japanese, Koreans, and Chinese as competent but cold; Mexicans, Africans, and undocumented are perceived as incompetent and cold; Irish and Italians are warm but incompetent; Americans, Europeans, and Canadians belong to competent and warm reference groups. Distinctive immigrant stereotypes could offer useful insights on hosts' preferences and reactions toward different immigrant subgroups (Lee & Fiske, 2006).

Other Entities That Have Intent

Not only human social groups fit the SCM: Because they are perceived as also having intent and capability, animals likewise appear to vary on warmth–competence dimensions (Sevillano & Fiske, 2016a, 2016b). Animals spread out across the SCM space: Pets such as dogs and cats appear in the competent and warm quadrant, while pests such as snakes and rats appear in the incompetent and cold quadrant. Predators such as tigers and lions are in the competent but cold space, while edible farm animals such as sheep and ducks are seen as nice but incompetent (Sevillano & Fiske, 2016b).

Also resembling human social group perceptions are images of brands or corporations. Brands seem like intention-having entities, such that consumers differentiate brands through the lens of warmth–competence social perceptions, eliciting predictable emotions and behavioral tendencies toward different brands (Kervyn, Bergsieker, et al., 2012; Kervyn, Fiske, & Malone, 2012).

Cultural Variations

Data from over 47 countries and regions have investigated the SCM (Cuddy et al., 2009; Durante et al., 2013, 2017; Grigoryan et al., 2020; Wu et al., 2018). Samples include 12 Western European countries (Belgium, Denmark, England, Finland, Germany, Greece, Italy, Norway, Portugal, Spain, Sweden, Switzerland), eight Eastern European post-Soviet countries (Armenia, Georgia, Belarus, Kazakhstan, Russia, Ukraine, Uzbekistan, Kosovo), nine Middle Eastern countries (Afghanistan, Egypt, Iran, Iraq, Israel, Jordan, Lebanon, Pakistan, Turkey), six Asian countries/regions (India, Malaysia, South Korea, Japan, Hong Kong, China), three African countries (Kenya, South Africa, Uganda), two Southwest Pacific countries (Australia,

New Zealand), two North American countries besides the United States (Canada, Mexico), and four South and Central American countries (Bolivia, Chile, Costa Rica, Peru).

First, international samples have verified SCM warmth and competence space, such that perceived warmth and competence consistently distinguish social groups in each tested society. Second, qualitative similarities and differences characterize the social groups listed across countries. For instance, commonly mentioned groups are age, gender, socioeconomic status, race/ethnicity, and religious groups; culturally idiosyncratic groups are various indigenous groups and occupations. Third, some groups end up being perceived more similarly across societies, but others may differ a lot. For example, the rich are often competent but cold, migrants are often low-low, elders are often warm but incompetent, and citizens are often high-high—all with exceptions, of course. However, other groups' stereotypes are exceptionally variable: For example, homosexuals are dispersed, from low-low to high-high competence, depending on their society.

Specific cultural variables reveal some patterns: Comparing individualistic versus collectivistic countries, three Asian samples do not show high-high ingroup/reference group clusters as Europeans and Americans do (Cuddy et al., 2009). Collectivistic norms such as modesty, humility, and harmony may moderate the positive evaluations of the societal ingroups.

To expand cultural comparisons from different angles, Durante and colleagues examined how socioecological factors of income inequality (2013) and conflict (2017) influence people's psychological perceptions of others, in the shape of the SCM. One cross-national study (Durante et al., 2013) explored the possibility that societies display different degrees of ambivalent stereotypes (high on one dimension, while low on the other) as related to the societies' levels of income inequality. A negative linear relation between ambivalence (indexed by the overall warmth–competence correlation) and inequality (indexed by Gini coefficients) supports the hypothesis (i.e., the more unequal societies show more ambivalent stereotypes). As if unequal societies have more explaining to do, they separate stereotypes into deserving and undeserving poor, deserving and undeserving rich.

Another cross-national study (Durante et al., 2017) investigated the relations between peaceful–conflictual societal environment and stereotype ambivalence. Using the Global Peace Index to measure conflict, a quadratic relationship between ambivalence and conflict demonstrates that both extremely peaceful (e.g., Denmark) and extremely conflictual (e.g., Pakistan) countries display less ambivalence (i.e., they show greater us vs. them polarity), whereas intermediately conflictual countries (United States) exhibit higher ambivalence. At both extremes, societies must define ingroup boundaries, but for different reasons: under peace, to protect those who qualify for the social safety net (e.g., compared to ineligible refugees) and under war, to defend the ingroup and attack the enemy outgroup. Intermediate peaceful–conflictual places no such demands to simplify the intergroup space.

Recently, the SCM has suggested how people adapt to diversity. In comparisons replicating at three levels (nations, U.S. states, and individuals), people in homogenous settings paradoxically differentiate among societal groups, spreading them out across the warmth–competence space. People in Wyoming and Vermont (the two Whitest states) have distinct images of Mexicans and Chinese they have never met. New Yorkers and Hawaiians, in their diverse settings, realize the variety in groups they see all the time, and they cluster everybody into an ingroup clump, the melting pot ("We're all New Yorkers"; Bai, Ramos, & Fiske, 2020). Nondiverse settings show the usual SCM dispersion of stereotypes—with the change to one ingroup cluster as diversity increases. This explains how diversity may generate initial discomfort, but people adjust over time with exposure (Ramos, Bennett, Massey & Hewstone, 2019).

At a macro level, thus, national indices describe the shape of the SCM cluster-analysis cloud of points: the warmth–competence correlation, ranging from low (circular cloud, incorporating ambivalence) to high (more of an oblong vector, low-low to high-high), predicted by inequality and peace–conflict. Dispersion of groups across the space—differentiated stereotypes—are predicted by *less* exposure to diversity.

Competing Frameworks: Convergence and Divergence

Besides the historical precedents to the SCM reviewed earlier, more contemporary approaches have complemented and diverged from the SCM in a variety of ways. These competing frameworks sometimes originated from fields in person perception other than the stereotyping domain (e.g., Abele & Wojciszke, 2007), while others have been a direct response to the SCM (e.g., Koch, Imhoff, Dotsch, Unkelbach, & Alves, 2016). Below we summarize these alternative approaches to the study of stereotype content.

The Dual-Perspective Model of Agency and Communion

The dual-perspective model of agency and communion (DPM-AC; Abele & Wojciszke, 2014) aims to be a general framework for the study of the content of person perception. The first difference from the SCM is evident in the name of the model, as it uses the concepts of agency (akin to competence) and communion (akin to warmth) to describe the "Big Two" of social cognition content. Whereas the SCM borrows these terms directly from classic studies on person perception (Asch, 1946) and the loading of trait names in early studies on the two main factors (Fiske et al., 1999), the DPM-AC proponents have argued that "communion" and "agency" (1) are broader terms that better account for the content covered by each dimension, (2) align better with terms used in other psychological fields, and (3) are less likely to be confused with lay interpretations (Abele & Wojciszke, 2014). However, with a few exceptions (see the following section), the dimensions are equivalent (Abele, Ellemers, Fiske, Koch, & Yzerbyt, 2020).

The DPM-AC makes three main claims about the two dimensions of social cognition content: (1) It posits, in line with the SCM, that communion/warmth has priority as a dimension. However, and crucially, it proposes that the relevance of content is moderated by perspective, such that (2) communion/warmth is particularly important when considering the perspective of the observer or recipient of a social behavior, while (3) agency/competence is more important when thinking from the perspective of self or the actor of a social behavior.

Support for the general primacy of communion/warmth comes from multiple studies showing that, for example, communion/warmth accounts for more variance than agency/competence does (Abele & Wojciszke, 2007), communal/warm words are recognized faster (Ybarra, Chan, & Park, 2001), and they are mentioned earlier in descriptions of others (Abele & Bruckmüller, 2011). Support for the increased role of communion/warmth in the observer perspective comes from studies showing, for example, that global impressions of targets are more affected by information about their communion/warmth than their agency/competence (e.g., Wojciszke, Bazinska, & Jaworski, 1998), and that observers' emotional responses to others' behaviors is more directly linked to communion/warmth than agency/competence (Wojciszke & Szymkow, 2003).

Support for the increased relevance of agency/competence from the actor perspective comes from findings such as people choosing to receive training on developing skills related to agency/competence over those related to communion/warmth (Abele & Wojciszke, 2007). Also, self-esteem is better predicted by self-rated agency/competence than self-rated communion/warmth (Wojciszke, Baryla, Parzuchowski, Szymkow, & Abele, 2011; however, see Gebauer, Wagner, Sedikides, & Neberich, 2013, who found high variability in this effect).

Largely, the DPM-AC perspective moderation does not conflict with the SCM, but provides additional considerations about the interplay of self- and other- perspectives. As we discuss later, such interaction of perspectives has become relevant to conceptions of stereotyping arising from newer stereotype content research.

Subdimensions

The SCM has focused on the two dimensions of warmth and competence. However, a number of authors have argued that these two factors are too broad and that additional insights can be gained by considering their subcomponents.

An early line of research on the topic argued that additional attention should be paid to morality-related traits (e.g., *trustworthy, sincere*) that together with sociability-related traits (e.g., *friendly, warm*) form the SCM's dimension of warmth. For example (Leach et al., 2007), people self-report that their group's morality is more important to them than their group's sociability or competence, and higher group identification predicts ascriptions of morality (but not sociability or competence) to the group. Furthermore, only experimental manipulations of a group's morality (and not of its sociability or competence) lead to higher group pride and lower perceptions of group variability.

Similarly, a primacy of morality emerges in evaluations of outgroups (e.g., Brambilla, Sacchi, Rusconi, Cherubini, & Yzerbyt, 2012). Global impressions of targets are also more closely related to morality than sociability (Goodwin, Piazza, & Rozin, 2014). In measures of information gathering, for example, morality is weighed more heavily than sociability (and competence) when deciding which facts to learn about a target (Brambilla, Rusconi, et al., 2011). A number of other findings support the importance of morality over all other proposed contents in topics varying from the elicitation of *Schadenfreude* (i.e., pleasure at others' misfortunes; Brambilla & Riva, 2017) to group norms' influence (Ellemers et al., 2008). As facets of warmth/communion, morality is more significant than sociability, probably because it has more depth and predicts intent better.

In terms of the competence dimension of the SCM, little research has differentiated between potential subcomponents. An exception comes recently, from the development of the Agency–Communion Inventory (AC-IN; Abele et al., 2016). Although a two-factor model of agency/competence and communion/warmth fit well, fit improved with a four-factor model composed of morality and sociability as facets of the larger communion/warmth factor, and assertiveness and ability as facets of the larger agency/competence factor (see Figure 20.4).

As just discussed, some research shows the unique importance of morality, but sociability also predicts unique outcomes, such as a person's extraversion (Abele et al., 2016). More relevantly, distinguishing between ability and

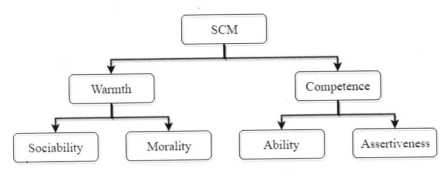

FIGURE 20.4. Warmth, competence, and their facets, inspired by Abele, Wojciszke, and Ellemers, consistent with SCM studies (see text).

assertiveness, both combined in the broader competence dimension of the SCM, allows for unique predictions in outcomes such as personality and self-esteem.

Much of the research just reviewed originates from the person perception literature and might not be as relevant to stereotype content. Or it might apply equally, adding to evidence for the generality of these two dimensions. However, these suggestions to consider facets of the SCM's warmth and competence dimensions will be relevant for future research, and we have incorporated it into some of our recent studies reviewed here.

Finally, consider one additional proposed facet of agency/competence: status. Although the SCM treats a group's status as a precursor to judgments of competence, the initial ABC (agency–beliefs–communion) model (Koch et al., 2016) incorporates the concept of status into its agency component (and excludes ability from it). This status + assertiveness criterion for agency came from the principal components that emerged from ratings of social groups in a variety of traits. The main difference, besides the method of analysis (e.g., principal component analysis vs. factor analysis; Fiske et al., 1999), was that Koch and colleagues (2016) used a more data-driven approach that incorporated traits outside of the expected warmth and competence space, whereas others (e.g., Fiske et al., 1999) used a theory-driven approach to test for traits that were hypothesized to fall within the warmth and competence space. The degree to which status, a relatively objective structural factor, should be considered in the same light as more subjective psychological traits

is already the focus of further inquiry. Warmth is clearly more personal than competence/status (Koch et al., in press).

The ABC Model of Stereotype Content

As just discussed, the SCM and other models of social cognition content made a number of theory-driven choices during their development (e.g., the SCM dimensions are based on functionalist theories about their usefulness in social life). However, a relatively recent model proposed by Koch and colleagues (2016), the ABC model of stereotype content, used a more data-driven approach to arrive at dimensions of group stereotyping. Research on the ABC model employed a series of steps to minimize the use of assumptions in the creation of their model. For example, they used traits that fell outside of the traditional warmth and competence semantic space, as noted. In addition, they elicited social groups from participants using minimal instructions that did not hint at specific social categories (e.g., the SCM instructions suggest ethnicity and gender, among other cues). They also had each individual rater compare as many as 80 groups at a time. (The SCM has a limit of 10–15 groups per rater, intended to increase rating quality.) Crucially, the ABC procedure to determine content dimensions used similarity metrics and multidimensional scaling to find content dimensions, another relatively data-driven step in the design.

The ABC model uses two dimensions to represent intergroup similarity, which (when correlated with group ratings on several traits) represent the groups in terms of their agency (socioeconomic status) and liberal–conservative beliefs (a novel dimension in their model). In contrast to the SCM and the DPM-AC, their 2016 model did not show evidence of warmth/communion as a main dimension. Instead, it emerged as centrality, such that groups that were closer to the midpoint of both dimensions were seen as most warm/communal—with decreasing warmth/communion as groups moved toward polarized extremes of either the agency or beliefs dimensions.

The finding that warmth/communion decreases as competence/agency and beliefs become more extreme and is highest for moderate levels is similarly dealt with in a development of the ABC model (Imhoff & Koch, 2017), in which the authors argue that the pattern is manifested in curvilinear relationships between the dimensions. Groups' warmth/communion is inferred from the rater's similarity to their agency/competence and their beliefs, unless warmth/communion is directly available. Thus, for parsimony, warmth/communion should not be processed preferentially (as proposed by the SCM and other models of person perception), but should follow processing of agency/competence information, which would in turn facilitate warmth/communion processing. This perspective differs from that of the SCM and other models that distinguish warmth as a more complex dimension (e.g., consisting of different facets) and differs from global evaluations of social targets (as in the semantic differential, reviewed earlier).

The ABC model (Koch et al., 2016) and the associated claims (Imhoff & Koch, 2017) constitute the most directly relevant challenge to the SCM. However, many of their claims are preliminary (a fact they readily admit in their papers) and contradict a large literature on the topic of person perception. For example, although the curvilinear relationship between warmth/communion and competence/agency appears robust, it does not necessarily follow from this finding that competence/agency would be given priority in cognitive processing (e.g., the findings are correlational). Additionally, the absence in their model of warmth/communion, a dimension found to account for large amounts of variance in other paradigms and considered primary in the SCM, calls for further clarification of how their novel approach differs from existing ones.

Thus, with the purpose of shedding some light on the nature of these discrepancies, several researchers in the tradition of the SCM and the proponents of the ABC model have been engaged in a series of adversarial collaborations. We review in the next sections how findings from these collaborations and other projects may advance research into stereotype content. These projects are in progress, so we present only the main findings that are guiding our collaboration.

Content Consensus

The ABC model team has been exploring the degree to which the warmth, competence, and beliefs dimensions are consensual. This project originated from the observation that the methods in the original ABC paper (Koch et al., 2016) averaged responses across participants. While this is widespread practice in psychology (including the SCM paradigm), researchers have been warned to be cautious with interpretations about mean patterns across individuals when the process of interest is intraindividual (Speelman & McGann, 2013; this problem might be even more pronounced in some dimension-reduction approaches such as those used in Koch et al., 2016). This may be problematic if dealing with dimensions of differing consensus across individuals and groups. Thus if, say, ascriptions of warmth to targets are idiosyncratic, with more interindividual variation than ascriptions of beliefs or competence, then warmth will be averaged out to a larger extent than beliefs or competence. To illustrate, imagine that liberals rate liberals as warmer than conservatives, and conservatives rate conservatives as warmer than liberals, but both rate liberals as more liberal and conservatives as more conservative. When averaging these ratings of conservatives and liberals across participants, only ratings of warmth will cancel each other out because of individual differences in judging which groups are warm.

Why would warmth show lower consensus between individuals? A potential explanation comes from the ABC model team's research on the curvilinear relationship between competence (or beliefs) and warmth (Imhoff & Koch, 2017), as well as research showing that similarity predicts trusting or liking (e.g., Klohnen & Luo, 2003). Specifically, we could expect that people varying in competence or beliefs will rate as warmer those targets who are more similar to themselves in terms of beliefs or competence.

Eight studies (Koch et al., 2020) tested this idea across cultures and used a variety of approaches. Warmth/communion depended on target–rater similarity. In particular, participants high on status (or conservative beliefs) rated targets similar to themselves as high on warmth, while the opposite was true for those low on status or conservative beliefs. This interaction effect was larger for the beliefs (vs. competence/status) dimension.

Following the logic that warmth requires considering interindividual variation, when replicating the original ABC model results using data at the individual level, warmth emerged as a dimension highly correlated with intergroup similarity.

Thus, the discrepancy between the SCM and the ABC model in terms of the warmth dimension was lessened as a result of these studies. However, note that this does not suggest that warmth is entirely determined by rater–target similarity on beliefs and competence/status. In fact, these effects explained less than 10% of the variance on warmth ratings. Additionally, the results are correlational, preventing the determination of causality. Thus, understanding of the degree of "primacy" of these dimensions (cf. Imhoff & Koch, 2017) is pending further research.

Other differences between the models remain, including the ABC model's proposal that the beliefs dimension emerges alongside warmth/communion and competence/status. With the purpose of shedding some additional light on potential moderating variables that could lead to differential use of the different dimensions, an additional adversarial collaboration focuses on information gathering; an ad-ditional project seeks to approach spontaneous stereotypes from an alternative approach to the ABC model's approach.

Information Gathering

In addition to stereotyping, the "Big Two" dimensions of warmth and competence operate in multiple person perception tasks, including the search for information about others (i.e., information gathering). Information gathering is crucial to social behavior because inferring the traits of others in as few dimensions as possible is an efficient way to organize behavior toward those targets. Thus, understanding which dimensions take priority for people seeking information about a stranger elucidates their fundamental role in social cognition.

Previous research has compared the use of warmth and competence on information gathering (finding, e.g., that warmth/communion is the most important dimension when forming global impressions of others; Wojciszke, 2005). However, given the novelty of the beliefs dimension, previous studies on information gathering had not included it as a point of comparison with other dimensions.

Furthermore, a comparison of the methods and assumptions of the SCM and the ABC model suggests that the SCM uses a more interpersonal/psychological approach, while the ABC model takes a more abstract/sociological perspective. For example, the SCM is based on functional theories about interpersonal interaction and is based solely on direct rating of a few groups. On the other hand, the data-driven approach of the ABC model asks participants to think about many different groups from the abstract perspective of "intergroup similarities," which might lead to a more sociological organization of social groups. Thus, in order to address these issues, an SCM-led project conducted several studies in collaboration with the ABC model team (Nicolas, Fiske, et al., 2020).

Two studies showed participants a vignette asking them to imagine that either their neighborhood newspaper or their national newspaper (between-subjects condition) described a new kind of people recently increasing in the neighborhood/nation—then asked, what did they want to learn more about them? In a third study, participants instead imagined that they themselves were moving to either a new neighborhood or a new nation and wanted to learn about the people there. The rationale for this manipulation was that neighborhoods and nations differ on their degree of potential for interpersonal contact versus abstract analysis, respectively, at the psychological versus sociological level. If the SCM dimensions are more interpersonal and psychological, they should be more appealing in the neighborhood condition. Similarly, if the ABC model dimensions are more abstract/sociological, they should be more appealing in the nation condition. Another study showed that the neighborhood elicits more relational goals, leading to direct manipulations of a more relational versus structural analysis goal.

The dependent variable changed from study to study and included both ratings of different dimensions and free responses that were then categorized into the dimensions. For these studies, the dimensions included the two facets of warmth (sociability and morality), the two facets of competence (ability and assertiveness), beliefs, and status.

Results across studies showed that regardless of the manipulation, participants were more interested in learning about warmth than about the other dimensions, adding to previous similar findings by showing that this priority effect persists even when including beliefs in the comparison, and when subdividing the dimensions into their facets. Furthermore, the manipulation showed the expected pattern, with participants being relatively more interested in sociability in the neighborhood (psychological), relational conditions, and relatively more interested in ability, agency, and beliefs (with some differences across studies) in the nation (sociological) condition. Morality remained a dimension of high interest across conditions.

In summary, information-gathering studies provide evidence for a moderator that could help explain differences between the SCM and the ABC model dimensions. Specifically, although warmth (sociability and morality) is the most important dimension across conditions, a more abstract/sociological perspective increases the importance of the ABC model dimension of beliefs, as well as competence.

Converging Collaborations

Another aspect studied in this adversarial collaboration is the role of instruction on the sampling of groups. The ABC model asked participants to name 40–80 social groups, and studies from this collaboration suggest that asking for such a large number of groups leads to biased sampling. Specifically, as compared to people who were just asked to name as many social groups as came to mind, when asked for a long list, people relied more on strategies (name an exhaustive list of religions), and they used more status and beliefs to select the social groups. This in turn could have led to differences between the models, which used different samples of groups. However, later studies on the ABC model paper (Koch et al., 2016) made use of a minimalist sample and still found the same pattern as that with the more structured sampling.

Spontaneous Stereotype Content and Other Research

One of the main claims in the ABC model's original paper (Koch et al., 2016) was that, given their relatively data-driven method, it measured *spontaneous* stereotype content. The final project discussed here took a different approach to spontaneity, namely, open-ended responses. Our reasoning was that if giving participants pre-specified dimensions to rate groups (as the SCM does) explained why beliefs could not have emerged as a dimension (see Koch et al., 2016), then asking for free responses would circumvent that issue. Given that open-ended responses are variable and complex, techniques from machine learning and natural language processing coded and analyzed the open-ended data. Here, we present the results from dictionaries designed to measure multiple dimensions, including sociability, morality, ability, assertiveness, status, and beliefs (Nicolas, Bai, & Fiske, 2020).

Three studies asked participants to provide the first characteristics they thought about in relation to a series of social groups. Our dictionaries accounted for over 80% of the responses, indicating that they were able to account for the vast majority of stereotype content. More importantly, an examination of the response distributions indicated that warmth and competence were used more than twice as frequently as beliefs dimensions. A subsequent study asked participants to label their own responses into different dimensions and found convergent evidence.

We are currently working on expanding these studies by looking at the primacy of the different dimensions in terms of order of processing (e.g., whether some dimensions are mentioned earlier than others), how spontaneous valence varies across different content dimensions (the results above collapse across positive and negative responses), and how spontaneous content may vary cross-culturally. This line of research may provide an alternative lens to understand spontaneous stereotypes and further clarify differences between the SCM and the ABC model. In addition, the methods used here can be extrapolated to the study of stereotype content outside the laboratory, particularly as data from social media and other large corpora become increasingly available to researchers.

Conclusions and Future Directions

Healthy debate over competing models suggests some shared principles: The agency/competence/status dimension reliably appears in various models, assessed by various methods. It combines capability and assertiveness. And it especially matters to self-perception. In other-perception, competence/agency follows from perceived societal status. In the SCM, this dimension predicts upward-comparison emotions (admiration or envy, respectively, for warm or cold targets); competence-agency also predicts downward-comparison emotions (pity or disgust; again, which emotion then depends on the warmth dimension). Behaviors predicted by perceived competence are passive help or passive harm, again depending on warmth. Status and competence correlate strongly, and judgments of them seem relatively consensual and even perhaps objective.

The warmth/communion dimension most comprehensively includes both sociability and morality/trustworthiness. It appears in most models especially important to perceivers making sense of others with whom they expect to interact. Warmth outranks competence in other perception. Perceived interdependence (cooperation/competition) predicts warmth. Warmth predicts positive emotions (pity or admiration) and active helping; low warmth predicts negative emotions (disgust or envy) and active harm (attack). Cooperation/competition and warmth are correlated but seem more subjective than status and competence, so consensus is more variable.

So far, the beliefs dimension appears only in the ABC model data, especially when raters are operating in an abstract, sociological, impersonal level of analysis. Understanding this dimension is the subject of ongoing research, some of it as a mutually respectful, adversarial collaboration.

Other future directions include open-ended data, analyzed through natural language processing, described earlier. Some related work will examine open-ended descriptions of category mash-ups that combine group memberships across SCM space, reminiscent of earlier efforts (e.g., Kunda, Miller, & Claire, 1990), but including the warmth dimension, neglected by previous work on contradictory categories for one person.

Finally, conceptual refinements will follow from data and ongoing debate among related models. A joint theoretical statement is one potential result (Abele, Ellemers, Fiske, Koch, & Yzerbyt, 2020), showing that adversarial positions can reconcile and advance science, being collectively both warm and competent.

REFERENCES

Abele, A. E., & Bruckmüller, S. (2011). The bigger one of the "Big Two"?: Preferential processing of communal information. *Journal of Experimental Social Psychology, 47,* 935–948.

Abele, A., Ellemers, N., Fiske, S., Koch, A., & Yzerbyt, V. (2020). *Navigating the social world: Shared horizontal and vertical evaluative dimensions.* Manuscript under review.

Abele, A. E., Hauke, N., Peters, K., Louvet, E., Szymkow, A., & Duan, Y. (2016). Facets of the fundamental content dimensions: Agency with competence and assertiveness–communion with warmth and morality. *Frontiers in Psychology, 7,* 1–17.

Abele, A. E., & Wojciszke, B. (2007). Agency and

communion from the perspective of self versus others. *Journal of Personality and Social Psychology, 93*(5), 751–763.

Abele, A. E., & Wojciszke, B. (2014). Communal and agentic content in social cognition: A dual perspective model. In J. M. Olson & M. P. Zanna (Eds.), *Advances in experimental social psychology* (pp. 195–255). San Diego, CA: Academic Press.

Alexander, M. G., Brewer, M. B., & Hermann, R. K. (1999). Images and affect: A functional analysis of out-group stereotypes. *Journal of Personality and Social Psychology, 77*(1), 78–93.

Allport, G. W. (1954). *The nature of prejudice.* Reading, MA: Addison-Wesley.

Asch, S. E. (1946). Forming impressions of personality. *Journal of Abnormal and Social Psychology, 46,* 303–314.

Bai, X., Ramos, M. R., & Fiske, S. T. (2020). As diversity increases, people paradoxically perceive social groups as more similar. *Proceedings of the National Academy of Sciences of the USA, 117*(23), 12741–12749.

Bales, R. F. (1950). *Interaction process analysis: A method for the study of small groups.* Reading, MA: Addison-Wesley.

Bergsieker, H. B., Leslie, L. M., Constantine, V. S., & Fiske, S. T. (2012). Stereotyping by omission: Eliminate the negative, accentuate the positive. *Journal of Personality and Social Psychology, 102*(6), 1214–1238.

Bergsieker, H. B., Shelton, J. N., & Richeson, J. A. (2010). To be liked versus respected: Divergent goals in interracial interactions. *Journal of Personality and Social Psychology, 99*(2), 248–264.

Brambilla, M., Carnaghi, A., & Ravenna, M. (2011). Status and cooperation shape lesbian stereotypes: Testing predictions from the stereotype content model. *Social Psychology, 42*(2), 101–110.

Brambilla, M., & Riva, P. (2017). Self-image and Schadenfreude: Pleasure at others' misfortune enhances satisfaction of basic human needs. *European Journal of Social Psychology, 47,* 399–411.

Brambilla, M., Rusconi, P., Sacchi, S., & Cherubini, P. (2011). Looking for honesty: The primary role of morality (vs. sociability and competence) in information gathering. *European Journal of Social Psychology, 41,* 135–143.

Brambilla, M., Sacchi, S., Rusconi, P., Cherubini, P., & Yzerbyt, V. Y. (2012). You want to give a good impression? Be honest!: Moral traits dominate group impression formation. *British Journal of Social Psychology, 51,* 149–166.

Burkley, E., Durante, F., Fiske, S. T., Burkley, M., & Andrade, A. (2017). Structure and content of Native American stereotypic subgroups: Not just

(ig)noble. *Cultural Diversity and Ethnic Minority Psychology, 23*(2), 209–219.

Cikara, M., Botvinick, M. M., & Fiske, S. T. (2011). Us versus them: Social identity shapes neural responses to intergroup competition and harm. *Psychological Science, 22,* 306–313.

Cikara, M., Bruneau, E. G., & Saxe, R. R. (2011). Us and them: Intergroup failures of empathy. *Current Directions in Psychological Science, 20*(3), 149–153.

Cikara, M., & Fiske, S. T. (2012). Stereotypes and Schadenfreude: Affective and physiological markers of pleasure at outgroup misfortunes. *Social Psychological and Personality Science, 3*(1), 63–71.

Clausell, E., & Fiske, S. T. (2005). When do subgroup parts add up to the stereotypic whole?: Mixed stereotype content for gay male subgroups explains overall ratings. *Social Cognition, 23*(2), 161–181.

Cuddy, A. J., Fiske, S. T., & Glick, P. (2007). The BIAS map: Behaviors from intergroup affect and stereotypes. *Journal of Personality and Social Psychology, 92*(4), 631–648.

Cuddy, A. J., Fiske, S. T., Kwan, V. S., Glick, P., Demoulin, S., Leyens, J. P., et al. (2009). Stereotype content model across cultures: Towards universal similarities and some differences. *British Journal of Social Psychology, 48*(1), 1–33.

Cuddy, A. J., Norton, M. I., & Fiske, S. T. (2005). This old stereotype: The pervasiveness and persistence of the elderly stereotype. *Journal of Social Issues, 61*(2), 267–285.

Dupree, C. H., & Fiske, S. T. (2019). Self-presentation in interracial settings: The competence downshift by white liberals. *Journal of Personality and Social Psychology, 117*(3), 579–604.

Durante, F., Fiske, S. T., Gelfand, M. J., Crippa, F., Suttora, C., Stillwell, A., et al. (2017). Ambivalent stereotypes link to peace, conflict, and inequality across 38 nations. *Proceedings of the National Academy of Sciences of the USA, 114*(4), 669–674.

Durante, F., Fiske, S. T., Kervyn, N., Cuddy, A. J., Akande, A. D., Adetoun, B. E., et al. (2013). Nations' income inequality predicts ambivalence in stereotype content: How societies mind the gap. *British Journal of Social Psychology, 52*(4), 726–746.

Durante, F., Tablante, C. B., & Fiske, S. T. (2017). Poor but warm, rich but cold (and competent): Social classes in the stereotype content model. *Journal of Social Issues, 73*(1), 138–157.

Eckes, T. (2002). Paternalistic and envious gender stereotypes: Testing predictions from the stereotype content model. *Sex Roles, 47*(3–4), 99–114.

Ellemers, N., Pagliaro, S., Barreto, M., & Leach, C. W. (2008). Is it better to be moral than smart?: The effects of morality and competence norms on the decision to work at group status improvement. *Journal of Personality and Social Psychology, 95,* 1397–1410.

Fiske, S. T. (1998). Stereotyping, prejudice, and discrimination. In D. T. Gilbert, S. T. Fiske, & G. Lindzey (Eds.), *Handbook of social psychology* (4th ed., Vol. 2, pp. 357–411). New York: McGraw-Hill.

Fiske, S. T. (2015). Intergroup biases: A focus on stereotype content. *Current Opinion in Behavioral Sciences, 3,* 45–50.

Fiske, S. T., Bergsieker, H. B., Russell, A. M., & Williams, L. (2009). Images of Black Americans: Then, "them," and now, "Obama!" *Du Bois Review: Social Science Research on Race, 6*(1), 83–101.

Fiske, S. T., Cuddy, A. J. C., Glick, P., & Xu, J. (2002). A model of (often mixed) stereotype content: Competence and warmth respectively follow from perceived status and competition. *Journal of Personality and Social Psychology, 82*(6), 878–902.

Fiske, S. T., Xu, J., Cuddy, A. J. C., & Glick, P. (1999). (Dis)respecting versus (dis)liking: Status and interdependence predict ambivalent stereotypes of competence and warmth. *Journal of Social Issues, 55,* 473–491.

Gebauer, J., Wagner, J., Sedikides, C., & Neberich, W. (2013). Agency–communion and self-esteem relations are moderated by culture, religiosity, age, and sex: Evidence for the "self-centrality breads self-enhancement" principle. *Journal of Personality, 81,* 261–275.

Glick, P., & Fiske, S. T. (1996). The Ambivalent Sexism Inventory: Differentiating hostile and benevolent sexism. *Journal of Personality and Social Psychology, 70,* 491–512.

Goodwin, G. P., Piazza, J., & Rozin, P. (2014). Moral character predominates in person perception and evaluation. *Journal of Personality and Social Psychology, 106*(1), 148–168.

Grigoryan, L., Bai, X., Durante, F., Fiske, S. T., Berdyna, E. M., Fabrykant, M., et al. (2020). Stereotypes as historical accidents: Social class stereotypes in post-communist versus capitalist societies. *Personality and Social Psychology Bulletin, 46*(6), 927–943.

Harris, L. T., & Fiske, S. T. (2009). Dehumanized perception: The social neuroscience of thinking (or not thinking) about disgusting people. In M. Hewstone & W. Stroebe (Eds.), *European review of social psychology* (Vol. 20, pp. 192–231). London: Wiley.

Holoien, D. S., & Fiske, S. T. (2013). Downplaying positive impressions: Compensation between warmth and competence in impression management. *Journal of Experimental Social Psychology, 49*(1), 33–41.

Imhoff, R., & Koch, A. (2017). How orthogonal are the Big Two of social perception?: On the curvilinear relation between agency and communion. *Perspectives on Psychological Science, 12,* 122–137.

Jones, E. E. (1990). *Interpersonal perception.* New York: Freeman.

Judd, C. M., James-Hawkins, L., Yzerbyt, V., & Kashima, Y. (2005). Fundamental dimensions of social judgment: Understanding the relations between judgments of competence and warmth. *Journal of Personality and Social Psychology, 89*(6), 899–913.

Katz, D., & Braly, K. (1933). Racial stereotypes of one hundred college students. *Journal of Abnormal and Social Psychology, 28,* 280–290.

Kervyn, N., Bergsieker, H. B., & Fiske, S. T. (2012). The innuendo effect: Hearing the positive but inferring the negative. *Journal of Experimental Social Psychology, 48*(1), 77–85.

Kervyn, N., Fiske, S. T., & Malone, C. (2012). Brands as intentional agents framework: How perceived intentions and ability can map brand perception. *Journal of Consumer Psychology, 22*(2), 166–176.

Kervyn, N., Fiske, S. T., & Yzerbyt, V. Y. (2013). Integrating the stereotype content model (warmth and competence) and the Osgood semantic differential (evaluation, potency, and activity). *European Journal of Social Psychology, 43*(7), 673–681.

Kervyn, N., Fiske, S., & Yzerbyt, V. (2015). Forecasting the primary dimension of social perception. *Social Psychology, 46,* 36–45.

Kervyn, N., Yzerbyt, V. Y., & Judd, C. M. (2011). When compensation guides inferences: Indirect and implicit measures of the compensation effect. *European Journal of Social Psychology, 41*(2), 144–150.

Klohnen, E. C., & Luo, S. (2003). Interpersonal attraction and personality: What is attractive—self similarity, ideal similarity, complementarity or attachment security? *Journal of Personality and Social Psychology, 85,* 709–722.

Koch, A., Dorrough, A., Glöckner, A., & Imhoff, R. (2020). The ABC of society: Perceived similarity in agency/socioeconomic success and conservative-progressive beliefs increases intergroup cooperation. *Journal of Experimental Social Psychology, 90.*

Koch, A., Imhoff, R., Dotsch, R., Unkelbach, C., & Alves, H. (2016). The ABC of stereotypes about groups: Agency/socio-economic success, conservative-progressive beliefs, and communion. *Journal of Personality and Social Psychology, 110,* 675–709.

Koch, A., Imhoff, R., Unkelbach, C., Nicolas, G.,

Fiske, S. T., Terache, J., et al. (in press). Groups' warmth is a personal matter: Understanding consensus on stereotype dimensions reconciles adversarial models of social evaluation. *Journal of Experimental Social Psychology.*

Kunda, Z., Miller, D. T., & Claire, T. (1990). Combining social concepts: The role of causal reasoning. *Cognitive Science, 14*(4), 551–577.

Leach, C. W., Ellemers, N., & Barreto, M. (2007). Group virtue: The importance of morality (vs. competence and sociability) in the positive evaluation of in-groups. *Journal of Personality and Social Psychology, 93,* 234–249.

Lee, T. L., & Fiske, S. T. (2006). Not an outgroup, not yet an ingroup: Immigrants in the stereotype content model. *International Journal of Intercultural Relations, 30*(6), 751–768.

Macrae, C. N., & Bodenhausen, G. V. (2000). Social cognition: Thinking categorically about others. *Annual Review of Psychology, 51,* 93–120.

Nicolas, G., Bai, X., & Fiske, S. T. (2020). *Spontaneous stereotype content model: Taxonomy and process.* Manuscript under review.

Nicolas, G., Fiske, S. T., Koch, A., Imhoff, R., Unkelbach, C., Terache, J., et al. (2020). *Relational versus structural goals moderate social information-gathering priorities.* Manuscript under review.

Pettigrew, T. F. (1979). The ultimate attribution error: Extending Allport's cognitive analysis of prejudice. *Personality and Social Psychology Bulletin, 5*(4), 461–476.

Osgood, C. E., Suci, G. J., & Tannenbaum, R. H. (1957). *The measurement of meaning.* Urbana: University of Illinois Press.

Ramos, M. R., Bennett, M. R., Massey, D. S., & Hewstone, M. (2019). Humans adapt to social diversity over time. *Proceedings of the National Academy of Sciences of the USA, 116*(25), 12244–12249.

Rosenberg, S., Nelson, C., & Vivekananthan, P. S. (1968). A multidimensional approach to the structure of personality impressions. *Journal of Personality and Social Psychology, 9*(4), 283–294.

Ross, L. (1977). The intuitive psychologist and his shortcomings: Distortions in the attribution process. In *Advances in experimental social psychology* (Vol. 10, pp. 173–220). New York: Academic Press.

Russell, A. M. T., & Fiske, S. T. (2008). It's all relative: Competition and status drive interpersonal perception. *European Journal of Social Psychology, 38*(7), 1193–1201.

Sevillano, V., & Fiske, S. T. (2016a). Animals as so-

cial objects: Groups, stereotypes, and intergroup threats. *European Psychologist, 21*(3), 206–217.

Sevillano, V., & Fiske, S. T. (2016b). Warmth and competence in animals. *Journal of Applied Social Psychology, 46*(5), 276–293.

Speelman, C. P., & McGann, M. (2013). How mean is the mean? *Frontiers in Psychology, 4,* 451.

Swencionis, J. K., & Fiske, S. T. (2016). Promote up, ingratiate down: Status comparisons drive warmth-competence tradeoffs in impression management. *Journal of Experimental Social Psychology, 64,* 27–34.

Tajfel, H., & Turner, J. C. (1986). The social identity theory of intergroup behavior. In S. W. Worchel & W. G. Austin (Eds.), *The psychology of intergroup relations* (pp. 7–24). Chicago: Hall.

Talaska, C. A., Fiske, S. T., & Chaiken, S. (2008). Legitimating racial discrimination: A meta-analysis of the racial attitude–behavior literature shows that emotions, not beliefs, best predict discrimination. *Social Justice Research: Social Power in Action, 21,* 263–296.

Wojciszke, B. (2005). Morality and competence in person and self perception. *European Review of Social Psychology, 16,* 155–188.

Wojciszke, B., Baryla, W., Parzuchowski, M., Szymkow, A., & Abele, A. E. (2011). Self-esteem is dominated by agentic over communal information. *European Journal of Social Psychology, 41,* 617–627.

Wojciszke, B., Bazinska, R., & Jaworski, M. (1998). On the dominance of moral categories in impression formation. *Personality and Social Psychology Bulletin, 24,* 1245–1257.

Wojciszke, B., & Szymkow, A. E. (2003). Emotions related to others' competence and morality. *Polish Psychological Bulletin, 34,* 135–142.

Wu, S. J., Bai, X., & Fiske, S. T. (2018). Admired rich or resented rich?: How two cultures vary in envy. *Journal of Cross-Cultural Psychology, 49*(7), 1114–1143.

Ybarra, O., Chan, E., & Park, D. (2001). Young and old adults' concerns about morality and competence. *Motivation and Emotion, 25,* 85–100.

Yzerbyt, V. Y., Kervyn, N., & Judd, C. M. (2008). Compensation versus halo: The unique relations between the fundamental dimensions of social judgment. *Personality and Social Psychology Bulletin, 34*(8), 1110–1123.

Yzerbyt, V., Provost, V., & Corneille, O. (2005). Not competent but warm . . . really?: Compensatory stereotypes in the French-speaking world. *Group Processes and Intergroup Relations, 8*(3), 291–308.

CHAPTER 21

Perceiving Others as Group Members

Basic Principles of Social Categorization Processes

Kerry Kawakami
Kurt Hugenberg
Yarrow Dunham

The implications of categorizing people into groups have long been a focal theme of research in social psychology (Allport, 1954) and there is no denying the broad impact of categorization on downstream social judgments. Besides leading to a general overestimation of perceived within-category similarity and between-category differences (Corneille & Judd, 1999; Krueger & Clement, 1994), construing targets as members of a social group activates corresponding group-specific knowledge structures. This activation can influence evaluations of the targets (Dunham, 2011; Kawakami, Phills, Steele, & Dovidio, 2007), the characteristics that we attribute to them (Amodio, 2014; Kawakami, Dovidio, Moll, Hermsen, & Russin, 2000), and the extent to which we associate the self with targets (Greenwald & Farnham, 2000; Phills, Kawakami, Tabi, Nadolny, & Inzlicht, 2011). These processes, in turn, have consequences for emotion identification (Bijlstra, Holland, Dotsch, Hugenberg, & Wigboldus, 2014; Friesen et al., 2019; Hugenberg & Bodenhausen, 2003, 2004), empathy with targets and responses to intergroup bias (Cikara, Botvinick, & Fiske, 2011; Karmali, Kawakami, & Page-Gould, 2017; Kawakami, Dunn, Karmali, & Dovidio,

2009), interpersonal behaviors such as social distancing (Amodio & Devine, 2006; Dovidio, Kawakami, Johnson, Johnson, & Howard, 1997), and support for public policy aimed at reducing discrimination (Hardin & Banaji, 2013; Lai et al., 2016).

Whereas this research has examined a wide range of *outcomes* related to social categorization, of late, the *process* of social categorization itself has also come under scrutiny. Our primary goal in this chapter is to describe current theory and research related to how and when people are categorized as members of a social group (Freeman & Ambady, 2011; Freeman, Stolier, & Brooks, 2020). Specifically, we outline four basic principles of this initial person construal phase, while also highlighting the primary methodologies used in this broad research domain.

There are four basic principles of social categorization:

- *Principle 1:* Social categorization begins in early infancy and develops throughout childhood.
- *Principle 2:* Social categorization is dynamic and influenced by both bottom-up target cues and top-down perceiver characteristics.

411

- *Principle 3:* Social categorization is not inevitable.
- *Principle 4:* Social categorization is influenced by cultural norms.

In our discussion of these four principles, we focus on categorization from the first year of life onward, while also highlighting recent advances in specific techniques that researchers employ to measure categorization and its downstream consequences. Although a comprehensive review of theory, methods, and findings in social categorization is beyond the scope of this chapter (see Kawakami, Amodio, & Hugenberg, 2017), our goal is to describe current theorizing and to include some of the most common methods used to study a variety of different target categories (e.g., gender, race) and participant populations (e.g., infants, children, adults).

Principle 1: Social Categorization Begins in Early Infancy and Develops throughout Childhood

The general premises that categorization is a foundation for intergroup processes and that categorization is culturally bounded are two of the oldest active ideas in social psychology. Indeed, Lippman's (1922) original definition of stereotypes as a simplifying schema—a "picture or image in a person's mind, not based on personal experience but derived culturally"—presumes both an act of social categorization and that these category distinctions are learned through socialization (Dunham & Olson, 2008). Subsequent theorizing by Allport (1954) and Tajfel and Turner (1979; see also Dunham, 2018) on the "normality" of categorization underlines the notion that intergroup bias may be part of an early and general tendency for humans to make us–them differentiations.

From birth, babies are drawn to faces and face-like stimuli, orienting toward and looking longer at them than otherwise matched non-face-like displays (Pascalis & Slater, 2003). This visual attention guides babies toward engagement with their primary caregivers and facilitates the recognition of mothers and familiar others. The early extraction of individual identity from faces, however, quickly gives rise to a broader bias for specific *kinds* of faces

(Kawakami, Friesen, & Vingilis-Jaremko, 2018). For example, infants begin to show longer looking toward same-race faces and female faces by 3 months of age (Bar-Haim, Ziv, Lamy, & Hodes, 2006; Quinn, Yahr, Kuhn, Slater, & Pascalis, 2002). These effects appear to be based on greater exposure to same-race and female primary caregivers, as they reverse in infants who were cross-racially adopted or who have a male primary caregiver. Interestingly, these effects of familiarity extend beyond mere attention and appear to reflect the construction of broader face prototypes, as well as superior same-race face discrimination. Indeed, younger infants are better at distinguishing other-race faces and even other-species faces than their older counterparts (Kelley et al., 2007, Pascalis, 2002). These processes, which closely parallel changes in phonological development (in which early abilities to distinguish non-native phonemes are lost over the first year of life; Kuhl, 1999), appear to reflect perceptual tuning designed to increase sensitivity to the most frequently encountered class of stimuli, in this case, the sorts of faces that characterize one's cultural group. As in the phonemic domain, better precision in the target domain has trade-offs, namely, a declining ability to distinguish outgroup (or outspecies) faces.

Toward the end of the first year of life, infants' responses begin to go beyond preferential attention and come to resemble categorization processes, in that babies familiarized to faces of one race will show renewed interest, dishabituation, to other-race faces (Anzures, Quinn, Pascalis, Slater, & Lee, 2010). Similar results emerge for gender when depicted visually or even auditorially via gender-typical voices (Miller, 1983; Quinn et al., 2002). Still, caution is warranted in interpreting these findings. The two primary methods used in infant research are preferential looking and habituation–dishabituation paradigms. Although both have been immensely informative, they have limitations that should be clearly acknowledged.

In a standard *preferential looking paradigm,* two stimuli are presented, and attention toward each is measured, with greater attention for one class of stimulus indicating some form of differentiation. Importantly, however, biases in *attention* are not necessarily evidence of positive social attitudes. Indeed, while somewhat older babies continue to attend more to same-race compared to other-race adult faces, they are not more likely to socially engage with or take food from same-race adults. This is not because they never engage in those richer forms of group-based preference; they do show both greater looking time and partiality in social engagement for speakers of their native language (Kinzler, Dupoux, & Spelke, 2012; Shutts, Kinzler, McKee, & Spelke, 2009). Furthermore, as we do not generally know what features of faces draw the attention of babies, it would be hasty to conclude that whatever differentiation babies are engaged in maps directly onto adult social categories such as race or gender.

Habituation methodologies present the possibility of stronger inferences. In a standard habituation paradigm, an infant might be shown a lengthy sequence of distinct female faces, for example, until they appear to grow disinterested, as evidenced by a decline in looking toward the new face. A male face is then interspersed into the sequence. If the infant recovers from habituation by orienting to the male face, it provides evidence that the child must have categorized the string of female targets as one category, then noted the change when the male face appeared. But again, it is difficult to know what features infants were attending to and how other details of the study design influenced attention. For example, infants may have habituated to long hair and responded to a change to short hair. Although this feature surely correlates with the category of sex or gender, it is not equivalent to this category. Ruling out such potential confounds requires careful work. Furthermore, even if infants can extract a category from a series of stimuli, it does not necessarily follow that they spontaneously make use of those categories in everyday life or that these categories are activated and used in ways typical of adults.

So when do children make explicit category judgments by placing targets into race and gender categories in ways that dovetail with adult classifications? Successful explicit categorization of photographs by gender appears to emerge just after the second birthday (Campbell, Shirley, & Caygill, 2002), with the spontaneous use of gendered language also emerg-

ing around this time (Zosuls et al., 2009). The case with race is somewhat more controversial. Early work suggested competencies that are in place by around ages 3–4, with high levels of categorization ability appearing soon thereafter (e.g., Hraba & Grant, 1970). However, this work tended to use very simple dichotomous forced-choice tasks with highly prototypical stimuli, which may have overestimated early abilities. More recent work suggests that development of race-based categorization is related to more complex perceptual learning that continues at least into early adolescence, with younger children's judgments dominated by skin color over other featural cues (Dunham, Dotsch, Clark, & Stepanova, 2016; Dunham, Stepanova, Dotsch, Todorov, 2015).

Whereas the latter research focuses on social categorization that is directly elicited by an experimental task, also of interest are more spontaneous processes that occur in the flow of ordinary behavior. Although there is a relative scarcity of work investigating spontaneous categorization in children, researchers have utilized the "Who said what?" paradigm to examine more implicit processes (Taylor, Fiske, Etcoff, & Ruderman, 1978). In this paradigm, participants are typically presented with statements made by a number of different individuals. In a subsequent surprise memory test, they are instructed to identify the person who made each statement. The results typically demonstrate greater intracategory errors (i.e., confusing members within one group) than intercategory errors (i.e., confusing members between two groups). For example, something said by a woman will be misattributed to another woman at higher rates than it is misattributed to a man. Although these methods were pioneered with adult populations, extensions to developmental populations indicate the automatic encoding of gender by around age 4, with more mixed results for the spontaneous categorization of race, which does not emerge until several years later (Bennet & Sani, 2003; Weisman, Johnson, & Shutts, 2015). Thus, gender appears to be more salient than race in children's early lives, despite their ability to use both, and their tendency to show social biases on the basis of both. While the reasons for this difference are not yet wholly clear, the fact that most children experience gender-differentiated caregiving as well as rich linguistic input marking gender boundaries seems to be particularly relevant (Bigler & Liben, 2007).

Learning Associations with Social Categories

Children also gradually internalize cultural associations about groups. By preschool, children know the stereotypes of gender, believing that same-gender children will like the same kinds of toys and activities (Berndt & Heller, 1986; Biernat, 1991). They also believe that a girl raised in an environment in which she is surrounded by boys will still grow up to have stereotypically female properties (and vice versa for boys; Taylor, Rhodes, & Gelman, 2009), which may indicate that gender is essentialized. However, children at these ages do not hold similarly rich expectations about the inductive potential and stability of race (Rhodes & Gelman, 2009). Indeed, knowledge of consensual racial stereotypes does not reliably emerge until at least middle childhood (Pauker, Ambady, & Apfelbaum, 2010). Children do, however, tend to essentialize at least some ethnic/racial social categories, assuming that members of the same social category will share characteristics and attitudes (Diesendruck & HaLevi, 2006; Kalish & Lawson, 2008; Waxman, 2010).

Distinct from stereotypes, which require learning culturally held category-associated characteristics, children generally show an ingroup bias. For example, by the preschool years, children (at least in higher-status majority groups) express positive views of ingroup members and negative views of outgroup members with respect to race (Kinzler, Schutts, & Spelke, 2012; Rutland, Cameron, Bennett, & Ferrell, 2005), gender (Halim, Ruble, Tamis-LeMonda, Shrout, & Amodio, 2017; Hilliard & Liben, 2010), religion (Heiphetz, Spelke, & Banaji, 2013), and nationality (Barrett, 2005).

As suggested by these results, how we categorize people has important implications for not only targets but also the self. One of the most basic forms of bias is the belief that members of outgroups are different from the self (Phills et al., 2011; Phills, Kawakami, Krusemark, & Nyguen, 2019). Perceiving other peo-

ple as being a part of a group in which we are not members (outgroup) compared to a group in which we are members (ingroup) can have significant consequences for impression formation processes and intergroup relations (Tajfel & Turner, 1979; Turner, Hogg, Oakes, Reicher, & Wetherell, 1987). Although in general, people may assume similarity with others, if a person is categorized as a member of a social group different than the perceiver's, he or she may be expected to share few similarities with the perceiver (Danyluck & Page-Gould, 2018; Insko, Nacoste, & Moe, 1983; Mallett, Wilson, & Gilbert, 2008; Rokeach, Smith, & Evans, 1960; Vorauer, Main, & O'Connell, 1998; Vorauer & Sakamoto, 2006; West, Magee, Gordon, & Gullett, 2014).

Research has investigated the impact of ingroup and outgroup distinctions with groups that are perceived to be socially relevant as well as with groups that are quite arbitrary (e.g., based on dot-estimations or random category assignment). This work indicates that both children and adults often react to these novel, experimentally created, minimal groups (Dunham, 2018) in ways that are similar to societally meaningful social categories. For example, adults and children as young as 3 prefer others assigned to their minimal ingroup on measures of liking, friendship preference, and even implicit measures such as the Implicit Association Test (IAT; Baron & Dunham, 2015; Dunham, Baron, & Banaji, 2008; Dunham, Baron, & Carey, 2011; Richter, Over, & Dunham, 2016).

Children are also attuned to social hierarchies within and between groups. Indeed, they generally seem to prefer individuals and groups in higher-status positions. This phenomenon is most clearly visible when we compare the intergroup attitudes of children from higher-status majority groups (e.g., White Americans) and children from lower-status minority groups (e.g., Black or Latino Americans). In such cases, the modal pattern is that members of minority groups show diminished ingroup biases, at least when comparing themselves to the dominant majority (Dunham, Baron, & Banaji, 2007; Newheiser & Olson, 2012). These findings are generally interpreted as the internalization of social status and power (Dunham et al., 2008;

Steele, George, Williams, & Tay, 2018). Thus, attention to us and them, as well as to social hierarchies, provides children with a rich set of building blocks, which they use to build a sophisticated map of their culturally determined social order.

Principle 2: Social Categorization Is Dynamic and Influenced by Both Bottom-Up Target Cues and Top-Down Perceiver Characteristics

At first glance, social categorization may seem to be a process that is switched on or off in a wholesale manner by the presence or absence of a single categorical feature. However, both past and recent theorizing suggest a more complex process in which categorization processes are a function of both top-down perceiver characteristics and bottom-up cues from the target. For example, Higgins (1996) proposed that the categorization of stimuli might be related to the accessibility of a categorical construct (a property of the perceiver) and the fit between this stored knowledge and the stimuli (a property of the target). In terms of intergroup processes, a social category that is readily accessible through chronic or momentary activation, expectations, or goals is more likely to be used when the attended features of the target are applicable to the accessible category information. For example, according to this theorizing, if a perceiver has recently read a novel about conservative ideologies, the perceiver would be more likely to categorize an individual male as a Republican, if his facial and body features fit expectations related to this category (e.g., middle-aged or elderly and White). Similarly, perceivers who see the same Asian woman may be more likely to think of her in terms of her gender when seeing her putting on makeup (a female stereotypical behavior) than when eating noodles with chopsticks (an Asian stereotypical behavior; Macrae, Bodenhausen, & Milne, 1995).

More recent theorizing proposes that the coactivation of targets' physical attributes and perceivers' associations, expectations, and goals interact *dynamically* over time to constrain which of many potential categories will ultimately be used as a basis for person perception (Freeman & Ambady, 2011; Freeman et al., 2020). Specifically, this model suggests that although early perceptual information from a target may be partially consistent and inconsistent with multiple categories, an interplay between bottom-up target cues and top-down perceiver characteristics that activate in parallel a variety of category-relevant information is ongoing until one category dominates the process, resulting in the stable construal of the target as a member of a specific group.

Research utilizing a novel *mouse tracking* paradigm provides evidence for this latter model related to a parallel constraint process. In this task, researchers use computer mouse trajectories over time to infer the activation of category-related content during person construal. In particular, participants are typically presented with a human face and move the mouse from the bottom center of the screen to the top left or top right of the screen to indicate the relevant social category. For example, participants may be instructed to categorize a target face as male or female. When male faces include both feminine and masculine characteristics (e.g., long hair and strong jaw), the mouse trajectory may "pull" more strongly toward the female category than when male faces include primarily male characteristics (e.g., short hair and strong jaw). In short, the coactivation of the female and male category for the former faces will result in a larger arc than the more direct mouse trajectory related to the latter faces (Freeman, Ambady, Rule, & Johnson, 2008). Although both types of faces may result in the ultimate classification of the target as a man at similar rates, the process itself is affected by competing cues that can subtly affect the dynamics of social categorization.

Social Categorization Is Influenced by Bottom-Up Cues

In line with both classic and recent models of social categorization, the preceding mouse-tracking example underlines the importance of perceptual qualities of the target in this process (Freeman & Johnson, 2016; Macrae & Bodenhausen, 2000). In particular, bottom-up cues related to facial features, body shapes, and movement activate category content, which is then integrated to determine person construal.

Face Perception

Because faces are a rich source of social information, they are processed in special ways and are singularly influential when forming impressions of others (Hugenberg & Wilson, 2013; Zebrowitz, 2006). Specifically, faces are processed in face-specialized regions of the brain (Haxby, Hoffman, & Gobbini, 2000; Kanwisher, McDermott, & Chun, 1997) and in a more Gestalt manner than are most other objects (Maurer, Le Grand, & Mondloch, 2002; Tanaka & Gauthier, 1997). Numerous facial features (e.g., skin tone, facial roundness, nose or eye shape) can provide important cues to category membership (Stepanova & Strube, 2012). Furthermore, face processing related to visually obvious social groups occurs very early in the perceptual stream (Ebner, He, Fichtenholtz, McCarthy, & Johnson, 2011; Mouchetant-Rostaing, Girard, Bentin, Aguera, & Pernier, 2000) and continues to impact how we construe others throughout interactions (Freeman & Ambady, 2011; Kawakami et al., 2017).

Body Perception

Beyond faces, perceivers can also extract cues to others' social categories from their bodily shapes and movements (Cutting, 1978; Johnson & Iida, 2013). Although it is probably of no surprise that sex can be categorized from bodily shapes relatively easily and accurately, men and women's different morphology also creates sexually dimorphic kinematics—men and women move differently. Indeed, Cutting's (1978) early work used *point-light displays* to demonstrate that perceivers can differentiate between male and female point-light walkers, absent body shape. Point-light displays are visual images, and typically videos, of multiple dots of light moving against a dark background. By highlighting human joints with glowing dots at a walking figure's feet, knees, hips, shoulders, elbows, and wrists, one can provide the immediate impression of a walking form, without showing the morphology of the body.

Johnson and Tassinary (2005, 2007) have demonstrated that perceivers simultaneously use both body shape and body movement to make their judgments of targets' sex. In this work, perceivers watched computer-animated

human bodies that varied both in sex-typical shape (waist-to-hip ratio) and sex-typical motion (hip sway and shoulder swagger). Participants' sex category decisions relied heavily on body shape, however, judgments of targets' masculinity and femininity relied both on sex-typical body shape and motion. Interestingly, these researchers found that when perceivers already believed that they knew the target's sex, their visual scan patterns changed, focusing far less on the waist and hip regions of the target. Importantly, this work demonstrates that both bottom-up cues from the targets' body form and body movement interact with perceivers' top-down beliefs to influence the search for category diagnostic information and ultimate classification.

Cues related to bodies and bodily motion are also used to classify members of other social categories, such as age, race, and even sexual orientation. For example, Montepare and Zebrowitz-McArthur (1988) created point-light displays of elderly and youthful walkers and found that not only were perceivers able to accurately categorize targets according to age, but that these categorizations led to a commonplace outcome of categorization—stereotyping. In accordance with common associations (e.g., feeble, fragile, helpless, bitter, lonely) related to the elderly (Chasteen, Schwarz, & Park, 2002), point-light displays of elderly individuals were believed to be less powerful and less happy than their more youthful counterparts. Race categories, too, may be extractable from bodily motion. For example, Lick, Golay, and Johnson (2014) found that point-light displays created from White and Asian walkers could be discriminated by race at better-than-chance accuracy based on the belief that Asians move in more feminine ways than Whites.

Concealable Categories

Although categories such as race, sex, and age are often readily extracted from targets' faces and bodies, not all categories may be as easy to discern. For example, so-called "concealable categories" such as religious or political affiliation, or sexual orientation, may have less obvious physical markers of category membership. Despite this, perceivers appear capable of categorizing targets of such groups at above-chance levels (Rule, Garrett, & Ambady, 2010; Tskhay & Rule, 2013). For example, in a typical *"thin slice" paradigm* (Ambady, Hallahan, & Conner, 1999), participants including heterosexual men and women, gay men, and lesbians were presented with 10-second silent video clips, 1-second silent video clips, or still photographs of heterosexual men and women, gay men, and lesbians discussing their balance between extracurricular and academic activities. Participants were instructed to rate the extent to which they thought each target was homosexual and heterosexual. The results demonstrated that participants were able to judge sexual orientation at above-chance levels and that accuracy was greater for video clips that included dynamic nonverbal behavior compared to still photographs.

Extending these findings, computer programs have recently been developed that claim to be able to categorize the sexual orientation of targets from facial cues. In particular, Wang and Kosinski (2018) used 35,326 images from public profiles on a U.S. dating website to train and test a "sexual orientation detector." Notably, they reported 71% accuracy for lesbians and 81% accuracy for gay men using this classification algorithm. The possibility that perceivers (both human and computer) are capable of classifying ostensibly concealable categories with some degree of accuracy suggests that cues must be present that signal membership status (Agüera y Arcas, Mitchell, & Todorov, 2017; Alaei & Rule, 2016; Rule, Ambady, Adams, & Macrae, 2008). The question remains, however, as to whether these cues are related to stable differences in targets' facial structure and body or to more superficial transient differences in image quality, grooming, style, and expressions (Agüera y Arcas, Todorov, & Mitchell, 2018; Cox, Devine, Bischmann, & Hyde, 2015).

Ambiguous or Complex Categories

In addition to membership in more-or-less concealable categories, targets may display cues typical of multiple categories. Categorizing such targets (e.g., targets whose features are phenotypically related to multiple racial categories) may not only be more difficult but also result in a different type of process (Chen & Hamilton, 2012; Pauker, Meyers, Sanchez, Gaither,

& Young, 2018). For example, research using a mouse-tracking task (Freeman, Pauker, Apfelbaum, & Ambady, 2010) demonstrated that categorizing targets who were less prototypical of only one category (e.g., light skinned Black exemplars and dark skinned White exemplars) along racial lines resulted in more attraction to the nondominant category (operationalized as larger arcs) than faces that were more prototypical of a specific race (e.g., dark-skinned Blacks exemplars and light-skinned White exemplars). These results suggest that for biracial targets, White and Black categories may have initially been simultaneously activated before an ultimate racial categorization was reached.

Furthermore, research has demonstrated that the ultimate categorization of biracial targets may be more malleable and vary across perceivers, situations, and time (Chen, Moons, Gaither, Hamilton, & Sherman, 2014; Pauker et al., 2009, 2018). For example, the same target may be perceived in different ways by different people or in different contexts. Part of this instability may be related to a greater influence of top-down factors on categorization processes (Freeman & Ambady, 2011; Higgins, 1996; Kawakami, Amodio, et al., 2017), a topic to which we turn next.

Social Categorization Is Influenced by Top-Down Characteristics

Although initial categorization is constrained by bottom-up cues related to features of the target, these cues interact with top-down characteristics of the perceiver to influence person construal in fundamental ways. In line with Bruner's (1957) classic argument that categorization is, in part, a function of perceivers' readiness to categorize a stimulus, a growing body of research suggests that perceivers' motivations and expectations can affect even the early stages of categorizing social stimuli (Bernstein, Young, Brown, Sacco, & Claypool, 2008; Freeman, Ma, Han, & Ambady, 2013; Ratner & Amodio, 2013). For example, because of cultural stereotypes associating Blacks with the working class and Whites with white-collar jobs, the same racially ambiguous target may be categorized as White more often when wearing a business suit and Black more often when wearing a janitor's uniform (Freeman, Penner,

Saperstein, Scheutz, & Ambady, 2011). Furthermore, holding stereotypes that Blacks are aggressive can lead high-prejudice Whites to categorize the same racially ambiguous face as Black more often when it is angry than when it is happy (Hugenberg & Bodenhausen, 2004; but see Dunham, 2011).

Personal attitudes and beliefs can also influence social categorization. For example, an affinity for group-based hierarchies can interact with threat to generate a stronger tendency to categorize racially ambiguous targets as Black rather than White (Ho, Sidanius, Cuddy, & Banaji, 2013). Believing that traits are immutable (Eberhardt, Dasgupta, & Banaszynski, 2003) can have similar effects on memory. In particular, entity theorists (i.e., people who believe traits are fixed) misremember faces as more racially prototypical than do incremental theorists (i.e., people who believe traits are malleable; see also Corneille, Huart, Becquart, & Brédart, 2004). Likewise, beliefs about economic scarcity can influence categorization. For example, using a *point of subjective equality (PSE)* paradigm, Krosch and Amodio (2014) presented non-Black participants with a series of morphed faces ranging in appearance from predominantly Black prototypical features to predominantly White prototypical features. The participants' task was simply to classify each face as either Black or White. In general, targets were categorized as Black if their faces represented 47% or more Black features. More importantly, the threshold for categorizing a target as Black decreased as scarcity became salient, such that even faces that were predominantly White (with only 35% Black features) were categorized as Black. This pattern was demonstrated both when scarcity was chronically accessible, such as when perceivers believed that Blacks and Whites were in a zero-sum economic competition, and when scarcity was made temporarily accessible, such as when participants were subliminally primed with economic scarcity-related words.

Together these results demonstrate the strong influence that perceiver expectations and beliefs can have on categorization processes. These top-down perceiver characteristics can interact with bottom-up target cues to activate a variety of category-relevant information that

impacts not only the ultimate categorization (e.g., Black vs. White) but also how the process unfolds.

Principle 3: Social Categorization Is Not Inevitable

From our review so far, it should be obvious that categories can become activated and employed in a variety of contexts, even absent perceiver intent. Furthermore, attention to low-level perceptual characteristics of faces that signal social membership related to race, sex, and age can occur quickly. Event-related potential (ERP) studies (Amodio & Bartholow, 2011; Ebner et al., 2011; Mouchetant-Rostaing et al., 2000) and other procedures (Amodio, Bartholow, & Ito, 2013; Kubota & Ito, 2007) provide evidence that we respond to categorical cues very early in the processing stream. For example, Ito and Urland (2003) investigated electrophysiological responses by instructing participants to categorize target faces by race or sex and found that the visual system extracted information related to these perceptually obvious groups within 200 milliseconds. Notably, even when participants were instructed to categorize based on gender, early neural responses to race occurred. Furthermore, these basic categories may become activated even when target faces are presented suboptimally (Cloutier, Mason, & Macrae, 2005; Macrae, Quinn, Mason, & Quadflieg, 2005), subliminally (Bargh, Chen, & Burrows, 1996; Macrae & Martin, 2007), and without intent to categorize (Cañadas, Rodríguez-Bailón, Milliken, & Lupiáñez, 2013; Taylor et al., 1978).

Nonetheless, even in the presence of these initial percepts, neither the activation nor the use of social categories in forming impressions is inevitable. Indeed, in some cases, the category representation does not become active due to contextual or motivational factors, and in other cases, perceivers are able to focus instead on noncategorical, *individuating* information when forming impressions of others.

Failing to Activate Categories

As noted earlier, the process of categorization is influenced dynamically not only by attention to features of the target but also top-down characteristics of the perceiver. These latter factors influence which category will come to dominate the process, as well as the extent or likelihood that a target will be perceived according to a social group (Macrae & Bodenhausen, 2000). Research by Quinn and Macrae (2005), for example, demonstrated that recently activated categories or expectations can affect the strength or relevance of specific categories. Using a *repetition priming paradigm,* these researchers examined whether a prior sex categorization task would influence the speed of subsequent sex categorizations. Specifically, they manipulated whether participants either passively viewed or actively categorized male and female faces by sex. In a subsequent task, participants viewed all of the faces again and were instructed to categorize them by sex as quickly and accurately as possible. The results demonstrated that participants were faster at distinguishing between the sexes if they had categorized the targets' sex in the first task compared to passively viewing the stimuli. In accordance with prior research, these finding suggest that repeated prior knowledge activation reliably increases accessibility (see Higgins, 1996, for a review). Thus, repeated categorization or contextual relevance might be one factor that leads a category to dominate the construal process.

Similarly, perceivers' familiarity with targets can play a role in influencing initial category activation (Bruce, Dench, & Burton, 1993; Bruce & Valentine, 1985). For example, Quinn, Mason, and Macrae (2009) employed a *sequential priming task,* in which they showed participants a series of two faces. They manipulated the sequence of target sex, sometimes presenting sex-congruent faces (e.g., a woman followed by another woman) and sometimes sex-incongruent faces (e.g., a woman followed by a man). Participants were instructed to categorize the second target by sex as quickly and accurately as possible. Not surprisingly, the second target in a sex-congruent pair was categorized more quickly than the second target in a sex-incongruent pair. However, this sequential priming effect did not occur when the second target was highly familiar (i.e., a famous person). Even when participants were instructed to process targets according to sex, presenting a same-sex target before a highly familiar face

did not reduce the speed of categorization, indicating that categorizing targets according to sex for familiar faces was not inevitable. Instead, for familiar others, individuated processing may dominate construals.

Finally, although previous research has demonstrated that attention to categorical features and categorization can occur without intent (Cañadas et al., 2013; Ito & Urland, 2003; Taylor et al., 1978), this process can still be influenced by perceiver goals, motives, and cognitive capacity. Instantiating nonsocial goals or shallow processing may divert attention away from social group memberships and therefore inhibit spontaneous categorization processes. For example, instructing participants to attend to a dot on a stimulus face or to the mere presence of any competing stimulus (both social and nonsocial) can reduce category activation (Macrae, Bodenhausen, Milne, Thorn, & Castelli, 1997). Similarly, when perceivers are cognitively busy during initial encoding, this too can undermine initial category activation (Gilbert & Hixon, 1991). Thus, the activation of even well-learned and often salient social categories may not occur under some processing goals or perceiver states.

Although research indicates that the activation of and attention to certain visible categories (e.g., sex, race, age) can often be fast and unintentional, whether targets are ultimately perceived as members of a category may not be inevitable. Top-down factors such as personal experiences, familiarity, available cognitive capacity, and activated goals are just some of the variables that can influence the final person construal.

Individuating Targets

Even in situations where perceivers may activate categories, categorization need not dominate impressions. Indeed, theorists have long proposed two major approaches to impression formation. One is a category-oriented approach in which impressions are based on membership in social groups and the other is an attribute-oriented approach in which impressions are based on unique characteristics of individuals (Fiske & Neuberg, 1990; Hugenberg, Young, Bernstein, & Sacco, 2010; Macrae & Bodenhausen, 2000). Although categorization can be a powerful cognitive default (Brewer, 1988; Freeman &

Ambady, 2011), theorists propose that at times people also form impressions according to individuation processes (Fiske & Neuberg, 1990). For example, when meeting a septuagenarian for the first time, one's judgments may be primarily related to his or her age (the category *elderly*) or to distinctive individual behavior (e.g., his or her witty and fun banter).

Recently, *eye-tracking* techniques have been employed to investigate individuation and categorization processes. For example, Kawakami and colleagues (2014) presented White participants with a series of faces of Black and White targets, and monitored their attention to the targets' specific facial features. The results demonstrated that White participants attended more to the eyes of ingroup White than outgroup Black faces. Because the eyes easily differentiate between targets (Henderson, Williams, & Falk, 2005), attention to this area may be indicative of individuated processing. In a subsequent study, when White participants were paid to individuate Black targets, perceivers spontaneously attended more to the eyes of Black faces. Notably, in the original study, participants also attended more to the noses and mouths of Black compared to White faces, features that are prototypical of the category Black (Stepanova & Strube, 2012) and indicative of categorical processing. In an additional experiment, no attentional bias was found toward the nose and mouth of faces of minimal groups, in which perceptual features are not related to category membership. However, participants in this study did focus more on the eyes of ingroup relative to outgroup members, providing further evidence for the special role of this feature in intergroup face processing.

In general, these findings indicate how basic intergroup motives may play a role in both the allocation of visual attention and individuation. In accordance with previous theorizing (Hugenberg et al., 2010; Levin, 2000), these results suggest that White participants may be more motivated to process White compared to Black targets as individuals and thereby focus on the eyes. Furthermore, these results suggest that White participants may be more motivated to process Black compared to White targets as category exemplars and therefore focus on category prototypical features such as the nose and mouth. However, these findings also indicate that when sufficiently motivated (e.g., monetary rewards), they are able to overcome these biases (see also Hugenberg, Miller, & Claypool, 2007).

Whereas some models propose a sequential process in which an initial categorization phase is followed by individuation, other models suggest the possibility of the parallel activation of categorical and individuating processes. For example, the continuum model suggests that individuated processing can supplant the categorization of targets when perceivers are sufficiently motivated and able to attend to distinctive target features (Fiske & Neuberg, 1990). Other theories (e.g., Kunda & Thagard, 1996), however, propose that categorical and individuating processes may be co-activated, and at times interact to form a single impression. Supporting this view, Kawakami, Friesen, and Vingilis-Jaremko (2020) discovered independent effects of category information (e.g., race) and individuating information (e.g., perceived interpersonal similarity between the target and self) in person perception using an *Own-Group Bias (OGB)* face memory task.

The OGB task has been used to measure categorization versus individuation processes and the extent to which people are able to recognize members of social groups. In this task, participants are typically first presented with a series of ingroup and outgroup faces. In a subsequent phase, they are once again presented with faces from the previous phase (i.e., old faces) as well as novel faces (i.e., new faces), and they are instructed to simply identify each face as "old" or "new." Whereas the classic finding in the OGB literature is that perceivers are better able to distinguish between old and new ingroup than outgroup faces, instructions to individuate outgroup members can reduce this ingroup advantage (Hugenberg et al., 2007; Kawakami et al., 2014). These latter findings suggest that one reason why people are better at recognizing members of their own group is because they spontaneously process own-group targets as individuals and other-group targets as category members, thereby focusing on identity diagnostic features for ingroup members and category diagnostic features for outgroup faces (Hugenberg & Sacco, 2008; Hugenberg et al., 2010; Levin, 2000; Rhodes, Locke, Ewing, &

Evangelista, 2009; Vingilis-Jaremko, Kawakami, & Friesen, in press). Notably, recent work has indicated that training perceivers to shift attention toward identity diagnostic information, rather than category diagnostic information, can also reduce the OGB (Lebrecht, Pierce, Tarr, & Tanaka, 2009; Qian et al., 2017).

In accordance with past OGB research, Kawakami and colleagues (2020) demonstrated that White participants showed better recognition for faces of White than Black targets (i.e., typical ingroup–outgroup categorization effects). However, these researchers also found that manipulating the extent to which a target was ostensibly more or less similar to the participant on a personality test also influenced recognition. In accordance with early studies showing that for White participants, perceived similarity was related to more liking and a greater willingness to work with both Black and White targets (Byrne & McGraw, 1964; Byrne & Wong, 1962; Insko et al., 1983; Rokeach et al., 1960), the results of the Kawakami and colleagues experiments indicated that as similarity increased, recognition accuracy also increased, regardless of the race of the target. In short, whereas participants continued to show better recognition for ingroup over outgroup faces, perceived similarity improved the processing of individual ingroup and outgroup faces. These findings suggest that participants may have been responding to outgroup targets both in terms of outgroup membership *and* interpersonal similarity, with no evidence that these processes directly interacted.

Taken together, this research provides evidence that in construing others, categorization is not inevitable. Certain targets and goals can impact this process. Although ingroup members and similar others may be construed according to more interpersonal characteristics than outgroup members, motivating people to reduce categorical processing, through such processes as individuation, can be effective in decreasing intergroup biases.

Principle 4: Social Categorization Is Influenced by Cultural Norms

Despite the long history of research on social categorization, there is a relative scarcity of cross-cultural work investigating how culture influences the content and process of social categorization. There is no questioning, however, the fact that these processes are culturally bound. Cultures determine not only whether we will categorize others, but also which cues and categories will be given prominence in this process; that is, cultures provide us with the features to be used as the basis of social classifications, the evaluative and semantic associations with those categories (i.e., prejudices and stereotypes), and the ways in which members of those groups are treated (i.e., norms for behavior).

It is clear that very early in life, children are prolific users of social categories, rapidly learning about the people and groups that populate their environment (Bigler & Liben, 2007). Thus, in many ways a discussion of how culture dictates categorization (our fourth principle) must be rooted in development (our first principle). As we noted earlier, in early infancy, children begin to figure out which determinants related to people and groups are socially meaningful and should therefore garner attention. This process should be considered a specific instantiation of their more general goal of developing a sense of shared reality with their cultural elders (Higgins, 2016). Whereas some categories, such as sex, are perceived to be relevant across cultures (either due to cross-cultural invariance or biological preparation), the importance of many other social categories is more culturally specific. Children also adeptly learn traits, positive or negative evaluations, status, objects, and contexts associated with particular social groups in a given culture (Pauker et al., 2010; Taylor et al., 2009). These associations can directly impact the cultural meaningfulness of a social category. In this section, we explore several potential reasons for cultural variations in how and who we categorize. Some of these reasons are related to differences in specific cultural histories and category associations, whereas other variations have deeper roots in broader cultural processes about how the self is represented.

First, a culture or nation's history can have a large impact on determinants of social categorization and the cultural significance of specific categories. For example, given the unique histories of the United States and Canada, the relevance of categories such as Latino or Hispanic and their use in construal processes differ in each country. Specifically, based on immigration trends and their relationship with Mexico and Latin America, these ethnic categories may be more meaningful in the United States than in Canada. Furthermore, given the importance of changing norms over time, the relevance of specific categories even within a culture will adapt. For example, the significance of the category "Irish" as meaningfully distinct from the category "White" has changed dramatically over the last 200 years in the United States. During the 18th and 19th centuries, the category "Irish" was considered a unique racial category that was quite distinct from the broader category "White" and was highly stigmatized. Over time, the category "Irish" has largely become amalgamated with this broader omnibus category (Ignatiev, 1995). Looking forward, other category representations may be changing as well. For example, given the rapidly shifting attitudes toward gay men and lesbians, the use of this characteristic in the future may also lose its significance as a basis for categorization.

Furthermore, it is not just that different categories are more salient or culturally relevant cross-culturally; *how* categories are represented can also differ. For example, whereas countries like the United States and Brazil may seem to have many cultural, historical, and geographic commonalities, the unique histories of race relations in each country have impacted how they conceive of race (Chen, Couto, Sacco, & Dunham, 2018). In particular, U.S. perceivers generally engage in hypodescent—categorizing mixed-race individuals in terms of the lower-status non-White group. U.S. perceivers also heavily weight parentage information when determining category membership, even over and above phenotypic cues of the target individual. Thus, in the United States, a biracial child of a Black and a White parent is considered Black. By contrast, Brazilian perceivers do not engage in hypodescent and do not use parentage information to make race decisions. Instead, Brazilians use appearance cues, and especially skin color, to determine a target's race. Notably, racial categorization by Brazilians (but not Americans) is influenced by economic cues as

well, perhaps reflecting the internalization of the Brazilian adage "money Whitens."

Recent research has also demonstrated the importance of cultural stereotypes and norms in categorization processes. Specifically, Karasawa, Maass, Rakić, and Kato (2014) demonstrated culture differences in the extent to which age differences in targets were used in spontaneous categorization. Given the importance of age-related status in Japanese culture, these researchers predicted that Japanese but not Italian participants would spontaneously categorize along small differences in age. Using the "Who said what?" paradigm, Japanese and Italian participants were presented with statements associated with a specific number. Half of the participants were told that the number referred to the favorite number of the speaker, and the other participants were told that it referred to the age of the speaker. Importantly, for these latter participants, the ages of the targets were slightly younger (16, 17, and 18) or slightly older (24, 25, and 26) than the participants. The results demonstrated that only when Japanese participants believed the numbers represented age and not just numbers, did they make more within- than between-age errors. In contrast, Italian participants, for whom minor age differences are less meaningful and less related to social status norms, showed no differences in errors across conditions.

Finally, there is extensive research demonstrating that the self is represented differently across cultures. In comparison to individualistic cultures such as the United States, collectivist cultures such as Japan often view the self in relation to others, making group membership generally more accessible (Markus & Kitayama, 1991). This distinction can have potentially important implications for social categorization processes. On the one hand, members of collectivist cultures tend to see social groups as more cohesive, leading them to more readily make stereotype-based inferences about group members (Spencer-Rodgers, Williams, Hamilton, Peng, & Wang, 2007). On the other hand, members of collectivist cultures may be somewhat more selective in deciding to affiliate with groups. For example, some work has shown that members of these cultures show less ingroup bias when assigned to arbitrary minimal groups but more bias with respect to real-world groups (Falk, Heine, & Takemura, 2013; Fischer & Derham, 2016). This seeming tension between a strong versus weak tendency to categorize and demonstrate bias may be resolved by considering the perceived social obligations related to belonging to a group in a collectivist culture. Because of these obligations, members of collectivist cultures may be more reticent in assigning social importance to new potential social identities (Dunham, 2018).

Together these examples highlight the importance of history, global politics, stereotypes, and within-culture norms in dictating and constraining the way in which basic social categorization processes play out. Future research, however, is clearly needed to investigate variations in categorization between and within cultures. In particular, comparing and contrasting how categorization develops in children and how these processes unfold among adults across cultures would be particularly informative in discovering how societies influence basic ingroup and outgroup processes.

Conclusions

Our initial construal of others as members of social categories has important consequences for how we judge and interact with them. We all understand from experience the importance of perceiving someone else, or indeed ourselves, as old or young, Black or White, or male or female. In this chapter, we have described four general principles of social categorization processes. These principles reflect current theorizing and research on the learning of category content and the development of social categorization processes in ways that are often culturally specific. They describe a dynamic process involving the fast and spontaneous activation of categories, determined by both bottom-up cues of targets and top-down expectations and motives of perceivers. In describing these principles, we have also attempted to provide a window into the current state of the field in terms of methodology. Taken together, these principles help to provide a broad but brief overview of how others are categorized as members of social groups based on initial perceptions.

REFERENCES

Agüera y Arcas, B., Mitchell, M., & Todorov, A. (2017). Physiognomy's new clothes. Retrieved from *https://medium.com/@blaisea/physiognomys-new- clothes-f2d4b59fdd6a*.

Agüera y Arcas, B., Todorov, A., & Mitchell, M. (2018). Do algorithms reveal sexual orientation or just expose our stereotypes? Retrieved from *https://medium.com/@blaisea/do-algorithms-reveal-sexual-orientation-or-just-expose-our-stereotypes-d998fafdf477*.

Alaei, R., & Rule, N. O. (2016). Accuracy of perceiving social attributes. In J. A. Hall, M. Schmid Mast, & T. V. West (Eds.), *The social psychology of perceiving others accurately* (pp. 125–142). Cambridge, UK: Cambridge University Press.

Allport, G. W. (1954). *The nature of prejudice.* Washington, DC: Perseus.

Ambady, N., Hallahan, M., & Conner, B. (1999). Accuracy of judgments of sexual orientation from thin slices of behavior. *Journal of Personality and Social Psychology, 77*, 538–547.

Amodio, D. M. (2014). The neuroscience of prejudice and stereotyping. *Nature Reviews Neuroscience, 15*, 670–682.

Amodio, D. M., & Bartholow, B. D. (2011). Event-related potential methods in social cognition. In A. Voss, C. Stahl, & C. Klauer (Eds.), *Cognitive methods in social psychology* (pp. 303–339). New York: Guilford Press.

Amodio, D. M., Bartholow, B. D., & Ito, T. A. (2013). Tracking the dynamics of the social brain: ERP approaches for social cognitive and affective neuroscience. *Social Cognitive and Affective Neuroscience, 9*, 385–393.

Amodio, D. M., & Devine, P. G. (2006). Stereotyping and evaluation in implicit race bias: Evidence for independent constructs and unique effects on behavior. *Journal of Personality and Social Psychology, 91*, 652–661.

Anzures, G., Quinn, P. C., Pascalis, O., Slater, A. M., & Lee, K. (2010). Categorization, categorical perception, and asymmetry in infants' representation of face race. *Developmental Science, 13*, 553–564.

Bar-Haim, Y., Ziv, T., Lamy, D., & Hodes, R. M. (2006). Nature and nurture in own-race face processing. *Psychological Science, 17*, 159–163.

Bargh, J. A., Chen, M., & Burrows, L. (1996). Automaticity of social behavior: Direct effects of trait construct and stereotype activation on action. *Journal of Personality and Social Psychology, 71*, 230–244.

Baron, A. S., & Dunham, Y. (2015). Representing "us" and "them": Building blocks of intergroup cognition. *Journal of Cognition and Development, 16,* 780–801.

Barrett, M. (2005). Children's understanding of, and feelings about, countries and national groups. In M. Barrett & E. Buchanan-Barrow (Eds.), *Children's understanding of society* (pp. 251–285). Hove, UK: Psychology Press.

Bennett, M., & Sani, F. (2003). The role of target gender and race in children's encoding of category-neutral person information. *British Journal of Developmental Psychology, 21,* 99–112.

Berndt, T. J., & Heller, K. A. (1986). Gender stereotypes and social inferences: A developmental study. *Journal of Personality and Social Psychology, 50,* 889–898.

Bernstein, M. J., Young, S. G., Brown, C. M., Sacco, D. F., & Claypool, H. M. (2008). Adaptive responses to social exclusion: Social rejection improves detection of real and fake smiles. *Psychological Science, 19,* 981–983.

Biernat, M. (1991). Gender stereotypes and the relationship between masculinity and femininity: A developmental analysis. *Journal of Personality and Social Psychology, 61,* 351–365.

Bigler, R. S., & Liben, L. S. (2007). Developmental intergroup theory: Explaining and reducing children's social stereotyping and prejudice. *Current Directions in Psychological Science, 16,* 162–166.

Bijlstra, G., Holland, R. W., Dotsch, R., Hugenberg, K., & Wigboldus, D. H. J. (2014). Stereotype associations and emotion recognition. *Personality and Social Psychology Bulletin, 40,* 567–577.

Brewer, M. B. (1988). A dual process model of impression formation. In T. K. Srull & R. S. Wyer, Jr. (Eds.), *Advances in social cognition: Vol. 1. A dual process model of impression formation* (pp. 1–36). Hillsdale, NJ: Erlbaum.

Bruce, V., Dench, N., & Burton, M. (1993). Effects of distinctiveness, repetition and semantic priming on the recognition of face familiarity. *Canadian Journal of Experimental Psychology, 47,* 38–60.

Bruce, V., & Valentine, T. (1985). Identity priming in the recognition of familiar faces. *British Journal of Psychology, 76,* 373–383.

Bruner, J. S. (1957). On perceptual readiness. *Psychological Review, 64,* 123–152.

Byrne, D., & McGraw, C. (1964). Interpersonal attraction towards Negroes. *Human Relations, 17,* 201–213.

Byrne, D., & Wong, T. J. (1962). Racial prejudice, interpersonal attraction, and assumed dissimilarity of attitudes. *Journal of Abnormal and Social Psychology, 65,* 246–253.

Campbell, A., Shirley, L., & Caygill, L. (2002). Sex-typed preferences in three domains: Do two-year-

olds need cognitive variables? *British Journal of Psychology, 93,* 203–217.

Cañadas, E., Rodríguez-Bailón, R., Milliken, B., & Lupiáñez, J. (2013). Social categories as a context for the allocation of attentional control. *Journal of Experimental Psychology: General, 142,* 934–943.

Chasteen, A. L., Schwarz, N., & Park, D. C. (2002). The Activation of Aging Stereotypes in Younger and Older Adults. *Journal of Gerontology B: Psychological Science, 57,* 540–647.

Chen, J. M., Couto, M. C. P. de P., Sacco, A. M., & Dunham, Y. (2018). To be or not to be (Black or Multiracial or White): Cultural variation in racial boundaries. *Social Psychological and Personality Science, 9,* 763–772.

Chen, J. M., & Hamilton, D. L. (2012). Natural ambiguities: Racial categorization of multiracial individuals. *Journal of Experimental Social Psychology, 48,* 152–164.

Chen, J. M., Moons, W. G., Gaither, S. E., Hamilton, D. L., & Sherman, J. W. (2014). Motivation to control prejudice predicts categorization of multiracials. *Personality and Social Psychology Bulletin, 40,* 590–603.

Cikara, M., Botvinick, M. M., & Fiske, S. T. (2011). Us versus them: Social identity shapes neural responses to intergroup competition and harm. *Psychological Science, 22,* 306–313.

Cloutier, J., Mason, M. F., & Macrae, C. N. (2005). The perceptual determinants of person construal: Reopening the social-cognitive toolbox. *Journal of Personality and Social Psychology, 88,* 885–894.

Corneille, O., Huart, J., Becquart, E., & Brédart, S. (2004). When memory shifts toward more typical category exemplars: Accentuation effects in the recollection of ethnically ambiguous faces. *Journal of Personality and Social Psychology, 86,* 236–250.

Corneille, O., & Judd, C. M. (1999). Accentuation and sensitization effects in the categorization of multifaceted stimuli. *Journal of Personality and Social Psychology, 77,* 927–941.

Cox, W. T. L., Devine, P. G., Bischmann, A. A., & Hyde, J. (2015). Inferences about sexual orientation: The role of stereotypes, faces, and the gaydar myth. *Journal of Sex Research, 53,* 157–171.

Cutting, J. E. (1978). Generation of synthetic male and female walkers through manipulation of a biomechanical invariant. *Perception, 7,* 393–405.

Danyluck, C., & Page-Gould, E. (2018). Intergroup dissimilarity predicts physiological synchrony and affiliation in intergroup interaction. *Journal of Experimental Social Psychology, 74,* 111–120.

Diesendruck, G., & HaLevi, H. (2006). The role of

language, appearance, and culture in children's social category-based induction. *Child Development, 77,* 539–553.

Dovidio, J. F., Kawakami, K., Johnson, C., Johnson, B., & Howard, A. (1997). On the nature of prejudice: Automatic and controlled processes. *Journal of Experimental Social Psychology, 33,* 510–540.

Dunham, Y. (2011). An angry = outgroup effect. *Journal of Experimental Social Psychology, 47,* 668–671.

Dunham, Y. (2018). Mere membership. *Trends in Cognitive Sciences, 22,* 780–793.

Dunham, Y., Baron, A. S., & Banaji, M. R. (2007). Children and social groups: A developmental analysis of implicit consistency in Hispanic Americans. *Self and Identity, 6,* 238–255.

Dunham, Y., Baron, A. S., & Banaji, M. R. (2008). The development of implicit intergroup cognition. *Trends in Cognitive Sciences, 12,* 248–253.

Dunham, Y., Baron, A. S., & Carey, S. (2011). Consequences of "minimal" group affiliations in children. *Child Development, 82,* 793–811.

Dunham, Y., Dotsch, R., Clark, A. R., & Stepanova, E. V. (2016). The development of White–Asian categorization: Contributions from skin color and other physiognomic cues. *PLoS ONE, 11,* e0158211.

Dunham, Y., & Olson, K. R. (2008). The importance of origins: Why cognitive development is central to a mature understanding of social cognition. *Open Psychology Journal, 1,* 59–65.

Dunham, Y., Stepanova, E. V., Dotsch, R., & Todorov, A. (2015). The development of race-based perceptual categorization: Skin color dominates early category judgments. *Developmental Science, 18,* 469–483.

Eberhardt, J. L., Dasgupta, N., & Banaszynski, T. L. (2003). Believing is seeing: the effects of racial labels and implicit beliefs on face perception. *Personality and Social Psychology Bulletin, 29,* 360–370.

Ebner, N. C., He, Y., Fichtenholtz, H. M., McCarthy, G., & Johnson, M. K. (2011). Electrophysiological correlates of processing faces of younger and older individuals. *Social, Cognitive, and Affective Neuroscience, 6,* 526–535.

Falk, C. F., Heine, S. J., & Takemura, K. (2013). Cultural variation in the minimal group effect. *Journal of Cross-Cultural Psychology, 45,* 265–281.

Fischer, R., & Derham, C. (2016). Is in-group bias culture-dependent? A meta-analysis across 18 societies. *SpringerPlus, 5,* 1–9.

Fiske, S. T., & Neuberg, S. L. (1990). A continuum of impression formation, from category-based to individuating processes: Influences of information and motivation on attention and interpretation. In M. P. Zanna (Ed.), *Advances in experimental social psychology* (Vol. 23, pp. 1–67). San Diego, CA: Academic Press.

Freeman, J. B., & Ambady, N. (2011). A dynamic interactive theory of person construal. *Psychological Review, 118,* 247–279.

Freeman, J. B., Ambady, N., Rule, N. O., & Johnson, K. L. (2008). Will a category cue attract you?: Motor output reveals dynamic competition across person construal. *Journal of Experimental Psychology: General, 137,* 673–690.

Freeman, J. B., & Johnson, K. L. (2016). More than meets the eye: Split-second social perception. *Trends in Cognitive Sciences, 20,* 362–374.

Freeman, J. B., Ma, Y., Han, S., & Ambady, N. (2013). Influences of culture and visual context on real-time social categorization. *Journal of Experimental Social Psychology, 49,* 206–210.

Freeman, J. B., Pauker, K., Apfelbaum, E., & Ambady, N. (2010). Continuous dynamics in the real-time perception of race. *Journal of Experimental Social Psychology, 46,* 179–185.

Freeman, J. B., Penner, A. M., Saperstein, A., Scheutz, M., & Ambady, N. (2011). Looking the part: Social status cues shape race perception. *PLoS ONE, 6,* e25107.

Freeman, J. B., Stolier, R. M., & Brooks, J. A. (2020). Dynamic interactive theory as a domain general account of social perception. In J. M. Olsen (Ed.), *Advances in experimental social psychology* (Vol. 61, pp. 239–286). Cambridge, MA: Academic Press.

Friesen, J. P., Kawakami, K., Vingilis-Jaremko, L., Caprara, R., Sidhu, D. M., Williams, A., et al. (2019). Perceiving happiness in an intergroup context: The role of race and attention to the eyes in differentiating between true and false smiles. *Journal of Personality and Social Psychology, 116,* 375–395.

Gilbert, D. T., & Hixon, H. J. (1991). The trouble of thinking: Activation and application of stereotypic beliefs. *Journal of Personality and Social Psychology, 60,* 509–517.

Greenwald, A. G., & Farnham, S. D. (2000). Using the implicit association test to measure self-esteem and self-concept. *Journal of Personality and Social Psychology, 79,* 1022–1038.

Greenwald, A. G., McGhee, D. E., & Schwartz, J. L. K. (1998). Measuring individual differences in implicit cognition: The Implicit Association Test. *Journal of Personality and Social Psychology, 74,* 1464–1480.

Halim, M. L. D., Ruble, D. N., Tamis-LeMonda, C. S., Shrout, P. E., & Amodio, D. M. (2017). Gender attitudes in early childhood: Behavioral consequences and cognitive antecedents. *Child Development, 88,* 882–899.

Hardin, C. D., & Banaji, M. R. (2013). The nature of implicit prejudice: Implications for personal and public policy. In E. Shafir (Ed.), *The behavioral foundations of public policy* (pp. 13–31). Princeton University Press.

Haxby, J., Hoffman, E., & Gobbini, M. (2000). The distributed human neural system for face perception. *Trends in Cognitive Sciences, 4,* 223–232.

Heiphetz, L., Spelke, E. S., & Banaji, M. R. (2013). Patterns of implicit and explicit attitudes in children and adults: Tests in the domain of religion. *Journal of Experimental Psychology: General, 142,* 864–879.

Henderson, J. M., Williams, C. C., & Falk, R. J. (2005). Eye movements are functional during face learning. *Memory and Cognition, 33,* 98–106.

Higgins, E. T. (1996). Knowledge activation: Accessibility, applicability, and salience. In E. T. Higgins & A. W. Kruglanski (Eds.), *Social psychology: Handbook of basic principles* (pp. 133–168). New York: Guilford Press.

Higgins, E. T. (2016). Shared-reality development in childhood. *Perspectives on Psychological Science, 11,* 466–495.

Hilliard, L. J., & Liben, L. S. (2010). Differing levels of gender salience in preschool classrooms: Effects on children's gender attitudes and intergroup bias. *Child Development, 81,* 1787–1798.

Ho, A. K., Sidanius, J., Cuddy, A. J. C., & Banaji, M. R. (2013). Status-boundary enforcement and the categorization of Black–White biracials. *Journal of Experimental Social Psychology, 49,* 940–943.

Hraba, J., & Grant, G. (1970). Black is beautiful: A reexamination of racial preference and identification. *Journal of Personality and Social Psychology, 16,* 398–402.

Hugenberg, K., & Bodenhausen, G. V. (2003). Facing prejudice: Prejudice and the perception of facial threat. *Psychological Science, 14,* 640–643.

Hugenberg, K., & Bodenhausen, G. V. (2004). Ambiguity in social categorization: The role of prejudice and facial affect in race categorization. *Psychological Science, 15,* 342–345.

Hugenberg, K., Miller, J., & Claypool, H. M. (2007). Categorization and individuation in the cross-race recognition deficit: Toward a solution to an insidious problem. *Journal of Experimental Social Psychology, 43,* 334–340.

Hugenberg, K., & Sacco, D. F. (2008). Social categorization and stereotyping: How social categorization biases person perception and face memory. *Social and Personality Psychology Compass, 2,* 1052–1072.

Hugenberg, K., & Wilson, J. P. (2013). Faces are central to social cognition. In D. E. Carlston (Ed.), *The Oxford handbook of social cognition* (pp. 167–193). New York: Oxford University Press.

Hugenberg, K., Young, S. G., Bernstein, M. J., & Sacco, D. F. (2010). The categorization-individuation model: An integrative account of the other-race recognition deficit. *Psychological Review, 117,* 1168–1187.

Ignatiev, M. (1995). *How the Irish became White.* New York: Routledge.

Insko, C. A., Nacoste, R. W., & Moe, J. L. (1983). Belief congruence and racial discrimination: Review of the evidence and critical evaluation. *European Journal of Social Psychology, 13,* 153–174.

Ito, T. A., & Urland, G. R. (2003). Race and gender on the brain: Electrocortical measures of attention to the race and gender of multiply categorizable individuals. *Journal of Personality and Social Psychology, 85,* 616–626.

Johnson, K. L., & Iida, M. (2013). *Person (mis) perception: On the functional biases that derail construal of others.* In K. L. Johnson & M. Shiffrar (Eds.), *People watching: Social, perceptual, and neurophysiological studies of body perception* (pp. 203–219). New York: Oxford University Press.

Johnson, K. L., & Tassinary, L. G. (2005). Perceiving sex directly and indirectly: Meaning in motion and morphology. *Psychological Science, 16,* 890–897.

Johnson, K. L., & Tassinary, L. G. (2007). Compatibility of basic social perceptions determines perceived attractiveness. *Proceedings of the National Academy of Sciences USA, 104,* 5246–5251.

Kalish, C. W., & Lawson, C. A. (2008). Development of social category representations: Early appreciation of roles and deontic relations. *Child Development, 79,* 577–593.

Kanwisher, N., McDermott, J., & Chun, M. M. (1997). The fusiform face area: A module in human extrastriate cortex specialized for face perception. *Journal of Neuroscience, 17,* 4302–4311.

Karasawa, M., Maass, A., Rakić, T., & Kato, A. (2014). The emergent nature of culturally meaningful categorization and language use: A Japanese–Italian comparison of age categories. *Journal of Cross-Cultural Psychology, 45,* 431–451.

Karmali, F., Kawakami, K., & Page-Gould, E. (2017). He said what?: Physiological and cognitive responses to imagining and witnessing outgroup racism. *Journal of Experimental Psychology: General, 146,* 1073–1085.

Kawakami, K., Amodio, D. M., & Hugenberg, K. (2017). Intergroup perception and cognition: An integrative framework for understanding the causes and consequences of social categorization. In J. M. Olsen (Ed.), *Advances in experimental so-*

cial psychology (Vol. 55, 1–80). Cambridge, MA: Academic Press.

Kawakami, K., Dovidio, J. F., Moll, J., Hermsen, S., & Russin, A. (2000). Just say no (to stereotyping): Effects of training in the negation of stereotypic associations on stereotype activation. *Journal of Personality and Social Psychology, 78*, 871–888.

Kawakami, K., Dunn, E., Karmali, F., & Dovidio, J. F. (2009). Mispredicting affective and behavioral responses to racism. *Science, 323*, 276–278.

Kawakami, K., Friesen, J., & Vingilis-Jaremko, L. (2018). Visual attention to members of own and other groups: Preferences, determinants, and consequences. *Social Personality Psychology Compass, 12*, e12380.

Kawakami, K., Friesen, J., & Vingilis-Jaremko, L. (2020). *The impact similarity and race on the own race bias.* Manuscript under review.

Kawakami, K., Phills, C. E., Steele, J. R., & Dovidio, J. F. (2007). (Close) distance makes the heart grow fonder: Improving implicit racial attitudes and interracial interactions through approach behaviors. *Journal of Personality and Social Psychology, 92*, 957–971.

Kawakami, K., Williams, A., Sidhu, D., Choma, B. L., Rodriguez-Bailón, R., Cañadas, E., et al. (2014). An eye for the I: Preferential attention to the eyes of ingroup members. *Journal of Personality and Social Psychology, 107*, 1–20.

Kelly, D. J., Quinn, P. C., Slater, A. M., Lee, K., Ge, L., & Pascalis, O. (2007). The other-race effect develops during infancy: Evidence of perceptual narrowing. *Psychological Science, 18*, 1084–1089.

Kinzler, K. D., Dupoux, E., & Spelke, E. S. (2012). "Native" objects and collaborators: Infants' object choices and acts of giving reflect favor for native over foreign speakers. *Journal of Cognition and Development, 13*, 67–81.

Kinzler, K. D., Shutts, K., & Spelke, E. S. (2012). Language-based social preferences among children in South Africa. *Language Learning and Development, 8*, 215–232.

Krosch, A. K., & Amodio, D. M. (2014). Economic scarcity alters the perception of race. *Proceedings of the National Academy of Sciences USA, 111*, 9079–9084.

Krueger, J., & Clement, R. W. (1994). Memory-based judgments about multiple categories: A revision and extension of Tajfel's accentuation theory. *Journal of Personality and Social Psychology, 67*, 35–47.

Kubota, J. T., & Ito, T. A. (2007). Multiple cues in social perception: The time course of processing race and facial expression. *Journal of Experimental Social Psychology, 43*, 738–752.

Kuhl, P. K. (1999). Language, mind, and brain: Ex-

perience alters perception. In M. S. Gazzaniga (Ed.), *The new cognitive neurosciences* (Vol. 2, pp. 99–115). Cambridge, MA: MIT Press.

Kunda, Z., & Thagard, P. (1996). Forming impressions from stereotypes, traits, and behaviors: A parallel-constraint-satisfaction theory. *Psychological Review, 103*, 284–308.

Lai, C. K., Skinner, A. L., Cooley, E., Murrar, S., Brauer, M., Devos, T., et al. (2016). Reducing implicit racial preferences: II. Intervention effectiveness across time. *Journal of Experimental Psychology: General, 145*, 1001–1016.

Lebrecht, S., Pierce, L. J., Tarr, M. J., Tanaka, J. W. (2009). Perceptual other-race training reduces implicit racial bias. *PLoS ONE, 4*, e4215.

Levin, D. T. (2000). Race as a visual feature: Using visual search and perceptual discrimination tasks to understand face categories and the cross-race recognition deficit. *Journal of Experimental Psychology: General, 129*, 559–574.

Lick, D. J., Golay, A. E., & Johnson, K. L. (2014, February). *Race categorizations drawn from dynamic body motions: Accuracy, heuristics, and intersectional biases.* Poster presented at the annual meeting of the Society for Personality and Social Psychology, Austin, TX.

Lippmann, W. (1922). *Public opinion.* New York: Macmillan.

Macrae, C. N., & Bodenhausen, G. V. (2000). Social cognition: Thinking categorically about others. *Annual Review of Psychology, 51*, 93–120.

Macrae, C. N., Bodenhausen, G. V., & Milne, A. B. (1995). The dissection of selection in person perception: Inhibitory processes in social stereotyping. *Journal of Personality and Social Psychology, 69*, 397–407.

Macrae, C. N., Bodenhausen, G. V., Milne, A. B., Thorn, T. M. J., & Castelli, L. (1997). On the activation of social stereotypes: The moderating role of processing objectives. *Journal of Experimental Social Psychology, 33*, 471–489.

Macrae, C. N., & Martin, D. (2007). A boy primed Sue: Feature-based processing and person construal. *European Journal of Social Psychology, 37*, 793–805.

Macrae, C. N., Quinn, K. A., Mason, M. F., & Quadflieg, S. (2005). Understanding others: The face and person construal. *Journal of Personality and Social Psychology, 89*, 686–695.

Mallett, R. K., Wilson, T. D., & Gilbert, D. T. (2008). Expected the unexpected: Failure to anticipate similarities leads to an intergroup forecasting error. *Journal of Personality and Social Psychology, 94*, 265–277.

Markus, H. R., & Kitayama, S. (1991). Culture and the self: Implications for cognition, emotion, and motivation. *Psychological Review, 98,* 224–253.

Maurer, D., Le Grand, R., & Mondloch, C. J. (2002). The many faces of configural processing. *Trends in Cognitive Sciences, 6,* 255–260.

Miller, C. L. (1983). Developmental changes in male/female voice classification by infants. *Infant Behavior and Development, 6,* 313–330.

Montepare, J. M., & Zebrowitz-McArthur, L. A. (1998). Person perception comes of age: The salience and significance of age in social judgments. In M. P. Zanna (Ed.), *Advances in experimental social psychology* (Vol. 30, pp. 93–163). New York: Academic Press.

Mouchetant-Rostaing, Y., Girard, M. H., Bentin, S., Aguera, P. E., & Pernier, J. (2000). Neurophysiological correlates of face gender processing in humans. *European Journal of Neuroscience, 12,* 303–310.

Newheiser, A. K., & Olson, K. R. (2012). White and Black American children's implicit intergroup bias. *Journal of Experimental Social Psychology, 48,* 264–270.

Pascalis, O. (2002). Is face processing species-specific during the first year of life? *Science, 296,* 1321–1323.

Pascalis, O., & Slater, A. (2003). *The development of face processing in infancy and early childhood: Current perspectives.* Hauppauge, NY: Nova.

Pauker, K., Ambady, N., & Apfelbaum, E. P. (2010). Race salience and essentialist thinking in racial stereotype development. *Child Development, 81,* 1799–1813.

Pauker, K., Meyers, C., Sanchez, D. T., Gaither, S. E., & Young, D. M. (2018). A review of multiracial malleability: Identity, categorization, and shifting racial attitudes. *Social and Personality Psychology Compass, 12,* e12392.

Pauker, K., Weisbuch, M., Ambady, N., Sommers, S. R., Adams, R. B., Jr., & Ivcevic, Z. (2009). Not so Black and White: Memory for ambiguous group members. *Journal of Personality and Social Psychology, 96,* 795– 810.

Phills, C. E., Kawakami, K., Krusemark, D. R., & Nyguen, J. (2019). Does reducing prejudice increase outgroup identification?: The downstream consequences of associating positive concepts with racial categories. *Social Psychological and Personality Science, 10,* 26–34.

Phills, C. E., Kawakami, K., Tabi, E., Nadolny, D., & Inzlicht, M. (2011). Mind the gap: Increasing associations between the self and Blacks with approach behaviors. *Journal of Personality and Social Psychology, 100,* 197–210.

Qian, M. K., Quinn, P. C., Heyman, G. D., Pascalis, O., Fu, G., Lee, K. (2017). Perceptual individua-

tion training (but not mere exposure) reduces implicit racial bias in preschool children. *Developmental Psychology, 53,* 845–859.

Quinn, K. A., & Macrae, C. N. (2005). Categorizing others: The dynamics of person construal. *Journal of Personality and Social Psychology, 88,* 467–479.

Quinn, K. A., Mason, M. F., & Macrae, C. N. (2009). Familiarity and person construal: Individual knowledge moderates the automaticity of category activation. *European Journal of Social Psychology, 39,* 852–861.

Quinn, P. C., Yahr, J., Kuhn, A., Slater, A. M., & Pascalis, O. (2002). Representation of the gender of human faces by infants: A preference for female. *Perception, 31,* 1109–1121.

Ratner, K. G., & Amodio, D. M. (2013). Seeing "us vs. them": Minimal group effects on the neural encoding of faces. *Journal of Experimental Social Psychology, 49,* 298–301.

Rhodes, G., Locke, V., Ewing, L., & Evangelista, E. (2009). Race coding and the other-race effect in face recognition. *Perception, 38,* 232–241.

Rhodes, M., & Gelman, S. A. (2009). A developmental examination of the conceptual structure of animal, artifact, and human social categories across two cultural contexts. *Cognitive Psychology, 59,* 244–274.

Richter, N., Over, H., & Dunham, Y. (2016). The effects of minimal group membership on young preschoolers' social preferences, estimates of similarity, and behavioral attribution. Retrieved from *www.collabra.org/articles/10.1525/collabra.44/print.*

Rokeach, M., Smith, P. W., & Evans, R. I. (1960). Two kinds of prejudice or one? In M. Rokcach (Ed.), *The open and closed mind* (pp. 132–168). New York: Basic Books.

Rule, N. O., Ambady, N., Adams, R. B., Jr., & Macrae, C. N. (2008). Accuracy and awareness in the perception and categorization of male sexual orientation. *Journal of Personality and Social Psychology, 95,* 1019–1028.

Rule, N. O., Garrett, J. V., & Ambady, N. (2010). On the perception of religious group membership from faces. *PLoS ONE, 5,* e14241.

Rutland, A., Cameron, L., Bennett, L., & Ferrell, J. (2005). Interracial contact and racial constancy: A multi-site study of racial intergroup bias in 3–5 year old Anglo-British children. *Journal of Applied Developmental Psychology, 26,* 699–713.

Shutts, K., Kinzler, K. D., McKee, C. B., & Spelke, E. S. (2009). Social information guides infants' selection of foods. *Journal of Cognition and Development, 10,* 1–17.

Spencer-Rodgers, J., Williams, M. J., Hamilton, D.

L., Peng, K., & Wang, L. (2007). Culture and group perception: Dispositional and stereotypic inferences about novel and national groups. *Journal of Personality and Social Psychology, 93,* 525–543.

Steele, J. R., George, M., Williams, A., & Tay, E. (2018). A cross-cultural investigation of children's implicit attitudes toward White and Black racial outgroups. *Developmental Science, 21,* e12673.

Stepanova, E. V., & Strube, M. J. (2012). The role of skin color and facial physiognomy in racial categorization: Moderation by implicit racial bias. *Journal of Experimental Social Psychology, 48,* 867–878.

Tajfel, H., & Turner, J. C. (1979). An integrative theory of intergroup conflict. In W. G. Austin & S. Worchel (Eds.), *The social psychology of intergroup relations* (pp. 33–47). Monterey, CA: Brooks/Cole.

Tanaka, J. W., & Gauthier, I. (1997). Expertise in object and face recognition. In R. L. Goldstone, P. G. Schyns, & D. L. Medin (Eds.), *Psychology of learning and motivation* (Vol. 36, pp. 83–125). San Diego, CA: Academic Press.

Taylor, M. G., Rhodes, M., & Gelman, S. A. (2009). Boys will be boys; cows will be cows: Children's essentialist reasoning about gender categories and animal species. *Child Development, 80,* 461–481.

Taylor, S. E., Fiske, S. T., Etcoff, N. L., & Ruderman, A. J. (1978). Categorical and contextual bases of person memory and stereotyping. *Journal of Personality and Social Psychology, 36,* 778–793.

Tskhay, K. O., & Rule, N. O. (2013). Accuracy in categorizing perceptually ambiguous groups: A review and meta-analysis. *Personality and Social Psychology Review, 17,* 72–86.

Turner, J. C., Hogg, M. A., Oakes, P. J., Reicher, S. D., & Wetherell, M. S. (1987). *Rediscovering the social group: A self-categorization theory.* Cambridge, MA: Blackwell.

Vingilis-Jaremko, L., Kawakami, K., & Friesen, J. (in press). Other-groups bias effects?: Recognizing faces from outgroups. *Social Psychological and Personality Science.*

Vorauer, J. D., Main, K. J., & O'Connell, G. B. (1998). How do individuals expect to be viewed by members of lower status groups?: Content and implications of meta-stereotypes. *Journal of Personality and Social Psychology, 75,* 917–937.

Vorauer, J. D., & Sakamoto, Y. (2006). I thought we could be friends, but. . . . *Psychological Science, 17,* 326–331.

Wang, Y., & Kosinski, M. (2018). Deep neural networks are more accurate than humans at detecting sexual orientation from facial images. *Journal of Personality and Social Psychology, 114,* 246–257.

Waxman, S. R. (2010). Names will never hurt me?: Naming and the development of racial and gender categories in preschool-aged children. *European Journal of Social Psychology, 40,* 593–610.

Weisman, K., Johnson, M. V., & Shutts, K. (2015). Young children's automatic encoding of social categories. *Developmental Science, 18,* 1036–1043.

West, T. V., Magee, J. C., Gordon, S. H., & Gullett, L. (2014). A little similarity goes a long way: The effects of peripheral but self-revealing similarities on improving and sustaining interracial relationships. *Journal of Personality and Social Psychology, 107,* 81–100.

Zebrowitz, L. A. (2006). Finally, faces find favor. *Social Cognition, 24,* 657–701.

Zosuls, K. M., Ruble, D. N., Tamis-LeMonda, C. S., Shrout, P. E., Bornstein, M. H., & Greulich, F. K. (2009). The acquisition of gender labels in infancy: Implications for gender-typed play. *Developmental Psychology, 45,* 688–701.

CHAPTER 22

Intergroup Contact and Prejudice Reduction
Three Guiding Principles

Angelika Love
Miles Hewstone

> The scientist, by the very nature of his commitment, creates more and more questions, never fewer. Indeed the measure of our intellectual maturity . . . is our capacity to feel less and less satisfied with our answers to better and better problems.
>
> —GORDON ALLPORT (1955, p. 67)

The intergroup contact hypothesis proposes that positive face-to-face interactions between members of opposed groups can reduce intergroup prejudice (Allport, 1954). While this is a relatively intuitive proposition, the psychological underpinnings of contact effects continue to fascinate and sometimes puzzle researchers. In the spirit of Gordon Allport's description of science quoted above, intergroup contact continues to be studied in ever greater detail and, as a consequence, to be understood more comprehensively: from physiological changes throughout intergroup interactions to the influence of context and across a wide variety of conflict-laden and more benign intergroup settings.

Although contact research is a well-established part of the social psychology of intergroup conflict, it also remains innovative in its methodology and links to other disciplines. Still, social psychologists who study intergroup contact remain committed to contact experiences as essentially psychological: Contact between members of different groups affects individual thought and emotion toward whole *groups* and their members. It therefore exerts influence at a higher level of abstraction than the interaction between individual representatives of those groups would initially seem to suggest.

In this chapter, we provide an introductory overview of three guiding principles, or lessons learned, about when and how contact between members of different groups affects intergroup relations:

- *Principle 1:* The effect of intergroup contact depends primarily on the quality, rather than the quantity, of the experience.

- *Principle 2:* Contact affects intergroup relations through an interplay of affective and cognitive processes.
- *Principle 3:* Contact experiences extend beyond self–outgroup relations and are shaped by the social context.

Throughout this chapter, our aim is to draw the reader's attention to an overview, inevitably selective, of both classic and very recent findings, well-established as well as innovative methods, and old, unanswered as well as newly emerging research questions.

Principle 1: The Effect of Intergroup Contact Depends on the Quality of the Experience

This first principle of intergroup contact—that the effectiveness of cross-group interactions is contingent on the quality of contact—harks back to the formulation of the contact hypothesis by Allport (1954), who postulated that contact will reduce prejudice most effectively if "it is of a sort that leads to the perception of common interests and common humanity between members of the two groups" (p. 281) and if it is regarded as intimate rather than trivial (p. 263). Similarly, Cook (1962), distilling the growing research literature into essential hallmarks of successful intergroup contact, highlighted that contact experiences would reduce prejudice and improve outgroup attitudes "to the extent to which participation in a given situation with another individual implies that one is willing to accept him as a social equal, and, at least potentially, as a friend" (p. 75). Finally, in formulating a process-oriented contact theory, Pettigrew (1998) went as far as making "the opportunity to become friends" (p. 76) a core attribute of effective intergroup contact. From the outset, contact researchers have clearly not considered prejudice reduction an inevitable consequence of intergroup contact but have, rather, been sensitive to the *quality* of such interactions as a principal determinant of their effectiveness.

While the formulation of a contact hypothesis, and later contact theory, initially led to a proliferation of research on an ever-growing list of "ingredients" of efficacious contact, it is now clear that many types of intergroup experiences in many settings can improve intergroup relations—provided they are broadly positive experiences (Pettigrew & Tropp, 2006). To develop this first principle of intergroup contact, we begin by outlining research showing that contact quality takes precedence over contact quantity, then turn to intergroup friendship as the most potent form of contact, and finally address the long-neglected question of how negative contact affects intergroup relations. In considering these different measures of intergroup contact, it should be noted that contact is sometimes manipulated experimentally, but that most studies have used self-report measures; however, in more recent research, as we report, additional measures have been developed, including measures derived from social network analysis. In the subsections below, we include examples of some of the main measures of each type of contact assessed (for a detailed overview of measures, see Lolliot et al., 2014).

Quality over Quantity

Contact *quantity* relates to the frequency with which someone has direct intergroup encounters. Example items are the following (Islam & Hewstone, 1993):

How much contact do you have with [outgroup] ... (1 = *none at all* to 7 = *a great deal*)

1. ... at college?
2. ... as neighbors?
3. ... as close friends?

How often have you ... (1 = *not at all* to 7 = *very often*)

4. ... engaged in informal conversations with outgroup members?
5. ... visited the homes of outgroup members?

Contact *quality* reflects the extent to which face-to-face intergroup encounters are experienced positively or negatively. Example items are the following (Islam & Hewstone, 1993):

To what extent did you experience the contact with [outgroup] as ...

1. ... equal (1 = *definitely not* to 7 = *definitely yes*)
2. ... involuntary or voluntary (1 = *definitely involuntary* to 7 = *definitely voluntary*)

3. . . . superficial or intimate (1 = *very super-ficial* to 7 = *very intimate*)
4. . . . pleasant (1 = *not at all* to 7 = *very*)
5. . . . competitive or cooperative (1 = *very competitive* to 7 = *very cooperative*)

A wealth of contact research now supports the argument that the *quality* of a contact experience is a principal determinant of its effect on intergroup relations. Cross-sectional evidence for the importance of contact quality was provided by Hamberger and Hewstone (1997) who, using a large, multinational European dataset, compared the contact–prejudice association across several types of intergroup relationships. They found that the number of outgroup friends participants reported having was reliably associated with lowest levels of outgroup prejudice, whereas self-reported contact quantity at work was occasionally even associated with higher levels of prejudice. Using the same dataset, Pettigrew (1997) found that the stronger the affective tie between ingroup and outgroup member (e.g., friends vs. co-workers), the stronger the association between contact quantity and outgroup attitudes. In line with these findings, Tropp and Pettigrew (2005) reported that the number of outgroup friends but not acquaintances was reliably negatively associated with prejudice. Additionally, perceived closeness with one's outgroup contacts also predicted less prejudice. A more recent cross-sectional study by Hodson, Costello, and MacInnis (2013) further substantiated the claim that contact quality trumps quantity. Across a wide range of outgroups, these researchers found that contact quality always correlated positively with outgroup attitudes, whereas contact quantity was a less reliable and weaker positive predictor. Finally, although they did not explicitly compare effects of contact quality and contact quantity, Pettigrew and Tropp's (2006) seminal meta-analysis of intergroup contact research showed that the contact–prejudice association was strongest when contact took the form of cross-group friendship, a relationship that is (among other attributes outlined below) likely to be especially positive when compared to more trivial contact.

Pettigrew and Tropp's (2006) meta-analytic assessment of contact effects was limited by the relative paucity of experimental and longi-tudinal research that could identify directional effects of contact on prejudice, as opposed to selection effects, whereby less (more) preju-diced individuals seek (avoid) outgroup contact. Experimental manipulations of contact are the method of choice to identify causal effects in line with the contact hypothesis. For example, Bettencourt, Brewer, Croak, and Miller (1992) studied outgroup-directed behavior and evalu-ations of unknown outgroup members in a paradigm that assigned participants to experi-mentally created teams. When intergroup in-teractions had a personal (vs. task) focus and thus included greater self-disclosure of indi-vidual team members—a hallmark of friendly interactions (Davies, Tropp, Aron, Pettigrew, & Wright, 2011)—participants displayed less ingroup bias in reward allocation and attitudes, and perceived greater outgroup variability (see also Cook, 1978; Ioannou, Al Ramiah, & Hew-stone, 2018; Page-Gould, Mendoza-Denton, & Tropp, 2008). Recent experimental research on more indirect contact experiences, includ-ing computer-mediated contact (White, Abu-Rayya, Bliuc, & Faulkner, 2015), further sub-stantiated the claim that contact quality is a principal determinant of the effect of contact on intergroup relations.

Adding external validity to intergroup con-tact research, longitudinal survey research on intergroup contact has increased confidence in directional effects from contact to reduced prej-udice and the argument that the contact effects are contingent on contact quality.[1] For example, Levin, van Laar, and Sidanius (2003) used a five-wave longitudinal design to study the de-velopment of interracial friendship among col-lege students and how these friendships relate to participants' intergroup attitudes. While they found that intergroup anxiety and negative out-group biases predicted having fewer outgroup friends (see also Wölfer & Hewstone, 2018), being friends with outgroup members also re-duced ingroup bias and intergroup anxiety. Longitudinal contact effects were also found in the more conflict-laden context of post-Apart-heid South Africa (Swart, Hewstone, Christ, & Voci, 2011) and, more recently, in studies add-ing social network data to self-report measures of friendship quantity (Wölfer, Schmid, Hew-stone, & van Zalk, 2016). These longitudinal studies further substantiate the claim that the reliable association of intergroup contact quality and intergroup relations reflects, to a large extent, positive contact effects.

Why Friendship Contact Is the Most Potent Form of Intergroup Contact

Cross-group friendships are considered to be the strongest form of direct contact, impacting on a wide range of outcomes (Davies et al., 2011; Pettigrew & Tropp, 2006). The following brief scale to assess cross-group friendships (Turner, Hewstone, & Voci, 2007) illustrates the kinds of items used to assess friendship contact:

1. How many close friends do you have at school who are [outgroup]?
2. How many close friends do you have outside school who are [outgroup]?
3. How often do you spend time with [outgroup] friends when you are at school?
4. How often do you spend time with [outgroup] friends outside school?

(Scale for items 1 and 2: 1 = *none*, 2 = *one*, 3 = *between two and five*, 4 = *between five and 10*, 5 = *more than 10*; scale for items 3 and 4: 1 = *never*, 2 = *occasionally*, 3 = *sometimes*, 4 = *quite a lot*, 5 = *all the time*)

Research on cross-group friendship has provided insights into the mechanisms that make this form of intergroup contact so effective. First, although it may be challenging to initiate cross-group friendship when intergroup relations are fraught, once established, cross-group friendship can initiate a positively escalating process in which outgroup contact begets more outgroup contact. This is supported by several longitudinal analyses showing that the reliable effect of contact, for example, improved attitudes and reduced anxiety, reduces future contact avoidance (Levin et al., 2003; Swart et al., 2011).

Second, a recent meta-analysis by Davies and colleagues (2011) suggested that friendship contact can reduce prejudice to the extent that friendship interactions are time intensive and involve self-disclosure. In line with this pattern across the literature, Turner and colleagues (2007) found that intended self-disclosure mediated the effect of friendship contact on attitudes, and that this effect was further explained by the association of self-disclosure with empathy and trust.

Importantly, intimate contact must not be equated with chronically decategorized contact—interactions in which individuals are never aware of each other's group memberships. A large body of research on the effect of interpersonal experiences on intergroup relations shows that contact effects will generalize most from interactions with specific outgroup members to more positive intergroup relations if group membership is salient in the interactions (e.g., van Oudenhoven, Groenewoud, & Hewstone, 1996), that is, if the encountered outgroup member is sufficiently associated with a mental representation of the outgroup (see Brown & Hewstone, 2005). Outgroup contact is particularly effective at generalizing beyond the contact dyad to the outgroup more generally if contact partners disconfirm negative outgroup-directed beliefs but are, at the same time, typical enough of the outgroup to be associated with it in the first place (McIntyre, Paolini, & Hewstone, 2016; Wilder, Simon, & Faith, 1996; Wolsko, Park, Judd, & Bachelor, 2003). This may be difficult to achieve, yet cross-group friendship might be a type of interaction in which these seemingly contradictory conditions can co-occur because here contact unfolds over a longer period of time, reveals individuating information that could disconfirm negative outgroup-directed beliefs, and can also involve periods of heightened category salience (Davies et al., 2011; Pettigrew, 1998).

Negative Contact

We have outlined that while even less intimate (yet positive) forms of contact than friendship can help improve intergroup relations, contact quantity is sometimes unrelated to measures of intergroup relations. Failure to find effects of mere contact may reflect the previously neglected fact that some contact experiences are far from positive. Surprisingly, contact researchers have only recently begun to study negative contact more systematically. These studies now highlight that the principle that the quality of contact is paramount goes beyond questions of *how positive* contact is and also relates to the potentially detrimental effect of negative contact.

The simplest measure of "valenced" contact asks one item each for positive and negative contact (Barlow et al., 2012):

1. On average, how frequently do you have positive/good contact with [outgroup] people?
2. On average, how frequently do you have negative/bad contact with [outgroup] people?"

(1 = *never* to 7 = *extremely frequently*)

A recent, more detailed (but also more time-consuming) scale acknowledges that contact experiences may vary not only in their valence (i.e., whether they are positive or negative) but also in their intensity (i.e., how strongly positive or negative they are; see Hayward, Tropp, Hornsey, & Barlow, 2017).

There is now cross-sectional, experimental, and longitudinal research showing that negative contact is associated with, and can lead to, more negative explicit and implicit attitudes (Aberson & Gaffney, 2009). And although most studies suggest that negative contact is experienced less often than positive contact of a similar intensity (Dhont & Van Hiel, 2009; Graf, Paolini, & Rubin, 2014), negative contact might also be a more potent intergroup experience than positive contact (Barlow et al., 2012; Bekhuis, Ruiter, & Coenders, 2013; Dhont, Cornelis, & van Hiel, 2010). Some experimental research suggests that this valence asymmetry effect reflects heightened group membership salience during negative interactions (Paolini, Harwood, & Rubin, 2010; Paolini et al., 2014) and therefore greater person-to-group generalization, but other studies found positive contact to have a stronger effect on outgroup attitudes than negative contact (Aberson & Gaffney, 2009; Christ, Ullrich, & Wagner, 2008; Pettigrew, Tropp, Wagner, & Christ, 2011). Evidence for a stronger effect of negative than positive contact therefore remains at best inconclusive.

Rather than comparing the size of positive and negative contact effects, it is sensible to consider that contact experiences rarely happen in a vacuum. Rather, they are influenced by past experiences and expectations about future interactions. Positive and negative contact experiences are therefore not independent and ought to be studied in concert. First evidence for an interaction between positive and negative contact was provided by Paolini and colleagues (2014), who found that the category salience-heightening effect of experimentally induced negative contact was weaker among participants with more prior cross-group friendships. Prior positive experiences could therefore buffer the detrimental effects of negative contact, although other plausible interactions between positive and negative contact remain to be explored in depth.

As societal diversity increases, so do opportunities for not only positive but also negative contact (Laurence, Schmid, & Hewstone, 2018; Schmid, Tausch, Hewstone, Hughes, & Cairns, 2008). A concerted evaluation of positive and negative contact experiences is clearly especially relevant as contact researchers try to understand whether and how such diversity affects intergroup relations. Although there is strong evidence for the positive effect of positively valenced contact, especially cross-group friendship, additional research is required to understand when and how negative contact affects intergroup relations, and how positive and negative contact experiences interact.

Principle 2: Contact Affects Intergroup Relations through an Interplay of Affective and Cognitive Processes

The effect of positive intergroup contact, especially cross-group friendship, on a host of affective, cognitive, and behavioral measures of intergroup relations is now well established across a variety of intergroup contexts. More recently, intergroup contact research has been marked by a proliferation of studies on the processes that account for these effects and, conjunctively, the maturation of the original contact hypothesis into a more full fledged intergroup contact theory (Hewstone & Swart, 2011; Pettigrew, 1998). The wealth of studies on the processes, or mediators, whereby intergroup interactions help improve intergroup relations highlights a second principle of intergroup contact: Contact affects intergroup relations through an interplay of affective and cognitive processes.

Affective Processes

Pettigrew and Tropp's (2008) meta-analysis of key contact mediators suggested that changes in how individuals relate emotionally to the outgroup, especially reductions in intergroup anxiety and increases in outgroup empathy, lie at the heart of intergroup contact effects. Since then, researchers have studied a range of additional affective processes, including threat perception and the development of outgroup trust, which, in addition to anxiety and empathy, we briefly outline below.

Intergroup Anxiety

Intergroup anxiety describes a feeling of uncertainty and insecurity at the prospect of engaging with outgroup members (Stephan & Stephan, 1985). Intergroup anxiety is the most commonly considered process variable in intergroup contact research (see Paolini, Harris, & Griffin, 2016). Theoretically, anxiety affects intergroup relations in multifaceted ways: It narrows the focus of attention, increases stereotypical thinking, heightens awareness of behavioral norms, and is associated with a negativity bias that draws attention to stereotype-confirming information and biases the interpretation of ambiguous behaviors (Fox, Russo, Bowles, & Dutton, 2001; Stephan & Stephan, 1985; Wilder, 1993). Contact that lowers intergroup anxiety could therefore facilitate not only more positive evaluations of a contact partner but also the generalization of this experience to outgroup evaluations more widely.

Several longitudinal (e.g., Binder et al., 2009; Swart et al., 2011) and experimental (e.g., Page-Gould et al., 2008) studies now show that positive contact experiences help improve intergroup relations by reducing intergroup anxiety, including studies conducted in post-conflict intergroup settings such as Northern Ireland (Paolini, Hewstone, Cairns, & Voci, 2004) and South Africa (Swart et al., 2011), where intergroup relations often continue to be fraught. Intergroup anxiety reduction is associated with not only indicators of reduced affective prejudice (Tropp & Pettigrew, 2005) such as more positive outgroup-directed emotions and greater outgroup liking (Paolini, Hewstone, Voci, Harwood, & Cairns, 2006), but also indicators of reduced cognitive prejudice such as greater perceived outgroup variability (Islam & Hewstone, 1993; Swart et al., 2011). Importantly, anxiety reduction also contributes to the self-perpetuation of positive intergroup contact and has been associated with more positive expectancies about future contact (Gómez, Tropp, & Fernández, 2011) and less outgroup avoidance (Kenworthy et al., 2016). Furthermore, in a rare study on physiological markers of contact-related anxiety, Page-Gould and colleagues (2008) found that anxiety decreased throughout positive intergroup interactions, especially among the most prejudiced participants. These, in turn, were also the participants who later initiated most cross-group encounters outside the laboratory. Overall, research on intergroup anxiety highlights that although anxiety is usually considered an affective mediator, it is directly related to not only affective but also cognitive and even behavioral aspects of intergroup relations.

In light of the reliable and wide-reaching implications of intergroup anxiety for intergroup contact effects, it is unsurprising to find that it also contributes to the effect of extended contact on outgroup attitudes. *Extended contact* describes the experience of merely knowing about ingroup members' outgroup contact (Wright, Aron, McLaughlin-Volpe, & Ropp, 1997). In its simplest form, extended contact is assessed by a single question: "How many ingroup members do you know who have [outgroup] friends?" (1 = *none* to 6 = *all*). But wider forms of extended contact can also be studied by asking about the range of outgroup relations experienced by a variety of ingroup members (Tausch et al., 2011):

> How many of your ingroup [*neighbors* (excluding item 1 below)/*colleagues* (excluding item 2 below)/*friends/family members*] have . . .
>
> 1. . . . neighbors from [the outgroup]
> 2. . . . work colleagues from [the outgroup]
> 3. . . . close friends from [the outgroup]
> 4. . . . are married to someone from [the outgroup]
>
> (Scale: 1 = *none* to 6 = *all*)

As we outline in greater detail in our discussion of Principle 3, such indirect contact can both reduce prejudice and facilitate more direct contact. This is, in part, underpinned by the intergroup anxiety-reducing effect of a more passive introduction to the outgroup through extended contact (Gómez et al., 2011; Turner, Hewstone, Voci, & Vonofakou, 2008).

Threat

Threat perception is closely related to intergroup anxiety. However, whereas anxiety operates mainly on an individual level insofar as it describes the individual's uncertainty in intergroup situations, threat—the anticipation of negative consequences of the outgroup's presence for the ingroup—explicitly concerns the ingroup as a whole (Stephan & Stephan, 2000; Tausch, Hewstone, Kenworthy, Cairns, & Christ, 2007). In the intergroup context, research focuses mostly on symbolic threat (threat to ingroup values) and realistic threat (threat to ingroup status), although other forms of threat are also relevant (e.g., distinctiveness threat; see Schmid, Hewstone, Tausch, Cairns, & Hughes, 2009). Several laboratory studies on involuntary physiological markers of threat have shown that threat is more acute in intergroup than in intragroup encounters, and that intergroup contact may attenuate this effect (Blascovich, Mendes, Hunter, Lickel, & Kowai-Bell, 2001; Mendes, Blascovich, Lickel, & Hunter, 2002).

Research on threat as a mediator of contact effects highlights not only that threat reduction contributes to positive contact effects, but also that different contact mediators are more or less relevant for different individuals. In a cross-sectional sample of Northern Irish Catholics and Protestants, Tausch and colleagues (2007) found that symbolic threat was a stronger mediator of the contact–prejudice association among individuals who identified particularly strongly with the ingroup. Similarly, Asbrock, Christ, Duckitt, and Sibley (2012) found that threat mediated the association of contact and immigrant-directed prejudice only in participants with high right-wing authoritarianism (RWA) but not individuals with high social-dominance orientation (SDO). These findings suggest that people who avoid intergroup contact because they fear that ingroup cohesion and collective security will be undermined by outgroups (i.e., those high in RWA) benefit more from threat reduction than do people who seek to maintain a social hierarchy of power (SDO).

In addition to such individual differences, group status may also moderate which processes underpin contact effects. Some research suggests that anxiety (especially fear of embarrassment) accounts for contact effects among advantaged group members, whereas threat perception is more relevant among disadvantaged group members (Binder et al., 2009). However, both anxiety and threat have been shown to mediate contact effects among members of advantaged and disadvantaged groups (Swart et al., 2011; Tausch et al., 2007), and although their effects may be situationally determined, both contribute to contact effects across a broad range of intergroup contexts.

Trust

Trust has been described as "a psychological means to overcome uncertain social interactions by making benign assumptions about other people's behavior" (Kenworthy et al., 2016, p. 1044), including the expectation that others will not exploit vulnerability and will be cooperative (Kramer & Carnevale, 2003; Tam, Hewstone, Kenworthy, & Cairns, 2009). The satisfactory deescalations of conflict, reconciliation, and forgiveness after violent disputes are all predicated on mutual trust (Tam et al., 2009). However, trusting outgroup members implies a willingness to engage in potentially costly intergroup behavior rather than settling for separation and peaceful coexistence of groups (Kenworthy et al., 2016). Therefore, trust has been described as an intergroup contact-related process that is particularly challenging yet powerful, especially in contexts that have been scarred by conflict.

Cross-sectional and, more recently, some longitudinal research provides evidence for the implication of outgroup trust in intergroup contact processes. Turner, Hewstone, and Voci's (2007, Study 4) cross-sectional study on interethnic relations in the United Kingdom found that cross-group friendships could improve explicit outgroup attitudes by fostering the development of outgroup trust. Trust also mediated the association of positive contact with forgiveness (Cehajic, Brown, & Castano, 2008) and approach and avoidance tendencies (Tam et al., 2009). There is some correlational evidence that, like other affective processes, trust also mediates extended contact effects, although this effect seems to be weaker than its implication in direct contact processes (Capozza, Falvo, Favara, & Trifiletti, 2013; Dhont & Van Hiel, 2011; Tam et al., 2009). Finally, although Kenworthy and colleagues (2016) showed that, over time, positive contact increases trust, longitudinal and experimental research on intergroup contact and outgroup trust remains scarce.

Empathy

While anxiety, threat, and trust are nominally affective mediators with less commonly acknowledged cognitive facets, empathy is now recognized as a mediator with distinct affective and cognitive dimensions. Broadly, *affective empathy* can be described as "the capacity to experience affective reactions to the observed experience of others" (Davis, 1996, p. 45). *Cognitive empathy,* on the other hand, also called *perspective taking* (Batson, Early, & Salvarani, 1997; Harwood, Hewstone, Paolini, & Voci, 2005; Stephan & Finlay, 1999) is closely related to the notion that contact can help expand the sense of self to include the outgroup (Aron, Aron, & Norman, 2001; Tropp & Wright, 2001).

Studies covering a wide range of intergroup contexts, and operationalizing empathy in various ways, have shown that positive contact can improve intergroup relations by increasing empathy for the outgroup. Harwood and colleagues (2005), for example, studied intergenerational contact and found perspective taking to be a particularly powerful mediator of the contact–attitudes association. Similarly, Cehajic and colleagues' (2008) research in postconflict Bosnia–Herzegovina found that increased cognitive empathy partly accounted for the correlation of positive contact with a willingness to forgive and to engage in further contact. More indirect contact experiences have now also been shown to increase outgroup empathy (e.g., Vezzali, Hewstone, Capozza, Giovannini, & Wölfer, 2014).

In the first longitudinal study of contact to include a measure of affective empathy, Swart and colleagues (2011) found, over three waves, that empathy mediated the effect of contact on outgroup attitudes, behavioral intentions, and perceived outgroup variability. As prior research on other nominally affective mediators (e.g.,

anxiety; Islam & Hewstone, 1993) has done, Swart and colleagues highlighted that affective processes influence not only affective dimensions of prejudice but also cognitive and behavioral ones. Furthermore, Swart and colleagues found that empathy develops when anxiety is reduced, and thus emphasized the importance of studying the concerted action of multiple mediators within a longitudinal framework.

Interactions between several mediating processes also stand out when we consider research on cognitive mediators and their relation to mediators such as empathy, trust, threat, and anxiety. We now turn to research on such cognitive mediators, then revisit the distinction between affective and cognitive contact processes.

Cognitive Processes

Distinguishing cognitive from affective processes is challenging and, as we argue below, not always sensible. Here we address processes that may be described as cognitive insofar as they relate to changes in the cognitive representation of an individual's own social identity and the relationship between their[2] ingroup(s) and outgroup(s). Such processes were central to Pettigrew's (1998) influential deprovincialization hypothesis, which stated that intergroup contact can facilitate improved intergroup relations by facilitating a less provincial view of the ingroup. While most research on deprovincialization has focused on changes in ingroup identification, research on changes in perceived ingroup norms and possibly a more complex perception of one's own social identity could also be described as deprovincialization. We address these processes in turn.

Ingroup Identification

Theoretically, social identity theory (Tajfel & Turner, 1986) and self-categorization theory (Turner, Hogg, Oakes, Reicher, & Wetherell, 1987) have linked intergroup discrimination to ingroup identification and the need to positively distinguish the ingroup from the outgroup. If contact can weaken ingroup identification, it might therefore also weaken intergroup discrimination.

A number of cross-sectional and longitudinal studies support the argument that contact can reduce ingroup identification. Pettigrew (1997), for example, found that majority group members with more outgroup friends also showed less national pride. Similarly, Pettigrew (2009) found that Germans with more positive contact with foreigners had a weaker German identity (see also Van Laar, Levin, Sinclair, & Sidanius, 2005).

Although contact can reduce ingroup identification, this does not always translate into more positive intergroup relations (Tausch et al., 2010). As had been suggested by research on the role of threat perception and anxiety (Asbrock et al., 2012), Kauff, Schmid, Lolliot, Al Ramiah, and Hewstone (2016) argued that the significance of deprovincialization processes also depends on the origins of an individual's prejudice. Previous research showed that ingroup identification is only associated with more outgroup discrimination among individuals who are invested in strong group hierarchies. In line with this argument, Kauff and colleagues found that the ingroup identification-reducing effect of contact only translated into more positive outgroup attitudes among individuals with high SDO.

Social Identity Complexity

Deprovincialization has been conceptualized not only as reduced ingroup identification but also, more recently, as increased social identity complexity (SIC). SIC emphasizes an individual's awareness of their multiple ingroups and the extent to which they are interrelated in complex ways. Unlike ingroup identification, which has strong affective components, SIC is a particularly cognitive appraisal of ingroup identities (Roccas & Brewer, 2002). Although it concerns ingroup perceptions, greater SIC has been associated with more outgroup tolerance and less intergroup bias (Roccas & Brewer, 2002).

Intergroup contact could improve intergroup relations through increased SIC by highlighting points of overlap between ingroup and outgroup members, and by decreasing reliance on a single dimension of comparison to achieve optimal distinctiveness and a positive social identity. In line with this argument, Schmid and colleagues (2009), in a cross-sectional study of Catholics and Protestants in Northern Ireland, found that positive contact effects were mediated by in-

creases in SIC. By increasing the complexity of an individual's appraisal of their multiple ingroups, contact produced more positive outgroup and less positive ingroup evaluations.

Changed Perception of Group Norms

Contact can not only change how people relate to their social identities, but it can also alter their perception of the social norms that govern outgroup-directed behavior within their ingroup (ingroup norms), and ingroup-directed behavior among outgroup members (outgroup norms).

Norms are "attitudinal and behavioral uniformities or shared beliefs about the appropriate conduct for a group member" (Sharp, Voci, & Hewstone, 2011, p. 208) that are typically closely related to intergroup behavior (Jetten, Spears, & Manstead, 1996). Norms can be inferred from behavior observed among ingroup members (Christ et al., 2014) who thus act as sources of referent informational influence. Changes in perceived norms have therefore mostly been associated with extended contact (see below), and several longitudinal, cross-sectional, and experimental studies now show that extended contact can affect intergroup relations through a change in perceived ingroup and outgroup norms about intergroup behavior (e.g., De Tezanos-Pinto, Bratt, & Brown, 2010; Turner et al., 2008). A handful of cross-sectional studies have also tested the link between direct contact experiences and group norms, but there is to date little evidence to suggest an effect of direct contact on norms (e.g., Turner et al., 2008). Rather, more weight is placed on the argument that through extended contact, the perception of positive norms about intergroup contact can encourage direct intergroup contact (Wright et al., 1997).

Changed Social Categorization

Although studies on social categorization and intergroup contact are usually considered as separate research topics in social psychology (see Ellemers and de Gilder, Chapter 23, this volume), both fields are clearly linked theoretically and, occasionally, empirically. Theoretically, changes to social categorization patterns could mediate contact effects. Pettigrew (1998), for example, suggested that cross-group friendship could affect intergroup relations by facilitating recategorization of ingroup and outgroup members under a shared superordinate identity (see also Gaertner & Dovidio, 2000).

In line with this suggestion, a recent cross-sectional study by Reimer, Kamble, Schmid, and Hewstone (2020) in India, employing the triple crossed categorization task (van Dommelen, Schmid, Hewstone, Gonsalkorale, & Brewer, 2015), found that having more outgroup friends was associated with a heightened likelihood of describing the outgroup as "us" (vs. "not us"), whereas negative contact had the opposite effect. Including others in the ingroup was, in turn, associated with more favorable attitudes toward and less desired social distance from these individuals. These findings provide the first correlational evidence for a relation between positive contact and more inclusive social identities, which in turn may have positive implications for how we relate to people whose backgrounds differ from our own. However, while contact and categorization are complementary rather than competing perspectives on intergroup relations (e.g., Glasford & Dovidio, 2011), empirical evidence for contact effects that are mediated by changes in categorization is scant (see also Eller & Abrams, 2004).

Inclusion of the Outgroup in the Self

Inclusion of the outgroup in the self (IOS) describes the psychological distance that an individual perceives between themselves and an object, person, or group (Aron, Aron, & Smollan, 1992; Tropp & Wright, 2001). Research that suggests positive contact could increase the perceived similarity between self and outgroup, or between ingroup and outgroup, is closely related to the argument that contact could facilitate more inclusive social categorization.

Where IOS has been treated as a measure of self–outgroup overlap or, in extended contact research, as a measure of ingroup–outgroup overlap, evidence for mediation is mixed. Several cross-sectional studies on direct and extended contact suggest that extended contact effects are partially mediated by increased perception of self–outgroup overlap (Capozza, Falvo, Trifiletti, & Pagani, 2014; Gómez et al., 2011; Turner et al., 2008), while others do not (Capozza et al.,

2013; Hodson, Harry, & Mitchell, 2009). Longitudinal evidence for a mediating effect of IOS is also inconclusive at best. For example, Eller, Abrams, and Zimmermann (2011) found that extended contact increases IOS, but they did not find IOS to mediate extended contact effects.

The Cognitive–Affective Distinction

Much like prejudice has been divided into cognitive (e.g., stereotypes, beliefs) and affective (e.g., outgroup directed emotions, liking) dimensions (Tropp & Pettigrew, 2005), the processes underpinning contact effects on these outcome variables are often described as either cognitive or affective (e.g., Harwood et al., 2005; Vezzali et al., 2014). Our own organization of the abundant literature on mediation effects in this chapter illustrates how this distinction can help structure the growing number of known mediators. However, our review of research on contact mediators has also highlighted that organizing mediators this way overlooks the fact that many mediators have both cognitive and affective dimensions. Furthermore, cognitive and affective responses to contact experiences are in no way independent but are intricately related, sometimes causally. It may therefore be misleading to describe contact effects as either cognitive or affective.

Cognitive and affective processes are intimately intertwined, with cognition changing emotion and vice versa. Schmid and colleagues (2009), for example, found that the effect of contact on ingroup bias in terms of ingroup- and outgroup-directed warmth—an affective measure of prejudice—was mediated by SIC. Conversely, Swart and associates (2011) found that the effect of contact on perceived outgroup variability—a cognitive measure of prejudice— was mediated by empathy and anxiety.

The interplay between cognitive and affective processes is further highlighted by research that considers several mediators simultaneously. For example, Schmid and colleagues (2009) studied not only the relationship between contact and SIC but also the interplay of threat perception and SIC. They found that the effect of contact on ingroup bias was conjointly mediated by (distinctiveness) threat and SIC, and that SIC was diminished when individuals felt that the distinctiveness of their group was more threatened. Another example of the joint contribution of cognitive and affective processes to contact effects was provided by Verkuyten, Thijs, and Bekhuis (2010), who found that lower levels of threat were also associated with weaker ingroup identification, and by Tausch and colleagues (2007), whose findings suggest that the effects of threat and anxiety on outgroup attitudes are attenuated when ingroup identification is reduced.

Future research on the processes that underpin the effect of contact on a range of prejudice indicators will benefit from considering several mediators and their complex interrelationships simultaneously in a theory-led fashion and, in order to establish the sequence of processes that bring about contact effects, longitudinally. This, we argue, should take priority over expanding the list of mediators under consideration. Rather than risking another laundry-list approach to the study of intergroup contact (Pettigrew, 1986), focusing on the interactions of a set of core mediators, tested simultaneously, promises to provide exciting new insights into the psychological processes that explain intergroup contact effects.

Principle 3: Contact Experiences Extend beyond Self–Outgroup Relations

One of the key motivators for intergroup contact research over the past decade has been the promise that intergroup contact effects are constrained to the contact parties' personal attitudes and stereotypes about each other and, at best, each other's groups. There is now ample evidence to suggest a third principle of intergroup contact: that intergroup contact experiences extend beyond the well-established individual-to-group and cross-context generalization patterns that concerned earlier contact research (see Brown & Hewstone, 2005; Pettigrew & Tropp, 2006). Here, we focus on two additional generalization effects: (1) from one ingroup member's experience to fellow ingroup members' attitudes (extended contact effects) and (2) from the contact partner's outgroup to uninvolved outgroups (secondary transfer effects). We also briefly discuss the wider-reaching effects of contact beyond prejudice, which

are usually not described in terms of generalization but can be included under the umbrella of contact's wider ripple effects.

Extended Contact

Not everybody has the opportunity to engage in contact with outgroup members or is inclined to exploit those opportunities. However, research on indirect contact via fellow ingroup members now shows that the direct contact experiences of a handful of individuals can indirectly change how ingroup members who themselves do not engage in intergroup contact relate to the outgroup (Vezzali et al., 2014; Wright et al., 1997; Zhou, Page-Gould, Aron, Moyer, & Hewstone, 2019). In the first theory-led discussion of these indirect contact effects, Wright and colleagues (1997) distinguished between two forms: *observing* ingroup members having outgroup contact (vicarious contact) and *knowing* that ingroup members have outgroup contact (extended contact). Although extended and vicarious contact are often collectively referred to as *extended contact,* here we explicitly focus on extended contact in the original sense as the experience that is removed in both time and place from direct intergroup interactions.

Numerous experimental, cross-sectional, and longitudinal studies across different intergroup contexts show that extended contact affects many indices of intergroup relations, including blatant (Dhont, Roets, & Van Hiel, 2011) and implicit (Vezzali & Giovannini, 2011) measures of attitudes, stereotypes (Paolini et al., 2004), and behavioral intentions (Paolini, Hewstone, & Cairns, 2007; Vezzali, Stathi, & Giovannini, 2012). These effects emerge even when direct contact effects are statistically controlled.

A recent meta-analysis of extended contact research by Zhou and colleagues (2019) found extended contact to be similarly effective among advantaged and disadvantaged populations and, surprisingly perhaps, to yield an effect size equivalent to that of direct contact. Importantly, extended contact is also particularly effective among more prejudiced individuals, especially individuals with high levels of RWA (Dhont & Van Hiel, 2011). It has also been found to promote peaceful intergroup relations in post-conflict settings (Andrighetto, Mari, Volpato, & Behluli, 2012; Du Toit & Quayle, 2011, Tam et al., 2009). Although negative extended contact remains severely under-researched, available research on extended contact makes a strong case for positive direct contact interventions, even if they only initially reach a small number of people, because the effects of contact can be spread across people who themselves did not experience the contact directly.

As we have already outlined in our discussion of Principle 2, many cognitive and affective mediators of direct contact also conjointly account for extended contact effects (see Vezzali et al., 2014). However, as a passive experience, extended contact is by definition clearly distinct from direct contact. This distinction is also reflected in several proposed theoretical foundations of extended contact effects, including the need to reduce dissonance between the behavior and attitudes of ingroup members and the self (Cooper & Hogg, 2007) and the tendency to balance relationship triads in which it is not only true that "my friend's friend is my friend" (Aronson & Cope, 1968) but also that "my group member's friend's group is my friend" (Wright et al., 1997; also see Vezzali et al., 2014).

Social Network Analysis

Evidence for extended contact highlights how intergroup contact is best understood with reference to the wider relationship networks in which it occurs. Recently, social psychologists have turned to social network analysis (SNA) as a tool for studying contact. SNA is especially suited to the study of extended contact because it does justice to the definition of extended contact as a two-tiered association: (1) the relationship between an individual and their ingroup contacts and (2) the relationships between those ingroup contacts and outgroup members. Traditional measures of extended contact require participants to estimate their ingroup contacts' outgroup contact—a complex measure that is likely inaccurate, especially if the wider relationship network spans several distant social contexts. Such complex self-report measures of extended contact are also likely to suffer from additional biases (e.g., confirmation bias, whereby we report outgroup contact to match our attitudes; and projection bias, whereby people tend to project their own experience onto fellow ingroup members).

SNA can help circumvent these challenges by quantifying extended contact on the basis of the self-reported direct connections (e.g., friends) of all members of a circumscribed relationship network (e.g., students in a school class). Although SNA requires complex analytical and statistical techniques, it uses the simplest of measures that can be completed by even very young children. For example, every child in a school class is asked to nominate their five (or 10, or unlimited) "best friends," or to make similar nominations for a series of behaviors (e.g., "who you play with out of school"; "who is sometimes mean to you"; "who bullies you"). By going beyond an individual's immediate relationship network (e.g., person A's direct friendships with B and C) and collecting data on the direct relations of these contacts too (i.e., who else B and C are friends with), a more complete picture of the wider network can be established. If this network data is then integrated with information about the group membership of all network members (e.g., all students in a school class), extended contact can be quantified in a way that is more objective than purely self-report-reliant data (e.g., Munniksma, Stark, Verkuyten, Flache, & Veenstra, 2013; see also Wölfer & Hewstone, 2017).

More recently, researchers have begun to go beyond the constraints of the network boundary (e.g., the school class) by combining social network and self-report data. Wölfer and colleagues (2016) used social network data to quantify direct contact with ingroup members within the network boundary (i.e., ties with other ingroup members); then, additionally, they used these ingroup members' self-reports of outgroup contact outside of the network boundary. This methodological approach can help to quantify contact experiences that are likely to be truly indirect and overcomes the fact that people may lack adequate knowledge of the actual outgroup contact experiences of fellow ingroup members. Moreover, it removes the risk that people merely project their own contact experiences when asked to report on the outgroup contact of other ingroup members.

The Importance of Context

Research on indirect contact highlights that intergroup relations are shaped by the context in which they occur. The role of contextual variables was implicit in early formulations of the contact hypothesis, which stressed, among other factors, the importance of institutional support for contact (Allport, 1954). However, research on contextual moderators of contact is scarce (see also Paluck, Green, & Green, 2019). Methodologically, SNA can provide insight into the contribution of wider network parameters (e.g., the number of existing connections relative to the number of possible connections, or "network density") to individual-level processes. Notwithstanding, this application of SNA to the social psychology of intergroup contact is still nascent.

Conversely, multilevel analyses of survey data have now begun to shed light on the joint contribution of individual- and context-level processes to intergroup contact effects. For example, Christ and colleagues (2014) found that it is not just an individual's own positive contact experiences but also, additionally, the positive contact experiences occurring within their wider social environment that affect prejudice. This context-level effect was mediated by pro-diversity norms: Environments where intergroup contact is more common signal more positive norms around diversity, which contributes to prejudice reduction independently of individuals' direct contact experiences.

Further evidence for an interplay of an individual's own contact experiences and the contact experienced by others in their environment, was provided by research suggesting that extended contact effects are strongest when, due to segregation or low diversity, direct contact experiences are rare (Christ et al., 2010; Wölfer et al., 2016), and that indirect contact can facilitate direct contact by highlighting positive ingroup and outgroup norms (Mallett & Wilson, 2010; Schofield, Hausmann, Ye, & Woods, 2010; Vezzali et al., 2015) and reducing intergroup anxiety (Wölfer et al., 2019).

Secondary Transfer Effects

Research on secondary transfer effects (STEs) of contact provides further evidence for a ripple effect of contact beyond the individuals (and their groups) involved in the contact situation. While research on indirect contact shows that contact can affect uninvolved *ingroup* mem-

bers, research on STEs suggests that contact also changes how individuals relate to uninvolved *outgroups*. In other words, contact effects can transfer from primary outgroups (involved in the contact situation) to secondary outgroups (not involved in the contact situation) with whom contact may be negligible (Lolliot et al., 2013; Pettigrew, 2009).

In his formulation of the contact hypothesis, Allport (1954) anticipated the interrelatedness of attitudes toward different outgroups, stating that "if a person is anti-Jewish, he is likely to be anti-Catholic, anti-Negro, anti any out-group" (p. 66)—a prediction that finds empirical support in early research on intergroup relations (e.g., Hartley, 1946). That intergroup contact effects are not limited to the contact partner's outgroup was suggested first by Pettigrew's (1997) analysis of several European national probability samples, which suggested that contact predicted attitudes toward not only a contacted outgroup (the primary outgroup) but also outgroups that were not present in participants' countries (secondary outgroups). However, because this study did not include measures of direct contact to those secondary outgroups, and because of its cross-sectional design, Pettigrew's analyses of STEs remained speculative at first.

More recently, longitudinal studies have explicitly distinguished STEs from prejudice effects whereby more prejudiced people seek out less contact with a wide range of outgroups. For example, in a two-wave longitudinal study that controlled for secondary outgroup contact, Tausch and colleagues (2010, Study 4) found that attitudes predicted contact with neither the primary nor the secondary outgroup. This finding thus unequivocally attributes secondary transfer to contact rather than to prejudice effects. Furthermore, several studies that deliberately used a range of contact and attitude measures now also highlight that STEs cannot be solely attributed to methodological artifacts such as shared method variance (Pettigrew, 2009; Schmid, Hewstone, Küpper, Zick, & Wagner, 2012; Tausch et al., 2010).

Attitude Generalization

Research across various intergroup contexts suggests that STEs are greatest when the primary and the secondary outgroup are similar

(Van Laar et al., 2005; see also Lolliot et al., 2013). This finding supports the hypothesis that secondary transfer occurs primarily through a process of attitude generalization, whereby attitudes toward an attitude object (e.g., a group) generalize to other, similar objects (Shook, Fazio, & Eiser, 2007). In the case of the STE, contact with outgroup *A* changes attitude toward outgroup *B* via a change in attitude toward outgroup *A*. Several cross-sectional and longitudinal studies have indicated that the effect of contact with a primary outgroup on attitudes toward a secondary outgroup is mediated by attitudes toward the primary outgroup (Bowman & Griffin, 2012; Tausch et al., 2010).

Deprovincialization

In addition to changed appraisals of the primary outgroup, changes in ingroup appraisal ("deprovincialization") could also potentially underpin STEs (see Lolliot et al., 2013). However, evidence for this mechanism remains rare. Pettigrew (2009), for example, found that the effect of contact with immigrants on attitudes toward homosexuals and the homeless was mediated by German participants' reduced national identification. Furthermore, Tausch and colleagues' (2010, Study 1) cross-sectional study of contact between Turkish- and Greek-origin Cypriots also identified a measure of deprovincialization (lowered collective self-esteem) as a mediator of STEs. However, the strength of this finding is limited because Tausch and associates (Study 1) did not control for direct contact with secondary outgroups.

In a more carefully controlled study of STEs in Northern Ireland, Tausch and colleagues (2010, Study 4) also tested deprovincialization and found that neither ingroup-directed feelings nor collective self-esteem mediated STEs. Other conceptualizations of ingroup reappraisal, however, have been found to mediate STEs more reliably, including increased social identity complexity (Schmid & Hewstone, 2011), and greater endorsement of multicultural norms (see Lolliot et al., 2013).

Secondary transfer continues to be a relatively unexplored area of intergroup contact research, with outstanding issues including the role of negative contact (but see Brylka, Jasinskaja-Lahti, & Mähönen, 2016) and the

quality and durability of attitudes toward secondary outgroups. And whereas many studies on STEs now control for direct contact with the secondary outgroup, we are also not aware of research accounting for the potentially confounding contribution of extended contact with the secondary outgroup to STEs, too. Nevertheless, a growing body of research now suggests that contact with members of one outgroup has consequences for the intergroup relations more widely: Intergroup contact has ripple effects that affect not only other ingroup members (via extended and vicarious contact) but also the appraisal of uninvolved outgroups (via STEs).

Contact Effects Beyond Prejudice

Although most intergroup research has focused on prejudice reduction, there is now also a growing literature on the effect of contact on more distal measures of well-being and participation in civic life.

Mental and Physical Health

The experience of persistent group-based discrimination is associated with a range of outcomes that limit psychological and even physiological well-being, including heightened stress (Dion & Earn, 1975), anxiety (Landrine & Klonoff, 1996), low self-esteem, and negative mood (Branscombe, Schmitt, & Harvey, 1999). Laboratory and field experiments have also shown that the perception of threat (Chen & Matthews, 2001) and hostile intent (Flory, Matthews, & Owens, 1998), and being in a disadvantaged role (Mendelson, Thurston, & Kubzansky, 2008) are all associated with risk factors for cardiovascular disease (see Williams, Neighbors, & Jackson 2003). These pernicious links between discrimination and health suggest that prejudice reduction via intergroup contact could translate into improved mental and physical well-being. To date, few studies have focused directly on the effect of intergroup contact on well-being. In a recent, large-scale study, Ramos, Bennett, Massey, and Hewstone (2019) analyzed data across 22 years on religious diversity worldwide, and showed that increasing diversity is initially associated with lower self-reported quality of life, explained by decreased trust in others. However, these negative effects are compensated in the longer term by benefits of intergroup contact, which alleviates earlier negative effects.

Participation in Collective Action for Social Change

Critics of intergroup contact research have argued that the prejudice-reducing (or attitude-enhancing) effect of contact might at the same time have a "sedative" or demobilizing effect and undermine minority group members' efforts to increase social equality (Dixon, Levine, Reicher, & Durrheim, 2012; Reicher, 2007). According to this view of intergroup relations, positive contact may entrench the *status quo* by emphasizing the minority's commonalities with a majority, diverting their attention away from inequalities, and creating affective loyalties toward the majority outgroup which then discourage collective action (Çakal, Hewstone, Güler, & Heath, 2016; Saguy, Tausch, Dovidio, & Pratto, 2009; Tausch, Saguy, & Bryson, 2015).

However, contact could arguably also strengthen the desire for social change, for example, by making intergroup inequality more visible or by highlighting that advantaged majority members support social change (Pettigrew & Hewstone, 2017). Supporting this rebuttal of the demobilization hypothesis, Becker, Wright, Lubensky, and Zhou (2013) showed that contact does not undermine collective action by minority group members when majority outgroup partners explicitly denounce inequality as unjust. Moreover, milder forms of negative contact, which may be relatively common in diverse settings (Schmid, Al Ramiah, & Hewstone, 2014), may actually energize resistance to the status quo. In two recent studies (one cross-sectional, and one longitudinal), we found that negative contact with majority outgroup members increased the willingness of minority group members to take action for social change by drawing attention to group-based injustice (Reimer et al., 2017).

Contact also provides a potentially powerful opportunity for majority-group members to foster political solidarity with the minority group (Mallett, Huntsinger, Sinclair, & Swim, 2008). Consistent with this view, positive contact not only promotes majority support for policies that benefit a minority outgroup (Voci & Hewstone,

2003), but it can also energize participation in solidarity-based collective action on behalf of a disadvantaged minority group (Reimer et al., 2017; Selvanathan, Techakesari, Tropp, & Barlow, 2017).

Volunteering

Volunteering is a mostly proactive behavior that entails some commitment of time and effort to benefit another person, group, or organization, and is widely considered an important indicator of social capital and citizenship (Wilson, 2000). Volunteering is more common in communities where people trust their neighbors (Lim & Laurence, 2015). The trust-enhancing effect of intergroup contact, outlined in our discussion of Principle 2, could therefore indirectly translate into more positive citizenship behavior.

Social relations within and across groups also affect which organizations individuals choose to join. In their analysis of representative U.S. survey data, Savelkoul, Hewstone, Scheepers, and Stolle (2015) found that interethnic contact was associated with lower perceived threat and thus more involvement with volunteering organizations in which further interethnic contact was likely ("bridging" as opposed to "bonding" voluntary organizations; Putnam, 2007). By alleviating threat perceptions, contact could thus indirectly boost active participation in civic activities that further improve intergroup relations.

Conclusion

Throughout the chapter, we have outlined the many promises that positive intergroup contact holds both for individuals engaged in cross-group interactions and their social context more widely. Fifteen years ago, one of us (M. H.) argued that while contact holds much potential for improved intergroup relations, it is no panacea for prejudice (Hewstone, 2003). Since this assertion, intergroup contact research has flourished, revealing an impressive increase in numbers of studies published (see Dovidio, Love, Schellhaas, & Hewstone, 2017) and the sophistication of theory and research. A "hypothesis" has been developed into a substantive theory. We have learned that intergroup contact experiences have consequences that reach wider and go deeper than the intuitive proposition that positive contact improves intergroup relations initially suggested. This includes the processes that underpin contact effects and the wider ripple effects of contact.

Meta-analyses of direct (Pettigrew & Tropp, 2006) and extended (Zhou et al., 2019) contact, friendship contact (Davies et al., 2011), and contact through interventions aimed at improving relations across various intergroup settings (Lemmer & Wagner, 2015; Paluck et al., 2019) all point to the overall small to moderate effect of intergroup contact, and such small effects should not be misunderstood as unimportant, especially if they accumulate over time and their effects are multiplied across individuals and outgroups not directly involved in the intervention (see also Funder & Ozer, 2019). Over 65 years after Allport's (1954) influential statement of the "contact hypothesis," the field can take credit for exploring his ideas fully and providing a deeper analysis of social psychology's most significant contribution to reducing prejudice.

NOTES

1. It should be noted here that bidirectional effects are often found. However, for contact to be confirmed as providing a basis for prejudice-reducing social interventions, it is only necessary to show that contact promotes prejudice reduction (even if the reverse is also found).

2. In the chapter, we have given careful thought to pronoun use. In situations like this one in which pronoun use was needed and the gender identity of the person being referenced is unknown, we used "they/them/their" to indicate a gender-neutral pronoun.

REFERENCES

Aberson, C. L., & Gaffney, A. M. (2009). An integrated threat model of explicit and implicit attitudes. *European Journal of Social Psychology, 39,* 808–830.

Allport, G. W. (1954). *The nature of prejudice.* Cambridge/Reading, MA: Addison-Wesley.

Allport, G. W. (1955). *Becoming: Basic considerations for a psychology of personality.* New Haven, CT: Yale University Press.

Andrighetto, L., Mari, S., Volpato, C., & Behluli, B. (2012). Reducing competitive victimhood in Kosovo: The role of extended contact and common ingroup identity. *Political Psychology, 33,* 513–529.

Aron, A., Aron, E. N., & Norman, C. (2001). The self-expansion model of motivation and cognition in close relationships and beyond. In M. Clark & G. Fletcher (Eds.), *Blackwell handbook of social psychology* (Vol. 2, pp. 478–501). Malden, MA: Blackwell.

Aron, A., Aron, E. N., & Smollan, D. (1992). Inclusion of Other in the Self Scale and the structure of interpersonal closeness. *Journal of Personality and Social Psychology, 63,* 596–612.

Aronson, E., & Cope, V. (1968). My enemy's enemy is my friend. *Journal of Personality and Social Psychology, 8,* 8–12.

Asbrock, F., Christ, O., Duckitt, J., & Sibley, C. G. (2012). Differential effects of intergroup contact for authoritarians and social dominators: A dual process model perspective. *Personality and Social Psychology Bulletin, 38,* 477–490.

Barlow, F. K., Paolini, S., Pedersen, A., Hornsey, M. J., Radke, H. R. M., Harwood, J., et al. (2012). The contact caveat: Negative contact predicts increased prejudice more than positive contact predicts reduced prejudice. *Personality and Social Psychology Bulletin, 38,* 1629–1643.

Batson, C. D., Early, S., & Salvarani, G. (1997). Perspective taking: Imagining how another feels versus imaging how you would feel. *Personality and Social Psychology Bulletin, 23,* 751–758.

Becker, J. C., Wright, S. C., Lubensky, M. E., & Zhou, S. (2013). Friend or ally: Whether cross-group contact undermines collective action depends on what advantaged group members say (or don't say). *Personality and Social Psychology Bulletin, 39,* 442–455.

Bekhuis, H., Ruiter, S., & Coenders, M. (2013). Xenophobia among youngsters: The effect of interethnic contact. *European Sociological Review, 29,* 229–242.

Bettencourt, B. A., Brewer, M. B., Croak, M. R., & Miller, N. (1992). Cooperation and the reduction of intergroup bias: The role of reward structure and social orientation. *Journal of Experimental Social Psychology, 28,* 301–319.

Binder, J., Zagefka, H., Brown, R., Funke, F., Kessler, T., Mummendey, A., et al. (2009). Does contact reduce prejudice or does prejudice reduce contact?: A longitudinal test of the contact hypothesis among majority and minority groups in three European countries. *Journal of Personality and Social Psychology, 96,* 843–856.

Blascovich, J., Mendes, W. B., Hunter, S. B., Lickel,

B., & Kowai-Bell, N. (2001). Perceiver threat in social interactions with stigmatized others. *Journal of Personality and Social Psychology, 80,* 253–267.

Bowman, N. A., & Griffin, T. M. (2012). Secondary transfer effects of interracial contact: The moderating role of social status. *Cultural Diversity and Ethnic Minority Psychology, 18,* 35–44.

Branscombe, N. R., Schmitt, M. T., & Harvey, R. D. (1999). Perceiving pervasive discrimination among African Americans: Implications for group identification and well-being. *Journal of Personality and Social Psychology, 77,* 135–149.

Brown, R., & Hewstone, M. (2005). An integrative theory of intergroup contact. *Advances in Experimental Social Psychology, 37,* 255–343.

Brylka, A., Jasinskaja-Lahti, I., & Mähönen, T. A. (2016). The majority influence on interminority attitudes: The secondary transfer effect of positive and negative contact. *International Journal of Intercultural Relations, 50,* 76–88.

Çakal, H., Hewstone, M., Güler, M., & Heath, A. (2016). Predicting support for collective action in the conflict between Turks and Kurds: Perceived threats as a mediator of intergroup contact and social identity. *Group Processes and Intergroup Relations, 19,* 732–752.

Capozza, D., Falvo, R., Favara, I., & Trifiletti, E. (2013). The relationship between direct and indirect cross-group friendships and outgroup humanization: Emotional and cognitive mediators. *TPM—Testing, Psychometrics, Methodology in Applied Psychology, 20,* 383–398.

Capozza, D., Falvo, R., Trifiletti, E., & Pagani, A. (2014). Cross-group friendships, extended contact, and humanity attributions to homosexuals. *Procedia—Social and Behavioral Sciences, 114,* 276–282.

Cehajic, S., Brown, R., & Castano, E. (2008). Forgive and forget?: Antecedents and consequences of intergroup forgiveness in Bosnia and Herzegovina. *Political Psychology, 29,* 351–367.

Chen, E., & Matthews, K. A. (2001). Cognitive appraisal biases: An approach to understanding the relation between socioeconomic status and cardiovascular reactivity in children. *Annals of Behavioral Medicine, 23,* 101–111.

Christ, O., Hewstone, M., Tausch, N., Wagner, U., Voci, A., Hughes, J., et al. (2010). Direct contact as a moderator of extended contact effects: Cross-sectional and longitudinal impact on outgroup attitudes, behavioral intentions, and attitude certainty. *Personality and Social Psychology Bulletin, 36,* 1662–1674.

Christ, O., Schmid, K., Lolliot, S., Swart, H., Stolle, D., Tausch, N., et al. (2014). Contextual effect of positive intergroup contact on outgroup prejudice. *Proceedings of the National Academy of Sciences of the USA, 111,* 3996–4000.

Christ, O., Ullrich, J., Wagner, U. (2008, June). *The joint effects of positive and negative contact on attitudes and attitude strength.* Paper presented at the general meeting of the European Association of Experimental Social Psychology, Opatija, Croatia.

Cook, S. W. (1962). The systematic analysis of socially significant events: A strategy for social research. *Journal of Social Issues, 18,* 66–84.

Cook, S. W. (1978). Interpersonal and attitudinal outcomes in cooperating interracial groups. *Journal of Research and Development in Education, 12,* 97–113.

Cooper, J., & Hogg, M. A. (2007). Feeling the anguish of others: A theory of vicarious dissonance. *Advances in Experimental Social Psychology, 39,* 359–403.

Davies, K., Tropp, L. R., Aron, A., Pettigrew, T. F., & Wright, S. C. (2011). Cross-group friendships and intergroup attitudes: A meta-analytic review. *Personality and Social Psychology Review, 15,* 332–351.

Davis, M. H. (1996). *Empathy: A social psychological approach.* Boulder, CO: Westview Press.

De Tezanos-Pinto, P., Bratt, C., & Brown, R. (2010). What will the others think?: In-group norms as a mediator of the effects of intergroup contact. *British Journal of Social Psychology, 49,* 507–523.

Dhont, K., Cornelis, I., & Van Hiel, A. (2010). Interracial public–police contact: Relationships with police officers' racial and work-related attitudes and behavior. *International Journal of Intercultural Relations, 34,* 551–560.

Dhont, K., Roets, A., & Van Hiel, A. (2011). Opening closed minds: The combined effects of intergroup contact and need for closure on prejudice. *Personality and Social Psychology Bulletin, 37,* 514–528.

Dhont, K., & Van Hiel, A. (2009). We must not be enemies: Interracial contact and the reduction of prejudice among authoritarians. *Personality and Individual Differences, 46,* 172–177.

Dhont, K., & Van Hiel, A. (2011). Direct contact and authoritarianism as moderators between extended contact and reduced prejudice: Lower threat and greater trust as mediators. *Group Processes and Intergroup Relations, 14,* 223–237.

Dion, K. L., & Earn, B. M. (1975). The phenomenology of being a target of prejudice. *Journal of Personality and Social Psychology, 32,* 944–950.

Dixon, J., Levine, M., Reicher, S., & Durrheim, K. (2012). Beyond prejudice: Are negative evaluations the problem and is getting us to like one another more the solution? *Behavioral and Brain Sciences, 35,* 411–425.

Dovidio, J. F., Love, A., Schellhaas, F. M. H., & Hewstone, M. (2017). Reducing intergroup bias through intergroup contact: Twenty years of progress and future directions. *Group Processes and Intergroup Relations, 20,* 606–620.

du Toit, M., & Quayle, M. (2011). Multiracial families and contact theory in South Africa: Does direct and extended contact facilitated by multiracial families predict reduced prejudice? *South African Journal of Psychology, 41,* 540–551.

Eller, A., & Abrams, D. (2004). Come together: Longitudinal comparisons of Pettigrew's reformulated intergroup contact model and the common ingroup identity model in Anglo-French and Mexican-American contexts. *European Journal of Social Psychology, 34,* 229–256.

Eller, A., Abrams, D., & Zimmermann, A. (2011). Two degrees of separation: A longitudinal study of actual and perceived extended international contact. *Group Processes and Intergroup Relations, 14,* 175–191.

Flory, J. D., Matthews, K. A., & Owens, J. F. (1998). A social information processing approach to dispositional hostility: Relationships with negative mood and blood pressure elevations at work. *Journal of Social and Clinical Psychology, 17,* 491–504.

Fox, E., Russo, R., Bowles, R., & Dutton, K. (2001). Do threatening stimuli draw or hold visual attention in subclinical anxiety? *Journal of Experimental Psychology, 130,* 681–700.

Funder, D. C., & Ozer, D. J. (2019). Evaluating effect size in psychological research: Sense and nonsense. *Advances in Methods and Practices in Psychological Science, 2,* 156–168.

Gaertner, S. L., & Dovidio, J. F. (2000). *Reducing intergroup bias: The common ingroup identity model.* Philadelphia: Psychology Press.

Glasford, D. E., & Dovidio, J. F. (2011). E pluribus unum: Dual identity and minority group members' motivation to engage in contact, as well as social change. *Journal of Experimental Social Psychology, 47,* 1021–1024.

Gómez, A., Tropp, L. R., & Fernández, S. (2011). When extended contact opens the door to future contact: Testing the effects of extended contact on attitudes and intergroup expectancies in majority and minority groups. *Group Processes and Intergroup Relations, 14,* 161–173.

Graf, S., Paolini, S., & Rubin, M. (2014). Negative intergroup contact is more influential, but positive intergroup contact is more common: Assessing contact prominence and contact prevalence in five Central European countries: Influential negative but more common positive contact. *European Journal of Social Psychology, 44,* 536–547.

Hamberger, J., & Hewstone, M. (1997). Inter-ethnic contact as a predictor of blatant and subtle prejudice: Tests of a model in four West European nations. *British Journal of Social Psychology, 36,* 173–190.

Hartley, E. (1946). *Problems in prejudice.* Oxford, UK: King's Crown Press.

Harwood, J., Hewstone, M., Paolini, S., & Voci, A. (2005). Grandparent–grandchild contact and attitudes toward older adults: Moderator and mediator effects. *Personality and Social Psychology Bulletin, 31,* 393–406.

Hayward, L., Tropp, L., Hornsey, M., & Barlow, F. (2017). Toward a comprehensive understanding of intergroup contact: Descriptions and mediators of positive and negative contact among majority and minority groups. *Personality and Social Psychology Bulletin, 43,* 347–364.

Hewstone, M. (2003). Intergroup contact: Panacea for prejudice? *The Psychologist, 16,* 352–355.

Hewstone, M., & Swart, H. (2011). Fifty-odd years of inter-group contact: From hypothesis to integrated theory. *British Journal of Social Psychology, 50,* 374–386.

Hodson, G., Costello, K., & MacInnis, C. C. (2013). Is intergroup contact beneficial among intolerant people?: Exploring individual differences in the benefits of contact on attitudes. In G. Hodson & M. Hewstone (Eds.), *Advances in intergroup contact* (pp. 49–80). New York: Psychology Press.

Hodson, G., Harry, H., & Mitchell, A. (2009). Independent benefits of contact and friendship on attitudes toward homosexuals among authoritarians and highly identified heterosexuals. *European Journal of Social Psychology, 39,* 509–525.

Ioannou, M., Al Ramiah, A., & Hewstone, M. (2018). An experimental comparison of direct and indirect intergroup contact. *Journal of Experimental Social Psychology, 76,* 393–403.

Islam, M. R., & Hewstone, M. (1993). Dimensions of contact as predictors of intergroup anxiety, perceived out-group variability, and out-group attitude: An integrative model. *Personality and Social Psychology Bulletin, 19,* 700–710.

Jetten, J., Spears, R., & Manstead, A. S. R. (1996). Intergroup norms and intergroup discrimination: Distinctive self-categorization and social identity effects. *Journal of Personality and Social Psychology, 71,* 1222–1233.

Kauff, M., Schmid, K., Lolliot, S., Al Ramiah, A., & Hewstone, M. (2016). Intergroup contact effects via ingroup distancing among majority and minority groups: Moderation by social dominance orientation. *PLOS ONE, 11,* e0146895.

Kenworthy, J. B., Voci, A., Ramiah, A. A., Tausch, N., Hughes, J., & Hewstone, M. (2016). Building trust in a postconflict society: An integrative model of cross-group friendship and intergroup emotions. *Journal of Conflict Resolution, 60,* 1041–1070.

Kramer, R. M., & Carnevale, P. J. (2003). Trust and intergroup negotiation. In R. Brown & S. Gaertner (Eds.), *Blackwell handbook of social psychology: Intergroup processes* (pp. 431–450). Oxford, UK: Blackwell.

Landrine, H., & Klonoff, E. A. (1996). The schedule of racist events: A measure of racial discrimination and a study of its negative physical and mental health consequences. *Journal of Black Psychology, 22,* 144–168.

Laurence, J., Schmid, K., & Hewstone, M. (2018). Ethnic diversity, inter-group attitudes and countervailing pathways of positive and negative intergroup contact: An analysis across workplaces and neighbourhoods. *Social Indicators Research, 136,* 719–749.

Lemmer, G., & Wagner, U. (2015). Can we really reduce ethnic prejudice outside the lab?: A meta-analysis of direct and indirect contact interventions. *European Journal of Social Psychology, 45,* 152–168.

Levin, S., van Laar, C., & Sidanius, J. (2003). The effects of ingroup and outgroup friendships on ethnic attitudes in college: A longitudinal study. *Group Processes and Intergroup Relations, 6,* 76–92.

Lim, C., & Laurence, J. (2015). Doing good when times are bad: Volunteering behaviour in economic hard times. *British Journal of Sociology, 66,* 319–344.

Lolliot, S., Fell, B., Schmid, K., Wölfer, R., Swart, H., Voci, A., et al. (2014). Measures of intergroup contact. In G. J. Boyle, D. H. Saklofske, & G. Matthews (Eds.), *Measures of personality and social psychological constructs* (pp. 652–683). New York: Elsevier.

Lolliot, S., Schmid, K., Hewstone, M., Al Ramiah, A., Tausch, N., & Swart, H. (2013). Generalized effects of intergroup contact: The secondary transfer effects. In G. Hodson & M. Hewstone (Eds.), *Advances in intergroup contact* (pp. 81–112). Hove, UK: Psychology Press.

Mallett, R. K., Huntsinger, J. R., Sinclair, S., & Swim, J. K. (2008). Seeing through their eyes: When majority group members take collective action on behalf of an outgroup. *Group Processes and Intergroup Relations, 11,* 451–470.

Mallett, R. K., & Wilson, T. D. (2010). Increasing positive intergroup contact. *Journal of Experimental Social Psychology, 46,* 382–387.

McIntyre, K., Paolini, S., & Hewstone, M. (2016). Changing people's views of outgroups through

individual-to-group generalisation: Meta-analytic reviews and theoretical considerations. *European Review of Social Psychology, 27,* 63–115.

Mendelson, T., Thurston, R. C., & Kubzansky, L. D. (2008). Affective and cardiovascular effects of experimentally-induced social status. *Health Psychology, 27,* 482–489.

Mendes, W. B., Blascovich, J., Lickel, B., & Hunter, S. (2002). Challenge and threat during social interactions with White and Black men. *Personality and Social Psychology Bulletin, 28,* 939–952.

Munniksma, A., Stark, T. H., Verkuyten, M., Flache, A., & Veenstra, R. (2013). Extended intergroup friendships within social settings: The moderating role of initial outgroup attitudes. *Group Processes and Intergroup Relations, 16,* 752–770.

Page-Gould, E., Mendoza-Denton, R., & Tropp, L. R. (2008). With a little help from my cross-group friend: Reducing anxiety in intergroup contexts through cross-group friendship. *Journal of Personality and Social Psychology, 95,* 1080–1094.

Paluck, E. L., Green, S. A., & Green, D. P. (2019). The contact hypothesis re-evaluated. *Behavioural Public Policy, 3,* 129–158.

Paolini, S., Harris, N. C., & Griffin, A. S. (2016). Learning anxiety in interactions with the outgroup: Towards a learning model of anxiety and stress in intergroup contact. *Group Processes and Intergroup Relations, 19,* 275–313.

Paolini, S., Harwood, J., & Rubin, M. (2010). Negative intergroup contact makes group memberships salient: Explaining why intergroup conflict endures. *Personality and Social Psychology Bulletin, 36,* 1723–1738.

Paolini, S., Harwood, J., Rubin, M., Husnu, S., Joyce, N., & Hewstone, M. (2014). Positive and extensive intergroup contact in the past buffers against the disproportionate impact of negative contact in the present. *European Journal of Social Psychology, 44,* 548–562.

Paolini, S., Hewstone, M., & Cairns, E. (2007). Direct and indirect intergroup friendship effects: Testing the moderating role of the affective-cognitive bases of prejudice. *Personality and Social Psychology Bulletin, 33,* 1406–1420.

Paolini, S., Hewstone, M., Cairns, E., & Voci, A. (2004). Effects of direct and indirect cross-group friendships on judgments of Catholics and Protestants in Northern Ireland: The mediating role of an anxiety-reduction mechanism. *Personality and Social Psychology Bulletin, 30,* 770–786.

Paolini, S., Hewstone, M., Voci, A., Harwood, J., & Cairns, E. (2006). Intergroup contact and the promotion of intergroup harmony: The influence of intergroup emotions. In R. Brown & D. Capozza (Eds.), *Social identities: Motivational, emotional, and cultural influences* (pp. 209–238). Hove, UK: Psychology Press.

Pettigrew, T. F. (1986). The intergroup contact hypothesis reconsidered. In M. Hewstone & R. Brown (Eds.), *Contact and conflict in intergroup encounters* (pp. 169–195). Cambridge, MA: Blackwell.

Pettigrew, T. F. (1997). Generalized intergroup contact effects on prejudice. *Personality and Social Psychology Bulletin, 23,* 173–185.

Pettigrew, T. F. (1998). Intergroup contact theory. *Annual Review of Psychology, 49,* 65–85.

Pettigrew, T. F. (2008). Future directions for intergroup contact theory and research. *International Journal of Intercultural Relations, 32,* 187–199.

Pettigrew, T. F. (2009). Secondary transfer effect of contact: Do intergroup contact effects spread to noncontacted outgroups? *Social Psychology, 40,* 55–65.

Pettigrew, T. F., & Hewstone, M. (2017). The single factor fallacy: Implications of missing critical variables from an analysis of intergroup contact theory. *Social Issues and Policy Review, 11,* 8–37.

Pettigrew, T. F., & Tropp, L. R. (2006). A meta-analytic test of intergroup contact theory. *Journal of Personality and Social Psychology, 90,* 751–783.

Pettigrew, T. F., & Tropp, L. R. (2008). How does intergroup contact reduce prejudice?: Meta-analytic tests of three mediators. *European Journal of Social Psychology, 38,* 922–934.

Pettigrew, T. F., Tropp, L. R., Wagner, U., & Christ, O. (2011). Recent advances in intergroup contact theory. *International Journal of Intercultural Relations, 35,* 271–280.

Putnam, R. D. (2007). E pluribus unum: Diversity and community in the twenty-first century the 2006 Johan Skytte Prize Lecture. *Scandinavian Political Studies, 30,* 137–174.

Ramos, M., Bennett, M., Massey, D. S., & Hewstone, M. (2019). Humans adapt to social diversity over time. *Proceedings of the National Academy of Sciences of the USA, 116,* 12244–12249.

Reicher, S. (2007). Rethinking the paradigm of prejudice. *South African Journal of Psychology, 37,* 820–834.

Reimer, N. K., Becker, J. C., Benz, A., Christ, O., Dhont, K., Klocke, U., et al. (2017). Intergroup contact and social change: Implications of negative and positive contact for collective action in advantaged and disadvantaged groups. *Personality and Social Psychology Bulletin, 43,* 121–136.

Reimer, N. K., Kamble, S. V., Schmid, K., & Hewstone, M. (2020). *Intergroup contact fosters more inclusive social identities.* Manuscript submitted for publication.

Roccas, S., & Brewer, M. B. (2002). Social identity

complexity. *Personality and Social Psychology Review, 6,* 88–106.

Saguy, T., Tausch, N., Dovidio, J. F., & Pratto, F. (2009). The irony of harmony: Intergroup contact can produce false expectations for equality. *Psychological Science, 20,* 114–121.

Savelkoul, M., Hewstone, M., Scheepers, P., & Stolle, D. (2015). Does relative out-group size in neighborhoods drive down associational life of Whites in the U.S.?: Testing constrict, conflict and contact theories. *Social Science Research, 52,* 236–252.

Schmid, K., Al Ramiah, A., & Hewstone, M. (2014). Neighborhood ethnic diversity and trust the role of intergroup contact and perceived threat. *Psychological Science, 25,* 665–674.

Schmid, K., & Hewstone, M. (2011). Social identity complexity: Theoretical implications for the social psychology of intergroup relations. In R. M. Kramer, G. Leonardelli, & R. Livingston (Eds.), *Social cognition, social identity, and intergroup relations: A Festschrift in honor of Marilynn Brewer* (pp. 77–102). Philadelphia: Psychology Press.

Schmid, K., Hewstone, M., Küpper, B., Zick, A., & Wagner, U. (2012). Secondary transfer effects of intergroup contact: A cross-national comparison in Europe. *Social Psychology Quarterly, 75,* 28–51.

Schmid, K., Hewstone, M., Tausch, N., Cairns, E., & Hughes, J. (2009). Antecedents and consequences of social identity complexity: Intergroup contact, distinctiveness threat, and outgroup attitudes. *Personality and Social Psychology Bulletin, 35,* 1085–1098.

Schmid, K., Tausch, N., Hewstone, M., Hughes, J., & Cairns, E. (2008). The effects of living in segregated vs. mixed areas in Northern Ireland: A simultaneous analysis of contact and threat effects in the context of micro-level neighbourhoods. *International Journal of Conflict and Violence, 2,* 56–71.

Schofield, J. W., Hausmann, L. R. M., Ye, F., & Woods, R. L. (2010). Intergroup friendships on campus: Predicting close and casual friendships between White and African American first-year college students. *Group Processes and Intergroup Relations, 13,* 585–602.

Selvanathan, H. P., Techakesari, P., Tropp, L. R., & Barlow, F. K. (2017). Whites for racial justice: How contact with Black Americans predicts support for collective action among White Americans. *Group Processes and Intergroup Relations, 21,* 893–912.

Sharp, M., Voci, A., & Hewstone, M. (2011). Individual difference variables as moderators of the effect of extended cross-group friendship on prejudice: Testing the effects of public self-consciousness and social comparison. *Group Processes and Intergroup Relations, 14,* 207–221.

Shook, N. J., Fazio, R. H., & Eiser, J. R. (2007). Attitude generalization: Similarity, valence, and extremity. *Journal of Experimental Social Psychology, 43,* 641–647.

Stephan, W. G., & Finlay, K. (1999). The role of empathy in improving intergroup relations. *Journal of Social Issues, 55,* 729–743.

Stephan, W. G., & Stephan, C. W. (1985). Intergroup anxiety. *Journal of Social Issues, 41,* 157–175.

Stephan, W. G., & Stephan, C. W. (2000). An integrated threat theory of prejudice. In S. Oskamp (Ed.), *Reducing prejudice and discrimination* (pp. 23–45). New York: Psychology Press.

Swart, H., Hewstone, M., Christ, O., & Voci, A. (2011). Affective mediators of intergroup contact: A three-wave longitudinal study in South Africa. *Journal of Personality and Social Psychology, 101,* 1221–1238.

Tajfel, H., & Turner, J. C. (1986). The social identity theory of intergroup behavior. In S. Worchel & W. Austin (Eds.), *Psychology of intergroup relations* (pp. 33–48). Chicago: Nelson-Hall.

Tam, T., Hewstone, M., Kenworthy, J., & Cairns, E. (2009). Intergroup trust in Northern Ireland. *Personality and Social Psychology Bulletin, 35,* 45–59.

Tausch, N., Hewstone, M., Kenworthy, J., Cairns, E., & Christ, O. (2007). Cross-community contact, perceived status differences, and intergroup attitudes in Northern Ireland: The mediating roles of individual-level versus group-level threats and the moderating role of social identification. *Political Psychology, 28,* 53–68.

Tausch, N., Hewstone, M., Kenworthy, J. B., Psaltis, C., Schmid, K., Popan, J. R., et al. (2010). Secondary transfer effects of intergroup contact: Alternative accounts and underlying processes. *Journal of Personality and Social Psychology, 99,* 282–302.

Tausch, N., Hewstone, M., Schmid, K., Hughes, J., & Cairns, E. (2011). Extended contact effects as a function of closeness of relationship with ingroup contacts. *Group Processes and Intergroup Relations, 14,* 239–254.

Tausch, N., Saguy, T., & Bryson, J. (2015). How does intergroup contact affect social change?: Its impact on collective action and individual mobility intentions among members of a disadvantaged group. *Journal of Social Issues, 71,* 536–553.

Tropp, L. R., & Pettigrew, T. F. (2005). Differential relationships between intergroup contact and affective and cognitive dimensions of prejudice. *Personality and Social Psychology Bulletin, 31,* 1145–1158.

Tropp, L. R., & Wright, S. C. (2001). Ingroup identification as the inclusion of ingroup in the self. *Personality and Social Psychology Bulletin, 27,* 585–600.

Turner, J. C., Hogg, M. A., Oakes, P. J., Reicher, S. D., & Wetherell, M. S. (1987). *Rediscovering the social group: A self-categorization theory.* Oxford, UK: Blackwell.

Turner, R. N., Hewstone, M., & Voci, A. (2007). Reducing explicit and implicit outgroup prejudice via direct and extended contact: The mediating role of self-disclosure and intergroup anxiety. *Journal of Personality and Social Psychology, 93,* 369–388.

Turner, R. N., Hewstone, M., Voci, A., & Vonofakou, C. (2008). A test of the extended intergroup contact hypothesis: The mediating role of intergroup anxiety, perceived ingroup and outgroup norms, and inclusion of the outgroup in the self. *Journal of Personality and Social Psychology, 95,* 843–860.

van Dommelen, A., Schmid, K., Hewstone, M., Gonsalkorale, K., & Brewer, M. (2015). Construing multiple ingroups: Assessing social identity inclusiveness and structure in ethnic and religious minority group members. *European Journal of Social Psychology, 45,* 386–399.

Van Laar, C., Levin, S., Sinclair, S., & Sidanius, J. (2005). The effect of university roommate contact on ethnic attitudes and behavior. *Journal of Experimental Social Psychology, 41,* 329–345.

Van Oudenhoven, J. P., Groenewoud, J. T., & Hewstone, M. (1996). Cooperation, ethnic salience and generalization of interethnic attitudes. *European Journal of Social Psychology, 26,* 649–661.

Verkuyten, M., Thijs, J., & Bekhuis, H. (2010). Intergroup contact and ingroup reappraisal: Examining the deprovincialization thesis. *Social Psychology Quarterly, 73,* 398–416.

Vezzali, L., & Giovannini, D. (2011). Intergroup contact and reduction of explicit and implicit prejudice toward immigrants: A study with Italian businessmen owning small and medium enterprises. *Quality and Quantity, 45,* 213–222.

Vezzali, L., Hewstone, M., Capozza, D., Giovannini, D., & Wölfer, R. (2014). Improving intergroup relations with extended and vicarious forms of indirect contact. *European Review of Social Psychology, 25,* 314–389.

Vezzali, L., Stathi, S., & Giovannini, D. (2012). Indirect contact through book reading: Improving adolescents' attitudes and behavioral intentions toward immigrants. *Psychology in the Schools, 49,* 148–162.

Vezzali, L., Stathi, S., Giovannini, D., Capozza, D., &

Visintin, E. P. (2015). "And the best essay is . . . ": Extended contact and cross-group friendships at school. *British Journal of Social Psychology, 54,* 601–615.

Voci, A., & Hewstone, M. (2003). Intergroup contact and prejudice toward immigrants in Italy: The mediational role of anxiety and the moderational role of group salience. *Group Processes and Intergroup Relations, 6,* 37–54.

White, F. A., Abu-Rayya, H. M., Bliuc, A.-M., & Faulkner, N. (2015). Emotion expression and intergroup bias reduction between Muslims and Christians: Long-term Internet contact. *Computers in Human Behavior, 53,* 435–442.

Wilder, D. A. (1993). The role of anxiety in facilitating stereotypic judgments of outgroup behavior. In D. M. Mackie & D. L. Hamilton (Eds.), *Affect, cognition and stereotyping: Interactive processes in group perception* (pp. 87–109). San Diego, CA: Academic Press.

Wilder, D. A., Simon, A. F., & Faith, M. (1996). Enhancing the impact of counterstereotypic information: Dispositional attributions for deviance. *Journal of Personality and Social Psychology, 71,* 276–287.

Williams, D. R., Neighbors, H. W., & Jackson, J. S. (2003). Racial/ethnic discrimination and health: Findings from community studies. *American Journal of Public Health, 93,* 200–208.

Wilson, J. (2000). Volunteering. *Annual Review of Sociology, 26,* 215–240.

Wölfer, R., Christ, O., Schmid, K., Tausch, N.,

Vuchallik, F. M., Vertovec, S., et al. (2019). Indirect contact predicts direct contact: Longitudinal evidence and the mediating role of intergroup anxiety. *Journal of Personality and Social Psychology, 116,* 277–295.

Wölfer, R., & Hewstone, M. (2017). Beyond the dyadic perspective: 10 reasons for using social network analysis in intergroup contact research. *British Journal of Social Psychology, 56,* 609–617.

Wölfer, R., & Hewstone, M. (2018). What buffers ethnic homophily?: Explaining the development of outgroup contact in adolescence. *Developmental Psychology, 54,* 1507–1518.

Wölfer, R., Schmid, K., Hewstone, M., & van Zalk, M. (2016). Developmental dynamics of intergroup contact and intergroup attitudes: Long-term effects in adolescence and early adulthood. *Child Development, 87,* 1466–1478.

Wolsko, C., Park, B., Judd, C. M., & Bachelor, J. (2003). Intergroup contact: Effects on group evaluations and perceived variability. *Group Processes and Intergroup Relations, 6,* 93–110.

Wright, S. C., Aron, A., McLaughlin-Volpe, T., & Ropp, S. A. (1997). The extended contact effect: Knowledge of cross-group friendships and prejudice. *Journal of Personality and Social Psychology, 73,* 73–90.

Zhou, S., Page-Gould, E., Aron, A., Moyer, A., & Hewstone, M. (2019). The extended contact hypothesis: A meta-analysis on 20 years of research. *Personality and Social Psychology Review, 23,* 132–160.

CHAPTER 23

Categorization and Identity as Motivational Principles in Intergroup Relations

Naomi Ellemers
Dick de Gilder

Mechanisms relating to categorization and identity are perceived as lying at the root of many tensions between groups in society. Recruiters of organizations that fail to diversify their workforce are accused of too easily categorizing others into groups—excluding them because of negative group stereotypes instead of learning about their individual qualifications. Social unrest and political polarization are explained by arguing that people from different social or cultural origins have incompatible identities. It is important to gain insight in the origins, nature, and implications of categorization and identity to understand the motivational processes guiding intergroup relations.

The analysis provided here relies on the notion that people can have a "group self" in addition to a personal self (Ellemers, 2012). Of course, when introducing oneself at a social event, one may choose to focus on one's personal identity by emphasizing individual skills, beliefs, or character traits that one sees as self-defining and distinguishing one from other individuals in that situation. However, people are just as likely—if not more likely—to communicate to others who they are by referring to group-based identities and by noting features they share with others, for instance by virtue of their profession, city of residence, or family status. Considering oneself and others in terms of such shared features and group-based identities (e.g., as a Southerner, as a musician) has far-reaching implications. It reveals motivational forces that cannot be fully understood from individual-level motives, such as the conviction that people cooperate with others only to secure individual outcomes, or that people direct their efforts to those goals that offer personal benefit.

Defining oneself as a Southerner, for instance, may prompt people to defend the views and actions of others living in the South, even when they don't personally know these individuals or personally approve of what they do. Thinking of oneself as a musician can motivate one to support other musicians, by lending them instruments, or sponsoring their performances, even if it is clear these other musicians will not be able to reciprocate such favors. In this chapter, we consider the mechanisms through which people may develop different perceptions, emotions, and behaviors in situations in which their group-based identities and the features they share with others are more important to them than their personal characteristics or the features that set themselves apart from other members of their group.

These phenomena can be understood from theory and research about *social categorization and social identity*. This approach goes beyond notions of interdependence and self-interest. It convincingly argues for the existence of a more *symbolic* value people can attach to group memberships as a source of loyalty that merits self-sacrifice. It also explains the experience of empathy and vicarious emotions due to the plight of others that do not directly affect the self. Understanding the basic principles of categorization and identity explains when and how group affiliations impact on the way people relate to each other, in ways that cannot be explained from individual-level concerns. Categorization and identity principles explain when and why we are often inclined to distinguish "us" from "them," why we find it difficult to trust people just because they have a different skin color or country of origin, and what can be done to build a sense of common purpose and collaborate with others.

The key to understanding these issues is the notion that the same individual can be motivated to act in different ways depending on the categorization that is activated in a particular situation. Thinking of oneself as a Dutch national may raise suspicion of migrant workers; thinking of oneself and others as fellow professionals working in the same company may alleviate such feelings. Thus, learning about the psychological mechanisms involved in categorization and identity helps us understand how this affects people's sense of involvement with others and the goals they find important, depending on how these relate to important indicators of their identity.

In this chapter, we draw on important principles relating to social identity and self-categorization that are usually indicated as "the social identity approach." Since the seminal publication specifying the origins of this school of thought (Tajfel & Turner, 1979), four decades of theorizing and empirical studies by many different researchers have led to further elaboration and refinement of this approach, which we apply here to explain and understand the behavior of individuals and groups (see also Ellemers & Haslam, 2011; Haslam, Ellemers, Reicher, Reynolds, & Schmitt, 2010).

Categorization and Identity as Basic Principles

Categorization

In processing information about their surroundings, people organize situations, objects, and creatures, trying to capture their essential features by categorizing them into groups. Categorization is important to human perception because it offers important information about unknown stimuli that can be used to adequately deal with new situations. It is useful to know whether a bottle with a colorful liquid contains soap or lemonade, without having to taste it. When in a strange country, we quickly find out which features to look out for to be able to distinguish a billboard from a bus stop, or a private car from a taxi that can be hailed, even though they come in different shapes, sizes, and colors. This strategy to derive information and anticipate the likely properties of objects by categorizing them into groups is also applied in our interactions with other people: This is commonly referred to as *social* categorization. We learn that the uniforms individuals wear tell us something about their professional roles and likely skills, and if we need help to carry a heavy load, we look out for someone we can classify as a young adult, preferably male, instead of a child or senior citizen.

Deciding who belongs to which category can yield useful information, as we indicated earlier. However, the very act of boundary drawing in itself has far-reaching implications, as placing an object or individual in a particular category also *influences* the way the object or person is perceived (Lamont & Molnár, 2002). For example, knowing that you have a new colleague called Robin is not very helpful before you know whether this is a male or a female. Only then are you able to imagine what this person will be like and which types of activities you might share. Thus, category-based perception not only emerges from *bottom-up* processing of objective features (Robin's hobbies or preferences). It also implies imposing a *top-down* structure, in which the category label and its characteristic properties are used to make inferences about individual qualities. You may hope a man called Robin will join you in watching the football game; you may expect a woman called Robin to join you in shopping for shoes—even if this is unwarranted.

This tendency of our brain to "fill in" missing information by relying on category-based expectations happens immediately—even before we realize that we do this or can consciously decide this is not what we want. Furthermore, this tendency is very pervasive; it is used even if this does not accurately reflect key features of the object or person under consideration (Cikara & Van Bavel, 2014). Robin, the man, may hate football; Robin, the woman, may loathe shopping. As we explain in more detail below, such category-based expectations may nevertheless have far-reaching consequences, for instance, for the career opportunities people receive, the life-choices they make, and how these affect their physical and mental well-being (see also Ellemers, 2018).

As soon as we place separate objects or individuals in the same category, we tend to focus on the properties they have in common, while we exaggerate the way they differ from stimuli placed in other categories. The now classic demonstration of this phenomenon was first described by Tajfel and Wilkes (1963), who asked people to estimate the length of eight different lines that were presented to them, and discovered that even perceptions of such objective features are distorted by category-based expectations. When each line was randomly paired with a letter (A or B), research participants were able to accurately estimate the length of each line that was presented to them. This was the control condition. However, some research participants saw the four shortest lines paired with letter A, and the four longest lines, with letter B. This manipulation constituted the "categorization" condition, as it implicitly allowed research participants to categorize individual lines that were presented to them as "short" (A) versus "long" (B). An important consequence was that now participants apparently inferred that lines accompanied by the letter A should clearly be shorter than lines with the letter B, and this "knowledge" about the properties of these two categories of lines distorted the accuracy of their perceptual judgments. Thus, results from this study revealed that line lengths were estimated relatively accurately when the letter codes were not related to their length. However, when the letter codes facilitated categorizing lines as "short" versus "long," participants' estimates exaggerated similarities within categories and differences between categories (see Figure 23.1). Over the years, similar effects of other types of categorizations on the way in-

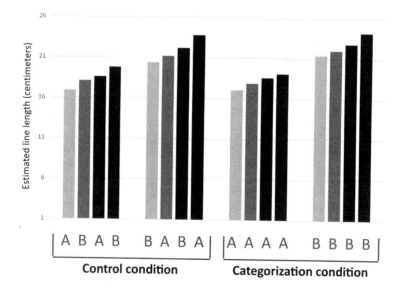

FIGURE 23.1. Perceptions are guided by categorization processes. The figure illustrates the effects of allowing people to classify lines into Category *A* ("short lines") and Category *B* ("long lines") on perception of individual line length. Based on Tajfel and Wilkes (1963).

dividual properties of different types of objects and stimuli are perceived have been demonstrated many times (for a review, see Corneille, Klein, Lambert, & Judd, 2002).

In summary, categorization offers an efficient and indispensable strategy to deal with novel and complex information. Even if people have no specific motivation to do so, the often felt need to quickly process information about many stimuli by lumping them together in meaningful categories leads them to inaccurately perceive properties of—or to form judgments about—specific individuals by relying on group-level characteristics. At the *group* level, this quick and dirty information-processing strategy is likely to result in relatively accurate inferences that facilitate adequate responses in many situations (e.g., on average, men are stronger than women). However, the categorization process also implies that differences between individual exemplars within a single category are not fully processed and appreciated (some men are weak; some women are strong). This causes people to misrepresent individuals or objects that deviate from the prototype, as they fail to acknowledge qualities that do not match group-based expectations (e.g., in the case of a female athlete). Thus, relying on social categorizations to evaluate *specific individuals* can result in faulty judgments. At the same time, such category-based representations—even if they are inaccurate—guide which information about others we seek and remember, influence the way we interpret their actions and intentions, and determine the way we behave toward them (see Table 23.1). As a result, one might unthinkingly challenge a woman in a bar to a game of arm wrestling, and only regret this once her companions point out she is a professional body builder. Below, we elaborate on the range of implications the categorization process has for motivational mechanisms relevant to relations between groups of people in society.

Identity

The basic mechanisms we use to categorize objects (e.g., private cars vs. taxis) are similar to

TABLE 23.1. Implications of Categorization

Process	Categorization	Perception	Attribution	Anticipated intent	Behavior
Key mechanism and central outcome	Drawing boundaries in society	Overestimate differences between groups	Stereotype consistency due to individual	Same category: constructive intent	Same category: cooperative
	Classify individuals into us versus them	Underestimate differences within groups	Stereotype inconsistency due to situation	Different category: harmful intent	Different category: competitive (or indifferent)
Implications for *others*	Organize information about individuals	Stereotyping, outgroup homogeneity	Stereotype maintenance	Outcome focus Infrahumanization	Stereotype enactment
Implications for *ingroup–outgroup*	Search for distinctiveness and group pride	Emphasize positive ingroup features Social creativity	Ingroup favoritism Communicating intergroup bias	Relation focus Ingroup trust	Ingroup favoritism Outgroup neglect
Implications for *self*	Self-categorization, search for intragroup respect	Self-stereotyping, claim positive group features	Self-confidence, self-efficacy	Sensitivity to ingroup norms and feedback	Group value endorsement
	Assigning individuals to groups →	*Selecting relevant features* →	*Interpreting past behavior* →	*Expecting future behavior* →	*Deciding how to behave* →

the ones we use to classify people into groups (e.g., nurses vs. doctors in "social categorization"). While the act of object categorization, as well as social categorization, can help us to infer useful information, as indicated earlier, in both cases mistakes are also made: Individual exemplars can be misclassified, and category-based inferences can be incorrect. However, compared to object categorization, social categorization is different in that it is a more recursive and interactive process; that is, the classifications we use, the category-based inferences we make, and the resulting (inaccurate) perception of individual properties not only impact how we perceive and approach *others* but also shape the way we define *ourselves* and how others perceive and approach us. Hence, social categorizations influence the nature of the interaction that unfolds, as well as the self-views we develop: our sense of *identity* (see also Ellemers, 2018). As we explain further below, group-based identities not only *describe* the features individuals are *likely* to have but they also are seen to *prescribe* how individual group members *should* behave. Those who behave in stereotype-consistent ways can rely on social approval, while those who deviate from the stereotype run the risk of being misunderstood and devalued by others. People are generally aware that such group-based expectations guide what others find appropriate or inappropriate behaviors for them. These expectations in turn may set in motion a self-fulfilling prophecy when people feel compelled to behave in ways that are seen as appropriate for the groups with which they identify.

In addition to referring to unique, individual physical (e.g., length, eye color) and psychological features (e.g., personal preferences, character traits) that define our "personal identity," we also use social categories to anchor and define our sense of self. This is referred to as our "social identity" (Tajfel, 1978; Tajfel & Turner, 1979), and indicates which categories (do not) include us, as a way to locate ourselves in the social structure (e.g., as a man or a woman, as a psychologist or a physicist, as a Dutch or U.S. citizen). Thus, our identities not only comprise collections of unique individual features but also reflect a category-based anchoring of our place in the social world. When introducing

ourselves to others, we use references to social categories such as our profession to indicate who we are and where we belong. We declare our social identities to communicate to others how we would like them to consider us. We also use these identities as sources of information for ourselves: Observing the behavior of people like us provides useful cues about how to behave in new situations and how to approach others, depending on whether their identity is similar or different than ours (Ellemers & Haslam, 2011; Ellemers, Kortekaas, & Ouwerkerk, 1999). For instance when talking to the teacher of your children, you might emphasize that you are familiar with the professional issues she faces by saying, "At the University I am a teacher, too." Thus, our social identities inform our behaviors and attitudes, indicate what to expect from others, and guide us in how to present ourselves to others (in dress or language use), and how we think of ourselves (in terms of key values or symbolic acts).

Initial insights on social identity theory (e.g., Tajfel & Turner, 1979) were based on experimental studies in which individuals randomly assigned to groups started to attach meaning and adapt their behavior according to these group memberships. These so-called "minimal" group experiments offered important proof of the principle that social categorizations and group-level concerns can overrule individual dispositions or interpersonal relations. However, later studies conducted with natural groups in different social contexts clarified that the categorization of individuals into groups will only be used as an anchor to think of the self and others, when it offers information that is relevant to the situation at hand, and is experienced as meaningful to the self (see also Turner, 1985).

A social identity (e.g., as an urban professional) typically comprises at least three components (Ellemers et al., 1999; Leach et al., 2008). We establish who we are through processes of *self-categorization* ("To which group do I belong?"), *group commitment* ("How important is this group to me?"), and *collective self-esteem* ("What is the value of this group?"). These different components often go together and can influence each other (e.g., we tend to value more positively the groups that include us (*in-*

groups) than the groups that do not include us (*outgroups*). Yet research has revealed that each component depends on different group features and has distinct implications for people's self-views, behaviors, and well-being, respectively (Ellemers et al., 1999). Importantly, the willingness to exert oneself toward the achievement of shared goals is driven primarily by a sense of affective *commitment* to the group and what it stands for (Ellemers, de Gilder, & Haslam, 2004; Ellemers, Platow, Van Knippenberg, & Haslam, 2003; Ouwerkerk, Ellemers, & de Gilder, 1999; see Figure 23.2).

Each of the three components of identity thus raises different questions that people ask themselves implicitly or explicitly. Deciding where you (want to) belong and how this makes you different from others satisfies *self-categorization* concerns. Questions of *self-esteem* prompt people to find out how much they are valued and what they can do to secure their sense of self-worth. *Affective commitment* to specific groups helps people decide which people they care about and what they can do to achieve key shared goals. The fact that there are three different components of identity also implies that there can be discrepancies between them, and that they may not always pull people in the same

direction. Even when individuals clearly see themselves as members of a particular group (e.g., self-categorizing as a Jew), this does not necessarily imply that they subscribe to the goals that characterize this group (e.g., feel a commitment to Zionism). Even if group belongingness only raises ridicule, stigma, or even self-loathing (e.g., the low collective esteem of some homosexuals), this does not necessarily preclude individuals from embracing and communicating identities they see as self-defining (e.g., self-categorization as a homosexual). Below, we explain in more detail how the social identities to which people subscribe and the implications this has for their self-views, goal commitment, and sense of social worth, impact on their behavioral motivations, and how this affects relationships between different groups in society.

Motivational Implications of Categorization and Identification

Shared Values as a Source of Motivation

Social categorization processes that inform people's identities impact the way people think of themselves in relation to others. Ideally,

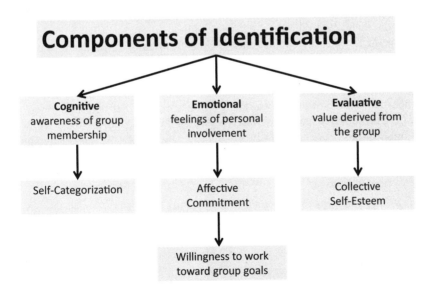

FIGURE 23.2. Components of identity. Based on Ellemers, Kortekaas, and Ouwerkerk (1999); Ellemers, Platow, Van Knippenberg, and Haslam (2003); and Ouwerkerk, Ellemers, and de Gilder (1999).

social categorizations and identities act as a source of *positive* inspiration and coordinated effort because they clarify important goals and key values individuals share with others. This is the case when vegetarians join forces to lobby more successfully for policies that help protect the environment by limiting the production of meat. Thus, their shared identity can facilitate goal alignment between individuals and help direct and sustain efforts to achieve them, even at the expense of personal outcomes or well-being. The motivation to think well of the self as a good group member who pursues important goals guides such efforts, benefiting group commitment and joint achievement.

However, no group exists in isolation, and there often are social costs when people celebrate the superior values and distinctive goals of the group and its members. Indeed, when vegetarians argue for the importance of their mission by emphasizing that their values are superior to those of individuals or groups that prioritize economic efficiency over animal well-being, this elicits antagonism and strife (Minson & Monin, 2012). Group leaders often exploit and encourage such sentiments to keep individual group members in the fold and to strengthen their own position by pointing out that others outside the group undermine the achievement of valued goals (Ellemers & Jetten, 2013).

Thus, on the one hand, shared values are a source of positive motivation that guides individuals to coordinate their efforts toward the achievement of shared goals and the enactment of values that distinguish the group from others. This is an important source of self-worth and social meaning. On the other hand, this often has negative implications. Feeling morally superior to other groups and excluding those who don't meet moral standards of the group raises antagonism, social exclusion, and intergroup conflict. Thus, even when the goals and values that bind people together into groups are virtuous and inspirational, the comparative way in which social categories and identities are defined also tend to have *negative* implications as they elicit a sense of *identity threat* in others.

Identity Threats as a Source of Motivation

Identity threats that people commonly experience relate to the two basic functions of categorization and identity (Figure 23.3; see also Branscombe, Ellemers, Spears, & Doosje, 1999). First, people seek to interpret and understand social situations. This activates the *meaning-seeking* function, which prompts people to determine the group to which they belong, and how this provides themselves and others with information about who they are in relation to others. Additionally, people have a general desire to think well of themselves, which causes them to find out how their group memberships can contribute to a sense of *social worth*.

In addressing each of these functions, people cannot freely pursue their personal preferences. Instead, they are limited by reality constraints—sometimes rooted in very real and unmalleable individual characteristics. For instance, physical features or formally registered parenthood limit the degrees of freedom people have in choosing their ethnicity. Furthermore, because of the *social* functions of the mechanisms we consider, self-defined categories or identities count for little unless they are acknowledged and validated by others. Discrepancies between

Seeking meaning	Seeking social worth
Guiding question: Which group do I belong to?	Guiding question: Can I think well of myself?

• Categorization threat:
  Do others acknowledge my sense of self?
	• Acceptance threat:
	  Am I a worthy group member?

• Distinctiveness threat:
  How is my group different from other groups?
	• Value threat:
	  Is my group a source of esteem?

FIGURE 23.3. Key concerns relating to categorization and identity. Based on Branscombe, Ellemers, Spears, and Doosje (1999).

self-views and perceptions of others represent sources of threat that invite motivated efforts to bring (social) realities in line with self-preferred views. This can happen to second-generation migrants who think of themselves as natives of the society in which they were born, even when others infer from their family name that they must be foreigners or assume from their skin color they do not speak the language.

When entering an unknown situation, for instance, when starting a new job or meeting new neighbors, attempts to interpret how individuals relate to each other can be incompatible with their self-views. For instance, young men may suffer from *categorization threat* when they meet people they do not know. Since #MeToo, many of them fear to be viewed as sexual predators when encountering women at social events or meeting new colleagues, and they feel that others expect the worst of them by virtue of their gender alone. To alleviate the sense of threat that ensues, individuals may become very careful not to act in any ways that might be in line with the group stereotype or to confirm negative expectations others may have of them when they categorize them according to their gender.

Even if the categorization of the individual as a member of the group is adequate to the situation and in line with one's self-views, one may still experience threat when others fail to acknowledge essential features that characterize one's group as different from other groups. The neglect of key characteristics that are seen as essential to the group may cause *distinctiveness threat*. This has been documented, for instance, among successful career women, whose colleagues sometimes assume they are unlikely to be ambitious. Instead of acknowledging that successful career women form a specific subgroup and must have organized their lives accordingly, people often assume that they should prioritize their families, just like other women.

Once it is clear which categorization applies, and even if this matches with self-defined identities and their characteristic features, additional concerns are likely to emerge as motivational forces due to the sense of social *worth* implied in people's group memberships and their ensuing identity. When others question one's loyalty or contributions to the group, this raises *acceptance threat*. This happens, for instance, when migrant workers who have acquired legitimate citizenship repeatedly are questioned about their "deviant" religious background or cultural practices. This conveys that they are not respected as proper and worthy fellow nationals and reminds them that others may challenge their inclusion in the group (van Laar, Derks, & Ellemers, 2013). As a result, they may feel compelled to explicitly denounce habits, speech styles, or forms of dress that may call into question their status as legitimate group members, and to clearly champion and visibly enact practices that are seen as beneficial for the group (Ellemers & Jetten, 2013).

A final form of identity threat may occur when others fail to validate the group as a source of pride and social esteem. This happens when others neglect positive contributions of the group or downplay the worthiness and importance of characteristic group features or achievements. This is referred to as a *value threat* to the group and its members and is commonly felt by members of groups with low status and those that are traditionally stigmatized in society. Here, too, the experience of threat is an important source of motivation that drives the way people present their group-based identity to others as well as the way they direct their efforts. For instance, those working in low status and underpaid professions (garbage collectors, primary school teachers) may argue for a re-assessment of the burden of their work as well as the importance of their contributions to a well-functioning society.

In summary, social categorizations and identities impact on the way people place themselves in the world, and how they interact with others. How they enact important values and cope with threats relating to their identity determines what people aim for, how hard they try, and when they give up. The goals on which people focus, the strength of their efforts, and the likelihood that they will persist together indicate the *motivation* raised by categorization and identity processes (Ellemers et al., 2004; Pinder, 2008). Understanding how these basic mechanisms work elucidates how members of different groups in society relate to each other, when they will be inclined to cooperate peacefully, and why they sometimes become entwined in irresolvable conflicts (Riek, Mania, & Gaertner, 2006). We now consider these implications in more detail.

The Impact of Categorization and Identification

As displayed in Table 23.1, social categorization and identification processes and the mechanisms they elicit can have far-reaching implications for others, for how ingroup–outgroup relations develop, and for the self. This affects the boundaries we draw to classify individuals into categories, the way we perceive individuals and groups, how we explain their actions and anticipate their intents, and how we behave toward them. Even though these different responses and implications are often interrelated, we discuss them in turn below.

Categorization of Individuals into Groups

One may be tempted to think that categorizing people into groups is undesirable, as this always implies an underestimation of differences between individuals and thus a simplification of social reality. When the categorization is not obviously relevant to the situation (e.g., distinguishing between men and women at work), this can have detrimental consequences, as the boundaries that are drawn separate people who are supposed to work together toward shared goals. However, in itself, categorization is a neutral process that helps people make sense of social situations. Assigning individuals to groups helps to *organize information* about them and defines their relation to the self. Furthermore, is it an implicit process that often happens outside our awareness or conscious control, and it is almost impossible to prevent. Some categorizations based on visible characteristics such as sex, race, physical features, or clothing styles easily stand out. We cannot avoid seeing them, the categorization is instantaneous, and we feel uncomfortable when we encounter an individual who cannot immediately be classified in this way. However, people may also actively seek out category markers that are less visible. Indeed, organizing individuals in terms of their profession, sexual orientation, or team membership can carry relevant informational value and define how people relate to each other.

Each of these social categories that can be used to draw boundaries between individuals helps to classify them into meaningful groups. This also helps people decide who does and does not share the same category membership as they do, classifying them into *ingroups* and *outgroups*. Considering some as ingroup members and others as outgroup members is an important tool that people use in their *search for distinctiveness and group pride,* in order to establish and maintain a positive social identity. This can happen even in relatively large and ill-defined groups such as their work organization or their university, where they often consider themselves as part of a group whose members they may not like or do not even know. They are particularly motivated to do this when group-level features can afford them a positive identity. For instance, in work settings, high prestige attributed to the organization by outsiders has been found to influence self-conceptions of employees and to enhance their identification with the organization (Smidts, Pruyn, & van Riel, 2001).

Individuals can think of themselves as part of a group even when they cannot rightfully claim a role in achieving group-level prestige. This phenomenon was first observed in an examination of how performance of a university sports team affected the way other students at that university categorized themselves. This revealed that after the sports team had won, students were much more likely to consider themselves part of the university than when the team had lost. They communicated this, for instance, by wearing clothes displaying the university colors and team logo, or by using the pronoun *we* in describing the team's victory—while descriptions of team failure maintained that "they" lost (Cialdini et al., 1976). A more recent study among professionals working in an organization with a poor image showed that they redefined the relevant categorization at a different level (Frandsen, 2012); that is, they embraced their professional identity, which presumably afforded them with a sense of group pride, rather than acknowledging their inclusion in the organization that would reflect negatively upon them. Apparently, their affiliation with the organization represented a *categorization threat* to which they responded by dissociating the self from the negative group image and reverting to another categorization instead. In fact, those who thought of themselves as high-status individuals in a low-status organization even referred to the organization in which they worked as an outgroup (Frandsen, 2012).

Another reason to redraw group boundaries occurs when an individual does not live up to the group's behavioral standards. The deviant behavior of a single individual may harm the positive identity of the ingroup, as it calls into question the values and moral standing of the whole group, thus representing a *group value threat*. In cases such as these, people may redraw group boundaries to exclude the deviant ingroup member from the group, or deny him or her full group membership to protect the group's positive identity (Van der Lee, Ellemers, Scheepers, & Rutjens, 2017). This phenomenon has become known as the "black sheep effect" (Marques, Yzerbyt, & Leyens, 1998). A particularly sad example occurred when the perpetrator accused of abusing and killing a child turned out to be a policeman. When the event was brought up in interviews among his colleagues, a common reaction of the interviewees was that "he was not a *real* policeman," thus excluding him from the group. Likewise, recent revelations of ongoing abuse in the Catholic Church eventually have led to the public denouncement of some culprits. Denying these individuals the right of considering themselves true group members by declaring them "black sheep" or excluding them as "bad apples" may help protect the image of the ingroup. This is a strategy often advised by legal counsel and it is often observed in the way business leaders (for instance at Volkswagen, FIFA, or ING banking) try to avert responsibility even for large-scale rule transgressions, corruption, or fraud. Thus, whereas redrawing group boundaries to exclude those who display problem behavior can help protect the image of the ingroup, it also prevents the group from addressing more systemic factors or revealing more widespread practices that contributed to the emergence or continuation of these excesses.

Considering the *self* as part of a group instead of as a unique individual can also have important motivational implications. For instance, most victims of sexual harassment are reluctant to publicize their experiences. They consider what happened to them as a personal misfortune—or worse, they experienced shame and often take (part of) the blame for what happened upon themselves. As these events mostly occur in private, one-on-one situations, it may not be self-evident to victims that others may have suffered similar experiences. However, from the stories emerging in the #MeToo discussion, it suddenly became clear how often this happened and was an experience shared by many like them. This allowed victims to redefine their personal experience as symptomatic of a more widespread social problem relating to power asymmetries between men and women. Categorizing victims and perpetrators in this way offered a different interpretation of the situation, and empowered victims even after many years to break the silence and join forces to combat sexually transgressive behavior.

Strategically categorizing the self as included in some groups and not in others also allows individuals to position themselves in groups that afford them with a sense of *intragroup respect*. Such a process was revealed in a study examining a merger between a large, high-status airline and a small, low-status domestic airline. Individual workers were more willing to identify with the merged organization when they perceived an opportunity to obtain an attractive position within the organization after the merger (Terry, Carey, & Callan, 2001). All these examples reveal the motivational mechanisms that guide social categorization processes, as well as resulting from them, and illustrate how the act of group boundary drawing to assign individuals to groups can be strategically used to protect the self from identity threat and facilitate the experience of pride and respect.

Perception of Relevant Group Features

Although categorization itself can be a neutral process, it often elicits biased perceptions. This happens when people use category memberships to apply stereotypical information and neglect individual features. Indeed, due to categorization processes, category-based expectations and stereotype-consistent information can drive the way people perceive others. This elicits the tendency to overemphasize similarities within groups and to exaggerate difference between groups. As a result of ingroup–outgroup asymmetries, they are tempted to think that "all foreigners are alike," while they are more attentive and mindful of the unique and distinctive features of ingroup members. Even though such perceived *outgroup homogeneity* occurs quite frequently, it is driven by motivational concerns instead of the inability to understand or process individuating information about outgroup members. Indeed, in situations that call for a clear and unified image of the ingroup (e.g., under the *distinctiveness threat*), people may also come to perceive their ingroup as more homogeneous than the outgroup (Doosje, Spears, Ellemers, & Koomen, 1999).

The application of group-based stereotypes to guide perceptions of *others* may result in judgments that are clearly wrong; however, this occurs even when more correct factual information is available. This has been documented extensively in educational and work settings in which the stereotype is that women are less competent and ambitious than men (see Ellemers, 2018, for an overview). For instance, one study revealed that, in biology classes, the performance of male students is perceived as being better than the performance of their female classmates, even when the women in the class actually have higher grades (Grunspan et al., 2016). Stereotypical judgments of the academic abilities of men and women are also found in other areas of science and predict the likelihood that women are present in these disciplines (*www.sciencemag.org/content/347/6219/262. short*). Female professors also apply these stereotypes, as they were found to underestimate the career motivation of female PhD students, and to have higher expectations of male PhDs. This study additionally showed this was due to group-based perceptions, as self-reports revealed that these female PhD students actually indicated being more committed to their careers than did male PhD students (Ellemers, van den Heuvel, de Gilder, Maass, & Bonvini, 2004). In commercial businesses, too, gender stereotypes rather than factual information guide important perceptions. This was demonstrated in a study using archival data to show that investors underestimated the objective value of companies with women on company boards, to their own detriment, of course, as this might lead them to

make less valid investment decisions (Haslam, Ryan, Kulich, Trojanowski, & Atkins, 2010).

Such misperceptions of reality and objective facts are probably unintentional and may influence people's judgments outside their awareness. Indeed, examinations of brain activity suggests that they do not necessarily result from deliberate decisions but instead reflect involuntary or "automatic" tendencies in information processing; that is, event-related potentials (ERPs) in the brain (P600, associated with detection of grammatical errors or syntactical anomalies) reveal that it is easier for people to comprehend information that is consistent with the gender stereotype (she is a nurse) than counterstereotypical information (she is an architect; Canal, Garnham, & Oakhill, 2015). Results such as these clearly show how hard it is to suppress or change existing stereotypes, even in the face of stereotype-disconfirming information. This explains why group-based perceptions of individual features are quite pervasive. In fact, they may even color the way people think of their own abilities, performance, and potential, as a result of *self-stereotyping*. This was revealed, for instance, even in a situation in which clear and objective performance indicators were present and explicitly known. In this study, female research participants who endorsed gender stereotypes consistently underestimated the marks they had actually received in high school mathematics, and overestimated their marks in language and arts. At the same time, male research participants who endorsed gender stereotypes recalled their math grades as being higher than they actually had been. Thus, even in their self-perceptions, members of both groups reproduced beliefs about what is characteristic for the gender stereotype, instead of reporting their actual grades (Chatard, Guimond, & Selimbegovic, 2007).

When the self is implicated in category-based perceptions of ingroup versus outgroup members, the motivation to establish a positive social identity easily tempts people to prioritize positive features in considering the groups to which they belong. When objective information about the group is unfavorable, there is a range of *social creativity* strategies that can be used to maintain a positive *perception* of the ingroup and of the self as a part of that group, – even if one has no option to improve objective outcomes for the group. Different forms of socially creative perceptions have been documented, for instance, in organizational settings in which employees do "dirty work" or have low-prestige jobs. Here, employees may reframe—and thereby reject—outsiders' negative perceptions of their work by focusing on the positive contributions to important societal outcomes in their perceptions of the group. For instance, they may acknowledge the stresses and unattractive features of their work but also claim indispensability by arguing that "without undertakers/cleaners/garbage collectors the world would be a mess, and health threats would occur" (Ashforth & Kreiner, 1999; Kreiner, Ashforth, & Sluss, 2006). Likewise, a qualitative study of the way medical staff dealt with medical incidents in their hospital revealed that medical doctors patronized nurses and looked down on them as colleagues with lower status. However, the nurses emphasized their crucial role in avoiding incidents and providing good health care (van Os, de Gilder, van Dyck, & Groenewegen, 2015). These nurses thus redefined perceptions of their group to maintain a positive sense of self.

In contexts in which intergroup comparisons are made, a derogatory description of one's group can be countered at the perceptual level without challenging its accuracy, for instance, by adopting a derogatory label as an honorary nickname. Hillary Clinton's reference to Trump supporters as "a basket of deplorables" in the 2016 U.S. presidential campaign was seen by her opponents as expressing contempt for unfortunate Americans. This prompted middle-class Americans who had lost their jobs or homes to repeat this statement again and again, in the process redefining the incident as reflecting badly on Hillary Clinton instead of themselves. Derogatory names can also be turned around in this way and come to constitute a key element of group pride ("Black is beautiful"). For instance, in the Dutch national soccer competition, a team from a rural town derided as "peasants" after a while started taking pride in referring to themselves as "superpeasants." Likewise, a team that was booed by supporters of other teams seeking to offend them as "Jews" now proudly refer to themselves as "Super-Jews," with fans who wave the Israeli flag in the stadium, even though the team actually has no connection at all to Jewry or to Israel.

Sometimes, ingroup and outgroup members *cooperate* in adapting their perceptions to mutually affirm positive views of both groups. This happens in contexts in which multiple dimensions of value are available. Here, ingroup and outgroup members may cooperate to appreciate each other's unique characteristics, allowing each of them to *claim positive ingroup features*. Such mutual appreciation of each other's qualities was observed, for instance, in an organizational merger. Members of the lower-status organization entering the merger accepted their evidently lower status on status-relevant dimensions (e.g., being less technologically advanced). At the same time, they emphasized their special qualities on alternative dimensions (e.g., having friendly relations among colleagues). Their perceptions were endorsed by members of the higher-status organization entering the merger, implying that the two merged organizations cooperated in mutually validating each other's status on different dimensions (Terry & Callan, 1998), a clear example of *social creativity*.

On the one hand, such cognitive (social creativity) strategies may be psychologically beneficial for individual group members, as they avert different types of identity threat. Moreover, cooperative efforts to afford each group a positive identity contribute to avoiding societal clashes between groups (Yzerbyt, 2016; Yzerbyt & Cambon, 2017). At the same time, as we explained earlier, the lack of action implied in such cognitive redefinitions of the status quo may lead to the maintenance of group stereotypes that bias perceptions of people's actual characteristics and achievements. Furthermore, it may result in a continuation of societally undesirable practices. For instance, some jobs that are important in society (nursing, teaching) continue to receive low prestige and low pay, and are seen as unattractive career options, even if members of these groups are socially valued for being caring and kind. Thus, social creativity may not only protect perceptions of group value and feelings of group pride but also undermine behavior aiming to address the real causes of social identity threat, and prevent individuals from engaging in collective action to achieve social change (Becker, 2012; Vaast & Levina, 2015).

Attribution of Behavior

Categorization and perception processes help people to make sense of social reality. They often occur quickly and do not always involve deliberate thinking. However, people do engage—and often have to engage—in more cognitive activity as they try to understand the origins and meaning of their own behavior and that of others. Indeed, many social situations are complex and ambiguous, making it difficult to clearly establish a single cause underlying a particular behavior or outcome. For instance, in dangerous traffic situations, people tend to attribute the danger to the behavior displayed by other drivers, not to themselves. However, others present in the situation do this, too—the cause of many irritations and mutual accusations of being "a Sunday driver," "aggressive," or "antisocial."

In general, when observing behavior of *others* that is unexpected—for instance, because the individual does not conform to the group stereotype—people tend to seek an explanation, frequently in a way that somehow preserves or restores stereotypical expectations about the group. They do this by attributing stereotypically inconsistent behavior to temporary situational circumstances, the exception to the rule, while attributing stereotypically consistent behavior to more enduring qualities of the individual—even if these are not rooted in factual information. As a result, when two people display exactly the same behavior, this may still be interpreted differently, depending on their category membership and the stereotypical expectations this evokes. When the behavior of an individual seems to be consistent with the group stereotype, this tends to be attributed to the individual, whereas stereotypically inconsistent behavior is more frequently attributed to the situation, leading to *stereotype maintenance*.

This was demonstrated in a study in which mathematics teachers reflected on the performance of their male and female students. Good test results of male students were seen as indicating their ability for logical reasoning. However, when an identical high performance was shown by a female student, this was attributed to their exceptional effort—not their mathematical talent. For students who did not perform well, this was seen as indicating a lack of effort by male students, implicitly conveying that they might still improve their performance if only they put in more work. However, the same performance was seen as a sign of insufficient ability for female students (Tiedemann, 2000). Thus, regardless of the actual performance that was displayed by the boys and girls in the class, the inferences their teachers made actually maintained the stereotype that girls are less good at math—even though "mountains of research" have not revealed reliable gender differences in math ability (Hyde, 2014).

The general motivation to maintain a more positive image of one's group in *ingroup–outgroup* comparisons can come to the fore relatively subtly in the attributions they make. Indeed, research consistently shows that the inferences we make about the causes for the behaviors of other individuals not only reflect stereotypical expectations we hold about members of different groups but can also reveal *ingroup favoritism*, as the same behavior is ascribed to different causes, depending on whether it is displayed by an ingroup member or an outgroup member (Hewstone, 1990). Literature on the linguistic category bias shows that people have subtle ways to *communicate intergroup bias* in choosing the words to think of and describe the behaviors and achievements of ingroup and outgroup members. When an ingroup member has done well, this is consistent with positive expectations about the ingroup, whereas undesirable behavior or an unfavorable outcome achieved by an ingroup member threatens positive ingroup views. This influences the attributions that are made, and the language that is being used to describe what happened (Wigboldus, Semin, & Spears, 2000). Behaviors and achievements that reflect positively on the ingroup are described with generalizing, abstract language (e.g., "He is such a great person"; "We are the best"), whereas ingroup behaviors or outcomes that might damage the group's positive image are described with language referring to the specific and temporary nature of this outcome, and the rarity of such an event (e.g., "He had a bad day"; "The referee was biased"). For outgroup members, the opposite occurs: Behaviors and outcomes that would help the motivation to think of the outgroup as doing less well are attributed to enduring characteristics of the individual or essential features of the group and its members (e.g., "They are not very good at this" or "He is a loser"). An unexpectedly good result or outcome achieved by an outgroup member is dismissed by invoking situational features or temporary circumstances (e.g., "They were lucky" or "She worked really hard"; Roberson & Stevens, 2006).

Stereotype-consistent and ingroup-favoring attributions for actual performance shown are not innocent: They also impact the way targets of such attributions think about the *self* and interpret their own achievements and performance. This can easily elicit a self-fulfilling cycle affecting *self-efficacy* and self-confidence to encourage some, while undermining motivation and resulting in self-defeat among others. The example detailed earlier illustrates this, as the attribution patterns observed among math teachers (Tiedemann, 2000) make it less likely that they encourage their female students to try again when they fail, or even that they acknowledge the talent of female students who actually do well. Other research also shows that the way others interpret and communicate about people's abilities and achievements impact on the encouragement and support people receive, the way they come to think of their own performance and potential, and the task engagement and performance they display over time (e.g., Derks, van Laar, & Ellemers, 2006). There is by now overwhelming evidence that we all tend to evaluate the talents of individuals and communicate about them by relying on stereotypical attributions and biased communications, instead of simply reflecting their actual performance. This has been demonstrated most frequently in educational and work contexts, and has been documented as a plausible cause for diverging personal and professional choices and differential career success, for instance, of men and women (see Ellemers, 2018, for a review).

Anticipated Intentions

Social categorizations and group-based identities—and the perceptual and attributional patterns these elicit—also affect how we anticipate the behavior of *others* in the future and the intentions we expect them to have. In fact, categorizations are even used to determine whose intentions we are willing to attend to, and whose inner states we prefer to ignore. Categorizing people who are cold and hungry out on the street as "homeless" makes us less likely to see them as real humans. Research indicates that we simply fail to activate the part of our brains that we use for social perception when looking at them, and experience disgust instead of empathizing with their plight (Harris & Fiske, 2006). This process of *infrahumanization,* causing us to see other people as animals, machines, or objects, implies that we do not take into account their mental state or perspective. A range of studies indicates that this can happen to sexually objectified women (Heflick & Goldenberg, 2009), enemy prisoners (Viki, Osgood, & Phillips, 2013), or war refugees (Esses, Veenvliet, Hodson, & Mihic, 2008), and makes us ignore their ability to experience more complex emotions, deny them a sense of agency, and be less likely to think they will experience pain. Even individuals who are caring, helpful, friendly, or altruistic use category boundaries in this way to be able to limit the circle of people they care for and to protect themselves from suffering from the plight of all those who are less fortunate (Ellemers, 2017). Thus, the mere fact that we assign individuals to groups and draw boundaries between them also has implications for our inclination to consider their needs, desires, and intentions, as well as our willingness to empathize with their misfortune and pain. Excluding individuals from the group of "real humans" justifies aggression against them, legitimizes their exploitation and abuse, makes us less affected by their suffering, and generally prevents us from empathizing with their plight (Skitka & Mullen, 2003).

In *ingroup–outgroup* comparisons, we are more willing to make an effort to understand and explain intentions of ingroup members, and show more willingness to see things from their perspective or to take into account their needs. As a result, behavior displayed by ingroup members tends to be seen as more benevolent and well intentioned, even when the behavior itself is unpleasant. Such effects can occur for categories and identities defined at a very abstract or macro level. This was demonstrated by Hornsey and Imani (2004) in a study showing that criticism about Australia from foreigners (the outgroup) is taken less well than similar comments are made by fellow Australians (the ingroup). This study additionally showed that the greater openness to criticism from fellow ingroup members indeed was mediated by the assumption of positive intent and perceived constructiveness of the comments made. No support was found for the alternative explanation that ingroup critics were taken more seriously because they presumably had more expertise and experience with the actual situation in Australia.

In interactions with others, people frequently give and receive corrections and feedback, and hope this will help them improve. Sometimes they are even *expected* to or comment critically on the behavior or others, for instance, when they act in a leadership role at work. Research shows, however, that responses to such work-related corrections may differ depending on the group membership of the individual providing the correction, and their anticipated intent (see also leader–member exchange (LMX; Scandura, 1999) theory. This was demonstrated in research examining how subordinates responded when their decisions were overruled and corrected by the group leader. In general, this is not a pleasant experience, as this also implies criticism of the subordinate and his or her decisions. However, this study revealed that when the leader was categorized as an ingroup member, subordinates were more inclined to see such behavior as indicating good intent and meant to help the team perform well. Accordingly, even after having their decisions overruled, subordinates were still willing to display cooperative behavior toward an ingroup leader who requested help. This was not the case when their decisions had been overruled by an outgroup leader, displaying differential *sensitivity to feedback* (Bruins, Ellemers, & de Gilder, 1999).

Studies in other contexts also reveal that people's willingness to accept unpleasant messages or authorities' unfavorable decisions depends on whether they categorize these others as ingroup or outgroup members, and the intent they infer accordingly. Studies reveal that ingroup authorities elicit a *relation focus* and raise *in-group trust*. We are interested in maintaining good relations with them and have confidence in their benevolent intentions toward us. As long as the procedures they use seem fair, we rely on their good intentions and are willing to accept their decisions, even if they are unfavorable for us (Ståhl, Vermunt, & Ellemers, 2008a). However, in the case of outgroup authorities, relational concerns are less important, and we are less ready to assume we will be treated fairly. Indeed, we tend to adopt an *outcome focus* when considering decisions made by outgroup authorities, and accept decisions that are favorable for us, while rejecting unfavorable outcomes, regardless of the fairness of the procedure that was followed (Ståhl, Vermunt, & Ellemers, 2008b).

All the mechanisms we have reviewed explain that anticipated intent and expectations about the future behavior of others—driven by categorizations and ingroup–outgroup distinctions—also have implications for the *self*. The relational focus raised when interacting with ingroup members and the confidence in the validity of their concerns and intentions enhances our *sensitivity to ingroup norms*. Indeed, a series of studies indicates that we are quite willing to accept and adapt our behavior to what other ingroup members tell us is the right way to behave, while we are less likely to follow behavioral norms imposed upon us by outgroup members (Pagliaro, Ellemers, & Barreto, 2011). This reluctance to follow norms set by people we see as representing a different group also explains the limited impact of comments made by the general public, or even of recommendations by outside experts, whenever they see reason to criticize the behavior or general practices of a particular professional or cultural group.

Behavioral Implications

The literature on the behavioral consequences of categorization and identity processes is extensive, and we provide only a few selected examples here. Even though the behavioral consequences of the previously discussed categorizations, perceptions, attributions, and perceived intent may seem obvious by now, it is the *behavior* resulting from these mechanisms that is most consequential for ourselves and other ingroup–outgroup members and can have far-reaching implications for the broader society. The general tendency displayed in all the research on this topic is that individuals tend to show *cooperative* behavior toward those who share the same category membership (ingroup members), whereas they tend to show *competitive* behavior toward those who represent a different category (outgroup members). These cooperative and competitive behaviors can take many shapes and forms, ranging from allocations of valued outcomes in experimental simulations to help provided to others and displays of citizenship in organizations.

An important behavioral implication affecting *others* is the phenomenon of *stereotype enactment*; that is, group-based stereotypes, and the perceptions and attributions they elicit, may prompt people to act in ways that reinforce and perpetuate the stereotype. This was shown, for instance, in experiments revealing how gender stereotypes affect individual employment and funding decisions; that is, merely changing the name on the CV of a job applicant ("John" vs. "Jennifer") who allegedly created an architectural design, or the name of the teacher of an online course, was shown to raise different perceptions of the individual's competence, effectiveness, and creativity (MacNell, Driscoll, & Hunt, 2015; Proudfoot, Kay, & Koval, 2015). Importantly, this also affected the likelihood that the applicant actually was offered the job, as well as the pay rate received (Moss-Racusin, Dovidio, Brescoll, Graham, & Handelsman, 2012). Obviously, these are far-reaching implications of imaginary differences in individual competence derived from category-based stereotypes.

Behavior in contexts in which both *ingroup* and *outgroup* members are present is also affected, as group members tend to display ingroup favoritism and *outgroup neglect*. This extends beyond the more obvious readiness or reluctance to empathize and extend help and support to others. A multitude of studies indicate that less attention is generally paid to communications received from outgroup members than to those from the ingroup members (Mackie, Worth, & Asuncion, 1990; Van Knippenberg, & Wilke, 1992); that is, experiments manipulating ingroup–outgroup membership show that persuasive messages from ingroup members are remembered better, are seen as more convincing, and are generally more likely to achieve the intended change in people's attitudes and behaviors than messages from outgroup members. This is true also when outgroup messages include criticism of the ingroup. This "intergroup sensitivity effect," as is has been dubbed, demonstrates that outsiders making such critical comments are rejected, irrespective of the quality of their arguments (Esposo, Hornsey, & Spoor, 2013). For instance, Elsbach and Kramer (1996) showed that business school students ignored unfavorable rankings of the business school they attended, claiming that these were made by outsiders, and instead emphasized dimensions that were not recognized in the rankings.

The tendency to ignore important information when this seems to come from outgroup members can be quite risky when ingroup–outgroup categorizations are derived from power differentials. Results from different studies show that even random assignment to a powerful position makes people consider those with less power as outgroup members. As a result, they show less interest in relevant information others provide (e.g., Goodwin, Gubin, Fiske, & Yzerbyt, 2000), and take less advice from others below them (See, Morrison, Rothman, & Soll, 2011), even when these are the true experts (Tost, Gino, & Larrick, 2012). To the extent that power differences are based on differential expertise, rejecting potential contributions of outgroup members may be justified. However, even then, rejecting alternative views, legitimate criticism, and complementary expertise hinders reform and positive change for the ingroup or even for society (Hornsey, 2005). This can have outright detrimental effects, as shown, for instance, in a case study on the management of a large project. Here it was revealed that members of a project team withheld their knowledge of evident risks in an infrastructure project, as they regarded this as threatening their identity and stature as experts (van Os, van Berkel, de Gilder, van Dyck, & Groenewegen, 2015).

Behavioral implications for the *self* ensue when people engage in *group value endorsement,* through their actions, as they act in line with important goals that characterize the group. This was observed among soldiers on a peacekeeping mission: Teams in which soldiers felt more respected, included, and valued by their team mates were more motivated to invest in the team, and displayed more action readiness as observed by their team supervisors (Ellemers, Sleebos, Stam, & de Gilder, 2013). However, behavioral endorsement of important group goals and values may also emerge to counter threats to one's identity as a good group member. This is often the case among successful career women, who have been exposed to gender stereotypes throughout their career. They generally cope with the threat this implies to their professional identity by displaying the masculine behaviors that are so highly valued in the organization but also set them apart from other women. As a result, they often are reluctant to invest in mentoring or other efforts to help more junior women (Derks, van Laar, & Ellemers, 20016; Schmitt, Ellemers, & Branscombe, 2003). However, women who manage to achieve positions of leadership without suffering from such gender-related professional identity threats are generally quite willing to support other women to achieve similar career advancement (Derks, Ellemers, van Laar, & de Groot, 2011).

Those who experience a threat to their identity as a good group member may go to great lengths to defer such threat. It is easy to understand that some simply retaliate by aggressing against their colleagues and showing harmful behavior toward the organization (Aquino & Douglas, 2003). Others, however, try to establish their status as a true group member by acting in line with group norms and trying to important group goals. This may happen even when the resulting behavior seems undesirable from a broader societal point of view, for instance, when it leads employees to lie to their customers (Leavitt & Sluss, 2015) or engage in other unethical behaviors that show their willingness to help the organization (Umphress, Bingham, & Mitchell, 2010).

To the extent that a spoiled identity is not immediately visible, individuals can choose to behave in ways that hide their devalued identity. They often hope to avoid the stigma associated with their group membership in this way. Some lesbian, gay, bisexual, transgender, and/or intersex (LGBTI) workers who prefer not to reveal

their sexual preference to their colleagues at work do this, for fear of being ridiculed or devalued. At first sight, this seems a viable strategy that is sometimes even formally advocated by organizations (as in the U.S. military, "Don't ask, don't tell"). However, research shows that the cognitive efforts needed to successfully hide a stigmatized identity, and the guilt and shame people experience as a result, may also be detrimental (Barreto, Ellemers, & Banal, 2006). Trying to conceal one's membership in a stigmatized group impairs the quality of social interactions, deprives individuals of the social support of others like them, and prevents them from gaining access to special provisions developed to assist them (Barreto & Ellemers, 2015).

Threats to the value of the group that cannot be met by distancing the self from the group or redefining the value of the group through social creativity strategies can raise anger at the position of their group in society, leading them to join forces to achieve social change (Van Zomeren, Postmes, & Spears, 2008). Individuals who strongly identify with the group may invest substantial efforts, resources, future opportunities, and even their health while they engage in collective action, for instance, when they engage in union activities or political protest (Veenstra & Haslam, 2000). Again, other examples abound, with suicide terrorist making the ultimate self-sacrifice to achieve goals that are important for the group. Clearly, such behaviors can only be addressed by applying insights on the motivational mechanisms of categorization and identity.

Conclusion: How Categorization and Identification Affect Relations between Groups

In this chapter we have argued that relations between groups in society cannot be fully understood from individual-level character traits (e.g., altruism) or from instrumental motives to join forces with others to achieve valued outcomes. Instead, we have shown how conflict and cooperation between groups in society are often rooted in symbolic differences and reflect shared or diverging values. Those who are excluded from important groups in society—as these groups fail to respect their distinctive talents or to acknowledge their achievements—experience a threat to their identity as valued members of society. When their efforts to cope with this identity threat fail, this only leads to mutual rejection and frustration. The research we have reviewed here also shows that relatively subtle situational variations impact on behavior in ways that are not easily explained by other approaches.

Thinking of others as lesser humans and denying them even basic concern for their needs and well-being, to secure our own values and justify our privileges only serves to sustain and intensify intergroup conflicts. Many see this as an inevitable outcome of increased globalization and (class) migration. However, the same mechanisms that are so often use to exclude and antagonize others can also be recruited to resolve such tensions. Finding higher-order categories that connect different groups, defining shared values that motivate them to work together, and acknowledging complex identities that incorporate multiple groups may all help to make people change their perceptions, attributions, perceived intentions and behaviors toward others. This seems a viable strategy to reconnect and reconcile people with different identities, even after a long history of violent conflict (Maloku, Derks, van Laar, & Ellemers, 2016), as this allows them to move away from negative motivations instigated by feelings of threat, toward positive motivations to enact shared values guiding the way they relate to members of other groups in society.

REFERENCES

Aquino, K., & Douglas, S. (2003). Identity threat and antisocial behavior in organizations: The moderating effects of individual differences, aggressive modeling, and hierarchical status. *Organizational Behavior and Human Decision Processes, 90*(1), 195–208.

Ashforth, B. E., & Kreiner, G. E. (1999). "How can you do it?": Dirty work and the challenge of constructing a positive identity. *Academy of Management Review, 24*(3), 413–434.

Barreto, M., & Ellemers, N. (2015). Detecting and experiencing prejudice: New answers to old questions. *Advances in Experimental Social Psychology, 52*, 139–219.

Barreto, M., Ellemers, N., & Banal, S. (2006). Work-

ing under cover: Performance-related self-confidence among members of contextually devalued groups who try to pass. *European Journal of Social Psychology, 36*, 337–352.

Becker, J. C. (2012). The system-stabilizing role of identity management strategies: Social creativity can undermine collective action for social change. *Journal of Personality and Social Psychology, 103*(4), 642–647.

Branscombe, N., Ellemers, N., Spears, R., & Doosje, B. (1999). The context and content of identity threat. In N. Ellemers, R. Spears, & B. Doosje (Eds.), *Social identity: Context, commitment, content* (pp. 35–58). Oxford, UK: Blackwell.

Bruins, J., Ellemers, N., & de Gilder, D. (1999). Power use and differential competence as determinant of subordinates' evaluation and behavioural responses in simulated organizations. *European Journal of Social Psychology, 29*, 843–870.

Canal, P., Garnham, A., & Oakhill, J. (2015). Beyond gender stereotypes in language comprehension: Self sex-role descriptions affect the brain's potentials associated with agreement processing. *Frontiers in Psychology, 6*, 1–17.

Chatard, A., Guimond, S., & Selimbegovic, L. (2007). "How good are you in math?": The effect of gender stereotypes on students' recollection of their school marks. *Journal of Experimental Social Psychology, 43*(6), 1017–1024.

Cialdini, R. B., Borden, R. J., Thorne, A., Walker, M. R., Freeman, S., & Sloan, L. R. (1976). Basking in reflected glory: Three (football) field studies. *Journal of Personality and Social Psychology, 34*(3), 366–375.

Cikara, M., & Van Bavel, J. J. (2014). The neuroscience of intergroup relations: An integrative review. *Perspectives on Psychological Science, 9*(3), 245–274.

Corneille, O., Klein, O., Lambert, S., & Judd, C. M. (2002). On the role of familiarity with units of measurement in categorical accentuation: Tajfel and Wilkes (1963) revisited and replicated. *Psychological Science, 13*(4), 380–383.

Derks, B., Ellemers, N., van Laar, C., & de Groot, K. (2011). Do sexist organizational cultures create the Queen Bee? *British Journal of Social Psychology, 50*(3), 519–535.

Derks, B., van Laar, C., & Ellemers, N. (2006). Striving for success in outgroup settings: Effects of contextually emphasizing ingroup dimensions on stigmatized group members' social identity and performance styles. *Personality and Social Psychology Bulletin, 32*, 576–588.

Derks, B., van Laar, C., & Ellemers, N. (2016). The Queen Bee phenomenon: Why women leaders distance themselves from junior women. *Leadership Quarterly, 27,* 456–469.

Doosje, B., Spears, R., Ellemers, N., & Koomen, W. (1999). Group variability in intergroup relations: The distinctive role of social identity. *European Review of Social Psychology, 10,* 41–74.

Ellemers, N. (2012). The group self. *Science, 336*(6083), 848–852.

Ellemers, N. (2017). *Morality and the regulation of social behavior: Groups as moral anchors.* Milton Park, UK: Routledge.

Ellemers, N. (2018). Gender stereotypes. *Annual Review of Psychology, 69,* 275–298.

Ellemers, N., de Gilder, D., & Haslam, S. A. (2004). Motivating individuals and groups at work: A social identity perspective on leadership and group performance. *Academy of Management Review, 29*(3), 459–478.

Ellemers, N., & Haslam, S. A. (2011). Social identity theory. In P. Van Lange, A. Kruglanski, & T. Higgins (Eds.), *Handbook of theories of social psychology* (pp. 379–398). London: SAGE.

Ellemers, N., & Jetten, J. (2013). The many ways to be marginal in a group. *Personality and Social Psychology Review, 17*(1), 3–21.

Ellemers, N., Kortekaas, P., & Ouwerkerk, J. (1999). Self-categorization, commitment to the group and social self-esteem as related but distinct aspects of social identity. *European Journal of Social Psychology, 29*(2–3), 371–389.

Ellemers, N., Platow, M., Van Knippenberg, D., & Haslam, A. (2003). Social identity at work: Definitions, debates, and directions. In A. Haslam, D. Van Knippenberg, M. Platow, & N. Ellemers (Eds.), *Social identity at work: Developing theory for organizational practice* (pp. 3–28). New York: Psychology Press.

Ellemers, N., Sleebos, E., Stam, D., & de Gilder, D. (2013). Feeling included and valued: How perceived respect affects positive team identity and willingness to invest in the team. *British Journal of Management, 24*(1), 21–37.

Ellemers, N., van den Heuvel, H., de Gilder, D., Maass, A., & Bonvini, A. (2004). The underrepresentation of women in science: Differential commitment or the queen bee syndrome? *British Journal of Social Psychology, 43*(3), 315–338.

Elsbach, K. D., & Kramer, R. M. (1996). Members' responses to organizational identity threats: Encountering and countering the *Business Week* rankings. *Administrative Science Quarterly, 41*(3), 442–476.

Esposo, S. R., Hornsey, M. J., & Spoor, J. R. (2013). Shooting the messenger: Outsiders critical of your group are rejected regardless of argument quality. *British Journal of Social Psychology, 52*(2), 386–395.

Esses, V., Veenvliet, S., Hodson, G., & Mihic, L. (2008). Justice, morality, and the dehumanization of refugees. *Social Justice Research, 21,* 4–25.

Frandsen, S. (2012). Organizational image, identification, and cynical distance: Prestigious professionals in a low-prestige organization. *Management Communication Quarterly, 26*(3), 351–376.

Goodwin, S. A., Gubin, A., Fiske, S. T., & Yzerbyt, V. Y. (2000). Power can bias impression processes: Stereotyping subordinates by default and by design. *Group Processes and Intergroup Relations, 3*(3), 227–256.

Grunspan, D. Z., Eddy, S. L., Brownell, S. E., Wiggins, B. L., Crowe, A. J., & Goodreau, S. M. (2016). Males under-estimate academic performance of their female peers in undergraduate biology classrooms. *PLOS ONE, 11*(2), e0148405.

Harris, L., & Fiske, S. T. (2006). Dehumanizing the lowest of the low: Neuroimaging responses to extreme out-groups. *Psychological Science, 17,* 847–853.

Haslam, A., Ellemers, N., Reicher, S., Reynolds, K., & Schmitt, M. (2010). The social identity perspective today: The impact of its defining ideas. In T. Postmes & N. R. Branscombe (Eds.), *Rediscovering social identity: Core sources* (pp. 341–356). New York: Psychology Press.

Haslam, S. A., Ryan, M. K., Kulich, C., Trojanowski, G., & Atkins, C. (2010). Investing with prejudice: The relationship between women's presence on company boards and objective and subjective measures of company performance. *British Journal of Management, 21*(2), 484–497.

Heflick, N. A., & Goldenberg, J. L. (2009). Objectifying Sarah Palin: Evidence that objectification causes women to be perceived as less competent and less fully human. *Journal of Experimental Social Psychology, 45,* 598–601.

Hewstone, M. (1990). The "ultimate attribution error"?: A review of the literature on intergroup causal attribution. *European Journal of Social Psychology, 20,* 311–335.

Hornsey, M. J. (2005). Why being right is not enough: Predicting defensiveness in the face of group criticism. *European Review of Social Psychology, 16*(1), 301–334.

Hornsey, M. J., & Imani, A. (2004). Criticizing groups from the inside and the outside: An identity perspective on the intergroup sensitivity effect. *Personality and Social Psychology Bulletin, 30*(3), 365–383.

Hyde, J. S. (2014). Gender similarities and differences. *Annual Review of Psychology, 65,* 373–398.

Kreiner, G. E., Ashforth, B. E., & Sluss, D. M. (2006). Identity dynamics in occupational dirty work: Integrating social identity and system justification perspectives. *Organization Science, 17*(5), 619–636.

Lamont, M., & Molnár, V. (2002). The study of boundaries in the social sciences. *Annual Review of Sociology, 28*(1), 167–195.

Leach, C. W., Van Zomeren, M., Zebel, S., Vliek, M., Pennekamp, S. F., Doosje, B., et al. (2008). Group-level self-definition and self-investment: A hierarchical (multicomponent) model of in-group identification. *Journal of Personality and Social Psychology, 95*(1), 144–165.

Leavitt, K., & Sluss, D. M. (2015). Lying for who we are: An identity-based model of workplace dishonesty. *Academy of Management Review, 40*(4), 587–610.

Mackie, D. M., Worth, L. T., & Asuncion, A. G. (1990). Processing of persuasive in-group messages. *Journal of Personality and Social Psychology, 58*(5), 812–822.

MacNell, L., Driscoll, A., & Hunt, A. N. (2015). What's in a name: Exposing gender bias in student ratings of teaching. *Innovative Higher Education, 40*(4), 291–303.

Maloku, E., Derks, B., van Laar, C., & Ellemers, N. (2016). Building national identity in newborn Kosovo: Challenges of integrating national identity with ethnic identity among Kosovar Albanians and Kosovar Serbs. In S. McKeown, R. Haji, & N. Ferguson (Eds.), *Understanding peace and conflict through social identity theory: Contemporary and world-wide perspectives* (pp. 245–260). New York: Springer.

Marques, J. M., Yzerbyt, V. Y., & Leyens, J. P. (1988). The "black sheep effect": Extremity of judgments towards ingroup members as a function of group identification. *European Journal of Social Psychology, 18*(1), 1–16.

Minson, J. A., & Monin, B. (2012). Do-gooder derogation: Disparaging morally motivated minorities to defuse anticipated reproach. *Social Psychological and Personality Science, 3*(2), 200–207.

Moss-Racusin, C. A., Dovidio, J. F., Brescoll, V. L., Graham, M. J., & Handelsman, J. (2012). Science faculty's subtle gender biases favor male students. *Proceedings of the National Academy of Sciences of the USA, 109*(41), 16474–16479.

Ouwerkerk, J., Ellemers, N., & de Gilder, D. (1999). Group commitment and individual effort in experimental and organizational contexts. In N. Ellemers, R. Spears, & B. Doosje (Eds.), *Social identity: Context, commitment, content* (pp. 184–204). Oxford, UK: Blackwell.

Pagliaro, S., Ellemers, N., & Barreto, M. (2011). Sharing moral values: Anticipated ingroup respect as a determinant of adherence to morality-based (but not competence-based) group norms.

Personality and Social Psychology Bulletin, 37, 1117–1129.

Pinder, C. C. (2008). *Work motivation in organizational behavior.* New York: Psychology Press.

Proudfoot, D., Kay, A. C., & Koval, C. Z. (2015). A gender bias in the attribution of creativity: Archival and experimental evidence for the perceived association between masculinity and creative thinking. *Psychological Science, 26*(11), 1751–1761.

Riek, B. M., Mania, E. W., & Gaertner, S. L. (2006). Intergroup threat and outgroup attitudes: A meta-analytic review. *Personality and Social Psychology Review, 10*(4), 336–353.

Roberson, Q. M., & Stevens, C. K. (2006). Making sense of diversity in the workplace: Organizational justice and language abstraction in employees' accounts of diversity-related incidents. *Journal of Applied Psychology, 91*(2), 379–391.

Scandura, T. A. (1999). Rethinking leader–member exchange: An organizational justice perspective. *Leadership Quarterly, 10,* 25–40.

Schmitt, M. T., Ellemers, N., & Branscombe, N. R. (2003). Perceiving and responding to gender discrimination at work. In S. A. Haslam, D. Van Knippenberg, M. J. Platow, & N. Ellemers (Eds.), *Social identity at work: Developing theory for organizational practice* (pp. 277–292). New York: Psychology Press.

See, K. E., Morrison, E. W., Rothman, N. B., & Soll, J. B. (2011). The detrimental effects of power on confidence, advice taking, and accuracy. *Organizational Behavior and Human Decision Processes, 116*(2), 272–285.

Skitka, L. J., & Mullen, E. (2003). The dark side of moral conviction. *Analysis of Social Issues and Public Policy, 2,* 35–41.

Smidts, A., Pruyn, A. T. H., & van Riel, C. B. (2001). The impact of employee communication and perceived external prestige on organizational identification. *Academy of Management Journal, 44*(5), 1051–1062.

Ståhl, T., Vermunt, R., & Ellemers, N. (2008a). For love or money?: How activation of relational versus instrumental concerns affects reactions to allocations by authorities. *Journal of Experimental Social Psychology, 44,* 80–94.

Ståhl, T., Vermunt, R., & Ellemers, N. (2008b). Reactions to outgroup authorities' decisions: The role of expected bias, procedural fairness and outcome favorability. *Group Processes and Intergroup Relations, 11,* 281–299.

Tajfel, H. (1978). Social categorization, social identity, and social comparison. In H. Tajfel (Ed.), *Differentiation between social groups: Studies in the social psychology of intergroup relations* (pp. 61–76). New York: Academic Press.

Tajfel, H., & Turner, J. C. (1979). An integrative theory of intergroup conflict. In W. G. Austin & S. Worchel (Eds.), *The social psychology of intergroup relations* (pp. 33–47). Monterey, CA: Brooks/Cole.

Tajfel, H., & Wilkes, H. (1963). Classification and quantitative judgment. *British Journal of Psychology, 54*(2), 101–114.

Terry, D. J., & Callan, V. J. (1998). In-group bias in response to an organizational merger. *Group Dynamics: Theory, Research, and Practice, 2*(2), 67–81.

Terry, D. J., Carey, C. J., & Callan, V. J. (2001). Employee adjustment to an organizational merger: An intergroup perspective. *Personality and Social Psychology Bulletin, 27*(3), 267–280.

Tiedemann, J. (2000). Gender-related beliefs of teachers in elementary school mathematics. *Educational Studies in Mathematics, 41*(2), 191–207.

Tost, L. P., Gino, F., & Larrick, R. P. (2012). Power, competitiveness, and advice taking: Why the powerful don't listen. *Organizational Behavior and Human Decision Processes, 117*(1), 53–65.

Turner, J. C. (1985). Social categorization and the self-concept: A social cognitive theory of group behaviour. In E. J. Lawler (Ed.), *Advances in group processes* (Vol. 2, pp. 77–122). Greenwich, CT: JAI Press.

Umphress, E. E., Bingham, J. B., & Mitchell, M. S. (2010). Unethical behavior in the name of the company: The moderating effect of organizational identification and positive reciprocity beliefs on unethical pro-organizational behavior. *Journal of Applied Psychology, 95*(4), 769–780.

Vaast, E., & Levina, N. (2015). Speaking as one, but not speaking up: Dealing with new moral taint in an occupational online community. *Information and Organization, 25*(2), 73–98.

van der Lee, R. A., Ellemers, N., Scheepers, D. T., & Rutjens, B. (2017). In or out?: How the morality (vs. competence) of prospective group members affects acceptance and rejection. *European Journal of Social Psychology, 47*, 748–762.

van Knippenberg, D., & Wilke, H. (1992). Prototypicality of arguments and conformity to ingroup norms. *European Journal of Social Psychology, 22*, 141–155.

van Laar, C., Derks, B., & Ellemers, N. (2013). Motivation for education and work in young muslim women: The importance of value for ingroup domains. *Basic and Applied Psychology, 35*, 64–74.

van Os, A., de Gilder, D., van Dyck, C., & Groenewegen, P. (2015). Responses to professional identity threat: Identity management strategies in incident narratives of health care professionals. *Journal of Health Organization and Management, 29*(7), 1011–1028.

van Os, A., van Berkel, F., de Gilder, D., van Dyck, C., & Groenewegen, P. (2015). Project risk as identity threat: Explaining the development and consequences of risk discourse in an infrastructure project. *International Journal of Project Management, 33*(4), 877–888.

Van Zomeren, M., Postmes, T., & Spears, R. (2008). Toward an integrative social identity model of collective action: A quantitative research synthesis of three socio-psychological perspectives. *Psychological Bulletin, 134*(4), 504–535.

Veenstra, K., & Haslam, S. A. (2000). Willingness to participate in industrial protest: Exploring social identification in context. *British Journal of Social Psychology, 39*(2), 153–172.

Viki, G. T., Osgood, D., & Phillips, S. (2013). Dehumanization and self-reported proclivity to torture prisoners of war. *Journal of Experimental Social Psychology, 49*, 325–328.

Wigboldus, D. H., Semin, G. R., & Spears, R. (2000). How do we communicate stereotypes?: Linguistic bases and inferential consequences. *Journal of Personality and Social Psychology, 78*(1), 5–18.

Yzerbyt, V. Y. (2016). Intergroup stereotyping. *Current Opinion in Psychology, 11*, 90–95.

Yzerbyt, V. Y., & Cambon, L. (2017). The dynamics of compensation: When ingroup favoritism paves the way for outgroup praise. *Personality and Social Psychology Bulletin, 43*(5), 587–600.

CHAPTER 24

Culture and Intergroup Relations

Yoshihisa Kashima
Michele Gelfand

Culture is an essential part of human psychology. Humanity's success as a biological species is in no small measure thanks to the human ability to form, maintain, and transform complex culture, and adapt to and alter natural and human-made environments. Intergroup context is one of the critical aspects of the human-made environment, which shapes culture. However, culture can also be a driver of intergroup dynamics. We outline in this chapter the basic model of cultural dynamics (e.g., Kashima, Bain, & Perfors, 2019)—formation, maintenance, and transformation of culture over time—and its implications for intergroup relations. In a nutshell, we argue that culture and intergroup relations are mutually constitutive in many cases and discuss contemporary challenges of the 21st century through this perspective.

Niche Constructionism, Culture, and Human-Made Environment

Culture here is conceptualized as the set of *socially transmittable* (i.e., by learning from others; e.g., Boyd & Richerson, 1985; Cavalli-Sforza & Feldman, 1981; Tomasello, Kruger, & Ratner, 1993) information in a population, which can potentially influence cognition, affect, and behavior. Cultural information, therefore, contrasts with genetic information, in channel of transmission—the latter is nonsocially but genetically transmittable. Cultural information typically includes ideas and practices (i.e., what something is and how something is done). Cultural ideas can be about inanimate objects and substance, plants, animals, humans, spirits, and gods, or abstract concepts such as liberty, equality, and fraternity, as well as government and law, rights and obligations, and good and evil. Cultural practices can vary from relatively simple (e.g., shaking hands, rubbing noses, or bowing to greet) to complex and sophisticated (e.g., making bows and arrows, participating in religious rituals, solving differential equations). Cultural information can be represented not only in the brain and body (and therefore behavior) but also in the artifacts produced by people (e.g., tools, technologies, books, apps and websites). To the extent that someone can interpret it, make use of it, or transmit it to someone else, it can be regarded as meaningful cultural information and can potentially form part of a human population's culture (e.g., Kashima, 2016).

Foundational to this perspective is *population thinking,* that is, not thinking in terms of any particular individuals, but in terms of a population of individuals as a whole and the cultural information available to this population (Claidière, Scott-Phillips, & Sperber, 2014; Lewens, 2015). Depending on the scope of one's theory and research, a population of humans may be geographically localized, distributed over a wide spatial geographical area or virtual area such as the Internet, or even the totality of humanity. According to niche constructionism (e.g., Laland, Odling-Smee, & Feldman, 2000; Yamagishi, 2011), a human population constructs its *niche* (i.e., physical and social environment) in which to live, through which its members adapt to the surrounding natural environment. This niche is the *human-made environment* of the population. Humans have two channels of information transmission—genetic and social—that enable them to construct their human-made environment. We discuss the meaning of environment more extensively later in this chapter. However, as humans go about the business of constructing their human-made environment, their culture too changes in adaptation to the human-made and natural environments. It is this dynamic process of niche construction and adaptation that drive the cultural dynamics (i.e., the formation, maintenance, and transformation of culture over time) and their impact on human thoughts, feelings, and action.

This conceptualization of culture is congruent with many others' in psychology (C.-Y. Chiu & Hong, 2013), anthropology and cognitive science (e.g., Boyd & Richerson, 1985; Sperber, 1996), and biology (e.g., Cavalli-Sforza & Feldman, 1981; Dawkins, 1976). This type of thinking is often called *cultural evolution* (e.g., Claidière et al., 2014; Lewens, 2015; Mesoudi, 2011); however, we here call it *cultural dynamics* in order to avoid any confusion with theories of social evolution of the late 19th and early 20th centuries (see Kashima, 2019, for a brief discussion of evolutionism in culture and psychology).

Processes of Cultural Dynamics

Three main processes are involved in cultural dynamics: (1) introduction of novel cultural information to a population, (2) transmission of cultural information among individuals in the population, and (3) processes that affect the prevalence of cultural information in the population.

Introduction of Novel Cultural Information

Cultural information becomes available to a focal human population through two possible processes. One is *invention*—novel cultural information, which has not existed in the focal population—is endogenously produced within the population. Simonton (2011) suggests that novel ideas and practices are often generated by combining existing cultural ideas and practices blindly. Compatible with this line of thinking is what Kauffman (1993) called *adjacent possible,* in which invention is conceptualized as a stochastic exploration of cultural space, such that a novel idea is generated adjacent to the existing cultural ideas and practices. Recent research has provided empirical support for this theorizing in innovations in cultural materials such as online music catalogs and Wikipedia (Tria, Loreto, Servedio, & Strogatz, 2014). It is possible that some inventions are a result of intentional processes, in that people may intentionally try to invent novel cultural ideas and practices. In these cases, inventions may be guided by their goals and conscious thoughts. Nonetheless, some theorists have argued that even these consciously guided thoughts are blindly generated (e.g., Dennett, 1996).

Another process is *importation*—cultural information invented elsewhere in a different population is brought into the focal population. Although the importing population may accept the imported cultural information as is, more often than not, it exhibits a variety of short-term reactions to imported cultural information, partly as a function of the attitudes held by the importing population toward the exporting culture (e.g., Morris, Chiu, & Liu, 2015). First, imported information may be assimilated into the preexisting cultural information. Bartlett (1932) called it *conventionalization*—a cultural material foreign to people that is transformed into a form and content conventional to the receiving people. For instance, in his classic experiments, Bartlett found that English readers in the early 20th-century United Kingdom turned *The War of the Ghosts,* an Amerindian story about raiding worriers in canoes, into soldiers going to a battle in boats (see Kashima, 2000a, 2000b). Second, the imported information may be rejected (e.g., Chiu & Cheng, 2007). For instance, U.S. participants who were shown a photograph of an Independence Day march with American soldiers hoisting a Chinese dragon reacted to the image with disgust (Cheon, Christopoulos, & Hong, 2016). Third, exposure to foreign cultural information may trigger invention (e.g., Leung, Maddux, Galinsky, & Chiu, 2008), raising the possibility that cultural innovation may occur in a zone in which different cultures interface with each other and generate the experience of ambiguous in-betweenness, which Victor Turner (1969) called *liminality*.

Social Transmission of Cultural Information

Cultural information, once introduced into a population, needs to be socially transmitted from individuals to others in order for it to spread in the focal population. We call social transmission of cultural information *cultural transmission,* of which Tomasello and colleagues (1993) distinguished three types: instruction, imitation, and collaboration. *Instruction* occurs when the sender of information intentionally gives that information to its receiver; *imitation* occurs when the receiver learns information from the sender not necessarily with the latter's intent to give the information; and *collaboration* occurs when both sender and receiver collaboratively exchange information. Cultural information may be transmitted from one generation to the next. When it occurs from parents to their offspring, it is called *vertical transmission*; when it occurs between those without a genetic relationship, it is called *oblique transmission* (Cavalli-Sforza & Feldman, 1981). When information travels horizontally within the same generation, all three forms are possible.

There is voluminous research in social sciences about how cultural information is transmitted and diffuses through a population (see Kashima, Peters, & Whelan, 2008, for a brief review). However, more micro-level analyses of cultural transmission have been conducted particularly in psychology (for a review, see e.g., Kashima, Bratanova, & Peters, 2017). Importantly, the latter models draw a distinction between neutral and biased transmission at this point. Cultural transmission may be *neutral,* in

that individuals acquire cultural information by chance (i.e., randomly selected information from randomly selected others in the population). This is often regarded as a baseline null model of cultural transmission (e.g., Cavalli-Sforza & Feldman, 1981), analogous to neutral evolution in population genetics (e.g., Kimura & Crow, 1964). However, a variety of factors are known to *bias* cultural transmission (i.e., deviating from the neural transmission), including well-known tendencies such as conformity (i.e., one acquires prevalent cultural information more frequently than expected by chance), prestige bias (i.e., one acquires information endorsed and deployed by prestigious others), and the like. In fact, many of these biases have been documented in the social psychology of social influence (e.g., Cialdini & Goldstein, 2004).

Altering the Prevalence of Cultural Information

As cultural information is transmitted throughout a population and to next generations, its prevalence (i.e., people who adopt it at a given point in time) changes. The distribution of cultural information may change due to *selection*. If cultural information confers some advantage and benefit, its use is likely reinforced, and the likelihood of its future reuse increases. In contrast, if it incurs some disadvantage and cost, the likelihood of its future use is reduced. This logic is broadly consistent with Thorndike's (1927) law of effect and Skinner's (1981) behavior selection by consequence, whose intellectual roots can be found in Darwin's natural selection. These benefits and costs are often construed in terms of an increase or a decrease in *fitness*; fitness-enhancing (reducing) information is likely to increase (decrease) its prevalence. That is to say, cultural information is selected in to the extent that its use accrues benefits and selected out to the extent that its use incurs costs. And the costs and benefits for cultural information are largely dependent on the environments in which the cultural information is deployed. In the end, cultural information with greater benefits than costs in a given configuration of environmental factors becomes more prevalent. In this way, selection processes facilitate the retention of cultural information adaptive to the environments.

When cultural transmission is neutral, *cultural drift* can occur; that is, the prevalence of cultural information in a population changes randomly. Bentley, Hahn, and Shennan (2004) provided some evidence of cultural drift, showing that predictions based on the assumption of neutral transmission were largely borne out by data about popular baby names of the 20th-century U.S. census, pottery motifs from Neolithic Germany, and patents and their citations from the United States. For instance, parents may choose their babies' names fairly randomly from a set of popular names in the United States (e.g., Bob, Deborah, John, Sarah), and this random choice can generate a fluctuation in the prevalence of first names from one generation to the next.

Environments, Selection, and Adaptation

Culture is one of the most critical adaptation devices for humanity. Cultural information helps a population and individuals adapt by increasing overall fitness. It is, however, important to recognize that although fitness in biological evolution is measured in terms of reproductive success, cultural fitness can capture a far broader set of costs and benefits. For example, O'Dwyer and Kandler's (2017) analysis of a complete set of baby names from Australia found that the adoption of common baby names shows a cultural drift as in Bentley and colleagues' (2004) work on American baby names, but that there is a bias against unusual names, suggesting a possibility of selection at play. Parents may choose not to give "unusual" names, believing that names rare in a dominant culture (e.g., due to cultural differences in naming conventions) may socially disadvantage their children. In this case, "costs" may be due in part to reproductive success (e.g., children with unusual names may have difficulty finding mates), but may have more to do with social and economic success (e.g., popularity, jobs) and other types of outcomes. That is to say, cultural information such as a baby name may be associated with differential cultural fitness, but its fitness depends on a variety of outcomes in relation to a diverse array of environmental factors.

In line with this thinking, Kashima (2019) discussed a variety of fitness affecting environments (see Table 24.1). According to him, a human population constructs the *human-made environment* using available cultural informa-

tion in adaptation to the *natural environment*. The natural environment can consist of a broad set of things, including climate, land, water, and a variety of natural resources usable for human consumption, and constitute the local biosphere, including fauna and flora, and plants and animals that can be domesticated. In addition, it includes a microbial world made of microorganisms, including pathogenic ones. For example, Van de Vliert (2013) highlighted the importance of macro-level harshness of climate on individual freedom, Van Lange, Rinderu, and Bushman (2017) made a case for the effect of hot climate on aggression, and Gelfand and colleagues (2011) noted the importance of natural disaster prevalence on cultural tightness, whereas Fincher, Thornhill, Murray, and Schaller (2008) drew attention to the micro-world of pathogens—the pathogenic environment tends to encourage stranger avoidance (for a review of ecological perspective on psychology, see Oishi, 2014).

However, the human made environment itself presents environmental challenges to the human population. Consider Segall, Campbell, and Herskovits's (1966) carpentered world hypothesis. They argued that the residents of an urbanized *built environment* dominated by vertical and horizontal straight lines and 90-degree angles may grow up with the visual system adapted to this physical environment, such that they may be more susceptible to the Müller-Lyer illusion than those in the rural environment. Indeed, their data corroborate this conjecture. The human social environment including the economic, intergroup, and intragroup environments can present their own challenges. Kashima (2019) provides more detailed discussions about the variety of environments and cultural adaptation. We highlight the intergroup environment in this chapter.

Because there are many, diverse environmental demands, cultural information may be fitness enhancing for some environments but not for others. It is the overall net costs and benefits in adaptation to diverse environments that would shape the trajectory of cultural dynamics. It is important to remember that not everything that is cultural is adaptive; however, the mechanisms of generation, transmission, and selection of cultural ideas and practices can ex-

TABLE 24.1. A Variety of Environmental Challenges

Types of environments			Examples
Natural			Climate
			Pathogens
			Natural disasters
			Resource scarcity
Human made	Built		Carpentered world
	Social	Economic	Mode of production
		Intergroup	Competition
			War and territorial invasions
		Intragroup	Population density
			Residential mobility
	Psychological		Existential anxiety
			Cognition and communication

Note. Adapted from Kashima, Bain, and Perfors (2019). See Kashima (2019) for detailed discussions.

plain the adaptiveness of many, though not all, existing cultural ideas and practices in the population's environmental niche. In this sense, the processes of cultural dynamics may be Darwinian (Mesoudi, 2011; Richerson & Boyd, 2005).

While acknowledging that culture helps adaptation and selectionist mechanisms are at play, Sperber and his colleagues (e.g., Claidière et al., 2014; Sperber, 1996) have suggested that culture changes by *attraction* as well, which occurs when transmitted cultural information undergoes transformation and eventually moves towards attractors in the cultural space. Bloodletting as a treatment for illness may be an example (Miton, Claidière, & Mercier, 2015). The idea that a physical ailment can be cured by letting blood out from the same location (e.g., bloodletting from head to cure headache) appears to be widespread in diverse traditional cultures, and a story about bloodletting is more likely reproduced by American participants than other equally questionable treatments. Although its precise formulation is still to be worked out, whether it can be reformulated within a selectionist framework is yet to be determined. For instance, psychological attraction may be understood in terms of adaptation to the psychological environment. Nonetheless, it aspires to present an alternative metatheoretical perspective to the neo-Darwinian theory of cultural evolution.

Ultrasociality, Cooperation, and Culture

One of the most significant environments for a human population is the human-made environment that it has created for itself (e.g., D. Cohen, 2001). It is no coincidence that a significant aspect of any culture has to do with the regulation of human sociality (i.e., how humans in a population live with each other). As a biological species, however, humanity is peculiar in this respect. Don Campbell (1982) characterized this peculiarly human sociality in the following way:

Ultrasociality refers to the most social of animal organizations, with full time division of labor, specialists who gather no food but are fed by others, effective sharing of information about sources of food and danger, self-sacrificial effort in collective defense. This level has been achieved by ants, termites and humans in several scattered archaic city-states. . . . In the social insects, the further route to ultrasociality has been achieved by caste sterility, almost entirely removing genetic competition among the cooperators; this route has *not* been available for human urban societies. Instead, cultural evolution (including norms inhibiting human selfishness, deceitfulness and cowardice) has been required. (p. 160)

Ever since, theorists have noted this human sociality as a species-specific characteristic that enabled humanity to be successful as a biological species. It is the human ability to maintain large-scale cooperation among genetically un-related individuals.

Indeed, from the perspective of classical theories of rationality and evolution, large-scale human cooperation is puzzling. How can humans manage to cooperate even when they are always individually worse off if they cooperate? A paradigmatic case is the provision of public goods. By definition, *public goods* are goods and services to which everyone has access and are therefore collectively beneficial. Concrete examples include public parks, a public broadcaster, clean air, and waterways. However, because access to them cannot be denied once established, and their provision incurs cost to the contributor, a co-operator who contributes to the provision of a public good is always worse off than a non-cooperator who doesn't (often called *defector,* or *free rider,* in the game theoretic parlance). From the perspective of classical game theory, if an individual computes the overall benefit, it is rational not to cooperate. From the perspective of classical theory of evolution, if an individual's fitness equals the overall benefit, a cooperator has a lower level of fitness than a defector on average, and therefore is less likely to be reproductively successful and should go extinct in the long run. This is the problem of social dilemma (Dawes, 1980) or collective action (Olson, 1965).

The current consensus is that the evolutionary feat of human ultrasociality is largely culturally enabled (e.g., Richerson & Boyd, 1998; Turchin, 2013). Decades of theoretical and empirical research on cooperation has shown that even if the situation is highly competitive, there exist some mechanisms that can maintain cooperation (e.g., Kurzban, Burton-Chellew, & West, 2015; Nowak, 2006b). We suggest that these mechanisms have both genetic and cultural ingredients and are shaped and modified by socialization and situational variations. We highlight two mechanisms, *assortment* and *punishment* (and reward to some extent) that are most relevant in the context of culture and intergroup relationship. Both mechanisms modify the incentive structure of social interactions, such that cooperation becomes more beneficial (Taylor & Nowak, 2007). Assortment does so by structuring the pattern of social interaction

so that cooperators have a better than chance level of interacting with other cooperators; punishment does so by making defection less beneficial; therefore, cooperation is more beneficial in the long run.

Assortment and Partner Selection

A robust mechanism to sustain cooperation is *assortment.* When cooperative individuals have better than chance opportunities to interact with other cooperative individuals (i.e., assorting themselves into pairs and groups for interaction), cooperation can be sustained in a population (e.g., Eshel & Cavalli-Sforza, 1982; West, Griffin, & Gardner, 2007). There are a number of practices[1] that can increase assortment. The most obvious case is *kinship*-based assortment. If people cooperate with their kin, they increase not only inclusive fitness, thereby enhancing reproductive success in a broad sense (Hamilton, 1964a, 1964b), but also their overall cultural fitness. Beyond kinship, however, there is a mechanism that can *maintain* assortment once a relationship among people is established. A good example is *direct reciprocity,* in which one cooperates if one's partners cooperate (e.g., Trivers, 1971). Although Gouldner (1960) framed this tendency as a norm, implying its cultural origin, it is possible that some mechanisms involved in reciprocal exchange of cooperation have genetic components. There are some indications that genetic variability is associated with moral adherence across cultures (Mrazek, Chiao, Blizinsky, Lun, & Gelfand, 2013).

Nonetheless, a large-scale assortment requires mechanisms of *partner selection* (for a recent review, see Baumard, Andre, & Sperber, 2013), that is, mechanisms that enable cooperative individuals to select other cooperative individuals without kinship and form new social relationships, so that a mechanism such as direct reciprocity can maintain mutual cooperation. The complement to partner selection is *ostracism* (e.g., Williams, 2007), in which one excludes some from being potential partners for cooperative interaction. In combination, partner selection and ostracism can expand and maintain assortment and a cluster of cooperation.

One of the practices that can bootstrap cooperative relationship is an initial gesture of cooperation. That is to say, when one meets a stranger, one cooperates with him or her first, and observes what he or she does. If the partner cooperates, one cooperates; if the partner defects, one defects, and thereafter, direct reciprocity can maintain cooperation. This practice that couples initial cooperation with direct reciprocity is Amnon Rappaport's *tit-for-tat with initial cooperation* (Axelrod, 1984) and its variants (Nowak, 2006a), which tends to be able to keep fitness relative to many other practices.

Other practices of partner selection can extend cooperation beyond kinship and serendipitous encounters with strangers. One is based on *indirect reciprocity,* in which one selects a partner who has a good reputation as a cooperator (e.g., Nowak & Sigmund, 1998). Here, one does not personally know the potential partner but learns about the target via gossip (e.g., Sommerfeld, Krambeck, Semmann, & Milinski, 2007) or other means (e.g., ratings on an Internet site) and chooses to interact and cooperate with the target. In *network reciprocity,* one selects a partner who cooperates with one's cooperative partner (e.g., Fu, Hauert, Nowak, & Wang, 2008; Ohtsuki, Hauert, Lieberman, & Nowak, 2006). It is akin to "my friend's friend is my friend" as implied in Heider's (1958) balance theory. To the extent that there are enough

cooperators within an immediate social network, cooperation can be engendered and maintained. Another is *attribute-based cooperation,* in which one selects a partner who shares the same attribute as oneself (e.g., Riolo, Cohen, & Axelrod, 2001). An attribute can be ethnicity, religion, or even a green beard (Dawkins, 1976). To the extent that there is a shared practice to use any arbitrary attribute to select a partner and cooperate with this person, cooperation can evolve in a population.

It is worth noting that different partner selection practices can expand the *moral circle* to different extents. Moral circle (e.g., Laham, 2009; Singer, 1981) defines the outer bounds of the social world, inside which people treat each other morally. If cooperative interaction is a significant part of moral treatment, different partner selection practices are likely to influence the radius of the moral circle. First, indirect reciprocity can expand potential partners to everyone whose reputation one knows about. Network reciprocity can further expand potential partners by gathering reputational information from one's friends or using mutual friendship as a proxy for reputational information. Attribute-based cooperation can expand partnerships even further. The only thing that matters is whether a potential partner shares the same attribute or not (see Figure 24.1).

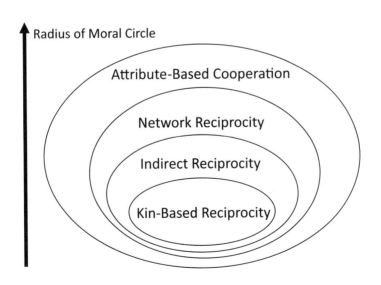

FIGURE 24.1. Partner selection practice and the moral circle.

Punishment and Reward

Punishment of an undesirable behavior can reduce the likelihood of its recurrence, whereas reward of a desirable behavior can increase it. Under many circumstances, punishment could keep the frequency of the undesirable behavior in a population at bay at least in principle (e.g., Boyd & Richerson, 1992). Punishment of noncooperative behavior and reward of cooperative behavior are no exception (e.g., Sigmund, Hauert, & Nowak, 2001). Punishing a noncooperative behavior (i.e., defector, free rider, cheater) can sustain cooperation (Fehr & Fischbacher, 2004a), and rewarding cooperation can also sustain cooperation (e.g., Panchanathan & Boyd, 2004) under some circumstances, especially when (1) an individual's action can be sufficiently accurately monitored, (2) his or her reputation can be made known to relevant others without bias, and (3) the action can be appropriately responded to (i.e., defection with punishment, avoidance, or exclusion and cooperation with reward, partner selection, or inclusion) (e.g., Ostrom, 2015).

Nevertheless, these conditions are not always met. The conditions of accurate monitoring and availability of unbiased reputational information may be relatively easily met if only a small number of individuals are involved and most actions occur in full view of everyone in the community (i.e., when reputation is common knowledge). However, when a large number of individuals are involved, these conditions are not always satisfied. As the group size increases, so does the cost and difficulty of monitoring action and management of reputational information. Furthermore, the third condition of appropriate social responses is not so easily achieved either. Take a scenario in which two individuals interact in a situation characterized by a prisoner's dilemma. One cooperates and the other defects. At this point, however, the scenario can take different turns, generating a complex array of possibilities and ramifications (see Figure 24.2; for discussion, Cushman, 2015; Sigmund, 2007). One possibility is that the cooperator punishes the defector. This type of punishment is called *second-party peer* punishment, in which a peer who has suffered from his or her partner's noncooperative behavior punishes the defector. However, this behavior may be costly and diminish the person's fitness in the long run.

Moreover, it may run into a problem of retaliation—the punished may retaliate against the punisher (i.e., counterpunishment; Nikiforakis, 2008), which could then be retaliated, and so forth, toward a downward spiral. Another course of possibilities is that the cooperator avoids the defector, so that he or she will not interact with the defector in the future. If everyone ends up avoiding the defector, this would be an exclusion or ostracism. However, if there are enough potential cooperators in the population that the defector can exploit, defection may be more beneficial for the defector in the end. In other words, punishment of defection can become a *second-order public good* (Yamagishi, 1986); if it is costlier to punish than to avoid, a peer may choose to avoid, but this avoidance can be construed as a kind of "defection" in that nonpunishment can encourage the noncooperation. This gives rise to the possibility of a *third-party peer punishment,* in which a third party who was not involved in the original interaction punishes the defector (Fehr & Fischbacher, 2004b). However, a third-party peer punishment can be sustained only under restricted social context (Roos, Gelfand, Nau, & Carr, 2014). Then, there is another, more insidious, possibility. Although the co-operator may be more likely to punish the defector, it is possible that the defector may punish the co-operator (Herrmann, Thöni, & Gächter, 2008). This is called *antisocial punishment,* and it can thwart cooperation (Rand & Nowak, 2011).

The role of rewards could be somewhat different from punishment. If cooperation is met by cooperation (i.e., reciprocity), then this can certainly sustain cooperation. Second- and third-party peer reward can further sustain cooperation; an upward spiral toward greater prosociality is presumably possible. A reward system may be able to avoid the issue analogous to the second-order social dilemma involving punishment – those who do not punish defectors need to be encouraged to engage in punishment, that is, by rewarding those who reward cooperators, especially when combined with a use of punishment in the form of punishing those who fail to reward cooperators (Kiyonari & Barclay, 2008). Nonetheless, there may be an antisocial

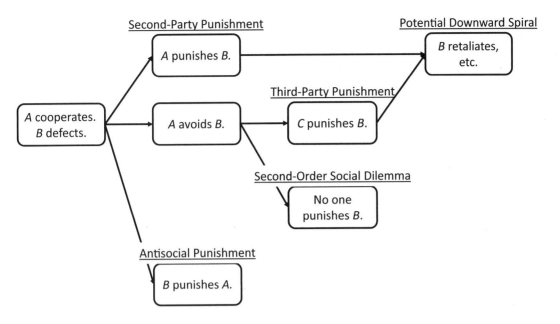

FIGURE 24.2. Punishment and its discontents.

reward (e.g., corruption, bribery, and inordinate ingratiation).

Religion and Moralizing Gods

One of the cultural mechanisms that may help sustain cooperation is religion, or more specifically, a belief in moralizing supernatural beings. Although beliefs in beings that have superhuman and supernatural capabilities (e.g., ability to read minds, in violation of folk psychology; ability to fly, defying folk physics) may be a type of exaptation based on a variety of human psychological adaptations (Atran & Norenzayan, 2004), sincere beliefs in the existence of supernatural beings that are concerned with human affairs have been argued to enable the formation and maintenance of a large-scale group (Norenzayan et al., 2016). Often dubbed "moralizing gods" (Roes & Raymond, 2003), beliefs in supernatural beings that are able and willing to monitor human conduct and to punish misbehavior or reward prosociality can deter believers from defection or free riding.

This cultural mechanism may be all the more powerful, especially if a group is large. As noted earlier, as group size increases, surveillance and sanction become more difficult,

and it is more difficult to provide public goods and maintain mutual cooperation. With beliefs in moralizing gods, people may be able to do just that, secure in thoughts that any wrongdoing is punished and defectors would get just desserts. Indeed, human groups with beliefs in moralizing gods tend to be larger in size (Roes & Raymond, 2003) and more enduring (Sosis & Alcorta, 2003) than those without them. World religions such as Christianity and Islam are good examples. More recently, in fieldwork with diverse small-scale communities, Purzycki and colleagues (2016) showed that those who believe that their deities are knowledgeable about people's thoughts and punitive toward moral violations tended to make a fairer allocation of resources to those who believe in the same deities but live far away. In other words, beliefs in moralizing gods appeared to expand their moral circle.

Institution

Another class of mechanisms that can sustain cooperation is *institutions,* that is, institutionalized mechanisms that monitor individuals' actions, and reward cooperation and punish defection (e.g., Sigmund, De Silva, Traulsen,

& Hauert, 2010; Yamagishi, 1986). Obvious examples are police, courts, and other mechanisms of law enforcement (punishment), as well as conferment of medals, decorations, and other forms of official recognitions of social contribution (reward).

A variety of sanctioning institutions has existed in different parts of the world at different points in human history; however, nation-states (e.g., France, the United States, Japan) are most prevalent in the contemporary world. The nation-state emerged as a form of social institution in Western and Central Europe. Its origin is often attributed to the Treaties of Westphalia, in 1648, which ended a prolonged and devastating religion-triggered intergroup conflict in Europe called the 30 Years' War. Since then, the nation-state as a model of governance has spread around the world over the past centuries. A social theorist, Anthony Giddens (1990) characterizes the nation-state as a form of governance that combines a highly sophisticated system of surveillance (i.e., monitoring) and a powerful means of violence (i.e., military, police). In the idealized prototypical form, the nation-state is combined with democracy as a mode of government selection and the rule of law as a mode of social regulation. Obviously, the nation-state is not the only actor dispensing institutional sanctions (e.g., International Court, United Nations, other nongovernment organizations, including militant or dissident ones such as ISIS), though other institutions usually have weaker surveillance and law enforcement mechanisms than many nation-states in the contemporary world.

Nation-states are institutions that, among other things, provide mechanisms of social control to ensure individuals under their jurisdiction sustain cooperation in a broad sense. If an individual does not interact with others in a cooperative or coordinated way, the states and their apparatuses are meant to exercise their powers to sanction those who violate their regulatory framework. Under this assurance, individuals can maintain an expectation of cooperation from others under state jurisdiction. This way, those who share the attribute of membership of a state (i.e., citizenship) constitute a *civil society,* and members of the civil society can be trusted to cooperate with each other and coordinate their actions under the same social regulatory umbrella (Rothstein & Stolle, 2008).

We suggest that if the institution of nation-states is well functioning, and combined with *universalism* (i.e., the cultural idea that institutional framework applies to everyone equally and universally), generalized trust (i.e., belief that people can be generally trusted to cooperate) can be sustained under the state's jurisdiction (Tabellini, 2008). In this sense, the nation-state provides social categories whose membership can act as an attribute for attribute-based partner selection. In addition, it also has a built-in mechanism of social control (punishment and reward) to maintain a large-scale cooperation among those who share its membership. Existing evidence suggests that people from Western Europe prefer institutional sanctions to peer sanctions (Traulsen, Rohl, & Milinski, 2012). However, it is possible that those who live under unfair and oppressive institutions show a different preference. This is because they may regard "taking the law into one's own hands" as preferable to arbitrarily exploitative institutions.

Cultural Dimensions: Collectivisms, Tightness, and Honor

Culture and psychology researchers have investigated three main cultural dimensions over the past few decades: collectivism, tightness, and honor. We suggest that each dimension can be conceptualized in terms of the prevalence of certain cultural ideas and practices, and their cultural dynamics.

Collectivisms

We suggest that different types of collectivism(s) imply different cultural practices that encourage people to select a particular type of partner and cultural ideas that support and justify the cultural practices, so that they assort themselves into cooperation (see Table 24.2).

Kin-based collectivism implies the cultural practices of partner selection practices that prescribe one to interact and cooperate with people of the same kin (i.e., kinsmen should help each other). Although the norms and practice of mutual help among kinsfolk appear to be widespread (e.g., Triandis, 1995), especially for life-and-death matters (Burnstein, Crandall, &

TABLE 24.2. A Variety of Collectivisms

Type	Subtype	Ideas and practices of partner selection
Kin-based		Family and kinship
Network-based		Non-kin social network ties (e.g., *guanxi*)
Attribute-based		Attributes (e.g., ethnicity, language, religion)
	Nation-state based (societal)	Nation-state or civil society

Kitayama, 1994), there are cultural differences in *familism* (Realo, Allik, & Greenfield, 2008), cultural practices of kinship-based assortment and cooperation. *Network-based* collectivism means partner selection practices that encourage one to interact and cooperate with one's partner's partner (i.e., "my friend's friend is my friend"), whereas in *attribute-based* collectivism, partner selection practices encourage one to interact with others who share the same attribute, such as a race, a nationality, an accent, a religion, an occupation, and so forth. An attribute can be anything publicly recognizable to those who are involved in interaction. We suggest that a special subtype of attribute-based collectivism is nation-state or civil society-based collectivism.

Network- and attribute-based collectivisms closely resemble what Brewer and Chen (2007) called relational and group collectivism. *Relational collectivism* emphasizes the maintenance of harmonious interpersonal relationships, whereas *group collectivism* emphasizes the significance of a social category-based membership. The former tends toward a cohesive and tightly knit small group, whereas the latter enables the formation and maintenance of a large-scale collective that shares a social identity and can also act as a basis for ingroup–outgroup differentiation and competition (Brewer & Yuki, 2007). There is evidence to suggest that network-based partner selection is more prevalent among East Asians than among North Americans (e.g., Ye & Ng, 2017; Yuki, Maddux, Brewer, & Takemura, 2005).

Tightness

Cultural tightness is concerned with cultural ideas and practices about norm following and reactions to norm violation. Tight cultures require that cultural ideas and normative practices in a population be closely followed, and deviations from the norms are to be punished (Pelto, 1968). In this sense, tightness is a meta-norm (i.e., a norm about cultural norms). Gelfand and her colleagues (2011) showed that countries around the world and U. S. states (Harrington & Gelfand, 2014) that have experienced a number of threats posed to groups and individuals by natural and human-made environments (e.g., invasions, natural disasters, pathogens, resource scarcity), tend to have tight culture. It has been theorized that tightness may be a cultural adaptation to threats to the social fabric of a group: Tightly following and enforcing norms that support cooperation and coordination among group members may enhance the likelihood of their survival when natural and human-made disasters threaten their livelihoods. Loose cultural groups, by contrast, have comparatively less threat and require less coordination to survive. Evolutionary game theoretic models have shown that evolution of cooperation, coordination, and punishment of defectors is based on either chronic threat or a temporary increase in threat (Roos, Gelfand, Nau, & Lun, 2015).

Consistent with this, neuroscience research suggests that individuals in tight societies have stronger neural responses to norm violations than do those in loose societies (Mu, Kitayama, Han, & Gelfand, 2015), and research using hyperscanning electroencephalography has shown that groups under threat are better able to coordinate their actions as mediated through increased brain synchrony on gamma (i.e., fear) waves (Mu, Han, & Gelfand, 2017).

The degree of tightness–looseness confers certain advantages and liabilities for groups. Tight groups tend to have more synchrony, greater monitoring, and higher degrees of self-control. Loose groups tend to be more disorganized, have lower monitoring, and experience a number of self-regulation problems (Gelfand, Harrington, & Jackson, 2017). Whereas loose groups are much more open to new ideas, people, and to change, tight groups tend to be more ethnocentric and resist new ideas and change (Gelfand et al., 2017). Evolutionary game theoretic models, for example, show that the introduction of novel cultural information—even if it has higher payoffs for a population—tends to be rejected more in tight than in loose groups, and that the former have lower exploration rates than the latter (De, Nau, & Gelfand, 2017). Other crowd-sourcing studies show that creativity is much higher within loose groups, and the importation of new ideas from other populations is much lower in tight groups (Chua, Roth, & Lemoine, 2015). These cultural dynamics result in higher cultural inertia in tighter groups, until a tipping point is crossed, when the culture may change rapidly to a new equilibrium (De, Nau, Pan, & Gelfand, 2018). The evolution of *ethnocentrism* (interacting with people with similar attributes) appears also to occur more strongly in tight groups that experience a lot of threat (Jackson et al., 2019).

Honor

A culture of honor can be thought of as a set of cultural ideas and practices to react aggressively against perceived or real threats to one's reputation or resources (e.g., Cohen, Nisbett, Bowdle, & Schwarz, 1996; Cross et al., 2014; Nisbett & Cohen, 1996). If other actors—be they individuals or groups—can take away one's resources or damage one's reputation, strong reactions to resource or reputational threats can help protect one's resources and reputation or act as a deterrent (e.g., Nisbett & Cohen, 1996). This is especially the case when an institutional protection of one's resources or reputation is absent (Nisbett & Cohen, 1996).

Computational models have shown that in contexts in which the police are unreliable and resources are scarce, honor agents evolve in part to thwart other aggressive agents in the population, in a predator–prey-like dynamic (Nowak, Gelfand, Borkowski, Cohen, & Hernandez, 2016). If there is a well-functioning impersonal institution (e.g., police, military,

judiciary) that can reliably protect individuals' and groups' resources, honor-based cultural practices do not need to be enacted. Honor cultures—having a strong reputation for both benevolence and strength—have been known to characterize some ancient societies, but they also apply to modern nations (e.g., the Middle East, Latin America) and states (the U.S. South) (Nisbett & Cohen, 1996; Nowak et al., 2016).

Culture and Intergroup Context

Culture and intergroup context are mutually constitutive. Cultural information can shape intergroup relationships, but the intergroup context, in turn, shapes cultural dynamics.

Intergroup Context Can Impact Culture

Intergroup context is an aspect of the human-made social environment (see Table 24.1); culture may then be formed, maintained, and transformed in adaptation to the intergroup context. Particularly pertinent here is the process of *group selection*. Suppose that there are many groups, each of which consists of a population of individuals. If cultural information that benefits a group (i.e., information that increases the average fitness of the group) is common within a group, this group is likely to be able to survive, but a group without this cultural information is likely to disintegrate and go extinct. Often attributed to Charles Darwin (1888), this notion has been critically scrutinized from a variety of perspectives, and the consensus is that this process can work only when groups are small in size and between-group migration is limited (e.g., Okasha, 2006).

However, it has been shown that if cultural information is assumed to be transmitted better within each group than between groups, so that between-group differentiation is maintained, group selection processes can effect cultural adaptation by group selection in the long run (e.g., Soltis, Boyd, & Richerson, 1995). In other words, to the extent that intergroup context is such that cultural dynamics maintains the group boundary, group selection processes may ensure the survival of a group with more group-beneficial cultural characteristics and the disintegration and extinction of a group with group-detrimental cultural characteristics. General orientation to cooperate with ingroup members (i.e., intragroup cooperation) is a significant psychological driver that can motivate the endorsement and enactment of group-beneficial ideas and practices. Richerson and Boyd (1998) and their colleagues have argued that there is sufficient evidence for the important role of group selection in the emergence of human ultrasociality (also see Richerson et al., 2016).

Intergroup Competition, Conflict, and Warfare

Intergroup competition, conflict, or warfare is likely to provide just such intergroup context. Realistic conflict theory (e.g., Sherif, Harvey, White, Hood, & Sherif, 1961) suggests that competition for limited resources can give rise to intergroup conflicts (i.e., symbolic or physical hostilities) or even outright wars (i.e., violent conflicts with armed combatants). Under these circumstances, group boundaries are likely to be tightly maintained by severely limiting open exchanges of goods, services, and information, and movements of people (Taylor & Moghaddam, 1994). As a consequence of this type of hostile intergroup context, group-beneficial cultural ideas and practices can be sustained within a group even if a large cost is incurred to an individual who contributes to the group.

Parochial altruism, perhaps the most dramatic example of this type of mechanism postulated to date (Bowles, 2012; Choi & Bowles, 2007), involves a combination of ideas and practices (1) to cooperate with ingroup members and punish those who don't cooperate and (2) to avoid cooperating with (García & van den Bergh, 2011) or even aggress against (Choi & Bowles, 2007) outgroups at the same time. Mathematical modeling and computer simulations have shown that parochial altruism can be maintained in a population when there is conflictful intergroup context (e.g., Choi & Bowles, 2007; García & van den Bergh, 2011). There is experimental evidence that adults in nonhostile tribes in the Western Highlands of Papua New Guinea (Bernhard, Fischbacher, & Fehr, 2006) as well as students (Abbink, Brandts, Herrmann, & Orzen, 2012), engage in parochially altruistic behavior in economic games. Furthermore, based on archaeological data and ethnographic reports of hunter–gatherers living

in the late Pleistocene or early Holocene epoch (i.e., when modern humans emerged), Bowles (2012) estimated that the fraction of total mortality due to warfare was sizable at approximately .12 to .14 on the average. Although he argued that parochial altruism could emerge and remain in human populations as a genetically coded trait, comparative studies of human hunter–gatherers and chimpanzees cast some doubt on the genetic basis of parochial altruism (Langergraber et al., 2011; Wrangham, Wilson, & Muller, 2006). Rusch (2014) provides a critical review of parochial altruism.

Symbolic Intergroup Differentiation

Even in the absence of overt intergroup competition and conflict, there can be symbolic differentiation between groups. Social identity theory (Tajfel, 1982; Tajfel & Turner, 1979) and self-categorization theory (Turner, 1987) suggest that when there exists an attribute dimension on which a clear differentiation can be made between groups, such that within-group similarities are greater than between-group similarities, social categories that differentiate the group members may emerge, and members of the groups may categorize themselves in terms of those categories. The self-categorizations may constitute significant aspects of individuals' social identities, which in turn can become a psychological basis of group formation and maintenance. Intergroup differentiations based on social identities can be marked by a variety of observable, often symbolic, characteristics such as ethnic markers (Boyd & Richerson, 1987), accent (Cohen et al., 2012), and others.

Not only can social identity—self–group relation—be a basis of symbolic intergroup differentiation, but cultural identity can also become a basis of intergroup differentiation. Cultural identity is based on individuals' identification with cultural artifacts, ideas, and practices (C.-Y. Chiu & Hong, 2013), rather than social groups per se. As we noted earlier, when a cultural element is imported into a group, the importing population responds to it differently (e.g., Morris et al., 2015). For instance, intergroup differentiations are symbolically maintained when the imported cultural information is rejected or negatively reacted to, just as when Americans were shown a picture of American soldiers carrying a Chinese dragon in an Independence Day march (Cheon et al., 2016).

Intergroup Context and Cultural Dimensions

Figure 24.3 outlines potential cultural implications of intergroup context. Symbolically well-differentiated intergroup context presents the human-made environment in which attribute-based collectivism and tight punishment mechanisms to avoid defection are likely to be adaptive. Be it an ethnic marker, a religion, or a skin color, an attribute that can be used to differentiate members of one's ingroup and outgroups can act as a way of keeping the groups separate, so that goods, information, and people do not move across group boundaries. At the same time, attribute-based collectivism can also foster intragroup cooperation. This is because it can facilitate the attribute-based assortment and help create the intragroup context in which mutual cooperation among group members can be beneficial in the long run.

Symbolically differentiated groups are not always in competition or in conflict, but they can be. In a competitive or conflictual intergroup context, outgroups can pose threats to a population, and this could increase cultural tightness, which has been theorized to help the group increase the intragroup cooperation and coordination. If members of a group tightly follow a set of group-beneficial normative ideas

and practices, groups are likely to be able to cooperate with one another and coordinate their actions, and the group would have a better chance of protecting itself against aggressors or hostile outgroups, or even of aggressing against outgroups to gain more resources. Under those circumstances in which groups are on the lookout for potential intergroup threats, honor-based ideas and practices may emerge as a possible cultural adaptation to the hostile intergroup environment, particularly when institutions are weak. By aggressively reacting to outgroups' transgressions, groups may be able to fend off aggressions or deter their future hostilities.

Nevertheless, it is important to recognize that there are other cultural ideas and practices that can prevent these things from happening. For instance, a sanctioning institution that can reduce intergroup threats and police intergroup relations can dampen these cultural dynamics.

Culture Can Shape Intergroup Relations

Just as the intergroup context can shape culture, culture can shape intergroup relations. In particular, we suggest that attribute-based collectivism can strengthen symbolic intergroup differentiation (Figure 24.3). When an attribute-based collectivism is in operation, intragroup cooperation can become a shared norm, there may emerge an expectation that others who share the group-differentiating attribute would

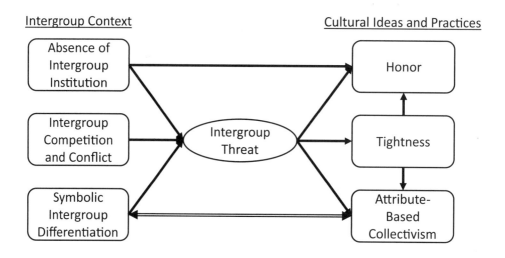

FIGURE 24.3. Mutual constitution of intergroup context and culture.

cooperate, and there is likely to be greater cooperation within a group than with outgroup members (Balliet, Wu, & De Dreu, 2014). This can set in motion a positive feedback loop of further intergroup differentiation by symbolic markers of group membership (e.g., McElreath, Boyd, & Richerson, 2003). These cultural dynamics can then further clarify which attributes are used to differentiate the groups. For instance, if religion (e.g., Catholic vs. Protestant, Christianity vs. Islam) and its markers symbolically differentiate groups, they may be further elaborated and strengthened to demarcate the group boundaries. Likewise, race or nationality may be able to have an analogous consequence.

Essentialism can symbolically differentiate groups further. It is a set of cultural ideas and practices that attribute an immutable essence that defines the membership of a category (Medin & Ortony, 1989). Applied to a social category that defines a social group, *essentializing* a group means to assume there is an unchangeable character to a member of the group and tends to result in exaggerated perceptions of group differences (Haslam, Bastian, Bain, & Kashima, 2006). When fortified with a somewhat misguided understanding of modern genetics, this can result in genetic essentialism (Dar-Nimrod & Heine, 2011), which can bias intergroup perceptions and actions. In light of the finding that intergroup attitudes can be improved by increasing the perception of group malleability (Goldenberg et al., 2018), essentialism that can increase the perceived immutability is likely to be a significant factor in the entrenchment of intergroup differentiation.

Existing evidence suggests symbolic intergroup differentiation is unlikely to be sufficient to generate outgroup derogation (Balliet et al., 2014; Brewer, 1979), hostility, and intergroup conflict. However, realistic conflict over scarce resources (e.g., territory) can cause intergroup competition and conflict (e.g., Sherif, Harvey, Hood, Sherif, & White, 1988), and culture of honor may increase the potential for intergroup conflict. This is because honor culture can amplify the possibility of aggressive reactions to real and perceived intergroup threats, which can further trigger the spiral of punishment and retaliatory punishment (see Figure 24.2) downward to an intergroup conflict. Although

intragroup communications about an outgroup may maintain shared stereotypes toward the outgroup (e.g., Kashima, 2000a), it is when emotionally charged negative information is shared between group members that they may coordinate their attitudes and actions toward the outgroup (e.g., Peters & Kashima, 2007). If there is an indication of intergroup conflict, cultural transmission within an ingroup may further exacerbate the perception of conflict in favor of the ingroup (Lee, Gelfand, & Kashima, 2014). Once there is a widespread perception of intergroup conflict, this may set in motion the cultural dynamics of further tightening of the cultural norm and strengthening of honor culture. In the absence of an institutional arrangement that can curtail intergroup competition and conflict, the mutual constitution of culture and intergroup context may continue.

Mutual Constitution of Intergroup Context and Culture

The theoretical analysis about the relation between intergroup context and culture can be summarized in the following five principles.

Cultural Dynamics

Culture is the set of socially transmittable information (e.g., cultural ideas and practices) available in a human population. *Cultural dynamics* are concerned with the stability and change in the distribution of cultural information in the population over time. Three main processes produce cultural dynamics: (1) introduction of novel cultural information to a population, (2) transmission of cultural information among individuals in the population, and (3) processes that affect the prevalence of cultural information in the population.

Cultural Selection

The prevalence of cultural information tends to increase if it generates benefits broadly conceived, but it tends to decrease if it incurs costs. The costs and benefits due to cultural information are largely dependent on the environments in which the cultural information is deployed, and environments can include both natural and human-made environments, such as intergroup context. Cultural information with greater benefits than costs in a given configuration of environmental factors becomes more prevalent.

Cooperation, Assortment, and Punishment

Cooperation, construed as a cultural practice, can become culturally prevalent even in an environment where cooperation is more costly and less beneficial than noncooperation, if cooperative individuals have a better chance of interacting with other cooperative individuals (assortment), or if noncooperation is reliably punished (or cooperation rewarded).

Cooperation and a Variety of Collectivisms

Different types of collectivism (kin-based, attribute-based, or network-based) are configurations of cultural ideas and practices that increase assortment, and thus can coevolve with cooperation.

1. Kin-based collectivism can increase assortment by kinship.
2. Attribute-based collectivism can increase assortment by a shared attribute such as religion, ethnicity, and nationality.
3. Network-based collectivism can increase assortment by relational ties.

Mutual Constitution of Culture and Intergroup Context

Culture and intergroup context are mutually constitutive.

1. Intergroup context shapes cultural dynamics.
   a. Symbolic intergroup differentiation, intergroup competition and conflict, and the absence of institutions that mitigate intergroup conflict increase the likelihood of intergroup threats.
   b. Intergroup threats tend to increase cultural tightness and attribute-based collectivism.
   c. Intergroup threats in the absence of institutions that mitigate intergroup conflict tend to encourage honor culture.
   d. Cultural tightness tends to strengthen norms, including attribute-based collectivism and honor culture.

2. Culture shapes intergroup relationships.
   a. Attribute-based collectivism tends to strengthen symbolic intergroup differentiation.
   b. Attribute-based collectivism may produce ingroup favoritism, but may not necessarily exacerbate outgroup hostility in and of itself.
   c. In the context of intergroup competition or conflict, intragroup cultural dynamics tend to exacerbate not only ingroup favoritism but also outgroup derogation or aggression.
   d. Honor culture may amplify the possibility of intergroup aggression and potential downward spiral due to the positive feedback loop of aggression and retaliation.

Let us reiterate the interpretation of these principles here. We are making a claim that (1) given a certain intergroup context, certain cultural ideas and practices are likely to confer advantages (or reduce disadvantages) to the individuals and groups on the average and therefore are likely to be transmitted within and between generations, and selected *in* to be retained and become widely available, accessible, and applied in the population; and that (2) given that a certain set of cultural ideas and practices is available, accessible, and applied in concrete situations, certain intergroup relationships are likely to ensue. Item 1 is statements about adaptation in the sense explicated earlier in the chapter, and item 2 is meaning-based explanations of behavior as described in Kashima (2015). Both types of statements come with the usual *ceteris paribus* clause. Other things can include different types of environments for item 1, and different types of cultural elements for item 2. We explicate these caveats later.

Is there evidence for this type of analysis? There is some historical research that gives credence. Turchin, Currie, Turner, and Gavrilets (2013) have examined the formation and dissipation of large-scale human groups that have occupied large territories (e.g., empires) from 1500 B.C.E. to 1500 C.E. in the Afroeurasian landmass that includes Africa, Asia, and Europe. They constructed a mathematical model based on the contemporary theories of cultural evolution, simulated its prediction over the three millennia, and compared the model prediction and available historical evidence of human population dynamics. Their model includes, among other things, an assumption of conflictful intergroup context, especially between nomadic groups living in steppes and agrarians living in cultivated lands; inventions and diffusion of military technologies, such as chariots and cavalry; and institutions of governance and cooperative norms that can maintain intragroup cooperation. The model could account for 64% of the variance in imperial density, that is, the frequency with which a large territorial area (100 km × 100 km cell) was occupied by a large-scale group within a 100-year interval. To put it crudely, this research can be interpreted to show that the rise and fall of empires in different parts of Afroeurasia could be explained partly in terms of the interplay between conflictful intergroup context and culture with norms of intragroup cooperation and societal institutions that ensure cooperative transactions within a large territorial group.

Caveats

There are many caveats we need to address. First, as Turchin and colleagues (2013) noted, their theory about the rise and fall of great empires of the Afroeurasian past does not mean the same dynamics operated in other parts of the world, for instance, in the Americas. Potential regional variability needs to be examined in future research. In particular, some characteristics of the intergroup environment, such as the possibility of mobility between groups, also affect how cultural dynamics intersect with intergroup processes. For example, high levels of mobility thwart the evolution of ethnocentrism, and the possibility of intergroup conflict (see De, Gelfand, Nau, & Roos, 2015). Second, even though this analysis may have applied in the past, it does not have to apply in the future (e.g., Bowles, 2009). There are other historical forces and institutional arrangements that can alter the trajectory of culture–intergroup dynamics.

More importantly, not all cultural dynamics are aligned with intergroup processes. Although attribute-based collectivism, tightness, and culture of honor may be particularly aligned with intergroup processes, other types of cultural

ideas and practices may not necessarily follow the same trajectories. For instance, network-based collectivism provides a different path for partner selection in which one seeks to partner with another who shares mutual partners. In principle, network-based partner selection can create intergroup social tie. For instance, consider a scenario where there are groups A and B, and suppose that a is a member of A and b, a member of B. If a has a friend, who is also a friend of b, an attribute-based partner selection practice may discourage a from making friends with b; however, a network-based partner selection practice can encourage the formation of an a–b relationship. To put it differently, attribute-based partner selection practices exacerbate the social separation between groups, whereas network-based partner selection practices are orthogonal to intergroup separation and may even facilitate cross-group friendships, which tend to lessen negative intergroup relations (e.g., Davies, Tropp, Aron, Pettigrew, & Wright, 2011).

Concluding Comments: Challenges of the 21st Century

Without a doubt, recent human history has been shaped by the interplay between culture and intergroup relations. The 21st century began with the September 11 attacks in 2001, ostensibly an event of intergroup hostility across the boundaries marked by culture and religion. However, even before then, intergroup relations across cultural boundaries animated many of the notable geopolitical events and trends—the rise of China as a superpower, tensions in the Middle East, and a dramatic increase in refugees and displacements of peoples around the world. In the years so far in this century, intercultural–intergroup issues have continued to drive headline events around the globe—the resurgence of Russia, activities of ISIS, refugee crises originating in Syria and surrounding areas, as well as Rohingya in Myanmar, not to mention the threats and anxiety about nuclear arms confrontations.

There are two megatrends that can exacerbate these ongoing processes. One is climate change. In 2001, the same year as the September 11th attacks, the Intergovernmental Panel on Climate Change (2001) released its third assessment, warning the world of a potentially catastrophic climate change. There is some evidence to suggest deepening global warming could exacerbate aggression and civil unrest (e.g., Hsiang, Burke, & Miguel, 2013), raising the possibility that climate change may exacerbate intergroup conflict. The other is globalization. Increasing interconnectivity, exchange of goods, services, and information, and movements of people across national boundaries have not only enhanced the possibility of cultural transmission across the globe but also highlighted the cultural differences hitherto unnoticed or largely ignored. One potential consequence is a rise of attribute-based collectivism and tightness as cultural ideas and practices. Does this mean its special case, nation-state-based collectivism and tightness or what one may call nationalism, is on the rise? At one level, this may be so—witness Brexit and the 2016 U.S. presidential election. Leaders around the globe (Putin, Duterte, Erdogan, Trump) indeed appear to be using the principles of cultural dynamics to maintain their power: They exaggerate threat in order to tighten their own societies. But at another level, this is not so—witness failed (or fragile) states such as South Sudan and Somalia, increasing human movements across national borders, and increasing prominence of nonstate actors around the globe.

Given these global megatrends, there is an urgent need for an examination of the interplay between culture and intergroup relations. We need to be able to forecast where human cultures are likely to go and how intergroup relations develop, so that the citizens of the world can be better prepared. But it is increasingly important to understand and investigate how cultural dynamics can be harnessed. Interdisciplinary translational sciences for cultural dynamics seem critically needed for this purpose. What shape they may take is a question for the future.

ACKNOWLEDGMENTS

The preparation of this chapter was facilitated by grants from the Australian Research Council (DP160102226 and DP160102231) to Yoshihisa Kashima and a U.S. Air Force Grant (FA9550-14-1-0020) to Michele Gelfand.

NOTE

1. These mechanisms are typically called *strategies* in the evolutionary game theoretic parlance. It is an unfortunate naming because *strategy* implies a conscious, intentional action when such is not intended by the theorists. Instead we use the terms *ideas* and *practices*.

REFERENCES

Abbink, K., Brandts, J., Herrmann, B., & Orzen, H. (2012). Parochial altruism in inter-group conflicts. *Economics Letters, 117*(1), 45–48.

Atran, S., & Norenzayan, A. (2004). Religion's evolutionary landscape: Counterintuition, commitment, compassion, communion. *Behavioral and Brain Sciences, 27*(6), 713–770.

Axelrod, R. (1984). *The evolution of cooperation.* New York: Basic Books.

Balliet, D., Wu, J., & De Dreu, C. K. W. (2014). Ingroup favoritism in cooperation: A meta-analysis. *Psychological Bulletin, 140*(6), 1556–1581.

Bartlett, F. C. (1932). *Remembering: A study in experimental and social psychology.* Cambridge, UK: Cambridge University Press.

Baumard, N., Andre, J. B., & Sperber, D. (2013). A mutualistic approach to morality: The evolution of fairness by partner choice. *Behavioral and Brain Sciences, 36*(1), 59–78.

Bentley, R. A., Hahn, M. W., & Shennan, S. J. (2004). Random drift and culture change. *Proceedings of the Royal Society of London B: Biological Sciences, 271,* 1443–1450.

Bernhard, H., Fischbacher, U., & Fehr, E. (2006). Parochial altruism in humans. *Nature, 442*(7105), 912–915.

Bowles, S. (2009). Did warfare among ancestral hunter–gatherers affect the evolution of human social behaviors? *Science, 324,* 1293–1298.

Bowles, S. (2012). Warriors, levelers, and the role of conflict in human social evolution. *Science, 336,* 876–879.

Boyd, R., & Richerson, P. J. (1985). *Culture and the evolutionary process.* Chicago: University of Chicago Press.

Boyd, R., & Richerson, P. J. (1987). The evolution of ethnic markers. *Cultural Anthropology, 2*(1), 65–79.

Boyd, R., & Richerson, P. J. (1992). Punishment allows the evolution of cooperation (or anything else) in sizable groups. *Ethology and Sociobiology, 13*(3), 171–195.

Brewer, M. B. (1979). In-group bias in the minimal intergroup situation: A cognitive–motivational analysis. *Psychological Bulletin, 86*(2), 307–324.

Brewer, M. B., & Chen, Y. R. (2007). Where (who) are collectives in collectivism?: Toward conceptual clarification of individualism and collectivism. *Psychological Review, 114*(1), 133–151.

Brewer, M. B., & Yuki, M. (2007). Culture and social identity. In S. Kitayama & D. Cohen (Eds.), *Handbook of cultural psychology* (pp. 307–322). New York: Guilford Press.

Burnstein, E., Crandall, C., & Kitayama, S. (1994). Some neo-Darwinian decision rules for altruism: Weighing cues for inclusive fitness as a function of the biological importance of the decision. *Journal of Personality and Social Psychology, 67*(5), 773–789.

Campbell, D. T. (1982). Legal and primary-group social controls. In M. Gruter & P. Bohannan (Eds.), *Law, biology and culture: The evolution of law* (pp. 59–171). San Diego, CA: Ross-Erikson.

Cavalli-Sforza, L. L., & Feldman, M. W. (1981). *Cultural transmission and evolution.* Princeton, NJ: Princeton University Press.

Cheon, B. K., Christopoulos, G. I., & Hong, Y. Y. (2016). Disgust associated with culture mixing: Why and who? *Journal of Cross-Cultural Psychology, 47*(10), 1268–1285.

Chiu, C.-Y., & Cheng, S. Y. (2007). Toward a social psychology of culture and globalization: Some social cognitive consequences of activating two cultures simultaneously. *Social and Personality Psychology Compass, 1*(1), 84–100.

Chiu, C.-Y., & Hong, Y.-Y. (2013). *Social psychology of culture*: New York: Psychology Press.

Choi, J. K., & Bowles, S. (2007). The coevolution of parochial altruism and war. *Science, 318*(5850), 636–640.

Chua, R. Y., Roth, Y., & Lemoine, J.-F. (2015). The impact of culture on creativity: How cultural tightness and cultural distance affect global innovation crowdsourcing work. *Administrative Science Quarterly, 60*(2), 189–227.

Cialdini, R. B., & Goldstein, N. J. (2004). Social influence: Compliance and conformity. *Annual Review of Psychology, 55,* 591–621.

Claidiere, N., Scott-Phillips, T. C., & Sperber, D. (2014). How Darwinian is cultural evolution? *Philosophical Transactions of the Royal Society of London B: Biological Sciences, 369,* Article 20130368.

Cohen, D. (2001). Cultural variation: Considerations and implications. *Psychological Bulletin, 127*(4), 451–471.

Cohen, D., Nisbett, R. E., Bowdle, B. F., & Schwarz, N. (1996). Insult, aggression, and the southern culture of honor: An "experimental ethnography." *Journal of Personality and Social Psychology, 70*(5), 945–960.

Cohen, E., Atkinson, Q. D., Dediu, D., Dingemanse, M. D., Kinzler, K., Ladd, D. R., et al. (2012). The evolution of tag-based cooperation in humans: The case for accent. *Current Anthropology, 53*(5), 588–616.

Cross, S. E., Uskul, A. K., Gercek-Swing, B., Sunbay, Z., Alozkan, C., Gunsoy, C., et al. (2014). Cultural prototypes and dimensions of honor. *Personality and Social Psychology Bulletin, 40*(2), 232–249.

Cushman, F. (2015). Punishment in humans: From intuitions to institutions. *Philosophy Compass, 10*(2), 117–133.

Dar-Nimrod, I., & Heine, S. J. (2011). Genetic essentialism: On the deceptive determinism of DNA. *Psychological Bulletin, 137*(5), 800–818.

Darwin, C. (1888). *The descent of man and selection in relation to sex* (Vol. 1). London: John Murray.

Davies, K., Tropp, L. R., Aron, A., Pettigrew, T. F., & Wright, S. C. (2011). Cross-group friendships and intergroup attitudes: A meta-analytic review. *Personality and Social Psychology Review, 15*(4), 332–351.

Dawes, R. M. (1980). Social dilemmas. *Annual Review of Psychology, 31*(1), 169–193.

Dawkins, R. (1976). *The selfish gene.* Oxford, UK: Oxford University Press.

De, S., Gelfand, M. J., Nau, D., & Roos, P. (2015). The inevitability of ethnocentrism revisited: Ethnocentrism diminishes as mobility increases. *Scientific Reports, 5,* Article No. 17963.

De, S., Nau, D. S., & Gelfand, M. J. (2017). *Understanding norm change: An evolutionary game-theoretic approach.* Paper presented at the Proceedings of the 16th Conference on Autonomous Agents and MultiAgent Systems, São Paulo, Brazil.

De, S., Nau, D. S., Pan, X., & Gelfand, M. J. (2018). Tipping points for norm change in human cultures. In R. Thomson, C. Dancy, A. Hyder, & H. Bisgin (Eds.), *SBP-BRiMS 2018: Social, cultural, and behavioral modeling* (Vol. 10899, pp. 61–69). Washington, DC: Springer.

Dennett, D. C. (1996). *Darwin's dangerous idea: Evolution and the meaning of life.* London: Penguin Books.

Eshel, I., & Cavalli-Sforza, L. L. (1982). Assortment of encounters and evolution of cooperativeness. *Proceedings of the National Academy of Sciences USA, 79*(4), 1331–1335.

Fehr, E., & Fischbacher, U. (2004a). Social norms and human cooperation. *Trends in Cognitive Sciences, 8*(4), 185–190.

Fehr, E., & Fischbacher, U. (2004b). Third-party punishment and social norms. *Evolution and Human Behavior, 25*(2), 63–87.

Fincher, C. L., Thornhill, R., Murray, D. R., &

Schaller, M. (2008). Pathogen prevalence predicts human cross-cultural variability in individualism/collectivism. *Proceedings. Biological Sciences, 275*, 1279–1285.

Fu, F., Hauert, C., Nowak, M. A., & Wang, L. (2008). Reputation-based partner choice promotes cooperation in social networks. *Physical Review E, 78*(2), Article No. 026117.

García, J., & van den Bergh, J. C. (2011). Evolution of parochial altruism by multilevel selection. *Evolution and Human Behavior, 32*(4), 277–287.

Gelfand, M. J., Harrington, J. R., & Jackson, J. C. (2017). The strength of social norms across human groups. *Perspectives on Psychological Science, 12*(5), 800–809.

Gelfand, M. J., Raver, J. L., Nishii, L., Leslie, L. M., Lun, J., Lim, B. C., et al. (2011). Differences between tight and loose cultures: A 33-nation study. *Science, 332*, 1100–1104.

Giddens, A. (1990). *The consequences of modernity.* Stanford, CA: Stanford University Press.

Goldenberg, A., Cohen-Chen, S., Goyer, J. P., Dweck, C. S., Gross, J. J., & Halperin, E. (2018). Testing the impact and durability of a group malleability intervention in the context of the Israeli–Palestinian conflict. *Proceedings of the National Academy of Sciences of the USA, 115*(4), 696–701.

Gouldner, A. W. (1960). The norm of reciprocity: A preliminary statement. *American Sociological Review, 25*, 161–178.

Hamilton, W. D. (1964a). The genetical evolution of social behaviour. I. *Journal of Theoretical Biology, 7*(1), 1–16.

Hamilton, W. D. (1964b). The genetical evolution of social behaviour. II. *Journal of Theoretical Biology, 7*(1), 17–52.

Harrington, J. R., & Gelfand, M. J. (2014). Tightness-looseness across the 50 United States. *Proceedings of the National Academy of Sciences of the USA, 111*(22), 7990–7995.

Haslam, N., Bastian, B., Bain, P., & Kashima, Y. (2006). Psychological essentialism, implicit theories, and intergroup relations. *Group Processes and Intergroup Relations, 9*(1), 63–76.

Heider, F. (1958). *The psychology of interpersonal relations.* Hillsdale, NJ: Erlbaum.

Herrmann, B., Thöni, C., & & Gächter, S. (2008). Antisocial punishment across societies. *Science, 319*, 1362–1367.

Hsiang, S. M., Burke, M., & Miguel, E. (2013). Quantifying the influence of climate on human conflict. *Science, 341*, Article No. 1235367.

Intergovernmental Panel on Climate Change. (2001). Climate change 2001: Synthesis report. Retrieved from *www.ipcc.ch/ipccreports/tar/vol4/english.*

Jackson, J. C., van Egmond, M., Choi, V. K., Ember,

C. R., Halberstadt, J., Balanovic, J., et al. (2019). Ecological and cultural factors underlying the global distribution of prejudice. *PLOS ONE, 14*(9).

Kashima, Y. (2000a). Maintaining cultural stereotypes in the serial reproduction of narratives. *Personality and Social Psychology Bulletin, 26*(5), 594–604.

Kashima, Y. (2000b). Recovering Bartlett's social psychology of cultural dynamics. *European Journal of Social Psychology, 30*(3), 383–403.

Kashima, Y. (2015). Causal and meaning-based explanation. In B. Gawronski & G. V. Bodenhausen (Eds.), *Theory and explanation in social psychology* (pp. 41–62). New York: Guilford Press.

Kashima, Y. (2016). Cultural dynamics. *Current Opinion in Psychology, 8,* 93–97.

Kashima, Y. (2019). What is culture for? In D. Matsumoto (Ed.), *Handbook of culture and psychology* (2nd ed., pp. 123–160). New York: Oxford University Press.

Kashima, Y., Bain, P., & Perfors, A. (2019). The psychology of cultural dynamics: What is it, what is known, and what is yet to be known? *Annual Review of Psychology, 70*, 499–529.

Kashima, Y., Bratanova, B., & Peters, K. (2018). Social transmission and shared reality in cultural dynamics. *Current Opinion in Psychology, 23*, 15–19.

Kashima, Y., Peters, K., & Whelan, J. (2008). Culture, narrative, and human agency. In R. M. Sorrentino & S. Yamaguchi (Eds.), *Handbook of motivation and cognition across cultures* (pp. 393–421). San Diego, CA: Academic Press.

Kauffman, S. A. (1993). *The origins of order: Self-organization and selection in evolution.* New York: Oxford University Press.

Kimura, M., & Crow, J. F. (1964). The number of alleles that can be maintained in a finite population. *Genetics, 49*(4), 725–738.

Kiyonari, T., & Barclay, P. (2008). Cooperation in social dilemmas: Free riding may be thwarted by second-order reward rather than by punishment. *Journal of Personality and Social Psychology, 95*(4), 826–842.

Kurzban, R., Burton-Chellew, M. N., & West, S. A. (2015). The evolution of altruism in humans. *Annual Review of Psychology, 66*, 575–599.

Laham, S. M. (2009). Expanding the moral circle: Inclusion and exclusion mindsets and the circle of moral regard. *Journal of Experimental Social Psychology, 45*(1), 250–253.

Laland, K. N., Odling-Smee, J. F., & Feldman, M. W. (2000). Niche construction, biological evolution, and cultural change. *Behavioral and Brain Sciences, 23*(1), 131–146.

Langergraber, K., Schubert, G., Rowney, C., Wrangham, R., Zommers, Z., & Vigilant, L. (2011). Genetic differentiation and the evolution of cooperation in chimpanzees and humans. *Proceedings of the Royal Society of London B: Biological Sciences, 278,* 2546–2552.

Lee, T. L., Gelfand, M. J., & Kashima, Y. (2014). The serial reproduction of conflict: Third parties escalate conflict through communication biases. *Journal of Experimental Social Psychology, 54*(1), 68–72.

Leung, A. K.-Y., Maddux, W. W., Galinsky, A. D., & Chiu, C. Y. (2008). Multicultural experience enhances creativity: The when and how. *American Psychologist, 63*(3), 169–181.

Lewens, T. (2015). *Cultural evolution.* Oxford, UK: Oxford University Press.

McElreath, R., Boyd, R., & Richerson, P. (2003). Shared norms and the evolution of ethnic markers. *Current Anthropology, 44*(1), 122–130.

Medin, D. L., & Ortony, A. (1989). Psychological essentialism. In S. Vosniadou & A. Ortony (Eds.), *Similarity and anlogical reasoning* (pp. 179–195). New York: Cambridge University Press.

Mesoudi, A. (2011). *Cultural evolution: How Darwinian theory can explain human culture and synthesize the social sciences.* Chicago: University of Chicago Press.

Miton, H., Claidière, N., & Mercier, H. (2015). Universal cognitive mechanisms explain the cultural success of bloodletting. *Evolution and Human Behavior, 36*(4), 303–312.

Morris, M. W., Chiu, C. Y., & Liu, Z. (2015). Polycultural psychology. *Annual Review of Psychology, 66,* 631–659.

Mrazek, A. J., Chiao, J. Y., Blizinsky, K. D., Lun, J., & Gelfand, M. J. (2013). The role of culture–gene coevolution in morality judgment: Examining the interplay between tightness–looseness and allelic variation of the serotonin transporter gene. *Culture and Brain, 1*(2–4), 100–117.

Mu, Y., Han, S., & Gelfand, M. J. (2017). The role of gamma interbrain synchrony in social coordination when humans face territorial threats. *Social Cognitive and Affective Neuroscience, 12*(10), 1614–1623.

Mu, Y., Kitayama, S., Han, S., & Gelfand, M. J. (2015). How culture gets embrained: Cultural differences in event-related potentials of social norm violations. *Proceedings of the National Academy of Sciences of the USA, 112*(50), 15348–15353.

Nikiforakis, N. (2008). Punishment and counter-punishment in public good games: Can we really govern ourselves? *Journal of Public Economics, 92*(1–2), 91–112.

Nisbett, R. E., & Cohen, D. (1996). *Culture of honor: The psychology of violence in the south.* Boulder, CO: Westview Press.

Norenzayan, A., Shariff, A. F., Gervais, W. M., Willard, A. K., McNamara, R. A., Slingerland, E., et al. (2016). The cultural evolution of prosocial religions. *Behavioral and Brain Sciences, 39,* 1–19.

Nowak, A., Gelfand, M. J., Borkowski, W., Cohen, D., & Hernandez, I. (2016). The evolutionary basis of honor cultures. *Psychological Science, 27*(1), 12–24.

Nowak, M. A. (2006a). *Evolutionary dynamics: Exploring the equations of life.* Cambridge, MA: Harvard University Press.

Nowak, M. A. (2006b). Five rules for the evolution of cooperation. *Science, 314,* 1560–1563.

Nowak, M. A., & Sigmund, K. (1998). Evolution of indirect reciprocity by image scoring. *Nature, 393*(6685), 573–577.

O'Dwyer, J. P., & Kandler, A. (2017). Inferring processes of cultural transmission: The critical role of rare variants in distinguishing neutrality from novelty biases. *Philosophical Transactions of the Royal Society of London B: Biological Sciences, 372,* Article No. 20160426.

Ohtsuki, H., Hauert, C., Lieberman, E., & Nowak, M. A. (2006). A simple rule for the evolution of cooperation on graphs and social networks. *Nature, 441,* 502–505.

Oishi, S. (2014). Socioecological psychology. *Annual Review of Psychology, 65,* 581–609.

Okasha, S. (2006). *Evolution and the levels of selection*: Oxford, UK: Oxford University Press.

Olson, M. (1965). *The logic of collective action: Public goods and the theory of groups.* Boston: Harvard University Press.

Ostrom, E. (2015). *Governing the commons.* Cambridge, UK: Cambridge University Press.

Panchanathan, K., & Boyd, R. (2004). Indirect reciprocity can stabilize cooperation without the second-order free rider problem. *Nature, 432,* 499–502.

Pelto, P. J. (1968). The differences between "tight" and "loose" societies. *Transaction, 5*(5), 37–40.

Peters, K., & Kashima, Y. (2007). From social talk to social action: Shaping the social triad with emotion sharing. *Journal of Personality and Social Psychology, 93*(5), 780–797.

Purzycki, B. G., Apicella, C., Atkinson, Q. D., Cohen, E., McNamara, R. A., Willard, A. K., et al. (2016). Moralistic gods, supernatural punishment and the expansion of human sociality. *Nature, 530,* 327–330.

Rand, D. G., & Nowak, M. A. (2011). The evolution of antisocial punishment in optional public goods games. *Nature Communications, 2,* Article No. 434.

Realo, A., Allik, J., & Greenfield, B. (2008). Radius of trust: Social capital in relation to familism and institutional collectivism. *Journal of Cross-Cultural Psychology, 39*(4), 447–462.

Richerson, P. J., Baldini, R., Bell, A. V., Demps, K., Frost, K., Hillis, V., et al. (2016). Cultural group selection plays an essential role in explaining human cooperation: A sketch of the evidence. *Behavioral and Brain Sciences, 39,* Article No. e30.

Richerson, P. J., & Boyd, R. (1998). The evolution of human ultrasociality. In I. Eibl-Eibisfeldt & F. Salter (Eds.), *Indoctrinability, ideology, and warfare* (pp. 71–95). New York: Berghahn Books.

Richerson, P. J., & Boyd, R. (2005). *Not by genes alone: How culture transformed human evolution.* Chicago: University of Chicago Press.

Riolo, R. L., Cohen, M., & Axelrod, R. (2001). Evolution of cooperation without reciprocity. *Nature, 414,* 441–443.

Roes, F. L., & Raymond, M. (2003). Belief in moralizing gods. *Evolution and Human Behavior, 24*(2), 126–135.

Roos, P., Gelfand, M., Nau, D., & Carr, R. (2014). High strength-of-ties and low mobility enable the evolution of third-party punishment. *Proceedings of the Royal Society of London B: Biological Sciences, 281,* Article No. 20132661.

Roos, P., Gelfand, M., Nau, D., & Lun, J. (2015). Societal threat and cultural variation in the strength of social norms: An evolutionary basis. *Organizational Behavior and Human Decision Processes, 129,* 14–23.

Rothstein, B., & Stolle, D. (2008). The state and social capital: An institutional theory of generalized trust. *Comparative Politics, 40*(4), 441–459.

Rusch, H. (2014). The evolutionary interplay of intergroup conflict and altruism in humans: A review of parochial altruism theory and prospects for its extension. *Proceedings of the Royal Society of London B: Biological Sciences, 281,* Article No. 20141539.

Segall, M. H., Campbell, D. T., & Herskovits, M. J. (1966). *The influence of culture on visual perception.* Indianapolis, IN: Bobbs-Merrill.

Sherif, M., Harvey, O. J., Hood, W. R., Sherif, C. W., & White, J. (1988). *The Robbers Cave experiment: Intergroup conflict and cooperation.* Middletown, CT: Wesleyan University Press.

Sherif, M., Harvey, O., White, B. J., Hood, W. R., & Sherif, C. W. (1961). *Intergroup cooperation and competition: The Robbers Cave experiment.* Norman, OK: University Book Exchange.

Sigmund, K. (2007). Punish or perish?: Retaliation and collaboration among humans. *Trends in Ecology and Evolution, 22*(11), 593–600.

Sigmund, K., De Silva, H., Traulsen, A., & Hauert, C. (2010). Social learning promotes institutions for governing the commons. *Nature, 466,* 861–863.

Sigmund, K., Hauert, C., & Nowak, M. A. (2001). Reward and punishment. *Proceedings of the National Academy of Sciences of the USA, 98*(19), 10757–10762.

Simonton, D. K. (2011). Creativity and discovery as blind variation: Campbell's (1960) BVSR model after the half-century mark. *Review of General Psychology, 15*(2), 158–174.

Singer, P. (1981). *The expanding circle.* Oxford, UK: Clarendon.

Skinner, B. F. (1981). Selection by consequences. *Science, 213,* 501–504.

Soltis, J., Boyd, R., & Richerson, P. J. (1995). Can group-functional behaviors evolve by cultural group selection?: An empirical test. *Current Anthropology, 36*(3), 473–494.

Sommerfeld, R. D., Krambeck, H. J., Semmann, D., & Milinski, M. (2007). Gossip as an alternative for direct observation in games of indirect reciprocity. *Proceedings of the National Academy of Sciences of the USA, 104*(44), 17435–17440.

Sosis, R., & Alcorta, C. (2003). Signaling, solidarity, and the sacred: The evolution of religious behavior. *Evolutionary Anthropology, 12*(6), 264–274.

Sperber, D. (1996). *Explaining culture: A naturalistic approach.* Oxford, UK: Blackwell.

Tabellini, G. (2008). Institutions and culture. *Journal of the European Economic Association, 6*(2–3), 255–294.

Tajfel, H. (1982). Social psychology of intergroup relations. *Annual Review of Psychology, 33*(1), 1–39.

Tajfel, H., & Turner, J. C. (1979). The social identity theory of intergroup behavior. In S. Worchel & L. W. Austin (Eds.), *Psychology of intergroup relations* (pp. 149–163). Chicago: Nelson-Hall.

Taylor, C., & Nowak, M. A. (2007). Transforming the dilemma. *Evolution, 61*(10), 2281–2292.

Taylor, D. M., & Moghaddam, F. M. (1994). *Theories of intergroup relations: International social psychological perspectives.* Westport, CT: Greenwood.

Thorndike, E. L. (1927). The law of effect. *American Journal of Psychology, 39*(1/4), 212–222.

Tomasello, M., Kruger, A. C., & Ratner, H. H. (1993). Cultural learning. *Behavioral and Brain Sciences, 16,* 495–511.

Traulsen, A., Rohl, T., & Milinski, M. (2012). An economic experiment reveals that humans prefer pool punishment to maintain the commons. *Proceedings of the Royal Society of London B: Biological Sciences, 279,* 3716–3721.

Tria, F., Loreto, V., Servedio, V. D. P., & Strogatz, S. H. (2014). The dynamics of correlated novelties. *Science Reports, 4,* Article No. 5890.

Triandis, H. C. (1995). *Individualism and collectivism.* Boulder, CO: Westview Press.

Trivers, R. L. (1971). The evolution of reciprocal altruism. *Quarterly Review of Biology, 46*(1), 35–57.

Turchin, P. (2013). The puzzle of human ultrasociality. In P. J. Richerson & M. H. Christiansen (Eds.), *Cultural evolution: Society, technology, language, and religion* (pp. 61–73). Cambridge, MA: MIT Press.

Turchin, P., Currie, T. E., Turner, E. A., & Gavrilets, S. (2013). War, space, and the evolution of Old World complex societies. *Proceedings of the National Academy of Sciences of the USA, 110*(41), 16384–16389.

Turner, J. C. (1987). *Rediscovering the social group.* Oxford, UK: Blackwell.

Turner, V. (1969). *The ritual process.* London: Routledge.

Van de Vliert, E. (2013). Climato-economic habitats support patterns of human needs, stresses, and freedoms. *Behavioral and Brain Sciences, 36*(5), 465–480.

Van Lange, P. A., Rinderu, M. I., & Bushman, B. J. (2017). Aggression and violence around the world: A model of climate, aggression, and self-control in humans (CLASH). *Behavioral and Brain Sciences, 40,* Article No. e75.

West, S. A., Griffin, A. S., & Gardner, A. (2007). Evolutionary explanations for cooperation. *Current Biology, 17*(16), R661–672.

Williams, K. D. (2007). Ostracism. *Annual Review of Psychology, 58,* 425–452.

Wrangham, R. W., Wilson, M. L., & Muller, M. N. (2006). Comparative rates of violence in chimpanzees and humans. *Primates, 47*(1), 14–26.

Yamagishi, T. (1986). The provision of a sanctioning system as a public good. *Journal of Personality and Social Psychology, 51*(1), 110–116.

Yamagishi, T. (2011). Micro-macro dynamics of the cultural construction of reality: A niche construction approach to culture. In M. J. Gelfand, C.-Y. Chiu, & Y.-Y. Hong (Eds.), *Advances in culture psychology* (Vol. 1, pp. 251–308). New York: Oxford University Press.

Ye, J. W., & Ng, S. H. (2017). An intermediary enhances out-group trust and in-group profit expectation of Chinese but not Australians. *International Journal of Psychology, 52*(3), 189–196.

Yuki, M., Maddux, W. W., Brewer, M. B., & Takemura, K. (2005). Cross-cultural differences in relationship-and group-based trust. *Personality and Social Psychology Bulletin, 31*(1), 48–62.

PART II

PRINCIPLES IN CONTEXT

CHAPTER 25

Helping, in Context

Predictors and Products of Prosocial Behavior

Lara B. Aknin
Deborah A. Small
Michael I. Norton

Although humans are capable of extraordinary acts of altruism when faced with people in need, it is also the case that they often attempt to shirk that duty. Indeed, perhaps the most classic research investigating altruism in social psychology—Darley and Latane's (1968) exploration of bystander intervention—focuses on how the presence of others leads to diffusion of responsibility, and, often, the failure of anyone offering to help. Even without others to take the blame, however, people are often skilled at avoiding altruism, both in actions and in rationalizations. For example, Andreoni, Rao, and Trachtman (2017) placed Salvation Army bell ringers at either one or both entrances to a supermarket, making it either easy or difficult to "avoid the ask." While making avoidance difficult did increase donations, it was also the case that many people chose to avoid the bell ringers altogether by entering through the unmanned door. Similarly, when faced with a decision either to split $10 with another participant, or simply take $9 instead (and leave the other person with $0), fully one-third of participants took the $9—provided that the recipient would never know about that choice (Dana, Cain, & Dawes, 2006).

People also go to great lengths to convince themselves that their selfish behavior is in fact fair and egalitarian (see Gino, Norton, & Weber, 2016). For instance, Batson, Kobrynowicz, Dinnerstein, Kampf, and Wilson (1997) asked participants in a laboratory experiment to distribute two tasks between themselves and another participant: a positive task (earning tickets to a raffle) and a negative task (described as "dull and boring"). Half of participants simply assigned the tasks, with some 90% giving themselves the positive task; more interestingly, half of participants decided to flip a coin to make the decision—except that 90% of these participants also won the positive task (despite the probability being 50/50). More disturbingly, although the latter group had in the end behaved as selfishly as the former group, flipping the coin led them to rate their actions as more moral. Most disturbingly, this pattern of hypocrisy appears to have a developmental trend: In one study of children ages 6–11, there was no developmental trend in how often children assigned themselves the positive task, but there was a developmental trend for hypocrisy, with older children far more likely to flip the coin than younger children (Shaw et al. 2014).

Given these barriers—both structural and psychological—it is not surprising that a large body of research attempts to explore when and why people actually choose to help. Below, we review research elucidating three basic principles of giving. The first principle suggests that consideration of the emotional reactions of would-be helpers is critical; we document how a wide range of emotions (both positive and negative) play a role both in producing giving and in shaping the experience of donors after having given. We also suggest that consideration of the social consequences of helping is critical, resulting in two different principles. The second principle centers on the importance of the human desire to connect with others—with not only recipients of help but also other donors. The third principle centers on the human desire to stand out from others, such as when gaining status and positive reputational benefits from prosocial behavior. When possible, we also note field experiments and other interventions that have leveraged these insights to increase giving. We then discuss how these principles that promote giving—emotional and social—also determine postgiving outcomes not for recipients of aid, but for donors themselves, with a focus on how the aftermath of giving is likely to influence people's proclivities to give again.

Emotional Predictors of Giving

As suggested by our first principle of giving, one key motivator of prosocial behavior documented in the literature is emotion (Aknin, Van de Vondervoort, & Hamlin, 2018). People's likelihood of providing assistance to others is influenced by their experience of both positive and negative emotional states. Below we survey the evidence linking a range of emotions with increased prosociality.

Generalized Positive Affect and Well-Being

Numerous correlational studies demonstrate a positive relationship between well-being and prosocial behavior. For instance, when Meier and Stutzer (2004) analyzed responses from approximately 22,000 German respondents collected from 1985 until 1999 as part of the German Socio-Economic Panel (GSOEP), they found that those who engaged in more frequent volunteer work also reported higher levels of life satisfaction. Importantly, this positive association held when controlling for a number of relevant variables, such as household income, age, gender, marital status, and education, suggesting that these individual differences are not responsible for the link between well-being and volunteer work. Beyond Germany, a similar pattern of results has been documented in other countries and distinct communities. For example, volunteering has been associated with greater happiness among Māori and non-Māori populations in New Zealand (Dulin, Gavala, Stephens, Kostick, & McDonald, 2012), and among 29 states in the United States (Borgonovi, 2008; see also Musick & Wilson, 2003; Thoits & Hewitt, 2001; Wheeler, Gorey, & Greenblatt, 1998; Whiteley, 2004). Critically, longitudinal evidence indicates that happiness and life satisfaction reported at initial surveys predict volunteer work at a later date. Indeed, Thoits and Hewitt (2001), who analyzed data from over 2,600 respondents in the America Changing Lives survey, found that individuals who were happier, who reported greater life satisfaction and lower depression at an initial survey, reported volunteering significantly more hours when surveyed 3 years later.

Moreover, experimental evidence indicates that positive affect and well-being have a causal impact on prosocial behavior. For instance, classic research (Isen, 1970) has demonstrated that individuals informed of their recent success (vs. failure) in a laboratory task, which presumably boosted their current mood, provided more money to charity and, in separate studies, were more likely to provide assistance to a confederate. Similar results have been observed in field experiments. Participants randomly assigned to receive a positive surprise—a gift of cookies or a dime in a pay phone—were subsequently more likely to provide help to a research assistant and spontaneously pick up fallen objects for a stranger in a mall (Isen & Levin, 1972). Finally, a number of additional experiments using more direct mood manipulations, such as those in which participants were asked to read positive statements, list positive thoughts, or imagine a dream vacation, yielded similar findings on a dependent variables, including blood donation, charitable giving, and interpersonal assistance (Aderman, 1972; O'Malley & Andrews, 1983; Rosenhan, Underwood, & Moore, 1974).

Other Positive Emotions: Awe, Elevation, Empathy, and Gratitude

In addition to positive affect and general well-being, several other positive emotional states have been shown to increase prosocial behavior. One example is *awe,* an emotion that people typically experience when they encounter vast perceptual stimuli, such as enormous fjords or craters. Because such stimuli may lead onlookers to feel small by comparison, awe has been proposed to reduce self-focused concerns and inspire prosocial behavior (Piff, Dietze, Feinberg, Stancato, & Keltner, 2015). Consistent with this logic, individuals who report a higher tendency to experience awe also demonstrate more prosocial behavior in economic games. In addition, participants randomly assigned to watch an awe-inducing nature film were more generous—giving more entries in a raffle ticket draw for $100 to an anonymous, unpaid partner—than participants assigned to watch an amusing nature film or a neutral film.

Elevation, another positive emotion shown to increase prosocial behavior, is defined as an emotion that one experiences when observing another person commit a kind or virtuous act on behalf of another (Algoe & Haidt, 2009; Haidt, 2003; Keltner & Haidt, 2003). Research has shown that elevation has a causal impact on prosociality. Participants randomly assigned to watch a short elevation-inducing video clip (vs. a neutral or humorous clip) reported higher levels of elevation afterward and were more likely to provide assistance on an optional, unpaid, and boring task (Schnall, Roper, & Fessler, 2010). In more intimate relationships, such as mother–infant dyads, elevation has been shown to increase several forms of maternal care. For instance, mothers randomly assigned to watch a short elevation-inducing clip (vs. a humorous clip) were more likely to nurse and hug their infant within several minutes of viewing (Silvers & Haidt, 2008).

A vast body of work has also shown that *empathy*—the tendency or ability to understand, share, and experience the emotions of others (Decety & Jackson, 2004; Zaki & Cikara, 2015)—increases prosociality. For instance, individual differences in trait empathy predict higher engagement in various forms of prosocial behavior, such as helping a teacher, sharing food, and comforting others (see Eisenberg & Miller, 1987, for review). Moreover, classic experiments indicate that individuals randomly assigned to high-empathy conditions, such as those presented with a high-need (vs. low-need) target, are more likely to provide help or assistance (Batson et al., 1991; Batson, Duncan, Ackerman, Buckley, & Birch, 1981; Toi & Batson, 1982). While some models argue that empathy can occur in a variety of contexts, such as when a target's emotion is salient, when the target is familiar, or when the observer has experience with the situation (Preston & de Waal, 2002), other accounts suggest that empathy is motivated and selective because it serves to build and maintain social bonds with individuals who are most likely to impact our safety and procreation (Anderson & Keltner, 2002; Zaki, 2014; Zaki & Cikara, 2015). Consistent with this logic, recent studies show human empathy is not always equitable and generous, more frequently directing aid to singular, similar, and attractive targets (Bloom, 2016; Slovic, Västfjäll, Erlandsson & Gregory, 2017; Zaki, 2014).

Finally, being grateful for the help we receive from others—experiencing *gratitude*—can boost prosocial action. For instance, in one experiment, participants were randomly assigned to either interact with a confederate or receive assistance from the same person. Those who received help reported more gratitude, which, in turn, predicted higher levels of aid directed to the helper and an unknown stranger (Bartlett & DeSteno, 2006; DeSteno, Bartlett, Baumann, Williams, & Dickens, 2010).

Negative States and Emotions

In addition to the well-documented relationship between various positive emotional states and prosociality, another line of research suggests that some negative emotions may also spur helping. The most well-known research conducted on the topic is that testing the negative state relief hypothesis (Baumann, Cialdini, & Kenrick, 1981; Cialdini & Kenrick, 1976), which proposes that some seemingly selfless acts of prosocial behavior, such as those mo-tivated by high levels of empathy for a needy target, may actually more accurately reflect a selfish desire to reduce one's personal sadness after seeing someone in peril. Supporting this proposition, Cialdini and colleagues (1987) found that individuals expressing higher levels of personal sadness, but not empathy, predicted help for a victim, and that participants led to be-lieve they could alleviate their sadness by tak-ing a drug (as opposed to helping) were inclined to do so. As such, these findings suggest that personal distress or sadness may also motivate prosociality as a means of improving one's per-sonal emotional state.

Social Predictors of Giving

In addition to emotional triggers for giving, a large body of research documents the power of the social context for prompting giving.

One key predictor of prosociality—suggested by our second principle of giving—is the pres-ence of a marked connection with the recipient(s) of aid (see Small, 2011, 2015). This connection can arise for a variety of reasons. First, people connect more with a specific target than with an abstract target, a phenomenon called the *iden-tifiable victim effect* (Schelling, 1968; Small & Loewenstein, 2003; Small, Loewenstein, & Slovic, 2007). Whereas it is difficult and un-natural to feel a connection to an abstract cause (e.g., poverty, cancer), it is comparatively more natural to connect to a specific case of a malady. The identifiable victim effect is even more pro-nounced when the identified recipient is a single individual compared to many identified individ-uals (Kogut & Ritov, 2005) but nonetheless per-sists for groups or other entities that comprise a defined unit (e.g., a single village; Smith, Faro, & Burson, 2013).

Beyond the identifiable victim effect, people feel stronger connections to recipients when they share a group identity—even minimally. Causal evidence for the effects of similarity on prosocial behavior comes from studies that use a minimal group paradigm, wherein a mere label that identifies people as members of dif-ferent inconsequential groups affects people's likelihood of helping another (Dovidio et al., 1997). Furthermore, in field data from the on-line micro-lending platform, Kiva.org, people tend to choose recipients who match themselves in terms of gender and occupation (Galak, Small, & Stephen, 2011).

Finally, personal experiences with misfortu-nate, such as experiencing a hurricane or hav-ing a loved one suffer from particular disease also fosters a sense of connection to others who suffer from that same misfortune (Small & Simonsohn, 2008). For example, family and friends of breast cancer victims are more likely to support breast cancer causes than are others without a history of personal experience. Impor-tantly, this personal experience does *not* extend to victims of other misfortunes. In other words, family and friends of breast cancer victims are no more generous toward victims or heart dis-ease, which supports the notion that the effect of personal experience on prosociality is through creating a connection between potential help-ers and recipients. Just as a person might feel a similarity and connection to a person who shares the same zip code or occupation, he or she might feel a greater similarity and connec-tion to a person whose experience is relatable.

Why does a personal connection drive pro-sociality? As a general principle, capturing at-tention and engagement serves as a precursor to creating an emotional response—suggesting a link between our first and second principles of giving. Seminal research on vividness high-lights how concrete and vivid targets evoke a stronger emotional reaction than do pallid, ab-stract targets (Nisbett & Ross, 1980; Piavio, 1969). So when a news article reports a tear-jerking personal story of a needy child, people attend to it, connect with it, and feel. (As we discussed earlier, such emotional reactions and empathy are often powerful triggers for proso-cial behavior.)

A field experiment by Grant and colleagues (2007) suggests the power of personal connec-tion in promoting prosocial behavior. In the ex-periment, some employees at a university's call center who were tasked with calling potential donors to the school received an unexpected visit: scholarship students who had benefited from the school's fundraising. Other call center employees did not receive this visit. This brief intervention—connecting people with the bene-ficiaries of their prosocial behavior—motivated employees to spend more time calling, resulting in increased donations from alumni.

Moreover, another field experiment suggests that the desire for social connection can prompt giving even when that connection is not with the recipients of charitable behavior, but with others engaged in that behavior. In Anik, Norton, and Ariely (2014), people who encountered an opportunity to commit to a recurring donation were more likely to donate when told that if, and only if, 75% of people committed to engage in charitable donations would matching funds kick in. Why? In part, because they felt a sense of responsibility to donors who had already given—and who might be disappointed if the 75% threshold was not reached.

The fact that observability—the possibility that others learn about or see your behavior—is a powerful predictor of prosociality offers support for our third principle of giving regarding the social benefits of prosocial behavior. Observable actions influence the actor's reputation and how likely others are to interact and cooperate with him or her in the future (Gintis, Smith, & Bowles, 2001; Glazer & Konrad, 1996). As a result, people are more likely to contribute to public goods (i.e., vote, donate blood, give to charity) when others are or may become aware (Bandiera, Barankay, & Rasul, 2005; Gerber, Green, & Larimer, 2008; Lacetera & Macis, 2010). For instance, in a relatively recent large-scale field experiment conducted with over 770,000 people, Americans were significantly more likely to vote in an upcoming election when their reminder letter stated, "We may call you after the election to ask about your voting experience" than when this statement was absent (Rogers, Ternovski, & Yoeli, 2016). These findings suggest that harnessing the human sensitivity for social connection can promote prosociality.

Emotional Consequences of Giving

Our first principle of giving holds that emotions serve as both predictors and products of giving. As noted earlier, a large body of correlational research has demonstrated a link between various forms of prosocial behavior, such as donating one's time or money, and well-being. While numerous studies reveal that greater well-being promotes prosociality, the well-being and generosity relationship is bidirectional, with a number of experiments demonstrating the causal impact of prosociality on happiness (see Curry et al., 2018, for a meta-analysis). For instance, Lyubomirsky, Sheldon, and Schkade (2005) found that participants randomly assigned to engage in five acts of kindness in a single day each week for 6 weeks reported higher subjective well-being relative to a control group that did not engage in prosocial behavior. More recently, Nelson, Layous, Cole, and Lyubomirsky (2016) reported that participants randomly assigned to one of two prosocial conditions, completing kind acts for other people or for the world, reported greater positive emotions and decreased negative emotions over a 6-week span than individuals randomly assigned to do a nice thing for themselves or simply keep track of their daily activities. Using a weeklong online compassion intervention, Mongrain, Chin, and Shapira (2011) found that helping others led to larger happiness gains over a 6-month period than completing a neutral task (see also Chancellor, Jacobs Bao, & Lyubomirsky, 2018; Pressman, Kraft, & Cross, 2015; but see Whillans, Seider, et al., 2016). Indeed, researchers have extended investigation of the potential benefits of prosociality to socially anxious individuals and report consistent findings. Specifically, Alden and Trew (2013) found that socially anxious students randomly assigned to complete three kind acts a day, 2 days a week for 4 weeks, reported higher levels of positive affect in comparison to socially anxious students assigned to a negative affect reduction or neutral control group.

Along similar lines, using one's financial resources to help others, called *prosocial spending,* is associated with and leads to higher well-being. For instance, data from a nationally representative sample of Americans indicate that people who spend more money on others in an average month through gift giving and charitable donations report greater happiness, but spending more on oneself through higher expenses and self-directed gifts does not (Dunn, Aknin, & Norton, 2008). Experimental studies provide converging causal evidence: Students randomly assigned to spend a windfall of either $5 or $20 on themselves or someone else by the end of the day were happier when directed to spend the money on others, regardless of whether they spent the smaller or the larger sum (Dunn et al., 2008; see also Geenen, Hohelüchter, Langhoff, & Walther, 2014). Importantly, the emotional rewards of prosocial spending have been detected in a recent high-powered, pre-registered replication (Aknin, Dunn, Proulx, Lok, & Norton, 2020) that adopts the field's highest standards for evidentiary value.

Evidence for the hedonic rewards of prosocial behavior is not limited to North American college students but has been observed in a variety of contexts. For instance, responses from over 230,000 individuals in 136 countries contacted as part of the Gallup World Poll indicate that those who have donated money to charity within the past month also tend to report higher levels of life satisfaction than those who have not donated (Aknin, Barrington-Leigh, et al., 2013). Moreover, students and adults from relatively rich and poor nations experience greater happiness after spending money on others or recalling a prosocial spending experience than do those assigned to spend on themselves or recall a previous instance of self-directed spending. Findings have even been replicated in small-scale traditional societies (Aknin, Broesch, Hamlin, & Van de Vondervoort, 2015), among criminal ex-offenders reporting elevated levels of antisocial and psychopathic tendencies (Hanniball, Aknin, Douglas, & Viljoen, 2019), and among children under the age of two (Aknin, Hamlin, & Dunn, 2012). Indeed, toddlers display significantly larger smiles when giving an edible treat away than when receiving an identical treat themselves (Aknin, Hamlin, & Dunn, 2012). Other forms of generous action appear to boost well-being outside of North America as well. Students in both the United States and South Korea displayed well-being gains from engaging in acts of kindness relative to a neutral control activity (Layous, Choi, Lee, & Lyubomirsky, 2013).

When is prosociality most likely to promote well-being? Four key factors have been identified. First, and in line with our second principle of giving, prosocial behavior yields the greatest emotional rewards when it facilitates social connection (Dunn, Aknin, & Norton,

2014). Humans are an extremely social species, and past research demonstrates that social relationships are some of the most important and robust predictors of happiness (Baumeister & Leary, 1995; Diener & Seligman, 2002; Lyubomirsky, King, & Diener, 2005). As such, acts that facilitate or strengthen social bonds should promote well-being, and prosocial behavior is no exception. For instance, individuals randomly assigned to spend a $10 gift card by the end of the day were happiest when they were assigned to spend the gift card on someone else in a way that required them to spend time with the recipient, rather than simply give the gift card away (Aknin, Dunn, Sandstrom, & Norton, 2013). Moreover, social connection may also explain why giving items that are closely tied to oneself, such as a previously owned item or blood, leads to greater commitment and subsequent generosity than giving gifts with minimized personal connection (Koo & Fischbach, 2016).

Prosocial action is also more likely to promote happiness when motivated by other-focused as opposed to self-focused concerns. Supporting this claim, correlational data indicate that volunteering predicts lower risk of mortality risk in older adults, but only when volunteering is motivated by other-oriented (as opposed to self-oriented) motives (Konrath, Fuhrel-Forbis, Lou, & Brown, 2012). Experimental evidence provides converging results. A series of studies indicates that participants randomly assigned to recall engaging in various forms of helping behavior reported higher positive emotions when their prosocial acts were motivated by concern for others as opposed to self-benefit (Wiwad & Aknin, 2017). This may be why introducing opportunity for self-benefit undermines the emotional rewards of giving. Indeed, Wang and Tong (2015) found that people report greater happiness after making private (as opposed to public) donations, potentially because public donations are more likely to be motivated by self-focused concerns.

Two final factors that make the benefits of giving more likely are volition and impact. When people feel that their kind behavior was strongly shaped by others or external forces, prosocial action does not predict happiness (Weinstein & Ryan, 2010). Indeed, Weinstein and Ryan found that students who provided larger donations to others reported greater happiness, but only when donation amounts were freely chosen; participants required to give preset donation amounts were no happier giving larger (vs. smaller) amounts, presumably because they did not experience a sense of free choice or self-determination. This is why most prosocial spending studies inject a sense of volition by allowing participants to choose what they buy and, more critically, whether they would like to abstain from completing a prosocial act. While participants rarely decline the opportunity to spend money on others, the ability to opt out can provide an illusion of volition, which is important for experiencing the emotional rewards of giving.

Finally, knowing that you have made a positive difference in the life of others also enhances the well-being benefits of giving. Simply put, when donors are provided with information explaining how their contribution will be used to help those in need, larger donations predict greater well-being (Aknin, Dunn, Whillans, Grant, & Norton, 2013). Importantly, however, when information about the impact of one's gift is absent, larger donations do not translate into larger emotional rewards (Aknin, Dunn, Whillans, et al., 2013). Knowing this, grateful recipients and charitable organizations may be well advised to explicate how the gifts they have received provide a direct benefit to a target in need.

In addition to boosting the giver's happiness, prosocial action may promote the giver's health as well. A number of investigations with diverse samples of community-dwelling adults demonstrate that individuals who help others experience greater health. For instance, Brown, Condesine, and Magai (2005) found that providing costly material or emotional help within the past 3 months predicted lower morbidity in a sample of older American adults while controlling for socioeconomic status (SES), age, gender, education, ethnicity, social network size, and marital status. Similarly, individuals who report engaging in higher levels of volunteer work displayed lower levels of cardiovascular diseases risk (Burr, Han, & Tavares, 2015) and greater self-reported health (Piliavin & Siegl, 2007).

Furthermore, prospective studies indicate that providing informal assistance to others, including one's spouse, family, and friends, has benefits for the care provider that are detectable months and years later (e.g., Poulin, Brown, Dillard, & Smith, 2013). Indeed, Brown, Nesse, Vinokur, and Smith (2003) studied a sample of older married adults and found that mortality rates were lower for individuals who provided greater instrumental support to family, friends, and neighbors, as well as emotional support to their spouse 5 years earlier (also see Schwartz & Sendor, 1999). Interestingly, *receiving* support did not predict morality above and beyond support provision and demographic variables, suggesting that the benefits of giving support may outweigh those of receiving support in some samples (see also Brown et al., 2005). Additional prospective studies demonstrate the potential health buffering benefits of formal volunteer work as well. For instance, Sneed and Cohen (2013) examined a nationally representative sample of community-dwelling older adults and found that individuals who had volunteered more than 200 hours in the past year were less likely to develop hypertension than were nonvolunteers. Importantly though, volunteers reporting lower levels of involvement (<200 hours within the past 12 months) did not show similar benefits (Sneed & Cohen, 2013). Even short studies with student samples yield consistent findings. For example, a small number of students provided with $10 and the opportunity to distribute these funds between themselves and an unpaid peer reported greater subjective well-being and displayed faster cortisol recovery after engaging in generous (vs. stingy) economic behavior (Dunn, Ashton-James, Hanson & Aknin, 2010).

Finally, recent experimental work demonstrates that the impact of prosocial spending has detectable and meaningful health benefits for actors. Whillans, Dunn, and colleagues (2016) randomly assigned a sample of older adults to spend $20 on themselves or others once a week, for 3 consecutive weeks. Analyses revealed that older adults assigned to spend on others had lower systolic and diastolic blood pressure after the intervention than the older adults assigned to spend on themselves. Intriguingly, the observed benefits of prosocial spending were similar to hypertension medication and exercise.

Social Consequences of Giving

Our third principle of giving—suggesting the importance of the social benefits of giving—is supported by a large body of research documenting that prosocial behavior boosts the giver's status and worth in the eyes of others (Flynn, 2003; Flynn, Reagans, Amanatullah, & Ames, 2006; Grant & Gino, 2010; Klein, Grossman, Uksul, Kraus, & Epley, 2015; Levine, Barasch, Rand, Berman, & Small, 2018; Willer, 2009). Indeed, the reputational benefits of generosity serve as an incentive to individuals to act generously (Benabou & Tirole, 2010; Ellingsen & Johannesson, 2011; Harbaugh, 1998; Kraft-Todd, Yoeli, Bhanot, & Rand, 2015; Nowak & Sigmund, 2005). Anecdotally, nonprofits "sell" naming rights to donors because the reputational value donors earn from having their name forever stamped on a building make the sacrifice of the donation worth it. Empirically, many studies show enhanced generosity when donations are visible to others compared to when they are kept private (Andreoni & Petrie, 2004; Ariely, Bracha, & Meier, 2009).

However, the reputational benefits of giving can be weakened when the observers become skeptical that prosocial behavior was driven by an ulterior motive rather than by genuine prosociality. It is as if observers are attempting to assess a target's moral character through not only his or her actions (e.g., a donation to charity) but also what motives they ascribe to those actions (e.g., genuine concern, to gain public recognition). If they perceive an action to be driven by ulterior motives, they are quick to discount that action and give the actor less credit for it. In fact, some studies have found that a person who benefits from acting generously is given less credit than a person who did not act generously, suggesting that the discount from a perceived ulterior motive is larger than the status boost from generous behavior (Newman & Cain, 2014). Relatedly, people give less credit to an actor who benefits from a generous act even when the benefit was unforeseen or unpredictable and thus could not logically serve as an incentive (Lin-Healy & Small, 2013). Specifically, a scenario study described a person who was entered into a raffle for donating to charity, then experimentally varied whether the person won or lost the raffle. Raffle winners were judged as less generous than raffle losers, even though the outcome was transparently random and thus could not have meaningfully differentiated winners and losers. Taken together, people seem to act as intuitive judges—going beyond behavioral observation and sharply penalizing actors with flagrant ulterior motives (Critcher & Dunning, 2011).

Therefore, to reap the status benefits of prosociality, a person must not only *act* generously but also demonstrate authentic motives. In a set of experiments that recruited volunteers to persuade others to donate and varied whether the persuaders were also *paid* as a function of how well they did (i.e., "For every $1 donated by someone who viewed your pitch, we will also pay you $1"), compared to persuaders who had no selfish incentive, incentivized persuaders were less effective, even though the prospective donors were unaware of the existence of incentives (Barasch, Berman, & Small, 2016). Presumably, the payment they received tainted their motives in a way that was conveyed to the target donors. Moreover, the one form of selfish benefit that is *not* discounted is emotional benefits: Actors who feel good about their prosocial behavior are given *more,* not less, credit, perhaps related to the fact that emotion expression represents an authentic expression of caring (Barasch, Levine, Berman, & Small, 2014).

Nonetheless, the appearance of authentic motivation can become a catch-22 for individuals when it comes to whether to publicize their generous acts or to keep them private (Berman, Levine, Barasch, & Small, 2015). If generous deeds are performed privately, givers cannot reap the social benefits; yet, if good deeds are publicized, they run the risk of appearing as if their motives are inauthentic—driven by the desire to gain reputational benefits. A paradox arises because advertising one's own good deed provides information about how one behaved, which has a positive effect on one's reputation. Yet it also provides information about one's motive (that it was inauthentic), which has a negative effect on one's reputation. The lesson of this paradox is that advertising generosity only pays off in situations in which people do not otherwise know about one's generosity. Only in those situations can there be a net positive effect of publicizing, in which learning about one's behavior (a positive) counteracts learning about one's motive (a negative). If one's behavior is already known or is observable in some way, then publicizing is only negative, sending a signal of an ulterior motive.

Another means by which individuals learn whether others are truly prosocial is through gossip (Feinberg, Willer, Stellar, & Keltner, 2012; Wu, Balliet, & Van Lange, 2016). Gossip serves to identify antisocial individuals and is most readily applied by the most prosocial. In this way, gossip helps spread social information about whom to trust as cooperative and whom to avoid. Indeed, people are *most* generous when a recipient or an observer is highly socially connected and thus any reputational effects (positive or negative) are largest (Wu et al., 2016).

Giving, in the Future

The research we have reviewed primarily focuses on single-shot giving: people being exposed to an opportunity to give framed with either emotional or social benefits (via both connection and status), choosing to give or not, then experiencing emotional and social outcomes.

Of course, of great interest to scholars (and the world) is the extent to which giving on one occasion can prompt subsequent giving: from giving to becoming a giver. While a large body of evidence demonstrates the role of individual differences such as social value orientation in predicting prosocial behavior over time (e.g., Van Lange, Schippers, & Balliet, 2011), surprisingly little research has been devoted to interventions designed to causally increase subsequent giving. On the emotional angle and related to our first principle of giving, Aknin, Dunn, and Norton (2012) offer evidence that to the extent that giving enhances people's happiness, they may be more likely to give again. On the social side, Gray, Ward, and Norton (2014) suggest that prosocial behavior can be propagated when people choose to "pay it forward": Having been treated generously by someone else, they can pay that generosity forward to a third party. (Note, however, that Gray and colleagues' results suggest that negative behavior, such as greed, is relatively more likely to be paid forward; colloquially, we are more likely to cut someone off in traffic after having been cut off than we are to let someone in ahead of us after someone did the same for us.)

It is troubling that some research on moral licensing suggests that, if anything, people who behave prosocially may feel licensed to behave less prosocially in the future, evidence of a negative feedback loop (Jordan, Mullen, & Murnighan, 2011; Merritt, Effron, & Monin, 2010). However, Gneezy, Imas, Brown, Nelson, and Norton (2011) demonstrate that while licensing effects can occur, they are most likely when people have merely stated an intention to behave prosocially. Gneezy and colleagues suggest that when people have actually incurred a cost to behave prosocially—in money, time, effort, or other currencies—they become more likely to behave prosocially; in short, costly giving seems more likely to signal to people that they have not just temporarily engaged in giving, but they have adopted the more stable identity of being a giver.

Clearly, however, more research is needed to explore how both triggers of giving and outcomes of giving (emotional, social, or otherwise) can be leveraged to increase prosocial behavior.

Conclusion

Our goals in this chapter have been twofold. First, and practically, we aimed to understand more deeply the many barriers to prosocial behavior—both structural and psychological—to inform more successful interventions to promote generosity. We reviewed the growing body of field experiments in both psychology and economics that document a wide array of psychologically informed, novel interventions. Second, at the theoretical level, we aimed to highlight and unpack the underlying psychology of three basic principles of giving. Relative to the first principle, we reviewed research demonstrating the need to consider the emotional reactions of would-be helpers, and documented the role that an array of emotions (from happiness to awe to discomfort) play as predictors and products of prosocial behavior. For the second and third principles, we reviewed research demonstrating the need to consider the social consequences of helping, including both the human desire to connect with similar others and the equally salient goal to demonstrate status and gain reputation. While not exhaustive, these considerations encompass a substantial segment of the social scientific research on charitable giving, and (we hope) serve as a springboard for researchers to delve more deeply into these principles—and discover more.

REFERENCES

Aderman, D. (1972). Elation, depression, and helping behavior. *Journal of Personality and Social Psychology, 24,* 91–101.

Aknin, L. B., Barrington-Leigh, C. P., Dunn, E. W., Helliwell, J. F., Burns, J., Biswas-Diener, R., et al. (2013). Prosocial spending and well-being: Cross-cultural evidence for a psychological universal. *Journal of Personality and Social Psychology, 104*(4), 635–652.

Aknin, L. B., Broesch, T., Hamlin, J. K., & Van de Vondervoort, J. W. (2015). Prosocial behavior leads to happiness in a small-scale rural society. *Journal of Experimental Psychology: General, 144*(4), 788–795.

Aknin, L. B., Dunn, E. W., & Norton, M. I. (2012). Happiness runs in a circular motion: Evidence for a positive feedback loop between prosocial spending and happiness. *Journal of Happiness Studies, 13*(2), 347–355.

Aknin, L. B., Dunn, E. W., Proulx, J., Lok, I., & Norton, M. I. (2020). Does spending money on others promote happiness?: A registered replication report. *Journal of Personality and Social Psychology.* [Epub ahead of print]

Aknin, L. B., Dunn, E. W., Sandstrom, G. M., & Norton, M. I. (2013). Does social connection turn good deeds into good feelings?: The value of putting the "social" in prosocial spending. *International Journal of Happiness and Development, 1*(2), 155–171.

Aknin, L. B., Dunn, E. W., Whillans, A., Grant, A. M., & Norton, M. I. (2013). Feeling like you made a difference: On the importance of perceived prosocial impact when giving to others. *Journal of Economic Behavior and Organization, 88,* 90–95.

Aknin, L. B., Hamlin, J. K., & Dunn, E. W. (2012). Giving leads to happiness in young children. *PLOS ONE, 7*(6), e39211.

Aknin, L. B., Van de Vondervoort, J. W., & Hamlin, J. K. (2018). Positive feelings reward and promote prosocial behavior. *Current Opinion in Psychology, 20,* 55–59.

Alden, L. E., & Trew, J. L. (2013). If it makes you happy: Engaging in kind acts increases positive affect in socially anxious individuals. *Emotion, 13*(1), 64–75.

Algoe, S. B., & Haidt, J. (2009). Witnessing excellence in action: The "other-praising" emotions of elevation, gratitude, and admiration. *Journal of Positive Psychology, 4*(2), 105–127.

Anderson, C., & Keltner, D. (2002). The role of empathy in the formation and maintenance of social bonds. *Behavioral and Brain Sciences, 25*(1), 21–22.

Andreoni, J., & Petrie, R. (2004). Public goods experiments without confidentiality: A glimpse into fund-raising. *Journal of Public Economics, 88*(7–8), 1605–1623.

Andreoni, J., Rao, J. M., & Trachtman, H. (2017). Avoiding the ask: A field experiment on altruism, empathy, and charitable giving. *Journal of Political Economy, 125,* 625–653.

Anik, L., Norton, M. I., & Ariely, D. (2014). Contingent match incentives increase donations. *Journal of Marketing Research, 51,* 790–801.

Ariely, D., Bracha, A., & Meier, S. (2009). Doing good or doing well?: Image motivation and monetary incentives in behaving prosocially. *American Economic Review, 99*(1), 544–555.

Bandiera, O., Barankay, I., & Rasul, I. (2005). Social preferences and the response to incentives: Evidence from personnel data. *Quarterly Journal of Economics, 120*(3), 917–962.

Barasch, A., Berman, J. Z., & Small, D. A. (2016). When payment undermines the pitch: On the persuasiveness of pure motives in fund-raising. *Psychological Science, 27*(10), 1388–1397.

Barasch, A., Levine, E. E., Berman, J. Z., & Small, D. A. (2014). Selfish or selfless?: On the signal value of emotion in altruistic behavior. *Journal of Personality and Social Psychology, 107*(3), 393–413.

Bartlett, M. Y., & DeSteno, D. (2006). Gratitude and prosocial behavior: Helping when it costs you. *Psychological Science, 17*(4), 319–325.

Batson, C. D., Batson, J. G., Slingsby, J. K., Harrell, K. L., Peekna, H. M., & Todd, R. M. (1991). Empathic joy and the empathy–altruism hypothesis. *Journal of Personality and Social Psychology, 61,* 413–426.

Batson, C. D., Duncan, B. D., Ackerman, P., Buckley, T., & Birch, K. (1981). Is empathic emotion a source of altruistic motivation? *Journal of Personality and Social Psychology, 40*(2), 290–302.

Batson, C. D., Kobrynowicz, D., Dinnerstein, J. L., Kampf, H. C., & Wilson, A. D. (1997). In a very different voice: Unmasking moral hypocrisy. *Journal of Personality and Social Psychology, 72*(6), 1335–1348.

Baumann, D. J., Cialdini, R. B., & Kenrick, D. T. (1981). Altruism as hedonism: Helping and self-gratification as equivalent responses. *Journal of Personality and Social Psychology, 40*(6), 1039–1046.

Baumeister, R. F., & Leary, M. R. (1995). The need to belong: Desire for interpersonal attachments as a fundamental human motivation. *Psychological Bulletin, 117*, 497–529.

Benabou, R., & Tirole, J. (2010). Individual and corporate social responsibility. *Economica, 77*(305), 1–19.

Berman, J. Z., Levine, E. E., Barasch, A., & Small, D. A. (2015). The Braggart's dilemma: On the social rewards and penalties of advertising prosocial behavior. *Journal of Marketing Research, 52*(1), 90–104.

Bloom, P. (2016). *Against empathy: The case for rational compassion.* New York: Random House.

Borgonovi, F. (2008). Doing well by doing good: The relationship between formal volunteering and self-reported health and happiness. *Social Science and Medicine, 66*(11), 2321–2334.

Brown, S. L., Nesse, R. M., Vinokur, A. D., & Smith, D. M. (2003). Providing social support may be more beneficial than receiving it: Results from a prospective study of mortality. *Psychological Science, 14*(4), 320–327.

Brown, W. M., Consedine, N. S., & Magai, C. (2005). Altruism relates to health in an ethnically diverse sample of older adults. *Journals of Gerontology B: Psychological Sciences and Social Sciences, 60*(3), P143–P152.

Burr, J. A., Han, S. H., & Tavares, J. L. (2015). Volunteering and cardiovascular disease risk: Does helping others get "under the skin"? *The Gerontologist, 56*(5), 937–947.

Chancellor, J. A., Jacobs Bao, K., & Lyubomirsky, S. (2018). The propagation of everyday prosociality in the workplace: The reinforcing benefits of giving, getting, and glimpsing. *Journal of Positive Psychology, 13*, 271–283.

Cialdini, R. B., & Kenrick, D. T. (1976). Altruism as hedonism: A social development perspective on the relationship of negative mood state and helping. *Journal of Personality and Social Psychology, 34*(5), 907–914.

Cialdini, R. B., Schaller, M., Houlihan, D., Arps, K., Fultz, J., & Beaman, A. L. (1987). Empathy-based helping: Is it selflessly or selfishly motivated? *Journal of Personality and Social Psychology, 52*(4), 749–758.

Critcher, C. R., & Dunning, D. (2011). No good deed goes unquestioned: Cynical reconstruals maintain belief in the power of self-interest. *Journal of Experimental Social Psychology, 47*, 1207–1213.

Curry, O. S., Rowland, L. A., Van Lissa, C. J., Zlotowitz, S., McAlaney, J., & Whitehouse, H. (2018). Happy to help?: A systematic review and meta-analysis of the effects of performing acts of kindness on the well-being of the actor. *Journal of Experimental Social Psychology, 76*, 320–329.

Dana, J., Cain, D. M., & Dawes, R. M. (2006). What you don't know won't hurt me: Costly (but quiet) exit in dictator games. *Organizational Behavior and Human Decision Processes, 100*(2), 193–201.

Darley, J. M., & Latane, B. (1968). Bystander intervention in emergencies: Diffusion of responsibility. *Journal of Personality and Social Psychology, 8*, 377–383.

Decety, J., & Jackson, P. L. (2004). The functional architecture of human empathy. *Behavioral and Cognitive Neuroscience Reviews, 3*(2), 71–100.

DeSteno, D., Bartlett, M. Y., Baumann, J., Williams, L. A., & Dickens, L. (2010). Gratitude as moral sentiment: Emotion-guided cooperation in economic exchange. *Emotion, 10*(2), 289–293.

Diener, E., & Seligman, M. E. (2002). Very happy people. *Psychological Science, 13*(1), 81–84.

Dovidio, J. F., Gaertner, S. L., Validzic, A., Matoka, K., Johnson, B., & Frazier, S. (1997). Extending the benefits of recategorization: Evaluations, self-disclosure, and helping. *Journal of Experimental Social Psychology, 33*(4), 401–420.

Dulin, P. L., Gavala, J., Stephens, C., Kostick, M., & McDonald, J. (2012). Volunteering predicts happiness among older Māori and non-Māori in the New Zealand health, work, and retirement longitudinal study. *Aging and Mental Health, 16*(5), 617–624.

Dunn, E. W., Aknin, L. B., & Norton, M. I. (2008). Spending money on others promotes happiness. *Science, 319*, 1687–1688.

Dunn, E. W., Aknin, L. B., & Norton, M. I. (2014). Prosocial spending and happiness: Using money to benefit others pays off. *Current Directions in Psychological Science, 23*(1), 41–47.

Dunn, E. W., Ashton-James, C. E., Hanson, M. D., & Aknin, L. B. (2010). On the costs of self-interested economic behavior: How does stinginess get under the skin? *Journal of Health Psychology, 15*(4), 627–633.

Eisenberg, N., & Miller, P. A. (1987). The relation of empathy to prosocial and related behaviors. *Psychological Bulletin, 101*(1), 91–119.

Ellingsen, T., & Johannesson, M. (2011). Conspicuous generosity. *Journal of Public Economics, 95*(9/10), 1131–1143.

Feinberg, M., Willer, R., Stellar, J., & Keltner, D. (2012). The virtues of gossip: Reputational information sharing as prosocial behavior. *Journal of*

Personality and Social Psychology, 120(5), 1015–1030.

Flynn, F. J. (2003). How much should I give and how often?: The effects of generosity and frequency or favor exchange on social status and productivity. *Academy of Management Journal, 46*(5), 539–553.

Flynn, F. J., Reagans, R. E., Amanatullah, E. T., & Ames, D. R. (2006). Helping one's way to the top: Self-monitors achieve status by helping others and knowing who helps whom. *Journal of Personality and Social Psychology, 91*(6), 1123–1137.

Galak, J., Small, D. A., & Stephen, A. T. (2011). Microfinance decision making: A field study of prosocial lending [Special issue]. *Journal of Marketing Research, 48,* 130–137.

Geenen, N. Y. R., Hohelüchter, M., Langholf, V., & Walther, E. (2014). The beneficial effects of prosocial spending on happiness: Work hard, make money, and spend it on others? *Journal of Positive Psychology, 9,* 204–208.

Gerber, A. S., Green, D. P., & Larimer, C. W. (2008). Social pressure and voter turnout: Evidence from a large-scale field experiment. *American Political Science Review, 102*(1), 33–48.

Gino, F., Norton, M. I., & Weber, R. A. (2016). Motivated Bayesians: Feeling moral while acting egoistically. *Journal of Economic Perspectives, 30*(3), 189–212.

Gintis, H., Smith, E. A., & Bowles, S. (2001). Costly signaling and cooperation. *Journal of Theoretical Biology, 213*(1), 103–119.

Glazer, A., & Konrad, K. A. (1996). A signaling explanation for charity. *American Economic Review, 86*(4), 1019–1028.

Gneezy, A., Imas, A., Brown, A., Nelson, L. D., & Norton, M. I. (2011). Paying to be nice: Consistency and costly prosocial behavior. *Management Science, 58*(1), 179–187.

Grant, A. M., Campbell, E. M., Chen, G., Cottone, K., Lapedis, D., & Lee, K. (2007). Impact and the art of motivation maintenance: The effects of contact with beneficiaries on persistence behavior. *Organizational Behavior and Human Decision Processes, 103,* 53–67.

Grant, A. M., & Gino, F. (2010). A little thanks goes a long way: Explaining why gratitude expressions motivate prosocial behavior. *Journal of Personality and Social Psychology, 98*(6), 946–955.

Gray, K., Ward, A. F., & Norton, M. I. (2014). Paying it forward: Generalized reciprocity and the limits of generosity. *Journal of Experimental Psychology: General, 143*(1), 247–254.

Haidt, J. (2003). The moral emotions. In R. J. Davidson, K. R. Scherer, & H. H. Goldsmith (Eds.), *Handbook of affective sciences* (pp. 852–870). Oxford, UK: Oxford University Press.

Hanniball, K., Aknin, L. B., Douglas, K., & Viljoen, J. L. (2019). Does helping promote well-being in at-risk youth and ex-offender samples? *Journal of Experimental Social Psychology, 82,* 307–317.

Harbaugh, W. T. (1998). The prestige motive for making charitable transfers. *American Economic Review, 88*(2), 277–282.

Isen, A. M. (1970). Success, failure, attention, and reaction to others: The warm glow of success. *Journal of Personality and Social Psychology, 15*(4), 294–301.

Isen, A. M., & Levin, P. F. (1972). Effect of feeling good on helping: Cookies and kindness. *Journal of Personality and Social Psychology, 21*(3), 384–388.

Jordan, J., Mullen, E., & Murnighan J. K. (2011). Striving for the moral self: The effects of recalling past moral actions on future moral behavior. *Personality and Social Psychology Bulletin, 37,* 701–713.

Keltner, D., & Haidt, J. (2003). Approaching awe, a moral, spiritual, and aesthetic emotion. *Cognition and Emotion, 17*(2), 297–314.

Klein, N., Grossmann, I., Uskul, A. K., Kraus, A. A., & Epley, N. (2015). It pays to be nice, but not really nice: Asymmetric reputations from prosociality across 7 countries. *Judgment and Decision Making, 10*(4), 355–364.

Kogut, T., & Ritov, I. (2005). The "identified victim" effect: An identified group, or just a single individual? *Journal of Behavioral Decision Making, 18,* 157–167.

Konrath, S., Fuhrel-Forbis, A., Lou, A., & Brown, S. (2012). Motives for volunteering are associated with mortality risk in older adults. *Health Psychology, 31*(1), 87–96.

Koo, M., & Fishbach, A. (2016). Giving the self: Increasing commitment and generosity through giving something that represents one's essence. *Social Psychological and Personality Science, 7*(4), 339–348.

Kraft-Todd, G. T., Yoeli, E., Bhanot, S., & Rand, D. G. (2015). Promoting cooperation in the field. *Current Opinion Behavioral Science, 3,* 96–101.

Lacetera, N., & Macis, M. (2010). Social image concerns and prosocial behavior: Field evidence from a nonlinear incentive scheme. *Journal of Economic Behavior and Organization. 76*(2), 225–237.

Layous, K., Lee, H., Choi, I., & Lyubomirsky, S. (2013). Culture matters when designing a successful happiness-increasing activity: A comparison of the United States and South Korea. *Journal of Cross-Cultural Psychology, 44*(8), 1294–1303.

Levine, E. E., Barasch, A., Rand, D., Berman, J. Z., & Small, D. A. (2018). Signaling emotion and reason in cooperation. *Journal of Experimental Psychology: General, 145*(5), 702–719.

Lin-Healy, F., & Small, D. A. (2013). Nice guys finish last and guys in last are nice: The clash between doing well and doing good. *Social Psychological and Personality Science, 4*(6), 692–698.

Lyubomirsky, S., King, L., & Diener, E. (2005). The benefits of frequent positive affect: Does happiness lead to success? *Psychological Bulletin, 131*(6), 803–855.

Lyubomirsky, S., Sheldon, K. M., & Schkade, D. (2005). Pursuing happiness: The architecture of sustainable change. *Review of General Psychology, 9*(2), 111–131.

Meier, S., & Stutzer, A. (2004). Is volunteering rewarding in itself? *Economica, 75*(297), 39–59.

Merritt, A. C., Effron, D. A., & Monin, B. (2010). Moral self-licensing: When being good frees us to be bad. *Social and Personality Psychology Compass, 4*, 344–357.

Mongrain, M., Chin, J. M., & Shapira, L. B. (2011). Practicing compassion increases happiness and self-esteem. *Journal of Happiness Studies, 12*(6), 963–981.

Musick, M. A., & Wilson, J. (2003). Volunteering and depression: The role of psychological and social resources in different age groups. *Social Science and Medicine, 56*, 259–269.

Nelson, S. K., Layous, K., Cole, S. W., & Lyubomirsky, S. (2016). Do unto others or treat yourself?: The effects of prosocial and self-focused behavior on psychological flourishing. *Emotion, 16*(6), 850–861.

Newman, G. E., & Cain, D. M. (2014). Tainted altruism: When doing some good is evaluated as worse than doing no good at all. *Psychological Science, 25*(3), 648–655.

Nisbett, R. E., & Ross, L. (1980). *Human inference: Strategies and shortcomings of social judgment.* Englewood Cliffs, NJ: Prentice Hall.

Nowak, M. A., & Sigmund, K. (2005). Evolution of indirect reciprocity. *Nature, 437*, 1291–1298.

O'Malley, M. N., & Andrews, L. (1983). The effect of mood and incentives on helping: Are there some things money can't buy? *Motivation and Emotion, 7*(2), 179–189.

Paivio, A. (1969). Mental imagery and associative learning in memory. *Psychological Review, 76*, 241–263.

Piff, P. K., Dietze, P., Feinberg, M., Stancato, D. M., & Keltner, D. (2015). Awe, the small self, and prosocial behavior. *Journal of Personality and Social Psychology, 108*(6), 883–899.

Piliavin, J. A., & Siegl, E. (2007). Health benefits of volunteering in the Wisconsin longitudinal study. *Journal of Health and Social Behavior, 48*(4), 450–464.

Poulin, M. J., Brown, S. L., Dillard, A. J., & Smith, D. M. (2013). Giving to others and the association between stress and mortality. *American Journal of Public Health, 103*(9), 1649–1655.

Pressman, S. D., Kraft, T. L., & Cross, M. P. (2015). It's good to do good and receive good: The impact of a "pay it forward" style kindness intervention on giver and receiver well-being. *Journal of Positive Psychology, 10*(4), 293–302.

Preston, S. D., & de Waal, F. B. (2002). Empathy: Its ultimate and proximate bases. *Behavioral and Brain Sciences, 25*(1), 1–20.

Rogers, T., Ternovski, J., & Yoeli, E. (2016). Potential follow-up increases private contributions to public goods. *Proceedings of the National Academy of Sciences of the USA, 113*(19), 5218–5220.

Rosenhan, D. L., Underwood, B., & Moore, B. (1974). Affect moderates self-gratification and altruism. *Journal of Personality and Social Psychology, 30*(4), 546–552.

Schelling, T. C. (1968). The life you save may be your own. In S. B. Chase (Ed.), *Problems in public expenditure analysis* (pp. 127–162). Washington, DC: Brookings Institute.

Schnall, S., Roper, J., & Fessler, D. M. (2010). Elevation leads to altruistic behavior. *Psychological Science, 21*, 315–320.

Schwartz, C. E., & Sendor, R. M. (1999). Helping others helps oneself: Response shift effects in peer support. *Social Science and Medicine, 48*(11), 1563–1575.

Shaw, A., Montinari, N., Piovesan, M., Olson, K., Gino, F., & Norton. M. I. (2014). Children develop a veil of fairness. *Journal of Experimental Psychology: General 143*, 363–375.

Silvers, J. A., & Haidt, J. (2008). Moral elevation can induce nursing. *Emotion, 8*, 291–295.

Slovic, P., Västfjäll, D., Erlandsson, A., & Gregory, R. (2017). Iconic photographs and the ebb and flow of empathic response to humanitarian disasters. *Proceedings of the National Academy of Sciences of the USA, 114*(4), 640–644.

Small, D. A. (2011). "Sympathy biases and sympathy appeals: Reducing social distance to boost charitable contributions." In D. M. Oppenheimer & C. Y. Olivola (Eds.), *Experimental approaches to the study of charity* (pp. 149–160). New York: Taylor & Francis.

Small, D. A. (2015). "On the psychology of the identifiable victim effect." In G. Cohen, N. Eyal, & N. Daniels (Eds.), *Identifiable and statistical lives* (pp. 13–23). Oxford, UK: Oxford University Press.

Small, D. A., & Loewenstein, G. (2003). Helping *a* victim or helping *the* victim: Altruism and identifiabilty. *Journal of Risk and Uncertainty, 26*, 5–16.

Small, D. A., Loewenstein, G., & Slovic, P. (2007).

Sympathy and callousness: The impact of deliberative thought on donations to identifiable and
statistical victims. *Organizational Behavior and
Human Decision Processes, 102*(2), 143–153.

Small, D. A., & Simonsohn, U. (2008). Friends of
victims: The impact of personal relationships
with victims on generosity toward others. *Journal
of Consumer Research, 35,* 532–542.

Smith, R. W., Faro, D., & Burson, K. A. (2013). More
for the many: The influence of entitativity on
charitable giving. *Journal of Consumer Research,
39*(5), 961–976.

Sneed, R. S., & Cohen, S. (2013). A prospective
study of volunteerism and hypertension risk in
older adults. *Psychology and Aging, 28*(2), 578–
586.

Thoits, P. A., & Hewitt, L. N. (2001). Volunteer work
and well-being. *Journal of Health and Social Behavior, 42,* 115–131.

Toi, M., & Batson, C. D. (1982). More evidence that
empathy is a source of altruistic motivation. *Journal of Personality and Social Psychology, 43*(2),
281–292.

Van Lange, P. A. M., Schippers, M., & Balliet, D.
(2011). Who volunteers in psychology experiments?: An empirical review of prosocial motivation in volunteering. *Personality and Individual
Differences, 51,* 297–284.

Wang, X., & Tong, L. (2015). Hide the light or let
it shine?: Examining the factors influencing the
effect of publicizing donations on donors' happiness. *International Journal of Research in Marketing, 32*(4), 418–424.

Weinstein, N., & Ryan, R. M. (2010). When helping helps: Autonomous motivation for prosocial
behavior and its influence on well-being for the
helper and recipient. *Journal of Personality and
Social Psychology, 98*(2), 222–244.

Wheeler, J. A., Gorey, K. M., & Greenblatt, B.
(1998). The beneficial effects of volunteering
for older volunteers and the people they serve: A
meta-analysis. *International Journal of Aging and
Human Development, 47*(1), 69–79.

Whillans, A. V., Dunn, E. W., Sandstrom, G. M.,
Dickerson, S. S., & Madden, K. M. (2016). Is
spending money on others good for your heart?
Health Psychology, 35(6), 574–583.

Whillans, A. V., Seider, S. C., Chen, L., Dwyer, R.
J., Novick, S., Gramigna, K. J., et al. (2016). Does
volunteering improve well-being? *Comprehensive Results in Social Psychology, 1*(1–3), 35–50.

Whiteley, P. (2004). Press Release: The art of happiness: Is volunteering the blue-print for bliss?
Retrieved from *www.eurekalert.org/pub_releas-
es/2004-09/esr-tao091704.php.*

Wiwad, D., & Aknin, L. B. (2017). Motives matter:
The emotional consequences of recalled self- and
other-focused prosocial acts. *Motivation and
Emotion, 41*(6), 730–740.

Wu, J., Balliet, D., & Van Lange, P. A. M. (2016).
Reputation management: Why and how gossip enhances generosity. *Evolution and Human Behavior, 37*(3), 193–201.

Zaki, J. (2014). Empathy: A motivated account. *Psychological Bulletin, 140*(6), 1608–1647.

Zaki, J., & Cikara, M. (2015). Addressing empathic
failures. *Current Directions in Psychological Science, 24*(6), 471–476.

CHAPTER 26

Social Psychology and Law
Basic Principles in Legal Contexts

Kees van den Bos

The focus in this chapter is on the interface between social psychology and law. There are several reasons why it is important to study the intersection between these two scientific fields. One reason is that, upon reflection, it becomes clear that social psychology and law share many similarities. For example, the law as a system can be defined as a codified set of rules developed to regulate interactions and exchanges among people (Tyler & Jost, 2007). As such, the law constitutes an arrangement of rules and guidelines that are created and enforced through social and governmental institutions to regulate behavior. This regulation of behavior includes conflict resolution and sentencing decisions, and ideally takes place in such a way that a community shows respect to its members (Robertson, 2013).

Social psychology is the science of human behavior and how people think and feel in social contexts. More formally, it entails the scientific study of how people's thoughts, feelings, and behaviors are influenced by the actual, imagined, or implied presence of others (Allport, 1985). This chapter illustrates that insight into these issues is relevant for the understanding of how the law operates in courtrooms, how people perceive the law as a legal system, and how

officials function in several legal contexts, for example, in areas of legal decision making, law making, and law enforcement. In other words, this chapter seeks to show that social psychology is needed to understand how the law works (or *law in action*).

One could say that social psychology and law share a common interest in behavioral regulation such that whereas social psychology describes how human behavior *is* regulated, law as a discipline tends to focus on the issue of how behavior *should* be regulated. Of course, the two disciplines examine many more different issues, but this observation of *descriptive* versus *normative* accounts of behavioral regulation implies that legal scholars and legal practitioners can profit from the insights of the social psychological discipline to better understand how people's behaviors (and their associated thoughts and feelings) are, in fact, regulated. This implies that notions of how the law should work (or *law in the books*) can profit from an understanding of basic principles of social psychology.

Insight into social psychology in legal contexts is also important because it shows how important societal institutions can impact human behavior. This is an understudied issue in modern social psychology, which is surprising given social psychology's central orientation to the issue of how social contexts influence human reactions (Allport, 1985). This chapter is an attempt to fill this void. In doing so, I argue that studying in detail the basic principles of social psychology in legal contexts is not merely an instance of "applied social psychology." Rather, insights from the social psychology of law provide important nuances to (and hence feed into) basic social psychology, needed to make the social psychological discipline more robust, more fine-grained, and more relevant (see also Kruglanski, Chernikova, & Jasko, 2017).

This chapter fits into a growing—albeit not undisputed—trend in the legal discipline to pay attention to insights from the behavioral and societal sciences, including findings from empirical studies conducted in legal contexts. Because social psychology can be characterized as a hub science that bridges behavioral, societal, and other scientific disciplines by means of careful conceptual analysis and empirical study, it can well be argued that focusing on the social psychology of law is timely and important. In exploring this issue my aim in this chapter is twofold: (1) to provide a general overview of the topics that fit under the general umbrella of the "social psychology of law" and (2) to provide an overall conceptual framework for organizing these topics by affording a set of basic principles governing the social psychology of law.

Two Basic Principles and Two Contexts

Psychological science, including the science of social psychology, can be depicted as an exploded confetti factory, producing many colorful empirical findings and fascinating mini-theories (Ellemers, 2013). It can be difficult to figure out how the various ideas, research studies, phenomena, and domains in social psychology (including the social psychology of law) fit together (Stangor, 2011). In order to structure the burgeoning field of social psychology in legal contexts, I differentiate between two legal contexts and focus on two basic social psychological principles that I think are relevant for understanding what people think, feel, and do in these legal contexts. The chapter's focus is on the two basic principles that I distinguish in the social psychology of law.

The first social psychological principle that I distinguish has to do with the notion that people working in legal contexts are and should be busy with ascertaining the truth on which legal decisions should be based. An important corollary of this principle implies that the presence of bias in legal functioning and decision making warrants our close attention. In fact, a lot of legal psychology is oriented toward delineating these biases. This first principle includes the determination by people working in the legal domain of who is guilty or innocent in criminal law cases. The reliability of eyewitness testimony and to what extent we can trust human memory in criminal law is also important here. This basic principle also involves the striving for the absence of biases and discrimination, as well as the issue of individual and group decision making of judges and juries in various legal cases. In short, the first basic principle on which this chapter focuses examines *ascertaining the truth*. I label literature on this issue as *legal psychology*.

The second social psychological principle I put forward here focuses on the human justice judgment process that I assume is related to the first principle and that is important both inside and outside the courtroom. That is, the law is all about establishing justice. Thus, when people interpret their court hearings, perceive the legal system, and try to ascertain the truth in legal contexts, they rely on their judgments whether justice has prevailed and whether just treatment and just outcomes were established in the court hearings, by the law, and in the ascertainment of truth. I assume, therefore, that people's judgments of justice play a pivotal role in various legal contexts and in every topic thus far mentioned. This assumption implies that the justice judgment process warrants our special attention when studying the social psychology of law. I pay careful attention in this chapter to the process by which people form justice judgments. In fact, I propose the *justice judgment process* as the second principle and refer to this as the *social psychology of justice judgments* when examining this principle.

I note explicitly that the principles on which I focus do not operate in an autonomous manner, but often function in combination to shape thoughts, feelings, and behaviors in legal contexts. For example, one could say that justice in legal contexts is about establishing the truth of legal decisions. Therefore, the first and second principles are clearly related to each other. Nevertheless, it makes sense, I argue, to discuss these two principles separately, for reasons of emphasis and because different literatures provide meaningful input for the social psychology of these two principles.

I further propose that to understand the social psychology in legal contexts, it is pivotal to realize that there are many different legal contexts that vary in important ways from each other, both from legal and psychological perspectives. Lawyers distinguish, for example, between criminal law cases (pertaining to crimes and the appropriate punishment of those crimes), civil law cases (having to do with private relations between members of a community or organizations or businesses within that community), and constitutional or administrative law cases (referring to the relationship between individuals and the state). Many different categorizations are made by lawyers, and many nuances are important to understand the ins and outs of legal arrangements and different types of law cases. Thus, lawyers make relevant distinctions between various legal contexts.

Furthermore, although different legal systems tend to deal with similar basic issues, jurisdictions categorize and identify their legal subjects in different ways. As such, systems can differ widely across different countries (e.g., the United States vs. the United Kingdom vs. Continental Europe). The presence or absence of juries is one important difference. This is not the time and the place to review all the different legal categories and the various legal contexts that are distinguished in the legal literature. Here, I note that the psychological processes involved in different types of law cases may well vary between cases, in part because different types of litigants tend to be involved in the different cases and because different legal issues are at stake in these different cases. This is something the social psychology of law should pay more attention to.

Against this background, I distinguish between two different legal contexts, namely, what happens inside the courtroom and what occurs outside the courtroom (or courthouse). This simple distinction is often overlooked, yet studies conducted inside or outside the courtroom tend to examine different social psychological issues and processes. Whereas studies inside the courtroom examine legal decision making and how litigants respond to this decision making, studies done outside the courtroom tend to assess how the legal system is functioning and how people perceive the functioning of the legal system. Therefore, after having discussed the two basic social psychological principles on which this chapter focuses, I pay some attention to the social psychology of people's reactions to what happens inside versus outside the courtroom as two relevant legal contexts.

Ascertaining the Truth

The whole justice system, including the criminal justice system, is oriented toward determining the truth. This does not imply that the law as a system is always able or even good at finding the truth, and it also does not mean that "the" truth is always simple to uncover, but it does suggest that officials working for the law are and should be oriented toward ascertaining the truth. This basic principle of law is the part that many people first think of when reflecting on psychology and the law. And indeed it is a very important part of what psychological insight can offer to the field of law. In fact, the literature on this issue is huge, and is inspired to a large extent by cognitive psychology and the literature on social cognition (see, e.g., Ellsworth & Mauro, 1998; Kovera & Borgida, 2010). Here I can discuss only some instances of the literature on legal psychology. I focus on basic psychological insight regarding eyewitness testimonies, lie detection, expert evidence in the courtroom, judicial and jury decision making, biases, and false convictions.

One of the core areas of legal psychology is the groundbreaking research on eyewitness reports by Loftus (1975) and others. Rooted in the observation that human memory is often flawed (e.g., Loftus & Greenspan, 2017), it has been shown that the way questions are asked during interrogations and other interviews can have a dramatic impact on what people report to have seen (Loftus, 1975). The way that possible guilty individuals are lined up and presented to those who have to identify the guilty person is also influencing cognitive processes and the decisions of those who do the identification tasks (Wells & Turtle, 1986). In addition to system variables such as lineup composition, lineup instruction, and lineup presentation that all influence witness accuracy, own race, unconscious transference, and stress of the identifying person also affect the (un)reliability of eyewitness identifications (Kovera & Borgida, 2010).

The criminal law system has been reluctant to accept these conclusions and the implications that follow from them, but things now seem to be changing, resulting in eyewitness science paying off in the end (Loftus, 2013). Perhaps the biggest boost to public appreciation of eyewitness research came as a result of progress in forensic DNA testing. It was DNA that helped exonerate many wrongfully convicted individuals in the mid-1990s, and today over 300 innocent people owe their freedom to that testing. As a result, expert testimony has an easier time being admitted. Courts are commenting more favorably on eyewitness science (Loftus, 2013). And expert evidence on eyewitness reports has played a very important role in important law cases (e.g., Wagenaar, 1988). This slow-to-start but exponentially growing collaboration among psychologists, legal professionals, and others has done a great deal to change the justice landscape for people accused of crimes (Steblay & Loftus, 2013), although a lot still needs to be done (see, e.g., Vredeveldt, Hildebrandt, & Van Koppen, 2016; Wixted & Wells, 2017).

Another important issue in legal psychology is whether there are experts in deception detection. Bond (2008) presented videotaped statements produced by paroled felons to students and law enforcement personnel. Results suggested that those correctional officers who could be identified as experts were accurate in their assessment of the video statements over 80 or 90% of the trials. Experts showed high discrimination in signal-detection tasks and did not evidence biased responding. The experts relied on nonverbal cues to make fast and accurate decisions.

O'Sullivan, Frank, Hurley, and Tiwana (2009) note that although most people have a no better than chance probability of detecting deception, some groups of police professionals have demonstrated significant lie detection accuracy. One reason for not detecting expert deception may be that the types of lies police are asked to judge in scientific experiments often do not represent the types of lies they see in their profession. Across 23 studies, involving 31 different police groups in eight countries, police officers tested with lie detection scenarios using high-stakes lies (i.e., the lie was personally involving and/or resulted in substantial rewards or punishments for the liar) and were significantly more accurate than law enforcement officials tested with low-stakes lies.

Van Veldhuizen, Horselenberg, Landström, Granhag, and Van Koppen (2017) demonstrated that Swedish asylum officials mainly formulate open-ended and information-gathering questions. These types of questions are likely to elicit more elaborate and accurate answers than closed-ended and accusatory questions. In contrast, Dutch asylum officials primarily pose predominantly closed-ended and fact-checking questions, and thereby are likely to elicit short answers that make it more difficult to ascertain the truth (Van Veldhuizen, Maas, Horselenberg, & Van Koppen, 2018). Related to this, Vrij (1993) showed that in interrogations Dutch officers tend to misinterpret the "looking away" behavior of Black norm violators from Suriname as confirmatory of the crime ("They must have something to hide"), while the Suriname person regards some avoidance of eye contact as showing respect to the officer.

Vrij and colleagues (2008) argue that observers could improve their deceit detection performance by taking a more active approach to the task, specifically by asking interviewees to report their stories in reverse order. Vrij and coauthors suggest that this is particularly debilitating for liars because their cognitive resources have already been partially depleted by the cognitively demanding task of lying. The authors hypothesized and found that increased cognitive load would lead to the emergence of more nonverbal and verbal differences between liars and truth tellers in reverse-order interviews than in chronological interviews, and that this facilitates the observers' task of discriminating between them.

Another issue concerns when expert evidence is admissible in court. Quality science provides the foundation for applications of social psychological science to the law. To be admissible in court, expert testimony must be legally relevant to the case at hand and scientifically valid (Kovera & Borgida, 2010). In this respect, it is important that contemporary social psychologists generally base (or should base) their understanding of phenomena not on single studies but on large groups of studies that have been submitted to rigorous statistical analysis to examine the magnitude and consistency of their findings across samples and methods. Quality science thus obtained can provide meaningful input, such as the role of expert knowledge on social cognition in employment discrimination cases (Fiske & Borgida, 2008).

Legal psychology has been concentrating on decision making of judges, in part to find out whether the truth is ascertained by means of judicial decision making. Guthrie, Rachlinski, and Wistrich (2001) note that the quality of the judicial system depends on the quality of decisions that judges make. Even the most talented and dedicated judges surely commit occasional mistakes, but the public understandably expects judges to avoid systematic errors. This expectation, however, might be unrealistic. Psychologists who study human judgment and choice have learned that people frequently fall prey to cognitive illusions that produce systematic errors in judgment. Even though judges are experienced, well-trained, and highly motivated decision makers, they might be vulnerable to cognitive illusions. Guthrie and colleagues reported that five common cognitive illusions (anchoring, framing, hindsight bias, the representativeness heuristic, and egocentric biases) influence the decision-making processes of a sample of 167 federal magistrate judges. Although the judges were somewhat less susceptible to two of these illusions (framing effects and the representativeness heuristic) than lay decision makers, the findings suggest that judges are human, and that their judgment is affected by cognitive illusions that can produce systematic errors in judgment.

Related to this, Danziger, Levav, and Avnaim-Pesso (2011) studied extraneous factors in judicial decisions. Their research focused on whether judicial rulings are based solely on laws and facts. This is an important issue, as legal formalism holds that judges apply legal reasons to the facts of a case in a rational, mechanical, and deliberative manner. In contrast, legal realists argue that the rational application of legal reasons does not sufficiently explain the decisions of judges, and that psychological, political, and social factors influence judicial rulings. Legal realism is sometimes referred to as depicting justice as "what the judge ate for breakfast." To test this metaphor empirically, Danziger and colleagues recorded sequential parole decisions made by experienced judges before or after daily food breaks.

The Danziger and associates (2011) results indicate that the likelihood of a favorable ruling is greater at the beginning of the workday or after a food break than later in the sequence of cases. The likelihood of a ruling in favor of a prisoner spikes at the beginning of each session. The probability of a favorable ruling steadily declines from (approximately) .65 to nearly zero and jumps back up to .65 after a break for a meal. The authors interpret these findings by arguing that when judges make repeated rulings, they show an increased tendency to rule in favor of the status quo. This tendency can be overcome by taking a break to eat a meal, consistent with previous research demonstrating the effects of a short rest, positive mood, and glucose on mental resource replenishment. These findings add to the literature that documents how experts are not immune to the influence of extraneous irrelevant information. Indeed, the metaphor that justice is "what the judge ate for breakfast" might be an appropriate depiction of human decision making in general.

A research project by Cho, Barnes, and Guanara (2017) fits with this line of reasoning. These authors argue that sleep deprivation in judges increases the severity of their sentences. Taking advantage of the natural quasi-manipulation of sleep deprivation during the shift to daylight saving time in the spring and analyzing archival data from judicial punishment handed out in the U.S. federal courts, their results show that judges doled out longer sentences when they were sleep deprived.

Projects such as these raise the question how judges do judge. Do they apply law to facts in a mechanical and deliberative way, as the formalists suggest they do, or do they rely on hunches and gut feelings, as the realists maintain? Relying on empirical studies of judicial reasoning and decision making, Guthrie, Rachlinski, and Wistrich (2007) propose a new model of judging. This model accounts for the tendency of the human brain to make automatic, snap judgments, which are surprisingly accurate, but which can also lead to erroneous decisions. The authors argue that their model provides a more accurate explanation of judicial behavior. In line with this proposition, Ham, Van den Bos, and Van Doorn (2009) found that when forming justice judgments, unconscious thought can indeed lead to more accurate justice judgments than do both conscious thought and immediate judgment.

In legal contexts, not only individuals but also groups make important decisions; hence, group processes and group decision making plays an important role in the ascertainment of truth (Kovera & Borgida, 2010). For example, in jury decision making, jury size, jury unanimity, jury competence, and processes of jury deliberation all matter (Ellsworth & Mauro, 1998). A famous example of decision making by juries is the 1957 movie *Twelve Angry Men,* in which one (male) jury holdout attempts to prevent a miscarriage of justice by forcing his colleagues to reconsider the evidence.

Following-up on this, Salerno and Peter-Hagene (2013) investigated whether expressing anger increases social influence for men, but diminishes social influence for women, during group deliberation. In a deception paradigm, participants believed they were engaged in a computer-mediated mock jury deliberation about a murder case. In actuality, the interaction was scripted. The script included five other mock jurors who provided verdicts and comments in support of the verdicts. Four of these jurors agreed with the participant, and one was a "holdout" dissenter. Holdouts expressed their opinions with no emotion, anger, or fear and had either male or female names. Holdouts exerted no influence on participants' opinions when they expressed no emotion or fear. Participants' confidence in their own verdict dropped significantly, however, after male holdouts expressed anger. However, participants became

significantly more confident in their original verdicts after female holdouts expressed anger, even though they were expressing the exact same opinion and emotion as the male holdouts. This study has implications for group decisions in general, and jury deliberations in particular, by suggesting that expressing anger might lead men to gain influence, but women to lose influence on societally important decisions, such as jury verdicts.

Recent advances in DNA, blood type, and fingerprint testing have increased the likelihood that average citizens will confront complex scientific evidence when serving as jurors in civil and criminal cases. McAuliff, Kovera, and Nunez (2009) examined the ability of jury-eligible community members to detect internal validity threats in psychological science presented during a trial. Participants read a case summary in which an expert testified about a study that varied in internal validity (valid, missing control group, confound, and experimenter bias) and ecological validity (high, low). Variations in internal validity did not influence verdict or ratings of plaintiff credibility, and no differences emerged as a function of ecological validity. The authors argue that their findings suggest that training programs on statistics and research methodology for the judiciary and bar become increasingly important. Future research aimed at developing new programs or evaluating those already in place is greatly needed if we genuinely desire to help the legal system better accommodate jurors' reasoning skills in trials containing psychological science.

Group processes such as tunnel vision during police interrogations can also play an important role in the functioning of the legal system. Directive police interrogation tactics can even lead to false convictions and false confessions (Ellsworth & Gross, 2013; Kovera & Borgida, 2010). Kassin and colleagues (2010) summarize what is known about police-induced confessions. Interrogation tactics such as excessive interrogation time, presentation of false evidence, and as an interrogator trying to minimize the crime can lead suspects to see confession as an expedient means to escape the interrogation interview. The mandatory electronic recording of interrogations and the reform of interrogation practices can protect vulnerable suspect populations.

Group processes can also impact possible verdicts. For example, Glaser, Martin, and Kahn (2015) conducted a survey-embedded experiment with a nationally representative sample in the United States to examine the effect on verdicts of sentence severity as a function of defendant race, presenting respondents with a triple-murder trial summary that manipulated the race of the defendant. When respondents had been told that death was the maximum sentence, respondents presented with Black defendants were significantly more likely to convict (80.0%) than were those with White defendants (55.1%). The results indicate that the death penalty may be a cause of racial disparities in criminal justice and implicate threats to civil rights and to effective criminal justice.

Similarly, Schuller, Kazoleas, and Kawakami (2009) studied the impact of prejudice screening procedures on racial bias in legal contexts. Specifically, the authors examined the influence of the challenge for cause procedure and its effectiveness in curbing racial prejudice in trials involving Black defendants. Participants were provided with a trial summary of a defendant charged with either drug trafficking or embezzlement. The race of the defendant was either White or Black, with participants in the Black defendant condition receiving (prior to the trial presentation) either no challenge, a close-ended standard challenge, or a modified reflective pretrial questioning strategy. Overall, the results revealed an anti-Black bias in judgments. While the closed-ended challenge did little to reduce this bias, the reflective format demonstrated a reduction in racial bias, suggesting there might be some remedies to biases in legal judgments.

Besides race, other group categories play an important role in legal decision making. For instance, Herzog and Oreg (2008) linked the observation of earlier studies showing that female offenders frequently receive more lenient judgments than equivalent males to chivalry theories, which argued that such leniency is the result of paternalistic, benevolent attitudes toward women, in particular toward those who fulfill stereotypical female roles. Eight hundred forty respondents from a national sample of Israeli residents evaluated the seriousness of hypothetical crime scenarios with (traditional and nontraditional) female and male offenders. As hypothesized, hostile and benevolent sexism moderated the effect of women's "traditionality" on respondents' crime seriousness judgments and on the severity of sentences assigned.

To conclude, I have discussed in this section some studies examining the multifaceted literature on legal psychology. What I argue in the next section is that the ascertainment of truth, being a core topic in legal psychology, in essence, to a large degree boils down to the establishment of justice. The next section focuses in some detail on the issue of how people form justice judgments.

Forming Justice Judgments

Whether people think that officials working for the legal system are successful in ascertaining the truth (discussed in the previous section) and how legally interested parties make sense of what is happening in court hearings, and how individuals outside the courthouse evaluate the legal system (to be discussed in the next sections) are issues related to a second basic social psychological principle that I discuss in some detail here: how people form justice judgments. I think there are good reasons to propose that this psychological process is a common thread underlying many issues of the social psychology of law.

After all, people are interested in justice concerns when interpreting their court hearings, evaluating how the law works, and determining whether the truth is ascertained or biases are present in legal functioning and legal decision making. Indeed, law is a "discipline organized to design *just* rules of conduct and to determine when those rules have been broken" (Ellsworth & Mauro, 1998, p. 686; emphasis added). Thus, I argue that the perception of just or unjust behavior by judges in the courtroom and other legal professionals of the legal system, as well as perceived justice of the legal system and the absence (or presence) of bias in legal decision making, are linked strongly to just conduct.

However, what is just conduct? To examine this issue, social psychologists interested in law focus not only on law in the books but also on law in action, in particular on people's justice judgments. Finkel (1995) examined the relationship between "law in the books," as set down in the Constitution and developed in legal cases and legal decisions, and what he calls "commonsense justice," the ordinary citizen's notions of what is just and fair. Law is an essentially human endeavor, Finkel argues, a collection of psychological theories about why people think, feel, and behave as they do, and when and why we should find some of them blameworthy and punishable. But is it independent of community sentiment, as some would contend? Or, as Finkel suggests, do juries bring the community's judgment to bear on the moral blameworthiness of the defendant? When jurors decide that the law is unfair, or the punishment inappropriate for a particular defendant, they have sometimes nullified the law.

Research shows that justice judgments are important, for one thing because discrepancies may cause citizens to feel alienated from authority, and reduce their voluntary compliance with legal codes (Darley, 2001). Justice judgments are also important because they can create a link to legitimacy of the law in society (Tyler & Jost, 2007). And justice judgments are important as a goal of the legal system for their own sake or because of moral concerns. After all, the goal of law is to create justice in society (Ellsworth & Mauro, 1998). Furthermore, justice judgments are important because they can have real consequences (Van den Bos, 2018).

Before I examine this latter notion in detail, I would like to focus on the subjective quality of justice judgments. After all, although justice judgments are important for several reasons, they can also be susceptible to various subjective factors, which is an issue with which many lawyers may be uncomfortable. This is understandable, but it is good to know that social psychological science indicates how to understand this subjective quality

Not only in law but also in all scientific fields that have examined the justice concept there exists an ongoing controversy between "rationalist" and "intuitionist" accounts of justice. Rationalist theories emphasize that reasoning causes justice judgments to be constructed primarily in a deliberate, objective, and cognitive way, whereas intuitionist notions suggest that justice judgments are mainly the result of automatic or spontaneous evaluations and are strongly influ-

enced by subjective and affective factors (for an overview, see Beauchamp, 2001). As a result of this controversy, the social psychology of law is confronted with scholars and practitioners who explicitly or implicitly adhere to the notion (attributed to Aristotle) that "the law is reason, free from passion" versus those who work from the assumption that justice judgments are derived from feelings, not from reasoning (e.g., Hume, 1739–1740/1951) and that subjectivity and affectivity hence play an inescapable role in the forming of justice judgments and the working of the law.

Ever since the days of Aristotle and Plato, there have been arguments in philosophy and science that either rationalist or intuitionist conceptions of justice are true. A social psychological perspective on this controversy is important, I argue, because the discipline proposes that in some situations, people construct justice judgments in a careful way, weighing all relevant information carefully in an impartial manner, whereas in other circumstances, people's gut reactions lead to snap judgments that are colored by their feelings or their own interests. Thus, rather than continuing the ancient and ongoing impasse of believing in either rationalist or intuitionist conceptions, social psychology suggests that it makes more sense to adopt an integrative approach that studies social conditions that affect the relative importance of rationalist and intuitionist accounts (Van den Bos, 2003).

Testing this integrative social psychological account, I argued in a 2003 article that when forming justice judgments, it is not uncommon for people to lack information that is most relevant in the particular situation. In information-uncertain conditions, people may therefore construct justice judgments by relying on how they feel about the events they have encountered, and justice judgments may hence be strongly influenced by affect information. Findings indeed show that in information-uncertain conditions, people's prior affective states that are unrelated to the justice event in fact strongly influenced justice judgments. This suggests that in situations of information uncertainty, people's judgments of justice can be very subjective, susceptible to affective states that have no logical relationship with the justice judgments they are constructing. This insight may have important implications for the social psychology of law and the rationalist and intuitionist conceptions of justice in that literature (see also Bandes & Blumenthal, 2012). People may also adopt rationalistic or intuitionist mindsets, and this may have an impact on their justice judgments without people being aware of this effect (Maas & Van den Bos, 2009).

An insight that follows from the justice judgment literature is that besides issues of relative deprivation, equity of outcomes, and people's belief in a just world, a core aspect of people's justice judgments is the notion of perceived "procedural justice." Whereas in organizational and interpersonal contexts, perceived procedural justice may entail predominantly the fairness of the way people are treated (Van den Bos, 2005, 2015), due to its special and formal qualities, perceived procedural justice in legal contexts also included the fairness and justice of formal procedures and processes that are used, or should be used, by the legal system (Thibaut & Walker, 1975). Indeed, both formal and informal aspects of procedural justice constitute pivotal aspects of justice judgments in legal contexts and influence people's behavior and other reactions in these contexts (e.g., Hollander-Blumoff, 2011; Lind & Tyler, 1988; Tyler, 2006).

The importance of perceived procedural justice does not imply that other notions of justice do not affect people's reactions. For example, courtroom research shows that litigants' perceived procedural justice is positively associated with their trust in judges, and that this effect is there when outcomes of court hearings are relatively favorable and is even stronger when outcomes are relatively unfavorable (Grootelaar & Van den Bos, 2018). These findings fit with a line of reasoning that perceived procedural justice is especially important to people when they are trying to make sense of what is going on in their environments (Van den Bos & Lind, 2009), such as when outcomes are unfavorable (Brockner & Wiesenfeld, 1996).

The importance of judgments of justice and injustice is also seen in the disdain for law in processes of radicalization. Van den Bos (2018) proposes that judgments of injustice are closely associated with the process of delegitimization and the rejection of law and democratic principles that often constitutes a turning point in the radicalization process of many people (see also Moghaddam, 2005). In particular, the issue of people perceiving certain things in their worlds as profoundly unjust and unfair can influence why Muslims or those who identify with right-wing or left-wing politics can be tempted to engage in violent extremism and be sympathetic to terrorist acts. For example, radicalizing individuals may feel that their group is being treated in a blatantly unjust manner or they judge crucial moral principles to be violated. These judgments of injustice threaten people's sense of who they are and jeopardize their beliefs of how the world should look. Furthermore, these judgments can have a disastrous impact on people's perceptions of legitimacy of democratic values and the rule of law.

There is evidence that delegitimization of government, law, and other societal institutions plays a crucial role in the radicalization of Muslims, right-wing groups, and left-wing individuals (Van den Bos, 2018). Key to understanding the ontogenesis of violent extremism and terrorism may well be people's rejection of constitutional democracy and law. After all, when it is hard or impossible for you to work within principles of constitutional democracy, then you might easily get frustrated that your wishes and opinions are not put into action. Related to this, when you cannot really force yourself to be open minded about different opinions and at least be willing to tolerate them to such a degree that you try to make your case heard through majority rule or other democratic rules, then you are more likely to take action yourself to ensure that things will go your way. Furthermore, violent extremism and terrorism constitute illegal acts, and when one does not care about what the law says, or when one even sympathizes with illegal behavior, it is easier to prepare or prompt oneself to engage in illegal actions.

It is very difficult to predict in advance people's intentions to break the law and whether they will actually break the law. This noted, modern social psychological insights can be used to account for people's intentions to commit legal violations. When people perceive that it is easy or doable for them to perform the illegal behavior, and when they believe that other important people positively evaluate the behavior, then people are likely to form the intention to break the law. This indicates that the relevance of behavioral control and what others think of the behavior in question can be key variables predicting when people will actually engage in illegal behavior, such as violent extremism (Van den Bos, 2018).

I hasten to note that adherence to radical beliefs and ideas does not need to imply violent breaking of the law. Radicals who engage in civil disobedience and as a result of this break the law also provide an interesting example in this respect. I also note explicitly that the task of understanding and predicting the actual onset of violent extremism and terrorism is very difficult. This noted, the psychology of judgments of unfairness and injustice can help us to understand violent extremism and perhaps even ways of countering this by trying to nourish agreement with democratic values (Van den Bos, 2018).

All this is an illustration of the notion that if perceptions are real, they tend to have real consequences (Thomas & Thomas, 1928). Understanding perceptions in general, and perceptions of justice and injustice in particular, can be complex, in part because these perceptions can be biased in important ways. What is just and unjust is really in the eye of the beholder, but because injustice perceptions are deeply felt as real and genuine, they tend to have real consequences and can fuel radical beliefs and extremist and terrorist behaviors in important ways (Van den Bos, 2018).

Making Sense of Law Inside the Courtroom: Interpreting Our Own Court Hearings

Thus far I have not distinguished between different contexts and discussed findings obtained across different settings, as if the actual settings in which the findings were obtained did not matter. This adheres to a trend that can be seen in many modern treatments of psychological science, which is heavily focused on trying to discover general laws of human thinking, feeling, and behavior (Van den Bos, McGregor, & Martin, 2015). However, part of the reason why the study of law is so exciting and impor-

tant (also for basic psychological science) is that it makes clear that differences between contexts do matter a lot and influence people's thoughts, feelings, and behaviors in important ways. Issues at stake differ across legal contexts, for instance, and so do the psychological processes involved in these different contexts. In this chapter, I distinguish between how people (with direct concerns at stake) evaluate how their own cases are being treated inside the courtroom and how people outside the courtroom (with or without direct concerns at stake) evaluate the legal system.

Insights regarding how people interpret what happens both inside and outside the courtroom can profit from the robust social psychological notion that people are sense makers (see, e.g., Kruglanski, 1989; Van den Bos & Lind, 2013); that is, human beings are heavily interested in trying to make sense of what is going on in their environments. This is especially the case when what is happening in these environments has special importance to them. Obviously, when people with legal concerns at stake have to appear at court hearings, it is important to them which decisions will be made about their legal cases. Thus, because of outcome reasons, and because of how they are treated signals how they are valued by important figures of society (e.g., judges), people interpret what is going on in their court hearings. Therefore, I note that people are heavily interested in interpreting their own court hearings. They try to make sense of the law as enacted within their court hearings and to assess whether the trust is ascertained and justice is done.

Against this background, I note here that recent research suggests at least one basic psychological process plays an important role in how litigants make sense of their own court hearings. That is, in her PhD research Liesbeth Hulst (2017) argues that when litigants are requested to appear at court hearings, they try to make sense of what is going on at the hearings and the legitimate system in which these hearings are taking place. One of the issues people are trying to find out is whether they can trust the judges in their legal system, and whether they can assign legitimacy to those powerholders. We know from earlier research that in situations such as court hearings, procedural justice serves an important role in people's evaluation processes. After all, when people perceive that their cases have been treated in a fair manner, this has positive effects on their evaluations whether judges can be trusted and are legitimate powerholders. In contrast, unfair treatment of cases leads to lowered trust and lowered legitimate power of the judges involved in the legal system (Tyler, 2006).

Hulst, Van den Bos, Akkermans, and Lind (2017b) integrated this observation with insights from cognitive psychology and basic social psychology that when people are trying to interpret what is going on, they are inclined to pause momentarily ongoing action to allow for the processing of potentially useful information and cues about what is going on and how to behave (Van den Bos, 2015). In cognitive psychology, these pause-and-check reactions are termed "inhibition effects," since ongoing patterns of behavior are inhibited as information is checked and attitudes and behaviors are processed and relinked (Van den Bos & Lind, 2013). Indeed, there is now a body of psychological research and theory that suggests the behavioral inhibition system (Carver & White 1994; Gray & McNaughton, 2000) is a fundamental psychological system that facilitates sense-making processes (see, e.g., Gable, Reis, & Elliot, 2000; Van den Bos & Lind, 2013). Work on regulatory modes of assessment (i.e., looking and checking) and locomotion (i.e., acting) is also relevant here (e.g., Higgins, 2012; Pierro, Giacomantonio, Pica, Kruglanski, & Higgins, 2011), with the implication that assessment interrupts locomotion.

Based on this line of reasoning, Hulst and colleagues (2017b) proposed that litigants who appear at bankruptcy or criminal court hearings try to make sense of what is going on in the courtroom and whether they can trust and find legitimacy in the system's judges. Furthermore, the behavioral inhibition system is conducive for sense-making processes and is activated when people engage in novel or potentially unsettling or otherwise confusing situations (Van den Bos & Lind, 2013). Hulst and coauthors argued that being summoned to court to have your financial or criminal history discussed is an experience that for most litigants is novel or at least potentially unsettling.

Hulst and colleagues (2017b) assumed that procedural justice serves an important role in these sense-making processes. Thus, in this presumed state of behavioral inhibition, experiences of procedural justice encountered in the courtroom are assumed to be salient and to impact litigants' impressions of how much trust and legitimate power they can assign to judges in their country. Combining all this, Hulst and coauthors proposed that the behavioral inhibition system is likely to be activated when litigants are associating their experiences of procedural justice with their evaluations of trust and evaluations of judges.

Importantly, Hulst and associates (2017b) argued that if this line of reasoning has merit, then it should be the case that weakening the state of behavioral inhibition should attenuate the association between procedural justice and litigants' evaluations of judges. Thus, when an experimental manipulation would deactivate people's behavioral inhibition system (e.g., as can be done by experimentally reminding people about having acted without behavioral inhibitions), then litigants should be less likely to engage in sense-making processes and hence less likely to rely on salient situational cues such as their perceptions of procedural justice when forming trust and legitimacy evaluations of judges. Arguably, then, such an experimental manipulation that has been shown to deactivate people's behavioral inhibition system (see Van den Bos, Müller, & Van Bussel, 2009) should attenuate the positive association between perceived procedural justice and evaluations whether judges in the system can be trusted and should be assigned legitimate power.

Hulst and colleagues (2017b) tested this line of reasoning by means of experimental manipulation in two courtroom experiments. In these experiments, real litigants were (vs. those who were not) reminded about having acted without behavioral inhibitions, a manipulation that is known to deactivate people's behavioral inhibition system without affecting other potentially relevant constructs (Van den Bos et al., 2011). As predicted, findings indicate that this disinhibition manipulation reliably weakened the positive association between procedural justice (as experienced by the litigants during the court hearings) and trust in judges and legitimate power assigned to judges, compared to control conditions in which nothing was made salient or a control topic was made salient.

Thus, in two real-world contexts of the Dutch legal system in which courts take important decisions about bankruptcy or criminal sentences, Hulst and colleagues (2017b) provided evidence for the role of behavioral inhibition in litigants' making sense of court hearings by means of experimental manipulation. The research also suggested a new conceptual reason why there often is a link between perceived procedural justice and trust and legitimacy ratings (see also Hulst, Van den Bos, Akkermans, & Lind, 2017a).

Of course, these are pioneering experiments and much more needs to be done to understand the psychology of people interpreting court hearings in detail. One obvious suggestion for future research would be to examine the differences between people with no court experience and those with multiple experiences. In fact, most people (including the majority of Hulst's litigant participants) encounter a court hearing for the first time, and hence may be inhibited in their responses in their court hearings, but "repeat players" may not be so much inhibited by what is going on, also because of differences in background and the specific legal issues and law cases in which they are involved. Zooming in on these kinds of issues can provide important nuances, much needed for the field of social psychology, including the social psychology of law.

The behavioral inhibition system may also work in other legal contexts. For example, Fishbein and colleagues (2009) observed that many inmates do not respond favorably to standard treatments routinely offered in prison. Executive cognitive functioning and emotional regulation may play a key role in treatment responsivity. Findings indicate that inmates exhibiting a relative lack of behavioral inhibition were less likely to progress favorably in a standard correctional treatment program, more likely to drop out early, and less likely to report improvement in aggressive reactions to provocation. Thus, relative deficits in behavioral inhibition significantly predicted treatment outcomes, more so than background, psychological or behavioral variables, and other neurocognitive and emotional regulatory measures.

Of course, the behavioral inhibition system is certainly not the only factor that affects people's judgments and attributions in the court or of the legal system. Issues such as motivated cognition, need for closure, and need for cognition are important as well. How people attribute causes and responsibilities also plays an important role in court hearings (Borgida & Fiske, 2008). Indeed, "the study of psychology and law is characterized by a bewildering diversity of topics and approaches" (Ellsworth & Mauro, 1998, p. 720), and I can discuss here only some of these topics and approaches. In the next section I examine how people perceive the law outside the courtroom.

Making Sense of Law Outside the Courtroom: Perceiving the Legal System

In the domain of law, often a distinction is made between those who have direct interests at stake in a certain law case versus those who do not have direct interests at stake. From a judicial perspective, only those people with direct interests at stake are considered to be legally relevant, such that they can be involved in the handling of legal cases. This may be so, but even when people are not actively involved in legal cases themselves, they perceive the legal system and try to assess whether the system reveals the truth and serves justice. Furthermore, most people are never in their lives involved in a court case as a legal party with direct interests at stake in the case at hand. Nevertheless, even when not involved in legal cases directly, people scrutinize how the legal system is functioning.

After all, there are important material concerns associated with the working of the legal system. Furthermore, law is a crucial societal institution, and what officials affiliated with the law do has important symbolic value. And a well-functioning legal system conveys that one is living in a fair and just society where good outcomes will be delivered to good people who behave decently, and that those who do not behave in appropriate manners will be given their deserved outcomes. A primary function of law is the creation of legitimacy in society. As such, smooth and just functioning of the law increases objective (legal) and subjective (experienced or psychological) legitimacy of the societal system. In short, there are several reasons why people outside the courtroom (parties with and without direct legal concerns at stake) perceive the legal system and interpret the functioning of legal institutions (e.g., courts), officials constructing laws (e.g., politicians), those enacting the law (e.g., police officers), and people deciding about the law (e.g., judges) in their abilities to deliver justice.

The social psychology of the legal system examines the links between courts and their constituents. Understanding how people perceive the legal system is important, in part because the interconnections of courts/judges and public opinion seems to work in two ways: Some research posits that public preferences influence the behavior of judges and courts, while other studies test the hypothesis that courts and decisions by judges shape public opinion (Gibson, 2010). The social psychology of the legal system is also important because it is related to trust in the law and legitimacy of the law (Tyler, 2006).

The literature on courts and the public is diverse and too vast to cover in detail. I therefore focus on some topics that are relevant for the understanding basic social psychological principles in legal contexts, zooming in on citizens' trust in the law and their perceived legitimacy of the law and the officials working for this societal system. In doing so, I observe that trust in the law and legitimacy of the law is often studied from a macro point of view, examining whether people trust the societal system of law, hence studying issues of institutional trust and institutional legitimacy. Social psychology teaches us, however, that people are often much better and much more oriented toward determining the level of trust they can put in other people, such as judges who are actively handling real cases (Van den Bos, 2011). Thus, studying issues of personal trust is important in understanding trust in law and legitimacy of the law. I argue here that at least two social psychological concepts are relevant for understanding personalized trust in the law: people's social psychological distance from individuals working for the law and people's political and cultural values.

Social psychological distance from officials working for the law is important for how people perceive the legal system, in part because this is related to the amount of information people have about these officials. For example, compared to the mass public, lawyers admitted to federal appellate bars hold very high and robust levels of legitimacy in the Supreme Court, in part because they have much more information about the court and more access to relevant sources of information (Bartels, Johnston, & Mark, 2015). In contrast, only a small proportion of people come in contact with the law in a given year, meaning that most citizens gather and receive information about the law through other sources to form their impressions (Rosenbaum, Lawrence, Hartnett, McDevitt, & Posick, 2015).

In particular, when forming judgments of trust in law, citizens who have no legal education tend to rely on their judgments of trust in persons working for the law, such as judges. Social psychological distance plays an important role in forming these trust judgments. For example, extending observations indicating that the behavioral sciences tend to rely heavily on Western, Educated, Industrialized, Rich, and Democratic (WEIRD) participants (Henrich, Heine, & Norenzayan, 2010), Hulst (2017) argued that studies on trust in law and society may be missing crucial patterns of participant reactions because participants are tested by WEIRD interviewers. Field experiments designed specifically to test this assumption show that when answering questionnaires on degree of trust in law and society as given to them by interviewers presenting themselves as coming from law schools, lower-educated citizens in the Netherlands indicated that they hold high levels of trust in Dutch judges. This pattern replicates a finding that is often seen in trust surveys. Yet when the same interviewer was presented as coming from a lower-educated background, participants reported much less trust in judges.

These findings suggest that social psychological distance between the person observing the legal system and being interviewed about this system versus the perceived (legal authorities and others working for the legal system) and researchers studying trust in the system (e.g., university researchers) plays a crucial role in trust in law and society. In particular, when researchers studying trust in law and society are perceived to come from the same high-status and WEIRD background as those who represent the legal system, this may lead non-WEIRD participants to indicate higher levels of trust in law than they tend to indicate to non-WEIRD interviewers who are lower in societal status than university researchers. This is an important observation at a time of polarization within societies and discontent among groups of lower-educated citizens against the establishment. Lower-educated people perceive social psychological distance to judges and hold low trust in the system's judges, at least under some conditions. In a time when social psychological distance is a growing concern in many societies, this insight into ingroup–outgroup identities and law and social psychology merits future investigation, focusing on underinvestigated participants such as those with lower education.

Perceptions of procedural justice may lead people to accept the law as a system (see also Tyler, 2006). Symbols of judicial authority and legitimacy, such as the robe, the gavel, and the cathedral-like court building, may also help with that. For instance, using an experimental design and a nationally representative sample, Gibson, Lodge, and Woodson (2014) showed that exposure to judicial symbols strengthens the link between institutional support and acquiescence among those with relatively low prior awareness of the Supreme Court and severs the link between disappointment with a disagreeable Court decision and willingness to challenge the ruling. Perhaps repeated presentation of judicial symbols decreases the social psychological distance between citizens and the law, leading these symbols to influence citizens in ways that reinforce the legitimacy of courts.

People's impressions about the law can be subject to biases and hence be unreliable and misleading, particularly when they do not have much information about the working of the law (Rosenbaum et al., 2015). Why, then, would researchers, scholars, and practitioners care about how ordinary people think about the law? First, people are citizens, and their opinions about the legal system need to be considered when laws are passed. Second, when societies create legal codes that deviate from citizens' moral intuitions, citizens can move toward disrespect for the credibility of the legal codes, as they do

no longer feel that the laws are a good guide to right and wrong (Darley & Gromet, 2010). The current wave of protests in Poland and other countries concerning the role of the constitutional court are an example of citizens' discontent with what the authorities are doing with the law. These and other examples indicate the importance of the study of how people perceive the legal system.

The literature on moral psychology is also important in this respect. For example, the typical response to learning about a significant moral transgression is one of moral outrage, based on information about what offenders justly deserve for the wrongs committed. In other words, by default, people tend to focus on punishing the offender when responding to crime. Empirical studies also show, however, that people are willing to make reductions in punishment inflicted on the transgressor if this is conducive to restorative goals that are designed to restore harmony within a community or society. Related to this, the target on which respondents focus—the offender, victim, or community—influences which sanctions they select to achieve justice. Thus, there seems to be reliable evidence for the hypothesis that people's need for punishment does not preclude a desire for restorative sanctions that address repairing the harm to victims and communities caused by wrongdoing. These findings suggest that people view the satisfaction of multiple justice goals as an appropriate and just response to wrongdoing (Gromet & Darley, 2009).

Experimental research also shows that opinions of judicial leniency can be changed by providing respondents with an example of the typical case that comes before the court (Stalans & Diamond, 1990). This indicates that providing relevant information may have some impact on public dissatisfaction with perceived leniency of the criminal justice system (but see St. Amand & Zamble, 2001).

These findings are important, in part because people's political and cultural values influence how they perceive the law as a legal system. For example, people's religious and demographic variables are related to their attitudes toward death penalty and sentencing of verdicts (Miller & Hayward, 2008). Furthermore, liberal participants are more likely to overturn laws that decrease taxes than laws that increase taxes. The opposite pattern holds for conservative participants. This effect is there even when participants believe their policy preferences have no influence on their constitutional decisions (Furgeson, Babcock, & Shane, 2008).

In turn, judges tend to respond to the political and cultural values of citizens. For example, an aggregate time series analysis on a measure of opinion clarity based on multifaceted textual readability scores showed that when Supreme Court judges anticipate public opposition to their decisions, they write clearer opinions (Black, Owens, Wedeking, & Wohlfarth, 2016). Political and other preferences may also impact legal experts, at least to some extent. For example, lawyers and legal scholars tend to respond to anti-terrorist military practice of targeted killings by relying on both the facts of the case and their policy preferences (Sulitzeanu-Kenan, Kremnitzer, & Alon, 2016).

Concluding Remarks

I wrote this chapter based on my expertise as a social psychologist (specialized in experimental social psychology of fairness and justice judgments) and my experience working at a law school for some years now (focusing on empirical legal studies). Based on this expertise and this experience, my aim was to briefly review social psychology in legal contexts to a broad audience of students and teachers in law schools and psychology programs, as well as practitioners working in various legal domains and others who are interested in the bridge between social psychology and law.

Importantly, I note explicitly that in the current review of social psychology in legal contexts, I have not discussed several important topics relevant for the intersection of social psychology and law. What I have discussed is four areas of psychological research organized in two basic social psychological principles and two legal contexts. Taken together, these areas, principles, and contexts may provide a taxonomy of the social psychology of law. In this taxonomy, the principles and contexts on which I focused on are to some extent interrelated. For example, people perceiving the legal system often evaluate it in terms of whether the truth is revealed by the system and, hence, whether justice is being done. Nevertheless, I hope to have shown that trying to systematize the social psychology of law by breaking it into four areas of research with different foci and points of interest makes sense and can help to further the science and practice of law (see also Haney, 1980).

Importantly, insight into the social psychology of law is not merely an application of basic social psychological principles in legal contexts. Rather, it is my experience that studying social psychology and the law often provides insights that may well feed into basic social psychological research. For example, we have seen that behavioral inhibition processes serve an important role in processes of interpretation and sense making, and not only in anxiety, fear, and stress (Hulst et al., 2017b). We have discussed that "WEIRDness" and social psychological distance may be more important in survey interviews than we often realize (Hulst, 2017). Law and psychology have worked together beautifully to reveal the relevance and validity of eyewitness reports in important court hearings (Loftus, 1975, 2013). And we saw how judgments of injustice feel so real and genuine to people that these judgments can impact processes of radicalization (Van den Bos, 2018).

All these issues have obvious societal relevance and can be examined in research programs with high levels of both internal and external validity, which is something modern social psychology really needs (Kruglanski et al., 2017). Furthermore, there is a tendency in current social psychology to generalize too much on the basis of too small sets of research studies that rely too much on overstudied research participants (e.g., university students or participants from online platforms such as Mechanical Turk). The result sometimes is a rather feeble basis and on occasion too abstract or overgeneralized theoretical frameworks. In contrast, the study of law tends to focus strongly on particulars of specific contexts, and to refrain from generalizations across contexts. As such, the study of law can provide contextual nuances much needed for a more precise, more robust, and more relevant social psychological science. The study of law may also stimulate social psychologists to stop their overreliance on laboratory experimentation and start using other research methods such as archival and observation studies and qualitative in-depth interviews more actively, creating a more balanced treatment of research methodology.

With these positive notes on the integration of social psychology and law, I do not want to underestimate the important differences in assumptions, conventions, interests, and orientations of the two disciplines. For example, social psychologists are comfortable with aggregate data. In contrast, lawyers reason on a case-by-case basis, searching the record for particular cases that match the one at hand, and looking for ways to distinguish a case from apparently similar cases. Many lawyers resist having to decide a person's fate on the basis of empirical data drawn from other people, no matter how large or representative the sample. Furthermore, social psychologists are comfortable thinking in terms of probabilities and making explicit quantified probability judgments. Although most legal judgments are probabilistic, many legal scholars are uncomfortable about making the probabilities explicit. Moreover, social psychologists are comfortable thinking in terms of continuous variables. The law's task is to draw lines, to create what to a psychologist are suspect dichotomies: sane or insane, fit or unfit to be a parent, voluntary or involuntary (Ellsworth & Mauro, 1998).

Twining (2009) has argued that—for understandable reasons—a great deal of legal research with an empirical dimension has been oriented toward policy or law reform, or other kinds of immediate practical decision making. "Many such enquiries are particular rather than general, not illuminated by theory, do not claim to be explanatory or predictive, and their findings do not accumulate" (Twining, 2009, p. 50). By focusing on some basic principles of social psychology in legal contexts, I hope this chapter contributes to the conceptual and empirical development of the exciting social psychological science of law.

ACKNOWLEDGMENTS

I thank Lisa Ansems, Hilke Grootelaar, Arie Kruglanski, and Paul van Lange for their comments and suggestions on earlier versions of this chapter.

REFERENCES

Allport, G. W. (1985). The historical background of social psychology. In G. Lindzey & E. Aronson (Eds.), *The handbook of social psychology* (3rd ed., Vol. 1, pp. 1–46). New York: McGraw-Hill.

Bandes, S. A., & Blumenthal, J. A. (2012). Emotion and the law. *Annual Review of Law and Social Science, 8,* 161–181.

Bartels, B. L., Johnston, C. D., & Mark, A. (2015). Lawyers' perceptions of the U.S. Supreme Court: Is the court a "political" institution? *Law and Society Review, 49,* 761–794.

Beauchamp, T. L. (2001). *Philosophical ethics: An introduction to moral philosophy* (3rd ed.). Boston: McGraw-Hill.

Black, R. C., Owens, R. J., Wedeking, J., & Wohlfarth, P. C. (2016). The influence of public sentiment on Supreme Court opinion clarity. *Law and Society Review, 50,* 703–732.

Bond, G. D. (2008). Deception detection expertise. *Law and Human Behavior, 32,* 339–351.

Borgida, E., & Fiske, S. T. (Eds.). (2008). *Beyond common sense: Psychological science in the courtroom.* Malden, MA: Blackwell.

Brockner, J., & Wiesenfeld, B. M. (1996). An integrative framework for explaining reactions to decisions: Interactive effects of outcomes and procedures. *Psychological Bulletin, 120,* 189–208.

Carver, C. S., & White, T. L. (1994). Behavioral inhibition, behavioral activation, and affective responses to impending reward and punishment: The BIS/BAS scales. *Journal of Personality and Social Psychology, 67,* 319–333.

Cho, K., Barnes, C. M., & Guanara, C. L. (2017). Sleepy punishers are harsh punishers: Daylight saving time and legal sentences. *Psychological Science, 28,* 242–247.

Danziger, S., Levav, J., & Avnaim-Pesso, L. (2011). Extraneous factors in judicial decisions. *Proceedings of the National Academy of Sciences of the USA, 17,* 6889–6892.

Darley, J. M. (2001). Citizens' sense of justice and the legal system. *Current Directions in Psychological Science, 10,* 10–13.

Darley, J. M., & Gromet, D. M. (2010). The psychology of punishment: Intuition and reason, retribution and restoration. In D. R. Bobocel, A. C. Kay, M. P. Zanna, & J. M. Olson (Eds.), *The psychology of justice and legitimacy: The Ontario Symposium* (Vol. 11, pp. 229–250). New York: Psychology Press.

Ellemers, N. (2013). Connecting the dots: Mobilizing theory to reveal the big picture in social psychology (and why we should do this). *European Journal of Social Psychology, 43,* 1–8.

Ellsworth, P. C., & Gross, S. (2013). False convictions. In E. Shafir (Ed.), *The behavioral foundations of public policy* (pp. 163–180). Princeton, NJ: Princeton University Press.

Ellsworth, P. C., & Mauro, R. (1998). Psychology and law. In D. T. Gilbert, S. T. Fiske, & G. Lindzey (Eds.), *The handbook of social psychology* (4th ed., Vol. 2, pp. 684–732). Boston: McGraw-Hill.

Finkel, N. J. (1995). *Commonsense justice: Jurors' notions of the law.* Cambridge, MA: Harvard University Press.

Fishbein, D., Sheppard, M., Hyde, C., Hubal, R., Newlin, D., Serin, R., et al. (2009). Deficits in behavioral inhibition predict treatment engagement in prison inmates. *Law and Human Behavior, 33,* 419–435.

Fiske, S. T., & Borgida, E. (2008). Providing expert knowledge in an adversarial context: Social-cognitive science in employment discrimination cases. *Annual Review of Law and Social Science, 4,* 123–148.

Furgeson, J. R., Babcock, L., & Shane, P. M. (2008). Do a law's policy implications affect beliefs about its constitutionality?: An experimental test. *Law and Human Behavior, 32,* 219–227.

Gable, S. L., Reis, H. T., & Elliot, A. J. (2000). Behavioral activation and inhibition in everyday life. *Journal of Personality and Social Psychology, 78,* 1135–1149.

Gibson, J. L. (2010). Public images and understanding of courts. In P. Cane & H. M. Kritzer (Eds.), *The Oxford handbook of empirical legal research* (pp. 828–853). Oxford, UK: Oxford University Press.

Gibson, J. L., Lodge, M., & Woodson, B. (2014). Losing, but accepting: Legitimacy, positivity theory, and the symbols of judicial authority. *Law and Society Review, 48,* 837–866.

Glaser, J., Martin, K. D., & Kahn, K. B. (2015). Possibility of death sentence has divergent effect on verdicts for Black and White defendants. *Law and Human Behavior, 39,* 539–546.

Gray, J. A., & McNaughton, N. (2000). *The neuropsychology of anxiety: An enquiry into the functions of the septo-hippocampal system.* Oxford, UK: Oxford University Press.

Gromet, D. M., & Darley, J. M. (2009). Punishment and beyond: Achieving justice through the satisfaction of multiple goals. *Law and Society Review, 43,* 1–37.

Grootelaar, H. A. M., & Van den Bos, K. (2018). How litigants in Dutch courtrooms come to trust judges: The role of perceived procedural justice, outcome favorability, and other socio-legal moderators. *Law and Society Review, 52,* 234–268.

Guthrie, C., Rachlinski, J. J., & Wistrich, A. J. (2001). Inside the judicial mind. *Cornell Law Review, 86,* 777–830.

Guthrie, C., Rachlinski, J. J., & Wistrich, A. J. (2007). Blinking on the bench: How judges decide cases. *Cornell Law Review, 93,* 1–43.

Ham, J., Van den Bos, K., & Van Doorn, E. A. (2009). Lady Justice thinks unconsciously: Unconscious thought can lead to more accurate justice judgments. *Social Cognition, 27,* 509–521.

Haney, C. (1980). Psychology and legal change: On the limits of factual jurisprudence. *Law and Human Behavior, 4,* 147–199.

Henrich, J., Heine, S. J., & Norenzayan, A. (2010). The weirdest people in the world? *Behavioral and Brain Sciences, 33,* 61–83.

Herzog, S., & Oreg, S. (2008). Chivalry and the moderating effect of ambivalent sexism: Individual differences in crime seriousness judgments. *Law and Society Review, 42,* 45–74.

Higgins, E. T. (2012). *Beyond pleasure and pain: How motivation works.* New York: Oxford University Press.

Hollander-Blumoff, R. (2011). The psychology of procedural justice in the federal courts. *Hastings Law Journal, 63,* 127–178.

Hulst, L. (2017). *Experimental legal studies on perceived procedural justice and trust in law and society.* Unpublished doctoral dissertation, Vrije Universiteit Amsterdam, Amsterdam, the Netherlands.

Hulst, L., Van den Bos, K., Akkermans, A. J., & Lind, E. A. (2017a). On the psychology of perceived procedural justice: Experimental evidence that behavioral inhibition strenghtens reactions to voice and no-voice procedures. *Frontiers in Psychological and Behavioral Science, 6,* 1–12.

Hulst, L., Van den Bos, K., Akkermans, A. J., & Lind, E. A. (2017b). On why procedural justice matters in court hearings: Experimental evidence that behavioral disinhibition weakens the association between procedural justice and evaluations of judges. *Utrecht Law Review, 13*(3), 114–129.

Hume, D. (1951). *A treatise of human nature.* Oxford, UK: Clarendon. (Original work published 1739–1740)

Kassin, S. M., Drizin, S. A., Grisso, T., Gudjonsson, G. H., Leo, R. A., & Redlich, A. D. (2010). Police-induced confessions: Risk factors and recommendations. *Law and Human Behavior, 34,* 3–38.

Kovera, M. B., & Borgida, E. (2010). Social psychology and law. In S. T. Fiske, D. T. Gilbert, & G. Lindzey (Eds.), *Handbook of social psychology* (5th ed., Vol. 2, pp. 1343–1385). Hoboken, NJ: Wiley.

Kruglanski, A. W. (1989). *Lay epistemics and human knowledge: Cognitive and motivational bases.* New York: Plenum Press.

Kruglanski, A. W., Chernikova, M., & Jasko, K. (2017). Social psychology circa 2016: A field on steroids. *European Journal of Social Psychology, 47,* 1–10.

Lind, E. A., & Tyler, T. R. (1988). *The social psychology of procedural justice.* New York: Plenum Press.

Loftus, E. (1975). Leading questions and the eyewitness report. *Cognitive Psychology, 7,* 560–572.

Loftus, E. F. (2013). 25 years of eyewitness science . . . finally pays off. *Perspectives on Psychological Science, 8,* 556–557.

Loftus, E. F., & Greenspan, R. L. (2017). If I'm certain, is it true?: Accuracy and confidence in eyewitness memory. *Psychological Science in the Public Interest, 18,* 1–2.

Maas, M., & Van den Bos, K. (2009). An affective–experiential perspective on reactions to fair and unfair events: Individual differences in affect intensity moderated by experiential mindsets. *Journal of Experimental Social Psychology, 45,* 667–675.

McAuliff, B. D., Kovera, M. B., & Nunez, G. (2009). Can jurors recognize missing control groups, confounds, and experimenter bias in psychological science? *Law and Human Behavior, 33,* 247–257.

Miller, M. K., & Hayward, D. R. (2008). Religious characteristics and the death penalty. *Law and Human Behavior, 32,* 113–123.

Moghaddam, F. M. (2005). The staircase to terrorism: A psychological exploration. *American Psychologist, 60,* 161–169.

O'Sullivan, M., Frank, M. G., Hurley, C. M., & Tiwana, J. (2009). Police lie detection accuracy: The effect of lie scenario. *Law and Human Behavior, 33,* 530–538.

Pierro, A., Giacomantonio, M., Pica, G., Kruglanski, A. W., & Higgins, E. T. (2011). On the psychology of time in action: Regulatory mode orientations and procrastination. *Journal of Personality and Social Psychology, 101,* 1317–1331.

Robertson, G. (2013). *Crimes against humanity: The struggle for global justice* (4th ed.). New York: New Press.

Rosenbaum, D., Lawrence, D. S., Hartnett, S. M., McDevitt, J., & Posick, C. (2015). Measuring procedural justice and legitimacy at the local level: The police–community interaction survey. *Journal of Experimental Criminology, 11,* 335–366.

Salerno, J. M., & Peter-Hagene, L. C. (2013). The interactive effect of anger and disgust on moral outrage and judgments. *Psychological Science, 24,* 2069–2078.

Schuller, R. A., Kazoleas, V., & Kawakami, K. (2009). The impact of prejudice screening procedures on racial bias in the courtroom. *Law and Human Behavior, 33,* 320–328.

St. Amand, M. D., & Zamble, E. (2001). Impact of information about sentencing decisions on public attitudes toward the criminal justice system. *Law and Human Behavior, 25,* 515–528.

Stalans, L. J., & Diamond, S. S. (1990). Formation and change in lay evaluations of criminal sentencing. *Law and Human Behavior, 14,* 199–214.

Stangor, C. (2011). *Principles of social psychology.* Nyack, NY: Flat World Knowledge.

Steblay, N. K., & Loftus, E. F. (2013). Eyewitness identification and the legal system. In E. Shafir (Ed.), *The behavioral foundations of policy* (pp. 145–162). Princeton, NJ: Princeton University Press.

Sulitzeanu-Kenan, R., Kremnitzer, M., & Alon, S. (2016). Facts, preferences, and doctrine: An empirical analysis of proportionality judgment. *Law and Society Review, 50,* 348–382.

Thibaut, J., & Walker, L. (1975). *Procedural justice: A psychological analysis.* Hillsdale, NJ: Erlbaum.

Thomas, W. I., & Thomas, D. S. (1928). *The child in America: Behavior problems and programs.* New York: Knopf.

Twining, W. (2009). *General jurisprudence: Understanding law from a global perspective.* Cambridge, UK: Cambridge University Press.

Tyler, T. R. (2006). *Why people obey the law.* Princeton, NJ: Princeton University Press.

Tyler, T. R., & Jost, J. T. (2007). Psychology and the law: Reconciling normative and descriptive accounts of social justice and system legitimacy. In A. W. Kruglanski & E. T. Higgins (Eds.), *Social psychology: Handbook of basic principles* (2nd ed., pp. 807–825). New York: Guilford Press.

Van den Bos, K. (2003). On the subjective quality of social justice: The role of affect as information in the psychology of justice judgments. *Journal of Personality and Social Psychology, 85,* 482–498.

Van den Bos, K. (2005). What is responsible for the fair process effect? In J. Greenberg & J. A. Colquitt (Eds.), *Handbook of organizational justice: Fundamental questions about fairness in the workplace* (pp. 273–300). Mahwah, NJ: Erlbaum.

Van den Bos, K. (2011). *Vertrouwen in de overheid [Trust in government].* The Hague, the Netherlands: Ministry of the Interior and Kingdom Relations.

Van den Bos, K. (2015). Humans making sense of alarming conditions: Psychological insight into the fair process effect. In R. S. Cropanzano & M. L. Ambrose (Eds.), *Oxford handbook of justice in work organizations* (pp. 403–417). New York: Oxford University Press.

Van den Bos, K. (2018). *Why people radicalize: How unfairness judgments are used to fuel radical beliefs, extremist behaviors, and terrorism.* New York: Oxford University Press.

Van den Bos, K., & Lind, E. A. (2009). The social psychology of fairness and the regulation of personal uncertainty. In R. M. Arkin, K. C. Oleson, & P. J. Carroll (Eds.), *Handbook of the uncertain self* (pp. 122–141). New York: Psychology Press.

Van den Bos, K., & Lind, E. A. (2013). On sense-making reactions and public inhibition of benign social motives: An appraisal model of prosocial behavior. In J. M. Olson & M. P. Zanna (Eds.), *Advances in experimental social psychology* (Vol. 48, pp. 1–58). San Diego, CA: Academic Press.

Van den Bos, K., McGregor, I., & Martin, L. L. (2015). Security and uncertainty in contemporary delayed-return cultures: Coping with the blockage of personal goals. In P. J. Carroll, R. M. Arkin, & A. L. Wichman (Eds.), *Handbook of personal security* (pp. 21–35). New York: Psychology Press.

Van den Bos, K., Müller, P. A., & Van Bussel, A. A. L. (2009). Helping to overcome intervention inertia in bystander's dilemmas: Behavioral disinhibition can improve the greater good. *Journal of Experimental Social Psychology, 45,* 873–878.

Van den Bos, K., Van Lange, P. A. M., Lind, E. A., Venhoeven, L. A., Beudeker, D. A., Cramwinckel, F. M., et al. (2011). On the benign qualities of behavioral disinhibition: Because of the prosocial nature of people, behavioral disinhibition can weaken pleasure with getting more than you deserve. *Journal of Personality and Social Psychology, 101,* 791–811.

Van Veldhuizen, T. S., Horselenberg, R., Landström, S., Granhag, P. A., & van Koppen, P. J. (2017). Interviewing asylum seekers: A vignette study on the questions asked to assess credibility of claims about origin and persecution. *Journal of Investigative Psychology and Offender Profiling, 14,* 3–22.

Van Veldhuizen, T. S., Maas, R. P. A. E., Horselenberg, R., & Van Koppen, P. J. (2018) Establishing origin: Analysing the questions asked in asylum interviews. *Psychiatry, Psychology, and Law, 25,* 283–302.

Vredeveldt, A., Hildebrandt, A., & Van Koppen, P. J. (2016). Acknowledge, repeat, rephrase, elaborate: Witnesses can help each other remember more. *Memory, 24,* 669–682.

Vrij, A. (1993). An impression formation framework on police prejudice: An overview of experiments on perceptual bias in police-citizen interaction. *Police Studies: International Review of Police Development, 16,* 28–32.

Vrij, A., Mann, S. A., Fisher, R. P., Leal, S., Milne, R., & Bull, R. (2008). Increasing cognitive load to facilitate lie detection: The benefit of recalling an event in reverse order. *Law and Human Behavior, 32,* 253–265.

Wagenaar, W. A. (1988). *Identifying Ivan: A case study in legal psychology.* New York: Harvester-Wheatsheaf.

Wells, G. L., & Turtle, J. W. (1986). Eyewitness identification: The importance of lineup models. *Psychological Bulletin, 99,* 320–329.

Wixted, J. T., & Wells, G. L. (2017). The relationship between eyewitness confidence and identification accuracy: A new synthesis. *Psychological Science in the Public Interest, 18,* 10–65.

CHAPTER 27

Psychological Shortcomings
to Optimal Negotiation Behavior
Intrapersonal and Interpersonal Challenges

Martha Jeong
Julia Minson
Francesca Gino

A *negotiation* is defined as an interaction in which individuals with mixed motives are communicating with each other in order to resolve their perceived divergent interests and reach their individual goals (Ben-Yoav & Pruitt, 1984). Negotiations can be either informal or formal in nature and they govern almost all of our social relationships (Ben-Yoav & Pruitt, 1984). Given that an effective negotiation requires a delicate balance of both cooperation and competition with others (Pruitt, 1983), negotiators often fail to maximize on both their individual and joint outcomes for various reasons (Nadler, Thompson, & van Boven, 2003; Neale & Bazerman, 1991).

As consequential negotiations pervade both our personal and professional relationships, it is important to understand the common shortcomings that stand in the way of our ability to negotiate successfully. In this chapter, we review some basic psychological challenges that stand in the way of optimal negotiation behavior and outcomes. For a review of basic negotiation and psychology-related principles, please refer to Table 27.1. On the intrapersonal level, we examine a pervasive cognitive bias, as well as the role of affect, in influencing negotiation behavior

and outcomes. On the interpersonal level, we explore the extent to which social perceptions of our opponent's economic and noneconomic behavior drive our negotiation strategies.

Intrapersonal Challenge:
Cognitive Bias

One of the most common and pervasive cognitive biases that negatively influences a negotiator's attitude and subsequent behavior is the fixed-pie belief (Bazerman & Neale, 1983; Fisher, Ury, & Patton, 2011; Thompson & Hastie, 1990). It is the perception that one's own interests are completely and diametrically opposed to an opponent's interests (Bazerman & Neale, 1983; Fisher et al., 2011; Thompson & Hastie, 1990). It has been identified as a bias because negotiators often adopt this belief in situations in which it does not apply, resulting in suboptimal negotiation behavior. Why do we hold this self-defeating belief? What are the psychological mechanisms attributing to this bias? How common is it? What are the consequences that follow? Have researchers been able to identify any effective interventions?

TABLE 27.1. Summary of Negotiation and Psychological Principles

Negotiation principles

Distributive negotiation: Single-issue, competitive negotiations, in which one player's gains are in a direct inverse relationship to the other player's losses, such as a one-off sales negotiation between a buyer and seller (Thompson, 2009).

Integrative negotiation: Multi-issue negotiations, in which the negotiators' goals are both cooperative and competitive in nature, so that value creation is possible (Fisher et al., 2011; Lax & Sebenius, 1986; Pruitt, 1991; Thompson, 2009).

Logrolling: A negotiation strategy that involves making beneficial trades across issues based on understanding a counterpart's preferences (Pruitt & Rubin, 1986).

BATNA: The best alternative to a negotiated agreement (Raiffa, 1982; White & Neale, 1991).

Psychological principles

Fixed-pie belief: Perception that one's own interests are completely and diametrically opposed to an opponent's interests (Bazerman & Neale, 1983; Fisher et al., 2011; Thompson & Hastie, 1990).

Egocentrism: Heavily focused on one's own situation, interests, or preferences, so that one fails to appropriately recognize a counterpart's situation (Chambers & de Dreu, 2014).

Naive realism: Belief that we perceive the world objectively, while those who disagree with us are biased or irrational (Pronin, Gilovich, & Ross, 2004).

Fundamental attribution error: Tendency to attribute behavior to personality, rather than situational demands (Ross, 1977).

Correspondence bias: Drawing inferences about another person based on his or her behaviors and attributing them to a person's dispositions rather than the situation (Gilbert & Malone, 1995; Jones, 1990).

Before we dive into the intricacies of the fixed-pie bias, we must first distinguish between two different types of negotiations: distributive and integrative negotiations. *Distributive negotiations* are single-issue negotiations, in which motives are purely competitive in nature (Thompson, 2009). Two or more players can be seen as "splitting the pie," so that one player's gains are in a direct inverse relationship to the other player's losses. A typical distributive negotiation would be a one-time sales negotiation between a buyer and seller, in which the single issue at stake is the price of the item or service.

Integrative negotiations, on the other hand, are multi-issue negotiations, in which the negotiators' goals are both cooperative and competitive in nature (Fisher et al., 2011; Lax & Sebenius, 1986; Pruitt, 1991; Thompson, 2009). By cultivating a trusting relationship and sharing critical information with each other, negotiators can identify ways for value creation, so that joint benefits can be reached as the "size of the pie grows" (de Dreu, Weingart, & Kwon, 2000; Pruitt & Lewis, 1975). A common integrative

negotiation would be an employment agreement in which multiple issues can be discussed and decided, such as salary, vacation days, bonus payments, retirement plans, stock/equity interest, insurance, relocation costs, starting date, and so forth.

While the majority of our negotiations can be considered integrative in nature with a potential for a "win–win" situation, a common shortcoming is to perceive them as distributive (Deutsch, 1973). This faulty belief in seeing negotiations as a fixed pie stems from our psychological tendencies to be egocentric; to fail to perspective-take; and to act as naive realists (Chambers & de Dreu, 2014; de Dreu, Koole & Steinel, 2000; Galinsky, Ku, & Wang, 2005; Pronin, Gilovich, & Ross, 2004). Our egocentrism causes us to focus heavily on our own situation, interests, and preferences, and we fail to perspective-take by appropriately recognizing how our opponent's situation may differ from ours (Chambers & de Dreu, 2014). As naive realists, we perceive ourselves to be objective, so that when we see others acting differently than we would have expected them to, we infer that others are biased, unreasonable, or acting under questionable motivations (Pronin et al., 2004).

Consequently, in the negotiation context, our fixed-pie bias will have us believe that our opponent's interests similarly mirror our own interests; therefore, we see each other's interests as being completely opposed in nature (de Dreu et al., 2000). In this way, we may see more conflict than there really is and erroneously believe the negotiation needs to be more contentious. With this bias, we fail to properly consider the ways in which our opponent may have different priorities or interests that we can use to our advantage to "expand the pie."

When surveyed, the majority of negotiators believe that their interests are incompatible with those of their opponents, so that one person's gain will be felt as another person's loss (Thompson & Hastie, 1990). This fixed-pie bias that negotiations are "win–lose" by nature is particularly strong among untrained, naive negotiators (O'Connor & Adams, 1999). When novice negotiators were asked to describe a common negotiation scheme, they invoked negotiations that involved competitive, incompatible interests in which negotiators sequentially resolved issues (O'Connor & Adams, 1999). More expert negotiators, however, are better able to see negotiations in a broader sense, as something that involves problem solving between parties with both compatible and competitive goals where interests can be played off each other (O'Connor & Adams, 1999).

The fixed-pie bias makes negotiators feel that an impasse is imminent and cooperation is unnecessary, and it results in issues being resolved one at a time. Negotiators often make the mistake of thinking there is only one issue to resolve; therefore, they focus on one issue at a time, usually the most salient one. In reality there are often several issues that can be negotiated together; however, they can be "hidden" and only become known when efforts are made to uncover them. The fixed-pie bias is most often triggered in negotiations that involve resolving interests (e.g., time and money) that invoke concepts of winning or losing, compared to intellectual or evaluative negotiations in which individuals are discussing, resolving, and problem-solving cognitive or value conflicts (Harinck, de Dreu, & Van Vianen, 2000).

This fixed-pie mindset and resulting behavior are not helpful, however, because in order to come to mutually beneficial integrative agreements, a number of things must happen: (1) Issues of joint value must be identified and voiced and (2) "logrolling" of issues must occur (Pruitt & Rubin, 1986). In other words, negotiators must find compatible interests and trade-off issues in such a way that each negotiator achieves most of his or her preferred outcomes on substantial issues, in exchange for concessions on less important issues, a negotiation strategy known as "logrolling" (Froman & Cohen, 1970). These integrative strategies, however, will be hampered if at least one of the negotiators succumbs to the fixed-pie belief.

Negotiators who hold fixed-pie perceptions of the negotiation often commit two common errors in relation to information disclosure: They may seek out far less than they should about diagnostic information the counterpart holds, and they may erroneously believe that disclosing any of their own information will be harmful (Thompson, 1991, 2009).

Many negotiations in the real world involve asymmetry in the information known between the two parties (Wolfe & McGinn, 2005). The ability to reach mutual gains depends on the exchange of critical information (Thompson, 1991, 2009). Negotiators who are able to consider the constraints and goals of their counterpart by eliciting diagnostic information are more successful (Galinsky, Maddux, Gilin, & White, 2008). Given that negotiators operating under the fixed-pie bias mistakenly believe that they know their counterpart's interests, they fail to search further for relevant information, such as asking their partners pertinent questions about what they value (Pinkley, Griffith, & Northcraft, 1995).

The sharing of information related to underlying interests, priorities, and key facts is important for maximizing the pie (Thompson, 1991, 2009). This kind of information can reveal important differences the parties have on their valuations of certain issues, expectations of certain events happening, as well as differences in capabilities, attitudes toward risk, and also time preferences (Thompson, 1991, 2009). Knowing and capitalizing on these differences can lead to the discovery of mutually beneficial outcomes in integrative agreements; unfortunately, the fixed-pie belief stymies efforts to ask for and exchange relevant information in an effective manner. Not surprisingly, research indicates that negotiators with a fixed-pie belief come to agreements that are less than optimal (Pinkley et al., 1995; Thompson, 1991; Thompson & Hastie, 1990). Not only do negotiators holding this belief make errors in information availability (not asking or exchanging relevant information), but they also make errors in information processing (Pinkley et al., 1995). In other words, even when relevant information is available to them, the negotiators ignore and/or distort that information because they do not recognize its value (Carroll, Bazerman, & Maury, 1988; Neale & Northcraft, 1991; Pinkley et al., 1995).

Overall, researchers have found that, unfortunately, this cognitive bias in fixed-pie perceptions is not only common but also persistent relative to knowledge, general negotiation experience, and direct feedback (Thompson, 1990, 1991; Thompson & DeHarpport, 1994). The kind of interventions that have been identified as successful tend to be more nuanced in nature and attempt to defeat this persistent bias through either cognitive or motivational means.

For example, researchers have found that specific and recent experience with integrative strategies, such as logrolling, can assist negotiators in recognizing integrative potential in different negotiation contexts (Thompson, 1990). This cognitive approach suggests that negotiators who are regularly trained in integrative negotiation skills, such as asking questions about a counterpart's interests and priorities and revealing one's own, may be more apt in recognizing compatible interests and creating joint value in a future negotiation (Thompson, 1990). Negotiators who actively engage in cognitive perspective taking can also overcome the pitfalls of the fixed-pie bias. Attempting to see the world through a counterpart's eyes can reduce contentious tactics and improve coordination issues (Galinsky et al., 2005).

A motivational account has been found to be successful in reducing the fixed-pie bias (Carnevale & Isen, 1986; de Dreu et al., 2000). Negotiators who are instructed to justify their behavior are more likely to deliberately and systematically process information, leading them to overcome the more automatic fixed-pie approach to a negotiation (de Dreu et al., 2000). Negotiators who are prosocially motivated, in comparison to those who are egoistically or individually motivated, have often been found to reach integrative potential because they are more likely to revise their fixed-pie perceptions and focus on joint benefits (Carnevale & Isen, 1986).

Intrapersonal Challenge: The Role of Affect

In addition to the cognitive bias of the fixed-pie belief, which stems from our psychological tendencies to be egocentric, fail to perspective-take, and to act as naive realists, a negotiator's individual felt or expressed affect may also surprisingly and detrimentally shape negotiation behavior and outcomes. Both moods and emotions can affect negotiations in fundamental ways. Moods are characterized as being diffuse in nature, varying along a single dimension, ranging from a positive to negative valence (Forgas, 1998). Transient moods have been shown to materially affect a negotiator's behavior (Carnevale & Isen, 1986; Forgas, 1998). For example, positive moods such as incidental happiness triggered by the experimenter resulted in a negotiator being more cooperative in planned and reported bargaining strategies, in comparison to negative moods, such as sadness (Forgas, 1998). Similarly, a positive mood reduced the use of contentious bargaining tactics and increased the use of integrative negotiation strategies (Carnevale & Isen, 1986).

Emotions, on the other hand, are defined as being more discrete in nature and experienced for a shorter period of time (Smith & Ellsworth, 1985). Emotions that affect negotiations can arise from incidents unrelated to the negotiation or triggered from the negotiation itself (Lerner, Small, & Loewenstein, 2004). Emotions that affect negotiations can be *self-directed* (emotional states experienced only by the self but affecting negotiation behavior) or other-directed.

A common self-directed emotional state that has been identified as materially changing negotiation behavior is anxiety (Brooks & Schweitzer, 2011). Anxiety was identified by negotiators as one of the most commonly and strongly felt emotional states prior to entering a negotiation, and researchers have found that it negatively influences negotiation behavior and outcomes (Brooks & Schweitzer, 2011). Negotiators who felt anxious entering a negotiation were more likely to expect an inferior outcome, to make less ambitious first offers, to take less time to respond to offers, to exit negotiations early, and ultimately to suffer in obtaining optimal outcomes (Brooks & Schweitzer, 2011). One way this harmful anxiety can be mitigated, however, is to boost the anxious negotiator's sense of self-efficacy as a competent negotiator (Brooks & Schweitzer, 2011).

Much research has been directed at understanding the way in which other-directed emotions affect negotiations, where emotions are seen as serving specific social functions over the course of the negotiation (Morris & Keltner, 2000). Two commonly studied emotions in the negotiation context are anger and compassion (Allred, Mallozzi, Matsui, & Raia, 1997). Anger expression has been linked to both negative and positive outcomes in a negotiation. These conflicting results point to important moderating factors that determine whether anger can hurt or help in a negotiation. Strategic expressions of anger, as operationalized through facial and physical expressions and aggressive word choice, are associated with greater value claiming, but only when recipients of the anger have poor alternatives (Sinaceur & Tiedens, 2006).

Anger is theorized to elicit compliance because negotiators "track" each other's emotional states (Van Kleef, de Dreu, & Manstead, 2004). Negotiators are therefore more likely to concede when they interact with angry counterparts rather than happy counterparts because they feel the need to make concessions in order to avoid an impasse (Van Kleef et al., 2004). For example, research indicates that negotiators who expressed anger via electronic negotiation achieved higher individual outcomes than negotiators who expressed happiness (Belkin, Kurtzberg, & Naquin, 2013). Interestingly, as negotiators become limited in their motivation or ability to consider their counterpart's emotional states, these effects disappear (Van Kleef et al., 2004). Strategic expressions of anger can convey an upper hand in the negotiation and

therefore elicit compliance when the recipient infers the anger to signal a potential impasse and to the extent that the recipient fears an impasse because of poor alternatives.

Other empirical researchers have come to the opposite finding that positive emotions such as friendliness, cooperativeness, and empathy are more effective at eliciting compliance in a negotiation than negative emotions such as anger and aggression (Kopelman, Rosette, & Thompson, 2006). In the context of an ultimatum, negotiators are more effective in gaining concessions from the other side with positive emotional displays over negative ones (Kopelman et al., 2006). In order to make sense of these conflicting empirical findings, other scholars have presented a dual-process model to understand how strategic emotional expressions can help negotiators by extracting concessions but also hurt negotiators by eliciting competition (Van Kleef & Côté, 2007).

The dual-process model posits that two important factors in whether anger will hurt or help are the perceived appropriateness of the anger and the amount of power that the recipient of the anger has in the negotiation (Van Kleef & Côté, 2007). High-power negotiators are unaffected by inappropriate anger, whereas low-power negotiators concede to angry opponents regardless of the anger's inappropriateness (Van Kleef & Côté, 2007). Strategically expressing anger in a negotiation can be one way to use emotional displays to gain an upper hand in the negotiation. As negotiators think about using this strategy, however, they must take into account a number of factors that shape whether the anger expression will hurt or help their negotiation goals, including the appropriateness of the anger (as perceived by the counterpart), the type of negotiation at stake (one time vs. repeated interactions), and the extent to which their counterpart has good alternatives to the negotiation.

Interpersonal Challenge: Social Perception

The role of social perception in mixed-motive conflicts is interesting because of the ubiquitous nature of negotiations in our professional and personal lives, and because social psychologists have found interpersonal conflict to be a context in which individuals routinely perceive and attribute their counterpart's behavior to personality traits, which in turn affect reactions and conflict resolution strategies (Orvis, Kelley, & Butler, 1976; Thompson & Hastie, 1990). In general, our ability to recognize and enact the optimal strategies in a negotiation ultimately determines negotiation outcomes (Malhotra & Bazerman, 2008).

Theories on conflict resolution suggest that the strategies selected by the negotiators are often determined by the negotiator's perceptions and attributions of the counterpart's behavior (Schelling, 1980). The two fundamental dimensions by which we perceive and evaluate others have long been identified in social psychology as warmth and competence (Abele & Wojciszke, 2007; Asch, 1946; Bales, 1950; Fiske, Cuddy, & Glick, 2007; Rosenberg, Nelson, & Vivekananthan, 1968). These determinations have important consequences for whom we decide to cooperate with, befriend, and trust, as well as those we decide to compete against, hurt, and deceive. Our perceptions of warmth and competence, and the behaviors that stem from these impressions, are particularly salient in the context of negotiations, in which individuals are trying to fulfill their individual goals through both cooperation and competition with others (Pruitt, 1983; Pruitt & Carnevale, 1993).

Even though it has been argued that negotiation behavior is largely driven by a negotiator's economic bargaining situation rather than the negotiator's personality traits, individuals often attribute negotiation behavior to personality traits (Malhotra & Bazerman, 2008; Thompson, 2009; Wheeler, 2002). A bargaining situation can be understood in terms of the negotiator's alternatives, referred to as the best alternative to a negotiated agreement, or BATNA (Raiffa, 1982; White & Neale, 1991), which can vary in both its value and its riskiness; it has been argued that these factors are what determines a negotiator's bargaining behavior and style (Thompson, 2009).

The tendency to attribute bargaining behavior to personality rather than to situational demands has long been studied in social psychology and is referred to as the *fundamental attribution error* (Ross, 1977) or the *correspondence bias*

(Gilbert & Malone, 1995; Jones, 1990), in which individuals attribute the behaviors of others to certain corresponding traits and dispositions. Even when negotiators acknowledge externally imposed situational limitations on the counterpart, they continue to attribute their counterparts' bargaining behavior to personal intent, perceiving counterparts with larger constraints as having greater competitive intent (Kelley & Stahelski, 1970; Pruitt & Drews, 1969). While "hard" bargaining strategies, such as haggling, are more often caused by the negotiator's situational limitations, such as the value of his or her BATNA, the counterpart will perceive the haggling behavior as more indicative of the negotiator's disagreeable or competitive nature (Morris, Larrick, & Su, 1999).

Recent empirical research indicates that in addition to important perceptions being drawn from the value and timing of their counterparts' offers, negotiators also make important inferences from the format and specificity of the numerical offers themselves. For example, negotiators (in the role of a buyer) who made more specific first offers were seen as more knowledgeable (Mason, Lee, Wiley, & Ames, 2013). These inferences of competence made these specific first offers stronger anchors in the negotiation (Mason et al., 2013). On the other hand, when sellers opened a negotiation with a specific first offer price, buyers were less likely to want to enter into a negotiation with them (Lee, Loschelder, Schweinsberg, Mason, & Galinsky, 2018). This occurred because the specificity in the listed price was attributed to the seller's inflexibility as a negotiator (Lee et al., 2018). Also, contrary to traditional negotiation textbook advice, range offers have also been found to be more potent first offers because of a tandem anchoring effect (Ames & Mason, 2015). Range offer-makers were seen as less aggressive, less confident, and more flexible than point offer-makers (Ames & Mason, 2015). Recipients of range offers felt it was more impolite to turn down a range offer than a single value offer (Ames & Mason, 2015).

While the aggressiveness (and specificity) of first offers and counteroffers can be perceived as representing the negotiator's competencies in terms of both bargaining power and prowess, of course, these numerical values are not communicated in a vacuum. Instead, they are couched in words that communicate a variety of information that can convey different impressions of the negotiator making these numerical offers (Bowles & Babcock, 2013; Lee & Ames, 2017; Trötschel, Loschelder, Höhne, & Majer, 2015). For example, scholars have shown that the same counteroffer can be framed in several different ways that can result in different consequences. For example, an offer that is less than what your counterpart seeks can be framed as a constraint due to your own budgetary restriction, or it can be framed as the appropriate amount given some kind of criticism aimed at the object of negotiation (Lee & Ames, 2017). Constraint rationales were found to be more effective than disparagement rationales in yielding both desired economic results and positive interpersonal consequences because they were perceived as being more valid signals of a buyer's true economic limit (Lee & Ames, 2017).

In a similar vein, negotiators who employed the strategy of framing an economic value as something *offered* to their counterpart, as opposed to *requested* from their counterpart, were able to gain greater concessions (Trötschel et al., 2015). More advantageous economic and interpersonal consequences were obtained from negotiators who acknowledged and gave credit to their counterparts for concessions (Ward, Disston, Brenner, & Ross, 2008). Similarly, emphasizing the benefits of a concession from the perspective of the counterpart assisted negotiators in getting better deals and preserving positive relationships (Bhatia, Chow, & Weingart, 2016). In summary, framing and rationales are able to justify and sometimes soften the blow of less than ideal economic offers. In turn, this can lead to reciprocity, both economically and interpersonally, as counterparts are more open to accepting these offers and feel more positively about these negotiators.

Negotiators also make important inferences based on the level of interpersonal warmth that is communicated. Negotiation scholars and practitioners have long extolled the virtues of embracing an affiliational interpersonal style in integrative negotiation settings (Fisher et al., 2011; Lax & Sebenius, 1986; Pruitt, 1991). On the practitioner side, Ron Shapiro (2001), a well-regarded sports agent and founder of the

Shapiro Negotiation Institute, has devoted an entire book to this subject titled *The Power of Nice*. In This American Life's radio essay titled "Good Guys," producers Ben Calhoun (2014) and Ira Glass test the efficacy of appealing to salespeople with warm camaraderie in hopes of obtaining a "good guy discount."

A warm interpersonal style, defined by the literature and practitioners as being prosocial, cooperative, and nice, has been shown to improve financial outcomes by virtue of creating extra value for both parties. Cooperative negotiators trust each other and therefore exchange more critical information, which thereby allows them to come to more beneficial joint outcomes (de Dreu & Boles, 1998; de Dreu, Giebels, & Van de Vliert, 1998; de Dreu et al., 2000; Weingart, Bennett, & Brett, 1993).

On the other hand, researchers have found that competitively motivated negotiators are more likely to erroneously view the integrative negotiation as a fixed-pie situation and therefore withhold information, take more distributive tactics, and thereby lose out on opportunities to find joint gains (de Dreu et al., 2000; O'Connor, Arnold & Burris, 2005). At the extreme end, competitively motivated negotiators may find themselves engaging in deception in order to exploit their counterparts (Lewicki & Robinson, 1998; O'Connor & Carnevale, 1997). Given that detecting deception may be difficult, negotiators who utilize self-serving lies may find themselves at a competitive advantage in the short term but may ultimately pay the price in the long term when it comes to reputational concerns once their acts of deception are exposed (Murnighan, Babcock, Thompson, & Pillutla, 1999; Rogers, Zeckhauser, Gino, Norton, & Schweitzer, 2017). In this line of research, scholars find that the psychological principle of reciprocity governs negotiation motivations and behaviors, so that cooperatively motivated behaviors are returned in kind, as are competitively motivated ones (Brett, Shapiro, & Lytle, 1998).

The positive economic and interpersonal consequences of taking on a warm interpersonal style in negotiations has some important limitations. First and importantly, it applies to integrative negotiations, a fundamental feature of which is opportunity for value creation (Fisher et al., 2011; Lax & Sebenius, 1986; Pruitt,

1991). In these situations, warmth helps secure mutually beneficial gains because expanding the pie requires disclosure of critical information, and warmth helps build trust and rapport between the two parties, which enable the sharing of information (de Dreu & Boles, 1998; de Dreu et al., 1998, 2000; Weingart et al., 1993). Even within the context of integrative negotiations, however, a completely cooperative motivation is not always beneficial in cases where negotiators mistakenly believe that cooperation means concessions. This often leads negotiators to settle or split the difference, when it would be more beneficial for parties to think both about their interests and their counterpart's interests in ways that would lead to more mutually beneficial outcomes (Pruitt & Carnevale, 1993). This can only be done as parties reveal their interests, trade-off issues in a "logrolling" manner, and therefore "expand the pie."

Recent empirical research examining how dominant or deferential individuals are in a negotiation indicates that the most optimal integrative agreements are reached by negotiators who have complementary styles in expressing dominance (Wiltermuth, Tiedens, & Neale, 2015). This occurred because negotiators who were dominant were generally assertive in expressing what they wanted, while negotiators who were submissive generally asked questions in order to achieve what they wanted to know, so this complementarity resulted in information being exchanged optimally without conflict escalation, which ultimately led to more successful and mutually beneficial outcomes (Wiltermuth et al., 2015).

A notable feature of most of the empirical research showing the positive effects of a cooperative orientation versus a competitive one is that outcomes are measured at the dyadic level (de Dreu et al., 2000). In other words, a dyad of cooperative negotiators has been shown to create a final joint outcome that is more economically advantageous than that achieved by a dyad of competitive negotiators (de Dreu et al., 2000). What is less clear is how the advantages are divided up at the individual level. In other words, while a warm interpersonal style can result in a bigger pie, it is less clear whether a warm negotiator will end up with a smaller portion of that pie compared to more competitively oriented negotiators.

There is less empirical evidence on the consequence of warmth in distributive negotiations, but there is growing research to suggest that it can result in disadvantageous outcomes. Negotiators high in trait agreeableness were shown to do well in integrative settings but poorly in distributive ones when their agreeableness became a liability (Barry & Friedman, 1998). Similarly, negotiators who were more likely to adopt cooperative strategies in a salary negotiation achieved lower salary gains, as compared to negotiators who used competitive approaches (Marks & Harold, 2011). Taking on a warm communication style in a distributive negotiation hurt economic outcomes because counterparts to a warm negotiator responded with more aggressive counteroffers than counterparts to a tough negotiator (Jeong, Minson, Yeomans, Gino, 2019). Interestingly, counterparts reciprocate interpersonal warmth in their communication style but accompany this linguistic warmth with more aggressive economic behavior (Jeong et al., 2019). The proposed mechanism for this difference is perceived dominance: Negotiators who use a warm communication style characterized by high levels of politeness are perceived as less dominant; therefore, counterparts respond with more aggressive concessionary behavior than to tough, or less polite, negotiators who are perceived as higher in dominance (Jeong et al., 2019).

In addition to social perceptions arising from a negotiator's economic and noneconomic behavior, certain characteristics about the negotiator, such as gender and cultural background, or the negotiating situation, such as the medium in which the communication is taking place, can also affect negotiation behavior. Literature on gender stereotypes shows that women are expected to be more communal and less agentic than men (Bem, 1974; Fiske & Lee, 2008). When women exhibit behaviors that are inconsistent with their prescribed stereotypes, such as acting aggressively or dominantly, they are punished (Rudman & Glick, 2001). This holds true in negotiation contexts, where research shows that women who act in self-promoting ways during salary negotiations and job interviews receive negative backlash (Amanatullah & Tinsley, 2013; Babcock & Laschever, 2009; Bowles, Babcock, & Lai, 2007; Kray & Thompson,

2004; Rudman & Glick, 2001). Unfortunately, even when women act in stereotype-consistent ways in a negotiation, their accommodating behavior is not reciprocated by their counterparts (Ames, Lee, & Wazlawek, 2017).

Social perceptions of negotiation behavior are also affected by the cultural background of the negotiators. Cultural differences can often result in negotiators having a more difficult time reaching integrative agreements due to differences in norms surrounding how and when to communicate, bargain, disclose information, and come to mutually beneficial agreements (Brett, 2007; Cox, Lobel, & McLeod, 1991; Tinsley & Pillutla, 1998; Wade-Benzoni et al., 2002).

Finally, another consideration in thinking about social perceptions in negotiation communications is how the medium of negotiation affects these perceptions. As electronic negotiations become more common, researchers have looked at how communicating offers electronically versus face-to-face changes the psychological dynamic of the interaction. For example, negotiations conducted in person reduce incidents of impasse and are more likely to lead to integrative potential given that trust and rapport can be more easily built in face-to-face interactions (Naquin & Paulson, 2003; Valley, Moag, & Bazerman, 1998). Also, all electronic communications are not created equal—negotiators can communicate via e-mail that has a time lag or via online chats (i.e., instant messaging) that occur in real time. An interesting wrinkle is that depending on one's bargaining power, certain electronic media are more conducive to optimal outcomes. For example, researchers have found that negotiators with strong bargaining power perform better in real-time electronic chat negotiations in which they can take advantage of the more dynamic nature of the conversation, whereas those with weaker bargaining power perform better via e-mail, in which the time delay acts an important buffer (Loewenstein, Morris, Chakravarti, Thompson, & Kopelman, 2005).

Conclusion

While negotiations pervade both our personal and professional relationships, we often find ourselves reaching less than optimal negotia-

tion outcomes due to a number of psychological challenges, both at the intrapersonal and interpersonal levels. A negotiator aspiring to act rationally and effectively can enter a negotiation with all of the necessary tools, information, knowledge, and preparation, yet become detrimentally influenced in surprising ways. In this chapter, we have identified two common psychological influences that can affect a negotiator's behavior and subsequent outcome, at both cognitive and affective levels. We discussed a common cognitive bias known as the "fixed-pie belief," including its pervasiveness, the psychological underpinnings motivating it, the consequences for negotiation, as well as potential social and motivational interventions. We also discussed a multitude of affective states that can influence the negotiator, from transient moods to incidental or triggered emotions, as well as strategic emotional displays. Given that negotiations involve at least two individuals who are communicating together in order to cooperate and compete with each other, the social perceptions that arise from the interactions drive a number of important behaviors. Our interpersonal perceptions help us navigate our interactions by determining how we perceive people and, consequently, how we behave toward them. These perceptions are critical in negotiation contexts because how we perceive our counterparts affects the negotiation strategies we choose to adopt, which ultimately determine negotiation outcomes. Perceptions arise from how we bargain economically, the information we select to disclose, the emotional displays we signal, and the interpersonal warmth we choose to convey, as well as the framing and rationale we use to deliver our economic offers. A successful negotiator is one who navigates the intricate and consequential nature of social perception, while accounting for the nuances and complexities arising from the negotiation context.

REFERENCES

Abele, A. E., & Wojciszke, B. (2007). Agency and communion from the perspective of self versus others. *Journal of Personality and Social Psychology, 93*(5), 751–763.

Allred, K. G., Mallozzi, J. S., Matsui, F., & Raia,

C. P. (1997). The influence of anger and compassion on negotiation performance. *Organizational Behavior and Human Decision Processes, 70*(3), 175–187.

Amanatullah, E. T., & Tinsley, C. H. (2013). Punishing female negotiators for asserting too much . . . or not enough: Exploring why advocacy moderates backlash against assertive female negotiators. *Organizational Behavior and Human Decision Processes, 120*(1), 110–122.

Ames, D., Lee, A., & Wazlawek, A. (2017). Interpersonal assertiveness: Inside the balancing act. *Social and Personality Psychology Compass, 11*(6), e12317.

Ames, D. R., & Mason, M. F. (2015). Tandem anchoring: Informational and politeness effects of range offers in social exchange. *Journal of Personality and Social Psychology, 108*(2), 254–274.

Asch, S. E. (1946). Forming impressions of personality. *Journal of Abnormal and Social Psychology, 41*(3), 258–290.

Babcock, L., & Laschever, S. (2009). *Women don't ask: Negotiation and the gender divide.* Princeton, NJ: Princeton University Press.

Bales, R. F. (1950). *Interaction process analysis: A method for the study of small groups.* Cambridge, MA: Addison-Wesley.

Barry, B., & Friedman, R. A. (1998). Bargainer characteristics in distributive and integrative negotiation. *Journal of Personality and Social Psychology, 74*(2), 345–359.

Bazerman, M. H., & Neale, M. A. (1983). Heuristics in negotiation: Limitations to effective dispute resolution. In M. H. Bazerman & R. J. Lewicki (Eds.), *Negotiating in organizations* (pp. 51–67). Beverly Hills, CA: SAGE.

Belkin, L. Y., Kurtzberg, T. R., & Naquin, C. E. (2013). Signaling dominance in online negotiations: The role of affective tone. *Negotiation and Conflict Management Research, 6*(4), 285–304.

Bem, S. L. (1974). The measurement of psychological androgyny. *Journal of Consulting and Clinical Psychology, 42*(2), 155–162.

Ben-Yoav, O., & Pruitt, D. G. (1984). Resistance to yielding and the expectation of cooperative future interaction in negotiation. *Journal of Experimental Social Psychology, 20*(4), 323–335.

Bhatia, N., Chow, R. M., & Weingart, L. R. (2016). *Your cost or my benefit?: Effects of concession frames in distributive negotiations.* Manuscript submitted for publication.

Bowles, H. R., & Babcock, L. (2013). How can women escape the compensation negotiation dilemma?: Relational accounts are one answer. *Psychology of Women Quarterly, 37*(1), 80–96.

Bowles, H. R., Babcock, L., & Lai, L. (2007). Social

incentives for gender differences in the propensity to initiate negotiations: Sometimes it does hurt to ask. *Organizational Behavior and Human Decision Processes, 103*(1), 84–103.

Brett, J. M. (2007). *Negotiating globally: How to negotiate deals, resolve disputes, and make decisions across cultural boundaries.* San Francisco: Jossey-Bass.

Brett, J. M., Shapiro, D. L., & Lytle, A. L. (1998). Breaking the bonds of reciprocity in negotiations. *Academy of Management Journal, 41*(4), 410–424.

Brooks, A. W., & Schweitzer, M. E. (2011). Can Nervous Nelly negotiate?: How anxiety causes negotiators to make low first offers, exit early, and earn less profit. *Organizational Behavior and Human Decision Processes, 115*(1), 43–54.

Calhoun, B. (Producer). (2014, January 10). Good Guys [Radio broadcast episode]. Retrieved from *www.thisamericanlife.org/radio-archives/episode/515/good-guys.*

Carnevale, P. J., & Isen, A. M. (1986). The influence of positive affect and visual access on the discovery of integrative solutions in bilateral negotiation. *Organizational Behavior and Human Decision Processes, 37*(1), 1–13.

Carroll, J. S., Bazerman, M. H., & Maury, R. (1988). Negotiator cognitions: A descriptive approach to negotiators' understanding of their opponents. *Organizational Behavior and Human Decision Processes, 41*(3), 352–370.

Chambers, J. R., & de Dreu, C. K. (2014). Egocentrism drives misunderstanding in conflict and negotiation. *Journal of Experimental Social Psychology, 51*, 15–26.

Cox, T. H., Lobel, S. A., & McLeod, P. L. (1991). Effects of ethnic group cultural differences on cooperative and competitive behavior on a group task. *Academy of Management Journal, 34*(4), 827–847.

de Dreu, C. K., & Boles, T. L. (1998). Share and share alike or winner take all?: The influence of social value orientation upon choice and recall of negotiation heuristics. *Organizational Behavior and Human Decision Processes, 76*(3), 253–276.

de Dreu, C. K., Giebels, E., & Van de Vliert, E. (1998). Social motives and trust in integrative negotiation: The disruptive effects of punitive capability. *Journal of Applied Psychology, 83*(3), 408–422.

de Dreu, C. K., Koole, S. L., & Steinel, W. (2000). Unfixing the fixed pie: A motivated information-processing approach to integrative negotiation. *Journal of Personality and Social Psychology, 79*(6), 975–987.

de Dreu, C. W., Weingart, L. R., & Kwon, S. (2000). Influence of social motives on integrative negotiation: A meta-analytic review and test of two theories. *Journal of Personality and Social Psychology, 78*(5), 889–905.

Deutsch, M. (1991). Subjective features of conflict resolution: Psychological, social and cultural influences. In R. Väyrynen (Ed.), *New directions in conflict theory* (pp. 26–56). London: SAGE.

Fisher, R., Ury, W. L., & Patton, B. (2011). *Getting to yes: Negotiating agreement without giving in.* New York: Penguin.

Fiske, S. T., Cuddy, A. J., & Glick, P. (2007). Universal dimensions of social cognition: Warmth and competence. *Trends in Cognitive Sciences, 11*(2), 77–83.

Fiske, S. T., & Lee, T. L. (2008). Stereotypes and prejudice create workplace discrimination. In A. P. Brief (Ed.), *Diversity at work* (pp. 13–52). Cambridge, UK: Cambridge University Press.

Forgas, J. P. (1998). On feeling good and getting your way: Mood effects on negotiator cognition and bargaining strategies. *Journal of Personality and Social Psychology, 74*(3), 565–577.

Froman, L. A., Jr., & Cohen, M. D. (1970). Compromise and logroll: Comparing the efficiency of two bargaining processes. *Behavioral Science, 15*(2), 180–183.

Galinsky, A. D., Ku, G., & Wang, C. S. (2005). Perspective-taking and self-other overlap: Fostering social bonds and facilitating social coordination. *Group Processes and Intergroup Relations, 8*(2), 109–124.

Galinsky, A. D., Maddux, W. W., Gilin, D., & White, J. B. (2008). Why it pays to get inside the head of your opponent: The differential effects of perspective taking and empathy in negotiations. *Psychological Science, 19*(4), 378–384.

Gilbert, D. T., & Malone, P. S. (1995). The correspondence bias. *Psychological Bulletin, 117*(1), 21–38.

Harinck, F., de Dreu, C. K., & Van Vianen, A. E. (2000). The impact of conflict issues on fixed-pie perceptions, problem solving, and integrative outcomes in negotiation. *Organizational Behavior and Human Decision Processes, 81*(2), 329–358.

Jeong, M., Minson, J., Yeomans, M., & Gino, F. (2019). Communicating with warmth in distributive negotiations is surprisingly counter-productive. *Management Science, 65*, 5813–5837.

Jones, E. E. (1990). *Interpersonal perception.* New York: Freeman.

Kelley, H. H., & Stahelski, A. J. (1970). Social interaction basis of cooperators' and competitors' beliefs about others. *Journal of Personality and Social Psychology, 16*(1), 66–91.

Kopelman, S., Rosette, A. S., & Thompson, L. (2006). The three faces of Eve: Strategic displays of positive, negative, and neutral emotions in ne-

gotiations. *Organizational Behavior and Human Decision Processes, 99*(1), 81–101.

Kray, L. J., & Thompson, L. (2004). Gender stereotypes and negotiation performance: An examination of theory and research. *Research in Organizational Behavior, 26*, 103–182.

Lax, D. A., & Sebenius, J. K. (1986). *The managerial negotiator: Bargaining for cooperation and competitive gain.* New York: Free Press.

Lee, A. J., & Ames, D. R. (2017). "I can't pay more" versus "It's not worth more": Divergent effects of constraint and disparagement rationales in negotiations. *Organizational Behavior and Human Decision Processes, 141*, 16–28.

Lee, A. J., Loschelder, D. D., Schweinsberg, M., Mason, M. F., & Galinsky, A. D. (2018). Too precise to pursue: How precise first offers create barriers-to-entry in negotiations and markets. *Organizational Behavior and Human Decision Processes, 148*, 87–100.

Lerner, J. S., Small, D. A., & Loewenstein, G. (2004). Heart strings and purse strings: Carryover effects of emotions on economic decisions. *Psychological Science, 15*(5), 337–341.

Lewicki, R. J., & Robinson, R. J. (1998). Ethical and unethical bargaining tactics: An empirical study. *Journal of Business Ethics, 17*(6), 665–682.

Loewenstein, J., Morris, M. W., Chakravarti, A., Thompson, L., & Kopelman, S. (2005). At a loss for words: Dominating the conversation and the outcome in negotiation as a function of intricate arguments and communication media. *Organizational Behavior and Human Decision Processes, 98*(1), 28–38.

Malhotra, D., & Bazerman, M. H. (2008). *Negotiation genius: How to overcome obstacles and achieve brilliant results at the bargaining table and beyond.* New York: Bantam.

Marks, M., & Harold, C. (2011). Who asks and who receives in salary negotiation. *Journal of Organizational Behavior, 32*(3), 371–394.

Mason, M. F., Lee, A. J., Wiley, E. A., & Ames, D. R. (2013). Precise offers are potent anchors: Conciliatory counteroffers and attributions of knowledge in negotiations. *Journal of Experimental Social Psychology, 49*(4), 759–763.

Morris, M. W., & Keltner, D. (2000). How emotions work: The social functions of emotional expression in negotiations. *Research in Organizational Behavior, 22*, 1–50.

Morris, M. W., Larrick, R. P., & Su, S. K. (1999). Misperceiving negotiation counterparts: When situationally determined bargaining behaviors are attributed to personality traits. *Journal of Personality and Social Psychology, 77*(1), 52–67.

Murnighan, J. K., Babcock, L., Thompson, L., &

Pillutla, M. (1999). The information dilemma in negotiations: Effects of experience, incentives, and integrative potential. *International Journal of Conflict Management, 10*(4), 313–339.

Nadler, J., Thompson, L., & Boven, L. V. (2003). Learning negotiation skills: Four models of knowledge creation and transfer. *Management Science, 49*(4), 529–540.

Naquin, C. E., & Paulson, G. D. (2003). Online bargaining and interpersonal trust. *Journal of Applied Psychology, 88*(1), 113–120.

Neale, M. A., & Bazerman, M. H. (1991). *Cognition and rationality in negotiation*. New York: Free Press.

Neale, M. A., & Northcraft, G. B. (1991). Behavioral negotiation theory: A framework for conceptualizing dyadic bargaining. *Research in Organizational Behavior, 13,* 147–190.

O'Connor, K. M., & Adams, A. A. (1999). What novices think about negotiation: A content analysis of scripts. *Negotiation Journal, 15*(2), 135–148.

O'Connor, K. M., Arnold, J. A., & Burris, E. R. (2005). Negotiators' bargaining histories and their effects on future negotiation performance. *Journal of Applied Psychology, 90*(2), 350–362.

O'Connor, K. M., & Carnevale, P. J. (1997). A nasty but effective negotiation strategy: Misrepresentation of a common-value issue. *Personality and Social Psychology Bulletin, 23*(5), 504–515.

Orvis, B. R., Kelley, H. H., & Butler, D. (1976). Attributional conflict in young couples. *New Directions in Attribution Research, 1,* 353–386.

Pinkley, R. L., Griffith, T. L., & Northcraft, G. B. (1995). "Fixed Pie" a la mode: Information availability, information processing, and the negotiation of suboptimal agreements. *Organizational Behavior and Human Decision Processes, 62*(1), 101–112.

Pronin, E., Gilovich, T., & Ross, L. (2004). Objectivity in the eye of the beholder: Divergent perceptions of bias in self versus others. *Psychological Review, 111*(3), 781–799.

Pruitt, D. G. (1983). Strategic choice in negotiation. *American Behavioral Scientist, 27*(2), 167–194.

Pruitt, D. G. (1991). Strategy in negotiation. In V. A. Kremenyuk (Ed.), *International negotiation: Analysis, approaches, issues* (pp. 78–89). San Francisco: Jossey-Bass.

Pruitt, D. G., & Carnevale, P. J. (1993). *Negotiation in social conflict*. Pacific Grove, CA: Thomson Brooks/Cole.

Pruitt, D. G., & Drews, J. L. (1969). The effect of time pressure, time elapsed, and the opponent's concession rate on behavior in negotiation. *Journal of Experimental Social Psychology, 5*(1), 43–60.

Pruitt, D. G., & Lewis, S. A. (1975). Development of integrative solutions in bilateral negotiation. *Journal of Personality and Social Psychology, 31*(4), 621–633.

Pruitt, D. G., & Rubin, J. Z. (1986). *Social conflict: Escalation, impasse, and resolution.* Reading, MA: Addison-Wesley.

Raiffa, H. (1982). *The art and science of negotiation.* Cambridge, MA: Harvard University Press.

Rogers, T., Zeckhauser, R., Gino, F., Norton, M. I., & Schweitzer, M. E. (2017). Artful paltering: The risks and rewards of using truthful statements to mislead others. *Journal of Personality and Social Psychology, 112*(3), 456–473.

Rosenberg, S., Nelson, C., & Vivekananthan, P. S. (1968). A multidimensional approach to the structure of personality impressions. *Journal of Personality and Social Psychology, 9*(4), 283–294.

Ross, L. (1977). The intuitive psychologist and his shortcomings: Distortions in the attribution process. In L. Berkowitz (Ed.), *Advances in experimental social psychology* (Vol. 10, pp. 173–220). San Diego, CA: Academic Press.

Rudman, L. A., & Glick, P. (2001). Prescriptive gender stereotypes and backlash toward agentic women. *Journal of Social Issues, 57*(4), 743–762.

Schelling, T. (1980). *The strategy of conflict.* Cambridge, MA: Harvard University Press.

Shapiro, R. M. (2001). *The power of nice: How to negotiate so everyone wins—especially you!* New York: Wiley.

Sinaceur, M., & Tiedens, L. Z. (2006). Get mad and get more than even: When and why anger expression is effective in negotiations. *Journal of Experimental Social Psychology, 42*(3), 314–322.

Smith, C. A., & Ellsworth, P. C. (1985). Patterns of cognitive appraisal in emotion. *Journal of Personality and Social Psychology, 48*(4), 813–838.

Thompson, L. (1990). The influence of experience on negotiation performance. *Journal of Experimental Social Psychology, 26*(6), 528–544.

Thompson, L. L. (1991). Information exchange in negotiation. *Journal of Experimental Social Psychology, 27*(2), 161–179.

Thompson, L. (2009). *The mind and heart of the negotiator* (4th ed.). Upper Saddle River, NJ: Prentice Hall.

Thompson, L., & DeHarpport, T. (1994). Social judgment, feedback, and interpersonal learning in negotiation. *Organizational Behavior and Human Decision Processes, 58*(3), 327–345.

Thompson, L., & Hastie, R. (1990). Social perception in negotiation. *Organizational Behavior and Human Decision Processes, 47*(1), 98–123.

Tinsley, C. H., & Pillutla, M. M. (1998). Negotiating in the United States and Hong Kong. *Journal of International Business Studies, 29*(4), 711–727.

Trötschel, R., Loschelder, D. D., Höhne, B. P., & Majer, J. M. (2015). Procedural frames in negotiations: How offering my resources versus requesting yours impacts perception, behavior, and outcomes. *Journal of Personality and Social Psychology, 108*(3), 417–435.

Valley, K. L., Moag, J., & Bazerman, M. H. (1998). A matter of trust: Effects of communication on the efficiency and distribution of outcomes. *Journal of Economic Behavior and Organization, 34*(2), 211–238.

Van Kleef, G. A., & Côté, S. (2007). Expressing anger in conflict: When it helps and when it hurts. *Journal of Applied Psychology, 92*(6), 1557–1569.

Van Kleef, G. A., de Dreu, C. K., & Manstead, A. S. (2004). The interpersonal effects of anger and happiness in negotiations. *Journal of Personality and Social Psychology, 86*(1), 57–76.

Wade-Benzoni, K. A., Okumura, T., Brett, J. M., Moore, D. A., Tenbrunsel, A. E., & Bazerman, M. H. (2002). Cognitions and behavior in asymmetric social dilemmas: A comparison of two cultures. *Journal of Applied Psychology, 87*(1), 87–95.

Ward, A., Disston, L. G., Brenner, L., & Ross, L. (2008). Acknowledging the other side in negotiation. *Negotiation Journal, 24*(3), 269–285.

Weingart, L. R., Bennett, R. J., & Brett, J. M. (1993). The impact of consideration of issues and motivational orientation on group negotiation process and outcome. *Journal of Applied Psychology, 78*(3), 504–517.

Wheeler, M. (2002). *Negotiation analysis: An introduction.* Cambridge, MA: Harvard Business School.

White, S. B., & Neale, M. A. (1991). Reservation prices, resistance points, and BATNAs: Determining the parameters of acceptable negotiated outcomes. *Negotiation Journal, 7*(4), 379–388.

Wiltermuth, S., Tiedens, L. Z., & Neale, M. (2015). The benefits of dominance complementarity in negotiations. *Negotiation and Conflict Management Research, 8*(3), 194–209.

Wolfe, R. J., & McGinn, K. L. (2005). Perceived relative power and its influence on negotiations. *Group Decision and Negotiation, 14*(1), 3–20.

CHAPTER 28

How Prominent Features
of Organizational Life
Inform Principles of Social Psychology

Joel Brockner
Batia M. Wiesenfeld
Ilona Fridman

There are multiple ways to discuss the interface of social and organizational psychology. For one thing, theory and research in social psychology may help to explain people's behaviors and attitudes in organizational settings. For example, Brockner and Wiesenfeld (1993) delineated how a host of basic social psychological principles help to account for the variability in how layoffs affect the productivity and morale of the employees who remain ("survivors"). Another approach pertains primarily to establishing external validity. Studies with this purpose in mind seek to examine whether the results of basic research generalize to real-world organizations. For instance, initial laboratory research on the escalation of commitment to a failing course of action (e.g., Rubin & Brockner, 1975; Staw, 1976) was followed by field studies showing how escalation manifests itself in organizations (e.g., Ross & Staw, 1993). Given concerns about the replicability and generalizability of basic research findings, there is obvious value in examining whether the results found under controlled conditions emerge in actual organizational settings.

As useful as these approaches are, we believe it would be even more fruitful to take an approach that enables us to advance theory. We do so by considering how *prominent features of organizational settings have implications for conceptual principles and empirical findings in social psychology*. For example, some social psychological findings may be more versus less pronounced as a function of variations in prominent dimensions of organizational life. In other instances, empirical findings may even take different forms as a function of certain organizational conditions. In short, this chapter examines how prominent features of work organizations inform theory and research in social psychology. Along the way, we also explore a few instances of how research on social psychological principles may deepen our understanding of the prominent features of organizational life.

By "organizational life" we are referring primarily to work organizations, be they for-profit, public, or nonprofit. By "prominent features," we do not mean to suggest that they *only* reside within organizations. Rather, "prominent features" refer to important and salient aspects of organizations that, when considered separately, could also describe other social entities such as dyads, informal groups, and crowds, but that in combination may be especially descriptive of work organizations. We consider how five prominent organizational features (i.e., hierarchy, ongoing time frame, the salience of economic considerations, person–environment congruence, and agency) inform a wide array of social psychological principles.

Prominent Features of Organizational Life

What features of organizations stand out and collectively make work organizations distinctive? First, one of the most pervasive features of organizations is that they are hierarchically arranged. Those of higher rank usually have legitimate authority to call the shots, whereas those at lower levels are tasked with doing what needs to be done for the organization to accomplish its mission. Second, in organizational life, interactions and relationships between people transpire in an *ongoing* context. As such, events in the here and now are affected by both the past and the anticipation of future interaction (e.g., Tyler & Sears, 1977). This is different from, say, many laboratory studies in social psychology that examine people's reactions on more of a "one-off" basis.

A third prominent feature of life in work organizations is the salience of tangible economic considerations. Most people work to live. Consequently, pay is an important motivator for employees' involvement in organizations. Moreover, organization members have many other reminders of the importance of money and other economic considerations. In public companies, the stock price is continually updated and depends in large part on the company's balance sheet, directing the attention of every layer of an organization's leadership to revenues and costs. Profits and losses are a common metric that define effectiveness and shape decision making at every level of an organization, from large divisions to small projects.

Fourth, the principle of person–environment congruence is prominent in organizational life. At a macro level, how well an organization functions depends on the fit between its strategy and various organizational arrangements such as structure, culture, and the configuration of tasks (Nadler & Tushman, 1982). The same

principle holds true at a micro level: Employees' work attitudes and behaviors depend on how much their personal attributes (e.g., values, traits, and abilities) fit with important features of their work environments. A fifth prominent feature of work environments is that they elicit the psychology of agency, which refers to acting on behalf of others. In their roles as agents, decision makers are expected to act in the best interests of various organizational stakeholders, which may require them to put aside their own interests and beliefs as bases of action. These features of hierarchy, continuity, salience of economic considerations, person–environment congruence, and agency combine to make work organizations distinctive. Moreover, each feature on its own can provide insight into basic social psychological principles. Hence, we now discuss how these five prominent features of work organizations inform social psychological principles residing in many literatures, including trust, justice, social hierarchy, ethics, the self, regulatory fit, behavioral decision making, and negotiations.

Organizations Are Hierarchical

Building on the age-old adage that people care about not only what is done but also how things are done, Brockner and Wiesenfeld (1996) reviewed a large body of studies showing that people's beliefs and behaviors are interactively influenced by the favorability of their outcomes and the fairness of the process used to arrive at those outcomes. One way to state this "process–outcome interaction effect" is that the typical tendency for people to react better when they receive more favorable outcomes is reduced considerably when the process is fairer. Also embedded within the interaction effect is the finding that a fair process can go a long way toward taking the sting out of "tough decisions" (i.e., those in which people did not receive the outcome they wanted). For example, people are much more likely to accept whatever decision authorities arrive at (even unfavorable ones) if they believe that their views were seriously considered (Lind & Tyler, 1988) or if they believe that they were given a good explanation of why the decision was made (Bies, 1987). One reason why a fair process reduces the effect of outcome favorability is that a fair process signals that the decision-maker can be trusted (Brockner, Siegel, Daly, Tyler, & Martin, 1997). Knowing that the process is fair, people are likely to believe that they will receive their share of favorable outcomes over the long haul. As a result, they assign less importance to, and hence are less affected by, the favorability of their current outcomes.

The pivotal role of trust in the decision-making authority suggests that people's hierarchical position also may have implications for the process–outcome interaction. People in lower hierarchical positions are likely to assign greater importance to determining how much to trust their higher-ups because their subordinate roles may cause them to feel insecure. As Kramer (1996) put it, "From the standpoint of those on the bottom, decisions regarding how much trust should be conferred on a particular relationship become simultaneously more *consequential* and more problematic. . . . Those on the bottom of a hierarchical relationship routinely encounter both vulnerability and uncertainty, and these are the conditions that *make salient concerns about trust*" (p. 223, emphasis added).

The process–outcome interaction is more likely to be shown by those who see themselves as lower in the hierarchy because they assign greater importance to determining how much to trust authorities and may therefore be more sensitive to trust-relevant information, such as the authorities' process fairness. If high process fairness generally reduces the effect of outcome favorability, it stands to reason that it will do so even more among those who assign greater importance to process fairness information. In fact, though not explicitly mentioned by Brockner and Wiesenfeld (1996), a common feature of the studies they reviewed is that the person on the receiving end of the decision always was lower in rank than the party making the decision. Many of the studies were conducted in work organizations in which the participants were employees who reacted to decisions made by their bosses that made employees either better off or worse off (outcome favorability) and were accompanied by a process varying in its degree of fairness. Whereas other studies in the Brockner and Wiesenfeld review were not done in work organizations, participants still were

in a lower hierarchical position relative to the party who had influence over outcome favorability and process fairness. For instance, some studies examined citizens' reactions to their encounters with legal authorities (the police and courts), whereas others examined participants in the laboratory reacting to decisions made by the experimenter, who is typically the higher-ranking party in that context. As Orne (1962) put it in his classic piece titled "On the Social Psychology of the Psychological Experiment," "a particularly striking aspect of the typical experimenter–subject relationship is the extent to which the subject will play his role and place himself under the control of the experimenter" (p. 777).

Indeed, subsequent research showed that being in the lower hierarchical position was a necessary precondition for producing the interactive relationship between outcome favorability and process fairness. For instance, it is possible for people on the receiving end to occupy a higher hierarchical position than those making the decision. In one study, people came from groups varying in status and negotiated with another party (Chen, Brockner, & Greenberg, 2003). Of particular relevance was how people in the mixed-status pairing (one higher, the other lower) reacted to the negotiation as a function of the favorability of the outcome and the extent to which the other party exhibited a fair process. The dependent variable was how much people wanted to have additional business dealings with their negotiation counterpart. The negotiator from the group lower in rank showed the typical process–outcome interaction effect: Being treated with high process fairness by the other negotiator reduced the positive relationship between outcome favorability and their desire for additional business dealings, relative to when process fairness was low.

Interestingly enough, people from the group in the higher-status position did not simply show less of the typical process–outcome interaction: They actually responded with an entirely different interactive pattern of their own. For them, high process fairness *heightened* the positive relationship between outcome favorability and desire for additional business dealings, relative to when process fairness was low. One explanation of the reactions of people from the higher-ranking group is that they have different motivations than do people from the lower-ranking group in their dealings with people. Rather than needing to determine the trustworthiness of the other party (which is a predominant concern of those lower in the hierarchy), people at higher ranks may be looking to maintain their relatively privileged positions. Hence, how much they want to have additional business dealings may depend on what the outcome and process information says about maintaining their privileged position.

Studies have indicated that people are more likely to make self-attributions for outcomes that are accompanied by fair rather than unfair processes (e.g., van den Bos, Bruins, Wilke, & Dronkert, 1999). Favorable outcomes accompanied by a fair process are self-enhancing, whereas unfavorable outcomes accompanied by a fair process are self-threatening. Hence, for people looking to maintain their higher position, outcome favorability will be strongly positively related to their desire for future business dealings provided that the other party engages in a fair process. A favorable outcome paired with a fair process affirms the status of the higher-ranking individual, whereas an unfavorable outcome accompanied by a fair process threatens the status of the higher-ranking individual. When the other party shows less process fairness, then the outcomes people receive are less likely to be attributed to themselves, making the favorability of the outcomes less relevant to people's concern with maintaining their privileged position. This may explain why outcome favorability had less of an effect on higher-ranked people's desire for future business dealings with their lower-status counterpart when the latter exhibited lower process fairness.

Admittedly, the reasons why people in the higher position behaved differently from those in the lower position are speculative; they need to be pinned down in future research. For now, however, we can conclude with greater certainty that the mechanism accounting for the process–outcome interaction differs for those lower versus higher in the hierarchy. The oft-replicated pattern reviewed elsewhere (Brockner & Wiesenfeld, 1996) is more likely to emerge when the recipient is in a lower hierarchical position, something that would not have been known until hierarchical position was examined as an independent variable in subsequent research.

Differentiating Power from Status

More recent theory and research on social hierarchy have shown that there is considerable value in differentiating between the dimensions of power and status (Magee & Galinsky, 2008). Whereas the two often covary, status and power are conceptually distinct. *Power* refers to how much people have control over valued resources, whereas *status* is how much people are seen by others as prestigious, respected, and worthy of their esteem. A key differentiator between having status and having power is the extent to which it fosters dependence on, and correspondingly the amount of attention people pay to, others. Status is socially conferred; ultimately, it is up to others to see the focal actor as worthy of respect and esteem. Consequently, having status makes people "concerned about the impressions they cultivate with social targets, to consider these parties' perspectives, and to act in ways that will be regarded as respectable and commendable" (Blader & Chen, 2012, p. 995). In contrast, when people have power, it liberates them "from social and normative pressures, leading them to shift their focus inward and towards their own goals and dispositions" (Blader & Chen, p. 996). Organizational scholars have recently amassed considerable evidence showing how this fundamental distinction between status and power leads to different effects on work behaviors and attitudes. Working from the basic principle that people at upper echelons of a social hierarchy behave differently or are perceived differently relative to people at lower levels of the hierarchy, we need to distinguish whether people's placement in the hierarchy is borne of status or of power, as recent studies have shown.

One line of research has shown how status and power lead to differing relationships with organizational justice. Within this line, some studies have examined the differential effects of felt power versus felt status on people's tendencies to behave fairly (Blader & Chen, 2012). Others have looked at the effects of people's tendencies to behave more versus less fairly on observers' judgments of their power and status (Rothman, Wheeler-Smith, Wiesenfeld, & Galinsky, 2020). Blader and Chen (2012) induced people to experience a high level of status or a high level of power. Relative to a control condition in which people were not induced to experience either high status or high power, those in the high-status condition behaved with greater distributive and procedural fairness, whereas those in the high-power condition behaved with lower distributive and procedural fairness. As further evidence that people's attentional focus is a key driver of the different effects of status and power on the expression of fairness, Blader and Chen found that the tendency for those in the high-power condition to behave less fairly than those in the control condition was attenuated among people who were dispositionally higher in their other-directedness.

Rothman and colleagues (2020) manipulated whether decision-makers exhibited various forms of process fairness (e.g., voice, informational fairness and interpersonal fairness) while carrying out decisions. Decision-makers who behaved fairly were perceived to have greater status, as well as lower power, relative to their counterparts who behaved less fairly. Moreover, perceptions of the decision-makers' attentional focus accounted for these findings. The positive effect of fairness on perceptions of status was mediated by how much decision-makers were seen as other-directed; fair leaders were seen as more other-directed, which in turn led to judgments of greater status. Moreover, the negative effect of fairness on perceptions of power was mediated by how much decision-makers were seen as self-focused; fair leaders were seen as less self-focused and, as a result, less powerful.

Power and Status Interact

Additional evidence of the distinction between power and status may be gleaned from studies showing that they combine interactively to influence people's behavior. When people experience low status and high power, they are especially likely to be interpersonally cantankerous, relative to all other combinations of status and power. People who are in low-status positions but who wield power within those positions have both the motivation and the ability to be interpersonally nasty. Motivationally speaking, as Fast, Halevy, and Galinsky (2012) suggested, "lacking status . . . makes people feel

disrespected and unappreciated, which can trigger aggressive compensatory behaviors aimed at boosting self-worth" (p. 391). Whereas those who experience low levels of status may be inclined to lash out, there are good reasons for them to be inhibited from doing so. However, the experience of power has disinhibiting effects (Keltner, Gruenfeld, & Anderson, 2003), freeing people up (or enabling them) to act in a manner consistent with their internal states and feelings. Fast and colleagues (2012) orthogonally manipulated status and power and examined their effects on people's tendencies to behave in a demeaning manner toward others. An interaction effect emerged, such that people were much more interpersonally demeaning when they experienced low status and high power. Anicich, Fast, Halevy, and Galinsky (2015) replicated these results and extended them to a different form of counterproductive interpersonal behavior: the tendency to initiate relationship conflict. Participants rated how much they felt status and power in their jobs, while also indicating the extent to which they experienced interpersonal conflict at work. Not only did status and power behave differently as main effects, such that status (power) was negatively (positively) related to conflict, but also status and power interacted: The highest level of interpersonal conflict was experienced when participants reported being low in status and high in power.

Blader and Chen (2012) also examined the interactive effect of felt status and felt power on people's tendencies to behave fairly. They found that the positive relationship between manipulated status and fairness was stronger among people who experienced lower levels of power. One interpretation of these findings emanates from the notion that lower-power people do not feel as free to act on their inner states or personal inclinations. Instead, lower-power people may be more reliant on external cues for appropriate behavior. Pitesa and Thau (2013) found, for instance, that people who were lower in power were more likely to conform to the behavior of others in deciding how to respond to an ethical dilemma, relative to those who experienced higher levels of power. In like fashion, given that experimental manipulations of higher status induce people to behave more fairly, lower-power people were shown to be more influenced by the situational cue of degree of status, whereas those with higher power were more likely to do their own thing regardless of whether they were in the higher- or lower-status condition.

In summary, theory and research emanating from the pervasive tendency for organizations to use hierarchies have advanced how we conceptualize the two fundamental bases of hierarchy, namely, status and power. The experience of status versus power leads to diametrically opposite effects on the expression of fairness. Further evidence of why it is useful to distinguish between status and power is provided by studies showing that status and power combine interactively to influence various interpersonal behaviors.

Implications of Macro Changes in Hierarchy for Principles

Another way to consider the relationship between prominent features of organizational life and social psychological principles is to evaluate how macro-level changes in the former affect the latter. For example, there is considerable evidence that organizational hierarchies are becoming flatter. One large-scale study showed that, 30 years ago, CEOs had four direct reports, whereas now they have an average of seven (Rajan & Wulf, 2003). More generally, there are fewer layers between people at the top and those at the bottom. If organizational hierarchies are becoming flatter, does this mean that the concept of hierarchy has less of a role in explaining people's work attitudes and behaviors?

We think not. For example, the tendency for organizational hierarchies to become flatter may have profound implications for the *voice effect,* which refers to people's tendencies to react more positively to decisions, decision-makers, and institutions when they have provided input into the decision. The voice effect has been shown in multiple areas in social and organizational psychology, including the justice literature (e.g., van den Bos, 2005) and the literature on perceived control (e.g., Deci & Ryan, 1985). We surmise that the voice effect in the workplace is likely to apply to growing numbers of people as social hierarchies become flatter. The flattening of hierarchies implies that

rank in the hierarchy is less important, and the ability to provide meaningful input is more important as a basis for the legitimacy of voice. As a result, with flatter hierarchies, more people may come to expect and/or want to have voice in a decision-making process, and therefore be more affected by how much they actually experienced voice in the decision process.

Evidence consistent with this reasoning comes from a series of studies examining how cultural differences in power distance moderate people's reactions to having voice (Brockner et al., 2001; van den Bos, Brockner, van den Oudenalder, Kamble, & Nasabi, 2013). *Power distance* refers to the extent to which less powerful members of a culture expect and accept unequal distribution of decision-making power. In a culture high in power distance, those in the less powerful position accept a hierarchical order in which all people have their place, with no further justification needed. In a culture low in power distance, people expect and want more equal distribution of decision-making power. In one series of studies Brockner and colleagues (2001) examined the voice effect in countries known to vary in power distance; high power distance countries included China and Mexico, whereas low power distance countries included the United States and Germany. The results showed that the voice effect was more pronounced in the low power distance countries than in the countries high in power distance. Moreover, when participants were sorted on the basis of their power distance beliefs (rather than their country of origin) the voice effect was found to be significantly more pronounced among those with lower power distance beliefs. In fact, as evidence of "mediated moderation," it was shown that the moderating influence of national culture on the voice effect disappeared once participants' power distance beliefs were statistically controlled.

Organizations Have a Past, Present, and Future

Unlike many studies in social psychology that examine people's actions at a single point in time, the ongoing nature of exchanges and relationships in organizations allows us to examine how principles play out over time. We do so in three ways in this section. First, we examine *behavioral sequence* effects, which refer to how taking an action at time 1 influences the action people take at time 2. Second, we consider how self-processes accounting for one behavioral sequence effect (and other noteworthy effects) can take different forms. Third, we discuss how people's experience of their current treatment may be influenced by the way they have been treated in the past.

Behavioral Sequence Effects

A classic example of a behavioral sequence effect is the foot-in-the-door influence technique, which showed that if people can be induced to take a small step in a certain direction, they are more likely to take a bigger step in that same direction than if they had not taken the initial small step (Freedman & Fraser, 1966). Theory and research on the escalation of commitment also have shown that once people embark on a particular course of action, they may be more likely to stay the course, even when the returns from the initial course of action are unfavorable (Brockner, 1992; Staw, 1976).

By way of illustrating a potential downside of scholars not taking behavioral sequence effects into account, consider the classic research by Milgram (1974) on obedience to authority. Defying the predictions of experts in human behavior, Milgram found that more than 60% of participants were willing to deliver what they believed to be painful electric shock to the "learner" in the study. By varying a host of situational factors in follow-up experiments, such as the location in which the study was conducted (i.e., on the campus of prestigious Yale University vs. in a rundown section of Bridgeport, Connecticut), or the psychological distance between the experimenter and the participants, Milgram demonstrated that unethical behavior was due to the situation rather than to participants' dispositional tendencies.

An important implication of Milgram's research is that by altering the situational factors that drive unethical behavior, it may be possible to elicit more ethical behavior in organizational settings. However, this line of reasoning fails to consider complexities introduced by behavioral sequence effects; that is, even if a relatively enduring aspect of a restructured work environ-

ment leads people to behave more ethically at time 1, does behaving more ethically at time 1 make them more likely to do so at time 2?

Indeed, a long-standing question in social psychology is how people's behaviors influence their subsequent actions. Dissonance theory (Festinger, 1957) and self-perception theory (Bem, 1972) posited that engaging in a course of action made people more likely to behave in a manner consistent with that course of action, especially when people saw themselves as free to act rather than coerced by external forces. Contemporary scholars have a very different perspective on behavioral consistency. Recent evidence suggests that engaging in a course of action can induce people to behave inconsistently with the initial course of action. For example, behaving ethically at time 1 has been shown to make people *less* likely to behave ethically at time 2 (Monin & Miller, 2001). Noting the inconsistency in the moral behavior of the two main actors in his novella, Robert Louis Stevenson dubbed it, "The *Strange Case* of Dr. Jekyll and Mr. Hyde" (emphasis added). Recent empirical evidence suggests that perhaps we should not be so surprised by inconsistency in moral behavior: Behaving ethically (like Dr. Jekyll) instigates psychological processes that make people likely to behave unethically (like Mr. Hyde).

A study by Lin, Ma, and Johnson (2016) showed that supervisors who behaved ethically on one day were more likely to behave abusively toward their subordinates the very next day. Two processes were shown to account for this relationship, one pertaining to moral licensing (Merritt, Effron, & Monin, 2010) and the other to ego depletion (Baumeister, Bratslavsky, Muraven, & Tice, 1998). In moral licensing, the initial act allowed people to see themselves as ethical, thereby enabling them to believe that they are "free" to engage in less ethical or more self-interested behaviors. A sample item measuring moral licensing is "My previous good deeds earned me credit as a moral person." In ego depletion, the initial act may have required people to exert self-control (e.g., to resist the temptation they may have felt to behave self-interestedly or unethically), thereby making them less able to withstand the temptation to behave unethically the next time. A sample item measuring ego depletion is "Right now, I feel my willpower is gone."

A recent study by Yam, Klotz, He, and Reynolds (2017) showed conceptually analogous results. Employees who engaged in extra work on behalf of the organization (organizational citizenship behavior, or OCB) at time 1 felt a sense of entitlement and were therefore more likely at time 2 to behave badly toward their coworkers (e.g., by making fun of them) or the organization (e.g., by taking property that did not belong to them). Unlike the study by Lin and colleagues (2016), in which the interval between time 1 and time 2 was merely 1 day, the interval between time 1 and time 2 in the Yam and colleagues study was considerably longer: 2 weeks. Moreover, how much people saw their OCB as externally motivated moderated the relationship between engaging in OCB at time 1 and behaving badly at time 2, such that the relationship was stronger among those who saw their OCB as more externally motivated. For instance, employees who said that they engaged in OCB "because I'll get in trouble if I don't," or "because others will reward me" were especially likely to behave badly at time 2 after engaging in OCB at time 1.

Moreover, the mediating role played by the experience of psychological entitlement may be related to the constructs of moral licensing and/ or ego depletion that Lin and colleagues (2016) found to account for the tendency of good behavior at time 1 to lead to bad behavior at time 2. The entitlement measure consisted of items that could be interpreted as tapping extremely positive self-evaluations (e.g., "I demand the best because I'm worth it"). Thus, engaging in OCB for external reasons may have led to extremely positive self-evaluations, which employees may have believed gave them license to behave badly. Alternatively, engaging in OCB for external reasons may have required people to exert particularly high levels of self-control. After all, doing the *extra* work entailed in OCB at time 1 is hardly a path of least resistance; it may require people to muster self-control resources. Moreover, this may be particularly true when engaging in OCB at time 1 comes from an externally rather than internally motivated place. As a result, those who engaged in OCB at time 1 for external reasons may have

had fewer self-control resources needed to not behave badly at time 2.

Milgram's (1974) research showed that unethical behavior is driven by situational factors to a considerable extent. However, behavioral sequence effects made possible by the ongoing nature of social encounters in organizations suggest that Milgram's situational analysis of unethical behavior may be only part of the story. Certainly, work environments can and should be restructured to make people more likely to behave ethically. However, ethical behavior at time 1 may not engender more of the same at time 2 and may even lead to less of the same at time 2. Hence, a matter of considerable theoretical and practical significance is not only how to bring about more ethical behavior in the first place but also how to *maintain* it.

Insights into this question may be found in a useful piece by Mullen and Monin (2016), who summarized research delineating the conditions under which behaving ethically at time 1 made people more likely to behave ethically at time 2 (a consistency effect) or less likely to behave ethically at time 2 (a licensing effect). Across multiple studies, consistency effects tend to emerge when people connect their behavior at time 1 to enduring aspects of themselves (e.g., values, traits, or attitudes). Whereas Mullen and Monin suggest that the disparate elicitors of licensing effects may be less conceptually coherent, there are several conditions under which behaving ethically at time 1 makes people less likely to behave ethically at time 2. For example, behavior seen as representing progress toward the goal of morality (rather than as commitment to the goal of morality) is more likely to lead to less ethical behavior at time 2.

More work is needed to delineate when and why behavior enacted at time 1 predisposes people to show more of the same (consistency) versus less of the same (licensing, a form of inconsistency) at time 2. Moreover, within the realm of inconsistency effects, thus far we have only discussed how enacting positively valenced (e.g., ethical) behavior can lead to negatively valenced (e.g., unethical) behavior. Mullen and Monin (2016) also considered an opposite tendency toward inconsistency known as *compensation,* in which unethical behavior at time 1 makes people more likely to behave ethically at time 2. A more complete understanding of inconsistency in behavioral sequence effects might be achieved if we were to specify the processes not only through which Dr. Jekyll can become Mr. Hyde but also how Mr. Hyde can become Dr. Jekyll.

We also encourage more ecologically valid studies. The research included in the Mullen and Monin (2016) review consisted of studies in which the interval between time 1 and time 2 was quite brief. Moreover, in many of those studies, participants did not even engage in behavior at time 1. Instead, they were merely asked to recall or think about a previous behavior; its impact on a subsequent action was then assessed. Such studies may be less informative of the nature of behavioral sequencing effects when actual rather than recalled behavior is the point of departure at time 1. Moreover, whereas Yam and colleagues (2017) found a licensing effect when the interval was 2 weeks, it is an open question whether the presence and form of such an effect may differ when the interval is even longer, which may be examined in organizations given the ongoing nature of social encounters and relationships transpiring within them.

Different Self-Processes, and Transitioning from One to the Other

Whereas the behaviors to which we alluded in the preceding section were quantitatively different from one another (e.g., more ethical behavior at time 1 led to less ethical behavior at time 2), the ongoing nature of exchanges and relationships in organizational settings suggests that there also may be qualitative differences in underlying processes over time. For example, consider the two factors that Lin and colleagues (2016) found to account for the relationship between ethical behavior at time 1 and abusive supervision at time 2: moral licensing and ego depletion. These processes are exemplars of two different ways in which the self exerts influence: as object and as subject. The difference between the self-as-object (SAO) and the self-as-subject (SAS) is certainly not new, harkening back to the distinction William James (1890) made between the "me-self" and the "I-self," respectively. As discussed elsewhere (Brockner & Wiesenfeld, 2016), SAO refers to

processes in which people reflect upon themselves. It is well established that people strive to see themselves in a positive light (Sedikides & Gregg, 2008). For example, according to self-affirmation theory (Steele, 1988), people want to see themselves as "competent, good, coherent, unitary, stable, capable of free choice and capable of controlling important outcomes" (p. 262). Moral licensing is an SAO process. Behaving virtuously at time 1 allows people to see themselves favorably, thereby freeing them up to behave in ways that are less virtuous at time 2.

The SAS refers to self-regulatory processes in which people seek to align their behaviors and beliefs with meaningful standards. For example, the exercise of executive control ("mental processes that enable us to plan, focus attention, remember instructions, and juggle multiple tasks successfully"; Brockner & Wiesenfeld, 2016, p. 36) is an SAS process. The ego depletion explanation of how behaving ethically at time 1 made managers more abusive at time 2 (Lin et al., 2016) is therefore based on the SAS. To the extent that managers had to exert self-control to behave ethically at time 1, it left them with fewer self-regulatory resources to do so at time 2, thereby leading to abusive behavior at that later point in time.

A related example of how unethical behavior results from ego depletion was discovered by Kouchaki and Smith (2014), which they dubbed the "morning morality effect." The results showed that people were more likely to behave unethically in a laboratory experiment conducted later in the day rather than earlier in the day. Kouchaki and Smith surmised that life's self-regulatory activities, such as resisting the temptation to have a second delicious piece of cake at lunch, or not overreacting to a coworker who behaves badly toward them, requires people to exert self-control cumulatively as the day wears on. As a result, they have fewer self-regulatory resources that may be needed to withstand the temptation to behave unethically later in the day.

In their test of multiple mediation, Lin and colleagues (2016) found that moral licensing and ego depletion accounted for the relationship between managers' ethical behavior at time 1 and abusive supervision at time 2; moreover, the two mediators were themselves empirically distinct ($r = .00$). Whereas Lin and associates found the two mediators to differ empirically, they did not discuss how the two differ conceptually. Moreover, the fact that moral licensing and ego depletion *can* account for the tendency of ethical behavior at time 1 to lead to unethical behavior at time 2 (the "ethical dropoff effect") raises the important question of when one mediating process may be more prominent than the other. When behaving ethically at time 1 requires people to exert high levels of self-control (e.g., when they would have had much to gain by behaving unethically instead and when it was unlikely they would have been found out if they did), then the ethical dropoff effect is likely to be explained by ego depletion. On the other hand, when behaving ethically at time 1 was enacted while people were in a more self-reflective mode (e.g., shortly after receiving a performance review) then the ethical dropoff effect may be explained by moral licensing.

Moreover, there are theoretical reasons to believe that the magnitude of the ethical dropoff effect may be influenced by a combination of the mediating process (e.g., moral licensing vs. ego depletion) and the length of time elapsed since the initial ethical act. More specifically, ego depletion may be more likely to dissipate over time than moral licensing. According to ego depletion theory, rest allows people to recuperate from the loss of energy elicited by the exertion of self-control (Baumeister, 2002). Therefore, to the extent that ethical behavior at time 1 elicited ego depletion, we would expect the tendency to behave unethically at time 2 to be less pronounced when there is a greater interval between time 1 and time 2, which would better allow people to restore their ego resources.

Moral licensing and ego depletion are exemplars of the different ways in which people's selves influence their beliefs and behaviors. Given the meaningful difference between the SAO and the SAS, another important question to be examined in future research is what causes people to shift from one self-process to the other. Once again, the study of such transitions (and the factors that elicit them) are facilitated by examining them in a context of ongoing interactions and exchanges, which include (but are not limited to) organizational settings.

The exigencies of everyday life require ongoing self-regulation. Hence, it seems plausible that the default mode for the operation of self-processes is the SAS. Self-regulatory activities are likely to be periodically punctuated, however, by experiences or events that induce people to take themselves as the object of attention. For example, when faced with important decisions (e.g., for individuals, what job or career to pursue, or, for managers in the workplace, which strategic direction to take), a well-thought-out process typically includes a self-reflective component (Janis & Mann, 1977). As people consider their alternatives, they need to ask themselves questions, such as "Which one is most congruent with who I am (we are)" or "Which one is likely to make me (us) feel good about myself (ourselves)?" Moreover, when the external environment is perceived to be undergoing change, thereby inducing decision-makers to (re)-evaluate the utility of their status quo behaviors, they may shift from doing (engaging in self-regulatory activity) to reflecting on who they are as a precursor to subsequent self-regulatory activity.

The environment also may shift in ways that induce people to transition from reflecting on themselves to engaging in self-regulation. For example, suppose a senior management team embarked on a multiday offsite retreat to determine its vision and strategy for the next 3 years. If done properly, such discussions should include a consideration of how the team thinks about its (and by extension, the organization's) identity. Suppose, further, that midway through the offsite retreat, the team caught wind of information that put it in crisis mode. Responses to crises typically do not afford one the luxury of being preceded and therefore informed by a self-reflective process. The emphasis is on *doing* what is required for successful self-regulation. To the extent that SAO processes are enacted in relation to crises, they are likely to occur at a later point in time, after the crisis has passed and decision-makers have the space to engage in a self-reflective afteraction review (Brockner & James, 2008).

How Others' Previous Actions Inform the Meaning of Their Present Behavior

Yet another way in which the ongoing nature of organizational life enriches understanding of social psychological principles is by capturing the reality that people's reactions to their current experiences are colored by their previous experiences. This truism allows us to extend what may be learned from "snapshot" studies of people's reactions to a one-time event, which is the form that many social psychology studies take. One conceptual framework from the justice literature that takes historical influences into account is fairness heuristic theory (FHT; Lind, 2001). According to this viewpoint, people use fairness information to evaluate the extent to which they can trust decision-making authorities. Moreover, once fairness judgments of the authorities have been formed, they become the default option (or heuristic) that guides people's perceptions of and reactions to subsequent encounters with the authorities. After all, it would be psychologically taxing for people to have to evaluate whether authorities can be trusted if they engaged in this process every time they were exposed to fairness-relevant information. Rather, in response to new or updated information, it would be far simpler for them to either (1) not engage in a fairness judgment process or (2) interpret the incoming information in a manner consistent with the extant fairness judgment, also known as an *assimilation effect*.

When either process or outcome information deviates from prior expectations but the other one does not, then assimilation is likely; the overall experience is unlikely to be felt as very different from prior expectations. However, when both forms of fairness-relevant information (i.e., outcomes and process) are at odds with people's expectations, then they are likely to reevaluate their expectations in the direction of the new information, also known as a *contrast effect*. For example, Bianchi and colleagues (2015) used employees' extant level of trust in the authority as a proxy for how fairly they expected to be treated; they then explored how process fairness and outcome fairness information affected employees' commitment to the organization. When process *and* outcome fairness information differed from employees' extant levels of trust, the combination led them to respond more in the direction of the incoming information. Thus, the subset of participants with higher levels of extant trust showed the greatest decline in commitment when

process and outcome fairness were relatively low, whereas those with lower levels of extant trust showed the greatest increase in commitment when process and outcome fairness were relatively high. Moreover, process fairness and outcome fairness combined interactively rather than additively; it was only when outcome *and* process were different from employees' extant levels of trust that their commitment shifted more in the direction of how fairly they had been treated. Perhaps this was because the combination of outcome fairness and process fairness represented the most clear-cut case of their experience contrasting with their prior expectations. If either process or outcome information differed from what their extant levels of trust led them to expect, whereas the other one did not, employees showed an assimilation effect rather than a contrast effect.

FHT and the Bianchi and colleagues (2015) findings also help us to understand the self-perpetuating nature of relationships characterized by high and low levels of trust. More often than not, incoming information does not cause a reevaluation of the extant level of trust in the relationship; for instance, it is likely to be interpreted in a manner consistent with the extant level of trust. This may account for the virtuous cycle of the perception of high trust and also for the vicious cycle of the perception of low trust. Moreover, this reasoning provides insight into how to break the vicious cycle of low trust. When untrusted authorities behave in ways that recipients cannot assimilate to their prior beliefs, there is a chance that recipients will come to view them in a more positive light. Of course, this is unlikely to happen overnight. However, if untrusted authorities can provide *repeated* evidence that they have changed their ways, the contrast is likely to be more striking and credible, and therefore may be more apt to bring about positive change in the relationship.

Organizations Make Economic Considerations Salient

Money is the "coin of the realm" for many in work organizations and probably moreso than in other social contexts. There are some exceptions, such as in organizations that articulate a strong sense of moral purpose or among employees who develop close friendships with their coworkers. Nevertheless, pay, profits and losses, and economic value serve as a common unit of account shared by organization members and a variety of other stakeholders. Thus, another prominent feature of organizations is the salience of tangible economic outcomes in members' psychology. In particular, this involves thinking about money, using economic value as a metric on which to base social comparisons and to evaluate one's time (with attendant implications for subjective perceptions of scarcity), and more holistically using an economic mindset in decision making. How does this prominent feature influence social psychological principles?

A guiding assumption of social psychology is that people are social beings. Much theory and evidence suggest that people value their relationships with others (e.g., McClelland, 1985), judge their self-worth in large part with respect to the how much they are valued by others (e.g., Leary & Baumeister, 2000), and have a fundamental need to belong, that is, "form and maintain strong, stable interpersonal relationships" (e.g., Baumeister & Leary, 1995). The motivations associated with this inherent sociality, and the extent to which it shapes thoughts, feelings and behaviors, may be weakened by the heightened focus on tangible economic outcomes in organizational life. In particular, salient economic concerns may lead people to be less other-focused.

A growing body of evidence suggests that the salience of money shifts people's attention away from the social domain. For example, a number of studies have shown that when money has been made salient via priming, for example, by having people solve word scrambles referring to money or by physically handling money, they become more psychologically insensitive to social rejection (Zhou, Vohs & Baumeister, 2009), more self-reliant, and demonstrate a stronger preference for solitary activities, whether in work or leisure (Mogilner, 2010; Vohs, Mead & Goode, 2006). Relatedly, access to money in the form of higher income leads people to spend less time on social activities and more time on individual pursuits (Bianchi & Vohs, 2016).

Prosociality in the form of voluntary helping behaviors occurs when people value their relationships with others. Thus, it is more likely to occur when people are attuned to the feelings and needs of others, which is less apt to happen when money is salient (Vohs et al., 2008). Even in cultures with strong communal norms to help (e.g., India), reminders of money reduced the quality of help people were willing to provide and led people to feel a lower moral obligation to help those who need it (Savani, Mead, Stillman, & Vohs, 2016). Relatedly, economics majors are more likely to behave noncooperatively, such as by defecting in a prisoner's dilemma game, than are noneconomics majors (Frank, Gilovich, & Regan, 1993). Likewise, priming an economic schema has been found to reduce how compassionate people are when delivering bad news, in part because it reduces their feelings of empathy for others (Molinsky, Grant, & Margolis, 2012). To be sure, the effect of priming money on the harshness of people's social attitudes (e.g., how supportive they are of inequality, of socioeconomic differences, and of group-based discrimination) have not always been replicated (e.g., Rohrer, Pashler, & Harris, 2015). On balance, however, money priming shows consistent results, with over 165 studies demonstrating the negative effect of reminders of money on prosociality (Vohs, 2015).

Economic concerns are made salient in a particular way in work settings: Employees begin to think of their time in terms of its economic value. To be paid, people must devote working hours to their employer. Many jobs tighten the link between money and time by paying by the hour. Linking money and time through hourly pay strengthens the association between happiness and how much money people make (Devoe & Pfeffer, 2009), with some negative consequences for attention to social bases of happiness. A stream of research on the economic value of time at work reinforces the negative relationship between money and helping behavior by demonstrating that when people arc paid on an hourly basis, they are less willing to volunteer their time (DeVoe & Pfeffer, 2010). This is due, in part, to the fact that linking time to money leads employees to feel that their time (like money) is scarce (DeVoe & Pfeffer, 2011).

Not only does the salience of money decrease prosociality, but also it increases the likelihood that people will focus their attention on pursuits that interfere with collaboration and helping, such as competition. For example, making money salient leads people to allocate more effort toward performing challenging tasks that are solitary and position them well competitively (Vohs et al., 2008). Organizations are structured in ways that enhance competition because they combine salient economic rewards with social hierarchy, thus attaching economic value to social comparisons. Pay dispersion elicits social comparisons based on money, thus reinforcing not only the salience of money but also incorporating money into social relationships at work. Pay dispersion has been found to reduce harmony and cooperation by encouraging dysfunctional competition (Pfeffer & Langton, 1993). When pay dispersion exists within a team, it leads to lower performance due to lower collaboration, and this pattern has been found in teams ranging from lower levels to the top management team of a corporation (Siegel & Hambrick, 2005; Trevor, Reilly & Gerhart, 2012).

Pay dispersion may have even more insidious effects when people perceive themselves to be paid less than others. Given that people envy the wealth of others even when they are near the top of a pay scale (Gino & Pierce, 2009), they are likely to make negative comparisons between the income they receive and what they desire. This leads people to subjectively feel that their income is low or insufficient, thereby eliciting the psychology of scarcity (Mullainathan & Shafir, 2013). Subjective economic insufficiency has been found to lead to *cognitive tunneling*, which is when feelings of scarcity focus attention on the economic resources in short supply, increasing cognitive load. By reducing people's ability to cope with complexity, cognitive tunneling leads decision making to be experienced as more onerous, and the decisions made are more likely to be suboptimal (Mullainathan & Shafir, 2013). Given the earlier evidence suggesting that a focus on money reduces relationally oriented motivations, cognitive tunneling may exacerbate the effect even further by limiting cognitive ability. Money may be particularly likely to induce cognitive tunneling because it is a lower-order objective. Cognitive tunneling may be less likely when higher-order goals are pursued because higher-order goals

are more abstract and induce greater cognitive flexibility, while lower order goals narrow focus (Trope & Liberman, 2010). Thus, cognitive tunneling may be more likely when people perceive that they do not have enough money than when they perceive that their lives and work are not as psychologically meaningful as they would like them to be.

Making money salient not only reduces the value that people place on their social relationships, but it also selectively increases their reliance on other mental frames that are less consistent with the pursuit of rich and rewarding social relationships. Among the more noteworthy casualties of these ways of thinking are ethics and morality, which are vital to social cohesion. For example, mere exposure to money increases the likelihood that people will utilize a "business decision frame," in which economic costs and benefits are the most salient criteria for decision making (Kouchaki, Smith-Crowe, Brief, & Sousa, 2013). Likely because of the focus on measurable costs and benefits, making money salient increases certain kinds of unethical behavior that are designed to maximize economic rewards for the self, such as cheating (Gino & Mogilner, 2014; Kouchaki et al., 2013). Reductions in morality and ethics also arise from subjective feelings of economic insufficiency. When people feel financially deprived, they lower their moral standards, exhibit reductions in moral judgment, and are more likely to cheat (Pitesa & Thau, 2014; Sharma, Mazar, Alter, & Ariely, 2014).

Person–Environment Congruence Determines Organizational Outcomes

Another prominent feature of organizational life is the principle of *congruence*: Employees' attitudes and behaviors depend on the degree of fit between various aspects of themselves (e.g., values, traits, and attitudes) and various elements of their work environments (e.g., the nature of the work, the personal qualities of their coworkers, and the organization's culture; Kristof, 1996). Employees who perceived having a greater fit with their jobs and organizational environment showed greater commitment, better job performance, and stronger job satisfaction (Greguras & Diefendorff, 2009).

While these findings suggest that fit often yields positive outcomes, a persistent theme in organizational research is that flexibility and creativity may be promoted by non-fit, and that the comfort, efficiency, and stability of congruence may not promote innovation and change, and may even inhibit it (e.g., March, 1991).

The effects of congruence have been well established in social psychological research as well. Higgins (2000) introduced the notion of regulatory fit as an extension of regulatory focus theory that distinguishes between two motivational orientations: promotion and prevention. Promotion-oriented individuals experience fit if they operate in an environment that matches their primary concerns of growth and advancement. In contrast, prevention-oriented individuals experience fit if they operate in an environment that matches their primary concerns of safety and security. Regulatory fit makes individuals feel more motivated, engaged with their tasks, and confident in their decisions (Higgins, 2005).

Regulatory fit has been shown to account for unique variance in work behaviors after researchers control for personality, motivation, and attitudes (Lanaj, Chang, & Johnson, 2012). For instance, promotion (prevention) employees feel more valued if their leaders have a promotion (prevention) focus (Hamstra, Sassenberg, Van Yperen, & Wisse, 2014). The more organizational characteristics match employees' promotion and prevention focus, the more they perceive their organization as being fair (Roczniewska, Retowski, & Higgins, 2017). Employees' experience of regulatory fit also is positively associated with commitment and motivation at work (Johnson, Chang, & Yang, 2010).

The implicit assumptions in most social psychological research on fit are that (1) fit and non-fit are opposites of one another and (2) the effects of fit are simply the mirror image of the effects of non-fit. Organizational research drawing attention to the beneficial effects of both fit and non-fit suggests that these assumptions should be reconsidered. Evidence suggests that it may be useful to separate the effects of fit from the effects of non-fit (e.g., Levine, Alexander, Wright, & Higgins, 2016). Under certain conditions, significant results may be due more

to the presence or degree of non-fit, whereas in other instances, the "action" may be due more to the presence or degree of fit. For example, a series of studies suggest that whereas performance on traditional tasks is enhanced by regulatory fit, performance on tasks that require creativity and a fresh perspective are enhanced by non-fit (Avnet & Higgins, 2020). Non-fit also may be especially consequential when people are strongly opposed to exhibiting a certain course of action. For example, suppose that an organization wanted to introduce a change in policy to which employees are likely to be resistant. If the organization's communications about the change fit with employees' regulatory focus orientations (i.e., emphasizing the benefits to be reaped when communicating with those with a promotion focus, or emphasizing the costs to be avoided when addressing those with a prevention focus), employees are likely to feel more committed to whatever they are doing or experiencing (Higgins, 2005). Quite plausibly, among those experiencing resistance, regulatory fit may induce people to be even more committed to their resistance to the change (i.e., the experience of regulatory fit may cause them to dig their heels in even further).

However, and somewhat ironically, a change might be accepted more if employees became less committed to their resistance. One way to lower commitment is by creating conditions of regulatory non-fit. The results of several recent studies are consistent with this possibility. Along with our colleagues Sara Feldman, Tory Higgins, and Zhi Liu, two of us (I. F. and J. B.) recently conducted a study in which participants were asked to imagine that they were cancer patients faced with a particularly undesirable course of action toward which they were likely to be resistant: being placed in hospice care. Participants were experimentally induced to be promotion or prevention focused and were then randomly assigned to read one of three communications encouraging them to consider hospice. The first emphasized the benefits (gains) of being in hospice, the second focused on the costs they could avoid (non-losses) by being in hospice, and the third (or control) condition said nothing about benefits or costs.

In the fit conditions, (1) promotion participants were told of the benefits of being in hospice care and (2) prevention participants were told of the costs they could avoid by being in hospice. In the non-fit conditions, (1) prevention participants were told of the benefits of being in hospice care and (2) promotion participants were told of the costs they could avoid by being in hospice. The primary dependent variable was their change in attitude towards hospice care (i.e., how much their resistance to being placed in hospice was reduced). The results showed an effect of regulatory non-fit but no effect of regulatory fit. Relative to the control condition, non-fit reduced participants' opposition to being placed in hospice presumably because it lowered commitment to their high level of resistance. In contrast, the attitudes of those in the fit condition were no different from those in the control condition, presumably because it was unlikely for the greater commitment elicited by regulatory fit to increase their already high level of resistance.

A second study examined in a very different context whether regulatory non-fit lowers people's likely resistance to a course of action. Participants were child welfare workers asked to decide whether children who were being maltreated by their parents should be placed in foster care. It is reasonable to assume that participants would be generally resistant to leave maltreated children under the care of their parents, and therefore would be at least somewhat inclined to recommend the maltreated children be placed in foster care. Independent variables in this study included the nature of the maltreatment (abuse vs. neglect) and the regulatory focus orientations of the child welfare workers.

A key difference between abuse and neglect is that abuse involves the presence of harmful action, while neglect involves the (also harmful) absence of positive action. Regulatory focus theory differentiates sensitivity to a harmful action as opposed to the absence of a positive action. The theory suggests that harmful action is a prevention focus failure, while the absence of a positive action is a promotion focus failure (Higgins & Silberman, 1998). It therefore stands to reason that abuse may be (1) more upsetting to child welfare workers who are higher rather than lower in prevention focus, due to the greater regulatory fit relevance of abuse for those higher than lower in prevention focus, and/or

(2) less upsetting to child welfare workers who are higher rather than lower in promotion focus, due to the greater regulatory non-fit of abuse among those higher than lower in promotion focus. In contrast, neglect may be (1) more upsetting to child welfare workers who are higher rather than lower in promotion focus, due to the greater regulatory fit relevance of neglect for those higher rather than lower in promotion focus, and/or (2) less upsetting to investigators who are higher rather than lower in prevention focus, due to the greater regulatory non-fit of neglect among those higher rather than lower in prevention focus.

Whereas this reasoning suggests that the decision to recommend foster care could have been elicited by regulatory fit and/or non-fit, we only found evidence of the latter; that is, under conditions of non-fit (neglect-prevention and abuse-promotion) we found significant negative relationships between participants' regulatory focus orientations and how strongly they recommended the children to be placed in foster care. In the case of abuse, those higher in promotion focus may have been less likely to recommend placement in foster care than those lower in promotion focus because higher promotion constituted greater non-fit that produced less commitment and a concomitant deintensification of distress about the maltreatment. In the case of neglect, those higher in prevention focus may have been less likely to recommend placement in foster care than those lower in prevention focus because higher prevention constituted greater non-fit and reduced commitment, which led to greater de-intensification of distress about the maltreatment. In short, non-fit may have lessened participants' commitment to their resistance to returning maltreated children to their parents, which could explain why those higher in promotion were less likely to recommend foster care than those lower in promotion in the case of abuse and those higher in prevention were less likely to recommend foster care than those lower in prevention in the case of neglect.

Motivation refers to *what* people are inclined to do and the *intensity* with which they are inclined to do it. Knowing these two things may provide insight into when significant effects are more likely to be driven by fit versus non-fit.

Strong opposition to a course of action may be reduced by the experience of non-fit because it reduces commitment to the opposition. Greater fit would have little impact because of a "ceiling effect" on commitment. On the other hand, low to moderate support for a course of action may be heightened by the experience of fit because fit may intensify people's commitment to their initial position. Greater non-fit would have little influence because of a "floor effect" on commitment. More generally, the prominent organizational feature of person–environment congruence has recently given rise to theory and research suggesting that fit and non-fit are not simply mirror images of one another (Avnet & Higgins, 2020).

Organizations Elicit a Sense of Agency

Agency, which refers to the process of acting on behalf of others, is inherent to the role of decision-makers at various levels within organizations. Outside of their work organizations, people often believe that they can act for themselves, engaging in their own endeavors and guided by their own goals, but inside their organizations, people have contractual obligations to enact a defined role, regardless of their personal identities or desires. Organizational systems and structures offer frequent reminders to members of their legal and fiduciary responsibilities to act on behalf of others, including investors, customers, direct reports, and team members. Organization members are compensated for enacting the role of agent, setting aside their own interests, preferences, and even values, while bearing the tensions and conflicts associated with this predicament.

Whether people are agents or acting on their own behalf has been shown to affect several well-established principles. For example, multiple literatures in social psychology, such as reactance theory (e.g., Brehm & Brehm, 1981) and perceived control (Deci & Ryan, 1985; Seligman, 1975) have shown that people prefer having a sense of choice about their behavior. More recent theory and research have suggested, however, that there may be such a thing as having too much choice (Iyengar, 2010; Schwartz, 2004). When people are given a large

number of alternatives to choose from (e.g., 35 different colors of watches; Polman, 2012a), they show evidence of "choice overload," in which they find the act of choosing overwhelming and therefore not very satisfying, which in turn leads them to have lower commitment to the chosen alternative.

A series of studies, however, has shown that the choice overload effect manifests itself when people are choosing on behalf of themselves, but not when they are choosing on behalf of others (Polman, 2012a). In fact, when choosing on behalf of others, people react more positively when they have a large number of choices than when they have few. This is because choosing for oneself versus choosing for others has different effects on people's regulatory focus orientations (Higgins, 1997). When choosing for themselves (others) people tend to be more prevention (promotion) focused. Hence, when choosing for themselves, people find that *many* choices confronts them with the discomfiting prospect that they may not be making the right choice; that is, they may be making an error of commission, which prevention-focused people are especially motivated to avoid (Crowe & Higgins, 1997).

A very different psychology is elicited among people choosing on behalf of others as a function of whether they have few or very many choices. For those acting as agents, the presence of *few* choices makes salient the discomfiting possibility that they may not be making the right choice; that is, they may be making an error of omission, which promotion-focused people are highly motivated to avoid (Crowe & Higgins, 1997). Put differently, when agents have many alternatives to choose from, their concomitant promotion focus makes them less likely to believe that they are making an error of omission, thereby leading to a reversal of the choice overload effect.

Other research by Polman (2012b) demonstrated that agency also has implications for the prominent principle of decision theory known as loss aversion. *Loss aversion* refers to people's general tendency to react more strongly to negative events than to positive events of an equal magnitude. Research on loss aversion has shown, for instance, that losing $100 feels worse than winning $100 feels good (Thaler, 1999), or, as Kahneman and Tversky (1984) put it, "losses loom larger than gains." Loss aversion has implications for many foundational effects in behavioral decision theory, such as the prospect theory notion that people are risk-averse when choosing between gains but are risk-seeking when choosing between losses, and the endowment effect in which people need to be paid more to part with an item than they are willing to pay for that same item when it is not in their possession (Thaler, 1980).

Polman's (2012b) research suggests that the influence of agency may be accounted for by a host of factors. Across eight studies, he found that decision-makers exhibited less loss aversion when they were acting as agents than when they were deciding for themselves. Moreover, Polman showed that a host of psychological factors that have been shown to influence loss aversion can account for the tendency of agency to make people less loss averse, including regulatory focus, construal level, and sense of power. Elsewhere, it has been shown that people have less loss aversion when (1) they are promotion rather than prevention focused (Idson, Liberman, & Higgins, 2000), (2) they construe events abstractly rather than concretely (Malkoc & Zauberman, 2006), and (3) their sense of power is relatively high (Inesi, 2010). Polman (2012b) found that each of these factors moderated the relationship between agency and loss aversion. Among those individuals whose psychological orientations predisposed them to be more loss averse (those with a prevention focus, a tendency to construe concretely, and a lower sense of power), people were indeed more loss averse when choosing on their own behalf than when they were acting as agents. However, people whose psychological orientations reduced their loss aversion (those with a promotion focus, a tendency to construe abstractly, and a higher sense of power) were no more loss averse when choosing for themselves than when they were acting as agents.

Organization members not only make decisions on behalf of others but also they often negotiate on behalf of others. Amanatullah and Morris (2010) found an intriguing interactive effect of participants' gender and whether they were negotiating on their own or others' behalf on the assertiveness of their behavior. When

negotiating on their own behalf, women were much less assertive than men. However, this difference was eliminated when people were negotiating on behalf of others. To state the interaction effect differently, women were much more assertive when negotiating on others' rather than on their own behalf, whereas men's negotiation behavior did not vary as a function of whether they were negotiating on their own or others' behalf.

By way of explanation, Amanatullah and Morris (2010) reasoned that women varied their behavior across conditions because they were acting in accordance with gender-stereotypical norms that mandate them to behave communally. When negotiating on behalf of themselves, women anticipated a backlash if they acted assertively; after all, it is not very communal for them to negotiate assertively. However, when negotiating on behalf of others, the communal thing to do is to act assertively (doing what is best for "us"). Freed from the role-incongruent perception of appearing selfish and/or encouraged by the norm of doing what is best for the collective, women negotiating as agents behaved more assertively.

Research on the choice overload effect, loss aversion, and gender differences in negotiations show that when people act as agents, they behave quite differently than when deciding for themselves. These differences can be accounted for by multiple factors. Further research is needed to delineate the conditions under which a given factor is likely to be particularly influential. For now, however, we can conclude that the prominent organizational feature of agency has important implications for social psychological principles.

Conclusion

We have considered how five prominent features of organizational life shed light on empirical regularities and theoretical principles in social psychology. Numerous studies have shown that the form or magnitude of certain effects are influenced by the prominent features. To cite a few examples:

1. The nature of the interactive relationship between outcome favorability and process

fairness depends on recipients' rank relative to the other party (hierarchy).

2. How people behave at time 1 may cause them to behave in an opposite manner at time 2, something that would only be known by examining people over time (the ongoing nature of organizational life).
3. Various manifestations of sociality, such as the value that people assign to their encounters and relationships with others, are lower when economic considerations are more salient.
4. The principle of loss aversion is reduced when people are acting as agents rather than on their own behalf (agency).

Looking to the future, we encourage efforts that further refine our understanding of the mechanisms through which prominent features of organizations affect empirically based principles of social psychology. For example, whereas moral licensing and ego depletion *can* explain why behaving ethically at time 1 makes people less likely to do so at time 2, it would be theoretically as well as practically worthwhile to delineate the organizational conditions that make one mechanism more relevant than the other.

Finally, an additional benefit of examining the implications of prominent features of organizations for social psychological principles is a deeper understanding of the prominent features themselves. For example, whereas the two bases of social hierarchy (power and status) are related, they are not only conceptually but also empirically distinguishable. The experience of power causes decision-makers to behave less fairly, whereas the experience of status causes them to behave more fairly. Further evidence of the utility of differentiating between power and status is that they combine interactively to influence people's tendencies to behave fairly as well as nastily toward others. Research presented in the section on person–environment congruence offers insight into how we think about the constructs of fit and non-fit. Contrary to the prevailing view that they are simply mirror images of one another, fit and non-fit may have separate effects of their own. We have also offered an informed speculation (that needs to be tested in future research) about the conditions under which people's experience of fit versus

non-fit is likely to be more influential; that is, fit may elicit change in the presence of a low to moderate level of prior support for a course of action, while non-fit may elicit change in the presence of a high level of prior resistance. In conclusion, much has been learned from theory and research residing at the interface between prominent features of organizations and social psychological principles. In the truest sense, the relationship between these two sets of considerations is reciprocal: Prominent features inform the principles, and analyses of the principles may inform our understanding of the prominent features.

REFERENCES

Amanatullah, E. T., & Morris, M. W. (2010). Negotiating gender roles: Gender differences in assertive negotiating are mediated by women's fear of backlash and attenuated when negotiating on behalf of others. *Journal of Personality and Social Psychology, 98*(2), 256–267.

Anicich, E. M., Fast, N. J., Halevy, N., & Galinsky, A. D. (2015). When the bases of social hierarchy collide: Power without status drives interpersonal conflict. *Organization Science, 27*(1), 123–140.

Avnet, T., & Higgins, E. T. (2020). *Fit and non-fit: Seeing the full picture versus the big picture.* Manuscript under review.

Baumeister, R. F. (2002). Ego depletion and self-control failure: An energy model of the self's executive function. *Self and Identity, 1,* 129–136.

Baumeister, R. F., Bratslavsky, E., Muraven, M., & Tice, D. M. (1998). Ego depletion: Is the active self a limited resource? *Journal of Personality and Social Psychology, 74*(5), 1252–1265.

Baumeister, R. F., & Leary, M. R. (1995). The need to belong: Desire for interpersonal attachments as a fundamental human motivation. *Psychological Bulletin, 117*(3), 497–529.

Bem, D. J. (1972). Self-perception theory. In L. Berkowitz (Ed.), *Advances in experimental social psychology* (Vol. 6, pp. 1–62). New York: Academic Press.

Bianchi, E. C., Brockner, J., van den Bos, K., Seifert, M., Moon, H., van Dijke, M., & De Cremer, D. (2015). Trust in decision-making authorities dictates the form of the interactive relationship between outcome fairness and procedural fairness. *Personality and Social Psychology Bulletin, 41*(1), 19–34.

Bianchi, E. C., & Vohs, K. D. (2016). Social class and social worlds: Income predicts the frequency and nature of social contact. *Social Psychological and Personality Science, 7*(5), 479–486.

Bies, R. J. (1987). The predicament of injustice: The management of moral outrage. In L. L. Cummings & B. M. Staw, (Eds.), *Research in organizational behavior* (Vol. 9, pp. 289–319). Greenwich, CT: JAI Press.

Blader, S. L., & Chen, Y. R. (2012). Differentiating the effects of status and power: A justice perspective. *Journal of Personality and Social Psychology, 102*(5), 994–1014.

Brehm, S. S., & Brehm, J. W. 1981. *Psychological reactance: A theory of freedom and control.* New York: Academic Press.

Brockner, J. (1992). The escalation of commitment to a failing course of action: Toward theoretical progress. *Academy of Management Review, 17*(1), 39–61.

Brockner, J., Ackerman, G., Greenberg, J., Gelfand, M., Francesco, A. M., Chen, Z. X., et al. (2001). Culture and procedural justice: The influence of power distance on reactions to voice. *Journal of Experimental Social Psychology, 37,* 300–315.

Brockner, J., & James, E. H. (2008). Toward an understanding of when executives see crisis as opportunity. *Journal of Applied Behavioral Science, 44*(1), 94–115.

Brockner, J., Siegel, P. A., Daly, J. P., Tyler, T., & Martin, C. (1997). When trust matters: The moderating effect of outcome favorability. *Administrative Science Quarterly, 42,* 558–583.

Brockner, J., & Wiesenfeld, B. M. (1993). Living on the edge (of social and organizational psychology): The effects of layoffs on those who remain. In J. K. Murnighan (Ed.), *Social psychology in organizations: Advances in theory and research* (pp. 119–140). Englewood Cliffs, NJ: Prentice Hall.

Brockner, J., & Wiesenfeld, B. M. (1996). An integrative framework for explaining reactions to decisions: Interactive effects of outcomes and procedures. *Psychological Bulletin, 120*(2), 189–208.

Brockner, J., & Wiesenfeld, B. M. (2016). Self-as-object and self-as-subject in the workplace. *Organizational Behavior and Human Decision Processes, 136,* 36–46.

Chen, Y. R., Brockner, J., & Greenberg, J. (2003). When is it "a pleasure to do business with you?": The effects of relative status, outcome favorability, and procedural fairness. *Organizational Behavior and Human Decision Processes, 92*(1–2), 1–21.

Crowe, E., & Higgins, E. T. (1997). Regulatory focus and strategic inclinations: Promotion and prevention in decision-making. *Organizational Behavior and Human Decision Processes, 69*(2), 117–132.

Deci, E. L., & Ryan, R. M. (1985). *Intrinsic motiva-tion and self-determination in human behavior.* New York: Plenum Press.

DeVoe, S. E., & Pfeffer, J. (2009). When is happiness about how much you earn?: The effect of hourly payment on the money–happiness connection. *Personality and Social Psychology Bulletin, 35*(12), 1602–1618.

DeVoe, S. E., & Pfeffer, J. (2010). The stingy hour: How accounting for time affects volunteering. *Personality and Social Psychology Bulletin, 36*(4), 470–483.

DeVoe, S. E., & Pfeffer, J. (2011). Time is tight: How higher economic value of time increases feelings of time pressure. *Journal of Applied Psychology, 96*(4), 665–676.

Fast, N. J., Halevy, N., & Galinsky, A. D. (2012). The destructive nature of power without status. *Journal of Experimental Social Psychology, 48*(1), 391–394.

Festinger, L. (1957). *A theory of cognitive dissonance.* Stanford, CA: Stanford University Press.

Frank, R., Gilovich, T., Regan, D. (1993). Does studying economics inhibit cooperation? *Journal of Economic Perspectives, 7*(2), 159–171.

Freedman, J. L., & Fraser, S. C. (1966). Compliance without pressure: The foot-in-the-door technique. *Journal of Personality and Social Psychology, 4*(2), 195–202.

Gino, F., & Mogilner, C. (2014). Time, money, and morality. *Psychological Science, 25*(2), 414–421.

Gino, F., & Pierce, L. (2009). The abundance effect: Unethical behavior in the presence of wealth. *Organizational Behavior and Human Decision Processes, 109,* 142–155.

Greguras, G. J., & Diefendorff, J. M. (2009). Different fits satisfy different needs: Linking person–environment fit to employee commitment and performance using self-determination theory. *Journal of Applied Psychology, 94*(2), 465–477.

Hamstra, M. R., Sassenberg, K., Van Yperen, N. W., & Wisse, B. (2014). Followers feel valued when leaders' regulatory focus makes leaders exhibit behavior that fits followers' regulatory focus. *Journal of Experimental Social Psychology, 51,* 34–40.

Higgins, E. T. (1997). Beyond pleasure and pain. *American Psychologist, 52*(12), 1280–1300.

Higgins, E. T. (2000). Making a good decision: Value from fit. *American Psychologist, 55*(11), 1217–1230.

Higgins, E. T. (2005). Value from regulatory fit. *Current Directions in Psychological Science, 14*(4), 209–213.

Higgins, E. T., & Silberman, I. (1998). Development of regulatory focus: Promotion and prevention as ways of living. In J. Heckhausen & C. S. Dweck

(Eds.), *Motivation and self-regulation across the life span* (pp. 78–113). New York: Cambridge University Press.

Idson, L. C., Liberman, N., & Higgins, E. T. (2000). Distinguishing gains from non-losses and losses from non-gains: A regulatory focus perspective on hedonic intensity. *Journal of Experimental Social Psychology, 36*(3), 252–274.

Inesi, M. E. (2010). Power and loss aversion. *Organizational Behavior and Human Decision Processes, 112*(1), 58–69.

Iyengar, S. S. (2010). *The art of choosing.* New York: Twelve.

James, W. (1890). The hidden self. *Scribner's Magazine, 7*(3), 361–373.

Janis, I. L., & Mann, L. (1977). *Decision making: A psychological analysis of conflict, choice, and commitment.* New York: Free Press.

Johnson, R. E., Chang, C. H., & Yang, L. Q. (2010). Commitment and motivation at work: The relevance of employee identity and regulatory focus. *Academy of Management Review, 35*(2), 226–245.

Kahneman, D., & Tversky, A. (1984). Choices, values, and frames. *American Psychologist, 39,* 341–350.

Keltner, D., Gruenfeld, D. H., & Anderson, C. (2003). Power, approach, and inhibition. *Psychological Review, 110*(2), 265–268.

Kouchaki, M., & Smith, I. (2014). The morning morality effect: The influence of time of day on unethical behavior. *Psychological Science, 25*(1), 95–102.

Kouchaki, M., Smith-Crowe, K., Brief, A. P., & Sousa, C. (2013). Seeing green: Mere exposure to money triggers a business decision frame and unethical outcomes. *Organizational Behavior and Human Decision Processes, 121*(1), 53–61.

Kramer, R. M. (1996). Divergent realities and convergent disappointments in the hierarchic relation: Trust and the intuitive auditor at work. In R. M. Kramer & T. R. Tyler (Eds.), *Trust in organizations: Frontiers of theory and research* (pp. 216–246). London: SAGE.

Kristof, A. L. (1996). Person–organization fit: An integrative review of its conceptualizations, measurement, and implications. *Personnel Psychology, 49*(1), 1–49.

Lanaj, K., Chang, C. H., & Johnson, R. E. (2012). Regulatory focus and work-related outcomes: A review and meta-analysis. *Psychological Bulletin, 138*(5), 998–1034.

Leary, M. R., & Baumeister, R. F. (2000). The nature and function of self-esteem: Sociometer theory. In M. P. Zanna (Ed.), *Advances in experimental social psychology* (Vol. 32, pp. 1–62). San Diego, CA: Academic Press.

Levine, J. M., Alexander, K. M., Wright, A. G., & Higgins, E. T. (2016). Group brainstorming: When regulatory non-fit enhances performance. *Group Processes and Intergroup Relations, 19*(2), 257–271.

Lin, S. H. J., Ma, J., & Johnson, R. E. (2016). When ethical leader behavior breaks bad: How ethical leader behavior can turn abusive via ego depletion and moral licensing. *Journal of Applied Psychology, 101*(6), 815–830.

Lind, E. A. (2001). Fairness heuristic theory: Justice judgments as pivotal cognitions in organizational relations. In J. Greenberg & R. Cropanzano (Eds.), *Advances in organizational justice* (pp. 56–88). Stanford, CA: Stanford University Press.

Lind, E. A., & Tyler, T. R. (1988). *The social psychology of procedural justice.* New York: Plenum Press.

Magee, J. C, & Galinsky, A. D. (2008). Social hierarchy: The self-reinforcing nature of power and status. *Academy of Management Annals, 2,* 351–398.

Malkoc, S. A., & Zauberman, G. (2006). Deferring versus expediting consumption: The effect of outcome concreteness on sensitivity to time horizon. *Journal of Marketing Research, 43*(4), 618–627.

March, J. G. (1991). Exploration and exploitation in organizational learning. *Organization Science, 2*(1), 71–87.

McClelland, D. C. (1985). *Human motivation.* Glenview, IL: Scott, Foresman.

Merritt, A. C., Effron, D. A., & Monin, B. (2010). Moral self-licensing: When being good frees us to be bad. *Social and Personality Psychology Compass, 4*(5), 344–357.

Milgram, S (1974). *Obedience to authority: An experimental view.* New York: Harper & Row.

Mogilner, C. (2010). The pursuit of happiness: Time, money, and social connection. *Psychological Science, 21,* 1348–1354.

Molinsky, A. L., Grant, A. M., & Margolis, J. D. (2012). The bedside manner of homo economicus: How and why priming an economic schema reduces compassion. *Organizational Behavior and Human Decision Processes, 119*(1), 27–37.

Monin, B., & Miller, D. T. (2001). Moral credentials and the expression of prejudice. *Journal of Personality and Social Psychology, 81*(1), 33–43.

Mullainathan, S., & Shafir, E. (2013). *Scarcity: Why having too little means so much.* New York: Holt.

Mullen, E., & Monin, B. (2016). Consistency versus licensing effects of past moral behavior. *Annual Review of Psychology, 67,* 363–385.

Nadler, D. A., & Tushman, M. (1982). Frameworks for organizational behavior. *Organizational Dynamics, 9,* 35–51.

Orne, M. T. (1962). On the social psychology of the

psychological experiment: With particular reference to demand characteristics and their implications. *American Psychologist, 17*(11), 776–783.

Pfeffer, J., & Langton, N. (1993). The effect of wage dispersion on satisfaction, productivity, and working collaboratively: Evidence from college and university faculty. *Administrative Science Quarterly, 38*(3), 382–407.

Pitesa, M., & Thau, S. (2013). Compliant sinners, obstinate saints: How power and self-focus determine the effectiveness of social influences in ethical decision making. *Academy of Management Journal, 56,* 635–658.

Pitesa, M., & Thau, S. (2014). A lack of material resources causes harsher moral judgments. *Psychological Science, 25,* 702–710.

Polman, E. (2012a). Effects of self–other decision making on regulatory focus and choice overload. *Journal of Personality and Social Psychology, 102*(5), 980–993.

Polman, E. (2012b). Self–other decision making and loss aversion. *Organizational Behavior and Human Decision Processes, 119,* 141–150.

Rajan, R., & Wulf, J. (2003). *The flattening firm: Evidence from panel data on the changing nature of corporate hierarchies* (NBER Working Paper No. 9633). Cambridge, MA: National Bureau of Economic Research.

Roczniewska, M., Retowski, S., & Higgins, E. T. (2017). How person–organization fit impacts employees' perceptions of justice and well-being. *Frontiers in Psychology, 8,* 1–17.

Rohrer, D., Pashler, H., & Harris, C. R. (2015). Do subtle reminders of money change people's political views? *Journal of Experimental Psychology: General, 144*(4), e73–e85.

Ross, J., & Staw, B. M. (1993). Organizational escalation and exit: Lessons from the Shoreham nuclear power plant. *Academy of Management Journal, 36,* 701–732.

Rothman, N. B., Wheeler-Smith, S., Wiesenfeld, B. M., & Galinsky, A. (2020). *Gaining power but losing status: Why unfair leaders are selected over fair leaders.* Manuscript in preparation.

Rubin, J. Z., & Brockner, J. (1975). Factors affecting entrapment in waiting situations: The Rosencrantz and Guildenstern effect. *Journal of Personality and Social Psychology, 31,* 1054–1063.

Savani, K., Mead, N. L., Stillman, T., & Vohs, K. D. (2016). No match for money: Even in intimate relationships and collectivistic cultures, reminders of money weaken sociomoral responses. *Self and Identity, 15*(3), 342–355.

Schwartz, B. (2004). *The paradox of choice: Why more is less.* New York: HarperCollins.

Sedikides, C., & Gregg, A. P. (2008). Self-enhance-

ment: Food for thought. *Perspectives on Psychological Science, 3*(2), 102–116.

Seligman, M. E. (1975). *Helplessness: On depression, development, and death.* New York: Freeman.

Sharma, E., Mazar, N., Alter, A. L., & Ariely, D. (2014). Financial deprivation selectively shifts moral standards and compromises moral decisions. *Organizational Behavior and Human Decision Processes, 123*(2), 90–100.

Siegel, P. A., & Hambrick, D. C. (2005). Pay disparities within top management groups: Evidence of harmful effects on performance of high-technology firms. *Organization Science, 16*(3), 259–274.

Staw, B. M. (1976). Knee-deep in the big muddy: A study of escalating commitment to a chosen course of action. *Organizational Behavior and Human Performance, 16*(1), 27–44.

Steele, C. M. (1988). The psychology of self-affirmation: Sustaining the integrity of the self. In L. Berkowitz (Ed.), *Advances in experimental social psychology* (Vol. 21, pp. 261–302). New York: Academic Press.

Thaler, R. (1980). Toward a positive theory of consumer choice. *Journal of Economic Behavior and Organization, 1*(1), 39–60.

Thaler, R. H. (1999). Mental accounting matters. *Journal of Behavioral Decision Making, 12*(3), 183–207.

Trevor, C. O., Reilly, G., & Gerhart, B. (2012). Reconsidering pay dispersion's effect on the performance of interdependent work: Reconciling sorting and pay inequality. *Academy of Management Journal, 55*(3), 585–610.

Trope, Y., & Liberman, N. (2010). Construal-level theory of psychological distance. *Psychological Review, 117*(2), 440–463.

Tyler, T. R., & Sears, D. O. (1977). Coming to like obnoxious people when we must live with them. *Journal of Personality and Social Psychology, 35*(4), 200–211.

van den Bos, K. (2005). What is responsible for the fair process effect? In J. Greenberg & J. A. Colquitt (Eds.), *Handbook of organizational justice* (pp. 273–300). New York: Psychology Press.

van den Bos, K., Brockner, J., van den Oudenalder, M., Kamble, S. V., & Nasabi, A. (2013). Delineating a method to study cross-cultural differences with experimental control: The voice effect and countercultural contexts regarding power distance. *Journal of Experimental Social Psychology, 49*(4), 624–634.

van den Bos, K., Bruins, J., Wilke, H. A. M., & Dronkert, E. (1999). Sometimes unfair procedures have nice aspects: On the psychology of the fair process effect. *Journal of Personality and Social Psychology, 77*(2), 324–336.

Vohs, K. D. (2015). Money priming can change people's thoughts, feelings, motivations, and behaviors: An update on 10 years of experiments. *Journal of Experimental Psychology: General, 144*(4), e86–e93.

Vohs, K. D., Mead, N. L., & Goode, M. R. (2008). Merely activating the concept of money changes personal and interpersonal behavior. *Current Directions in Psychological Science, 17*(3), 208–212.

Yam, K. C., Klotz, A. C., He, W., & Reynolds, S. J. (2017). From good soldiers to psychologically entitled: Examining when and why citizenship behavior leads to deviance. *Academy of Management Journal, 60*(1), 373–396.

Zhou, X., Vohs, K. D., & Baumeister, R. F. (2009). The symbolic power of money: Reminders of money alter social distress and physical pain. *Psychological Science, 20*(6),700–706.

CHAPTER 29

Political Extremism

Katarzyna Jasko
David Webber
Arie W. Kruglanski

Political violence is often portrayed as a means of last resort. Thus, there is a perception among those who use political violence that this tactic has a chance to succeed where others have failed. Extant evidence, however, suggests the contrary. For instance, a comparison of 323 violent and nonviolent campaigns from 1900 to 2006 revealed that violent campaigns only achieved their political goals 26% of the time, whereas nonviolent campaigns succeeded 50% of the time (Chenoweth & Stephan, 2011). Similarly, an assessment of 125 campaigns of foreign terrorist organizations revealed that only 30% were successful in at least partially achieving their stated political goals (Abrahms, 2012). When analyses were limited to assess the effectiveness of terrorist attacks that targeted civilians (vs. the military), the success rate dropped to under 5%. Further support comes from an analysis of transitions from authoritarian to democratic systems between 1973 and 2005 (Karatnycky & Ackerman, 2005), wherein peaceful tactics such as boycotts, mass protests, strikes, and civil disobedience were a central component in a majority (50 out of 67) of successful transitions.

In part, violence is less effective because violent campaigns mobilize fewer people than do nonviolent campaigns. Whereas the average nonviolent campaign mobilized 200,000 people, the average violent campaign mobilized only 50,000 people (Chenoweth & Stephan, 2011). Fewer participants exert less pressure on the target (e.g., government), signal lower importance of the cause, and are easier to fight back. Moreover, when political extremist campaigns initiate violence, the response is more likely retaliation in kind. Governments more easily justify violent counterattacks against armed insurgents than against peacefully protesting activists.

Violence also degrades public support for participants and their campaigns. Indeed, a series of studies revealed that although self-identified political activists believed that violence was an effective way to recruit popular support, the reality was that violence decreased popular support by way of reducing the extent to which individuals identified with the political movement (Feinberg, Willer, & Kovacheff, 2017). Even protesters with otherwise high levels of public support (i.e., antiracist activists counterprotesting a gathering of White nationalists) can lose it by using violence (Simpson, Willer, & Feinberg, 2018). In this vein, Thomas and Louis (2014) showed that a nonviolent protest was more supported and more effective in changing public perception than a violent one, and its participants were viewed with lower hostility than violent protesters.

Though these findings suggest that political violence is inimical to political success, its practice across the globe shows no signs of relenting. In this chapter we turn to social psychology for answers. Specifically, we review theories and empirical evidence addressing this phenomenon. We begin by defining basic constructs pertinent to the study of political violence and political extremism. We then describe the theoretical model that explains political extremism by identifying its basic motivational determinants. We conclude by functionally interrelating this model to models that focused on the progression toward extremism. We finish with recapitulating the state of the knowledge that research on political activism and political violence has managed to contribute, and we identify practical implications of this knowledge for solving the problem of violent extremism.

Defining Extremism

Extremism as Motivational Imbalance

Extremism of any kind can be defined in contrast to moderation or normality, concepts that imply a (more or less) balanced satisfaction of individuals' basic needs (e.g., Fiske, 2003; Higgins, 2012; Maslow, 1943). In a state of moderation, basic needs constrain one another, so that people tend to avoid behaviors that serve some needs but frustrate others. (In fact, one dictionary definition of moderation is "restraint" [*Bartlett's Roget's Thesaurus,* 1996, p. 1126]). For instance, an individual might decline a prestigious job offer that would best fulfill his or her strivings for personal achievement, if accepting that position required a relocation that harmed his or her ability to manage important social relationships. Similarly, one's need to be respected and admired might be served by engaging in dangerous physical exploits and daredevil adventures. However, concerns for safety and comfort may constrain the risks one might be willing to tolerate and curb one's enthusiasm about dangerous undertakings. In like fashion,

people may typically refrain from violent political action because it requires a commitment to beliefs and behaviors, and the devotion of time and resources that threatens one's ability to fulfill other needs. Carrying out a violent attack for a cause might fulfill a need to feel valuable but simultaneously endanger one's life and increase susceptibility to arrest and imprisonment that would strip one of freedoms. Many people may be reluctant to make those sacrifices.

We propose that extremism occurs when a given need acquires such intensity that it dominates and overshadows other basic concerns. Exaggerated investment of individual resources in a dominant need involves the conscious or unconscious inhibition of alternative needs (Shah, Friedman, & Kruglanski, 2002). When that happens, the constraints these latter needs usually exercise on behavior are relaxed. This frees a broader set of previously constrained behaviors serving the dominant need and allows them to be considered as options. Often, the very behaviors that undermine (i.e., are *counterfinal* to) those other concerns are viewed as particularly effective ways of serving the dominant need (Kruglanski et al., 2014; Schumpe Bélanger, Giacomantonio, Nisa, & Brizi, 2018), and are then selected as means of its pursuit. Because most individuals strive to have all their basic needs gratified, they are normally likely to eschew counterfinal means that satisfy the dominant need while frustrating others. Typically, then, majorities of people exhibit a motivational balance and moderation. Enactment of counterfinal behaviors or adoption of counterfinal beliefs is thus likely to be infrequent, in correspondence to a common view of extremism as rare and deviant from general patterns of behavior.

Political Extremism

As with extremism writ large, *political extremism* is defined by placing one need above the rest. Extremists strive to fulfill one need, knowing that in so doing, they are impairing or sacrificing other concerns. Political extremists are therefore willing to do whatever it takes to fulfill their focal goal, even if the behavior at stake sacrifices things that matter. Their intense commitment to their dominant concern sets them apart from most people and accounts for their deviance from general behavioral norms. An important line of research that demonstrates the consequences for political engagement of an imbalanced motivational structure is work on passion (Rip, Vallerand, & Lafrenière, 2012). According to the dualistic model of passion (Vallerand, 2010) two forms of passion— harmonious and obsessive—can be identified. Harmonious passion depicts the case wherein an individual works toward an important value or task, while leaving time to focus on other important needs. This is akin to an individual who is motivationally balanced. Obsessive passion pertains to the case wherein an individual obsessively strives toward the satisfaction of a given concern, leaving little mental resources for other concerns. This is akin to the notion of motivational imbalance discussed earlier. Research among both Quebec Sovereignty activists and devout Muslims showed that participants who were motivationally balanced endorsed democratic and peaceful forms of activism (Rip et al., 2012). In contrast, the motivationally imbalanced ones endorsed political extremism and aggression. Similarly, research has linked this imbalanced form of passion to support for violence and endorsement of radical behaviors in service of environmental causes (Bélanger et al., 2019; Gousse-Lessard, Vallerand, Carbonneau, & Lafrenière, 2013).

Behavioral and Ideological Extremism

Political extremism does not manifest itself exclusively in overt action; it also includes the upholding of extreme ideas, the latter of which also involves sacrifices of various sorts. Commitment to extreme or downright prohibited ideas of religious or political natures may risk social opprobrium, if not a more severe punishment. History is replete with examples in which people were persecuted for their faith. For instance, the treatment of Early Christians in ancient Rome, Jews under the Spanish Inquisition, and U.S. Communists in the McCarthy era strikingly exemplify the price that people were made to pay for their beliefs. Endorsement of unpopular ideas also destroys a sense of shared reality within a larger community, thereby frustrating a need for belonging and social connec-

tion (Hardin & Higgins, 1996). The degree of sacrifice entailed by subscribing to given ideas depends on the social and historical context at issue. For example, people who supported same-sex marriage would be socially shunned and considered extreme in the United States of the 1950s and to this day across the Middle East (Inglehart, 2017), but not so in the United States in 2019 (Rosenfeld, 2017). In contrast to such contextual relativity, beliefs that include support for violent means to pursue ideological goals are considered extreme in most societies given the widespread rejection of political violence by most cultures and religions. A belief that under most circumstances, harming others is morally wrong seems to be a human universal (Schein & Gray, 2018).

Often ideological extremism has behavioral consequences. In fact, violent behavior typically is guided by ideologies that identify what needs to be done in order to advance valued objectives. Nonetheless, one can refrain from radical actions, while still subscribing to ideologically extreme beliefs. The pyramid model proposed by McCauley and Moskalenko (2008) is informative in this regard. As we move from the base of the pyramid to the apex, the level of commitment required by an individual increases. Individuals who both endorse an extreme political ideology and act upon it comprise the apex of the pyramid. Terrorists who use violence and radicals who use nonviolent yet still illegal means reside here. Activists are located directly below the radicals. These individuals, like those above them, endorse an extreme political ideology but constrain their extreme political participation to actions that are nonviolent and legal. Finally, the broad base of the pyramid comprises individuals who are supporters or sympathizers of the political cause (i.e., they believe the extreme ideology), but they do not participate in extreme behavior. This is exemplified by individuals who agree with ISIS's goal to establish a global caliphate but think that this goal should not be achieved with violence. Likewise, it pertains to the masses of people in Western countries who fear immigration and believe that it threatens to eradicate people of White ancestry. They might demonstrate their support for these beliefs by voting for right-wing political parties, but they may not support the violent campaigns undertaken by far-right radicals in response to the situation.

Even though these individuals at the base of the pyramid do not engage in extreme political behavior, they should not be ignored. Extreme beliefs have the power to influence the political agenda and set the tone of the discussion. They influence voting decisions and create a political climate that influences individual behaviors. Eventually, people who believe in radical ideas may gradually increase their commitment to include extreme behaviors, if they believe that sufficient progress has not been made in achieving these political goals. Research on radicalized individuals in the United States confirmed that a strong relationship between ideological commitment and engagement in political violence exists (Jasko & LaFree, 2019). Importantly, as implied in the labels assigned by the pyramid model, these ideologically committed individuals provide a broad base of support that enables the radicals and terrorists to continue their extreme campaigns. Seeing that others believe in their objectives provides a powerful social justification for radical actions and reduces discomfort and guilt that such actions normally induce (Webber, Schimel, Martens, Hayes, & Faucher, 2013).

Finally, the distinction between ideological and behavioral extremism is important when discussing the rehabilitation of political extremists. Experts distinguish between two possible outcomes: disengagement and deradicalization (e.g., Horgan, 2009; Horgan & Braddock, 2010). On the one hand, a terrorist who has deradicalized is one who has disavowed both extreme behavior and the extreme political beliefs that justified those actions; that is, the individual has shed the toxic beliefs that justified extreme behavior, and no longer has a reason to engage in violence. Interviews with former right-wing members in Germany, for instance, revealed that these individuals commonly came to question whether violence was appropriate or effective, or they questioned the dehumanizing narrative about minorities that increased their willingness to inflict harm on minorities (Kruglanski, Webber, & Koehler, 2019). A terrorist who has disengaged, on the other hand,

has only disavowed political violence. This individual retains (some of) the beliefs that justify extreme actions, but for various reasons, has decided that he or she no longer wishes to engage in those actions.

Although deradicalization is more likely to lead to longer-term desistance than disengagement, disengagement is seen by some experts as a sufficient and more attainable outcome given the difficulty experienced in attempting to change entrenched beliefs (e.g., Dalgaard-Nielsen, 2013). This is particularly true in societies in which freedom of speech is protected and people are free to hold extreme attitudes as long as they do not act on those attitudes in a manner that may cause harm to others. Reducing engagement in extreme behaviors is therefore given priority in efforts to reduce violent extremism in society.

It is also possible to envision situations in which individuals engage in radical behaviors without holding radical beliefs. The most obvious examples include persons conscripted into terrorist organizations. Boko Haram in Nigeria and ISIS, for instance, are notorious for their forced recruitment of youth, whether through kidnapping, purchases from human traffickers, or policies that require adult members of the organization also to enlist their children (Melotti, Martins, Garms, & Peschke, 2017). Youth are forced into battle as child soldiers, or in more extreme cases, suicide bombers. Psychological theory suggests that being forced to engage in violent and extreme behavior provides sufficient (external) justification for so doing. Cognitive dissonance from engaging in immoral actions should therefore not arise, and the actors involved should have less need to endorse the extreme ideology to internally justify their actions (Festinger & Carlsmith, 1959). However, the separation between one's actions and beliefs might be difficult to maintain over a prolonged time, in part due to the motivation to create shared reality with close others. Indeed, empirical evidence shows that even under such enforced circumstances, increased identification with a violent group might occur (Littman, 2018), demonstrating that ideological and behavioral commitment to extremism are interrelated.

Determinants of Political Extremism

Precursors of the Motivational Imbalance

What might be the precursors of an imbalanced focus on political goals and the adoption of extreme behaviors as means to those goals? Some of the earliest psychological approaches toward understanding why individuals become terrorists and political extremists focused on identifying characteristics that would demarcate people who are politically extreme from those who are not. This effort proposed that individuals would only engage in violent behavior if they were psychologically abnormal in some way, for instance, if they suffered from a mental illness or psychological disorder that prevented them from following societal moral prescriptions against violence and impaired their ability to relate to others.

One commonly referenced disorder was what is now labeled as antisocial personality disorder (Cooper, 1978; Pearce, 1977). Psychoanalytic perspectives proposed that some form of traumatic experience in childhood prevented terrorists from forming healthy personalities and self-concepts (Crayton, 1983; Hubbard, 1971; Olsson, 1988; Post, 1998). Although these early approaches were popular and are consistent with popular lay views, evidence never materialized to support their claims (Crenshaw, 1981; Victoroff, 2005). Consequently, terrorism researchers came to overwhelmingly disregard the importance of individual psychopathologies as causes of extremism, and sought other, situational explanations of this phenomenon. This abrupt reactionary response, however, caused many to outright reject individual differences and mental illness as potentially relevant to extremism, rather than promoting an examination of these variables as potential risk factors that, in conjunction with other variables, may impact the political radicalization process (Gill & Corner, 2017). For instance, sensation seeking (Pauwels & Schils, 2016), need for cognitive closure (Kruglanski, 2004), prevention focus (Zhang, Cornwell, & Higgins, 2014), and other stable personal characteristics are some of the individual traits that could dispose individuals to "freeze" on a momentarily activated concern to the exclusion of other considerations,

thereby inducing a motivational imbalance that fosters extremism. This approach is illustrated by research findings that in contrast to promotion-oriented individuals, prevention-oriented individuals with strong moral convictions are more likely to justify hostile forms of collective action, even when they perceive those actions to be immoral (Zaal, Laar, Ståhl, Ellemers, & Derks, 2011).

Motivational Underpinnings of Political Extremism

The Quest for Significance

Granting that extremism is driven by a motivational imbalance in which a given need is privileged over others, we address a specific candidate need that is likely to become imbalanced in the case of political extremism. Based on empirical research and conceptual considerations, we propose the need for *personal significance,* which represents the universal human desire to feel respected, valued, and important (Kruglanski, Chen, Dechesne, Fishman, & Orehek, 2009; Kruglanski et al., 2014; Kruglanski, Jasko, Chernikova, Dugas, & Webber, 2017). It echoes other motivational constructs such as self-esteem, and the cravings for achievement, status, competence, and meaning (Anderson, Hildreth, & Howland, 2015; Frankl, 1969; Maslow, 1943). We conceive of it as an overarching motivation within which other kindred needs can be subsumed. Simply, the latter needs represent specific manifestations or ways in which one can gain or lose significance. It is noteworthy that individuals do not have to be cognizant that their self-sacrificial behavior is a means of fulfilling the significance need. To recognize that one's noble sacrifices for a cause are motivated by one's personal need is to diminish their significance-bestowing effect and cast them as "selfish." Instead, significance-seeking persons may believe that their actions are selflessly driven by socially valued causes.

As with all motives, the quest for significance may be situationally activated, and hence elevated in the appropriate circumstances for most persons. Such activation may be prompted by (1) one's loss of significance stemming from personal failings or an affront to one's social identity (e.g., one's religious, ethnic, national, or political group) or (2) an opportunity to gain special significance through performance of socially valued actions. For instance, an individual who is relatively well to do and generally successful may seize the opportunity to sacrifice for a hallowed cause in hopes that this will elevate his or her sense of significance to the status of a celebrated hero or martyr. The quest for significance may also be chronically active in some persons. Some people are generally more desirous of significance and more "ambitious" than others. Finally, situations might interact with certain individual predispositions. For instance, loss of significance might resonate more strongly with prevention-focused individuals (Scholer, Zou, Fujita, Stroessner, & Higgins, 2010), while an opportunity for significance gain might be more relevant to a promotion-focused individual.

Personal loss of significance that consequently prompted extremism is exemplified by cases of Palestinian women who volunteered for a suicidal mission following a disgrace that they personally suffered, either due to infertility, divorce, extra marital relations, or disfiguration of some sort (Kruglanski, Bélanger, & Gunaratna, 2019; Pedhazur, 2005). Personally disgraced individuals are likely to adopt a group cause (i.e., a value cherished by a group) and carry out extreme acts on its behalf. These group causes typically concern a collective grievance arising from a sense that the group has been treated unfairly and discriminated against. Perceived injustice and dishonor accorded to one's group may be a common reason why individuals who have been personally successful and prosperous may (surprisingly) radicalize. Indeed, as we discuss later, one of the most researched underpinnings of extreme political action has been collective grievances and relative deprivation.

A growing body of research has examined the role of the significance motive in political extremism. One such study examined the significance quest motivation of suicide bombers by identifying both negative circumstances in their lives that would induce feelings of insignificance, and evidence that these individuals were looking to gain significance, for instance, by explicitly stating they wished to become martyrs

(Webber, Klein, Kruglanski, Brizi, & Merari, 2017). The results revealed that suicide bombers with a stronger quest for significance caused a greater number of casualties in their attacks. Presumably, this was the case because a more successful attack would bring a greater sense of significance to the perpetrator. Research looking at political extremists in the United States revealed that extremists with experiences of significance loss in the domains of close relationship (e.g., with experiences of romantic rejection) or work (e.g., chronically unemployed) were more likely to have used violence, relative to nonviolence, in their attacks (Jasko, LaFree, & Kruglanski, 2017). Other researchers have more directly assessed the significance quest with survey methodologies and demonstrated that higher self-reported feelings of insignificance were positively correlated with political extremism (Webber, Babush, et al., 2018; Webber, Chernikova, et al., 2018). As an example, a study among Muslim immigrants revealed that their feelings of discrimination were related to greater sense of insignificance, which were subsequently related to greater support for radical interpretations of Islam and greater support for a hypothetical extremist group (Lyons-Padilla, Gelfand, Mirahmadi, Farooq, & van Egmond, 2015). This study demonstrates how insults to one's social identity may induce the experience of significance loss. Such a collective mode of humiliation is present in the theory of relative deprivation, which we consider next.

Relative Deprivation and the Quest for Significance

Relative deprivation theory (Gurr, 2015; Runciman, 1966) proposes that negative experiences such as discrimination or poverty do not always lead individuals to engage in behavior designed to address that grievance. An individual who experiences discrimination but views that treatment as warranted, fair, or consistent with expectations, is unlikely to rebel in order to remedy the situation. If, on the other hand, individuals perceive unequal treatment as unjust and undeserved, they are motivated to redress the perceived injustice. Indeed, a meta-analysis of 210 studies with 186,073 respondents confirmed that relative deprivation leads to actions aimed at reducing it, an effect that is stronger when the deprivation is perceived as unjust and hence evokes anger (Smith, Pettigrew, Pippin, & Bialosiewicz, 2012). Similarly, a meta-analysis of the collective action literature revealed a positive relationship between a sense of injustice and actions aimed at restoring the position of one's ingroup (van Zomeren, Postmes, & Spears, 2008). In line with this result, research showed that group-based anger systematically predicts willingness to engage and actual participation in collective action (Miller, Cronin, Garcia, & Branscombe, 2009; Tausch & Becker, 2013).

Whereas the foregoing studies did not differentiate between moderate and extreme radical action, other lines of research demonstrated relationships between collective grievances and relative deprivation on the one hand and support for political violence on the other. For example, a comparison of Western-born Muslims with those who were foreign-born showed that the former were more supportive of extremism and that the sense of group-based relative deprivation accounted for these differences (Obaidi, Bergh, Akrami, & Anjum, 2019). Likewise, greater emotional hostility and endorsement of punitive measures against the offending group was shown by individuals who felt that their social group had been dehumanized (Kteily & Bruneau, 2017). Unsurprisingly, terrorism researchers have consistently identified collective grievances as important determinants of terrorist behavior. For instance, Agnew (2010) applied the general strain theory to terrorism. Strains are stressors, including the presence of negative events and the inability to achieve valued goals, that have been identified to contribute to criminal behavior. Strains that are collective (i.e., directed toward members of an identifiable group), perceived as unjust, and inflicted by more powerful entities are believed to contribute to terrorism. Likewise, Sageman (2008) proposed that Western individuals often turn to Islamic extremism when they have personal experiences of discrimination that resonate with discrimination that has been inflicted on Muslims as a group, and Horgan (2005) discussed multiple risk factors for terrorism, including feelings of alienation and disenfranchisement.

In present terms, the latter feelings are likely to feed a sense of humiliation and insignificance. Studies that examined predictors of terrorism at a state level similarly found that attacks were more frequent in regions where minorities felt discriminated against (Piazza, 2006). More recently, an extensive set of pathway analyses, designed to examine 10 different variables assumed to promote political extremism, found that collective grievances were one of two variables whose presence in the model was necessary to explain acts of terrorism (Jensen, Seat, & James, 2018).

Deradicalization

Importantly, too, researchers have looked into the role of personal significance in the deradicalization of former terrorists (Webber, Chernikova, et al., 2018). Theoretically, there are multiple ways in which the significance motive can be co-opted to draw people out of extremism. This involves reversing the logic of the motivational imbalance. Specifically, if extremism results from a motivational imbalance, then restoring motivational balance should reduce the appeal of extremism. Interviews with former members of the right-wing movement in Germany revealed that one way this often happens is by increasing the salience of a different need, which in this case was the need for safety (Kruglanski, Webber, et al., 2019). When extremists came to fear for the safety of themselves or their family, whether at the hands of their political enemies, authorities, or other right-wing members, this motivated them to leave the movement. Motivational balance could also be restored through the provision of significance. This would remove the deficit that instated the imbalance, thereby reducing the dominance of the significance need and lessening its impact on directing behavior. To examine this notion, researchers surveyed terrorists who had been detained in rehabilitation facilities in Sri Lanka (Webber, Chernikova, et al., 2018). Some of the facilities offered detainees programming designed to educate, provide job skills, and provide psychological competency via psychosocial counseling—all tactics that should help individuals attain a sense of mattering and significance. Analyses comparing the facilities that offered these programs to those that did not revealed significantly greater reduction in the endorsement of political extremism. Moreover, detainees who reported participating in a greater number of rehabilitation activities subsequently reported lower feelings of insignificance, and thus lower endorsement of political extremism.

Alternative Needs: Thrill Seeking

In addition to the significance motive, other psychological needs have been identified as important in motivating political extremism. One such need is *sensation seeking,* which refers to the need to seek adventure, thrills, or novel experiences (Zuckerman 1994, 2007). To be sure, sensation seeking is not exclusively related to political extremism, but rather seems to encourage various types of extreme behavior. Thus, sensation seeking was invoked as a determinant of criminal behavior (e.g., Horvath & Zuckerman, 1993); alcohol and drug use among adolescents (e.g., Crawford, Pentz, Chou, Chaoyang, & Dwyer, 2003); participation in extreme sports such as whitewater rafting, mountain climbing, and skydiving (e.g., Jack & Ronan, 1998); and a proclivity for football hooliganism (e.g., Russell, 1995). Moreover, 78% of active duty military personnel were categorized as sensation seekers (Bray et al., 2009).

Research within the domain of political extremism has likewise found that traits consistent with sensation seeking were present among former members of armed combatant groups in Colombia (Nussio, 2017). In another study examining the relationship between exposure to extremist content and engagement in extremist behavior, self-reported thrill seeking was found to be predictive of self-reported political violence against property (e.g., political graffiti, arson, or other forms of politically motivated property damage; Pauwels & Schils, 2016). Finally, a series of studies revealed that self-reported sensation seeking was positively related to support for a violent political group, and this effect was mediated by the perception that this activist group was exciting (Schumpe et al., 2020).

In a related vein, boredom—one of the four factors that comprise sensation seeking (Zuck-

erman, 1971)—has been linked to political extremism. Writing in 1951, Hoffer suggested boredom as a predictor of joining a revolutionary movement. As he put it: "There is perhaps no more reliable indicator of a society's ripeness for a mass movement than the prevalence of unrelieved boredom" (pp. 51–52). While this is probably an overstated claim, a series of recent studies indicated that bored individuals are more likely to be politically extreme, and that boredom induced via experimental manipulation causes individuals to report more extreme political orientations (van Tilburg & Igou, 2016).

Whereas, on the surface, boredom and thrill seeking may seem different than the quest for significance, the two may be intimately related. Boredom arises when individuals experience a lack of meaningful engagement and perceive their manner of being as insufficiently challenging (Csikszentmihalyi, 1997) and lacking in purpose (Barbalet, 1999). Such perceptions motivate behavior aimed toward the pursuit of greater purpose and significance (Barbalet, 1999; van Tilburg & Igou, 2013; van Tilburg, Igou, & Sedikides, 2013). This idea was confirmed in a study in which self-reported proneness to boredom was positively related to political extremism, but that this relationship was mediated by increased search for meaning in life (van Tilburg & Igou, 2016). In this sense, boredom initiates a motivational imbalance that privileges personal significance over other common concerns such as safety or comfort. Similarly, Schumpe and colleagues (2020) showed that need for meaning in life was positively related to sensation seeking and through that mechanism to support for extreme political actions and groups.

Alternative Needs: The Need for Cognitive Closure

A final psychological need related to political extremism is the need for *closure,* that is, a desire for decisive answers and the eschewal of ambiguity (e.g., Kruglanski, 2004; Kruglanski & Webster, 1996; Webster & Kruglanski, 1994). Whereas the need for significance pertains to the contents of one's beliefs (i.e., that one is worthy and deserving), the need for closure pertains to their absolutistic form that divides the universe into neat, certainty affording, dichotomies (i.e., "us" vs. "them," "good" vs. "bad," "right" vs. "wrong"). A characteristic feature of political extremists is the absolutism of their beliefs and their firm conviction that they are right and alternative perspectives are wrong (van Prooijen & Krouwel, 2017). Political extremists tend to think about important political issues in dogmatic and simplistic terms (Conway et al., 2016), and to conceptualize political issues and stimuli in clearly defined and homogenous categories (Lammers, Koch, Conway, & Brandt, 2017). Such preference for simplicity and coherence among individuals on the political extremes has been linked to the endorsement of conspiracy theories (van Prooijen, Krouwel, & Pollet, 2015).

Relatedly, the need for closure has been linked to support for violence that benefits from absolutistic demonization of one's (real or imagined) adversary. In this vein, the need for closure has been associated with support for military action in Iraq among persons high in national attachment (Federico, Golec, & Dial, 2005), and has been found to promote ingroup glorification and support for extreme measures against one's group's enemies (Dugas et al., 2018). Research further indicates that instilling a feeling of uncertainty (which should activate the need for cognitive closure) in study participants increases the appeal of extreme groups (Hogg, Sherman, Dierselhuis, Maitner, & Moffitt, 2007), leads participants to react more extremely toward members of an outgroup (van den Bos, Euwema, Poortvliet, & Maas, 2007), and increases ideological extremism in the form of religious zeal (McGregor, Zanna, Holmes, & Spencer, 2001). Extremist groups tend to hold beliefs that are black and white, and devoid of ambiguity (Hogg, Kruglanski, & van den Bos, 2013). These groups also provide members with a group identity that is distinctive and clearly defined (Hogg, 2014), as well as being portrayed as good, virtuous but often underappreciated. These factors increase the appeal of political extremism to individuals seeking closure.

Studies have also investigated how the need for closure affects people's responses to grievances. In this vein, Doosje, Loseman, and van den Bos (2013) found that among Dutch youth, greater perceptions of collective grievance were related to increased feelings of uncertainty, which were subsequently related to extreme political attitudes in the form of increasing perceptions of ingroup superiority. In yet another set of studies conducted with imprisoned terrorists, feelings of insignificance were positively related to the need for closure, which was subsequently predictive of endorsement of ideological extremism (Webber, Babush, et al., 2018). The authors also conducted a series of experiments with American participants. Participants induced to feel insignificant (vs. those in a control condition) reported a higher need for closure, and that closure was predictive of increased endorsement of extreme political beliefs. These studies suggest that when individuals experience an insignificance-inducing grievance, it induces a state of uncertainty (McGregor et al., 2001). Presumably, these grievances violate the basic expectations people have with regard to their environment, thus activating the need for cognitive closure and increasing the appeal of extreme beliefs and groups that lend them certainty and self-worth.

The Extremist Narrative

People's quest for significance may be satisfied in multiple ways, but the specific way that is ultimately chosen depends on an individuals' subscription to a socially shared *narrative* that identifies specific actions as means to cherished values. Extreme (i.e., sacrificial) actions for a collective cause affirm one's commitment to social values whose endorsement and/or protection lends one a sense of personal significance (Olivola & Shafir, 2013; Steele & Liu, 1983). Often, these actions offer a direct way of addressing the collective grievance that caused one's loss of significance, by allowing the individual a way to strike back at the perpetrator responsible for the grievance, thus leveling the "playing field" and asserting one's mattering and power.

Moralization of Extremism

People typically avoid violent and extreme behaviors because those behaviors are denounced as immoral, wrong, and punishable. Not all forms of violence are subjected to these rules, however, with state-sponsored forms of violence (i.e., interstate warfare) being viewed as acceptable, and those who engage in this violence (i.e., soldiers) rewarded for their violent actions with commendation and heroism. Thus, a critical function of the extremist narrative is to justify the hardships and sacrifices entailed by embracing and acting on the narrative. A major mode of such justification involves the moralization of political objectives and their portrayal as serving supreme values. This should increase the perceived importance of the political cause, help suppress alternative concerns, and increase willingness to commit to a violent course of action. Fiske and Rai (2014), in their provocative book on violence, suggest that people engage in violence despite their reluctance to do so because most perpetrators of violence feel they are doing what they should do in this situation. In other words, from their subjective perspective, political aggressors believe that the violence they use is a morally justified and laudable course of action under the circumstances.

Various lines of research support this analysis. They converge on the notion that once a goal or action is associated with moral beliefs, individuals are unwilling to compromise on that goal/action, and relentlessly defend that value, come what may. Those who moralize political issues in this way are both more willing to use violence and perceive violence as a legitimate strategy toward goal attainment (Skitka, 2010). Studies conducted across various social contexts indicate that moral convictions predicted both intended and actual willingness to engage in collective action on behalf of various causes (Skitka, & Bauman, 2008; Skitka & Wisneski, 2011; van Zomeren, Postmes, & Spears, 2012). Other studies indicate that holding moral convictions is related to more hostility toward those with different political attitudes, and less respect for legitimate authorities (i.e., Supreme Court) that yield decisions inconsistent with observers' moral preferences (Ryan, 2014). In the context of the conflict between Israel and Palestine, politically left and right Jewish–Israelis surveyed after the Gaza War expressed more polarized opinions when their positions were high in moral conviction (Tagar, Morgan, Halperin, & Skitka, 2014).

Research into what has been termed *sacred values* echoes these sentiments (e.g., Atran & Ginges, 2012; Ginges, Atran, Medin, & Shikaki, 2007; Tetlock, 2003). This perspective differentiates values that are sacred from those that are profane/secular. Sacred values cannot be compromised and cannot mingle with the profane. Accordingly, individuals are loath to put a material value on things that they see as sacred. This dynamic makes individuals unamenable to negotiations involving these values, which might seem irrational to outside observers. In one set of studies, participants were presented with a hypothetical negotiation to end violent conflict (Ginges et al., 2007). These negotiations required participants to compromise on some value (i.e., Palestinians' right to a homeland) in return for monetary compensation. Individuals who held given values as sacred responded to the negotiation with emotional outrage and increased support for violence, relative to those that did not hold this value as sacred. Likewise, Tetlock, Kristel, Elson, Green, and Lerner (2000) found that when participants read about this manner of compromise to their sacred values, they responded with moral outrage and wished to engage in moral cleansing (i.e., volunteer for a good cause to remove the bad feeling caused by the compromise). A similar experiment examining political beliefs pertaining to the preservation of the environment revealed that participants exposed to a taboo negotiation reacted with increased political participation, that is, made larger donations to environmental causes (Stikvoort, Lindahl, & Daw, 2016). Taken together, this literature suggests that political extremism is more likely to be linked to deontological rather than to utilitarian reasoning. In line with this reasoning, Ginges and Atran (2011) demonstrated that decisions about political violence are less sensitive to utilitarian concerns (i.e., the number of people who could be saved by a course of action) than were decisions about nonviolent, diplomatic solutions.

One recent study examined the importance of moralization as it directly pertains to the perpetration of political violence (Mooijman, Hoover, Lin, Ji, & Dehghani, 2018). Researchers analyzed Twitter communications during a 2015 protest in Baltimore that turned violent. Analyses revealed that moral rhetoric in social media increased during days when more aggressive protests took place. More importantly, the frequency of tweets with a stronger moral intensity predicted the frequency of arrests and violence during the protests. This result indicates that the frequency with which people refer to morality when they think about a political issue is related to extreme political behavior. In other words, when people define a political issue in terms of ultimate moral values, they are more willing to approve of and use violence in their name.

Moral Values and Personal Significance

The moralization of political objectives lends value and significance to individuals whose actions are undertaken in the service of those objectives. In other words, a person who serves an important value and is willing to undergo sacrifices for its sake, is thereby a "good" person worthy of admiration and respect, even if it is just self-respect. In that sense, the literature on moralization and sacred values jibes with the quest for significance assumed to constitute a typical motivation of political extremists of various kinds. Indeed, recent research examined the extent to which political participation on behalf of cherished values provides individuals with a sense of significance. Six studies among different groups of political activists showed that when activists engage in political actions on behalf of important social values, they gain a sense of personal significance (Jasko, Szastok, Grzymala-Moszczynska, Maj, & Kruglanski, 2019). As a result of these significance feelings, they are more willing to self-sacrifice for the cause in the future. Moreover, those who engage in more demanding forms of sacrifice for a cause experience proportionately more significance gains from their involvement. Similarly, significance quest predicted the readiness to engage in difficult behaviors for an environmental cause, but less so in easy ones that were less sacrificial (Molinario et al., 2019). These findings suggest that

costly behaviors on behalf of a valued cause may be particularly appealing because they afford greater significance gain.

The Extremist Network

A motivational imbalance in which several basic concerns are sacrificed to satisfy a single dominant need is difficult to sustain. Thus, to buttress one's commitment to extremism, it is important to have such commitment validated. Such validation is typically performed by a reference group, a social network of significant others who embrace the imbalanced narrative and reward the members (with respect and appreciation) for implementing it in action. As research on shared reality demonstrates, it is often critical for one's worldview to be socially validated (Higgins, 2019). Especially where the narrative deviates from common norms of mainstream society, it is important to have a cohesive group of like-minded individuals who support the narrative. Indeed, understanding political extremism is nearly impossible without accounting for the social context in which extreme beliefs are held and extreme actions are undertaken. These beliefs and actions pertain to a collective cause that is cherished by a group to which one belongs, and hence closely tied to the shared reality of that group. The role of social networks in promoting violent extremism has been often highlighted in previous work on political violence. In this section, we focus on group and intergroup processes through which individuals are led to commit to and act on behalf of political goals.

Social Interactions

The first form of evidence for the role of social processes demonstrates that direct contact with radical others often facilitates one's own radicalization. Research from a variety of contexts consistently shows that just having a friend engaged in a radical course of action is positively related to individuals' personal involvement in that cause. For instance, a longitudinal study demonstrated that adolescents whose peers had been involved in illegal political behavior were more likely to get involved in such behavior themselves (Dahl & van Zalk, 2014).

Having connections to violent friends has been associated with engagement in tribal violence (Glowacki et al., 2016), becoming an ISIS foreign fighter (Holman, 2016), joining Al-Qaeda (Sageman, 2008), using violence among political extremists in the United States (Jasko et al., 2017), and supporting violent extremism among Tamils in Sri Lanka (Webber, Chernikova, et al., 2018). Finally, research with participants from six major religions showed that regular attendance at religious services (but not regular prayer) was related to support for outgroup hostility and violent martyrdom (Ginges, Hansen, & Norenzayan, 2009). This pattern of results was also confirmed with experimental data (Ginges et al., 2009).

Social Identity and Politicized Identity

Evidence conducted from within the perspective of social identity theory extends the role of groups beyond immediate interactions (Tajfel & Turner, 1979). Specifically, this research suggests that merely thinking of oneself as member of a social group is enough to influence political opinions and actions. A great deal of evidence has consistently found that the more a person identifies with a group, the higher are the chances that they will participate in collective action on behalf of that group (De Weerd & Klandermans, 1999; Simon & Klandermans, 2001; Simon et al., 1998). Research has further identified specific types of social identities that are particularly strongly related to extreme motivation on behalf of the collective cause. One such identity, called a *politicized identity,* is defined as an awareness of power dynamics in society and willingness to participate in changing those power dynamics. Simon and Klandermans (2001) proposed that when people become involved in a power struggle, they become more aware and more sensitive to power divisions in society, sharply demarcating those who possess power from those who are deprived of power. Politicizations sensitize people to grievances that certain groups experience, as well as motivate them to determine who should be blamed for those grievances. When one possesses a politicized collective identity, the social environment is restructured into victims and oppressors, op-

ponents and allies. Indeed, a meta-analysis of the social identity literature found that the effects on collective action are stronger for politicized (vs. nonpoliticized) identities (van Zomeren et al., 2008).

Group Fusion

Recent research into group processes has focused on the construct of group fusion (Swann, Jetten, Gómez, Whitehouse, & Bastian, 2012). Fusion represents a particularly strong form of attachment to one's group. According to the theory, when people are fused with a group, they come to endorse the goals of the group as their own, while also coming to view their group members in terms of familial bonds (i.e., like brothers and sisters). As a result, strongly fused persons are more likely to support fighting and dying for their ingroup (e.g., Besta, Gómez, & Vázquez, 2014; Gómez et al., 2011; Gómez, Morales, Hart, Vázquez & Swann, 2011; Swann, Gómez, Seyle, Morales, & Huici, 2009; Swann et al., 2012).

Empirical research offers support for this idea. For example, those who fused their personal identity with their American identity were more willing to donate blood to help victims of terrorist attacks (Buhrmester et al., 2015). A study on revolutionary Libyan groups looked at the extent to which individuals were fused with their battalion groups (Whitehouse, McQuinn, Buhrmester, & Swann, 2014). The study compared individuals in fighting and nonfighting roles. Nearly half of the fighters felt a higher sense of fusion with their battalion than with their own families, whereas just over one-fourth of the nonfighters felt this way. Research by Jong, Whitehouse, Kavanagh, and Lane (2015) further suggests that fusion is more likely to occur during times of crisis. Thus, priming individuals to think about the collective suffering of their ingroup (i.e., priming Northern Irelanders with suffering that occurred during the conflict between the nationalists and unionists, or priming Bostonians with memories of the 2013 Boston Marathon bombings) increased fusion with that ingroup. Interestingly, there is evidence that a sense of oneness experienced in a state of fusion can also be extended to outgroups. When it occurs, it can motivate extreme actions in solidarity with distant outgroups (Kunst et al., 2018).

Collective Narcissism

One last area of research pertinent to understanding the role of group processes examines *collective narcissism,* which is the belief that one's group possesses an extraordinary value that is unrecognized by others (Golec de Zavala, Cichocka, Eidelson, & Jayawickreme, 2009). People who are attached to their group in a narcissistic way are more prone to believe that the group has been insulted, humiliated, or discriminated against. Although collective narcissists declare positive attitudes toward the group on an explicit level, they seek constant validation and recognition of their group by others. When validation is not received, they feel threatened and react with intergroup hostility. For instance, among Portuguese participants, collective narcissism was associated with support for aggressive actions toward Germans in reaction to perceived dominance of Germany in the European Union (Golec de Zavala, Peker, Guerra, & Baran, 2016). Similarly, Mexican participants high in collective narcissism were more likely to perceive American border security operations as insulting to Mexicans, thus leading to increased desire to engage in destructive actions against the United States (Golec de Zavala et al., 2009). Thus, it seems that insecure attachment to one's group might lead to more extreme political action on the group's behalf because it offers an avenue to enhance such attachment. Taken together, this literature shows that when people perceive that their ingroup does not receive the respect and recognition it deserves, this may motivate extreme political action.

Mediating Group Processes

Several processes suggest the unique role that group membership may play in spawning extremism. First, when people are strongly identified with their group, they feel collective grievances more strongly; that is, they feel insulted, disrespected, and outraged when their group is treated unfairly, even if they do not experience those grievances firsthand. Indeed, a me-

ta-analysis revealed that the strength of one's social identity is related to a stronger sense of injustice (van Zomeren et al., 2008). These individuals are also more likely to interpret their individual situation through the lens of their collective situation and attribute the causes of their individual suffering and misfortunes to collective causes.

Second, group processes influence the choice of means used to address a collective cause. A study we cited earlier demonstrated that individuals who perceive political issues in moral terms are more supportive of violence at protests when they are convinced that other people agree with their position than when they see no such convergence (Mooijman et al., 2018). Likewise, a series of studies compared the responses from participants residing in social contexts that were more or less radical (Jasko, Webber, Kruglanski, Taufiqruhman, & Gelfand, 2020). The results indicated that radical social contexts strengthen the link between the quest for (collective) significance and support for political violence. Groups can make extreme means easier to carry out by offering approval for their implementation. For instance, research suggests that the use of violence by other group members decreases the moral burden associated with violence (Webber et al., 2013).

In addition to validating the extremist narrative, groups reward individuals who implement it in action. Specifically, groups value members who make sacrifices for the collective cause, by ascribing to them higher status, and affording them greater interpersonal influence (Willer, 2009). This mechanism is self-reinforcing, as those who received status for their contributions subsequently contributed more and viewed the group more positively. Moreover, in justifying one's extreme commitment, individuals may increase their loyalty to the group. Indeed, several studies documented the effects of participation in radical action on increased social identification. For example, Littman (2018) showed that among ex-combatants in Liberia and Uganda, engagement in violence during conflicts was correlated with their degree of identification with the violent group. Another study confirmed that participation in radical collective action fosters disidentification with the moderate group but enhances political identification with the radical subgroup (Becker, Tausch, Spears, & Christ, 2011).

Finally, by validating the extremist narrative and rewarding individuals for adhering to it, social groups perpetuate the motivational imbalance and allow it to endure. Specifically, this process creates behavioral norms that de-emphasize and/or delegitimize alternative goals and hence reduce the temptation to desist from extreme behaviors.

Progression to Extremism

Our discussion thus far has isolated various factors that have been hypothesized and/or empirically supported to constitute determinants of political extremism. Alternative conceptions have depicted the progression toward extremism in terms of processes or stages leading to extremism (e.g., Borum, 2003; Moghaddam, 2005; Precht, 2007; Silber & Bhatt, 2007; Wiktorowicz, 2005). Here, different phases of radicalization are identified. After progressing through all stages sequentially, an individual reaches the final stage to the point of being willing to engage in violent political extremism.

As an example, consider Moghaddam's (2005) influential staircase model of terrorism, wherein individuals are assumed to progress through six stages before they are willing to carry out an act of terrorism. In order, these stages include (1) interpreting material conditions as unfair, (2) perceiving that there are no legal or nonviolent options to fight this unfair treatment, (3) displacing aggression onto an outgroup, (4) moralizing political goals, (5) solidifying categorical thinking, and (6) engaging in terrorism. Masses of people start at the first stage, and as they proceed through each subsequent step, people drop out, ending with a small minority of individuals who actually engage in terrorism. From this description, it should be clear that this model combines many of the factors discussed in this chapter. Moghaddam's first stage involves relative deprivation, his third stage highlights group processes, his fourth stage highlights the importance of sacred values and moral convictions, and his fifth stage highlights the importance of the certainty motive. In another well-known "progression"

model, Sprinzak (1991) argues that extremist (i.e., terrorist) groups have a long preterroristic history, and that the path to terrorism involves a prolonged process of deviance from the mainstream and delegitimation by the establishment. In Sprinzak's framework, the journey into radicalization is partitioned into smaller, consecutive ideological and behavioral stages labeled as the *crisis of confidence, conflict of legitimacy,* and *crisis of legitimacy.*

It is of interest to note the relation of the progression models of extremism to the motivational imbalance view of extremism described earlier. Because extremism entails sacrifices that people generally seek to avoid, the road to extremism may involve a series of progressive steps that gradually, rather than abruptly, commit individuals to the extreme worldview and its action implications. With every successive step, the individual may find it relatively easier to proceed to the next incremental step of engagement, such that the ultimate embracement of violence may appear as a natural consequence of the preceding phase rather than an immense sacrifice. Due to the individual predispositions that we discussed earlier, some people might be more likely to follow this progressive path to extremism.

Finally, it is important to note that the progression models of radicalization are generally meant as approximations, a characterization of what typically takes place rather than invariably. In that sense they are not incompatible with cases of *sudden* radicalization in which the need, narrative, and network factors converge powerfully to convert a former moderate into a radical "overnight" as it were.

Concluding Comments

In this chapter, we have depicted political extremism as a special case of extremism writ large, that is, as a process that it shares with other extremisms in varied domains. We characterized extremism broadly in terms of a motivational imbalance in which a given need assumes dominance over alternative concerns, thus implying sacrifice as a defining feature of extremism. Because political extremism is characterized by the actors' devotion to a cherished value, we have hypothesized that it serves the need to feel significant and worthy (a feeling that is satisfied by serving an important value). Viewed in this way, extremism is a matter of degree, reflecting the extent of sacrifice that the politically involved individual is making. Furthermore, because most people are loath to sacrifice their basic concerns, extremism is rather rare and typically short-lived, representing a mere "radical phase" in a person's life. Extremism can be made more enduring through a compelling narrative that an individual may embrace that justifies the motivational imbalance. Commitment to extremism is additionally strengthened if such a narrative is validated by the individual's network of significant others who are willing to applaud and reward it by their respect and admiration for the extremist's devotion and sacrifice. Finally, because the degree of extremism is defined by the extent of sacrifice, individuals typically progress to high degrees of extremism piecemeal, via a sequence of graduated steps. The foregoing depiction of extremism is consistent with the considerable body of research findings we have cited. The basic principles of political extremism are summarized below.

1. Political extremism is a special case of a motivated behavior directed at an important goal. Extremism occurs when a given goal acquires such intensity that it dominates alternative concerns. A motivationally imbalanced individual is willing to do whatever it takes to achieve the goal, including the use of violence and other radical measures.

2. The need for personal significance has been identified as the psychological need underlying political extremism. Two forms of the need for significance can be distinguished: the quest for individual significance that is a result of personal experiences, and the quest for collective significance rooted in the perception that one's social group has been humiliated, discriminated, or disrespected. Alternative needs include thrill seeking and the need for epistemic certainty.

3. When a strong motivational imbalance is present, it releases constraints on means that serve the focal goal. Thus, when people are extremely committed to a political goal, they are willing to use any means perceived as instrumental to satisfying the goal, even if those means have adverse effects on other personal goals. These means, while extreme and sacrificial, do not need to be violent, and the nature of these means is dependent on additional factors such as ideological narratives and social networks in one's environment.

4. Ideological narratives that moralize political goals increase the perception that these goals are highly important and unamenable to compromise, thus approving the use of any means necessary in service of the goal and contributing to political extremism.

5. Social context influences political extremism through several paths. It elevates the importance of the cause, identifies the appropriate means to satisfy quest for significance, and makes effortful means, such as violence, easier to enact.

6. Individual differences in sensitivity to situations that induce the quest for individual or collective significance play a role in the radicalization process (e.g., prevention focus, need for cognitive closure, sensation seeking, social identification).

7. Political extremism does not manifest exclusively in behavior but includes the endorsement of extreme ideas. While behavioral extremism and ideological extremism are often interrelated, it is important to consider them separately. Progression to violent extremism often involves subscribing to extreme ideology first and engaging in violent actions next.

Practical Applications

Our analysis of political extremism in terms of the motivational imbalance suggests several avenues through which the imbalance can be redirected in a nonviolent direction, or through which the appeal of goals that motivate extremism can be reduced.

First, if we assume that political extremism is a result of an imbalanced goal structure that prioritizes the need for significance, then addressing the circumstances that induced this imbalance should remove the drive to prioritize the significance need (via political extremism). This might include removing the sources of individual or collective frustrations to decrease one's willingness to engage in extreme behaviors motivated by those frustrations. It might also involve promoting alternative ways to satisfy the significance needs that do not entail a painful sacrifice. Making salient alternative needs that the extremist mindset has tended to suppress should also have a similar effect. However, it is important to note that extreme engagement for a political cause is often socially valued and even desirable. For instance, with regard to pressing issues such as climate change or global economic inequalities, it is not necessarily in the general interest to suppress political engagement that aims to solve these issues. What is in the general interest is to reduce the appeal of violent means that some politically involved individuals might consider.

In order to decrease the appeal of violent means, alternative nonviolent means should be made available and convincingly portrayed as effective strategies of goal attainment. The least desirable situation occurs when people feel that they have nothing but violence at their disposal to satisfy their frustrated needs. Research demonstrates that people are more likely to support violence when they perceive that alternative means are beyond their reach or nonexistent (Jackson, Huq, Bradford, & Tyler, 2013; Saab, Spears, Tausch, & Sasse, 2016; Schumpe et al., 2018). When peaceful actions prove to be equally or more effective in satisfying the psychological need, the appeal of violence decreases.

Theoretically, nonviolent means of goal attainment can be made salient and viable through the same social psychological mechanisms that increase the viability of violence: ideological narratives and social networks. However, we caution that strong moralization of political conflict might interfere with that goal. While it is true that invoking moral values mobilizes action on behalf of those values, it might also induce categorical thinking in terms of moral imperatives that are impossible to compromise. The more the political conflict is represented as a zero-sum game over sacred values, the greater the likelihood of violence. From a social network perspective, it is important to support social networks that reject violence and offer alternative forms of political involvement. Dis-

rupting contacts with violent individuals and strengthening networks that are peaceful should thus reduce the propensity to use violence.

In the opening paragraphs of this chapter we asked why political violence is so rampant given that it is generally ineffective. Examination in the preceding pages of the underlying psychology of political extremism offers a possible answer to this query: Devotion to the cause and self-denying sacrifices on behalf of the cause bring psychological rewards that may be appealing to individuals seeking respect, glory, meaning, and personal significance, irrespective of the ultimate objective consequences and/or success.

ACKNOWLEDGMENT

Katarzyna Jasko was supported by a grant from the National Science Center (Grant No. 2015/17/D/HS6/00362).

REFERENCES

Abrahms, M. (2012). The political effectiveness of terrorism revisited. *Comparative Political Studies, 45,* 366–393.

Agnew, R. (2010). A general strain theory of terrorism. *Theoretical Criminology, 14,* 131–153.

Anderson, C., Hildreth, J. A. D., & Howland, L. (2015). Is the desire for status a fundamental human motive?: A review of the empirical literature. *Psychological Bulletin, 141*(3), 574–601.

Atran, S., & Ginges, J. (2012). Religious and sacred imperatives in human conflict. *Science, 336,* 855–857.

Barbalet, J. M. (1999). Boredom and social meaning. *British Journal of Sociology, 50*(4), 631–646.

Becker, J. C., Tausch, N., Spears, R., & Christ, O. (2011). Committed dis(s)idents: Participation in radical collective action fosters disidentification with the superordinate group but enhances political identification. *Personality and Social Psychology Bulletin, 37,* 1104–1116.

Bélanger, J. J., Schumpe, B. M., Nociti, N., Moyano, M., Dandeneau, S., Chamberland, P. E., et al. (2019). Passion and moral disengagement: Different pathways to political activism. *Journal of Personality, 87*(6), 1234–1249.

Besta, T., Gómez, Á., & Vázquez, A. (2014). Readiness to deny group's wrongdoing and willingness to fight for its members: The role of the Poles' identity fusion with the country and religious group. *Current Issues in Personality Psychology, 2*(1), 49–55.

Borum, R. (2003). Understanding the terrorist mindset. *FBI Law Enforcement Bulletin, 72,* 7–10.

Bray, R. M., Pemberton, M. R., Hourani, L. L., Witt, M., Olmsted, K. L., Brown, J. M., et al. (2009). *Department of Defense survey of health related behaviors among active duty military personnel.* Research Triangle Park, NC: RTI International.

Buhrmester, M. D., Fraser, W. T., Lanman, J. A., Whitehouse, H., & Swann, W. B., Jr. (2015). When terror hits home: Identity fused Americans who saw Boston bombing victims as "family" provided aid. *Self and Identity, 14*(3), 253–270.

Chenoweth, E., & Stephan, M. J. (2011). *Why civil resistance works: The strategic logic of nonviolent conflict.* New York: Columbia University Press.

Conway, L. G., III, Gornick, L. J., Houck, S. C., Anderson, C., Stockert, J., Sessoms, D., et al. (2016). Are conservatives really more simple-minded than liberals?: The domain specificity of complex thinking. *Political Psychology, 37*(6), 777–798.

Cooper, H. H. A. (1978). Psychopath as terrorist: A psychological perspective. *Legal Medical Quarterly, 2,* 253–262.

Crawford, A. M., Pentz, M. A., Chou, C. P., Li, C., & Dwyer, J. H. (2003). Parallel developmental trajectories of sensation seeking and regular substance use in adolescents. *Psychology of Addictive Behaviors, 17*(3), 179–192.

Crayton, J. W. (1983). Terrorism and the psychology of the self. In L. Z. Freedman & Y. Alexander (Eds.), *Perspectives on terrorism* (pp. 33–41). Wilmington, DE: Scholarly Resources.

Crenshaw, M. (1981). The causes of terrorism. *Comparative Politics, 13,* 379–399.

Csikszentmihalyi, M. (1997). *Finding flow: The psychology of engagement with everyday life.* New York: Basic Books.

Dahl, V., & van Zalk, M. (2014). Peer networks and the development of illegal political behavior among adolescents. *Journal of Research on Adolescence, 24*(2), 399–409.

Dalgaard-Nielsen, A. (2013). Promoting exit from violent extremism: Themes and approaches. *Studies in Conflict and Terrorism, 36*(2), 99–115.

De Weerd, M., & Klandermans, B. (1999). Group identification and political protest: Farmers' protests in the Netherlands. *European Journal of Social Psychology, 29,* 1073–1095.

Doosje, B., Loseman, A., & van Den Bos, K. (2013). Determinants of radicalization of Islamic youth in the Netherlands: Personal uncertainty, perceived injustice, and perceived group threat. *Journal of Social Issues, 69*(3), 586–604.

Dugas, M., Schori-Eyal, N., Kruglanski, A. W., Klar,

Y., Touchton-Leonard, K., McNeill, A., et al. (2018). Group-centric attitudes mediate the relationship between need for closure and intergroup hostility. *Group Processes and Intergroup Relations, 21*(8), 1155–1171.

Federico, C. M., Golec, A., & Dial, J. L. (2005). The relationship between the need for closure and support for military action against Iraq: Moderating effects of national attachment. *Personality and Social Psychology Bulletin, 31*(5), 621–632.

Feinberg, M., Willer, R., & Kovacheff, C. (2017). Extreme protest tactics reduce popular support for social movements (Rotman School of Management Working Paper No. 2911177).

Festinger, L., & Carlsmith, J. M. (1959). Cognitive consequences of forced compliance. *Journal of Abnormal and Social Psychology, 58*(2), 203–210.

Fiske, A. P., & Rai, T. S. (2014). *Virtuous violence: Hurting and killing to create, sustain, end, and honor social relationships.* Cambridge, UK: Cambridge University Press.

Fiske, S. T. (2003). Five core social motives plus or minus five. In S. J. Spencer & S. Fein (Eds.), *Motivated social perception: The Ontario Symposium* (Vol. 9, pp. 233–246). Mahwah, NJ: Erlbaum.

Frankl, V. E. (1969). *The will to meaning: Foundations and applications of logotherapy.* New York: Random House.

Gill, P., & Corner, E. (2017). There and back again: The study of mental disorder and terrorist involvement. *American Psychologist, 72*(3), 231–241.

Ginges, J., & Atran, S. (2011). War as a moral imperative (not just practical politics by other means). *Proceedings of the Royal Society of London B: Biological Sciences, 278*(1720), 2930–2938.

Ginges, J., Atran, S., Medin, D., & Shikaki, K. (2007). Sacred bounds on rational resolution of violent political conflict. *Proceedings of the National Academy of Sciences of the USA, 104,* 7357–7360.

Ginges, J., Hansen, I., & Norenzayan, A. (2009). Religion and support for suicide attacks. *Psychological Science, 20,* 224–230.

Glowacki, L., Isakov, A., Wrangham, R. W., McDermott, R., Fowler, J. H., & Christakis, N. A. (2016). Formation of raiding parties for intergroup violence is mediated by social network structure. *Proceedings of the National Academy of Sciences of the USA, 113,* 12114–12119.

Golec de Zavala, A. G., Cichocka, A., Eidelson, R., & Jayawickreme, N. (2009). Collective narcissism and its social consequences. *Journal of Personality and Social Psychology, 97*(6), 1074–1096.

Golec de Zavala, A., Peker, M., Guerra, R., & Baran, T. (2016). Collective narcissism predicts hypersensitivity to in-group insult and direct and indirect retaliatory intergroup hostility. *European Journal of Personality, 30*(6), 532–551.

Gómez, A., Brooks, M. L., Buhrmester, M. D., Vázquez, A., Jetten, J., & Swann, W. B., Jr. (2011). On the nature of identity fusion: Insights into the construct and a new measure. *Journal of Personality and Social Psychology, 100,* 918–933.

Gómez, Á., Morales, J. F., Hart, S., Vázquez, A., & Swann, W. B., Jr. (2011). Rejected and excluded forevermore, but even more devoted: Irrevocable ostracism intensifies loyalty to the group among identity-fused persons. *Personality and Social Psychology Bulletin, 37,* 1574–1586.

Gousse-Lessard, A. S., Vallerand, R. J., Carbonneau, N., & Lafrenière, M. A. K. (2013). The role of passion in mainstream and radical behaviors: A look at environmental activism. *Journal of Environmental Psychology, 35,* 18–29.

Gurr, T. R. (2015). *Why men rebel.* London: Routledge.

Hardin, C. D., & Higgins, E. T. (1996). Shared reality: How social verification makes the subjective objective. In R. M. Sorrentino & E. T. Higgins (Eds.), *Handbook of motivation and cognition, Vol. 3. The interpersonal context* (pp. 28–84). New York: Guilford Press.

Higgins, E. T. (2012). *Beyond pleasure and pain: How motivation works.* Oxford, UK: Oxford University Press.

Higgins, E. T. (2019). *Shared reality: What makes us strong and tears us apart.* Oxford, UK: Oxford University Press.

Hoffer, E. (1951). *The true believer.* New York: Harper & Row.

Hogg, M. A. (2014). From uncertainty to extremism: Social categorization and identity processes. *Current Directions in Psychological Science, 23*(5), 338–342.

Hogg, M. A., Kruglanski, A. W., & van den Bos, K. (2013). Uncertainty and the roots of extremism. *Journal of Social Issues, 69,* 407–418.

Hogg, M. A., Sherman, D. K., Dierselhuis, J., Maitner, A. T., & Moffitt, G. (2007). Uncertainty, entitativity, and group identification. *Journal of Experimental Social Psychology, 43,* 135–142.

Holman, T. (2016). "Gonna get myself connected": The role of facilitation in foreign fighter mobilizations. *Perspectives on Terrorism, 10*(2), 2–23.

Horgan, J. (2005). *The psychology of terrorism.* London: Routledge.

Horgan, J. G. (2009). *Walking away from terrorism: Accounts of disengagement from radical and extremist movements.* London: Routledge.

Horgan, J., & Braddock, K. (2010). Rehabilitating the terrorists?: Challenges in assessing the effec-

tiveness of de-radicalization programs. *Terrorism and Political Violence, 22*(2), 267–291.

Horvath, P., & Zuckerman, M. (1993). Sensation seeking, risk appraisal, and risky behavior. *Personality and Individual Differences, 14*(1), 41–52.

Hubbard, D. G. (1971). *The skyjacker: His flights of fantasy.* New York: Macmillan.

Inglehart, R. (2017). Changing values in the Islamic world and the West. In M. Moaddel & M. Gelfand (Eds.), *Values and political action in the Middle East* (pp. 3–24). New York: Oxford University Press.

Jack, S. J., & Ronan, K. R. (1998). Sensation seeking among high-and low-risk sports participants. *Personality and Individual Differences, 25*(6), 1063–1083.

Jackson, J., Huq, A. Z., Bradford, B., & Tyler, T. R. (2013). Monopolizing force?: Police legitimacy and public attitudes toward the acceptability of violence. *Psychology, Public Policy, and Law, 19*(4), 479–497.

Jasko, K., & LaFree, G. (2019). Who is more violent in extremist groups?: A comparison of leaders and followers. *Aggressive Behavior, 46,* 141–150.

Jasko, K., LaFree, G., & Kruglanski, A. W. (2017). Quest for significance and violent extremism: The case of domestic radicalization. *Political Psychology, 38,* 815–831.

Jasko, K., Szastok, M., Grzymala-Moszczynska, J., Maj, M., & Kruglanski, A. W. (2019). Rebel with a cause: Personal significance from political activism predicts willingness to self-sacrifice. *Journal of Social Issues, 75*(1), 314–349.

Jasko, K., Webber, D., Kruglanski, A. W., Taufiqruhman, M., & Gelfand, M. J. (2019). Social context moderates the effect of quest for significance on violent extremism. *Journal of Personality and Social Psychology.* [Epub ahead of print]

Jensen, M. A., Seate, A. A., & James, P. A. (2018). Radicalization to violence: A pathway approach to studying extremism. *Terrorism and Political Violence.* [Epub ahead of print]

Jong, J., Whitehouse, H., Kavanagh, C., & Lane, J. (2015). Shared negative experiences lead to identity fusion via personal reflection. *PLoS ONE, 10*(12), e0145611.

Karatnycky, A., & Ackerman, P. (2005). *How freedom is won: From civic resistance to durable democracy.* New York: Freedom House.

Kruglanski, A. (2004). *The psychology of closed mindedness.* New York: Psychology Press.

Kruglanski, A. W., Bélanger, J. J., Gelfand, M., Gunaratna, R., Hettiarachchi, M., Reinares, F., et al. (2013). Terrorism—A (self) love story: Redirecting the significance quest can end violence. *American Psychologist, 68,* 559–575.0

Kruglanski, A. W., Bélanger, J. J., & Gunaratna, R. (2019). *The three pillars of radicalization: Needs, narratives, and networks.* New York: Oxford University Press.

Kruglanski, A. W., Chen, X., Dechesne, M., Fishman, S., & Orehek, E. (2009). Fully committed: Suicide bombers' motivation and the quest for personal significance. *Political Psychology, 30,* 331–557.

Kruglanski, A. W., Gelfand, M. J., Bélanger, J. J., Sheveland, A., Hetiarachchi, M., & Gunaratna, R. (2014). The psychology of radicalization and deradicalization: How significance quest impacts violent extremism. *Political Psychology, 35,* 69–93.

Kruglanski, A. W., Jasko, K., Chernikova, M., Dugas, M., & Webber, D. (2017). To the fringe and back: Violent extremism and the psychology of deviance. *American Psychologist, 72*(3), 217–230.

Kruglanski, A. W., Webber, D., & Koehler, D. (2019). *The radical's journey: German Neo-Nazis' voyage to the edge and back.* Oxford, UK: Oxford University Press.

Kruglanski, A. W., & Webster, D. M. (1996). Motivated closing of the mind: "Seizing" and "freezing." *Psychological Review, 103,* 263–283.

Kteily, N., & Bruneau, E. (2017). Backlash: The politics and real-world consequences of minority group dehumanization. *Personality and Social Psychology Bulletin, 43*(1), 87–104.

Kunst, J. R., Boos, B., Kimel, S. Y., Obaidi, M., Shani, M., & Thomsen, L. (2018). Engaging in extreme activism in support of others' political struggles: The role of politically motivated fusion with out-groups. *PLoS ONE, 13*(1), e0190639.

Lammers, J., Koch, A., Conway, P., & Brandt, M. J. (2017). The political domain appears simpler to the politically extreme than to political moderates. *Social Psychological and Personality Science, 8*(6), 612–622.

Littman, R. (2018). Perpetrating violence increases identification with violent groups: Survey evidence from former combatants. *Personality and Social Psychology Bulletin, 44*(7), 1077–1089.

Lyons-Padilla, S., Gelfand, M. J., Mirahmadi, H., Farooq, M., & Van Egmond, M. (2015). Belonging nowhere: Marginalization and radicalization risk among Muslim immigrants. *Behavioral Science and Policy, 1*(2), 1–12.

Maslow, A. H. (1943). A theory of human motivation. *Psychological Review, 50*(4), 370–396.

McCauley, C., & Moskalenko, S. (2008). Mechanisms of political radicalization: Pathways toward terrorism. *Terrorism and Political Violence, 20*(3), 415–433.

McGregor, I., Zanna, M. P., Holmes, J. G., & Spencer, S. J. (2001). Compensatory conviction in the face of personal uncertainty: Going to extremes and being oneself. *Journal of Personality and Social Psychology, 80,* 472–488.

Melotti, G., Martins, A., Garms, U., & Peschke, K. (2017). Handbook on children recruited and exploited by terrorist and violent extremist groups: The role of the justice system. Retrieved from *www.unodc.org/documents/justice-and-prison-reform/child-victims/handbook_on_children_recruited_and_exploited_by_terrorist_and_violent_extremist_groups_the_role_of_the_justice_system.e.pdf.*

Miller, D. A., Cronin, T., Garcia, A. L., & Branscombe, N. R. (2009). The relative impact of anger and efficacy on collective action is affected by feelings of fear. *Group Processes and Intergroup Relations, 12*(4), 445–462.

Moghaddam, F. M. (2005). The staircase to terrorism: A psychological exploration. *American Psychologist, 60,* 161–169.

Molinario, E., Kruglanski, A. W., Bonaiuto, F., Bonnes, M., Cicero, L., Fornara, F., et al. (2019). Motivations to act for the protection of nature biodiversity and the environment: A matter of "significance." *Environment and Behavior.* [Epub ahead of print]

Mooijman, M., Hoover, J., Lin, Y., Ji, H., & Dehghani, M. (2018). Moralization in social networks and the emergence of violence during protests. *Nature Human Behaviour, 2*(6), 389–396.

Nussio, E. (2017). The role of sensation seeking in violent armed group participation. *Terrorism and Political Violence, 32,* 1–19.

Obaidi, M., Bergh, R., Akrami, N., & Anjum, G. (2019). Group-based relative deprivation explains endorsement of extremism among Western-born Muslims. *Psychological Science, 30*(4), 596–605.

Olivola, C. Y., & Shafir, E. (2013). The martyrdom effect: When pain and effort increase prosocial contributions. *Journal of Behavioral Decision Making, 26*(1), 91–105.

Olsson, P. A. (1988). The terrorist and the terrorized: Some psychoanalytic consideration. *Journal of Psychohistory, 16,* 47–60.

Pauwels, L., & Schils, N. (2016). Differential online exposure to extremist content and political violence: Testing the relative strength of social learning and competing perspectives. *Terrorism and Political Violence, 28*(1), 1–29.

Pearce, K. I. (1977). Police negotiations. *Canadian Psychiatric Association Journal, 22,* 171–174.

Pedahzur, A. (2005). *Suicide terrorism.* Cambridge, UK: Polity Press.

Piazza, J. A. (2006). Rooted in poverty?: Terrorism,

poor economic development, and social cleavages. *Terrorism and political Violence, 18*(1), 159–177.

Post, J. M. (1998). Terrorist psycho-logic: Terrorist behavior as a product of psychological forces. In W. Reich (Ed.), *Origins of terrorism: Psychologies, ideologies, theologies, states of mind* (pp. 25–40). Washington, DC: Woodrow Wilson Center Press.

Precht, T. (2007). Home grown terrorism and Islamist radicalisation in Europe: From conversion to terrorism. Retrieved from_*www.justitsministeriet.dk/sites/default/files/media/arbejdsomraader/forskning/forskningspuljen/2011/2007/home_grown_terrorism_and_islamist_radicalisation_in_europe_-_an_assessment_of_influencing_factors_2_.pdf.*

Rip, B., Vallerand, R. J., & Lafrenière, M. A. K. (2012). Passion for a cause, passion for a creed: On ideological passion, identity threat, and extremism. *Journal of Personality, 80*(3), 573–602.

Rosenfeld, M. J. (2017). Moving a mountain: The extraordinary trajectory of same-sex marriage approval in the United States. *Socius, 3.* [Epub ahead of print]

Runciman, W. G. (1966). *Relative deprivation and social justice: A study of attitudes to social inequality in 20th century England.* London: Routledge & Kegan Paul.

Russell, G. W. (1995). Personalities in the crowd: Those who would escalate a sports riot. *Aggressive Behavior, 21*(2), 91–100.

Ryan, T. J. (2014). Reconsidering moral issues in politics. *Journal of Politics, 76*(2), 380–397.

Saab, R., Spears, R., Tausch, N., & Sasse, J. (2016). Predicting aggressive collective action based on the efficacy of peaceful and aggressive actions. *European Journal of Social Psychology, 46*(5), 529–543.

Sageman, M. (2008). *Leaderless jihad: Terror networks in the twenty-first century.* Philadelphia: University of Pennsylvania Press.

Schein, C., & Gray, K. (2018). The theory of dyadic morality: Reinventing moral judgment by redefining harm. *Personality and Social Psychology Review, 22,* 32–70.

Scholer, A. A., Zou, X., Fujita, K., Stroessner, S. J., Higgins, E. T. (2010). When risk-seeking becomes a motivational necessity. *Journal of Personality and Social Psychology, 99,* 215–231.

Schumpe, B. M., Bélanger, J. J., Giacomantonio, M., Nisa, C. F., & Brizi, A. (2018). Weapons of peace: Providing alternative means for social change reduces political violence. *Journal of Applied Social Psychology, 48*(10), 549–558.

Schumpe, B. M., Bélanger, J. J., Moyano, M., & Nisa, C. F. (2020). The role of sensation seeking in political violence: An extension of the significance quest theory. *Journal of Personality and Social Psychology, 118*(4), 743–761.

Shah, J. Y., Friedman, R., & Kruglanski, A. W. (2002). Forgetting all else: On the antecedents and consequences of goal shielding. *Journal of Personality and Social Psychology, 83*(6), 1261–1280.

Silber, M. D., & Bhatt, A. (2007). *Radicalization in the West: The homegrown threat.* New York: New York City Police Department.

Simon, B., & Klandermans, B. (2001). Politicized collective identity: A social psychological analysis. *American Psychologist, 56*(4), 319–331.

Simon, B., Loewy, M., Stürmer, S., Weber, U., Freytag, P., Habig, C., et al. (1998). Collective identification and social movement participation. *Journal of Personality and Social Psychology, 74*(3), 646–658.

Simpson, B., Willer, R., & Feinberg, M. (2018). Does violent protest backfire?: Testing a theory of public reactions to activist violence. *Socius, 4.* [Epub ahead of print]

Skitka, L. J. (2010). The psychology of moral conviction. *Social and Personality Psychology Compass, 4,* 267–281.

Skitka, L. J., & Bauman, C. W. (2008). Moral conviction and political engagement. *Political Psychology, 29,* 29–54.

Skitka, L. J., & Wisneski, D. C. (2011). Moral conviction and emotion. *Emotion Review, 3,* 328–330.

Smith, H. J., Pettigrew, T. F., Pippin, G. M., & Bialosiewicz, S. (2012). Relative deprivation: A theoretical and meta-analytic review. *Personality and Social Psychology Review, 16*(3), 203–232.

Sprinzak, E. (1991). The process of delegitimation: Towards a linkage theory of political terrorism. *Terrorism and Political Violence, 3*(1), 50–68.

Steele, C. M., & Liu, T. J. (1983). Dissonance processes as self-affirmation. *Journal of Personality and Social Psychology, 45*(1), 5–19.

Stikvoort, B., Lindahl, T., & Daw, T. M. (2016). Thou shalt not sell nature: How taboo trade-offs can make us act pro-environmentally, to clear our conscience. *Ecological Economics, 129,* 252–259.

Swann, W. B., Jr., Gómez, A. M., Seyle, D. C., Morales, J. F., & Huici, C. (2009). Identity fusion: The interplay of personal and social identities in extreme group behavior. *Journal of Personality and Social Psychology, 96*(5), 995–1011.

Swann, W. B., Jr., Jetten, J., Gómez, Á., Whitehouse, H., & Bastian, B. (2012). When group membership gets personal: A theory of identity fusion. *Psychological Review, 119*(3), 441–456.

Tagar, M. R., Morgan, G. S., Halperin, E., & Skitka, L. J. (2014). When ideology matters: Moral conviction and the association between ideology and policy preferences in the Israeli–Palestinian conflict. *European Journal of Social Psychology, 44*(2), 117–125.

Tajfel, H., & Turner, J. C. (1979). An integrative theory of intergroup conflict. In S. Worchel & W. G. Austin (Eds.), *The social psychology of intergroup relations* (pp. 33–47). Monterey, CA: Brooks/Cole.

Tausch, N., & Becker, J. C. (2013). Emotional reactions to success and failure of collective action as predictors of future action intentions: A longitudinal investigation in the context of student protests in Germany. *British Journal of Social Psychology, 52*(3), 525–542.

Tetlock, P. E. (2003). Thinking the unthinkable: Sacred values and taboo cognitions. *Trends in Cognitive Sciences, 7*(7), 320–324.

Tetlock, P. E., Kristel, O. V., Elson, S. B., Green, M. C., & Lerner, J. S. (2000). The psychology of the unthinkable: Taboo trade-offs, forbidden base rates, and heretical counterfactuals. *Journal of Personality and Social Psychology, 78*(5), 853–870.

Thomas, E. F., & Louis, W. R. (2014). When will collective action be effective?: Violent and non-violent protests differentially influence perceptions of legitimacy and efficacy among sympathizers. *Personality and Social Psychology Bulletin, 40*(2), 263–276.

Vallerand, R. J. (2010). On passion for life activities: The dualistic model of passion. In M. P. Zanna (Ed.), *Advances in experimental social psychology* (Vol. 42, pp. 97–193). San Diego, CA: Academic Press.

van den Bos, K., Euwema, M. C., Poortvliet, P. M., & Maas, M. (2007). Uncertainty management and social issues: Uncertainty as an important determinant of reactions to socially deviating people. *Journal of Applied Social Psychology, 37,* 1726–1756.

van Prooijen, J. W., & Krouwel, A. P. (2017). Extreme political beliefs predict dogmatic intolerance. *Social Psychological and Personality Science, 8*(3), 292–300.

van Prooijen, J. W., Krouwel, A. P., & Pollet, T. V. (2015). Political extremism predicts belief in conspiracy theories. *Social Psychological and Personality Science, 6*(5), 570–578.

van Tilburg, W. A., & Igou, E. R. (2013). On the meaningfulness of behavior: An expectancy × value approach. *Motivation and Emotion, 37*(3), 373–388.

van Tilburg, W. A., & Igou, E. R. (2016). Going to political extremes in response to boredom. *European Journal of Social Psychology, 46*(6), 687–699.

van Tilburg, W. A., Igou, E. R., & Sedikides, C. (2013). In search of meaningfulness: Nostalgia as an antidote to boredom. *Emotion, 13*(3), 450–461.

van Zomeren, M., Postmes, T., & Spears, R. (2008). Toward an integrative social identity model of collective action: A quantitative research synthesis of three socio-psychological perspectives. *Psychological Bulletin, 134*(4), 504–535.

van Zomeren, M., Postmes, T., & Spears, R. (2012). On conviction's collective consequences: Integrating moral conviction with the social identity model of collective action. *British Journal of Social Psychology, 51*(1), 52–71.

Victoroff, J. (2005). The mind of the terrorist: A review and critique of psychological approaches. *Journal of Conflict Resolution, 49*(1), 3–42.

Webber, D., Babush, M., Schori-Eyal, N., Vazeou-Niewenhuis, A., Hettiarachchi, M., Bélanger, J. J., et al. (2018). The road to extremism: Field and experimental evidence that significance loss-induced need for closure fosters radicalization. *Journal of Personality and Social Psychology, 114*(2), 270–285.

Webber, D., Chernikova, M., Kruglanski, A. W., Gelfand, M. J., Hettiarachchi, M., Gunaratna, R., et al. (2018). Deradicalizing detained terrorists. *Political Psychology, 39*(3), 539–556.

Webber, D., Klein, K., Kruglanski, A. W., Brizi, A., & Merari, A. (2017). Divergent paths to martyrdom and significance among suicide attackers. *Terrorism and Political Violence, 29*(5), 852–874.

Webber, D., Schimel, J., Martens, A., Hayes, J., & Faucher, E. H. (2013). Using a bug-killing paradigm to understand how social validation and invalidation affect the distress of killing. *Personality and Social Psychology Bulletin, 39*(4), 470–481.

Webster, D. M., & Kruglanski, A. W. (1994). Individual differences in need for cognitive closure. *Journal of Personality and Social Psychology, 67,* 1049–1062.

Whitehouse, H., McQuinn, B., Buhrmester, M., & Swann, W. B., Jr. (2014). Brothers in arms: Libyan revolutionaries bond like family. *Proceedings of the National Academy of Sciences of the USA, 111*(50), 17783–17785.

Wiktorowicz, Q. (2005). *Radical Islam rising: Muslim extremism in the West.* Oxford, UK: Rowman & Littlefield.

Willer, R. (2009). Groups reward individual sacrifice: The status solution to the collective action problem. *American Sociological Review, 74,* 23–43.

Zaal, M. P., Laar, C. V., Ståhl, T., Ellemers, N., & Derks, B. (2011). By any means necessary: The effects of regulatory focus and moral conviction on hostile and benevolent forms of collective action. *British Journal of Social Psychology, 50*(4), 670–689.

Zhang, S., Cornwell, J. F., & Higgins, E. T. (2014). Repeating the past: Prevention focus motivates repetition, even for unethical decisions. *Psychological Science, 25,* 179–187.

Zuckerman, M. (1971). Dimensions of sensation seeking. *Journal of Consulting and Clinical Psychology, 36*(1), 45–52.

Zuckerman, M. (1994). *Behavioral expressions and biosocial bases of sensation seeking.* Cambridge, UK: Cambridge University Press.

CHAPTER 30

Achievement Goals and Self-Regulation in the Sport Context

Nico W. Van Yperen

Sports offer a compelling context in which social psychological principles make an important contribution to understanding human emotion, judgment, and behavior. In sports,

> the rules of the game are understood by all participants and enforced in a purportedly unbiased manner. There are clear winners and losers. Different teams and players are easily recognized by their distinctive uniforms and unique numbers or by their particular territorial boundaries. And to top things off, individual and team performance records are meticulously kept. . . . Sport offers a type of controlled "living laboratory" to study individuals and groups. (Day, Gordon, & Fink, 2012, pp. 398–399)

Because of these features, the sport context is different from other performance contexts such as work, school, and art. However, there are also commonalities. One of the purposes of this chapter is to mine those connections, similarities, and convergences to help us to understand how and why performers think, feel, and act as they do in different performance contexts (for a discussion on this generalizability issue, see Hays, 2012).

Social psychological research in the sports context began at the end of the 19th century, when Norman Triplett (1898) observed that racing cyclists performed faster in a competitive context (i.e., when racing against another racer) than when racing against the clock alone. In follow-up studies, he discovered that simply the presence of others (i.e., an audience) had the same effect, a social psychological principle that we now know as *social facilitation* (Allport, 1924; Zajonc, 1965). Since then, the social psychological research in the sports context cannot be exhaustively reviewed in a single chapter. Hence, this chapter focuses and elaborates on the following basic social psychological principles of high performance and effective self-regulation that are central in sports and other performance contexts:

- *Principle 1:* Enhance performance and self-regulation through goal setting.
- *Principle 2:* Structure the multifaceted nature of achievement goal pursuit into a hierarchical goal system.
- *Principle 3:* Differentiate achievement goals on the basis of evaluative standard and valence.
- *Principle 4:* Set approach goals rather than avoidance goals.
- *Principle 5:* Develop interventions that focus on self-based and task-based approach goals.

- *Principle 6:* Delineate athletes' idiosyncratic developmental trajectories to better understand the process of goal attainment and self-regulation.
- *Principle 7:* Work on strengths and weaknesses simultaneously.
- *Principle 8:* Distinguish between high pressure situations and athletes' psychological reactions to pressure.
- *Principle 9:* Accept fluctuating internal states and focus on goal-relevant cues and contingencies.
- *Principle 10:* Control the controllables.

By following these principles, coaches and their athletes likely increase athletes' chances to develop a successful sports career.

Principle 1. Enhance Performance and Self-Regulation through Goal Setting

Setting goals, or cognitive representations of a desired end point that impacts evaluations, emotions, and behaviors (Fishbach & Ferguson, 2007), is generally considered one of the most effective performance enhancement strategies in the behavioral sciences (Burton, Pickering, Weinberg, Yukelson, & Weigand, 2010; Locke & Latham, 1990, 2013). A core finding is that specific, difficult goals lead to higher performance than no goals or vague "do your best" goals. Specific and difficult goals determine the direction of an individual's behavior, level of intensity or effort, and level of persistence (Locke & Latham, 2013).

In sports, performance (e.g., score, time, pace, distance, points) is relatively easy to measure, so that discrepancies between the current situation and the desired end state can be relatively easily and objectively determined and monitored. This is one of the reasons why both short-term goals (e.g., master a skill) and long-term goals (e.g., qualify for the world championships) are ubiquitous in the sports context. Remarkably, however, early meta-analyses suggested that goal setting is less effective in enhancing performance in the sports context than in business settings, in which most of the goal-setting studies have been conducted (Burton, Naylor, & Holliday, 2001; Kyllo & Landers, 1995; Wil-

liams, 2013). One explanation was that because of the intrinsic nature of sports activities, goal interventions may not have incremental effects; that is, people choose to be involved in sports, but they have to work for a living (Hall & Kerr, 2001; Moran & Toner, 2017). In addition, sports-like tasks inherently provide intrinsic task feedback to the performer, so that spontaneous goal setting is likely to occur also in control conditions in intervention studies (Locke, 1991). In more recent studies in sports and physical activity contexts, controlling for such effects resulted in about equally strong goal-setting effects as typically observed in nonsports settings (Burton & Weiss, 2008); that is, in more than 80% of the goal-setting studies, moderate to strong goal-setting effects were observed (Williams, 2013). Note that the majority of goal-setting studies in sports and physical activity contexts used nonathlete or recreational samples. Only one-fourth of the studies relied on sports populations, and in these latter studies, high-level athletes were typically not represented (Burton et al., 2010). This is unfortunate because goal setting may become more valuable when goals become harder and take longer to attain, that is, when the competitive level increases and conditions become more demanding. For example, in a sample of 338 athletes from different sports who had a strong probability of making the next U.S. Summer Olympic team in 2 years, Burton et al. found that athletes highest in self-confidence and career success consistently perceived different types of goals as highly effective for themselves.

Principle 2: Structure the Multifaceted Nature of Achievement Goal Pursuit into a Hierarchical Goal System

The process whereby individuals activate and sustain behaviors, cognitions, and affects that are systematically oriented toward the attainment of their goals is known as *self-regulation* (Zimmerman, Schunk, & DiBenedetto, 2017). In this process, a major self-regulation challenge is how to cope with failures and losses. Athletes, including the most successful ones, share the experience of a negative balance between winning and losing. To illustrate, more than 11,000 athletes competed at the Olympics in Rio 2016, and only a handful returned home with a medal. A specific example is Ranomi Kromowidjojo, Dutch triple Olympic champion (50 m, 100 m, and 4 × 100 m freestyle) and multiple world record holder (50 m, 4 × 50 m, 4 × 100 m, and 4 × 200 m freestyle Short Course). At the World Aquatics Championships 2017, she finished fifth, with a personal best of 52.7. At the press conference after the race, Ranomi reflected on her race and explicitly addressed the issue of how to cope with her loss:

> When are you satisfied with your performance? When you win gold, or when you achieve a personal best? At the London Olympic Games I managed to secure a gold medal. It wasn't my best race ever, but I was happy with my time of 53.0 seconds. Now I did very well and reached my potential, but I am disappointed not to finish on the podium. (in Volkers, 2017).

Ranomi's mixed feelings about her performance reflect the multifaceted nature of achievement goal pursuit, and accordingly, the complex process of self-regulation. In the sports psychological goal-setting literature, three types of achievement goals are distinguished: *outcome goals, performance goals,* and *process goals* (Filby, Maynard, & Graydon, 1999; Hardy, 1997; Moran & Toner, 2017; Williams, 2013). Individuals with *outcomes goals* rely on social comparison (Festinger, 1954); that is, outcome goals (or other-based goals) are typically grounded in *inter*personal or normative standards such as winning a match or competition, or a particular position on a ranking. This type of goal represents the *why* of motivational processes (Filby et al., 1999; Moran & Toner, 2017). As humorously underlined by former Liverpool manager Bill Shankly, a defining feature of sports is competition: "Some people believe football is a matter of life and death, I am very disappointed with that attitude. I can assure you it is much, much more important than that" (MailOnline, 2009). This quote is clearly an overstatement, but sports are typically zero-sum games (i.e., the outcome is either win or lose). Hence, a *winning is all* mentality is almost automatically enforced in a sports context, and there is no doubt that *winning* is very much appreciated by any participant in any sports context.

From this perspective, Ranomi Kromowidjojo's feelings of disappointment and dissatisfaction are understandable. She did not manage to secure a medal position (i.e., a top 3 rank) at the 2017 World Aquatics Championships. She swam her best race ever, but her opponents performed (slightly) better. Indeed, the problem with *winning* as outcome goal is that athletes largely lack control over the outcome. Winning or losing is obviously a function of one's own talent and effort, but other variables also have substantial impact, including opponents, referees, game conditions, and chance. Therefore, from a self-regulation perspective, an outcome goal may be best considered a dream or desire. Like surfers who hope for sunshine and wind, athletes may hope that their own performance will ultimately be good enough for the victory. Like Ranomi, you may complete your perfect race but nevertheless lose because your opponents, who are also extremely talented and skilled, perform even better than you.

Accordingly, an exclusive focus on largely uncontrollable outcome goals may shift the athlete's attention away from the task through task-irrelevant interfering thoughts. Such thoughts typically undermine performance attainment and in the longer term make athletes vulnerable to structural frustration, chronic fear of failure, and burnout (e.g., Deffenbacher, 1980; Hatzigeorgiadis & Biddle, 2002; Sarason, Sarason, Keefe, Hayes, & Shearin, 1986). This does not imply that outcome goals should be neglected. In contrast, particularly among elite athletes, the goal to win inspires, energizes, and directs, and should be utilized at the right moment. For example, this strong motivational force may help athletes to deal with tough conditions (rain, cold, loneliness, pain) during training, inspire them before important matches, or cause them to give their all for the win at the final stage of a close race. However, for the maintenance of sports enjoyment, self-confidence, and long-term, sustainable development, it may be better to rely on the building blocks of outcome goals, namely, performance goals and process goals, which I discuss next.

A zero-sum *situation* does not imply exclusive zero-sum *motivation* (cf. Hays, 2012). In a competitive context, effective self-regulators pursue *performance goals* (or self-based goals) simultaneously, or subsequently. This type of goal represents *what* athletes are aiming to achieve. The standard is grounded in an *intra-personal* standard, that is, referring to a former version of oneself. Such a reliance on temporal comparison (Albert, 1977), which is largely under the athlete's own control, may refer to time ("Running the 100 m within 10 seconds"), distance or height ("To break the 8-meter [distance] or 2-meter [height] barrier"), technique ("Hitting draws and fades with a golf driver"), or effort ("Never give up in this match"). In the previous example, Ranomi's performance goal at the 2017 World Aquatics Championships was to post a personal best. Because swimming is a self-paced skill, no opponent could stop her from attaining her performance goal.

She additionally set process goals (or task-based goals) in service of her performance goal. *Process goals* refer to *how* athletes can achieve their performance and outcome goals. Process goals are set by breaking the performance goal down into manageable chunks and creating a plan to achieve it. Because process goals rely on standards that are inherent in the task itself, athletes receive direct, immediate, and ongoing feedback during their sports performances. This process facilitates learning and skills acquisition, enhances concentration and commitment, and makes flow states more likely to occur. In contrast, outcome and performance goals require the ability to cognitively represent two outcomes simultaneously (i.e., others' performances and one's own previous performances, respectively; Elliot, Murayama, & Pekrun, 2011), which may interfere with total absorption in the task.

The multiple goals athletes typically hold can be structured into a hierarchical goal system or framework (Williams, 2013). *Goal systems* are defined as the mental representations of motivational networks that comprise interconnected goals and means (Kruglanski et al., 2002). Specifically, superordinate outcome goals (*Why?*) should be used to flexibly organize performance goals (*What?*) and their means of attainment, or process goals (*How?*). These latter, lower-order goals, or tactics (Scholer & Higgins, 2008), are typically more numerous, context-specific, short-term (proximal), and substitutable (Duckworth & Gross, 2014). For example, at the 2017 World Aquatics Championships, Ranomi had a series of process goals with regard to start speed (15 m from signal), turn speed, finishing speed (last 5 m), swimming speed per lap, and stroke frequency and stroke length. Because she achieved all of her process goals, as well as her performance goal (a personal best), she was eventually pleased with her performance despite her unexpected and disappointing final rank. As an effective self-regulator, she acknowledged that she had achieved her performance and process goals over which she had personal control.

Although research on the effectiveness of goal hierarchies in sports is virtually nonexistent (Burton & Weiss, 2008; Williams, 2013), making goal systems visible and explicit likely helps athletes to effectively self-regulate and monitor their goal pursuit: It may increase athletes' awareness of what actions, means, and subgoals facilitate and inhibit their focal objective (Zimmerman et al., 2017). As illustrated by Ranomi's case, her process goals regarding speed (start, swimming, turn, and finish) and stroke (frequency and length) were the building blocks of her performance goal (a personal best), which should have led to achievement of her top-ranked but largely uncontrollable outcome goal (a spot on the podium).

When resources are limited, goal hierarchies may also help athletes to deactivate or inhibit rival goals that are deemed less important. Successful goal pursuit entails maintaining commitment to one's focal goals (e.g., Van Yperen, 2009), which is most likely to occur for individuals high in self-control and grit. *Self-control* refers to the capacity to regulate attention, emotion, and behavior in the presence of temptation (Baumeister, Schmeister, & Vohs, 2007); *grit* is the tenacious pursuit of a dominant superordinate goal despite setbacks (Duckworth, Peterson, Matthews, & Kelly, 2007). Thus, self-control is typically associated with attaining short-term process goals, whereas grit is more tightly coupled with achieving exceptional long-term outcome goals (Duckworth & Gross, 2014). Self-control and grit are particularly important in situations in which pursuing a negative subordinate proximal goal (e.g., training in wet and cold weather, accepting a nasty and selfish star player in your team) is required as a stepping-stone for attaining a positive superordinate distal goal (e.g., becoming world champion).

Principle 3: Differentiate Achievement Goals on the Basis of Evaluative Standard and Valence

The influential achievement goal approach to achievement motivation (Elliot & Hulleman, 2017) developed more or less independently of the goal-setting literature (Locke & Latham, 2013). Most noticeable (and confusing) about this development is that different labels are used for similar goals, and the same labels for different goals. Specifically, in the achievement goal approach, other-based outcome goals are referred to as *performance goals*. Self-based performance goals in the goal-setting literature are called *mastery goals* in the achievement goal approach. Even more confusing, achievement goal researchers in sports psychology tend to rely on a dichotomy of other-based *ego goals* versus self-based or task-based *task goals* (e.g., Duda, 2005). In the extant (achievement) goal literature, these different goals are operationalized as goal state, dispositional goal orientation, or perceived motivational climate (Biddle, Wang, Kavussanu, & Spray, 2003; Duda, 2005; Elliot, Jury, & Murayama, 2018).

Although self-based and task-based goal pursuits are closely related, these goals can be pursued independently. Hence, Elliot and colleagues (2011) identified three basic evaluative standards:

1. *Other-based standards* refer to others who are concrete and present in the achievement situation (as in face-to-face competition) or to aggregated normative information.
2. *Self-based standards* refer to one's personal performance trajectory.
3. *Task-based standards* refer to the absolute demands of the task (e.g., sinking a putt, lifting one's knees when running).

Following Elliot and colleagues (2011), in this chapter, the terms *other-based goal, self-based goal,* and *task-based goal* are used as labels throughout.

Achievement goals differ not just with respect to the evaluative standards individuals use. Another basic dimension is how competence is valenced, that is, as the individual's desired level of competence or undesired level of incompetence (for a recent review, see Elliot & Hulleman, 2017). Crossing the three standards used to define competence with how competence can be valenced yields a 3 × 2 achievement goal model (Elliot et al., 2011). Individuals may be focused on (1a) doing better than others or (1b) not doing worse than others, (2a) doing better than before or (2b) not doing worse than before, and (3a) doing the task correctly or (3b) not doing the task incorrectly. Mascret, Elliot, and Curry (2015) extended this 3 × 2 achievement goal model to the sports domain.

Principle 4: Set Approach Goals Rather Than Avoidance Goals

Few studies have examined differences between self-based and task-based goals (undifferentiated, known as "mastery goals"; Elliot & Hulleman, 2017), and particularly studies on negatively valenced self-based and task-based goals are underrepresented. Nevertheless, the quite consistent results of several meta-analyses suggest that particularly the valence dimension of achievement goals is important for performance attainment. Across achievement domains (i.e., sports, education, and work), approach goals (other, self, or task) are positively related to performance attainment, whereas avoidance goals (other, self, or task) are negatively related to performance attainment (Baranik, Stanley, Bynum, & Lance, 2010; Hulleman, Schrager, Bodmann, & Harackiewicz, 2010; Payne, Youngcourt, & Beaubien, 2007; Van Yperen, Blaga, & Postmes, 2014).

Particularly for sports psychologists and other applied scientists and practitioners, an important question is whether performance can be improved by achievement goal interventions. The observed positive links between approach goals and performance attainment in survey research are valuable and useful for providing ecologically valid information. However, in order to enhance performance, we need to know the *causal effects* of *assigned* achievement goals on performance and other outcomes of interest; that is, only findings from experimental achievement goal research provide a solid basis for the development of effective achievement goal interventions in applied settings. Note that in an experimental setting or practical intervention, typically, one particular achievement goal is assigned to the individual; this is assumed to be the individual's *dominant* achievement goal in that particular setting (Van Yperen, 2006).

A meta-analysis of experimental achievement goal research showed that the observed patterns in the rather small number of experimental studies are generally in line with the overall pattern found in correlational research; that is, relative to avoidance goals, approach goals enhance performance attainment (Van Yperen, Blaga, & Postmes, 2015). Self-regulation processes related to the positive, appetitive possibility of competence, including mental focus and feedback seeking, may explain the positive effect of approach goals, and self-based and task-based goals in particular, on performance (e.g., Anseel, Beatty, Shen, Lievens, & Sackett, 2015; Janssen & Van Yperen, 2004; Lee, Sheldon, & Turban, 2003). For example, in a meta-analysis of the antecedents and outcomes of feedback-seeking behavior, Anseel and colleagues (2015) showed that approach goals were positively associated with overall feedback seeking. These results suggest that approach-oriented individuals tend to view feedback seeking as a viable strategy for reaching their goal, either to improve on the task or to do better than others. However, individuals endorsing self-based or task-based goals may be particularly interested in information that helps them to improve, whereas individuals with other-based goals may find social comparison information most valuable (Janssen & Prins, 2007).

In contrast, avoidance forms of regulation tend to evoke negative outcomes, including lower levels of self-efficacy and performance (Payne et al., 2007), through increased levels of worry and intruding negative thoughts (e.g., Elliot & McGregor, 1999; Lee et al., 2003). For example, in two prospective studies, Pekrun, Elliot, and Maier (2006) showed that in contrast to approach goals, *other*-based avoidance goals were positive predictors of anxiety. In a longitudinal study, Lee and colleagues (2003) found a negative link between other-based avoidance goals and mental focus, which in turn was positively related to performance. These findings suggest that other-based avoidance goals may have undermined individuals' mental focus on the task and, accordingly, their performance on the task, due to worries or intruding thoughts about potential failure or other cognitive interferences.

Across studies in the sports domain, however, Van Yperen and colleagues (2014) did not observe a negative link between *other*-based avoidance goals and performance. Given that competition and social comparison are defining features of sports, an outcome-oriented sports climate may better fit with athletes' other-based goals; that is, athletes with other-based avoidance goals may not necessarily "feel bad" in a sports context, which may mitigate the decrease in task focus, effort, and persistence, and ultimately, performance deterioration, which is more often observed in other achievement domains. Furthermore, in sports contexts, an other-based avoidance goal may not have such a negative connotation because not performing worse than others, or not losing (i.e., a draw), may be perceived as a great achievement or a desired outcome (e.g., because the opponent is considered to be much stronger, or because not losing may be sufficient to qualify for the next round in a tournament or to become league champion).

Similarly, in achievement domains other than sports, *self*-based avoidance goals tend to have a negative impact on performance (Van Yperen, Blaga, & Postmes, 2015). This may be particularly true in a multiple-trial context, that is, a context that matches the intrapersonal evaluative focus of self-based avoidance goals (Van Yperen, Elliot, & Anseel, 2009). In such a context, an intrapersonal standard is highly diagnostic; that is, both the dimensions of comparison (the task itself, the conditions, etc.) and the comparison other (the self) are specific, clear, and unambiguous. Accordingly, doing worse than one did before on the same task under identical conditions can yield unequivocal negative feedback, which makes it hard to distort the undesired outcome in a self-enhancing manner and to find appropriate excuses for one's poor performance. Therefore, negative, interfering thoughts during task performance may even be stronger when pursuing a self-based avoidance goal relative to an other-based avoidance goal. Indeed, Sideridis (2008) showed that relative to other-based avoidance goals (and approach goals), self-based avoidance goals are associated with enhanced negative affect and increases in cognitive and somatic anxiety, as indicated using both self-report and physiological measures (cf. Preenen, van Vianen, & De Pater, 2014; Tanaka, Okuno, & Yamauchi, 2013).

In contrast, in sports contexts, athletes may be more likely to perceive a performance at their typical level (i.e., not performing worse than before) to be sufficient for a win or to finish at a particular rank. Especially among older athletes (30+), self-avoidance goals may not have such a negative effect on sport performance and related variables, since maintenance, loss-prevention, and self-based avoidance goals may be more prevalent in the final stage of one's sport career. In the work domain, there is some evidence that among employees in the final stage of their career (60+), self-based avoidance goals are positively associated with positively valenced variables, including well-being, task enjoyment, and work engagement (de Lange, Van Yperen, Van der Heijden, & Bal, 2010; Ebner, Freund, & Baltes, 2006; Senko & Freund, 2015). These findings are in line with the idea of regulatory fit: What works best for an individual depends on factors such as age, needs, and type of motivation (e.g., Unkelbach, Plessner, & Memmert, 2009).

Principle 5: Develop Interventions That Focus on Self-Based and Task-Based Approach Goals

A general conclusion based on experimental achievement goal research is that relative to avoidance goals, approach goals enhance task performance (Van Yperen et al., 2015). For the sports domain, the good news is that field research suggests that the negative link between avoidance goals and sports performance tends to be absent (Van Yperen et al., 2014). In the extant achievement goal research, the typical practical recommendation is to focus on *self*-based and *task*-based approach goals. The pursuit of these goals is generally considered to be the ideal type of competence-based regulation (Pintrich, 2000). Individuals pursuing these

goals have been found to be high in achievement motivation (Elliot & Church, 1997), intrinsic motivation (Rawsthorne & Elliot, 1999), task interest (Harackiewicz & Knogler, 2017), and agreeableness and conscientiousness (Day, Radosevich, & Chasteen, 2003; McCabe, Van Yperen, Elliot, & Verbraak, 2013). Furthermore, a focus on self-based and task-based goals tends to promote prosocial behavior, such as tolerance for opposing views (Darnon, Muller, Schrager, Pannuzzo, & Butera, 2006; Nederveen-Pieterse, van Knippenberg, & van Dierendonck, 2013) and sharing resources with others (Levy, Kaplan, & Patrick, 2004; Poortvliet, Janssen, Van Yperen, & Van de Vliert, 2007).

However, it is unrealistic to ignore other-based approach goals. Competition and social comparison are defining features of sports, so athletes rely primarily on social comparisons in their performance self-evaluations. This tendency exists in other performance contexts as well, even among individuals with dominant self-based approach goals (Van Yperen & Leander, 2014). The problem is that thoughts about (largely uncontrollable) other-based outcomes (either win or lose) tend to undermine athletes' mental focus on the task at hand, and, accordingly, their performance on the task, due to worries and other cognitive interferences. Other potential costs associated with other-based goals are a loss of interest (Harackiewicz & Knogler, 2017), anxiety, worry, negative affect (Elliot & McGregor, 2001; Pintrich, 2000), dissatisfaction (Van Yperen & Janssen, 2002), and neuroticism (Hendricks & Payne, 2007; McCabe et al., 2013). Other-based goals also tend to elicit unethical behaviors such as thwarting behavior and less accurate information-giving (Poortvliet, Anseel, Janssen, Van Yperen, & Van de Vliert, 2012), and cheating (Van Yperen, Hamstra, & van der Klauw, 2011), which should caution practitioners against their promotion (for reviews, see Ordóñez & Welsh, 2015; Van Yperen, 2017).

To optimize self-regulation, athletes should be aware of what actions, means, and subgoals facilitate and inhibit their other-based goal. This may be enhanced by (1) organizing athletes' goals into a hierarchical achievement goal system, (2) directing athletes' focus to the means rather than the outcomes, (3) emphasizing evaluation more in terms of progress and effort, (4) defining success more in terms of improvement, and (5) creating and maintaining a strong developmental climate in which athletes are stimulated to develop their technical, tactical, physical, and mental skills (cf. Ames, 1992). Directing athletes toward positively valenced self-based goals is likely to increase their perceived feasibility, whereas task-based goals may enhance their concentration and focus during task performance. To test the effectiveness of such goal-based interventions, repeated measures designs may be applied to athletes' self-based growth curves (i.e., patterns across time that are independent of others' performances). Remarkably, so far, this has rarely been done in achievement goal research (Da Motta Veiga & Turban, 2014; Yeo, Loft, Xiao, & Kiewitz, 2009).

Principle 6: Delineate Athletes' Idiosyncratic Developmental Trajectories to Better Understand the Process of Goal Attainment and Self-Regulation

Theoretical and practical progress in goal research can be made by examining, among other things, process-oriented explanations for goal attainment, and more generally, for developmental processes, such as becoming an elite athlete. Goals and performances likely develop out of structures of dynamically interacting (personal and environmental) factors or components, in the form of direct and indirect loops of reinforcement or diminishment (Den Hartigh, Van Dijk, Steenbeek, & Van Geert, 2016; Hill, Den Hartigh, Meijer, De Jonge, & Van Yperen, 2018). For example, the components of a competitive sports culture interact with athletes' goal-setting strategies and their ways of coping with the pressure to perform, losses, and disappointments (Den Hartigh, Van Yperen, & Van Geert, 2017). In such a dynamic network perspective, drops and rises in performance are not determined by a single component or event but by their interactions with time and other components in the athlete's network structure. Positive or negative events may trigger a boost or breakdown in the development of existing components and/or a reconfigura-

tion of connections between components, and then be repeatedly refueled or redirected by the same or other network components (cf. Cohen, Garcia, & Goyer, 2017). For example, Ranomi's unexpected loss discussed earlier may have resulted in even more focus, goal commitment, and motivation to succeed. A couple of months later, in December 2017, at the European Short Course Swimming Championships, she won four gold medals. In contrast, earlier in her career, she experienced a decline in performance because her coach left for another job in Australia. This latter event illustrates the occurrence of a negative developmental pattern due to the disappearance of a critical network component. To capture the dynamic and complex process of goal attainment, resilience, and athletes' development, different data sources may be used, including biographical data, (experimental) time-series data (e.g., by using wearables), and computer simulation data (Den Hartigh et al., 2016; Den Hartigh, Van Yperen, & Van Geert, 2017; Hill, Den Hartigh, Meijer, De Jonge, & Van Yperen, 2018). For example, to better understand the dynamics of psychological momentum, Den Hartigh, Gernigon, Van Yperen, Marin, and Van Geert (2014) asked rowing pairs to compete against a virtual opponent on rowing ergometers, while a screen in front of the team broadcast the ongoing race. The race was manipulated, so that the team's rowing avatar gradually progressed (positive momentum) or regressed (negative momentum) in relation to victory. The participants responded verbally to collective efficacy and task cohesion items appearing on the screen each minute. In addition, effort exertion and interpersonal coordination were continuously measured. This study revealed that relative to positive team momentum, negative momentum elicits stronger (opposite) psychological changes and accompanies different (less adaptive) behavioral regulation. In a follow-up study, Den Hartigh and colleagues (2016) demonstrated that rowers who had developed long-term positive psychological momentum after two successful races were less sensitive to a negative momentum scenario in the third race compared with athletes who had developed long-term negative momentum after two unsuccessful races. The asymmetry between positive and negative psychological team momentum dynamics, and the impact of both short- and long-term history of progress and regress, underlines the relevance of a dynamic system perspective.

Principle 7: Work on Strengths and Weaknesses Simultaneously

Another interesting goal-related issue is whether athletes' goals and effort should be directed toward enhancing their strengths or reducing their weaknesses? How are these assessed in the first place? To start with the latter question, individuals' self-evaluations are typically based on social comparison information (e.g., Van Yperen & Leander, 2014). However, when explicitly asked to indicate their relative weaknesses and strengths, individuals tend to use dimensional within-person comparisons as well (Möller & Marsh, 2013). For example, a soccer player may consider herself a better passer than header; that is, she considers passing a relative strength, and heading a relative weakness. As demonstrated in a meta-analytic investigation of within-person self-efficacy, self-efficacy is primarily a product of past performance (Sitzmann & Yeo, 2013). Therefore, relative to heading, the soccer player's self-efficacy with regard to passing is likely to be higher, which may positively affect subsequent performance. Indeed, a meta-analysis on the link between self-efficacy and performance in sports revealed an average correlation of .38 (Moritz, Feltz, Fahrbach, & Mack, 2000). Furthermore, research has shown that indices of self-efficacy are positively related to personal goal levels (Kane, Marks, Zaccaro, & Blair, 1996) and to intrinsic motivation and willingness to exert effort (e.g., Bandura & Locke, 2003; Hiemstra & Van Yperen, 2015; Latham & Pinder, 2005; Van Yperen, Den Hartigh, Visscher, & Elferink-Gemser, 2019), all of which may explain better subsequent performance. Thus, in an autonomous environment without constraints and extrinsic reinforcers such as money, credits, fame, and recognition, individuals may be most likely to work on their strengths because this reinforces their self-confidence.

In contrast, a focus on one's weaknesses may hamper one's self-confidence, but it may be deemed necessary to increase one's general effectiveness. For example, a tennis player with a technically vulnerable backhand is likely to be constantly bombarded on his backhand side by his opponents. He should improve his backhand technique to no longer feel shackled on his backhand wing, particularly under pressure. Research has shown that testing conditions (e.g., exams and competitions) may motivate individuals to invest more effort to meet the external standards, but they mostly enjoy working on their strengths (Hiemstra, Van Yperen, & Timmerman, 2019). To serve their distal, long-term, other-based goals (e.g., winning tournaments, becoming a champion), athletes' proximal process goals should be directed toward reducing their relative weaknesses (e.g., their backhand), but this may be more enjoyable when combined with drills and exercises that rely on their relative strengths. Such an approach serves both athletes' self-improvement and self-enhancement needs (Wood, 1989). A helpful tool in this regard may be performance profiling, a procedure that encourages athletes to identify, and reflect on, the qualities needed to be successful in their sport. Athletes are typically requested to indicate on a dartboard-like diagram "Where I am now?" and "Where I would like to be?" in those attributes, and next, to engage in deliberate practice to fill the gap (Butler & Hardy, 1992; Weston, Greenlees, & Thelwell, 2013). Although research has highlighted the range of beneficial impacts of profiling, rigorous empirical research on its efficacy is still lacking (Weston et al., 2013).

Principle 8: Distinguish between High-Pressure Situations and Athletes' Psychological Reactions to Pressure

When engaging in a zero-sum game (i.e., the outcome is either win or lose), athletes have the prospect of unequivocal normative evaluation. Particularly when the stakes are high, goal-committed athletes are likely to perceive performing in front of an audience as a high-pressure situation. Athletes cannot change this situation, but they can control and change their reaction to it. In other words, it is important to distinguish between a high-pressure situation and athletes' psychological reactions to pressure (Lazarus, 1991; Lazarus & Folkman, 1984), which have clear physiological underpinnings (Blascovich, 2008; Dienstbier, 1989).

High-pressure situations activate the sympathetic–adrenal–medullary (SAM) system, eliciting arousal (e.g., increased heart rate, dilated blood vessels, and higher levels of glucose) as an undifferentiated somatic state that mobilizes resources for vigorous action (i.e., "fight-or-flight" response; Blascovich, 2008; Jamieson, 2017; Whelan, Epkins, & Meyers, 1990). Performers' ("secondary") appraisal of their increased arousal level is determined, among other things, by their perceived abilities to cope effectively with the pressure situation (Lazarus & Folkman, 1984). When they feel they have the requisite physical, technical, tactical, and mental resources, they are likely to interpret their increased arousal level as a functional coping resource that aids rather than harms performance (Jamieson, 2017). Hence, they tend to perceive arousal as anticipatory excitement, which has been demonstrated to enhance subsequence performance (Jamieson, 2017; Moore, Vine, Wilson, & Freeman, 2015; Thomas, Mellalieu, & Hanton, 2009).

In contrast, performers who feel that they lack the skills to deal effectively with the high-pressure situation tend to perceive their increased levels of arousal as a hindrance rather than a help, and accordingly, are more likely to experience pressure, threat, and concomitant performance anxiety. Such an appraisal activates, in addition to the SAM system, the hypothalamic–pituitary–adrenocortical (HPA) system, resulting in the release of cortisol (Blascovich, 2008; Dienstbier, 1989). Furthermore, perceived threat increases vascular resistance, which limits blood flow to the periphery and produces high total peripheral resistance (TPR) scores. In contrast, low TPR scores reflect delivery of oxygenated blood to the brain and periphery, and are associated with perceived challenge (Jamieson, 2017; Seery, 2011).

The other related, yet distinct, component of performance anxiety has been referred to as anxious apprehension, worry, or cognitive concern about one's performance level and its implications for the self (Liebert & Morris, 1967; Nitschke, Heller, Imig, McDonald, & Miller, 2001). Performers high in anxious apprehension

have difficulties in keeping their performance efforts channeled toward task execution. Self-focus theories postulate that anxiety increases performers' self-consciousness, which hampers performance through their attempts to consciously monitor or control their previously automatic skills (Beilock, Schaeffer, & Rozek, 2017). Also, distraction theories such as attention control theory (ACT) state that anxious apprehension undermines performance through attentional control (Derakshan & Eysenck, 2009; Eysenck, Derakshan, Santos, & Calvo, 2007). Especially threat-related, interfering thoughts (e.g., thoughts about failure, negative evaluation, or losing) are assumed to reduce the cognitive resources available for processing and performing the task (Deffenbacher, 1980; Sarason et al., 1986). For example, Jordet and Hartman (2008) demonstrated that relative to an approach situation, in which a team win could be ensured immediately, in an avoidance situation, in which missing a penalty kick instantly produced a team loss, soccer players tended to respond more anxiously (e.g., by taking less time for their preparation).

Apparently, the outcome of a penalty shootout is a function of the immediate importance of the outcome, but the behavior of the goalkeeper may also have an effect. As demonstrated by Wood and Wilson (2010), under high-threat conditions, penalty takers found it more difficult to focus on their target (just inside the goal post) when the goalkeeper was arm-waving rather than stationary. *Choking under pressure* occurs when, in a high-stakes situation, the negative cognitive appraisal of arousal due to a lack of perceived control and self-presentational concerns leads to a dramatic and acute (rather than gradual) performance impairment, that is, a lower level of performance than one is capable of (Beilock et al., 2017; Hill, Hanton, Matthews, & Fleming, 2010).

Principle 9: Accept Fluctuating Internal States and Focus on Goal-Relevant Cues and Contingencies

As discussed in the previous section, performers may interpret increasing levels of arousal differently, which is likely a function of individual differences, time, and context. This also suggests that individuals can be educated and trained to restructure and reappraise increasing levels of arousal as an opportunity for growth, mastery, or gain, which likely leads to better performance (Jamieson, 2017; Lazarus & Folkman, 1984; Moore et al., 2015; Thomas et al., 2009). Whereas arousal reappraisal training is aimed at changing athletes' responses to increasing levels of arousal (Brooks, 2014; Crum, Salovey, & Achor, 2013), more traditional *psychological skills training (PST)*, including techniques such as imagery/mental rehearsal and self-talk, is typically targeted at controlling (e.g., eliminating or dampening) emotions, cognitions, and bodily states, which is assumed to create a psychological state for optimal performance (e.g., Hardy, Jones, & Gould, 1996). The ability to effectively regulate one's arousal level by using, for example, specific breathing and relaxation techniques may be helpful because beyond a particular point, even positively framed arousal levels may impair performance (e.g., Hanin, 2000; Hardy, Beattie, & Woodman, 2007; Yerkes & Dodson, 1908). Brown and Fletcher (2017) recently meta-analyzed randomized controlled trials on psychological, social, and psychosocial interventions with sports performers, focusing on variables relating to their athletic performance. Their conclusion was that these interventions have a moderate positive effect on sports performance, and this effect may last at least a month following the end of the intervention.

In contrast to PST, other types of psychological interventions are based on the assumption that changing, controlling, or reducing internal processes such as emotions (e.g., anxiety, uncertainty, fear of failure) and thoughts (e.g., thoughts about losing and quitting) is not the optimal strategy. For example, mindfulness–acceptance–commitment (MAC; Gardner & Moore, 2012) focuses primarily on athletes' ability to contact the present moment fully. Rather than reappraising, controlling, or self-regulating their internal processes (e.g., in high-pressure situations), athletes should engage in a nonjudging (i.e., not good, not bad, not right, not wrong), moment-to-moment awareness and acceptance of their internal states. In other words, MAC reinforces the idea that the natural ebb and flow of positive and negative thoughts,

emotions, and bodily sensations should be experienced without judgment or avoidance. Deliberate attempts to self-control or suppress such internal experiences, so-called *experiential avoidance* (Hayes, Wilson, Gifford, Follette, & Strosahl, 1996), are assumed to result in negative outcomes. For example, Wegner's (1994) ironic process theory proposes that efforts at self-regulation of thoughts lead to a rebound effect. Particularly under conditions of pressure, anxiety, fatigue, and mental load, attempts to block out unwanted thoughts (e.g., "Do not double-fault"; "Do not overshoot the hole") paradoxically make them more likely to surface. Their prominence in our consciousness may subsequently produce counterintentional outcomes. Presumably, this is due to an unconscious metacognitive scanning process that is automatically activated to monitor the effectiveness of the cognitive activity aimed at suppressing the unwanted emotions and thoughts, which are brought to awareness when detected (Moran & Toner, 2017). This cognitive activity interferes with consistent and effortful personal-values-driven commitment to behavioral actions and choices that support the person's athletic endeavors (Gardner & Moore, 2012). MAC training is geared toward athletes who want to learn to experience their internal states without judgment or avoidance, and to defuse or disconnect these states from their behavioral choices and actions. This behavioral flexibility is enhanced by teaching athletes how to align their behavior with their personal values and proximal and distal goals. They learn to accept fluctuating competitive demands and internal experiences and to (re)focus their attention to performance-relevant cues and contingencies that support their athletic endeavors (Gardner & Moore, 2012). After clinching his third grand slam title, the Swiss tennis player Stan Wawrinka (2016) unusually disclosed the following at the U.S. Open 2016 press conference:

> Today, before the final, I was really nervous like never before. I was shaking in the locker. When we start five minutes before the match talking, last few things with Magnus, I start to cry. I was completely shaking. But the only thing I was convinced with myself that my game was there. Physically I was there. My game was there. Put the fight on the court and you will have a chance to win.

The MAC approach, which emphasizes that so-called "negative" psychological processes do not necessarily hinder athletes' performance and well-being, has received promising empirical support across a variety of sports (e.g., Bernier, Thienot, Codron, & Fournier, 2009; Bühlmayer, Birrer, Röthlin, Faude, & Donath, 2017; Gardner & Moore, 2012; Henriksen, Hansen, & Larsen, 2019; Sappington & Longshore, 2015). A specific technique aimed at directly optimizing the performance process (rather than affecting the performer's internal state), is called *quiet eye*; this is discussed next.

Principle 10:
Control the Controllables

Attentional mechanisms are critical in understanding the relationship between performance anxiety and performance attainment (Wilson, 2012). Not only self-generated concerns arising from one's own thoughts and feelings, but also external distractors such as weather conditions, the click of a camera, or actions by opponents or parents, tend to impair attentional control, and accordingly, to negatively affect performance attainment. As discussed in the previous section, attempts to suppress such internal and external distractors, paradoxically, make them more likely to emerge. A more effective strategy is to *control the controllables,* that is, to focus on the task at hand and controllable actions.

An illustrative technique that directs performers' attention to the controllables is *quiet eye* (QE), which has been defined as the final fixation or tracking gaze that is located on a specific target or object prior to the onset of a critical movement (Vickers, 2007). Research has shown that experts have longer QE durations than nonexperts, and successful attempts have longer QE durations than unsuccessful attempts (Lebeau et al., 2016). Longer QE durations are associated with, for example, goaltender success in deflected ice hockey shots (Panchuk, Vickers, & Hopkins, 2017), golfers' improved putting performance on the course (Vine, Moore, & Wilson, 2011), and more perceived control and superior performance in a penalty shootout (Noël & Van der Kamp, 2012; Wood & Wilson, 2012). The extant QE literature suggests that ac-

tively maintaining effective gaze behavior (QE) alleviates the negative effects of anxiety on visual attentional control and subsequent performance (Vine, Moore, & Wilson, 2011; Wilson, 2012). Furthermore, timely information about targets from the gaze system (i.e., long QE duration) is proposed to increase the motor preparation period that involves the fine-tuning and accuracy of movement parameters responsible for motor programming. QE also provides the external focus of attention on process-related or task-relevant cues, which is believed to promote automatic behavior in skilled performers, and accordingly, helps in coping with distractors, including feelings of anxiety, negative thoughts, or the mechanics of skill execution (cf. Wulf, 2013). Finally, similar to a preperformance routine, QE helps the performer to create a more relaxed preperformance state, which becomes more and more profound with deliberate practice. Deliberate practice refers to engagement in practice activities assigned by a coach with a clear, specific goal of improvement and where the practice activities provide immediate feedback and opportunities for repetition to attain gradual improvement (Ericsson, Krampe, & Tesch-Römer, 1993; Ericsson, 2014). In general, engaging in deliberate practice to improve relevant technical, tactical, physical, and mental skills can be considered the key to success, also because adaptive, challenge-type responses to arousal are a function of athletes' perceived skills in dealing effectively with pressure situations.

Concluding Remarks

The main conclusion is that the last principle, control the controllables, can be considered an overarching principle of effective self-regulation. Athletes actually increase their control over actions, means, and subgoals when they (1) organize their goals into a hierarchical achievement goal system; (2) focus on self-based and task-based approach goals rather than other-based approach goals or avoidance goals; (3) work on both their strengths and weakness by engaging in deliberate practice; (4) accept fluctuating internal states; and (5) focus on goal-relevant cues and contingencies, particularly in high-pressure situations. Enhancing and developing personal control over goal attainment, but also accepting the uncontrollables, are indispensable mental skills to ultimately achieve the outcome that is happily welcomed by any sport performer: *coming out victorious.*

REFERENCES

Albert, S. (1977). Temporal comparison theory. *Psychological Review, 84,* 485–503.

Allport, F. H. (1924). *Social psychology.* Boston: Houghton Mifflin.

Ames, C. (1992). Classrooms: Goals, structures, and student motivation. *Journal of Educational Psychology, 84,* 261–271.

Anseel, F., Beatty, A. S., Shen, W., Lievens, F., & Sackett, P. R. (2015). How are we doing after 30 years?: A meta-analytic review of the antecedents and outcomes of feedback-seeking behavior. *Journal of Management, 41*(1), 318–348.

Bandura, A., & Locke, E. (2003). Negative self-efficacy and goal effects revisited. *Journal of Applied Psychology, 88,* 87–99.

Baranik, L. E., Stanley, L. J., Bynum, B. H., & Lance, C. E. (2010). Examining the construct validity of mastery-avoidance achievement goals: A meta-analysis. *Human Performance, 23,* 265–282.

Baumeister, R. F., Schmeister, B. J., & Vohs, K. D. (2007). Self-regulation and the executive function: The self as controlling agent. In A. W. Kruglanski & E. T. Higgins (Eds.), *Social psychology: Handbook of basic principles* (2nd ed., pp. 516–539). New York: Guilford Press.

Beilock, S. L., Schaeffer, M. J., & Rozek, C. S. (2017). Understanding and addressing performance anxiety. In A. J. Elliot, C. S. Dweck, & D. S. Yeager (Eds.), *Handbook of competence and motivation: Theory and application* (2nd ed., pp. 155–172). New York: Guilford Press.

Bernier, M., Thienot, E., Codron, R., & Fournier, J. F. (2009). Mindfulness and acceptance approaches in sport performance. *Journal of Clinical Sport Psychology, 3,* 320–333.

Biddle, S. J. H., Wang, J., Kavussanu, M., & Spray, C. M. (2003). Correlates of achievement goal orientations in physical activity: A systematic review of research. *European Journal of Sports Science, 3,* 1–19.

Blascovich, J. (2008). Challenge and threat. In A. J. Elliot (Ed.), *Handbook of approach and avoidance motivation* (pp. 431–445). New York: Psychology Press.

Brooks, A. W. (2014). Get excited: Reappraising preperformance anxiety as excitement. *Journal of Experimental Psychology: General, 143,* 1144–1158.

Brown, D. J., & Fletcher, D. (2017). Effects of psychological and psychosocial interventions on sport performance: A meta-analysis. *Sports Medicine, 47,* 77–99.

Bühlmayer, L., Birrer, D., Röthlin, P., Faude, O., & Donath, L. (2017). Effects of mindfulness practice on performance-relevant parameters and performance outcomes in sports: A meta-analytical review. *Sports Medicine, 47,* 2309–2321.

Burton, D., Naylor, S., & Holliday, B. (2001). Goal-setting in sport: Investigating the goal effectiveness paradox. In R. Singer, H. A. Hausenblas, & C. M. Janelle (Eds.), *Handbook of research on sport psychology* (2nd ed., pp. 497–528). New York: Wiley.

Burton, D., Pickering, M., Weinberg, R., Yukelson, D., & Weigand, D. (2010). The competitive goal effectiveness paradox revisited: Examining the goal practices of prospective olympic athletes. *Journal of Applied Sport Psychology, 22,* 72–86.

Burton, D., & Weiss, C. (2008). The fundamental goal concept: The path to process and performance success. In T. Horn (Ed.), *Advances in sport psychology* (3rd ed., pp. 339–376). Champaign, IL: Human Kinetics.

Butler, R. J., & Hardy, L. (1992). The performance profile: Theory and application. *The Sport Psychologist, 6,* 253–264.

Cohen, G. L., Garcia, J., & Goyer, J. P. (2017). Turning point: Targeted, tailored, and timely psychological intervention. In A. J. Elliot, C. S. Dweck, & D. S. Yeager (Eds.), *Handbook of competence and motivation: Theory and application* (2nd ed., pp. 657–686). New York: Guilford Press.

Crum, A. J., Salovey, P., & Achor, S. (2013). Rethinking stress: The role of mindsets in determining the stress response. *Journal of Personality and Social Psychology, 104,* 716–733.

Da Motta Veiga, S. P., & Turban, D. B. (2014). Are affect and perceived stress detrimental or beneficial to job seekers?: The role of learning goal orientation in job search self-regulation. *Organizational Behavior and Human Decision Processes, 125,* 193–203.

Darnon, C., Muller, D., Schrager, S. M., Pannuzzo, N., & Butera, F. (2006). Mastery and performance goals predict epistemic and relational conflict regulation. *Journal of Educational Psychology, 98*(4), 766–776.

Day, D. V., Gordon, S., & Fink, C. (2012). The sporting life: Exploring organizations through the lens of sport. *Academy of Management Annals, 6,* 397–433.

Day, E. A., Radosevich, D. J., & Chasteen, C. S. (2003). Construct- and criterion-related validity of four commonly used goal orientation instruments. *Contemporary Educational Psychology, 28,* 434–464.

de Lange, A. H., Van Yperen, N. W., Van der Heijden, B. I. J. M., & Bal, P. M. (2010). Dominant achievement goals of older workers and their relationship with motivation-related outcomes. *Journal of Vocational Behavior, 77,* 118–125.

Deffenbacher, J. L. (1980). Worry and emotionality in test anxiety. In I. G. Sarason (Ed.), *Test anxiety: Theory, research, and applications* (pp. 111–128). Hillsdale, NJ: Erlbaum.

Den Hartigh, R. J. R., Gernigon, C., Van Yperen, N. W., Marin, L., & Van Geert, P. L. C. (2014). How psychological and behavioral team states change during positive and negative momentum. *PLOS ONE, 9,* e97887.

Den Hartigh, R. J. R., Van Dijk, M. W., Steenbeek, H. W., & Van Geert, P. L. (2016). A dynamic network model to explain the development of excellent human performance. *Frontiers in Psychology, 7,* 532.

Den Hartigh, R. J. R., Van Geert, P. L. C., Van Yperen, N. W., Cox, R. F. A., & Gernigon, C. (2016). Psychological momentum during and across sports matches: Evidence for interconnected time scales. *Journal of Sport and Exercise Psychology, 38,* 82–92.

Den Hartigh, R. J. R., Van Yperen, N. W., & Van Geert, P. L. C. (2017). Embedding the psychosocial biographies of Olympic medalists in a (meta-)theoretical model of dynamic networks. *Progress in Brain Research, 232,* 137–140.

Derakshan, N., & Eysenck, M. W. (2009). Anxiety, processing efficiency, and cognitive performance: New developments from attentional control theory. *European Psychologist, 14,* 168–176.

Dienstbier, R. A. (1989). Arousal and physiological toughness: Implications for mental and physical health. *Psychological Review, 96,* 84–100.

Duckworth, A., & Gross, J. J. (2014). Self-control and grit: Related but separable determinants of success. *Current Directions in Psychological Science, 23,* 319–325.

Duckworth, A. L., Peterson, C., Matthews, M. D., & Kelly, D. R. (2007). Grit: Perseverance and passion for long-term goals. *Journal of Personality and Social Psychology, 92,* 1087–1101.

Duda, J. L. (2005). Motivation in sport: The relevance of competence and achievement goals. In A. J. Elliot & C. S. Dweck (Eds.), *Handbook of competence and motivation* (pp. 318–335). New York: Guilford Press.

Ebner, N. C., Freund, A. M., & Baltes, P. B. (2006). Developmental changes in personal goal orientation from young to late adulthood: From striving for gains to maintenance and prevention of losses. *Psychology and Aging, 21,* 664–678.

Elliot, A. J., & Church, M. A. (1997). A hierarchical model of approach and avoidance achievement motivation. *Journal of Personality and Social Psychology, 73,* 218–232.

Elliot, A. J., & Hulleman, C. S. (2017). Achievement goals. In A. J. Elliot, C. S. Dweck, & D. S. Yeager (Eds.), *Handbook of competence and motivation: Theory and application* (2nd ed., pp. 43–60). New York: Guilford Press.

Elliot, A. J., Jury, M., & Murayama, K. (2018). Trait and perceived environmental competitiveness in achievement situations. *Journal of Personality, 86,* 353–367.

Elliot, A. J., & McGregor, H. A. (1999). Test anxiety and the hierarchical model of approach and avoidance achievement motivation. *Journal of Personality and Social Psychology, 76,* 628–644.

Elliot, A. J., & McGregor, H. A. (2001). A 2 × 2 achievement goal framework. *Journal of Personality and Social Psychology, 80,* 501–519.

Elliot, A. J., Murayama, K., & Pekrun, R. (2011). A 3 × 2 achievement goal model. *Journal of Educational Psychology, 103,* 632–648.

Ericsson, K. A. (2014). Expertise. *Current Biology, 24,* 508–510.

Ericsson, K. A., Krampe, R. T., & Tesch-Römer, C. (1993). The role of deliberate practice in the acquisition of expert performance. *Psychological Review, 100,* 363–406.

Eysenck, M. W., Derakshan, N., Santos, R., & Calvo, M. G. (2007). Anxiety and cognitive performance: Attentional control theory. *Emotion, 7,* 336–353.

Festinger, L. (1954). A theory of social comparison processes. *Human Relations, 7,* 117–140.

Filby, W. C. D., Maynard, I. W., & Graydon, J. K. (1999). The effect of multiple-goal strategies on performance outcomes in training and competition. *Journal of Applied Sport Psychology, 11,* 230–246.

Fishbach, A., & Ferguson, M. J. (2007). The goal construct in social psychology. In A. W. Kruglanski & E. T. Higgins (Eds.), *Social psychology: Handbook of basic principles* (2nd ed., pp. 490–515). New York: Guilford Press.

Gardner, F. L., & Moore, Z. E. (2012). Mindfulness and acceptance models in sport psychology: A decade of basic and applied scientific advancements. *Canadian Psychology, 53,* 309–318.

Hall, H. K., & Kerr, A. W. (2001). Goal setting in sport and physical activity: Tracing empirical developments and establishing conceptual direction. In G. C. Roberts (Ed.), *Advances in motivation in sport and exercise* (pp. 183–233). Champaign, IL: Human Kinetics.

Hanin, Y. L. (2000). Individual zones of optimal functioning (IZOF) model: Emotion-performance relationships in sport. In Y. L. Hanin (Ed.). *Emotions in sport* (pp. 65–89). Champaign, IL: Human Kinetics.

Harackiewicz, J. M., & Knogler, M. (2017). Interest: Theory and application. In A. J. Elliot, C. S. Dweck, & D. S. Yeager (Eds.), *Handbook of competence and motivation: Theory and application* (2nd ed., pp. 334–352). New York: Guilford Press.

Hardy, L. (1997). The Coleman Roberts Griffith address: Three myths about applied consultancy work. *Journal of Applied Sport Psychology, 9,* 277–294.

Hardy, L., Beattie, S., & Woodman, T. (2007). Anxiety-induced performance catastrophes: Investigating effort required as an asymmetry factor. *British Journal of Psychology, 98,* 15–31.

Hardy, L., Jones, G., & Gould, D. (1996). *Understanding psychological preparation for sport: Theory and practice of elite performers.* New York: Wiley.

Hatzigeorgiadis, A., & Biddle, S. J. H. (2002). Cognitive interference during competition among volleyball players with different goal orientation profiles. *Journal of Sports Sciences, 20,* 707–715.

Hayes, S. C., Wilson, K. G., Gifford, E. V., Follette, V. M., & Strosahl, K. (1996). Experiential avoidance and behavioral disorders: A functional dimensional approach to diagnosis and treatment. *Journal of Consulting and Clinical Psychology, 64,* 1152–1168.

Hays, K. F. (2012). The psychology of performance in sport and other domains. In S. M. Murphy (Ed.), *The Oxford handbook of sport and performance psychology* (pp. 24–45). New York: Oxford University Press.

Hendricks, J., & Payne, S. (2007). Beyond the Big Five: Leader goal orientation as a predictor of leadership effectiveness. *Human Performance, 20,* 317–343.

Henriksen, K., Hansen, J., & Larsen, C. H. (Eds.). *Mindfulness and acceptance in sport: How to help athletes perform and thrive under pressure.* New York: Routledge.

Hiemstra, D., & Van Yperen, N. W. (2015). The effects of strength-based versus deficit-based self-regulated learning strategies on students' effort intentions. *Motivation and Emotion, 39,* 656–668.

Hiemstra, D., Van Yperen, N. W., & Timmerman, M. E. (2019). Students' effort allocation to their perceived strengths and weaknesses: The moderating effect of instructional strategy. *Learning and Instruction, 60,* 180–190.

Hill, D., Hanton, S. M., Matthews, N., & Fleming, S. (2010). Choking in sport: A review. *International Review of Sport and Exercise Psychology, 3,* 24–39.

Hill, Y., Den Hartigh, R. J. R., Meijer, R. R., De Jonge, P., & Van Yperen, N. W. (2018). Resilience in sports from a dynamical perspective. *Sport, Exercise, and Performance Psychology, 7,* 331–341.

Hulleman, C. S., Schrager, S. M., Bodmann, S. M., & Harackiewicz, J. M. (2010). A meta-analytic review of achievement goal measures: Different labels for the same constructs or different constructs with similar labels? *Psychological Bulletin, 136*(3), 422–449.

Jamieson, J. P. (2017). Challenge and threat appraisals. In A. J. Elliot, C. S. Dweck, & D. S. Yeager (Eds.), *Handbook of competence and motivation: Theory and application* (2nd ed., pp. 175–191). New York: Guilford Press.

Janssen, O., & Prins, J. (2007). Goal orientations and the seeking of different types of feedback information. *Journal of Occupational and Organizational Psychology, 80,* 235–249.

Janssen, O., & Van Yperen, N. W. (2004). Employees' goal orientations, the quality of leader–member exchange, and the outcomes of job performance and job satisfaction. *Academy of Management Journal, 47,* 368–384.

Jordet, G., & Hartman, E. (2008). Avoidance motivation and choking under pressure in soccer penalty shootouts. *Journal of Sport and Exercise Psychology, 30,* 452–459.

Kane, T. D., Marks, M. A., Zaccaro, S. J., & Blair, V. (1996). Self-efficacy, personal goals, and wrestlers' self-regulation. *Journal of Sport and Exercise Psychology, 18,* 36–48.

Kruglanski, A. W., Shah, J. Y., Fishbach, A., Friedman, R., Chun, W. Y., & Sleeth-Keppler, D. (2002). A theory of goal systems. *Advances in Experimental Social Psychology, 34,* 331–378.

Kyllo, L. B., & Landers, D. M. (1995). Goal-setting in sport and exercise: A research synthesis to resolve the controversy. *Journal of Sport and Exercise Psychology, 17*(2), 117–137.

Latham, G. P., & Pinder, C. C. (2005). Work motivation theory and research at the dawn of the twenty-first century. *Annual Review of Psychology, 56,* 485–516.

Lazarus, R. S. (1991). Progress on a cognitive–motivational–relational theory of emotion. *American Psychologist, 46,* 819–834.

Lazarus, R. S., & Folkman, S. (1984). *Stress, appraisal, and coping.* New York: Springer.

Lebeau, J., Liu, S., Saenz-Moncaleano, C., Sanduvete-Chaves, S., Chacon-Moscoso, S., Becker, B. J., & Tenenbaum, G. (2016). Quiet eye and performance in sport: A meta-analysis. *Journal of Sport and Exercise Psychology, 38,* 441–457.

Lee, F. K., Sheldon, K. M., & Turban, D. B. (2003). Personality and the goal-striving process: The influence of achievement goal patterns, goal level, and mental focus on performance and enjoyment. *Journal of Applied Psychology, 88,* 256–265.

Levy, I., Kaplan, A., & Patrick, H. (2004). Early adolescents' achievement goals, social status, and attitudes towards cooperation with peers. *Social Psychology of Education, 7,* 129–159.

Liebert, R. M., & Morris, L. W. (1967). Cognitive and emotional components of test anxiety: A distinction and some initial data. *Psychological Reports, 20,* 975–978.

Locke, E. A. (1991). Problems with goal-setting research in sports and their solution. *Journal of Sport and Exercise Psychology, 13*(3), 311–316.

Locke, E. A., & Latham, G. P. (1990). *A theory of goal setting and task performance.* Upper Saddle River, NJ: Prentice Hall.

Locke, E. A., & Latham, G. P. (2013). Goal setting theory. In E. A. Locke & G. P. Latham (Eds.), *New developments in goal setting and task performance* (pp. 3–15). New York: Routledge.

MailOnline. (2009, December 1). Bill Shankly: The top 10 quotes of a Liverpool legend 50 years to the day since he took over. Retrieved from *www.dailymail.co.uk/sport/football/article-1232318/bill-shankly-the-quotes-liverpool-legend-50-years-day-took-over.html.*

Mascret, N., Elliot, A. J., & Cury, F. (2015). Extending the 3 × 2 achievement goal model to the sport domain: The 3 × 2 Achievement Goal Questionnaire for Sport. *Psychology of Sport and Exercise, 17,* 7–14.

McCabe, K. O., Van Yperen, N. W., Elliot, A. J., & Verbraak, M. (2013). Big Five personality profiles of context-specific achievement goals. *Journal of Research in Personality, 47,* 698–707.

Möller, J., & Marsh, H. W. (2013). Dimensional comparison theory. *Psychological Review, 120,* 544–560.

Moore, L. J., Vine, S. J., Wilson, M. R., & Freeman, P. (2015). Reappraising threat: How to optimize performance under pressure. *Journal of Sport and Exercise Psychology, 37,* 339–343.

Moran, A., & Toner, J. (2017). *A critical introduction to sport psychology* (3rd ed.). New York: Routledge.

Moritz, S., Feltz, D., Fahrbach, K., & Mack, D. (2000). The relation of self-efficacy measures to sport performance: A meta-analytic review. *Research Quarterly for Exercise and Sport, 71,* 280–294.

Nederveen-Pieterse, A., van Knippenberg, D., & van Dierendonck, D. (2013). Cultural diversity and team performance: The role of team member goal orientation. *Academy of Management Journal, 56,* 782–804.

Nitschke, J. B., Heller, W., Imig, J. C., McDonald, R. P., & Miller, G. A. (2001). Distinguishing dimensions of anxiety and depression. *Cognitive Therapy and Research, 25*(1), 1–22.

Noël, B., & van der Kamp, J. (2012). Gaze behaviour during the soccer penalty kick: An investigation of the effects of strategy and anxiety. *International Journal of Sport Psychology, 43,* 326–345.

Ordóñez, L. D., & Welsh, D. T. (2015). Immoral goals: How goal setting may lead to unethical behavior. *Current Opinion in Psychology, 6,* 93–96.

Panchuk, D., Vickers, J. N., & Hopkins, W. G. (2017). Quiet eye predicts goaltender success in deflected ice hockey shots. *European Journal of Sport Sciences, 17,* 93–99.

Payne, S. C., Youngcourt, S. S., & Beaubien, J. M. (2007). A meta-analytic examination of the goal orientation nomological net. *Journal of Applied Psychology, 92,* 128–150.

Pekrun, R., Elliot, A. J., & Maier, M. A. (2006). Achievement goals and discrete achievement emotions: A theoretical model and prospective test. *Journal of Educational Psychology, 98,* 583–597.

Pintrich, P. R. (2000). An achievement goal theory perspective on issues in motivation terminology, theory, and research. *Contemporary Educational Psychology, 25,* 92–104.

Poortvliet, P. M., Anseel, F., Janssen, O., Van Yperen, N. W., & Van de Vliert, E. V. (2012). Perverse effects of other-referenced performance goals in an information exchange context. *Journal of Business Ethics, 106,* 401–414.

Poortvliet, P. M., Janssen, O., Van Yperen, N. W., & Van de Vliert, E. (2007). Achievement goals and interpersonal behavior: How mastery and performance goals shape information exchange. *Personality and Social Psychology Bulletin, 33,* 1435–1447.

Preenen, P., van Vianen, A., & de Pater, I. E. (2014). Challenging tasks: The role of employees' and supervisors' goal orientations. *European Journal of Work and Organizational Psychology, 23,* 48–61.

Rawsthorne, L. J., & Elliot, A. J. (1999). Achievement goals and intrinsic motivation: A meta-analytic review. *Personality and Social Psychology Review, 3,* 326–344.

Sappington, R., & Longshore, K. (2015). Systematically reviewing the efficacy of mindfulness-based interventions for enhanced athletic performance. *Journal of Clinical Sport Psychology, 9,* 232–262.

Sarason, I. G., Sarason, B. R., Keefe, D. E., Hayes, B. E., & Shearin, E. N. (1986). Cognitive interference: Situational determinants and traitlike characteristics. *Journal of Personality and Social Psychology, 51,* 215–226.

Scholer, A. A., & Higgins, E. T. (2008). Distinguishing levels of approach and avoidance: An analysis using regulatory focus theory. In A. J. Elliot (Ed.), *Handbook of approach and avoidance motivation* (pp. 489–503). Mahwah, NJ: Erlbaum.

Seery, M. D. (2011). Challenge or threat?: Cardiovascular indexes of resilience and vulnerability to potential stress in humans. *Neuroscience and Biobehavioral Reviews, 35,* 1603–1610.

Senko, C., & Freund, A. M. (2015). Are mastery-avoidance achievement goals always detrimental?: An adult development perspective. *Motivation and Emotion, 39,* 477–488.

Sideridis, G. D. (2008). The regulation of affect, anxiety, and stressful arousal from adopting mastery-avoidance goal orientations. *Stress and Health, 24*(1), 55–69.

Sitzmann, T., & Yeo, G. (2013). A meta-analytic investigation of the within-person self-efficacy domain: Is self-efficacy a product of past performance or a driver of future performance? *Personnel Psychology, 66,* 531–568.

Tanaka, A., Okuno, T., & Yamauchi, H. (2013). Longitudinal tests on the influence of achievement goals on effort and intrinsic interest in the workplace. *Motivation and Emotion, 37,* 457–464.

Thomas, O., Mellalieu, S. D., & Hanton, S. (2009). Stress management in applied sport psychology. In S. D. Mellalieu & S. Hanton (Eds.), *Advances in applied sport psychology: A review* (pp. 124–161). Abingdon, UK: Routledge.

Triplett, N. (1898). The dynamogenic factors in pacemaking and competition. *American Journal of Psychology, 9,* 507–533.

Unkelbach, C., Plessner, H., & Memmert, D. (2009). "Fit" in sports: Self-regulation and athletic performances. In J. P. Forgas, R. F. Baumeister, & D. M. Tice (Eds.), *Psychology of self-regulation: Cognitive, affective, and motivational processes* (pp. 93–105). Philadelphia: Psychological Press.

Van Yperen, N. W. (2006). A novel approach to assessing achievement goals in the context of the 2 × 2 framework: Identifying distinct profiles of individuals with different dominant achievement goals. *Personality and Social Psychology Bulletin, 32,* 1432–1445.

Van Yperen, N. W. (2009). Why some make it and others do not: Identifying psychological factors that predict career success in professional adult soccer. *The Sport Psychologist, 23,* 317–329.

Van Yperen, N. W. (2017). Competence and the workplace. In A. J. Elliot, C. S. Dweck, & D. S. Yeager (Eds.), *Handbook of competence and motivation: Theory and application* (pp. 635–654). New York: Guilford Press.

Van Yperen, N. W., Blaga, M., & Postmes, T. (2014).

A meta-analysis of self-reported achievement goals and nonself-report performance across three achievement domains (work, sports, and education). *PLOS ONE, 9*(4), e93594.

Van Yperen, N. W., Blaga, M., & Postmes, T. (2015). A meta-analysis of the impact of situationally induced achievement goals on task performance. *Human Performance, 28,* 165–182.

Van Yperen, N. W., Den Hartigh, R. J. R., Visscher, C., & Elferink-Gemser, M. T. (2019). Student-athletes' need for competence, effort, and attributions of success and failure: Differences between sport and school. *Journal of Applied Sport Psychology.* [Epub ahead of print]

Van Yperen, N. W., Elliot, A. J., & Anseel, F. (2009). The influence of mastery-avoidance goals on performance improvement. *European Journal of Social Psychology, 39,* 932–943.

Van Yperen, N. W., Hamstra, M. R. W., & van der Klauw, M. (2011). To win, or not to lose, at any cost: The impact of achievement goals on cheating. *British Journal of Management, 22,* S5–S15.

Van Yperen, N. W., & Janssen, O. (2002). Fatigued and dissatisfied or fatigued but satisfied?: Goal orientations and responses to high job demands. *Academy of Management Journal, 45,* 1161–1171.

Van Yperen, N. W., & Leander, N. P. (2014). The overpowering effect of social comparison information (TOESCI): On the misalignment between mastery-based goals and self-evaluation criteria. *Personality and Social Psychology Bulletin, 40,* 676–688.

Vickers, J. N. (2007). *Perception, cognition and decision training: The quiet eye in action.* Champaign IL: Human Kinetics.

Vine, S. J., Moore, L. J., & Wilson, M. R. (2011). Quiet eye training facilitates competitive putting performance in elite golfers. *Frontiers in Movement Science and Sport Psychology, 2,* 8.

Volkers, J. (2017, July 29). Met lege handen na de beste race ooit [Empty-handed after the best race ever]. Retrieved from *www.volkskrant.nl/sport/met-lege-handen-na-beste-race-ooit~a4508711.*

Wawrinka, S. (2016). Transcript of the press conference after the U.S. Open final. Retrieved from *www.asapsports.com/show_interview. php?id=123126.*

Wegner, D. M. (1994). Ironic processes of mental control. *Psychological Review, 101,* 34–52.

Weston, N., Greenlees, I., & Thelwell, R. (2013). A review of Butler and Hardy's (1992) performance profiling procedure. *International Review of Sport and Exercise Psychology, 6,* 1–21.

Whelan, J. P., Epkins, C., & Meyers, A. W. (1990). Arousal interventions for athletic performance: Influence of mental preparation and competitive experience. *Anxiety Research, 2,* 293–307.

Williams, K. J. (2013). Goal setting in sports. In E. A. Locke & G. P. Latham (Eds.), *New developments in goal setting and task performance* (pp. 375–396). New York: Routledge.

Wilson, M. R. (2012). Anxiety: Attention, the brain, the body, and performance. In S. Murphy (Ed.), *The Oxford handbook of sport and performance psychology* (pp. 173–190). New York: Routledge.

Wood, G., & Wilson, M. R. (2010). A moving goalkeeper distracts penalty takers and impairs shooting accuracy. *Journal of Sports Sciences, 28,* 937–946.

Wood, G., & Wilson, M. R. (2012). Quiet eye training, perceived control and performing under pressure. *Psychology of Sport and Exercise, 13,* 721–728.

Wood, J. (1989). Theory and research concerning social comparisons of personal attributes. *Psychological Bulletin, 106,* 231–248.

Wulf, G. (2013). Attentional focus and motor learning: A review of 15 years. *International Review of Sport and Exercise Psychology, 6,* 77e104.

Yeo, G., Loft, S., Xiao, T., & Kiewitz, C. (2009). Goal orientations and performance: Differential relationships across levels of analysis and as a function of task demands. *Journal of Applied Psychology, 94,* 710–726.

Yerkes, R. M., & Dodson, J. D. (1908). The relationship of strength of stimulus to rapidity of habit formation. *Journal of Comparative Neurology and Psychology, 18,* 459–482.

Zajonc, R. B. (1965). Social facilitation. *Science, 149,* 269–274.

Zimmerman, B. J., Schunk, D. H., & DiBenedetto, M. K. (2017). The role of self-efficacy and related beliefs in self-regulation of learning and performance. In A. J. Elliot, C. S. Dweck, & D. S. Yeager (Eds.), *Handbook of competence and motivation: Theory and application* (pp. 313–333). New York: Guilford Press.

Author Index

Subject Index

Page numbers followed by *f, n,* or *t* indicate a figure, note, or table.

628